P9-DEZ-662

Core Concepts in
Health

Paul M. Insel
Stanford University

Walton T. Roth
Stanford University

Jennifer D. Irwin
Western University

Shauna M. Burke
Western University

With contributions from

Heather M. Clarke Thomas, *Middlesex London Health Unit*

Tara Mantler, *Western University*

Don Morrow, *Western University*

Julie Parsons Tripp, *MD, CCFP*

Erin Pearson, *Lakehead University*

CORE CONCEPTS IN HEALTH
Second Canadian Edition

ISBN-13: 978-1-25-903071-0
ISBN-10: 1-25-903071-7

4 5 6 7 8 9 10   WEB 21 20 19 18 17

Printed and bound in Canada.

Director of Product Management: *Rhondda McNabb*
Product Manager: *Keara Emmett*
Senior Marketing Manager: *Margaret Greenfield*
Product Developer: *Jennifer Cressman / Brianna McIlwain*
Senior Product Team Associate: *Stephanie Giles*
Supervising Editor: *Stephanie Gay*
Photo/Permissions Editor: *Derek Capitaine*
Copy Editor: *Janice Dyer*
Plant Production Coordinator: *Michelle Saddler / Sarah Strynatka*
Manufacturing Production Coordinator: *Sheryl MacAdam*
Cover Design: *Mark Cruxton*
Interior Design: *Liz Harasymczuk*
Cover Image: *Cultura / Hugh Whitaker / Getty Images*
Page Layout: *Christopher Hudson*
Printer: *Webcom*

Dedication

For Don, Lily, and Benjamin, and to each and every student who has and will cross our paths; you inspire us to live fully, choose wisely, and be well. This book is for you.

About the Authors

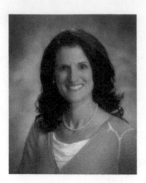

Jennifer D. Irwin, PhD

Jennifer D. Irwin is an Associate Professor in the Faculty of Health Sciences at Western University. She received her BA from Wilfrid Laurier University, MA from Dalhousie University, and PhD from the University of Waterloo. She specializes in health promotion from a behavioural perspective. In particular, her work focuses on behaviour change from a positive and empowering approach. Dr. Irwin is passionate about teaching and has received numerous accolades, including the Edward G. Pleva Award for Excellence in Teaching and Western University's Student Council/Alumni Teaching Award of Excellence. She is equally passionate about research and has authored or co-authored research papers and book chapters related to physical activity, obesity, stress, body image, nutrition, smoking cessation, and motivational interviewing/health-related coaching.

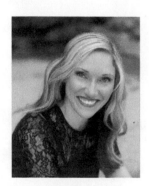

Shauna M. Burke, PhD

Shauna M. Burke is an Assistant Professor in the Faculty of Health Sciences at Western University. She received her Hons. BSc in Kinesiology from McMaster University, and her MA and PhD from Western University. Her primary research area is the psychology of health and physical activity, with a focus on childhood obesity and family health. In addition to over 100 presentations, workshops, and invited lectures at national and international scientific conferences, Dr. Burke has published several research articles and textbook chapters in the areas of childhood obesity, physical activity, group dynamics, and health. Since 2006, Dr. Burke has taught the Personal Determinants of Health course—the largest in the School of Health Studies—to about 500 first-year students each year. She has consistently received outstanding teaching evaluations and was recently nominated for two prestigious university teaching awards.

Brief Contents

Contents

PART 2
GETTING FIT

CHAPTER 4
Weight Management 118

CHAPTER 5
Nutrition Basics 164

Contents

CHAPTER 8
Cancer 312

CHAPTER 9
Immunity and Infection 358

PART 4
UNDERSTANDING SEXUALITY

CHAPTER 10
Healthy Relationships and Communication 400

Contents

CHAPTER 13
Sexually Transmitted Infections (STIs)   530

PART 5
MAKING RESPONSIBLE DECISIONS: SUBSTANCE USE AND ABUSE

CHAPTER 14
Drug Abuse and Addiction   568

CHAPTER 15
Alcohol Use and Alcoholism   608

Contents

PART 7
LIVING WELL IN THE WORLD

CHAPTER 19
Conventional and Complementary Medicine   744

CHAPTER 20
Personal Safety
ON CONNECT   784

CHAPTER 21
Environmental Health
ON CONNECT   826

Contents

Preface

Core Concepts in Health has maintained its leadership position in the field of personal health education for more than 30 years. Since Insel and Roth pioneered the concept of self-responsibility for personal health in 1976, millions of students have used the American-based book to become active, informed participants in their own health care. This history of excellence, combined with our own high opinion of the book, motivated us to create *Core Concepts in Health*, Second Canadian Edition. What follows is a book that we are both proud of and excited to use in our own classrooms.

Our Goals

Our goals and principles for *Core Concepts in Health*, Second Canadian Edition, are the following:
- To present scientifically based, accurate, up-to-date Canadian information in an accessible format
- To involve Canadian students in taking responsibility for their health and well-being
- To instill a sense of competence and personal power in Canadian students

The first of these goals means making expert knowledge about health and health care available to the individual. *Core Concepts in Health*, Second Canadian Edition, brings the most current, scientifically based, and accurate information to students about Canadian topics and issues that concern Canadians: exercise, stress, nutrition, weight management, contraception, intimate relationships, HIV infection, drugs, alcohol, and a multitude of others. Current, complete, and straightforward coverage is balanced with user-friendly features designed to make the text appealing. Written in an engaging, easy-to-read style and presented in a colourful, open format, *Core Concepts in Health*, Second Canadian Edition, invites students to read, learn, and remember. Boxes, tables, artwork, photographs, and many other features highlight areas of special interest throughout the book.

Our second goal is to involve students in taking responsibility for their health. *Core Concepts in Health*, Second Canadian Edition, uses innovative pedagogy and unique interactive features to get students thinking critically about how the material they are reading relates to their lives. We invite them to examine their emotions about the issues under discussion, consider their personal values and beliefs, develop their critical thinking skills, and analyze their health-related behaviours. Beyond this, for students who want to change behaviours that detract from a healthy lifestyle, we offer guidelines and tools, ranging from samples of health journals and personal contracts, to detailed assessments and behaviour change strategies.

Our third goal is perhaps the most important: to instill a sense of competence and personal power in students who read the book. Everyone has the ability to monitor, understand, and affect his or her health. Although medical and health professionals possess impressive skills and have access to a vast body of knowledge that benefits everyone in our society, people can help to optimize their health and minimize the amount of professional care they require in their lifetime by taking care of themselves—taking charge of their health—from an early age. Our hope is that *Core Concepts in Health*, Second Canadian Edition, will help Canadians make this exciting discovery—that they have the power to shape their futures.

Text Organization

The book is divided into seven parts. Part One, Establishing a Basis for Wellness, includes chapters on taking charge of your health (Chapter 1), psychological health (Chapter 2), and stress (Chapter 3).

Part Two, Getting Fit, includes a detailed discussion of weight management (Chapter 4), nutrition (Chapter 5), and exercise (Chapter 6).

Part Three, Protecting Yourself from Disease, deals with the most serious health threats facing Canadians today: cardiovascular disease (Chapter 7), cancer (Chapter 8), and infectious diseases (Chapter 9).

Part Four, Understanding Sexuality, opens with an exploration of communication and healthy relationships, including friendship, intimate partnerships, marriage, and family (Chapter 10) and then moves on to discuss physical sexuality, contraception, and abortion (Chapter 11), pregnancy and childbirth (Chapter 12), and sexually transmitted infections (Chapter 13).

Part Five, Making Responsible Decisions: Substance Use and Abuse, opens with a discussion of addictive behaviour and the different classes of psychoactive drugs (Chapter 14), followed by chapters on alcohol (Chapter 15) and tobacco (Chapter 16).

Part Six, Accepting Physical Limits, looks at aging (Chapter 17) and dying and death (Chapter 18).

Part Seven, Living Well in the World, explores conventional and complementary medicine (Chapter 19), personal safety (Chapter 20 on Connect), and environmental health (Chapter 21 on Connect).

Finally, the appendix (Nutritional Content of Popular Items from Fast-Food Restaurants) provides links to information on popular Canadian fast-food restaurants. Students can use this handy resource for making healthy food choices when eating out.

Taken together, the text content provides Canadian students with a complete guide to promoting and protecting their health, now and throughout their entire lives.

CHAPTER-by-CHAPTER CHANGES

Chapter 1
- Use of the most up-to-date Canadian statistics and information on the dimensions of wellness and major health challenges currently facing Canadians
- Inclusion of Social Determinants of Health
- Additional background on the Ottawa Charter for Health Promotion

Chapter 2
- Evidence-based information about psychological health, including self-esteem, and constructive approaches for dealing with issues of loneliness and anger
- Inclusion of new information from the Mental Health Commission of Canada

Chapter 3
- Updated information from Canada's campus survey of university and college students' experiences of stress
- More examples of challenges across Canadian college and university campuses

Chapter 4
- New information added on concepts such as the built/obesogenic environment, endocrine disrupting chemicals, and circumference measures

Chapter 5
- Inclusion of updated information reflecting current trends on dietary intake of proteins and sugars
- Additional relevant information about popular gluten-free diets and health implications of choosing to follow a gluten-free diet if not diagnosed with Celiac disease

Chapter 6
- Inclusion of updated physical activity and exercise guides for Canadians of all ages
- New information on high intensity interval training

Chapter 7
- New cholesterol guidelines and the inclusion of important CPR information
- Updated information about heart disease and stroke

Chapter 8
- Enhanced critical thinking and self-reflection opportunities
- Updated information about steps to reduce cancer risks and promote optimal health

Chapter 9

- New relevant information about immunity and reducing the spread of infection

Chapter 10

- Practical information about healthy relationships relevant for college and university students

Chapter 11

- New critical thinking and reflection questions to encourage students to think about their own views and decisions pertaining to healthy sexuality and sexual activity

Chapter 12

- Updated statistics and examples

Chapter 13

- New "In Focus" box including information from the Public Health Agency of Canada related to monitoring infections in Canada
- New photographs to provide a more realistic visual representation of many sexually transmitted infections (STIs)

Chapter 14

- New information pertaining to addiction, including an updated Canadian definition
- Updated information related to gambling disorder and substance use disorder from the Diagnostic and Statistical Manual of Mental Disorders, 5th Edition (DSM-5, 2013)
- New information regarding the use of "study drugs" by university students, as well as synthetic recreational drugs

Chapter 15

- Additional information related to alcohol use disorder (new in the DSM-5)
- Updated information about Canada's Low-Risk Alcohol Drinking Guidelines
- Updated Quick Stats boxes
- New section related to caffeinated alcoholic beverages (CABs)

Chapter 16

- Updated statistics
- New section on e-cigarettes

Chapter 17

- New brief "sexual functioning" section
- Additional information about dementia (symptoms, Lewy body dementia) and life expectancy for Canada's Aboriginal populations

Chapter 18

- Updated information related to physician-assisted death and palliative sedation
- New information about what students can do to support older family members as well as a new section, "When A Young Adult Loses a Friend"

Chapter 19

- Updated statistics and examples
- Extensive revisions to evidence-based decision-making guidelines for both conventional and complementary medicine

Chapter 20
- Updated information regarding the American Heart Association/Heart and Stroke Foundation of Canada CPR guidelines
- Additional information about the dangers of distracted driving
- New "Weather-Related Injuries" section and new information about the controversial Anti-Terrorism Act, 2015 (Bill C-51)

Chapter 21
- New "Environmental Threats of Extreme Energy Sources" and "Renewable Energy" sections
- Additional environmental examples, both Canadian and global

Key Features and Learning Aids

Core Concepts in Health, Second Canadian Edition, builds on the features that attracted and held readers' interest in past editions. One of the most popular features has always been the feature boxes, which allow for the exploration of a wide range of current topics in greater detail than is possible in the text itself. Each type of box is marked with a distinctive icon and label.

 In the News boxes focus on current Canadian-related health issues that have recently been highlighted in the media.

 Mind/Body/Spirit boxes focus on spiritual wellness and the close connections among people's feelings, states of mind, and their physical health.

 Take Charge boxes challenge students to take meaningful action toward personal improvement.

 Critical Consumer boxes help students develop and apply the critical thinking skills they need to make sound health-related choices.

 Dimensions of Diversity boxes give students the opportunity to identify specific health risks that affect them as individuals or as members of a group. One or more determinants of health, as defined by the Public Health Agency of Canada, are highlighted in each of these boxes.

 Gender Matters boxes highlight key gender differences related to wellness, as well as areas of particular concern to men or women. An overview of important gender-related wellness concerns is provided in Chapter 1.

 Assess Yourself boxes give students the opportunity to analyze their behaviour and identify ways that they can change their habits to improve their health.

 In Focus boxes highlight current wellness topics of particular interest.

 Thinking About the Environment boxes highlight specific environmental issues related to chapter topics.

Several additional features and learning aids are incorporated in the text:

Learning objectives labelled **Looking Ahead** appear on the opening page of each chapter, identifying major concepts and helping guide students in their reading and review of the text.

Each chapter begins with **Test Your Knowledge** —a set of multiple-choice and true-false questions with answers that emphasize important points, highlight common misconceptions, and spark debate on issues of relevance for Canadians.

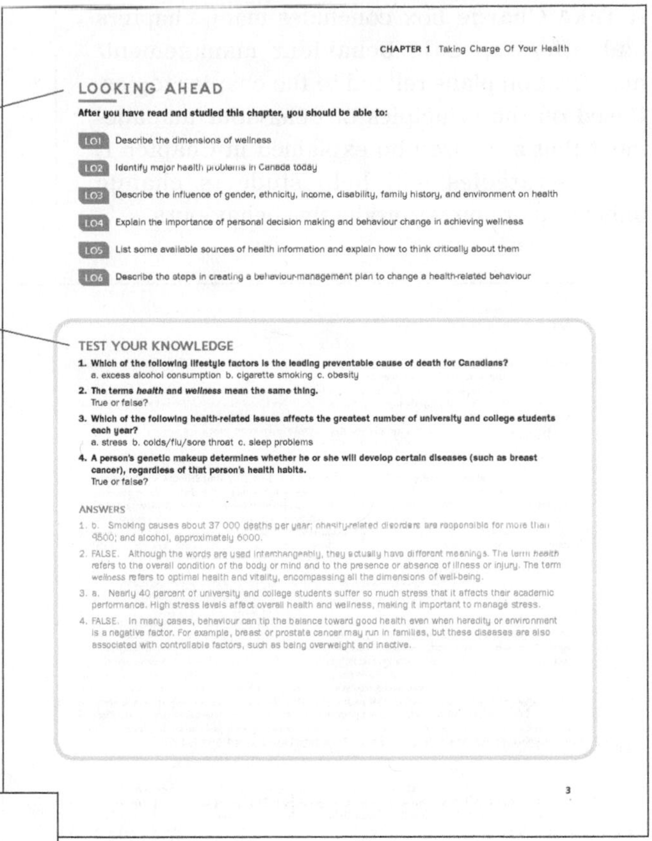

CHAPTER 1 Taking Charge Of Your Health

LOOKING AHEAD

After you have read and studied this chapter, you should be able to:

LO1   Describe the dimensions of wellness

LO2   Identify major health problems in Canada today

LO3   Describe the influence of gender, ethnicity, income, disability, family history, and environment on health

LO4   Explain the importance of personal decision making and behaviour change in achieving wellness

LO5   List some available sources of health information and explain how to think critically about them

LO6   Describe the steps in creating a behaviour-management plan to change a health-related behaviour

TEST YOUR KNOWLEDGE

1. **Which of the following lifestyle factors is the leading preventable cause of death for Canadians?**
   a. excess alcohol consumption   b. cigarette smoking   c. obesity
2. **The terms _health_ and _wellness_ mean the same thing.**
   True or false?
3. **Which of the following health-related issues affects the greatest number of university and college students each year?**
   a. stress   b. colds/flu/sore throat   c. sleep problems
4. **A person's genetic makeup determines whether he or she will develop certain diseases (such as breast cancer), regardless of that person's health habits.**
   True or false?

ANSWERS

1. b.   Smoking causes about 37 000 deaths per year; obesity-related disorders are responsible for more than 9500; and alcohol, approximately 6000.
2. FALSE.   Although the words are used interchangeably, they actually have different meanings. The term _health_ refers to the overall condition of the body or mind and to the presence or absence of illness or injury. The term _wellness_ refers to optimal health and vitality, encompassing all the dimensions of well-being.
3. a.   Nearly 40 percent of university and college students suffer so much stress that it affects their academic performance. High stress levels affect overall health and wellness, making it important to manage stress.
4. FALSE.   In many cases, behaviour can tip the balance toward good health even when heredity or environment is a negative factor. For example, breast or prostate cancer may run in families, but these diseases are also associated with controllable factors, such as being overweight and inactive.

3

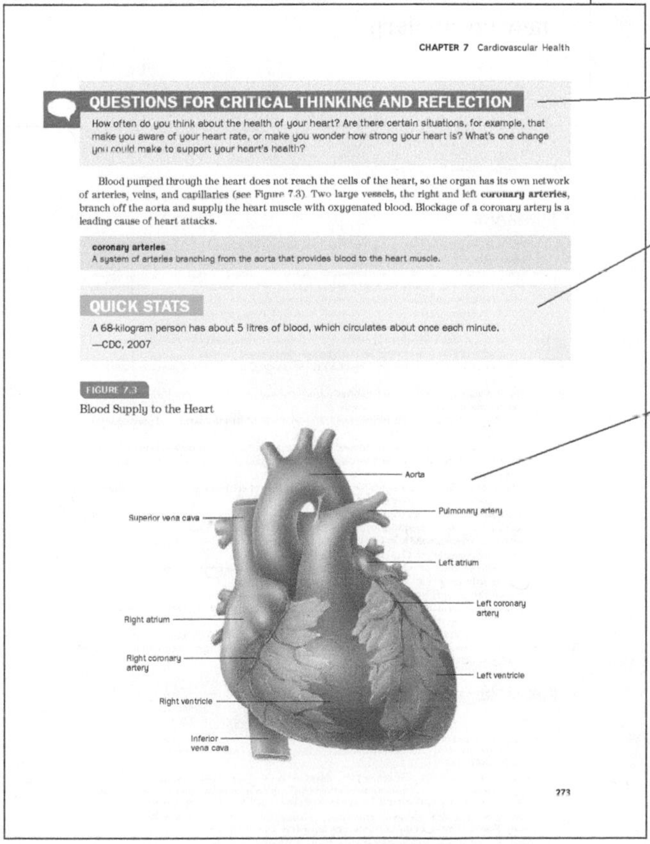

CHAPTER 7 Cardiovascular Health

💬 QUESTIONS FOR CRITICAL THINKING AND REFLECTION

How often do you think about the health of your heart? Are there certain situations, for example, that make you aware of your heart rate, or make you wonder how strong your heart is? What's one change you could make to support your heart's health?

Blood pumped through the heart does not reach the cells of the heart, so the organ has its own network of arteries, veins, and capillaries (see Figure 7.3). Two large vessels, the right and left **coronary arteries**, branch off the aorta and supply the heart muscle with oxygenated blood. Blockage of a coronary artery is a leading cause of heart attacks.

coronary arteries
A system of arteries branching from the aorta that provides blood to the heart muscle.

QUICK STATS

A 68-kilogram person has about 5 litres of blood, which circulates about once each minute.
—CDC, 2007

FIGURE 7.3
Blood Supply to the Heart

273

Questions for Critical Thinking and Reflection encourage critical reflection on students' own health-related behaviours.

Quick Stats highlight striking statistics related to the chapter content.

A wealth of attractive and informative **anatomical art**, prepared by medical illustrators, helps students understand important information, such as how blood flows through the heart, how the process of conception occurs, and how cholesterol moves throughout the body. These illustrations will particularly benefit students who learn best from visual images.

A **Take Charge** box concludes many chapters and offers specific behaviour management/modification plans related to the chapter topics. Based on the principles of behaviour management that are carefully explained in Chapter 1, these strategies will help students change unhealthy or counterproductive behaviours.

Important terms appear in boldface type in the text and are defined in a **running glossary**, helping students handle a large and complex new vocabulary.

Chapter summaries offer a concise review of the most important concepts in the chapter.

End-of-chapter **For More Information** sections contain annotated lists of books, newsletters, organizations, and websites that Canadian students can use to extend and broaden their knowledge or pursue subjects of interest. **Selected Bibliographies** can also be found at the end of every chapter.

Market Leading Technology

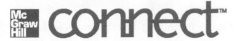

Learn without Limits

McGraw-Hill Connect® is an award-winning digital teaching and learning platform that gives students the means to better connect with their coursework, with their instructors, and with the important concepts that they will need to know for success now and in the future. With Connect, instructors can take advantage of McGraw-Hill's trusted content to seamlessly deliver assignments, quizzes, and tests online. McGraw-Hill Connect is a learning platform that continually adapts to each student, delivering precisely what they need, when they need it, so class time is more engaging and effective. Connect makes teaching and learning personal, easy, and proven.

Connect Key Features

SmartBook®

As the first and only adaptive reading experience, SmartBook is changing the way students read and learn. SmartBook creates a personalized reading experience by highlighting the most important concepts a student needs to learn at that moment in time. As a student engages with SmartBook, the reading experience continuously adapts by highlighting content based on what each student knows and doesn't know. This ensures that the student is focused on the content needed to close specific knowledge gaps, while simultaneously promoting long-term learning.

Connect Insight®

Connect Insight is Connect's new one-of-a-kind visual analytics dashboard—now available for instructors—that provides at-a-glance information regarding student performance, which is immediately actionable. By presenting assignment, assessment, and topical performance results together with a time metric that is easily visible for aggregate or individual results, Connect Insight gives instructors the ability to take a just-in-time approach to teaching and learning, which was never before available. Connect Insight presents data that helps instructors improve class performance in a way that is efficient and effective.

Simple Assignment Management

With Connect, creating assignments is easier than ever, so instructors can spend more time teaching and less time managing.
- Assign SmartBook learning modules.
- Edit existing questions and create new questions.
- Draw from a variety of text specific questions, resources, and test bank material to assign online.
- Streamline lesson planning, student progress reporting, and assignment grading to make classroom management more efficient than ever.

Smart Grading

When it comes to studying, time is precious. Connect helps students learn more efficiently by providing feedback and practice material when they need it, where they need it.
- Automatically score assignments, giving students immediate feedback on their work and comparisons with correct answers.
- Access and review each response; manually change grades or leave comments for students to review.

- Track individual student performance—by question, assignment, or in relation to the class overall—with detailed grade reports.
- Reinforce classroom concepts with practice tests and instant quizzes.
- Integrate grade reports easily with Learning Management Systems including Blackboard, D2L, and Moodle.

Instructor Library

The Connect Instructor Library is a repository for additional resources to improve student engagement in and out of the class. It provides all the critical resources instructors need to build their course.

- Access Instructor resources.
- View assignments and resources created for past sections.
- Post your own resources for students to use.

Instructor Resources

- The **Instructor's Manual** contains learning objectives, key terms with definitions, a detailed lecture outline, suggested Internet resources, and in-class activities.
- The **Test Bank** offers more than 3000 multiple-choice, true/false, and short essay questions. Each question is categorized according to learning objective and level of Bloom's taxonomy. The test bank is available in Word (rich text) format and through EZ Test Online—a flexible and easy-to-use electronic testing program that allows instructors to create tests from book-specific items.
- **Microsoft® PowerPoint® Lecture Slides** include key points and images from the text. They can be used as-is or you may modify them to fit your needs.

Superior Learning Solutions and Support

The McGraw-Hill Education team is ready to help instructors assess and integrate any of our products, technology, and services into your course for optimal teaching and learning performance. Whether it's helping your students improve their grades, or putting your entire course online, the McGraw-Hill Education team is here to help you do it. Contact your Learning Solutions Consultant today to learn how to maximize all of McGraw-Hill Education's resources.

For more information, please visit us online: http://www.mheducation.ca/he/solutions

Acknowledgements

The efforts of numerous people have gone into producing *Core Concepts in Health*, Second Canadian Edition. The book has benefited immensely from their thoughtful commentaries, expert knowledge and opinions, and many helpful suggestions. We are deeply grateful for their participation in the project.

Canadian Contributors

Erin Pearson, PhD
Weight Management

Heather M. Clarke Thomas, RD, MSc, PhD
Nutrition Basics

Julie Parsons Tripp, HBSc, MD, CCFP, DPD
Pregnancy and Childbirth

Tara Mantler, MSc, PhD
Toward a Tobacco-Free Self and Society

Don Morrow, BA(Hons), MA, PhD
Conventional and Complementary Medicine

Reviewers of the Second Canadian Edition

Darren Candow, *University of Regina*

Krista Carson, *Fanshawe College*

Jarold Cosby, *Brock University*

Sylvia Emmorey, *Durham College*

Leo Gallant, *St. Francis Xavier University*

Carly Hall, *Camosun College*

Cherie Hall, *Fanshawe College*

David G. Harper, *University of the Fraser Valley*

Matt Koller, *Humber College*

Renée MacPhee, *Wilfrid Laurier University*

Katherine McLeod, *University of Regina*

Courtney Newnham, *Western University*

Noel Quinn, *Sheridan College*

Jane Tyerman, *Trent University*

Finally, we would like to thank the members of the team at McGraw-Hill Ryerson. We are indebted to Jennifer Cressman for her dedication and steadfast excellence in the role of senior product developer for this edition. Thanks also to Brianna McIlwain, product developer; Keara Emmett, product manager; Stephanie Gay, supervising editor; Derek Capitaine, permissions editor; and Janice Dyer, copy editor. To all we express our deep appreciation.

Jennifer D. Irwin
Shauna M. Burke

Core Concepts in Health Disclaimer

The information in this text is for general educational purposes only. It does not and is not intended to provide medical advice, recommendations, diagnosis, or treatment. This text is a general resource for non-medical university students and does not qualify the reader to provide medical advice, recommendations, diagnosis, or treatment. It is not a substitute for professional medical advice, recommendations, diagnosis, or treatment, and readers should never disregard professional medical advice, or delay seeking such advice, because of information contained in this text.

General Disclaimer

While reasonable efforts have been made to ensure the accuracy, timeliness, and completeness of the information contained in this text at the time of its preparation, it may contain errors. More recent information may have become available that may make the information contained in this text incomplete or inaccurate.

The information contained in this text is provided "as is" without warranty of any kind. Neither McGraw-Hill Ryerson Limited, nor the authors, contributors, and/or editors, assume any responsibility for any errors, omissions, or inaccuracies in the information contained in this text or for the use of any information contained in this text. To the fullest extent permitted by law, McGraw-Hill Ryerson Limited and the authors, contributors, and/or editors disclaim all warranties, representations, and conditions of any kind, whether express or implied, including the implied warranties of merchantability and fitness for a particular purpose, with respect to the information contained in the text. In no event will McGraw-Hill Ryerson Limited, or any of the authors, editors, or contributors be liable for any damages of any kind (including, without limitation, direct, indirect, incidental, consequential, special, exemplary, and punitive damages), lost profits, personal injury (including death), fines, fees, penalties, or other liabilities, resulting from the use of the information contained in this text.

This text includes references to third party materials, including websites, papers, and other resources, for your convenience. Neither McGraw-Hill Ryerson Limited nor the authors, editors, or contributors is responsible for the content of third-party materials, and makes no representations as to their accuracy, timeliness, or completeness. Any reference to a product or service in this text is not an endorsement of or by such product or service.

CHAPTER 1

Taking Charge Of Your Health

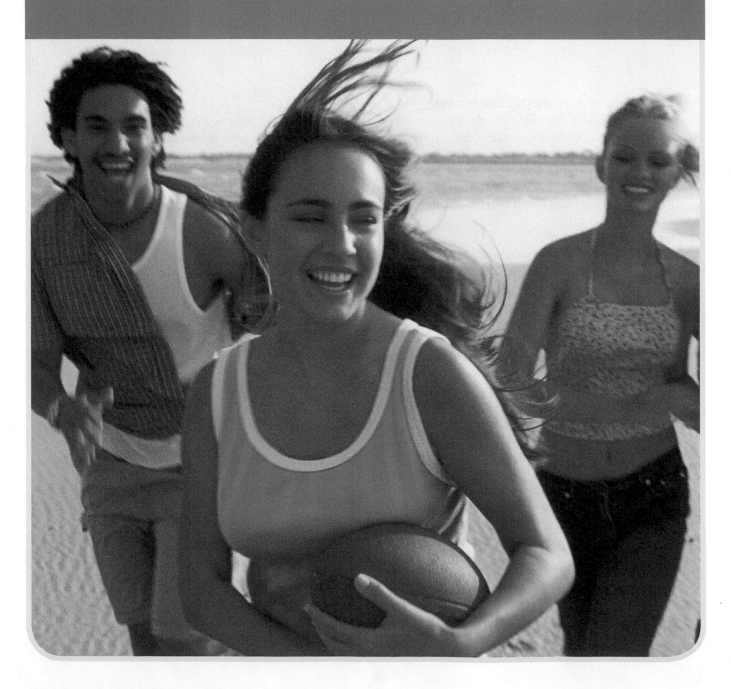

LOOKING AHEAD

After you have read and studied this chapter, you should be able to:

LO1 Describe the dimensions of wellness

LO2 Identify major health problems in Canada today

LO3 Describe the influence of gender, ethnicity, income, disability, family history, and environment on health

LO4 Explain the importance of personal decision making and behaviour change in achieving wellness

LO5 List some available sources of health information and explain how to think critically about them

LO6 Describe the steps in creating a behaviour-management plan to change a health-related behaviour

TEST YOUR KNOWLEDGE

1. **Which of the following lifestyle factors is the leading preventable cause of death for Canadians?**
   a. excess alcohol consumption b. cigarette smoking c. obesity

2. **The terms *health* and *wellness* mean the same thing.**
   True or false?

3. **Which of the following health-related issues affects the greatest number of university and college students each year?**
   a. stress b. colds/flu/sore throat c. sleep problems

4. **A person's genetic makeup determines whether he or she will develop certain diseases (such as breast cancer), regardless of that person's health habits.**
   True or false?

ANSWERS

1. b.   Smoking causes about 37 000 deaths per year; obesity-related disorders are responsible for more than 9500; and alcohol, approximately 6000.

2. FALSE.   Although the words are used interchangeably, they actually have different meanings. The term *health* refers to the overall condition of the body or mind and to the presence or absence of illness or injury. The term *wellness* refers to optimal health and vitality, encompassing all the dimensions of well-being.

3. a.   Nearly 40 percent of university and college students suffer so much stress that it affects their academic performance. High stress levels affect overall health and wellness, making it important to manage stress.

4. FALSE.   In many cases, behaviour can tip the balance toward good health even when heredity or environment is a negative factor. For example, breast or prostate cancer may run in families, but these diseases are also associated with controllable factors, such as being overweight and inactive.

A first year university student sets the following goals for herself:

- To manage her time to do all of her readings for classes each week
- To exercise every day
- To clean up garbage and plant trees in blighted neighbourhoods in her community

These goals may differ, but they have one thing in common: Each contributes, in its own way, to this student's health and well-being. Not satisfied merely to be free of illness, she wants more. She has decided to live actively and fully—not just to be healthy, but to pursue a state of overall wellness.

Wellness: The New Health Goal

Generations of people have viewed health simply as the absence of disease. That view largely prevails today; the word **health** typically refers to the overall condition of a person's body or mind and to the presence or absence of illness or injury. It's important to not become obsessed with our health as that, in itself, can be unhealthy. In fact, The Ottawa Charter for Health Promotion underscores the important distinction that health is a resource for living, not the objective of living. **Wellness** is a relatively new concept that expands our idea of health. Beyond the simple presence or absence of disease, wellness refers to optimal health and vitality—to living life to its fullest. Although we use the words *health* and *wellness* interchangeably in this text, two important differences exist between them:

health
The overall condition of body or mind and the presence or absence of illness or injury.

wellness
Optimal health and vitality, encompassing all the dimensions of well-being.

- Health—or some aspects of it—can be determined or influenced by factors beyond your control, such as your genes, age, the health care system, and the care you received as a young child (i.e., by some of the **social determinants of health**, see Table 1.1). For example, consider a 60-year-old man with a strong family history of prostate cancer, who lives in a rural community in the Northwest Territories, and who has limited access to cancer screening services. These factors place this man at a higher-than-average risk for developing prostate cancer himself.

social determinants of health
Factors that influence the health of individuals and groups.

- Wellness is largely determined by the decisions you make about how you live. That same 60-year-old man can reduce his risk of cancer by eating sensibly, exercising, and having screening tests when they are available. Even if he develops the disease, he may still rise above its effects to live a rich, meaningful life. This means choosing not only to care for himself physically, but also to maintain a positive outlook, keep up his relationships with others, challenge himself intellectually, honour his faith or spirituality, and nurture other aspects of his life.

Enhanced wellness, therefore, involves making conscious decisions to control **risk factors** that contribute to disease or injury. Age and family history are non-modifiable risk factors that you cannot control. Some behaviours, such as smoking, exercising, and eating a healthy diet, are modifiable factors. The Ottawa Charter for Health Promotion describes **health promotion** as a vehicle for achieving wellness; you must play an active role in the decisions related to each dimension of your wellness rather than deciding simply that your health status happens to you. And it is important to recognize that different people define their level of wellness differently.

risk factors
Conditions that increase a person's chances of disease or injury.

health promotion
A process of enabling people to increase control over and improve their health.

The Dimensions of Wellness

Experts have defined six dimensions of wellness:

- physical
- emotional
- intellectual
- interpersonal
- spiritual
- environmental

These dimensions are interrelated; each has an effect on the others, and researchers have found important connections between the wellness of the mind and that of the body (see Chapter 19). The process of achieving wellness is constant and dynamic (see Figure 1.1), and it involves change and growth. Wellness is not static; ignoring any dimension of wellness can have harmful effects on your life. The following sections briefly introduce the dimensions of wellness. Table 1.2 lists some of the specific qualities and behaviours associated with each dimension, and the Mind Body Spirit box discusses another important aspect of wellness.

TABLE 1.1

Social Determinants of Health

The Canadian Public Health Association identifies 14 key social determinants of health for both populations and individuals, the latter of which are the focus of this text. Some determinants are discussed throughout this chapter, and others are highlighted in the Dimensions of Diversity boxes throughout the entire text.

• Income and income distribution	• Social safety network
• Education	• Employment and working conditions
• Unemployment and job security	• Social exclusion
• Early childhood development	• Aboriginal status
• Food insecurity	• Race
• Housing	• Health services
• Gender	• Disability

Source: Raphael, D. (2009). *Social Determinants of Health:Canadian Perspectives*, 2nd edition. Toronto: Canadian Scholars' Press.

Physical Wellness

Your physical wellness includes not just your body's overall condition and the absence of disease, but also your fitness level and your ability to care for yourself. The higher your fitness level, the higher your level of physical wellness will be. Similarly, as you develop the ability to take care of your own physical needs, you ensure a greater level of physical wellness. To achieve optimum physical wellness, you need to make choices that will help you avoid illnesses and injuries. The decisions you make now, and the habits you develop over your lifetime, will largely determine the length and quality of your life.

Emotional Wellness

Your emotional wellness reflects your ability to understand and deal with your feelings. Emotional wellness involves attending to your own thoughts and feelings, monitoring your reactions, and identifying obstacles

FIGURE 1.1

The Wellness Continuum

The concept of wellness includes vitality in six interrelated dimensions, all of which contribute to overall wellness.

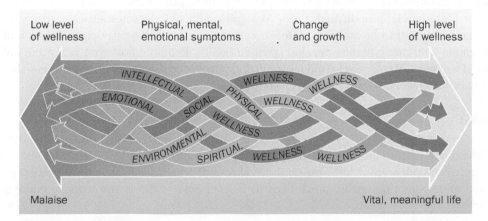

TABLE 1.2

Examples of Qualities and Behaviours Associated with the Dimensions of Wellness

Physical	Emotional	Intellectual	Interpersonal	Spiritual	Environmental
• Eating well • Exercising • Avoiding harmful habits • Practising safer sex • Recognizing symptoms of disease • Getting regular checkups • Avoiding injuries	• Optimism • Trust • Self-esteem • Self-acceptance • Self-confidence • Ability to understand and accept own feelings • Ability to share feelings with others	• Openness to new ideas • Capacity to question • Ability to think critically • Motivation to master new skills • Sense of humour • Creativity • Curiosity • Lifelong learning	• Communication skills • Capacity for intimacy • Ability to establish and maintain satisfying relationships • Ability to cultivate support system of friends and family	• Capacity for love • Compassion • Forgiveness • Altruism • Joy • Fulfillment • Caring for others • Sense of meaning and purpose • Sense of belonging to something greater than yourself	• Having abundant, clean natural resources • Maintaining sustainable development • Recycling whenever possible • Reducing pollution and waste

to emotional stability. Achieving this type of wellness means finding solutions to emotional problems, with professional help if necessary.

Intellectual Wellness

Those who enjoy intellectual (or mental) wellness constantly challenge their minds. An active mind is essential to wellness because it detects problems, finds solutions, and directs behaviour. People who enjoy intellectual wellness never stop learning; they continue trying to learn new things throughout their lifetime. They seek out and relish new experiences and challenges.

Interpersonal Wellness

Your interpersonal (or social) wellness is defined by your ability to develop and maintain satisfying and supportive relationships. Such relationships are essential to physical and emotional health. Social wellness requires participating in and contributing to your community and to society.

Spiritual Wellness

To enjoy spiritual wellness is to possess a set of guiding beliefs, principles, or values that give meaning and purpose to your life, especially in difficult times. The spiritually well person focuses on the positive aspects of life and finds spirituality to be an antidote for negative feelings, such as cynicism, anger, and pessimism. Organized religions help many people develop spiritual health. Religion, however, is not the only source or form of spiritual wellness. Many people find meaning and purpose in their lives on their own—through nature, art, meditation, or good works—or with their loved ones.

Environmental Wellness

Your environmental wellness is defined by the livability of your surroundings. Personal health depends on the health of the planet—from the safety of the food supply to the degree of violence in society. Your physical environment either supports your wellness or diminishes it. To improve your environmental wellness, you can learn about and protect yourself against hazards in your surroundings and work to make your world a cleaner and safer place.

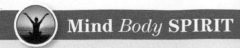 **Mind** *Body* **SPIRIT**

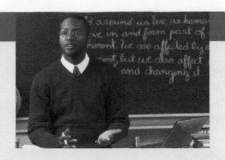

Occupational Wellness

Many experts contend that occupational (or career) wellness is a seventh dimension of wellness, in addition to the six dimensions described in this chapter. Whether or not occupational wellness appears on every list of wellness dimensions, a growing body of evidence suggests that our daily work has a considerable effect on our overall wellness.

Defining Occupational Wellness

The term *occupational wellness* refers to the level of happiness and fulfillment you gain through your work. Although high salaries and prestigious titles are nice, they alone do not generally bring about occupational wellness. Occupationally well people truly like their work, feel a connection to others in the workplace, and have opportunities to learn and be challenged.

Key aspects of occupational wellness include the following:
- enjoyable work
- job satisfaction
- recognition and acknowledgement from managers and colleagues
- feelings of achievement
- opportunities to learn and grow

An ideal job draws on your passions and interests, as well as your vocational skills, and allows you to feel that you are contributing to society in your everyday work.

Financial Wellness

Another important facet of occupational wellness is financial wellness. A person's economic situation is a key factor in overall well-being. People with low socioeconomic status have higher rates of death, injury, and disease; are less likely to have access to preventive health services; and are more likely to engage in unhealthy habits.

Although money and possessions in themselves won't necessarily make you happy, financial security can contribute to your peace of mind. If you are financially secure, you can worry less about daily expenses and focus on personal interests and your future. Conversely, money problems are a source of stress for individuals and families and are a contributing factor in many divorces and suicides.

You don't need to be rich to achieve financial wellness. Instead, you need to be comfortable with your financial situation. Financially well people understand the limits of their income and live within their means by keeping expenses in check. They know how to balance a chequebook and interpret their bank statements. The financially well person may not strive to be wealthy, but at least tries to save money for the future.

Achieving Occupational Wellness

How do you achieve such wellness? Career experts suggest setting career goals that reflect your personal values. For example, a career in sales may be a good way to earn a high income, but may not be a good career choice for someone whose highest values involve service to others. Such a person might find more personal satisfaction in teaching or nursing.

Aside from career choices, education is a critical factor in occupational and financial wellness. For starters, learn to manage money *before* you start making it. Classes on personal money management are available through many sources and can help you on your way to financial security, whether you dream of being wealthy or not.

New Opportunities, New Responsibilities

Wellness is a fairly new concept. A century ago, North Americans considered themselves lucky just to survive to adulthood (see Figure 1.2). A child born in 1900, for example, could expect to live only 47 years. Many people died from common **infectious diseases** (such as pneumonia, tuberculosis, or diarrhea) and poor environmental conditions (such as water pollution and poor sanitation).

infectious disease
A disease that can spread from person to person; caused by microorganisms, such as bacteria and viruses.

FIGURE 1.2

Public Health Achievements of the Twentieth Century

During the twentieth century, public health achievements greatly improved the quality of life for North Americans. A shift in the leading causes of death also occurred, with deaths from infectious diseases declining from 33 percent of all deaths to just 2 percent. Heart disease, cancer, and stroke are now responsible for more than half of all deaths among North Americans.

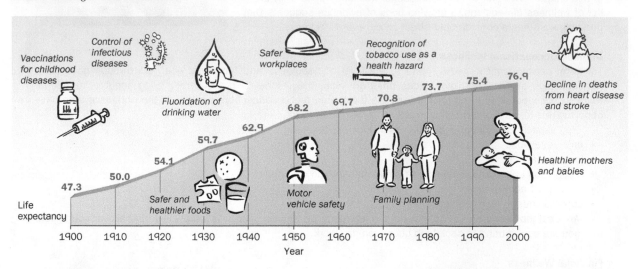

Sources: National Center for Health Statistics, Centers for Disease Control and Prevention. 1999. Ten great public health achievements—United States, 1900-1999. *Morbidity and Mortality Weekly Report* 48(50); U.S. Department of Health and Human Services. 2012. HealthCare.gov: Take Health Care into Your Own Hands, http://www.healthcare.gov: 1141; Statistics Canada. 2009. *Leading causes of death, total population, by age group and sex, Canada, CANSIM Table 102-0561*, http://www5.statcan.gc.ca/cansim/a2 6?lang=eng&retrLang=eng&id=1020561&paSer=&pattern=&stByVal=1&p1=1&p2=-1&tabMode=dataTable&csid= (retrieved March 4, 2015); and World Health Organization. 2011. Noncommunicable Diseases Country Profiles 2011. ISBN 978 92 4 150228.

Since 1900, however, life expectancy has nearly doubled, largely because of the development of vaccines and antibiotics to fight infections and because of public health measures to improve living conditions. Today, a different set of diseases has emerged as our major health threat: cancer, heart disease, and stroke are now the three leading causes of death for Canadians (see Table 1.3). Treating such **chronic diseases** is costly and difficult.

chronic diseases
Diseases that develop and continue over a long period, such as heart disease or cancer.

The good news is that people have some control over whether they develop chronic diseases. People make choices every day that increase or decrease their risks for such diseases. These **lifestyle choices** include many different behaviours, such as smoking, diet, exercise, and alcohol use. As Table 1.3 makes clear, lifestyle factors contribute to many deaths in Canada, and people can influence their own health risks.

lifestyle choices
Conscious behaviours that can increase or decrease a person's risk of disease or injury, such as eating a healthy diet, smoking, exercising, and others.

The need to make good choices is especially true for teens and young adults. For Canadians ages 15 to 24, for example, the top three causes of death are unintentional injuries (accidents), suicide, and cancer, as shown in Table 1.4.

TABLE 1.3

Ten Leading Causes of Death in Canada, 2011

Rank	Cause of Death	Number of Deaths	Percentage of Total Deaths	Death Rate*	Lifestyle Factors
	All causes	238 418	100.0	706.8	
	Total, ten leading causes of death	182 139	76.4		
1	Cancer	71 125	29.8	210.9	D I S A
2	Heart disease	49 271	20.7	146.1	D I S A
3	Stroke	14 105	5.9	41.8	D I S A
4	Chronic lower respiratory diseases	10 859	4.6	32.2	S
5	Unintentional injuries (accidents)	10 250	4.3	30.4	I S A
6	Diabetes mellitus	6 923	2.9	20.5	D I S
7	Alzheimer's disease	6 281	2.6	18.6	
8	Influenza and pneumonia	5 826	2.4	17.3	S
9	Intentional self-harm (suicide)	3 890	1.6	11.5	A
10	Kidney disease	3 609	1.5	10.7	D I S A

Source: Statistics Canada, *Leading Causes of Deaths in Canada*, 2009, CANSIM Table 102-0561, http://www.statcan.gc.ca/pub/84-215-x/2012001/table-tableau/tbl001-eng.htm (retrieved January 6, 2015).

Notes: D Diet plays a part; I Inactive lifestyle plays a part; S Smoking plays a part; A Excessive alcohol use plays a part

*Age-adjusted death rate per 100 000 people.

The Integrated Pan-Canadian Healthy Living Strategy

Wellness is a personal concern, but the Canadian government has humanitarian and financial interests in it, too. In addition to the enormous human suffering caused by our nation's leading chronic diseases, the estimated total cost in Canada of illness, disability, and death attributable to chronic diseases is more than $190 billion annually, with $68 billion going toward treatment and the rest to lost productivity.

The Integrated Pan-Canadian Healthy Living Strategy was created in 2002 when the federal, provincial, and territorial ministers of health sought a collaborative and coordinated approach to curbing our nation's non-communicable diseases. The goal was to address the diseases' common, preventable risk factors (physical inactivity, unhealthy diet, and tobacco use) and the underlying conditions in society that contribute to them, including income, employment, education, geographic isolation, social exclusion, and other factors. In 2010, the strategy was strengthened through two initiatives focused on making (a) the prevention of disease, disability and injury, and health promotion priorities, and (b) decreasing the prevalence of childhood obesity.

TABLE 1.4

Five Leading Causes of Death Among Canadians Ages 15 to 24

Rank	Cause of Death	Number of Deaths	Percentage of Total Deaths
	All causes	1781	
1	Accidents	822	46.2
2	Suicide	479	26.9
3	Cancer	165	9.3
4	Homicide	157	8.8
5	Heart disease	65	3.6

Source: Statistics Canada, *Leading Causes of Deaths in Canada, 2009*, CANSIM Tables 102-0561 and 102-0562, http://www.statcan.gc.ca/pub/84-215-x/2012001/table-tableau/tbl003-eng.htm (retrieved January 6, 2015).

The Strategy's vision is a healthy nation in which all Canadians experience the conditions that support the attainment of good health. Its goals were to improve overall health outcomes and reduce health disparities in meaningful ways by 2015. More specifically, the Strategy's aim was to increase healthy eating, physical activity, and healthy weights:

- *Healthy eating objective:* Increase by 20 percent the proportion of Canadians who make healthy food choices
- *Physical activity objective:* Increase by 20 percent the proportion of Canadians who participate in regular physical activity based on 30 minutes/day of moderate to vigorous activity (the amount needed for health benefits)
- *Healthy weights objective:* Increase by 20 percent the proportion of Canadians at a healthy body weight based on a body mass index (BMI) of 18.5 to 24.9

Information is collected for each objective to see if the targets are being met. If all Canadians improve these three areas of their lives, they will be better able to achieve their ideal level of wellness, and the nation as a whole will be much healthier. Table 1.5 outlines how each province and territory is attempting to meet the Strategy's goals. Table 1.6 summarizes the current eating and physical activity habits and smoking rates of each province's and territory's population.

Health Issues for Diverse Populations

Canadians are a diverse people. Over 200 ethnic origins were identified by those who completed the Canadian 2011 National Household Survey, and more than 1 million people were included in 13 of the ethnic origins. Even with such diversity, eight ethnic origins represent the majority of citizens (see Figure 1.3). We live in cities, suburbs, and rural areas and work at every imaginable occupation. We are at heart a nation of diversity, and though we often fall short of our goal, we strive for justice and equality for all.

When it comes to health, most differences among people are insignificant; most health issues concern us all equally. We all need to eat well, exercise, manage stress, and cultivate satisfying personal relationships. We need to know how to protect ourselves from heart disease, cancer, sexually transmitted infections (STIs), and injuries. We need to know how to use the health care system.

But some of our differences, as individuals and as members of groups, have important implications for health. Some of us, for example, have a genetic predisposition for developing certain health problems, such as high cholesterol. Some of us have grown up eating foods that raise our risk of heart disease or obesity. Some of us live in an environment that increases the chance that we will smoke cigarettes or abuse alcohol. These health-related differences among individuals and groups can be biological—determined genetically— or cultural—acquired as patterns of behaviour through daily interactions with our families, communities, and society. Many health conditions are a function of biology and culture combined. A person can have a genetic predisposition for a disease, for example, but won't actually develop the disease itself unless certain lifestyle factors are present, such as stress or a poor diet.

The Integrated Pan-Canadian Healthy Living Strategy Provincial and Territorial Healthy Living Targets

Province/Territory	Physical Activity Goal	Healthy Eating Goal	Healthy Weight Goal
British Columbia	↑ by 11.6 percentage points (from 58% to 69.6%)	↑ vegetable/fruit by 8 percentage points (from 40% to 48%)	↓ obesity and overweight by 8.4 percentage points (from 42.3% to 33.9%)
Alberta	↑ by 10 percentage points (from 52% to 62%)	↑ vegetable/fruit by 16 percentage points (from 34% to 50%)	↑ healthy weight by 8 percentage points (from 47% to 55%)
Saskatchewan	↑ by 10 percentage points	not specified	not specified
Manitoba	↑ by 10 percentage points	not specified	not specified
Ontario	↑ by 10 percentage points (to 55%)	not specified	not specified
Quebec	become more active	eat more healthily	get weight under control
Newfoundland and Labrador	↓ adult inactivity by 10 percentage points (from 64% to 54%) ↓ youth inactivity by 10 percentage points (33% to 23%)	not specified	↓ overweight by 5 percentage points (from 60% to 55%)
New Brunswick	↑ by 10%	↑ vegetable/fruit by 10%	↑ healthy weight from 36% to 46%
Nova Scotia	↑ % of active adults by 10 percentage points (from 44% to 54%) ↑ % of children and youth who are active	↑ vegetable/fruit from 29% to 34%	not specified
Prince Edward Island	↑ by 10 percentage points	↑ number with good nutritional health	not specified
Yukon	↑ by 10 percentage points	not specified	not specified
Northwest Territories	↑ by 10 percentage points	not specified	not specified
Nunavut	↑ by 10 percentage points	not specified	not specified

When we talk about health issues for diverse populations, we face two related dangers. The first is the danger of *stereotyping*, or talking about people as groups rather than as individuals. It's true that every person is an individual with a unique genetic endowment and unique life experiences. But many of these influences are shared with others of similar genetic and cultural background. Statements about these group similarities can be useful; for example, they can alert people to areas that may be of special concern for them and their families.

The second danger is that of *overgeneralizing*, or ignoring the extensive biological and cultural diversity that exists among peoples who are grouped together. Groups labelled Latino or Hispanic, for example, include Mexican Canadians, Puerto Ricans, people from South and Central America, and other Spanish-speaking people. Similarly, the population labelled Aboriginal peoples includes North American Indians, Métis, and Inuit, each with its own genetic and cultural heritage.

Health-related differences among groups can be identified and described in the context of several different dimensions. Well-accepted dimensions are gender, ethnicity, income and education, disability, geographic location, and sexual orientation.

TABLE 1.6

Eating Habits and Physical Activity and Smoking Levels Among Canadians

	Smoking* (%)	Healthy Eating Habits† (%)	Physically Active‡ (%)
British Columbia	11.0	42.0	62.3
Alberta	16.3	37.5	55.2
Saskatchewan	15.2	37.7	54.4
Manitoba	15.2	36.6	55.3
Ontario	14.2	39.6	54.7
Quebec	18.3	47.8	50.3
New Brunswick	18.5	32.1	55.3
Nova Scotia	17.7	33.5	56.2
Prince Edward Island	20.0	33.3	55.8
Newfoundland and Labrador	21.8	25.6	53.8
Yukon	22.5	40.2	67.5
Northwest Territories	28.3	37.5	55.2
Nunavut	47.1	25.8	47.5

Source: Statistics Canada. 2012. CANSIM Table I05-0503, "Health indicator profile, age-standardized rate, annual estimates, by sex, Canada, provinces and territories, occasional." (retrieved January 6, 2015)

* Refers to daily smokers

† Refers to consumption of five or more fruit or vegetables a day

‡ Refers to leisure-time activity level

FIGURE 1.3

The Ethnic Distribution of the Canadian Population

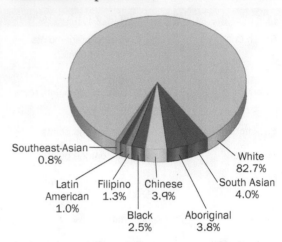

Sources: Statistics Canada. 2010. *Visible Minority Groups*, 2006 Counts, for Canada, Provinces and Territories—20% Sample Data, http://wwwI2.statcan.ca/census-recensement/2006/dp-pd/hlt/97-562/index.cfm?Lang=E (retrieved March 5, 2015); and Statistics Canada. 2010. *Aboriginal Identity Population by Age Groups, Median Age and Sex, 2006 Counts for Both Sexes, for Canada, Provinces and Territories—20% Sample Data*, http://wwwI2.statcan.ca/census-recensement/2006/dp-pd/hlt/97-558/index.cfm?Lang=E (retrieved January 14, 2015).

Sex and Gender

Sex and gender profoundly influence wellness. The World Health Organization (WHO) defines **sex** as the biological and physiological characteristics that define men and women; these characteristics are related to chromosomes and their effects on reproductive organs and the functioning of the body. Menstruation in women and the presence of testicles in men are examples of sex-related characteristics. **Gender** is defined as roles, behaviours, activities, and attributes that a given society considers appropriate for men and women. A person's gender is rooted in biology and physiology, but it is shaped by experience and environment—how society responds to individuals based on their sex. Examples of gender-related characteristics that affect wellness include higher rates of smoking and drinking among men and lower earnings among women (compared with earning for men doing similar work).

sex
The biological and physiological characteristics that define men and women.

gender
The roles, behaviours, activities, and attributes that a given society considers appropriate for men and women.

Both sex and gender have important effects on wellness, but they can be difficult to separate (see the Gender Matters box). For example, more women began smoking with changes in culturally defined ideas about women's behaviour (a gender issue). Because women are more vulnerable to the toxins in tobacco

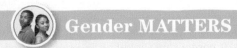 **Gender MATTERS**

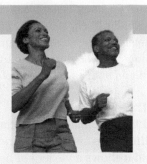

Women's Health/Men's Health

In terms of their health, women and men differ in many ways. They have different life expectancies, for one thing, and suffer from various diseases at different rates. Men and women tend to differ in some health-related behaviours, and they respond in dissimilar ways to some medications and medical treatments. The following table highlights some of the gender differences that can affect wellness.

Health Issues	Women	Men
Life expectancy	On average, live about 4.3 years longer but have higher rates of disabling health problems, such as arthritis, osteoporosis, and Alzheimer's disease	Shorter life expectancy but lower rates of disabling health problems
Height and weight	Shorter on average, with a lower proportion of muscle; tend to have a pear shape with excess body fat stored in the hips; obesity is more common in women than men	Taller on average, with a higher proportion of muscle; tend to have an apple shape with excess body fat stored in the abdomen
Skills and fluencies	Score better on tests of verbal fluency, speech production, fine motor skills, and visual and working memory	Score better on tests of visual-spatial ability (such as the ability to imagine the relationships between shapes and objects when rotated in space)
Heart attacks	Experience heart attacks about 10 years later than men, on average, with a poorer 1-year survival rate; more likely to experience atypical heart attack symptoms (such as fatigue and difficulty breathing) or silent heart attacks that occur without chest pain	Experience heart attacks about 10 years earlier than women, on average, with a better 1-year survival rate; more likely to have classic heart attack symptoms (such as chest pain)
Stroke	More likely to have a stroke or die from one, but more likely to recover language ability after a stroke that affects the left side of the brain	Less likely to die from a stroke, but more likely to suffer permanent loss of language ability after a stroke that affects the left side of the brain
Immune response	Stronger immune systems; less susceptible to infection by certain bacteria and viruses, but more likely to develop autoimmune diseases, such as lupus	Weaker immune systems; more susceptible to infection by certain bacteria and viruses, but less likely to develop autoimmune diseases
Smoking	Lower rates of smoking than men, but higher risk of lung cancer at a given level of exposure to smoke	Higher rates of smoking and spit tobacco use
Alcohol	Become more intoxicated at a given level of alcohol intake	Become less intoxicated at a given level of alcohol intake, but are more likely to use or abuse alcohol or to develop alcoholism
Stress	More likely to react to stress with a tend-and-befriend response that involves social support; may have a longevity advantage because of a reduced risk of stress-related disorders	More likely to react to stress with aggression or hostility, which may increase the rate of stress-related disorders
Depression	More likely to suffer from depression and to attempt suicide	Lower rates of depression than women and less likely to attempt suicide, but four times as likely to succeed at suicide
Headaches	More likely to suffer from migraine and chronic tension headaches	More likely to suffer from cluster headaches
Sexually transmitted infections (STIs)	More likely to be infected with an STI during a heterosexual encounter; more likely to suffer severe, long-term effects from STIs, such as chronic infection and infertility	Less likely to be infected with an STI during a heterosexual encounter

smoke (a sex issue), cancer rates also increased. A recent study shows that although men are more bio-logically likely than women to suffer from certain diseases (a sex issue), men are less likely to visit their physician for regular exams (a gender issue). As a result, only 70 percent of Canadian men, compared to almost 85 percent of Canadian women, were in contact with their doctor in the past year, and many say they wait as long as possible before seeing a doctor—even when they are sick.

Ethnicity

Although Canada is recognized for its diversity, little research has been done here about the specific health differences among the various ethnic groups. However, research from elsewhere in North America is relevant, and it shows a variety of health disparities among ethnic groups. These disparities result from a complex mix of genetic variations, environmental factors, and health behaviours.

Some diseases are concentrated in certain gene pools, the result of each ethnic group's relatively distinct history. For example, sickle-cell disease is most common among people of African ancestry. Tay-Sachs disease affects people of Eastern European Jewish heritage and French-Canadian heritage. Cystic fibrosis is more common among people of Northern European descent. In addition to biological differences, many cultural differences occur along ethnic lines. Ethnic groups may vary in their traditional diets; their family and interpersonal relationships; their attitudes toward tobacco, alcohol, and other drugs; and their health beliefs and practices. All these factors have implications for wellness. (See the Dimensions of Diversity box for more information.)

Within Canada, Aboriginal peoples have been relatively well studied, and these groups represent an important portion of the population in many ways, including cultural richness and historical prominence. Currently, about 4.3 percent (about 1.4 million) of Canadians are Aboriginal people, and approximately one in six can conduct a conversation in an Aboriginal language (Statistics Canada lists 13 different Aboriginal languages spoken in Canada, with over 60 different dialects). No single correct definition exists for the term *Aboriginal*, but Statistics Canada uses questions about ethnic origin (including ancestry), Aboriginal identity, Registered or Treaty Indian, and Band or First Nation membership to establish its definitions.

Compared with the non-Aboriginal population, Aboriginal people face additional health challenges. This population is about 13 years younger, on average, because of higher birth rates, but those living on reserves have a dramatically higher infant mortality rate than the general population, and even in adulthood have a shorter life expectancy. Additional serious health challenges affect First Nations, Inuit, and Aboriginal peoples more than non-Aboriginal Canadians, such as:

- about 1.5 to 2 times the rate heart disease
- three to five times the rate of type 2 diabetes mellitus among First Nations people (which is associated with overweight and obesity, a condition affecting about 17 percent of First Nations people living on-reserve, compared to 5 percent of non-Aboriginal people) and a rising rate among Inuit
- thirty times the rate of infection from tuberculosis (which is caused by a bacteria that is spread through the air) when living on-reserve

Lifestyle factors can affect these chronic diseases, including lack of physical activity, excessive alcohol consumption, and poor nutritional intake. For example, Figure 1.4a shows that First Nations people living on reserves struggle to achieve healthy levels of physical activity. And although abstaining from alcohol completely is more likely and overall alcohol consumption is less among First Nations than among the general population, First Nations people living on reserves report double the rate of heavy drinking and more than twice the rate of binge drinking once per week (16 percent versus 6 percent among non-Aboriginal people) (see Figure 1.4b).

Registered Indians on-reserve are also four times as likely to be unemployed and earn about one-half the income of non-Aboriginal Canadians. In the next section, we will highlight why the determinants of income and education are so vital to all Canadians' health status.

Recognizing the importance of reducing the health disparities among various group of Canadians, Health Canada's website states that the organization "is committed to closing the health status gap between First Nations people and Inuit and non-Aboriginal Canadians by working together to encourage healthy lifestyles, reduce and prevent diseases, and provide health care services."

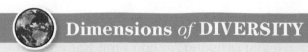

Dimensions *of* DIVERSITY

Health Disparities Among Ethnic Minorities

In studying the underlying causes of health disparities, it is often difficult to separate the many potential determinants or contributing factors.

Income and Education

Poverty and low educational attainment are the most important factors underlying health disparities. People with low incomes and less education have higher rates of death from all causes, especially chronic disease and injury, and they are less likely to have preventive health services, such as vaccinations and Pap tests. They are more likely to live in an area with a high rate of violence and many other environmental stressors. They also have higher rates of unhealthy behaviours.

Although ethnic disparities in health are significantly reduced when comparing groups with similar incomes and levels of education, they are not eliminated. For example, people living in poverty report worse health than people with higher incomes; but, within the latter group, minority populations often rate their health as worse than do whites. Infant mortality rates go down as the education level of mothers goes up; but among mothers who have received an education, Canadian Aboriginal peoples have significantly higher rates of infant mortality than whites. These variations point to the complexity of health disparities.

Access to Appropriate Health Care

People with low incomes are more likely to have problems arranging for transportation to access care. They are also more likely to lack information about services and preventive care. Ongoing studies continually find that racial minorities have less access to better health care (such as complex surgery at high-volume hospitals) and receive lower quality care than whites.

Factors affecting such disparities may include the following:

- *Local differences in the availability of high-tech health care and specialists*: Minorities, regardless of income, may be more likely to live in medically underserved areas.
- *Problems with communication and trust*: People whose primary language is not English or French are more likely to have trouble communicating with health care providers; they may also have problems interpreting health information from public health education campaigns. Language and cultural barriers may be exacerbated by an underrepresentation of minorities in the health professions.
- *Cultural preferences relating to health care*: Groups may vary in their assessment of when it is appropriate to seek medical care and what types of treatments are acceptable.

Culture and Lifestyle

As described earlier, ethnic groups may vary in health-related behaviours, such as diet, tobacco and alcohol use, coping strategies, and health practices, and these behaviours can have important implications, both positive and negative, for wellness. Some cultures' nutritional intake, for example, is influenced by their heritage and tradition, and this must be honoured and respected when helping groups engage in healthy eating practices. For instance, the Canadian Aboriginal Nutrition Network—a practice group of the Dietitians of Canada—focuses specifically on supporting Aboriginal nutrition. Being sensitive to traditional food preferences, cultural values, and peoples' spiritual connection with food is an essential part of facilitating healthy choices among Canada's various cultures.

Discrimination

Racism and discrimination are stressful events that can cause psychological distress and increase the risk of physical and psychological problems. Discrimination can contribute to lower socioeconomic status and its associated risks. Bias in medical care can directly affect treatment and health outcomes.

Conversely, recent research shows that better health care results when doctors ask patients detailed questions about their ethnicity. (Most medical questionnaires ask patients to put themselves in a vague racial or ethnic category, such as Asian or Caucasian). Armed with more information on patients' backgrounds, medical professionals may find it easier to detect some genetic diseases or to overcome language or cultural barriers.

Sources: U.S. Department of Health and Human Services, Agency for Healthcare Research and Quality. 2008. *2007 National Healthcare Disparities Report*. Rockville, Md.: U.S. Department of Health and Human Services, Agency for Healthcare Research and Quality, AHRQ Pub. No. 08-0041; National Center for Health Statistics. 2008. *Early Release of Selected Estimates Based on Data from the January–June 2008 National Health Interview Survey*, http://www.cdc.gov/nchs/about/major/nhis/released200812.htm (retrieved December 27, 2015); National Center for Health Statistics. 2007. *Health, United States, 2007, with Chartbook on Trends in the Health of Americans*. Hyattsville, Md.: National Center for Health Statistics; and Dietitians of Canada. 2005. *Registered Dietitians in Aboriginal Communities: Feeding Mind, Body and Spirit. Role Paper of the Dietitians of Canada Aboriginal Nutrition Network*, http://www.fsin.com/healthandsocial/childportal/images/Fedding%20Mind%20Body%20and%20Spirit.pdf (retrieved January 14, 2015).

Physical Activity Among First Nations People Living On Reserves

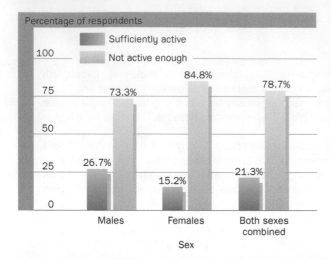

Heavy Drinking Among First Nations People Living On Reserves

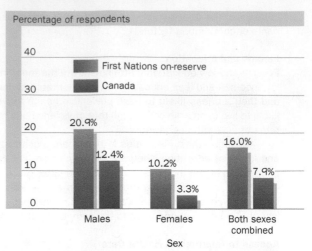

Sources: Figure 1.4A: Public Health Agency of Canada, *Prevalence of Self-Reported Obesity Among Males and Females 18 Years and Older, by Age Group, 2007—Obesity in Canada Snapshot,* 2006. Reproduced with the permission of the Minister of Health; Figure 1.4B: Survey 2002-03, *Results for Adults, Youth and Children Living in First Nations Communities.* Assembly of First Nations, November 2005; and Health Canada, *A Statistical Profile on the Health of First Nations in Canada: Determinants of Health, 1999 to 2003,* February 2009, HC Pub.: 3555 Cat: H34-193/1-2008E-PDF. ISBN: 978-0-662-48920-7 © Her Majesty the Queen in Right of Canada, 2009 Cat.: HP5-82/2009 ISBN: 978-0-662-06799-3.

Income and Education

Inequalities in income and education underlie many of the health disparities among Canadians. In fact, poverty and low educational attainment are far more important predictors of poor health than any ethnic factor. Income and education are closely related, and groups with the highest poverty rates and least education have the worst health status. These Canadians have higher rates of infant mortality, traumatic injury, and violent death, and many diseases, including heart disease, diabetes, tuberculosis, HIV infection, and some cancers. They are more likely to eat poorly, be overweight, smoke, drink, and use drugs. They are also exposed to more day-to-day stressors (such as the need to hold multiple jobs or deal with unreliable transportation).

A surprising finding from a 2006 study was that poor people living in wealthy neighbourhoods had higher mortality rates than poor people living in lower-income areas, perhaps because of the higher cost of living or psychosocial stressors.

Disability

People with disabilities have activity limitations, need assistance, or perceive themselves as having a disability. About one in ten Canadians aged 15 to 64 years and a third of Canadian seniors have some level of disability, and the rate is rising, especially among younger segments of the population. People with disabilities are more likely to be inactive and overweight. They also report more days of depression than people without disabilities.

Geographic Location

About one in five Canadians currently lives in a rural area—a place with fewer than 1000 residents and with less than 400 people per square kilometre. People living in rural areas have higher death rates and are less likely to be physically active, to use seat belts, or to obtain screening tests for preventive health care than are their urban counterparts. They are less likely to finish high school, have less access to timely emergency services, and have much higher rates of some diseases and injury-related death than people living in urban areas (see Figure 1.5). But living in a rural community is not all bad; rural Canadians are less likely to be diagnosed

Selected Health-Related Challenges of Rural Versus Urban Canadians

Rural dwellers tend to experience poorer health status and engage more often in health-detracting behaviours than urban habitants.

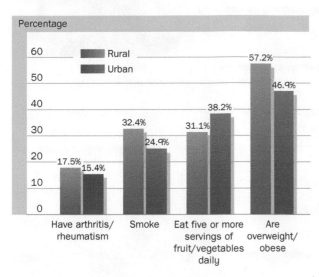

Source: Public Health Agency of Canada, "How Healthy Are Rural Canadians? An Assessment of Their Health Status and Health Determinants. *Canadian Institute for Health Information*, 2006. Adapted and reproduced with permission from the Minister of Health, 2011. © All Rights Reserved.

with cancer and report feeling less stressed, and have a stronger sense of community belonging than urban dwellers. It is clear that our neighbourhoods matter. In fact, children living in dangerous neighbourhoods—rural or urban—are four times as likely to be overweight as children living in safer areas.

Sexual Orientation

The 2 percent of Canadians aged 18 to 59 years who identify themselves as gay, lesbian, or bisexual make up a diverse community with varied health concerns. Their emotional wellness and personal safety are affected by factors relating to personal, family, and social acceptance of their sexual orientation. Gay, lesbian, bisexual, and transgender teens tend to experience increased social pressures, which may help to explain why research has found them to be more likely to engage in risky behaviours, such as unsafe sex and drug use; they are also more likely to be depressed and to attempt suicide. HIV/AIDS is a major concern for gay men, and gay men and lesbians may have higher rates of substance abuse, depression, and suicide.

Choosing Wellness

Wellness is something everyone can strive toward. Achieving it requires knowledge, self-awareness, motivation, and effort—but the benefits last a lifetime. Optimal health comes mostly from a healthy lifestyle, patterns of behaviour that promote and support your health now and as you get older. The next sections outline current information and provide suggestions you can use to build a better lifestyle. Of course, your individual health determinants make it easier or more challenging to make wellness-related decisions; it is important that you make the wellness-enhancing decisions that are within your control.

QUICK STATS

62% of Canadians ages 12 and older rate their health as either excellent or very good.
—Statistics Canada, 2012

Factors That Influence Wellness

Our behaviour, family health history, environment, and access to health care are all important influences on wellness. These factors, which vary for both individuals and groups, can interact in ways that produce either health or disease.

Health Habits

Scientific research is continually revealing new connections between our habits and health. For example, heart disease is associated with smoking, stress, hostile and suspicious attitudes, a poor diet, and a sedentary way of life. Unfortunately, poor health habits take hold before many Canadians reach adulthood. (See the In Focus box for more information on health habits and wellness concerns of university- and college-age North Americans.)

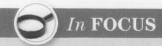 *In* FOCUS

Wellness Matters for Post-secondary Students

If you are like most post-secondary students, you probably feel pretty good about your health right now. Most university and college students are in their late teens or early twenties, lead busy lives, have plenty of friends, and look forward to a future filled with opportunity. With all these things going for you, why shouldn't you feel good?

A Closer Look

Although most university- and college-age people look healthy, appearances can be deceiving. Each year, thousands of students lose productive academic time to physical and emotional health problems—some of which can continue for life.

The table shows the top 10 health issues affecting students' academic performance, according to the 2013 National College Health Assessment of Canadian students.

Each of these issues is related to one or more of the six dimensions of wellness, and most can be influenced by choices students make daily. Although some troubles—such as the death of a friend—cannot be controlled, other physical and emotional concerns can be minimized by choosing healthy behaviours. For example, stress, the top health issue affecting students, can be managed in many ways. By reducing unhealthy choices (such as using alcohol to relax) and by increasing healthy choices (such as using time-management techniques), even busy students can reduce the impact of stress on their lives.

Health Issue	Students Affected (%)
Stress	38.7
Anxiety	28.5
Sleep difficulties	27.1
Cold/flu/sore throat	21.6
Internet use/computer games	21.1
Depression	17.2
Concern for a friend or family member	15.2
Relationship problems	12.9
Death of a friend or family member	6.9
Sinus or ear infection/bronchitis/strep throat	6.3

The survey also found that about 33 percent of university and college students reported being either overweight or obese. Although heredity plays a role in determining weight, lifestyle is also a factor in weight and weight management. In many studies over the past few decades, a large percentage of students have reported these types of behaviours:

- overeating
- snacking on junk food
- frequently eating high-fat foods
- using alcohol and binge drinking

Clearly, eating behaviours for students are often a matter of choice. Although students may not see (or feel) the effects of their dietary habits today, the long-term health risks are significant. Overweight and obese people run a higher-than-normal risk of developing diabetes, heart disease, and cancer later in life. We now know with certainty that improving your eating habits, even a little, can lead to weight loss and improved overall health.

Other Choices, Other Problems

Students commonly make other unhealthy choices. Here are some examples from the 2007 National College Health Assessment:

- Nearly 40 percent of students reported that they did not use a condom the last time they had vaginal intercourse.
- Almost 60 percent of students had three or more drinks the last time they partied, and of those, more than 20 percent had seven or more drinks.
- About 20 percent of students had used tobacco at least once during the past month.

What choices do you make in these situations? Remember: It's never too late to change. The sooner you trade an unhealthy behaviour for a healthy one, the longer you'll be around to enjoy the benefits.

Source: American College Health Association, *American College Health Association-National College Health Assessment II: Canadian Reference Group Data Reporting*, Spring 2013, Hanover, MD: American College Health Association.

Other habits, however, are beneficial. Regular exercise can help prevent heart disease, high blood pressure, diabetes, osteoporosis, and depression, and may reduce the risk of colon cancer, stroke, and back injury. A balanced and varied diet helps prevent many chronic diseases. As we learn more about how our actions affect our bodies and minds, we can make informed choices for a healthier life.

QUESTIONS FOR CRITICAL THINKING AND REFLECTION

How often do you feel exuberant? Vital? Joyful? What makes you feel that way? Conversely, how often do you feel downhearted, de-energized, or depressed? What makes you feel that way? Have you ever thought about how you might increase experiences of vitality and decrease experiences of discouragement?

Heredity and Family History

Your **genome** consists of the complete set of genetic material in your cells; it contains about 25 000 genes, half from each of your parents. **Genes** control the production of proteins that serve both as the structural material for your body and as the regulators of all your body's chemical reactions and metabolic processes. The human genome varies only slightly from person to person, and many of these differences do not affect health. However, some differences have important implications for health, and knowing your family health history can help you determine which conditions may be of special concern for you. Chapter 12 includes more information about creating a family health tree.

> **genome**
> The complete set of genetic material in an individual's cells.
>
> **genes**
> The basic units of heredity; sections of genetic material containing chemical instructions for making a particular protein.

Errors in our genes are responsible for about 3500 clearly hereditary conditions, including sickle-cell disease and cystic fibrosis. Altered genes also play a part in heart disease, cancer, stroke, diabetes, and many other common conditions. However, in these more common and complex disorders, genetic alterations serve only to increase an individual's risk, and the disease itself results from the interaction of many genes with other factors. An example of the power of behaviour and environment can be seen in the more than 100 percent increase in the incidence of diabetes that has occurred among Canadians since 1997. This huge increase is not due to any sudden change in our genes; it is the result of increasing rates of obesity caused by poor dietary choices and lack of physical activity.

QUICK STATS

5.2% of Canadians have been diagnosed with diabetes, but many more have it and don't know it.
—Statistics Canada, 2012

Environment

Your environment includes not only the air you breathe and the water you drink, but also substances and conditions in your home, workplace, and community. Are you frequently exposed to environmental tobacco smoke or the radiation in sunlight? Do you live in an area with poor air quality or high rates of crime and violence? Has alcohol or drug abuse been a problem in your family? These and other environmental factors all have an impact on wellness. (See the In the News box for more information on current environmental issues.)

Access to Health Care

Adequate health care helps improve both quality and quantity of life through preventive care and the treatment of disease. For example, vaccinations prevent many dangerous infections, and screening tests help

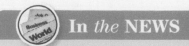

In *the* NEWS

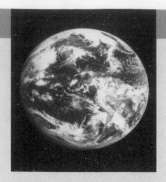

A Planet in Peril: Healing the Environment

Our treatment of the environment determines—to a far greater extent than many people want to believe—how Earth will treat us. This lesson has gradually become clear over several generations, but our troubled environment began attracting intensive worldwide attention only in the last few years. Today, the evidence is irrefutable: Our continuing abuse of the environment has led to a natural backlash that includes the extinction of entire species, shifts in global weather patterns, dying oceans, and the disappearance of polar ice fields.

Climate experts are now sounding the alarm. If we don't immediately begin reducing our impact on the environment, the damage may become irreversible. The compounded effects of humanity's environmental neglect could make our planet a much less hospitable and livable place, possibly within two or three decades.

The Root of the Problem

Pollution, of course, is not a new problem. People have contaminated the air by burning coal, wood, and oil for millennia. Age-old industries, such as forestry and mining, have laid waste to vast stretches of land, and such processes as tanning and printing have dumped untold amounts of lethal toxins into the ground and water. People began to take serious notice of pollution even before the Industrial Revolution, when a few scientists reported that the smoke from factories and trains was fouling the air, and that industrial runoff was polluting rivers.

Over time, improvements in technology made manufacturing easier and cheaper, while an increasing population and greater prosperity created an insatiable demand for manufactured goods. Industrial growth gave rise to explosive growth of urban areas—population centres that drove the need for transportation and electricity. As a result, industries and individuals consume ever-larger amounts of fuel and other resources, creating ever more waste and pollution in the process. Combine this with the pollution generated by our use of fossil-fuelled transportation, and the result is a recipe for global catastrophe.

Global Warming

Human practices affect the environment on every level. Our food chain is contaminated with pesticides, water must be cleaned of sewage and chemicals before we can drink it, and in some cities the air is so polluted with exhaust that it can actually be dangerous to breathe. But the most ravaging—and frightening—consequence of environmental abuse is the phenomenon known as global warming: the gradual rise in Earth's temperature that is causing polar ice caps to shrink, creating unfavourable weather patterns, and contributing to rapid devastation of land and oceans.

What causes global warming? As you will learn in Chapter 21, global warming is largely due to human activity. As we burn fossil fuels (such as coal, oil, and fuels derived from them) to power vehicles and factories, the process releases many kinds of waste gases into the skies. Some of these gases, chiefly carbon dioxide (CO_2), rise up into the air and stay there, acting as an invisible insulating blanket. These gases create a "greenhouse" effect by trapping some of the heat that radiates from Earth—heat that would normally dissipate through the atmosphere. By defeating the planet's natural temperature controls, CO_2 and other "greenhouse gases" are causing Earth to get warmer.

As already mentioned, this rise in temperature can wreak havoc on Earth, especially if temperatures increase unchecked over a long period. Experts are trying to determine how high Earth's temperature must climb before we reach the tipping point (when damage from climate change becomes irreversible) and how soon that point may be reached.

Reversing the Warming Trend

Until then, however, one fact is obvious. People, industries, societies, and governments must start taking action now to reduce their effect on the environment. Legislation, such as Ontario's Clean Water Act, has helped, but it is important to understand that pollution and global warming are not problems just for governments to solve. The environment affects every person in an individual way. The more we do as individuals, the more benefits will result from our collective efforts.

This is why *Core Concepts in Health*, Canadian edition, has been created with current environmental issues in mind. Not only does Chapter 21 examine the environment in detail, but every chapter also briefly addresses the environment's impact on a specific aspect of your well-being—including the way you exercise, the foods you eat, and your reproductive health. Each chapter includes a short feature called Thinking About the Environment. This feature relates the chapter's main theme to the environment and poses questions for you to consider or suggests actions you can take to improve the environment and promote your personal health and wellness.

identify key risk factors and diseases in their early, treatable stages. As described earlier in the chapter, inadequate access to the best health care is tied to various factors, such as low income. Cost is one of many issues surrounding the development of advanced health-related technologies.

Behaviour *Can* Make a Difference

In many cases, behaviour can tip the balance toward good health, even when heredity or environment is a negative factor. For example, breast cancer can run in families, but it also may be associated with being overweight, having poor nutrition, and being inactive. A woman with a family history of breast cancer is less likely to develop and die from the disease if she controls her weight, eats healthfully, exercises regularly, and has regular mammograms to help detect the disease in its early, most treatable stage.

Similarly, a young man with a family history of obesity can maintain a normal weight by being careful to choose healthier calories and to balance calorie intake against activities that burn calories. If your life is highly stressful, you can lessen the chances of heart disease and stroke by learning ways to manage and cope with stress. If you live in an area with severe air pollution, you can reduce the risk of lung disease by not smoking.

You can also take an active role in improving your environment. Behaviours like these enable you to make a difference in how great an impact heredity and environment will have on your health.

QUESTIONS FOR CRITICAL THINKING AND REFLECTION

We frequently hear news about the ways people harm the environment, but do you ever think about the ways your environment may be harming you? How would you describe the quality of the air you breathe (indoors and outdoors) and the water you drink? Is it easy to make healthy food choices in your neighbourhood? Do you find your home or school environment stressful?

Reaching Wellness Through Lifestyle Management

As you consider the behaviours that contribute to wellness—being physically active, choosing a healthy diet, and so on—you may be doing a mental comparison with your own behaviours. If you are like most young adults, you probably have some healthy habits and some habits that place your health at risk. For example, you may be physically active and have a healthy diet, but indulge in binge drinking on weekends. You may be careful to wear your seat belt in your car, but smoke cigarettes or use chewing tobacco. Moving in the direction of wellness means cultivating healthy behaviours and working to overcome unhealthy ones. This approach to lifestyle management is called **behaviour change**.

> **behaviour change**
> A lifestyle-management process that involves cultivating healthy behaviours and working to overcome unhealthy ones.

As you may already know from experience, changing an unhealthy habit can be hard. When you embark on a behaviour change plan, it may seem like too much work at first. But as you make progress, you will gain confidence in your ability to take charge of your life. You will also experience the benefits of wellness: more energy, greater vitality, deeper feelings of appreciation and curiosity, and a higher quality of life.

In the rest of this chapter, we outline a general process for changing unhealthy behaviours that is backed by research and that has worked for many people. We also offer many specific strategies and tips for change.

Getting Serious About Your Health

Before you can start changing a wellness-related behaviour, you have to know that the behaviour is problematic and that you *can* change it. To make good decisions, you need information about relevant topics and issues, including what resources are available to help you change.

Examine Your Current Health Habits

Have you considered how your current lifestyle is affecting your health today and how it will affect your health in the future? Do you know which of your current habits enhance your health and which detract from it? Begin your journey toward wellness with self-assessment: Think about your own behaviour, talk with friends and family members about what they've noticed about your lifestyle and your health, and take the quiz in the Assess Yourself box. Challenge any unrealistically optimistic attitudes or ideas you may hold—for example, "To protect my health, I don't need to worry about quitting smoking until I'm 40 years old," or "Being overweight won't put me at risk for diabetes." Health risks are very real, and health habits throughout life are important.

Many people start to consider changing a behaviour when friends or family members express concern, when a landmark event occurs (such as turning 30), or when new information raises their awareness of risk. If you find yourself reevaluating some of your behaviours as you read this text, take advantage of the opportunity to make a change in a structured way.

Choose a Target Behaviour

Changing any behaviour can be demanding. This is why it's a good idea to start small, by choosing one behaviour you want to change—called a **target behaviour**—and working on it until you succeed. Your chances of success will be greater if your first goal is simple, such as resisting the urge to snack between classes. As you change one behaviour, make your next goal a little more significant, and build on your success.

target behaviour
An isolated behaviour selected as the subject of a behaviour change program.

 Assess YOURSELF

Wellness: Evaluate Your Lifestyle

All of us want optimal health. But many of us do not know how to achieve it. Taking this quiz, adapted from one created by the U.S. Public Health Service, is a good place to start. The behaviours covered in the quiz are recommended for most North Americans. (Some of them may not apply to people with certain diseases or disabilities or to pregnant women, who may require special advice from their physician.) After you take the quiz, add up your score for each section.

	ALMOST ALWAYS	SOMETIMES	NEVER
Tobacco Use			
If you never use tobacco, enter a score of 10 for this section and go to the next section.			
1. I avoid using tobacco.	2	1	0
2. I smoke only low-tar/nicotine cigarettes *or* I smoke a pipe or cigars *or* I use smokeless tobacco.	2	1	0
Tobacco Score: _____			
Alcohol and Other Drugs			
1. I avoid alcohol or I drink no more than 1 (women) *or* 2 (men) drinks a day.	4	1	0
2. I avoid using alcohol or other drugs as a way of handling stressful situations or problems in my life.	2	1	0
3. I am careful not to drink alcohol when taking medications, such as for colds or allergies, or when pregnant.	2	1	0
4. I read and follow the label directions when using prescribed and over-the-counter drugs.	2	1	0
Alcohol and Other Drugs Score: _____			

Nutrition

		ALMOST ALWAYS	SOMETIMES	NEVER
1.	I eat a variety of foods each day, including 7 or more servings of fruits and vegetables.	3	1	0
2.	I limit the amount of total fat and saturated and trans fat in my diet.	3	1	0
3.	I avoid skipping meals.	2	1	0
4.	I limit the amount of salt and sugar I eat.	2	1	0

Nutrition Score: _____

Exercise and Fitness

1.	I engage in moderate exercise for 20–60 minutes, 3–5 times a week.	4	1	0
2.	I maintain a healthy weight, avoiding overweight and underweight.	2	1	0
3.	I do exercises to develop muscular strength and endurance at least twice a week.	2	1	0
4.	I spend some of my leisure time participating in physical activities, such as gardening, bowling, golf, or baseball.	2	1	0

Exercise and Fitness Score: _____

Emotional Health

1.	I enjoy being a student, and I have a job or do other work that I like.	2	1	0
2.	I find it easy to relax and express my feelings freely.	2	1	0
3.	I manage stress well.	2	1	0
4.	I have close friends, relatives, or others I can talk to about personal matters and call on for help.	2	1	0
5.	I participate in group activities (such as church and community organizations) or hobbies that I enjoy.	2	1	0

Emotional Health Score: _____

Safety

1.	I wear a seat belt while riding in a car.	2	1	0
2.	I avoid driving while under the influence of alcohol or other drugs.	2	1	0
3.	I obey traffic rules and the speed limit when driving.	2	1	0
4.	I read and follow instructions on the labels of potentially harmful products or substances, such as household cleaners, poisons, and electrical appliances.	2	1	0
5.	I avoid smoking in bed.	2	1	0

Safety Score: _____

Disease Prevention

1.	I know the warning signs of cancer, diabetes, heart attack, and stroke.	2	1	0
2.	I avoid overexposure to the sun and use a sunscreen.	2	1	0
3.	I get recommended medical screening tests (such as blood pressure checks and Pap tests), immunizations, and booster shots.	2	1	0
4.	I regularly examine my breasts/testicles.	2	1	0
5.	I am not sexually active *or* I have sex with only one mutually faithful, uninfected partner *or* I always engage in safer sex (using condoms) *and* I do not share needles to inject drugs.	2	1	0

Disease Prevention Score: _____

What Your Scores Mean

Scores of 9 and 10 Excellent! Your answers show that you are aware of the importance of this area to your health. More important, you are putting your knowledge to work for you by practicing good health habits. As long as you continue to do so, this area should not pose a serious health risk.

Scores of 6 to 8 Your health practices in this area are good, but there is room for improvement.

Scores of 3 to 5 Your health risks are showing.

Scores of 0 to 2 You may be taking serious and unnecessary risks with your health.

Learn About Your Target Behaviour

Once you have chosen a target behaviour, you need to learn its risks and benefits for you—both now and in the future. Ask these questions:

- How is your target behaviour affecting your level of wellness today?
- What diseases or conditions does this behaviour place you at risk for?
- What effect would changing your behaviour have on your health?

As a starting point, use this text and the resources listed in the For More Information section at the end of each chapter; see the Critical Consumer box for additional guidelines.

Find Help

Have you identified a particularly challenging target behaviour or mood, something like alcohol addiction, binge eating, or depression, that interferes with your ability to function or places you at a serious health risk? Help may be needed to change behaviours or conditions that are too deeply rooted or too serious for self-management. Don't be stopped by the seriousness of the problem; many resources are available to help you solve it. On campus, the student health centre or campus counselling centre can provide assistance. To locate community resources, consult your physician or the Internet.

Building Motivation to Change

Knowledge is necessary for behaviour change, but it isn't usually enough to make people act. Millions of people have sedentary lifestyles, for example, even though they know it's bad for their health. This is particularly true of young adults, who may not be motivated to change because they feel healthy in spite of their unhealthy behaviours. To succeed at behaviour change, you need strong motivation.

Examine the Pros and Cons of Change

Health behaviours have short-term and long-term benefits and costs. Consider the benefits and costs of an inactive lifestyle:

- In the short term, such a lifestyle allows you more time to watch TV and hang out with friends, but it leaves you less physically fit and less able to participate in recreational activities.
- In the long term, it increases the risk of weight gain, heart disease, cancer, stroke, and premature death.

To successfully change your behaviour, you must believe that the benefits of change outweigh the costs. Carefully examine the pros and cons of continuing your current behaviour and of changing to a healthier one. Focus on the effects that are most meaningful to you, including those that are tied to your personal identity and values. For example, if you see yourself as an active person who is a good role model for others, then adopting certain behaviours, such as engaging in regular physical activity and getting adequate sleep, will support your personal identity. If you value independence and control over your life, then quitting smoking will be consistent with your values and goals. To complete your analysis, ask friends and family members about the effects of your behaviour on them. For example, a younger sister may tell you that your smoking habit influenced her decision to take up smoking.

The short-term benefits of behaviour change can be an important motivating force. Although some people are motivated by long-term goals, such as avoiding a disease that may hit them in 30 years, most are more likely to be moved to action by shorter-term, more personal goals. Feeling better, looking better, doing better in school, improving at a sport, reducing stress, and increasing self-esteem are common short-term benefits of health behaviour change.

Many wellness behaviours are associated with immediate improvements in quality of life. For example, surveys of North Americans have found that non-smokers feel healthy and full of energy more days each month than do smokers, and they report fewer days of sadness and troubled sleep. The same is true when physically active people are compared with sedentary people. Over time, these types of differences add up to a substantially higher quality of life for people who engage in healthy behaviours.

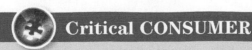

Critical CONSUMER

Evaluating Sources of Health Information

Believability of Health Information Sources

A recent survey indicated that university and college students are smart about evaluating health information. They trust the health information they receive from health professionals and educators and are skeptical about popular information sources.

How smart are you about evaluating health information? Here are some tips.

General Strategies

Whenever you encounter health-related information, take the following steps to make sure it is credible:

Rank	Source	Rank	Source
1	Health educators	8	Resident assistants or advisers
2	Health centre medical staff	9	Religious centres
3	Parents	10	Internet
4	Faculty or coursework	11	Friends
5	Leaflets, pamphlets, flyers	12	Magazines
6	Campus newspaper articles	13	Television
7	Campus peer educators	14	Other sources

- *Go to the original source.* Media reports often simplify the results of medical research. Find out for yourself what a study really reported, and determine whether it was based on good science. What type of study was it? Was it published in a recognized medical or health journal? Was it an animal study or did it involve people? Did the study include a large number of people? What did the authors of the study actually report?

- *Watch for misleading language.* Reports that tout "breakthroughs" or "dramatic proof" are probably hype. A study may state that a behaviour "contributes to" or is "associated with" an outcome; this does not prove a cause-and-effect relationship.

- *Distinguish between research reports and public health advice.* Do not change your behaviour based on the results of a single report or study. If an agency, such as the Canadian Cancer Society Research Institute, urges a behaviour change, however, you should follow its advice. Large, publicly-funded organizations issue such advice based on many studies, not a single report.

- *Remember that anecdotes are not facts.* A friend may tell you he lost weight on some new diet, but individual success stories do not mean the plan is truly safe or effective. Check with your physician before making any serious lifestyle changes.

- *Be skeptical.* If a report seems too good to be true, it probably is. Be wary of information contained in advertisements. An ad's goal is to sell a product, even if you have no need for it.

- *Make choices that are right for you.* Friends and family members can be a great source of ideas and inspiration, but you need to make health-related choices that work best for you.

Internet Resources

Online sources pose special challenges; when reviewing a health-related Web site, ask these questions:

- *What is the source of the information?* Web sites maintained by government agencies, professional associations, or established academic or medical institutions are likely to present trustworthy information. Many other groups and individuals post accurate information, but it is important to look at the qualifications of the people who are behind the site. (Check the home page or click the "About Us" link.)

- *How often is the site updated?* Look for sites that are updated frequently. Check the "last modified" date of any Web page.

- *Is the site promotional?* Be wary of information from sites that sell specific products, use testimonials as evidence, appear to have a social or political agenda, or ask for money.

- *What do other sources say about a topic?* Be cautious of claims or information that appears at only one site or comes from a chat room, bulletin board, or blog.

- *Does the site conform to any set of guidelines or criteria for quality and accuracy?* Look for sites that identify themselves as conforming to some code or set of principles, such as those set forth by the Health on the Net Foundation or the Canadian Medical Association. These codes include criteria, such as use of information from respected sources and disclosure of the site's sponsors.

Boost Self-Efficacy

When you start thinking about changing a health behaviour, a big factor in your eventual success is whether you have confidence in yourself and in your ability to change. **Self-efficacy** refers to your belief in your ability to successfully take action and perform a specific task. Strategies for boosting self-efficacy include developing an internal locus of control, using visualization and self-talk, and getting encouragement from supportive people.

> **self-efficacy**
> The belief in your ability to take action and perform a specific task.

LOCUS OF CONTROL   Who do you believe is controlling your life? Is it your parents, friends, or school? Is it fate? Or is it you? **Locus of control** refers to the figurative place a person designates as the source of responsibility for the events in his or her life. People who believe they are in control of their own lives are said to have an *internal locus of control.* Those who believe that factors beyond their control determine the course of their lives are said to have an *external locus of control.*

> **locus of control**
> The figurative place a person designates as the source of responsibility for the events in his or her life.

For lifestyle management, an internal locus of control is an advantage because it reinforces motivation and commitment. An external locus of control can sabotage efforts to change behaviour. For example, if you believe that you are destined to die from breast cancer because your mother died from the disease, you may view breast self-exams and regular checkups as a waste of time. In contrast, if you believe that you can take action to reduce your risk of breast cancer in spite of hereditary factors, you will be motivated to follow guidelines for early detection of the disease.

QUICK STATS

50–70% of Canadian university students are not physically active at the level needed for health benefits.
—Irwin, 2007; *National College Health Assessment II*, 2013

If you find yourself attributing too much influence to outside forces, gather more information about your wellness-related behaviours. List all the ways that making lifestyle changes will improve your health. If you believe you will succeed, and if you recognize that you are in charge of your life, you are on your way to wellness.

VISUALIZATION AND SELF-TALK   One of the best ways to boost your confidence and self-efficacy is to visualize yourself successfully engaging in a new, healthier behaviour. Imagine yourself going for an afternoon run three days a week or no longer smoking cigarettes. Also visualize yourself enjoying all the short-term and long-term benefits that your lifestyle change will bring. Create a new self-image: What will you and your life be like when you become a regular exerciser or a non-smoker?

You can also use self-talk, the internal dialogue you carry on with yourself, to increase your confidence in your ability to change. Counter any self-defeating patterns of thought with more positive or realistic thoughts: "I am a strong, capable person, and I can maintain my commitment to change." See Chapter 2 for more on self-talk.

ROLE MODELS AND OTHER SUPPORTIVE INDIVIDUALS   Social support can make a big difference in your level of motivation and your chances of success. Perhaps you know people who have reached the goal you are striving for; they could be role models or mentors for you, providing information and support for your efforts. Gain strength from their experiences, and tell yourself, "If they can do it, so can I." In addition, find a buddy who wants to make the same changes you do and who can take an active role in your behaviour change program. For example, Canadian research has found that an exercise buddy can provide companionship and encouragement when post-secondary students might be tempted to skip a workout.

IDENTIFY AND OVERCOME BARRIERS TO CHANGE   Don't let past failures at behaviour change discourage you; they can be a great source of information you can use to boost your chances of future success. Make a list of the problems and challenges you faced in any previous behaviour change attempts; to this, add the short-term costs of behaviour change that you identified in your analysis of the pros and cons of change. Once you have listed these key barriers to change, develop a practical plan for overcoming each one. For example, if you always smoke when you're with certain friends, decide in advance how you will turn down the next cigarette you are offered.

THINKING ABOUT THE ENVIRONMENT

As you think about target behaviours you may want to change, consider your behaviour toward the environment. By making simple changes to your daily routine or by using more environmentally friendly products, you can make a positive difference to the planet. For example, do you do any of the following?
- recycle paper, glass, plastic, and metal products
- use energy-efficient compact fluorescent light bulbs instead of standard incandescent bulbs
- keep your car well maintained to get the best possible gas mileage and emit the lowest possible amount of pollution
- avoid using aerosol products, pesticides, and other chemicals that could pollute the ground, air, or water

For more information on the environment and environmental health, see Chapter 21.

Enhancing Your Readiness to Change

The transtheoretical, or stages of change, model has been shown to be an effective approach to lifestyle self-management. According to this model, you move through distinct stages as you work to change your target behaviour. It is important to determine what stage you are in now so that you can choose appropriate strategies for progressing through the cycle of change. This approach can help you enhance your readiness and intention to change. Read the following sections to determine what stage you are in for your target behaviour. For ideas on changing stages, see the Take Charge box at the end of the chapter.

Precontemplation

People at this stage do not think they have a problem and do not intend to change their behaviour. They may be unaware of the risks associated with their behaviour or may deny them. They may have tried unsuccessfully to change in the past and may now think the situation is hopeless. They may also blame other people or external factors for their problems. People in the precontemplation stage believe that they have more reasons or more important reasons not to change than they do to change.

Contemplation

People at this stage know they have a problem and intend to take action within six months. They acknowledge the benefits of behaviour change, but are also aware of the costs of changing—to be successful, people must believe that the benefits of change outweigh the costs. People in the contemplation stage wonder about possible courses of action but don't know how to proceed. There may also be specific barriers to change that appear too difficult to overcome.

Preparation

People at this stage plan to take action within a month or may already have begun to make small changes in their behaviour. They may be engaging in their new, healthier behaviour but not yet regularly or consistently. They may have created a plan for change but may be worried about failing.

Action

During the action stage, people outwardly modify their behaviour and their environment. The action stage requires the greatest commitment of time and energy. People in this stage are at risk for reverting to old, unhealthy patterns of behaviour.

Maintenance

People at this stage have maintained their new, healthier lifestyle for at least six months. Lapses may have occurred, but people in maintenance have been successful in quickly reestablishing the desired behaviour. The maintenance stage can last a few months or many years.

Termination

For some behaviours, a person may reach the sixth and final stage of termination. People at this stage have exited the cycle of change and are no longer tempted to lapse back into their old behaviour. They have a new self-image and total self-efficacy with regard to their target behaviour.

FIGURE 1.6

The Stages of Change: A Spiral Model

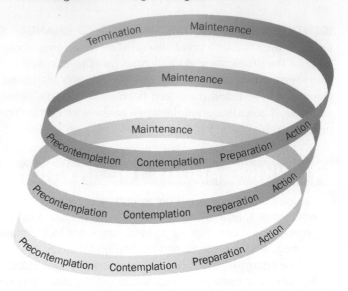

Source: Adapted from Prochaska, J. O., C. C. Diclemente, and J. C. Norcross. 1992. In Search of How People Change. *American Psychologist* 47(9): 1102–1114. Copyright © 1992 by the American Psychological Association. Reprinted by permission.

Dealing with Relapse

People seldom progress through the stages of change in a straightforward, linear way; rather, they tend to move to a certain stage and then slip back to a previous stage before resuming their forward progress. Research suggests that most people make several attempts before they successfully change a behaviour; four out of five people experience some degree of backsliding. For this reason, the stages of change are best conceptualized as a spiral, in which people cycle back through previous stages but are further along in the process each time they renew their commitment (see Figure 1.6).

QUICK STATS

More than 60% of Canadians who have ever smoked have now quit.

—Reid et al., 2012

If you experience a lapse—a single slip—or a relapse—a return to old habits—don't give up. Relapse can be demoralizing, but it is not the same as failure; failure means stopping before you reach your goal and never changing your target behaviour. During the early stages of the change process, it's a good idea to plan for relapse so you can avoid guilt and self-blame and get back on track quickly. Follow these steps:

1. *Forgive yourself.* A single setback isn't the end of the world, but abandoning your efforts to change could have negative effects on your life.
2. *Give yourself credit for the progress you have already made.* You can use that success as motivation to continue.
3. *Move on.* You can learn from a relapse and use that knowledge to deal with potential setbacks in the future.

If relapses keep occurring or if you can't seem to control them, you may need to return to a previous stage of the behaviour change process. If this is necessary, reevaluate your goals and your strategy. A different or less stressful approach may help you avoid setbacks when you try again.

Developing Skills for Change: Creating a Personalized Plan

Once you are committed to making a change, it's time to put together a plan of action. Your key to success is a well-thought-out plan that sets goals, anticipates problems, and includes rewards.

1. Monitor Your Behaviour and Gather Data

Keep a record of your target behaviour and the circumstances surrounding it. Record this information for at least a week or two. Keep your notes in a health journal or notebook or on your computer (see the sample journal entries in Figure 1.7). Record each occurrence of your behaviour, noting the following:
- what the activity was
- when and where it happened
- what you were doing
- how you felt at that time

2. Analyze the Data and Identify Patterns

After you have collected data on the behaviour, analyze the data to identify patterns. When are you most likely to overeat? What events trigger your appetite? Perhaps you are especially hungry at midmorning or when you put off eating dinner until 9 p.m. Perhaps you overindulge in food and drink when you go to a particular restaurant or when you are with certain friends. Note the connections between your feelings and external cues, such as time of day, location, situation, and the actions of others around you.

3. Be SMART About Setting Goals

If your goals are too challenging, you will have trouble making steady progress and will be more likely to give up altogether. If, for example, you are in poor physical condition, it will not make sense to set a goal of being ready to run a marathon within two months. If you set goals you can live with, it will be easier to stick with your behaviour change plan and be successful.

Experts suggest that your goals meet the SMART criteria; that is, your behaviour change goals should be the following:

FIGURE 1.7

Sample Health Journal Entries

If your goal is to start an exercise program, track your activities to determine how to make time for workouts.

Date November 5					Day M [TU] W TH F SA SU						
Time of day	M/S	Food eaten	Cals.	H	Where did you eat?	What else were you doing?	How did someone else influence you?	What made you want to eat what you did?	Emotions and feelings?	Thoughts and concerns?
7:30	M	250 mL Crispix cereal 150 mL skim milk coffee, black 250 mL orange juice	110 40 — 120	3	home	reading newspaper	alone	I always eat cereal in the morning	a little keyed up & worried	thinking about quiz in class today
10:30	S	1 apple	90	1	hall outside classroom	studying	alone	felt tired & wanted to wake up	tired	worried about next class
12:30	M	250 mL chili 1 roll 1 pat butter 1 orange 2 oatmeal cookies 1 soda	290 120 35 60 120 150	2	campus food court	talking	eating w/ friends; we decided to eat at the food court	wanted to be part of group	excited and happy	interested in hearing everyone's plans for the weekend
	M/S = Meal or snack			H = Hunger rating (0–3)						

- *Specific:* Avoid vague goals like "eat more fruits and vegetables." Instead, state your objectives in specific terms, such as "eat 500 millilitres of fruit and 750 millilitres of vegetables every day."
- *Measurable:* Recognize that your progress will be easier to track if your goals are quantifiable, so give your goal a number. You might measure your goal in terms of time (such as "walk briskly for 20 minutes a day"), distance ("run three kilometres, three days per week"), or some other amount ("drink five glasses of water every day").
- *Attainable:* Set goals that are within your physical limits. For example, if you are a poor swimmer, it might not be possible for you to meet a short-term fitness goal by swimming laps. Walking or biking might be better options.
- *Realistic:* Manage your expectations when you set goals. For example, it may not be possible for a long-time smoker to quit cold turkey. A more realistic approach might be to use nicotine-replacement patches or gum for several weeks while getting help from a support group.
- *Time frame specific:* Give yourself a reasonable amount of time to reach your goals, state the time frame in your behaviour change plan, and set your agenda to meet the goal within the given time.

Using these criteria, a sedentary person who wanted to improve his health and build fitness might set a goal of being able to run 5 kilometres in 30 minutes, to be achieved within 6 months. To work toward that goal, he might set a number of smaller, intermediate goals that are easier to achieve. Figure 1.8 shows an example of fitness goals.

Of course, it may not be possible to meet these goals, but you never know until you try. As you work toward meeting your long-term goal, you may find it necessary to adjust your short-term goals. For example, you may find that you can start running sooner than you thought, or you may be able to run farther than you originally estimated. In such cases, it may be reasonable to make your goals more challenging. Otherwise, you may want to make them easier to stay motivated.

FIGURE 1.8

Sample Fitness Goals

Week	Frequency (days/week)	Activity	Duration (minutes)
1	3	Walk < 2 km	10–15
2	3	Walk 2 km	15–20
3	4	Walk 2–3 km	20–25
4	4	Walk 3–4 km	25–30
5–7	3–4	Walk/run 2 km	15–20
.			
.			
.			
21–24	4–5	Run 4–5 km	25–30

QUICK STATS

Only about 15% of Canadian adults and 6% of Canadian children are meeting the current age-specific physical activity guidelines.

—Statistics Canada, *Health Measures Survey*, 2013

For some goals and situations, it may make more sense to focus on something other than your outcome goal. If you are in an early stage of change, for example, your goal may be to learn more about the risks associated with your target behaviour or to complete a cost-benefit analysis. If your goal involves a long-term lifestyle change, such as reaching a healthy weight, it is better to focus on developing healthy habits than to target a specific weight loss. Your goal in this case might be exercising for 30 minutes every day, reducing portion sizes, or eliminating late-night snacks.

4. Devise a Plan of Action

Develop a strategy that will support your efforts to change. Your plan of action should include the following steps:

- *Get what you need.* Identify resources that can help you. For example, you can join a community walking club or sign up for a smoking cessation program. You may also need to buy some new running shoes or nicotine-replacement patches. Get the items you need right away; waiting can delay your progress.

- *Modify your environment.* If cues in your environment trigger your target behaviour, try to control them. For example, if you normally have alcohol at home, getting rid of it can help prevent you from indulging. If you usually study with a group of friends in an environment that allows smoking, try moving to a non-smoking area. If you always buy a snack at a certain vending machine, change your route so you don't pass by it.

- *Control related habits.* You may have habits that contribute to your target behaviour; modifying these habits can help change the behaviour. For example, if you usually plop down on the sofa while watching TV, try putting an exercise bike in front of the set so you can burn calories while watching your favourite programs.

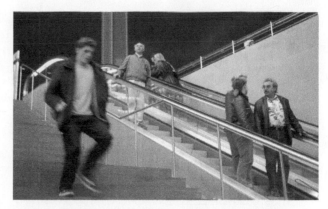

Your environment contains powerful cues for both positive and negative lifestyle choices. Identifying and using the healthier options available to you throughout the day is a key part of a successful behaviour change program.

- *Reward yourself.* Giving yourself instant, real rewards for good behaviour will reinforce your efforts. Plan your rewards; decide in advance what each one will be and how you will earn it. Tie rewards to achieving specific goals or subgoals. For example, you might treat yourself to a movie after a week of avoiding unhealthy snacks. Make a list of items or events to use as rewards; they should be special to you and preferably unrelated to food or alcohol.

- *Involve the people around you.* Tell family and friends about your plan, and ask them to help. To help them respond appropriately to your needs, create a specific list of dos and don'ts. For example, ask them to support you when you set aside time to exercise or avoid second helpings at dinner.

- *Plan for challenges.* Think about situations and people that might derail your program, and develop ways to cope with them. For example, if you think it will be hard to stick to your usual exercise program during exams, schedule short bouts of physical activity (such as a brisk walk) as stress-reducing study breaks.

5. Make a Personal Contract

A serious personal contract—one that commits you to your word—can result in a higher chance of follow-through than a casual, offhand promise. Your contract can help prevent procrastination by specifying important dates and can also serve as a reminder of your personal commitment to change.

Your contract should include a statement of your goal and your commitment to reaching it. The contract should also include details, such as the following:

- the date you will start
- the steps you will take to measure your progress
- the strategies you plan to use to promote change
- the date you expect to reach your final goal

Have someone—preferably someone who will be actively helping you with your program—sign your contract as a witness.

Figure 1.9 shows a sample behaviour change contract for someone who is committing to eating more fruit every day. You can apply the general behaviour change planning framework presented in this chapter to any target behaviour. Additional examples of behaviour change plans appear in the Behaviour Change Strategy sections at the end of many chapters in this text. In these sections, you will find specific plans for quitting smoking, starting an exercise program, and making other positive lifestyle changes.

Putting Your Plan into Action

The starting date has arrived, and you are ready to put your plan into action. This stage requires commitment, the resolve to stick with the plan no matter what temptations you encounter. Remember all the

FIGURE 1.9

A Sample Behaviour Change Contract

Behaviour Change Contract

1. I, _Tammy Lau_, agree to _increase my consumption of fruit from_ _250 mL per week to 500 mL per day._

2. I will begin on _10/5_ and plan to reach my goal of _500 mL_ _of fruit per day_ by _12/7_

3. To reach my final goal, I have devised the following schedule of mini-goals. For each step in my program, I will give myself the reward listed.

   I will begin to have 125 mL _____ 10/5 _____ see movie
   of fruit with breakfast

   I will begin to have 125 mL _____ 10/26 _____ new cd
   of fruit with lunch

   I will begin to substitute fruit _____ 11/16 _____ concert
   juice for pop 1 time per day

   My overall reward for reaching my goal will be _trip to beach_

4. I have gathered and analyzed data on my target behaviour and have identified the following strategies for changing my behaviour: _Keep the_ _fridge stocked with easy-to-carry fruit. Pack fruit in my backpack_ _every day. Buy lunch at place that serves fruit._

5. I will use the following tools to monitor my progress toward my final goal: _Chart on fridge door_ _Health journal_

   I sign this contract as an indication of my personal commitment to reach my goal: _Tammy Lau_   _9/28_

   I have recruited a helper who will witness my contract and _also increase_ _his consumption of fruit; eat lunch with me twice a week._
   _____ Eric March _____   _9/28_

A beautiful day and a spectacular setting contribute to making exercise a satisfying and pleasurable experience. Choosing the right activity and doing it the right way are important elements in a successful health behaviour change program.

reasons you have to make the change—and remember that *you* are the boss. Use all your strategies to make your plan work. Make sure your environment is change-friendly, and get as much support and encouragement from others as possible. Keep track of your progress in your health journal, and give yourself regular rewards. And don't forget to give yourself a pat on the back—congratulate yourself, notice how much better you look or feel, and feel good about how far you have come and how you have gained control of your behaviour.

Staying with It

As you continue with your program, don't be surprised when you run up against obstacles; they're inevitable. In fact, it's a good idea to expect problems and give yourself time to step back, see how you're doing, and make some changes before going on. If your program is grinding to a halt, identify what is blocking your progress. It may come from one of the sources described in the following sections.

Social Influences

Take a hard look at the reactions of the people you are counting on, and see if they are really supporting you. If they come up short, connect with others who will be more supportive.

A related trap is trying to get your friends or family members to change *their* behaviours. The decision to make a major behaviour change is something people come to only after intensive self-examination. You may be able to influence someone by tactfully providing facts or support, but that's all. Focus on yourself. When you succeed, you may become a role model for others.

Levels of Motivation and Commitment

You won't make real progress until an inner drive leads you to the stage of change at which you are ready to make a personal commitment to the goal. If commitment is your problem, you may need to wait until the behaviour you are dealing with makes you unhappier or unhealthier; then your desire to change it will be stronger. Or you may find that changing your goal will inspire you to keep going. For more ideas, see "Motivation Boosters" in the Library.

Choice of Techniques and Level of Effort

If your plan is not working as well as you thought it would, make changes where you are having the most trouble. If you have lagged on your running schedule, for example, maybe it's because you don't like running. An aerobics class might suit you better. There are many ways to move toward your goal. Or you may not be trying hard enough. You do have to push toward your goal. If it were easy, you wouldn't need a plan.

Stress Barrier

If you hit a wall in your program, look at the sources of stress in your life. If the stress is temporary, such as catching a cold or having a term paper due, you may want to wait until it passes before strengthening your efforts. If the stress is ongoing, find healthy ways to manage it (see Chapter 3). You may even want to make stress management your highest priority for behaviour change.

Procrastinating, Rationalizing, and Blaming

Be alert to games you might be playing with yourself, so you can stop them. Such games include the following:

- *Procrastinating:* If you tell yourself, "It's Friday already; I might as well wait until Monday to start," you're procrastinating. Break your plan into smaller steps that you can accomplish one day at a time.
- *Rationalizing:* If you tell yourself, "I wanted to go swimming today but wouldn't have had time to wash my hair afterward," you're making excuses. When you "win" by deceiving yourself, it isn't much of a victory.
- *Blaming:* If you tell yourself, "I couldn't exercise because Dave was hogging the elliptical trainer," you're blaming others for your own failure to follow through. Blaming is a way of taking your focus off the real problem and denying responsibility for your own actions.

Being Healthy for Life

Your first few behaviour change projects may never go beyond the planning stage. Those that do may not all succeed. But as you begin to see progress and changes, you will start to experience new and surprising positive feelings about yourself. You will probably find that you are less likely to buckle under stress. You may accomplish things you never thought possible—winning a race, climbing a mountain, quitting smoking. Being healthy takes extra effort, but the paybacks in energy and vitality are priceless.

Once you have started, don't stop. Remember that maintaining good health is an ongoing process. Tackle one area at a time, but make a careful inventory of your health strengths and weaknesses and lay out a long-range plan. Take on the easier problems first, and then use what you have learned to attack more difficult areas. Keep informed about the latest health news and trends; research is constantly providing new information that directly affects daily choices and habits.

Making Changes in Your World

You can't completely control every aspect of your health. At least three other factors—heredity, health care, and environment—play important roles in your well-being. After you quit smoking, for example, you may still be inhaling smoke from other people's cigarettes. Your resolve to eat better foods may suffer a setback when you can't find any healthy choices in vending machines.

QUESTIONS FOR CRITICAL THINKING AND REFLECTION

Think about the last time you made an unhealthy choice instead of a healthy one. How could you have changed the situation, the people in the situation, or your own thoughts, feelings, or intentions to avoid making that choice? What can you do in similar situations in the future to produce a different outcome?

But you can make a difference—you can help create an environment around you that supports wellness for everyone. You can help support non-smoking areas in public places. You can speak up in favour of more nutritious foods and better physical fitness facilities. You can include non-alcoholic drinks at your parties.

You can also work on larger environmental challenges: air and water pollution, traffic congestion, over-crowding and overpopulation, global warming and climate change, toxic and nuclear waste, and many others. These difficult issues need the attention and energy of people who are informed and who care about good health. On every level, from personal to planetary, we can all take an active role in shaping our environment.

What Does the Future Hold?

Sweeping changes in lifestyle have resulted in healthier Canadians in recent years, and could have even greater effects in the years to come. In your lifetime, you can choose to take an active role in the movement toward increased awareness, greater individual responsibility and control, healthier lifestyles, and a healthier planet. Your choices and actions will have a tremendous impact on your present and future wellness. The door is open, and the time is now—you simply have to begin.

QUESTIONS FOR CRITICAL THINKING AND REFLECTION

Have you tried to change a behaviour in the past, such as exercising more or quitting smoking? How successful were you? Do you feel the need to try again? If so, what would you do differently to improve your chances of success?

Take CHARGE

Tips for Moving Forward in the Cycle of Behaviour Change

Precontemplation
- *Raise your awareness.* Research your target behaviour and its effects.
- *Be self-aware.* Look at the mechanisms you use to resist change, such as denial or rationalization. Find ways to counteract these mechanisms.
- *Seek social support.* Friends and family members can help you identify target behaviours and understand their impact on the people around you.
- *Identify helpful resources.* These might include exercise classes or stress-management workshops offered by your school.

Contemplation
- *Keep a journal.* A record of your target behaviour and the circumstances that elicit the behaviour can help you plan a change program.
- *Do a cost-benefit analysis.* Identify the costs and benefits (both current and future) of maintaining your behaviour and of changing it. Costs can be monetary, social, emotional, and so on.

- *Identify barriers to change.* Knowing these obstacles can help you overcome them.
- *Engage your emotions.* Watch movies or read books about people with your target behaviour. Imagine what your life will be like if you don't change.
- *Create a new self-image.* Imagine what you'll be like after changing your target behaviour. Try to think of yourself in new terms right now.
- *Think before you act.* Learn why you engage in the target behaviour. Determine what sets you off, and train yourself not to act reflexively.

Preparation

- *Create a plan.* Include a start date, goals, rewards, and specific steps you will take to change your behaviour.
- *Make change a priority.* Create and sign a contract with yourself.
- *Practise visualization and self-talk.* These techniques can help prepare you mentally for challenging situations.
- *Take short steps.* Successfully practising your new behaviour for a short time—even a single day—can boost your confidence and motivation.

Action

- *Monitor your progress.* Keep up with your journal entries.
- *Change your environment.* Make changes that will discourage the target behaviour—for example, get rid of snack foods or don't stock the refrigerator with beer.
- *Find alternatives to your target behaviour.* Make a list of things you can do to replace the behaviour.
- *Reward yourself.* Rewards should be identified in your change plan. Give yourself lots of praise, and focus on your success.
- *Involve your friends.* Tell them you want to change, and ask for their help.
- *Don't get discouraged.* Real change can be difficult.

Maintenance

- *Keep going.* Continue using the positive strategies that worked in earlier stages.
- *Be prepared for lapses.* Don't let slip-ups set you back.
- *Be a role model.* Once you have successfully changed your behaviour, you may be able to help someone else do the same thing.

SUMMARY

- Wellness is the ability to live life fully, with vitality and meaning. Wellness is dynamic and multi-dimensional; it incorporates physical, emotional, intellectual, spiritual, interpersonal and social, and environmental dimensions.
- As chronic diseases have become the leading cause of death in Canada, people have recognized that they have greater control over, and greater responsibility for, their health than ever before.
- The Integrated Pan-Canadian Healthy Living Strategy's vision is good health for all Canadians. The broad goals of the Strategy are to improve healthy weights, physical activity, and healthy eating among Canadians.
- Health-related differences among people that have implications for wellness can be described in the context of gender, ethnicity, income and education, disability, geographic location, and sexual orientation.
- Although heredity, environment, and health care all play roles in wellness and disease, behaviour can mitigate their effects.
- To make lifestyle changes, you need information about yourself, your health habits, and resources available to help you change.

- You can increase your motivation for behaviour change by examining the benefits and costs of change, boosting self-efficacy, and identifying and overcoming key barriers to change.
- The stages of change model describes six stages that people move through as they try to change their behaviour: precontemplation, contemplation, preparation, action, maintenance, and termination.
- A specific plan for change can be developed by (1) monitoring behaviour by keeping a journal; (2) analyzing the recorded data; (3) setting specific goals; (4) devising strategies for modifying the environment, rewarding yourself, and involving others; and (5) making a personal contract.
- To start and maintain a behaviour change program, you need commitment, a well-developed plan, social support, and a system of rewards.
- Although we cannot control every aspect of our health, we can make a difference in helping create an environment that supports wellness for everyone.

FOR MORE INFORMATION

BOOKS

Duhigg, C. 2012. *The Power of Habit: Why We Do What We Do in Life and Business*. New York: Random House. An entertaining and intelligent exploration of how habits control our lives and how we can take charge of our habits to change our lives; includes both current research and a wealth of real-life stories.

Komaroff, A. L., ed. 2005. *Harvard Medical School Family Health Guide*. New York: Free Press. Consumer-oriented advice for the prevention and treatment of common health concerns.

Litin, S. C. (ed.). 2009. *Mayo Clinic Family Health Book*, 4th ed. New York: HarperCollins Publishers. A complete health reference for every stage of life, covering thousands of conditions, symptoms, and treatments.

Murat, B., and G. Stewart. 2009. *Do I Need to See the Doctor? The Home-Treatment Encyclopedia—Written by Medical Doctors—That Lets You Decide*, 2nd ed. New York: John Wiley & Sons. A fully illustrated, easy-to-read guide to hundreds of common symptoms and ailments to help consumers determine whether they can treat themselves or should seek professional medical attention.

Prochaska, J. O., J. C. Norcross, and C. C. DiClemente. 1995. *Changing for Good: The Revolutionary Program That Explains the Six Stages of Change and Teaches You How to Free Yourself from Bad Habits*. New York: Morrow. A model of behaviour change and suggestions and advice for each stage of change.

NEWSLETTERS

Consumer Reports on Health (800-274-7596; http://www.consumerreports.org/health/home.htm)

Harvard Health Publications (877-649-9457; http://www.health.harvard.edu)

Mayo Clinic Health Letter (800-333-9037; http://healthletter.mayoclinic.com)

University of California, Berkeley, Wellness Letter (800-829-9170; http://www.wellnessletter.com)

ORGANIZATIONS, HOTLINES, AND WEBSITES

The Internet addresses listed here were accurate at the time of publication.

Canadian Diabetes Association. Through phone, email, and the Internet, provides a wide variety of diabetes-related information and support.
http://www.diabetes.ca

Canadian Fitness and Lifestyle Research Institute. Conducts research, monitors trends, and makes recommendations to increase population levels of physical activity and improve the health of all Canadians.
http://www.cflri.ca

Canadian Institute for Health Information. Provides reports and data that inform health policies, support the effective delivery of health services, and raise awareness among Canadians of the factors that contribute to good health.
   http://www.cihi.ca

Centers for Disease Control and Prevention (CDC). Through phone, fax, and the Internet, provides a wide variety of health information.
   http://www.cdc.gov

Health Canada. Includes research articles, summaries, and general information for helping Canadians maintain and improve their health.
   http://www.hc-sc.gc.ca

Healthfinder. Provides a gateway to online publications, websites, support and self-help groups, agencies, and organizations that produce reliable health information.
   http://www.healthfinder.gov

MedlinePlus. Provides links to news and reliable information about health from government agencies and professional associations; includes a health encyclopedia and information on prescription and over-the-counter drugs.
   http://www.nlm.nih.gov/medlineplus/

National Wellness Institute. Serves professionals and organizations that promote optimal health and wellness.
   http://www.nationalwellness.org

National Women's Health Information Center. Provides information and answers to frequently asked questions.
   http://www.4woman.gov

Office of Minority Health Resource Center. Promotes improved health among racial and ethnic minority populations.
   http://minorityhealth.hhs.gov/omh/browse.aspx?lvl=1&lvlid=3

Public Health Agency of Canada. Provides Internet-based information to strengthen Canada's capacity to protect and improve the health of Canadians and to help reduce pressures on the health care system.
   http://www.publichealth.gc.ca

U.S. Federal Trade Commission: Consumer Protection—Health. Provides online brochures about a variety of consumer health topics, including fitness equipment, generic drugs, and fraudulent health claims.
   http://www.ftc.gov/bcp/menus/consumer/health.shtm

U.S. National Health Information Center. Puts consumers in touch with the organizations that are best able to provide answers to health-related questions.
   http://www.health.gov/nhic

U.S. National Institutes of Health. Provides information about all its activities as well as consumer publications, hotline information, and an A to Z listing of health issues with links to the appropriate institute.
   http://www.nih.gov

U.S. Surgeon General. Includes information on activities of the U.S. Surgeon General and the text of many key reports on such topics as tobacco use, physical activity, and mental health.
   http://www.surgeongeneral.gov

World Health Organization. Provides information about health topics and issues affecting people around the world.
   http://www.who.int

The following are just a few of the many sites that provide consumer-oriented information on a variety of health issues:
   CNN Health: http://www.cnn.com/health
   FamilyDoctor.Org: http://www.familydoctor.org
   Harvard Health Publications: www.health.harvard.edu
   MayoClinic.com: http://www.mayoclinic.org
   Medbroadcast: http://www.medbroadcast.com

MedlinePlus News: http://www.nlm.nih.gov/medlineplus/newsbydate.html
MedPage Today Medical News: http://www.medpagetoday.com
WebMD: http://www.webmd.com
Yahoo Health News: http://news.yahoo.com/health/

SELECTED BIBLIOGRAPHY

American Cancer Society. 2012. *Cancer Facts and Figures—2012.* Atlanta: American Cancer Society.

American College Health Association. 2013. *American College Health Association-National College Health Assessment II: Canadian Reference Group Data Reporting Spring 2013.* Hanover, MD: American College Health Association.

American Heart Association. 2012. *Heart Disease and Stroke Statistics—2012 Update.* Dallas: American Heart Association.

Barr, D. A. 2008. *Health Disparities in the United States: Social Class, Race, Ethnicity, and Health.* Baltimore: The Johns Hopkins University Press.

Canadian Diabetes Association. 2008. *The Prevalence and Costs of Diabetes,* http://www.diabetes.ca/files/prevalence-and-costs.pdf (retrieved March 6, 2015).

Canadian Fitness and Lifestyle Research Institute. 2009. *Kids CAN PLAY! Bulletin 1: Activity Levels of Canadian Children and Youth,* http://www.cflri.ca/eng/programs/canplay/documents/CANPLAY2009_Bulletin01_PA_levelsEN.pdf (retrieved March 6, 2015).

Canadian Public Health Association. *What are the Social Determinants of Health?* http://www.cpha.ca/en/programs/social-determinants/frontlinehealth/sdh.aspx (retrieved January 14, 2015).

Centers for Disease Control and Prevention. 2008. *Racial and Ethnic Approaches to Community Health (REACH U.S.): Finding Solutions to Health Disparities, 2008,* http://www.cdc.gov/nccdphp/publications/aag/pdf/reach.pdf (retrieved December 27, 2015).

Centers for Disease Control and Prevention. 2008. Racial/ethnic disparities in self-rated health status among adults with and without disabilities—United States, 2004–2006. *Morbidity and Mortality Weekly Report* 57(39), pp. 1069–1073.

Dietitians of Canada. 2005. *Registered Dietitians in Aboriginal Communities: Feeding Mind, Body and Spirit. Role Paper of the Dietitians of Canada Aboriginal Nutrition Network,* http://www.dietitians.ca/resources/resourcesearch.asp (retrieved September 3, 2015).

Finkelstein, E. A., et al. 2008. Do obese persons comprehend their personal health risks? *American Journal of Health Behaviour* 32(5), pp. 508–516.

First Nations Information Governance Centre. 2005. *First Nations Regional Longitudinal Health Survey (RHS) 2002/03: Results for Adults, Youth and Children Living in First Nations Communities,* http://www.fnigc.ca/sites/default/files/ENpdf/RHS_2002/rhs2002-03-technical_report.pdf (retrieved March 12, 2015).

Flegal, K. M., et al. 2007. Cause-specific excess deaths associated with underweight, overweight, and obesity. *Journal of the American Medical Association* 298(17), pp. 2028–2037.

Garriguet, D. 2008. Obesity and the eating habits of the Aboriginal population. *Health Reports* 19(1), pp. 21–35.

Gilmore, H. 2007. Physically active Canadians. *Health Reports* 18(3), pp. 45–67.

Gorman, B. K., and J. G. Read. 2006. Gender disparities in adult health: An examination of three measures of morbidity. *Journal of Health and Social Behaviour* 47(2), pp. 95–110.

Health Canada. 2009. *A Statistical Profile on the Health of First Nations in Canada: Determinants of Health, 1999 to 2003,* http://www.hc-sc.gc.ca/fniah-spnia/pubs/aborig-autoch/2009-stats-profil/index-eng.php (retrieved March 6, 2015).

Herd, P., et al. 2007. Socioeconomic position and health: The differential effects of education versus income on the onset versus progression of health problems. *Journal of Health and Social Behaviour* 48(3), pp. 223–238.

Horneffer-Ginter, K. 2008. Stages of change and possible selves: Two tools for promoting college health. *Journal of American College Health* 56(4), pp. 351–358.

How to keep those New Year's resolutions. 2006. *Harvard Health Letter,* January 31.

Irwin, J. D. 2007. The prevalence of physical activity maintenance in a sample of university students: A longitudinal study. *Journal of American College Health* 56(1), pp. 37–41.

Martin, G., and J. Pear. 2007. *Behaviour Modification: What It Is and How to Do It,* 8th ed. Upper Saddle River, N.J.: Prentice-Hall.

National Center for Health Statistics. 2007. *Health, United States, 2007, with Chartbook on Trends in the Health of Americans.* Hyattsville, Md.: National Center for Health Statistics.

National Center for Health Statistics. 2008. Deaths: Preliminary data for 2006. *National Vital Statistics Report* 56(16), http://www.cdc.gov/nchs/data/nvsr/nvsr56/nvsr56_16.pdf (retrieved March 6, 2015).

Nothwehr, F., et al. 2008. Age group differences in diet and physical activity related behaviors among rural men and women. *Journal of Nutrition, Health and Aging* 12(3), pp. 169–174.

Ogden, C. L., et al. 2006. Prevalence of overweight and obesity in the United States, 1999–2004. *Journal of the American Medical Association* 295(13), pp. 1549–1555.

O' Loughlin, J., et al. 2007. Lifestyle risk factors for chronic disease across family origin among adults in multiethnic, low-income, urban neighborhoods. *Ethnicity and Disease* 17(4), pp. 657–663

Secretariat for the Intersectoral Healthy Living Network in partnership with the F/P/T Healthy Living Task Group and the F/P/T Advisory Committee on Population Health and Health Security (ACPHHS). 2005. *The Integrated Pan-Canadian Healthy Living Strategy,* http://www.phac-aspc.gc.ca/hp-ps/hl-mvs/ipchls-spimmvs/pdf/ipchls-spimmvs-eng.pdf (retrieved April 17, 2015).

Statistics Canada. Leading Causes of Deaths in Canada, 2009, CANSIM Tables 102–0561 and 102–0562, http://www.statcan.gc.ca/pub/84-215-x/2012001/table-tableau/tbl003-eng.htm, (retrieved January 6, 2015).

Statistics Canada. 2009. *Population Urban and Rural, by Province and Territory,* http://www40.statcan.ca/l01/cst01/demo62a-eng.htm (retrieved March 6, 2015).

Statistics Canada. 2010. Visible Minority Groups, 2006 counts, for Canada, Provinces and Territories—20% Sample Data (table), http://www12.statcan.ca/census-recensement/2006/dp-pdhlt/97-562/pages/page.cfm?Lang=E&Geo=PR&Code=01&Table=1&Data=Count&StartRec=1&Sort=2&Display=Page (retrieved March 6, 2015).

Statistics Canada. 2012. Table105-0503 - Health indicator profile, age-standardized rate, annual estimates, by sex, Canada, provinces and territories, occasional, CANSIM (database) (retrieved January 6, 2015).

Song, J., et al. 2006. Gender differences across race/ethnicity in use of health care among Medicare-aged Americans. *Journal of Women's Health* 15(10), pp. 1205–1213.

Tjepkema, M., and M. Shields. 2004. *Nutrition. Findings from the Canadian Community Health Survey. Issue no.1. Measured Obesity: Adult Obesity in Canada.* Ottawa: Statistics Canada.

Transport Canada. 2008. *A Quick Look at Alcohol-related Crashes in Canada: Fact Sheet,* http://www.tc.gc.ca/eng/roadsafety/tp-tp2436-rs200809-menu-397.htm (retrieved March 6, 2015).

U. C. Berkeley. 2007. Do men get their fair share? University of California, *Berkeley, Wellness Letter,* April, 1–2.

U. C. Berkeley. 2008. *Evaluating Web Pages: Techniques to Apply and Questions to Ask,* http://www.lib.berkeley.edu/TeachingLib/Guides/Internet/Evaluate.html (retrieved December 27, 2015).

Walker, B., and C. P. Mouton. 2008. Environmental influences on cardiovascular health. *Journal of the National Medical Association* 100(1), pp. 98–102.

Walsh, T., et al. 2006. Spectrum of mutations in BRCA1, BRCA2, CHEK2, and TP53 in families at high risk of breast cancer. *Journal of the American Medical Association* 295, 99. 1379–1388.

World Health Organization. 2011. Noncommunicable Diseases Country Profiles 2011. ISBN 978 92 4 150228, http://www.who.int/nmh/publications/ncd_profiles_report.pdf (retrieved January 14, 2015).

CHAPTER 2

Psychological Health

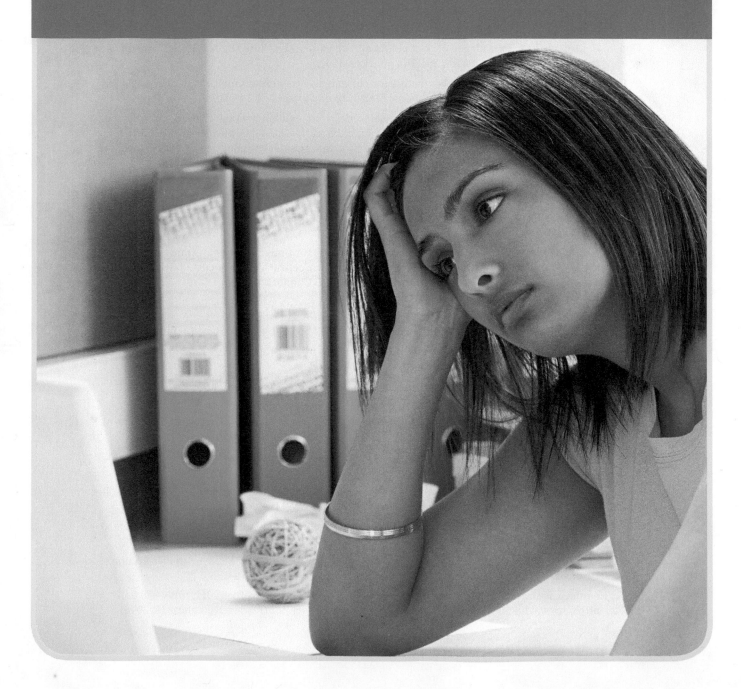

LOOKING AHEAD

After you have read and studied this chapter, you should be able to:

LO1 Describe what it means to be psychologically healthy

LO2 Explain how to develop and maintain a positive self-concept and healthy self-esteem

LO3 Discuss the importance of an optimistic outlook, good communication skills, and constructive approaches to dealing with loneliness and anger

LO4 Describe common psychological disorders

LO5 List the warning signs of suicide

LO6 Describe the different types of help available for psychological problems

TEST YOUR KNOWLEDGE

1. **Normality is a key component of psychological health.**
   True or false?

2. **Trying to think rationally about what bothers you won't get you very far, because psychological problems usually are due to emotions, not thinking.**
   True or false?

3. **About how many Canadians have a diagnosable psychological disorder at some time during their life?**
   a. 5% b. 10% c. 20%

4. **People with enough willpower can force themselves to snap out of their depression.**
   True or false?

5. **A person who attempts suicide but survives did not really intend to die.**
   True or false?

ANSWERS

1. FALSE. Normality simply means being close to average, and having unusual ideas or attitudes doesn't mean that a person has a mental illness. The fact that people's ideas are varied makes life interesting and helps people respond in creative ways to life's challenges.

2. FALSE. Research has shown that getting people to adopt more realistic attitudes and beliefs about themselves and others can alleviate depression.

3. c. According to the Mental Health Commission of Canada, about 6.7 million Canadians will have a diagnosable psychological disorder at some point.

4. FALSE. Depression, a disorder strongly linked to brain chemistry, can overcome whatever willpower people have and make it impossible for them to make decisions.

5. FALSE. A person may intend to die but miscalculate how to successfully commit suicide.

Psychological health (or mental health) contributes to every dimension of wellness. It can be very difficult to maintain emotional, social, or even physical wellness if you are not psychologically healthy.

> **psychological health**
> Mental health, defined either negatively as the absence of illness or positively as the presence of wellness.

Psychological health, however, is a broad concept—one that is as difficult to define as it is important to understand. That is why the first section of this chapter is devoted to explaining what psychological health is and is not. The rest of the chapter discusses a number of common psychological problems, their symptoms, and their treatments.

If life doesn't bring you the pleasure or happiness you think it should, or if you believe you should be functioning at a higher level, you should know that there are ways of getting help. This chapter will show you how.

Defining Psychological Health

Psychological or mental health can be defined as our capacity to think, feel, and behave in ways that contribute to our ability to enjoy life and manage challenges. Our psychological wellness can be supported or sabotaged by a variety of factors, such as dietary choices, sleep patterns, and relationship issues. With good psychological health, people have a positive sense of emotional and spiritual well-being that values fairness, culture, dignity, and interpersonal connections. That being said, we must be mindful that if we think of everyone who does not have a severe mental illness as being mentally healthy, we are ignoring common problems that can be addressed. For this reason, psychological health is sometimes defined more negatively as the absence of sickness. Clearly, freedom from disorders is only one factor in psychological wellness.

Maslow's Hierarchy: Striving Toward Self-Actualization

A positive definition—psychological health as the presence of wellness—is a more ambitious outlook that encourages us to fulfill our own potential.

During the 1960s, Abraham Maslow described such an ideal of mental health in his book *Toward a Psychology of Being*. According to Maslow, people have a *hierarchy of needs*, listed here in order of decreasing importance (see Figure 2.1):

- physiological needs
- safety
- being loved
- maintaining self-esteem
- self-actualization

When urgent (life-sustaining) needs—such as the need for food and water—are satisfied, less basic needs take priority. Most of us are well-fed and feel reasonably safe, and so we are driven by higher-level motives. Maslow's conclusions were based on his study of a group of visibly successful people who seemed to have lived, or be living, at their fullest. He stated that these people had achieved **self-actualization**; they had fulfilled

FIGURE 2.1

Maslow's Hierarchy of Needs

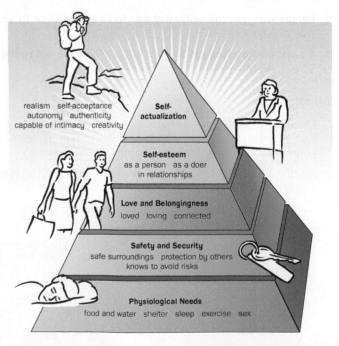

Source: Maslow, A. 1970. *Motivation and Personality*, 2nd ed. New York: Harper & Row.

a good measure of their human potential. Maslow suggested that self-actualized people all share certain qualities:

self-actualization
The highest level of growth in Maslow's hierarchy.

- *Realism:* Self-actualized people are realistic. They know the difference between what is real and what they want. As a result, they can cope with the world as it exists without demanding that it be different; they know what they can and cannot change. Just as important, realistic people accept evidence that contradicts what they want to believe. If the evidence is strong enough, they adapt their belief systems accordingly.
- *Acceptance:* Psychologically healthy people accept themselves as they are. Self-acceptance requires a positive **self-concept**, or *self-image:* a positive but realistic perception of yourself. Similarly, psychological health requires an appropriately high but realistic level of **self-esteem**. People with healthy self-esteem value themselves as people; they feel good about themselves and are likely to live up to their positive self-image and enjoy successes that in turn reinforce these good feelings. Self-acceptance also means being tolerant of your own imperfections, an ability that makes it easier to accept the imperfections of others.

self-concept
The ideas, feelings, and perceptions people have about themselves; also called self-image.

self-esteem
Satisfaction and confidence in yourself; the valuing of yourself as a person.

QUESTIONS FOR CRITICAL THINKING AND REFLECTION

Have you ever had a reason to feel concerned about your own psychological health? If so, what was the reason? Did your concern lead you to talk to someone about the issue or to seek professional help? If you did, what was the outcome, and how do you feel about it now?

- *Autonomy:* Psychologically healthy people are *autonomous*, meaning they can direct themselves and act independently of their social environment. **Autonomy** is more than physical independence; it is social, emotional, and intellectual independence, as well. Autonomous people are **inner-directed**, finding guidance from within, from their own rules and values. They have an internal locus of control and a high level of self-efficacy (see Chapter 1). By contrast, **other-directed** people often act only in response to what they feel as external pressure from others. Instead of speaking their true feelings, for example, other-directed people are more inclined to say what they believe will make other people happy.

autonomy
Independence; the sense of being self-directed.

inner-directed
Guided in behaviour by an inner set of rules and values.

other-directed
Guided in behaviour by the values and expectations of others.

- *Authenticity:* Autonomous people are not afraid to be themselves; sometimes, their capacity for being real may give them a certain childlike quality. They respond in a genuine, spontaneous way to whatever happens, without pretence or self-consciousness. Such people do not worry about being judged by others just for being themselves. This quality of genuineness is sometimes called **authenticity**.

authenticity
Genuineness.

- *Capacity for intimacy:* Healthy people can be physically and emotionally intimate. They are able to share their feelings and thoughts without fear of rejection. A psychologically healthy person is open to the pleasure of physical contact and the satisfaction of being close to others—but without being afraid of the risks involved in intimacy, such as the risk of getting hurt. (Chapters 10 and 11 discuss intimacy in more detail.)
- *Creativity:* Psychologically healthy people continually look at the world with renewed appreciation. Such appreciation can inform a person's creativity, which helps explain why so many mentally healthy people are creative. They may not be great poets or painters, but they live their everyday lives in creative ways. Creative people seem to see more and to be open to new experiences; they don't fear the unknown or avoid uncertainty.

Self-actualization is an ideal to strive for. Rather than dwelling on the past, we need to concentrate on meeting current challenges in ways that lead to long-term mental wellness. We must not consider ourselves failures if we do not achieve our full potential in every way or at every moment.

What Psychological Health Is Not

Psychological health is not the same as psychological **normality**. Being mentally normal simply means being close to average. We can define normal body temperature because a few degrees above or below this temperature means physical sickness. But your ideas and attitudes can vary tremendously without your losing efficiency or feeling emotional distress. In fact, psychological diversity—with the wide range of ideas, lifestyles, and attitudes it brings about—is a valuable asset to society.

normality
The psychological characteristics attributed to the majority of people in a population at a given time.

Never seeking help for personal problems does not prove you are psychologically healthy, any more than seeking help proves you have a mental illness. Unhappy people may avoid seeking help for many reasons, and people with a severe mental illness may not even realize they need help.

QUICK STATS

80% of all people who intend to commit suicide hint or make a comment to someone, usually a friend.
—Canadian Mental Health Association, 2011

Further, we can't say people have a mental illness or are mentally healthy based solely on the presence or absence of symptoms. Consider the symptom of anxiety, for example. Anxiety can help you face a problem and solve it before it becomes too big. Someone who shows no anxiety may be refusing to recognize problems or to do anything about them. A person who is anxious for good reason is likely to be judged more psychologically healthy in the long run than someone who is inappropriately calm.

Finally, we cannot judge psychological health from the way people look. All too often, a person who seems to be OK and even happy suddenly takes his or her own life. Usually, such people lack close friends who might have known their desperation. At an early age, we learn to conceal our feelings and even to lie about them. We may believe that our complaints put unfair demands on others. Although silence may sometimes be a virtue, it can also prevent the person from getting help.

Meeting Life's Challenges

Life is full of challenges—large and small. Everyone, regardless of heredity and family influences, must learn to cope successfully with new situations and new people. For emotional and mental wellness, each of us must continue to grow psychologically, developing new and more sophisticated coping mechanisms to suit our current lives. We must develop an adult identity that enhances our spiritual wellness, self-esteem, and autonomy. We must also learn to communicate honestly, handle anger and loneliness appropriately, and avoid being defensive.

> **QUICK STATS**
>
> Over 72% of Canadians report their mental health as excellent or very good.
> —*Statistics Canada*, 2012

Growing Up Psychologically

Our responses to life's challenges influence the development of our personality and identity. Psychologist Erik Erikson proposed that development proceeds through a series of eight stages that extend throughout life. Each stage is characterized by a major crisis or turning point—a time of increased vulnerability as well as increased potential for psychological growth (see Table 2.1).

TABLE 2.1

Erikson's Stages of Development

Age	Conflict	Important People	Task
Birth–1 year	Trust vs. mistrust	Mother or other primary caregiver	In being fed and comforted, developing the trust that others will respond to your needs
1–3 years	Autonomy vs. shame and self-doubt	Parents	In toilet training, locomotion, and exploration, learning self-control without losing the capacity for assertiveness
3–6 years	Initiative vs. guilt	Family	In playful talking and locomotion, developing a conscience (based on parental prohibitions) that is not too inhibiting
6–12 years	Industry vs. inferiority	Neighbourhood and school	In school and playing with peers, learning the value of accomplishment and perseverance without feeling inadequate
Adolescence	Identity vs. identity confusion	Peers	Developing a stable sense of who you are—your needs, abilities, interpersonal style, and values
Young adulthood	Intimacy vs. isolation	Close friends, sex partners	Learning to live and share intimately with others, often in sexual relationships
Middle adulthood	Generativity vs. self-absorption	Work associates, children, community	Doing things for others, including parenting and civic activities
Older adulthood	Integrity vs. despair	Humankind	Affirming the value of life and its ideals

Source: Erikson, E. 1963. *Childhood and Society.* New York: Norton.

The successful mastery of one stage is a basis for mastering the next; early failures can have repercussions in later life. Fortunately, life provides ongoing opportunities for mastering these tasks. For example, although the development of trust begins in infancy, it is refined as we grow older. We learn to trust people outside our immediate family and to limit our trust by identifying people who are untrustworthy.

Developing an Adult Identity

A primary task beginning in adolescence is the development of an adult identity: a unified sense of self, characterized by attitudes, beliefs, and ways of acting that are genuinely your own. People with adult identities know who they are, what they are capable of, what roles they play, and their place among their peers. They have a sense of their own uniqueness, but also appreciate what they have in common with others. They view themselves realistically and can assess their strengths and weaknesses without relying on the opinions of others. Achieving an identity also means being able to form intimate relationships with others while maintaining a strong sense of self.

Our identities evolve as we interact with the world and make choices about what we would like to do and who we would like to model ourselves after. Developing an adult identity is particularly challenging in a heterogeneous, secular, and relatively affluent society like ours, in which many roles are possible, many choices are tolerated, and ample time is allowed for experimenting and making up one's mind.

Early identities are often modelled after parents—or the opposite of parents, in rebellion against what they represent. Over time, peers, rock stars, sports heroes, and religious figures are added to the list of possible models. In high school and university or college, people often join cliques that assert a certain identity, such as the *jocks*, the *brains*, or the *slackers*. Although much of an identity is internal—a way of viewing ourselves and the world—certain aspects of it can be external, such as styles of talking and dressing, ornaments, such as earrings, and hairstyles.

Early identities are rarely permanent. A student who works for good grades and approval one year can turn into a class-skipping student devoted to wild parties a year later. At some point, however, most of us adopt a more stable, individual identity that ties together the experiences of childhood and the expectations and aspirations of adulthood. Erikson's theory does not suggest that one day we suddenly assume our final identity and never change after that. Life is more interesting for people who continue evolving into more distinct individuals, rather than being rigidly controlled by their pasts. Identity reflects a lifelong process, and it changes as a person develops new relationships and roles.

Developing an adult identity is an important part of psychological wellness. Without a personal identity, we begin to feel confused about who we are; Erikson called this situation an **identity crisis**. Until we have found ourselves, we cannot have much self-esteem, because a self is not firmly in place.

identity crisis
Internal confusion about who you are.

How far have you gotten in developing your adult identity? Create a list of characteristics you think a friend who knows you well would use to describe you. Rank them from the most to the least important. Your list might include such elements as gender, socioeconomic status, ethnic and religious identification, choice of university/college or major, parents' occupations, interests and talents, attitudes toward drugs and alcohol, style of dress, the kinds of people with whom you typically associate, your expected role in society, and aspects of your personality. Which elements of your identity do you feel are permanent, and which do you think may change over time? Are there any characteristics missing from your list that you would like to add?

Another aid to developing an adult identity is to identify possible role models. Who do you admire and want to be like? Which characteristics of that person do you want to emulate? How did that person acquire those characteristics, and how could you follow her or his example? Some role models might be willing to be mentors to you, spending time with you and sharing their wisdom.

Developing Intimacy

Erikson's developmental stages don't end with establishing an adult identity. Learning to live intimately with others and finding a productive role for yourself in society are other tasks of adulthood—to be able to love and work.

People with established identities can form intimate relationships and sexual unions characterized by sharing, open communication, long-term commitment, and love. Those who lack a firm sense of self may have difficulty establishing relationships because they feel overwhelmed by closeness and the needs of another person. As a result, they experience only short-term, superficial relationships with others and may remain isolated.

Developing Values and Purpose in Your Life

Erikson assigned his last two stages, generativity versus self-absorption and integrity versus despair, to middle adulthood and older adulthood. But these stages are concerned with values and purpose in life, issues that need to be addressed by young people and reexamined throughout life.

Values are criteria for judging what is good and bad; they underlie our moral decisions and behaviour. The first morality of the young child is to consider *good* to mean what brings immediate and tangible rewards, and *bad*, whatever results in punishment. An older child will explain right and wrong in terms of authority figures and rules. But the final stage of moral development, one that not everyone attains, is being able to conceive of right and wrong in more abstract terms, such as justice and virtue.

> **values**
> Criteria for judging what is good and bad, which underlie a person's moral decisions and behaviour.

As adults we need to assess how far we have evolved morally and what values we actually have adopted. Without an awareness of our personal values, our lives may be hurriedly driven forward by immediate desires and the passing demands of others. Living according to values means:

- considering your options carefully before making a choice;
- choosing between options without succumbing to outside pressures that oppose your values; and
- making a choice and acting on it rather than doing nothing.

Your actions and how you justify them proclaim to others what you stand for. A practical exercise for clarifying your values and goals is to write a draft of your obituary for a local newspaper. How would you like to be remembered? What would you like to have achieved? What will you have done to meet those goals? This obituary should not be a glorification, but rather an honest, realistic appraisal. End it by summarizing in a few sentences what was most important about your life. In reading what you have written, ask yourself, "How will I have to change to be the person I want to be?"

For more on discovering your values, see the Assess Yourself box.

Striving for Spiritual Wellness

Spiritual wellness is associated with greater coping skills and higher levels of overall wellness. It is a very personal wellness component, and it can be developed in many ways (see the Mind Body Spirit box). Researchers

 Assess YOURSELF

Assessing Your Values

Find out more about your core values by answering these questions:

- What personality traits or characteristics do you most value—for example, being friendly, patient, successful, outgoing, cooperative, loyal to family and friends? These can be characteristics you see in yourself or in others.
- What activities or accomplishments do you most value—for example, making lots of money, getting good grades, spending time with friends, making your own decisions? These can be accomplishments of your own or of others, or goals you have for the future.
- What social ideals, customs, and institutions do you value—for example, education, equality, freedom of speech, tolerance for diverse opinions?
- How well does your current lifestyle reflect your values? Can you think of some recent incidents in which you acted in accordance with your values or in ways that conflict with your values?

Mind *Body* SPIRIT

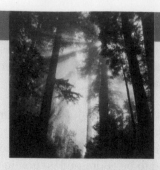

Paths to Spiritual Wellness

Spiritual wellness means different things to different people. For many, it involves developing a set of guiding beliefs, principles, or values that give purpose and meaning to life. It helps people achieve a sense of wholeness within themselves and in their relationships with others. Spiritual wellness influences people on an individual level, as well as on a community level, where it can bond people through compassion, love, forgiveness, and self-sacrifice.

Many paths to spiritual wellness exist. One of the most common in our society is organized religion. The major religions provide paths for transforming the self in ways that can lead to greater happiness and serenity and reduce feelings of anxiety and hopelessness. For example, in Christianity, salvation means turning away from the selfish ego and to God's sovereignty and grace, where a joy is found that frees the believer from anxious self-concern and despair. Islam represents a kind of self-surrender leading to peace with God. Buddhism teaches how to detach the self from selfish desire, leading to compassion for the suffering of others and freedom from fear-engendering illusions. Judaism emphasizes the social and ethical redemption members of the Jewish community can experience if they follow the laws of God.

Religions teach specific techniques for achieving these transformations of the self: prayer, both in groups and in private; meditation; the performance of rituals and ceremonies symbolizing religious truths; and good works and service to others. Religious organizations also usually offer social and material support to members who might otherwise be isolated.

Spiritual wellness does not require participation in organized religion. Many people find meaning and purpose in other ways. By spending time in nature or working on environmental issues, people can experience continuity with the natural world. Spiritual wellness can come through helping others in the community or by promoting human rights, peace, and harmony among people, and opportunities for human development on a global level. Other people develop spiritual wellness through art or through their personal relationships.

have linked spiritual wellness to longer life expectancy, reduced risk of disease, faster recovery, and improved emotional health. Although spirituality is difficult to study, and researchers aren't sure how or why spirituality seems to improve health, several explanations have been offered.

- *Social support:* Attending religious services or participating in volunteer organizations helps people feel that they are part of a community with similar values and promotes social connectedness and caring.
- *Healthy habits:* Some of the paths to spiritual wellness may encourage healthy behaviours, such as eating a vegetarian diet or consuming less meat and alcohol, and may discourage harmful habits, such as smoking.
- *Positive attitude:* Spirituality can give people a sense of meaning and purpose in life, and these qualities create a more positive attitude in people, which in turn helps them cope with life's challenges.
- *Moments of relaxation:* Spiritual practices, such as prayer, meditation, and immersion in artistic activities, can reduce stress by eliciting the relaxation response.

Spirituality provides an ethical path to personal fulfillment that includes connectedness with the self, others, and a higher power or larger reality. Spiritual wellness can make you more aware of your personal values and can help clarify them. Without an awareness of personal values, you might be driven by immediate desires and the passing demands of others. Living according to values means considering your options carefully before making a choice, choosing between options without succumbing to outside pressures that oppose your values, and making a choice and acting on it rather than doing nothing.

Achieving Healthy Self-Esteem

Having a healthy level of self-esteem means regarding your self, which includes all aspects of your identity, as good, competent, and worthy of love. It is a critical component of wellness.

Developing a Positive Self-Concept

Ideally, a positive self-concept begins in childhood, based on experiences both within the family and outside it. Children need to develop a sense of being loved and being able to give love and to accomplish their goals. If they feel rejected or neglected by their parents, they may fail to develop feelings of self-worth. They may grow to have a negative concept of themselves.

Another component of self-concept is *integration*. An integrated self-concept is one that you have made for yourself—not someone else's image of you or a mask that doesn't quite fit. Important building blocks of self-concept are the personality characteristics and mannerisms of parents, which children may adopt without realizing it. Later, they may be surprised to find themselves acting like one of their parents. Eventually, such building blocks should be reshaped and integrated into a new, individual personality.

A further aspect of self-concept is *stability*. Stability depends on the integration of the self and its freedom from contradictions. People who have received mixed messages about themselves from parents and friends may have contradictory self-images, which defy integration and make them vulnerable to shifting levels of self-esteem. At times they regard themselves as entirely good, capable, and lovable—an ideal self—and at other times they see themselves as entirely bad, incompetent, and unworthy of love. Neither of these extreme self-concepts allow people to see themselves or others realistically, and their

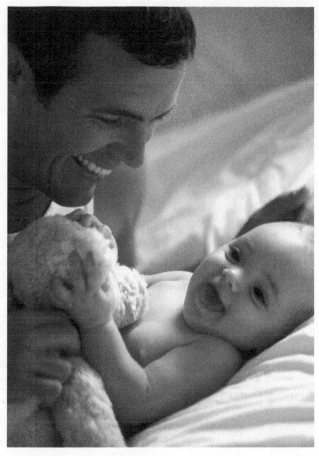

A positive self-concept begins in infancy. Knowing that he's loved and valued by his parents gives this baby a solid basis for lifelong psychological health.

relationships with other people are filled with misunderstandings and ultimately with conflict. The concepts we have about ourselves and others are an important part of our personalities. And all the components of our self-concept profoundly influence our interpersonal relationships.

How would you define spiritual wellness and its role in your life? What beliefs and practices do you associate with your sense of spiritual wellness? To achieve overall well-being, it is important to take time out to consider what you can do to help your spiritual side flourish.

Meeting Challenges to Self-Esteem

As an adult, you sometimes run into situations that challenge your self-concept. People you care about may tell you they don't love you or feel loved by you, for example, or your attempts to accomplish a goal may end in failure.

You can react to such challenges in several ways. The best approach is to acknowledge that something has gone wrong and try again, adjusting your goals to your abilities without radically revising your self-concept. Less productive responses are denying that anything went wrong and blaming someone else. These attitudes may preserve your self-concept temporarily, but in the end they keep you from meeting the challenge.

The worst reaction is to develop a lasting negative self-concept in which you feel bad, unloved, and ineffective—in other words, to become demoralized. Instead of coping, the demoralized person gives up, reinforcing the negative self-concept and setting in motion a cycle of bad self-concept and failure. In people who are genetically predisposed to depression, demoralization can progress to additional symptoms, which are discussed later in the chapter.

NOTICE YOUR PATTERNS OF THINKING One method for fighting demoralization is to recognize and test the negative thoughts and assumptions you may have about yourself and others. Try to note exactly when an unpleasant emotion—feeling worthless, wanting to give up, feeling depressed—occurs or gets worse, to identify the events or daydreams that trigger that emotion, and to observe whatever thoughts come into your head just before or during the emotional experience. It is helpful to keep a daily journal about such events.

AVOID FOCUSING ON THE NEGATIVE Imagine that you are waiting for a friend to meet you for dinner, but he's 30 minutes late. What kinds of thoughts go through your head when something like this happens? You might wonder what has happened to cause the delay: Perhaps he is stuck in traffic, you think, or needs to help a roommate who has the flu. This kind of reaction is healthy for several reasons:

- *You aren't jumping to a conclusion or blaming your friend for a failure of any kind.* After all, he probably hasn't forgotten about you or decided to ditch you.
- *You are being reasonable by giving your friend the benefit of the doubt.* Things happen. Your friend probably has a good reason for not being there. He deserves a chance to explain and may even need your help dealing with the situation that made him late.
- *You avoid personalizing the situation in such a way that you feel hurt or betrayed.* Jumping to a negative conclusion (such as "He isn't coming because he doesn't really like me") can make you feel bad unnecessarily. The same thing happens if you place blame—either on your friend or on yourself—without knowing all the facts.

By contrast, people who are demoralized tend to use all-or-nothing thinking. They overgeneralize from negative events. They overlook the positive and jump to negative conclusions, minimizing their own successes and magnifying the successes of others. They take responsibility for unfortunate situations that are not their fault, and then jump to more negative conclusions and more unfounded overgeneralizations. Patterns of thinking that make events seem worse than they are in reality are called **cognitive distortions**.

> **cognitive distortions**
> Patterns of negative thinking that make events seem worse than they are.

DEVELOP REALISTIC SELF-TALK When you react to a situation, an important piece of that reaction is your **self-talk**—the statements you make to yourself inside your own mind. To pick up on our earlier example, suppose your friend is late for a dinner date. As you wait for your friend to arrive, your self-talk has a profound effect on your reaction to his lateness. Someone who is demoralized or wrestling with a poor self-concept might immediately react with negative self-talk: *"He isn't coming. It's my fault; he probably doesn't like me because I'm boring. I bet he's with someone else."* This type of self-talk assigns blame (not just on your friend, but also on you), is judgmental, and jumps to an unverified conclusion about the meaning of your friend's lateness. In fact, you don't know why he is late or what he is thinking.

> **self-talk**
> The statements a person makes to himself or herself.

More rational thinking and self-talk will not only help get you through the situation without feeling upset, but will also help you avoid damaging your own self-concept. In this case, helpful self-talk is not negative, but neutral: *"He's never late for dinner. Something must be holding him up. I'll call him and make sure everything is all right."* This thinking recognizes that a problem may exist, but it does not judge or assign blame.

In your own fight against demoralization, it may be hard to think of a rational response until hours or days after the event that upset you. Responding rationally can be especially hard when you are having an argument with someone else, which is why people often say things they don't mean in the heat of the moment or develop hurt feelings even when the other person had no intention of hurting them.

Once you get used to noticing the way your mind works, however, you may be able to catch yourself thinking negatively and change the process before it goes too far. This approach to controlling your reactions is not the same as positive thinking—which means substituting a positive thought for a negative one. Instead, you simply try to make your thoughts as logical and accurate as possible, based on the facts of the situation as you know them, and not on snap judgments or conclusions that may turn out to be false.

Demoralized people can be tenacious about their negative beliefs—so tenacious that they make their beliefs come true in a self-fulfilling prophesy. For example, if you conclude that you are so boring that no one will like you anyway, you may decide not to bother socializing. This behaviour could make the negative belief become a reality.

For additional tips on changing distorted, negative ways of thinking, see the Take Charge box.

 Take **CHARGE**

Realistic Self-Talk

Do your patterns of thinking make events seem worse than they truly are? Do negative beliefs about yourself become self-fulfilling prophecies? Substituting realistic self-talk for negative self-talk can help you build and maintain self-esteem and cope better with the challenges in your life. Here are some examples of common types of distorted, negative self-talk, along with suggestions for more accurate and rational responses.

Cognitive Distortion	Negative Self-Talk	Realistic Self-Talk
Focusing on negatives	Babysitting is such a pain in the neck; I wish I didn't need the extra money so badly.	This is a tough job, but at least the money's decent and I can study once the kids go to bed.
Expecting the worst	I know I'm going to get an F in this course. I should just drop out of school now.	I'm not doing too well in this course. I should talk to my professor to see what kind of help I can get.
Overgeneralizing	My hair is a mess and I'm gaining weight. I'm so ugly. No one would ever want to date me.	I could use a haircut and should try to exercise more. This way I'll start feeling better about myself and will be more confident when I meet people.
Minimizing	It was nice of everyone to eat the dinner I cooked, even though I ruined it. I'm such a rotten cook.	Well, the roast was a little dry but they ate every bite. The veggies and rolls made up for it. I'm finally getting the hang of cooking!
Blaming others	Everyone I meet is such a jerk. Why aren't people more friendly?	I am going to make more of an effort to meet people who share my interests.
Expecting perfection	I cannot believe I flubbed that solo. They probably won't even let me audition for the orchestra next year.	It's a good thing I didn't stop playing when I hit that sour note. It didn't seem like anyone noticed it as much as I did.
Believing you're the cause of everything	Tom and Sara broke up and it's my fault. I shouldn't have insisted that Tom spend so much time with me and the guys.	It's a shame Tom and Sara broke up. I wish I knew what happened between them. Maybe Tom will tell me at soccer practice. At any rate, it isn't my fault; I've been a good friend to both of them.
Thinking in black and white	I thought that Mike was really cool, but after what he said today, I realize we have nothing in common.	I was really surprised that Mike disagreed with me today. I guess there are still things I don't know about him.
Magnifying events	I stuttered when I was giving my speech today in class. I must have sounded like a complete idiot. I'm sure everyone is talking about it.	My speech went really well, except for that one stutter. I bet most people didn't even notice it, though.

Being Less Defensive

Sometimes our wants come into conflict with people around us or with our conscience, and we become frustrated and anxious. If we cannot resolve the conflict by changing the external situation, we try to resolve the conflict internally by rearranging our thoughts and feelings. Some standard **defence mechanisms** are listed in Table 2.2. The drawback of many of these coping mechanisms is that they succeed temporarily, but make finding permanent solutions much harder.

defence mechanisms
Mental devices for coping with conflict or anxiety.

Recognizing your own defence mechanisms can be difficult because they have probably become habits, occurring unconsciously. But we each have some inkling about how our mind operates. By remembering the details of conflict situations you have been in, you may be able to figure out which defence mechanisms you used in successful or unsuccessful attempts to cope. Try to look at yourself as an objective, outside observer would and analyze your thoughts and behaviour in a psychologically stressful situation from the past. Having insight into what strategies you typically use can lead to new, less defensive, and more effective ways of coping in the future.

Being Optimistic

Many psychologists believe that pessimism is not just a symptom of everyday depression, but an important root cause, as well. Pessimists not only expect repeated failure and rejection, but also accept it as deserved. Pessimists do not see themselves as capable of success, and they irrationally dismiss any evidence of their own accomplishments. This negative point of view is learned, typically at a young age, from parents and other authority figures. But as an optimist would tell you, that means it also has the potential to be unlearned.

TABLE 2.2

Defence and Coping Mechanisms

Mechanism	Description	Example
Projection	Reacting to unacceptable inner impulses as if they were from outside the self	A student who dislikes his roommate feels that the roommate dislikes him
Repression	Expelling from awareness an unpleasant feeling, idea, or memory	The child of an alcoholic, neglectful father remembers him as a giving, loving person
Denial	Refusing to acknowledge to yourself what you really know to be true	A person believes that smoking cigarettes won't harm her because she's young and healthy
Passive-aggressive behaviour	Expressing hostility toward someone by being covertly uncooperative or passive	A person tells a co-worker, with whom she competes for project assignments, that she'll help him with a report but then never follows through
Displacement	Shifting your feelings about a person to another person	A student who is angry with one of his professors returns home and yells at one of his housemates
Rationalization	Giving a false, acceptable reason when the real reason is unacceptable	A shy young man decides not to attend a dorm party, telling himself he'd be bored
Substitution	Deliberately replacing a frustrating goal with one that is more attainable	A student having a difficult time passing courses in chemistry decides to change her major from biology to economics
Humour	Finding something funny in unpleasant situations	A student whose bicycle has been stolen thinks how surprised the thief will be when he or she starts downhill and discovers the brakes don't work

Psychologist Martin Seligman points out that we are more used to refuting negative statements, such as "The problem is going to last forever and ruin everything, and it's all my fault," when they come from others rather than from our own mind. But refuting such negative self-talk is exactly what a pessimist must learn to do to avoid chronic unhappiness. Pessimists must first recognize and then dispute the false, negative predictions they generate about themselves.

Maintaining Honest Communication

Another important area of psychological functioning is communicating honestly with others. It can be very frustrating for us and for people around us if we cannot express what we want and feel. Others can hardly respond to our needs if they don't know what those needs are. We must recognize what we want to communicate and then express it clearly. For example, how do you feel about going to the party instead of a movie? Do you care if your roommate talks on the phone late into the night?

Some people know what they want others to do but don't state it clearly because they fear denial of the request, which they interpret as personal rejection. Such people might benefit from **assertiveness** training: learning to insist on their rights and to bargain for what they want. Assertiveness includes being able to say no or yes depending on the situation.

assertiveness
Expression that is confident and direct but not hostile.

Communicating your feelings appropriately and clearly is important. For example, if you tell people you feel sad, they may have various reactions. If they feel close to you, they may express an intimate thought of their own, or they may feel guilty because they think you're implying they have caused your sadness. They may even be angry because they feel you expect them to cheer you up.

Depending on your intention and your prediction of how a statement will be taken, you may or may not want to make it. For example, if you say, "I feel like staying home tonight," you may also be implying something different. You could really be saying "Don't bother me," or opening a negotiation about what you would be willing to do that evening, given the right event or incentive. Although this approach may help you avoid a confrontation (or even a discussion) with someone else, it is unfair because you are not really being clear about what you want.

Good communication means expressing yourself clearly. You don't need any special psychological jargon to communicate effectively. (For tips, see the Take Charge box in Chapter 10.)

Dealing with Loneliness

It can be hard to strike the right balance between being alone and being with others. Some people are motivated to socialize by a fear of being alone—not the best reason to spend time with others. If you discover how to be happy by yourself, you will be better able to cope with periods when you are forced to be alone—for example, when you have just broken off a romantic relationship or when your usual friends are away on vacation.

Unhappiness with being alone may come from interpreting it as a sign of rejection—that others are not interested in spending time with you. Before you reach such a conclusion, be sure that you give others a real chance to get to know you.

Examine your patterns of thinking. You may harbour unrealistic expectations about other people—for example, that everyone you meet must like you and, if they don't, you must be terribly flawed. You might also consider the possibility that you expect too much from new acquaintances and, sensing this, they start to draw back, triggering your feelings of rejection. Not everyone you meet is a suitable and willing person for

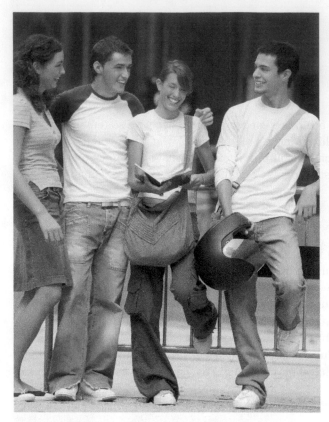

University or college offers many antidotes to loneliness, in the forms of clubs, organized activities, sports, and just hanging out with friends.

a close or intimate relationship. Feeling pressure to have such a relationship may lead you to take up with someone whose interests and needs are remote from yours or whose need to be cared for leaves you with little time of your own. You will have traded loneliness for potentially worse problems.

Loneliness is a passive feeling state. If you decide that you're not spending enough time with people, take action to change the situation. University or college life provides many opportunities to meet people. If you're shy, you may have to push yourself to join a group. Look for something you have enjoyed in the past or in which you have a genuine interest.

If your loneliness is the result of missing absent friends, remember that communication at a distance is cheaper and easier than ever before. For many people, email and cellphones are immediate and satisfying ways to keep up with people in their lives.

Dealing with Anger

Common wisdom holds that expressing anger is beneficial for psychological and physical health. However, recent studies have questioned this idea by showing that overtly hostile people seem to be at higher risk for heart attacks. Angry words or actions don't contribute to psychological wellness if they damage relationships or produce feelings of guilt or loss of control. Perhaps the best way to resolve this contradiction is to distinguish between a gratuitous expression of anger and a reasonable level of self-assertiveness.

At one extreme are people who never express anger or any opinion that might offend others, even when their own rights and needs are being jeopardized. They may be trapped in unhealthy relationships or chronically deprived of satisfaction at work and at home. If you have trouble expressing your anger, consider training in assertiveness and appropriate expressions of anger to help you learn to express yourself constructively.

At the other extreme are people whose anger is explosive or misdirected—a condition called *intermittent explosive disorder (IED)*. IED is often accompanied by depression or another disorder. Explosive anger or rage, like a child's tantrum, renders individuals temporarily unable to think straight or to act in their own best interest. During an IED episode, a person may lash out uncontrollably, hurting someone else or destroying property. Anyone who expresses anger this way should seek professional help.

Managing Your Own Anger

If you feel explosive anger coming on, consider the following two strategies to head it off. First, try to *reframe* what you're thinking at that moment. You will be less angry at another person if it is possible that his behaviour was not intentionally directed against you. Imagine that another driver suddenly cuts in front of you. You would certainly be angry if you knew the other driver did it on purpose, but you probably would be less angry if you knew he simply didn't see you. You might be even less upset if you consider that other mitigating factors may be present—for example, that the other driver was involved in an urgent situation of his own. If you're angry because you have just been criticized, avoid mentally replaying scenes from the past when you received similar unjust criticisms. Think about what is happening now, and try to act differently than you did in the past—less defensively and more analytically.

Second, until you're able to change your thinking, try to *distract* yourself. Use the old trick of counting to 10 before you respond, or start concentrating on your breathing. If needed, take a longer cooling-off period by leaving the situation until your anger has subsided. This does not mean that you should permanently avoid the issues and people who make you angry. When you have had a chance to think more clearly about the matter, return to it.

QUESTIONS FOR CRITICAL THINKING AND REFLECTION

Think about the last time you were truly angry. What triggered your anger? How did you express it? Do you typically handle your anger in the same manner? How appropriate does your anger-management technique seem?

Dealing with Anger in Other People

Anger can be infectious and disruptive to cooperation and communication. If someone you are with becomes very angry, respond asymmetrically by reacting not with anger, but with calm. Try to validate the other person by acknowledging that she has some reason to be angry. This does not mean apologizing if you don't think you're to blame, or accepting verbal abuse, which is always inappropriate. Try to focus on solving the problem by allowing the person to explain why she is so angry and what can be done to alleviate the situation. Finally, if the person cannot be calmed, it may be best to disengage, at least temporarily. After a time out, a rational problem-solving approach may become more successful.

Psychological Disorders

We have all felt anxious at times, and in dealing with the anxiety we may have avoided doing something that we wanted to do or should have done. Most of us have had periods of feeling down when we became pessimistic, less energetic, and less able to enjoy life. Many of us have been bothered at times by irrational thoughts or odd feelings. Such feelings and thoughts can be normal responses to the ordinary challenges of life, but when emotions or irrational thoughts start to interfere with daily activities and rob us of our peace of mind, they can be considered symptoms of a psychological disorder.

QUICK STATS

About 12% of Canadians have an anxiety disorder.
—Mental Health Commission of Canada, 2013

Psychological disorders are generally the result of many factors. Genetic differences, which underlie differences in how the brain processes information and experience, are known to play an important role, especially in certain disorders. However, exactly which genes are involved and how they alter the structure and chemistry of the brain is still under study. Learning and life events are important, too: Identical twins often don't have the same psychological disorders in spite of having identical genes. Some people have been exposed to more traumatic events than others, leading either to greater vulnerability to future traumas or, conversely, to the development of better coping skills. Further, what your parents, peers, and others have taught you strongly influences your level of self-esteem and how you deal with frightening or depressing life events (see the Dimensions of Diversity box).

Next we will examine some of the more common psychological disorders, including anxiety disorders, mood disorders, and schizophrenia.

Anxiety Disorders

Fear is a basic and useful emotion. Its value for our ancestors' survival cannot be overestimated; for modern humans, it provides motivation for self-protection and for learning to cope with new or potentially dangerous

Dimensions *of* **DIVERSITY**

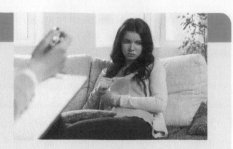

Ethnicity, Culture, and Psychological Disorders

Cultural and ethnic backgrounds shape the experience and expression of psychological health and disorders around the world. For example, how symptoms are interpreted and communicated, whether treatment is sought, and whether a social stigma is attached to a particular symptom or disorder can be affected by cultural differences.

Expression of Symptoms

People from different cultures or groups may manifest or describe symptoms differently. For example, in some cultures, people with social phobia may be more distressed about the imagined harm their social clumsiness causes to others than about their own embarrassment. In other cultures, depression may be expressed in ways that most Canadians would consider unusual, such as by taking on extra tasks. Some disorders, such as schizophrenia, may manifest with different delusions depending on the local culture.

Differing Attitudes

It is relatively easy for Canadians of northern European descent to regard emotional problems as psychological in nature and to therefore accept a psychological treatment. For other groups, symptoms of psychological distress may be viewed as a spiritual problem, best dealt with by religious figures.

People from some groups may have little hesitation about communicating intimate, personal problems to professional care providers. However, for others, particularly men and members of certain ethnic groups, loss of emotional control may be seen as a weakness.

In addition, the use of mental health services is viewed negatively in many cultures; this stigma may partly account for the fact that black Canadians and Asian Canadians are only about half as likely as whites to use any type of mental health service.

Assimilation

When people immigrate to Canada, raise their children here, and become more involved in their new community, they sometimes lose aspects of their own cultural heritage. When traditional values become less practiced, or are not honoured in the same ways as they once were, this assimilation can sometimes increase the likelihood for anxiety, depression, and substance abuse. Immigrants are the least likely to use mental health services in Canada.

Biological Risk Factors

Biology can also be a determinant of the differences seen among people of different ethnic groups. For example, psychotropic drugs are broken down in the body by a specific enzyme called CYP2C19. Reduction of the activity of this enzyme is caused by two mutations, one of which appears to be found only in Asian populations. These poor metabolizers are very sensitive to medications that are broken down by this enzyme. The percentage of poor metabolizers among Asians is between 15 and 30 percent; among Latinos, about 5 percent; and among whites, 3 percent. Asian people thus tend to have more adverse reactions to the doses of drugs standardized principally on white people.

Sources: Alegria, M., et al. 2007. Understanding differences in past year psychiatric disorders for Latinos living in the US. *Social Science & Medicine* 65(2): 214–230; Kleinman, A. 2004. Culture and depression. *New England Journal of Medicine* 351(10): 951–953; Kirmayer, L. J. 2001. Cultural variations in the clinical presentation of depression and anxiety: Implications for diagnosis and treatment. *Journal of Clinical Psychiatry* 62(13 Suppl.): 22–28; Lin, K. M. 2001. Biological differences in depression and anxiety across races and ethnic groups. *Journal of Clinical Psychiatry* 62(13 Suppl.): 13–19; Mood Disorders Society of Canada. 2009; *Quick Facts: Mental Illness and Addiction in Canada,* http://www.mooddisorderscanada.ca/page/quick-facts (retrieved January 17, 2015); and Wong, F.K and Edmond H. P. 2012. Ethnopsychopharmacology considerations for Asians and Asian Americans, *Asian Journal of Psychiatry* 5: 18-23.

environmental or social situations. Only when fear is out of proportion to real danger can it be considered a problem. **Anxiety** is another word for fear, especially a feeling of fear that is not in response to any definite threat. When anxiety is experienced almost daily or in life situations that recur and cannot be avoided, then anxiety can be called a disorder. Anxiety disorders are the most common of the psychological disorders among Canadians. This section provides brief descriptions of the major types of anxiety disorders.

> **anxiety**
> A feeling of fear that is not directed toward any definite threat.

Simple Phobia

The most common and most understandable anxiety disorder is a **simple (specific) phobia**, which is a fear of something definite, such as lightning or a particular animal or location. Nearly 13 percent of Canadians will have a specific phobia in their lifetime. Examples of commonly feared animals are snakes, spiders, and dogs; frightening locations are often high places or enclosed spaces. Simple phobias are believed to result from a combination of biological factors and life events. Sometimes, but not always, these fears originate in bad experiences, such as being bitten by a snake. A special kind of simple phobia is fear of blood, injections, or seeing injured people. These fears usually come from a tendency to faint or become nauseated in such situations.

> **simple (specific) phobia**
> A persistent and excessive fear of a specific object, activity, or situation.

Social Phobia

The 8 percent of Canadians with **social phobia** fear humiliation or embarrassment while being observed by others. Fear of speaking in public is perhaps the most common phobia of this kind. Extremely shy people can have social fears that extend to almost all social situations (see the In Focus box). People with these kinds of fears may not continue in school as far as they could and may restrict themselves to lower-paying jobs where they do not have to come into contact with new people.

> **social phobia**
> An excessive fear of being observed in public; speaking in public is the most common example.

Panic Disorder

People with **panic disorder** experience sudden unexpected surges in anxiety, accompanied by other symptoms, such as rapid and strong heartbeat, shortness of breath, loss of physical equilibrium, and a feeling of losing mental control. About 2 percent of Canadians experience a panic disorder in a given year, and 4 percent will experience it at some point in their lifetime. Such attacks usually begin in a person's early twenties and can lead to a fear of being in crowds or closed places or of driving or flying. These people fear that a panic attack will occur in a situation from which escape is difficult (such as while in an elevator), where the attack could be incapacitating and result in a dangerous or embarrassing loss of control (such as while driving a car or shopping), or where no medical help would be available if needed (such as when a person is alone away from home). Such fears lead to avoidance of situations that might cause trouble. The fears and avoidance may spread to a large variety of situations until a person is virtually housebound, a condition called **agoraphobia**. People with panic disorder can often function normally in feared situations if someone they trust accompanies them.

> **panic disorder**
> A syndrome of severe anxiety attacks accompanied by physical symptoms.
>
> **agoraphobia**
> An anxiety disorder characterized by fear of being alone, away from help, and avoidance of many different places and situations; in extreme cases, it results in a fear of leaving home.

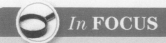

In FOCUS

Shyness

Shyness is a form of social anxiety, a fear of what others will think of our behaviour or appearance. Physical signs include a rapid heartbeat, an upset stomach, sweating, cold and clammy hands, blushing, dry mouth, a lump in the throat, and trembling muscles. Shy people are often excessively self-critical, and their self-talk can be very negative. Their feelings of self-consciousness, embarrassment, and unworthiness can be overwhelming.

To avoid situations that make them anxious, shy people may refrain from making eye contact or speaking up in public. They may shun social gatherings and avoid courses or job promotions that demand interpersonal interaction or public speaking.

Shyness is not the same thing as being introverted. Introverts prefer solitude to society. Shy people often long to be more outgoing, but their own negative thoughts prevent them from enjoying the social interaction they desire.

The consequences of severe shyness can include social isolation, loneliness, and lost personal and professional opportunities. Very shy people also have high rates of other anxiety and mood disorders and of substance abuse.

Shyness may be partly inherited. But for shyness, as for many health concerns, biology is not destiny. Many shy children outgrow their shyness, just as others acquire it later in life. Clearly, other factors are involved. The type of attachment between children and their caregiver is important, as are parenting styles. People's experiences during critical developmental transitions, such as starting school and entering adolescence, have also been linked to shyness. For adults, the precipitating factor may be an event, such as divorce or the loss of a job.

Shyness is very common, with 40 to 50 percent of North Americans describing themselves as shy. However, only about 3 percent of Canadian adults experience a severe form of shyness that interferes seriously with daily life. Recent surveys indicate that shyness rates may be rising in North America. With the advent of technologies, such as automatic teller machines, video games, voice mail, faxes, and email, the opportunities for face-to-face interaction are diminishing. Electronic media can be a wonderful way for shy people to communicate, but they can also allow us to hide from social interaction. In fact, one study found that greater use of the Internet was associated with a decline in participants' communication with family members, a reduction in the size of their social circles, and an increase in levels of depression and loneliness.

Shyness is often undiagnosed, but help is available. Shyness classes, assertiveness training groups, and public speaking clinics are available (see the Take Charge box at the end of the chapter). For the seriously shy, effective treatments include cognitive behavioural therapy and antidepressant drugs.

If you're shy, try to remember that shyness is widespread. Some degree of shyness has an upside. Shy people tend to be gentle, supportive, kind, and sensitive; they are often exceptional listeners. People who think carefully before they speak or act are less likely to hurt others' feelings. Shyness may also facilitate cooperation. For any group or society to function well, many roles are required, and quieter, more reflective individuals have a place.

Sources: American Psychological Association. 2007; 2011. *Painful Shyness in Children and Adults*, http://www.apa.org/helpcenter/shyness.aspx (retrieved January 25, 2015); Ebeling-Witte, S., et al. 2007. Shyness, Internet use, and personality. *Cyberpsychology and Behaviour* 10(5): 713–716; Rosenthal, J., et al. 2007. Beyond shy: When to suspect social anxiety disorder. *Journal of Family Practice* 56(5): 369–374; and Shields, M. 2004. Social anxiety disorder—Beyond shyness. *Health Reports* 15(Suppl.): 47–91.

Generalized Anxiety Disorder

A basic reaction to future threats is to worry about them. **Generalized anxiety disorder (GAD)** is experienced by about 2.6 percent of Canadians (ages 15 and older). This diagnosis is given to people whose worries have taken on a life of their own, pushing out other thoughts and refusing banishment by any effort of will. The topics of the worrying are ordinary concerns: Will I be able to pass the exam next Friday? Where will I get money to get my car fixed?

generalized anxiety disorder (GAD)
An anxiety disorder characterized by excessive, uncontrollable worry about all kinds of things and anxiety in many situations.

The worrying of the person with GAD is not completely unjustified—after all, thinking about problems can result in solving them. But this kind of thinking seems to just go around in circles, and the more they try to stop it, the more they feel at its mercy. The end result is a persistent feeling of nervousness, often accompanied by depression.

Obsessive-Compulsive Disorder

The diagnosis of **obsessive-compulsive disorder (OCD)** is given to about 2 percent of Canadians who may have obsessions or compulsions or both.

> **obsessive-compulsive disorder (OCD)**
> An anxiety disorder characterized by uncontrollable, recurring thoughts and the performing of irrational rituals.

- **Obsessions** are recurrent, unwanted thoughts or impulses. Unlike the worries of GAD, they are not ordinary concerns but improbable fears, such as of suddenly committing an antisocial act or of having been contaminated by germs.

> **obsessions**
> Recurrent, irrational, unwanted thoughts or impulses.

- **Compulsions** are repetitive, difficult-to-resist actions that are usually associated with obsessions. A common compulsion is handwashing, which is typically associated with an obsessive fear of contamination by dirt. Other compulsions are counting and repeatedly checking whether something has been done—for example, whether a door has been locked or a stove turned off.

> **compulsions**
> Irrational, repetitive, forced actions, usually associated with an obsession.

People with OCD feel anxious, out of control, and embarrassed. Their rituals can occupy much of their time and make them inefficient at work and difficult to live with.

Behavioural Addictions

In a **behavioural addiction**, such as to gambling, shopping, or sexual activity, the role of compulsion is small but significant. People experience intense urges to engage in the behaviour, which can create anxiety. The urge intensifies until they carry out the behaviour repeatedly, after which they usually feel relief and elation. As with substance addictions, the behaviour may have negative consequences, but the individual keeps returning to it in spite of them. The behaviour is both maladaptive and persistent. The Centre for Addiction and Mental Health offers treatment options for a wide variety of behavioural and substance-based addictions. (We discuss addiction in greater depth in Part V.)

> **behavioural addiction**
> An activity or a behaviour that is maladaptive and persistent despite the negative consequences.

Post-Traumatic Stress Disorder

People who have **post-traumatic stress disorder (PTSD)** are reacting to severely traumatic events (events that produce a sense of terror and helplessness), such as physical violence to themselves or loved ones. Trauma occurs in personal assaults (rape, military combat), natural disasters (floods, hurricanes), and tragedies (fires and airplane or car crashes).

> **post-traumatic stress disorder (PTSD)**
> An anxiety disorder characterized by reliving traumatic events through dreams, flashbacks, and hallucinations.

Symptoms include reexperiencing the trauma in dreams and in intrusive memories, trying to avoid anything associated with the trauma, and numbing of feelings. Hyperarousal, sleep disturbances, and other symptoms of anxiety and depression also commonly occur. Such symptoms can last months or even years. PTSD symptoms often decrease substantially within three months, and about half of individuals recover fully within six months. Unfortunately, others can experience symptoms for years. Recovery may be slower in those who have previously experienced trauma or who have ongoing psychological problems.

The terrorist attacks on September 11, 2001, brought PTSD into the spotlight. Among those affected were survivors, rescue workers, passersby, residents of Manhattan in general, and to some extent, television viewers around the world who saw countless repeated images of the devastation. An estimated 150 000 New Yorkers developed PTSD following the attacks; some were still experiencing symptoms five years later. Hurricane Katrina had a similarly devastating effect; in one survey, 19 percent of police officers and 22 percent of firefighters in the Gulf Coast states reported symptoms of PTSD. Canadian soldiers wounded in combat are also at risk for PTSD; among soldiers wounded in Iraq or Afghanistan, rates of PTSD increased during the first year after the injury, suggesting that the emotional impact deepens with time. When symptoms persist, and when daily functioning is disrupted, professional help is needed.

QUICK STATS

More than 25% of Canadian military officers experience high job strain.
—Statistics Canada, 2008

Treating Anxiety Disorders
Therapies for anxiety disorders range from medication to psychological interventions concentrating on a person's thoughts and behaviour. Both drug treatments and cognitive behavioural therapies are effective in panic disorder, OCD, and GAD. Simple phobias are best treated without drugs.

Mood Disorders

Daily, temporary mood changes typically don't affect our overall emotional state or level of wellness. A person with a **mood disorder**, however, experiences emotional disturbances that are intense and persistent enough to affect normal functioning. The two most common mood disorders are depression and bipolar disorder.

mood disorder
An emotional disturbance that is intense and persistent enough to affect normal function; two common types of mood disorders are depression and bipolar disorder.

Depression
The Mood Disorders Society of Canada estimates that **depression** affects about 11 percent of Canadians (ages 15 and older) at some point during their lifetime. Women are nearly twice as likely as their male counterparts to experience depression, at 14.1 percent compared to 8.5 percent, respectively.

depression
A mood disorder characterized by loss of interest, sadness, hopelessness, loss of appetite, disturbed sleep, and other physical symptoms.

Depression affects all ethnic groups, although not equally. For example, only 3.1 percent of Inuit have experienced a major depressive episode, while 16 percent of First Nations people have experienced major depression.

Depression takes different forms, but usually involves demoralization and can include the following:
- a feeling of sadness and hopelessness
- loss of pleasure in doing usual activities

- poor appetite and weight loss
- insomnia or disturbed sleep
- restlessness or, alternatively, fatigue
- thoughts of worthlessness and guilt
- trouble concentrating or making decisions
- thoughts of death or suicide

A person experiencing depression may not have all these symptoms. Sometimes instead of poor appetite and insomnia, the opposite occurs: eating too much and sleeping too long. (Depression may contribute to weight gain in young women.) People can have most of the symptoms of depression without feeling depressed, although they usually experience a loss of interest or pleasure in things (see the Assess Yourself box).

QUICK STATS

The cost of untreated and undiagnosed mental health issues in Canada is $51 billion annually.

—Canadian Mental Health Association, 2012

 ## Assess YOURSELF

Could You Have a Mood Disorder?

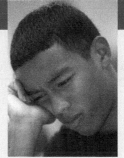

You should be evaluated by a professional if you have any symptoms that are significant enough to interfere with your life, if you have had five or more of the following symptoms for more than two weeks, or if any single symptom causes such a big change that you can't keep up your usual routine.

When You're Depressed

_____ You feel sad or cry a lot, and it doesn't go away.
_____ You feel guilty for no reason; you feel you're no good; you've lost your confidence.
_____ Life seems meaningless, or you think nothing good is ever going to happen again.
_____ You have a negative attitude a lot of the time, or it seems as if you have no feelings.
_____ You don't feel like doing a lot of the things you used to like to do—listening to music, playing sports, being with friends, going out, and so on—and you want to be left alone most of the time.
_____ It's hard to make decisions.
_____ You forget lots of things, and it's hard to concentrate.
_____ You get irritated often. Little things make you lose your temper; you overreact.
_____ Your sleep pattern changes: You start sleeping a lot more or you have trouble falling asleep at night; or you wake up really early most mornings and can't get back to sleep.
_____ Your eating pattern changes: You've lost your appetite or you eat a lot more.
_____ You feel restless and tired most of the time.
_____ You think about death or feel as if you're dying or have thoughts about committing suicide.

When You're Manic

_____ You feel high as a kite, like you're on top of the world.
_____ You get unrealistic ideas about the great things you can do—things that you really can't do.
_____ Thoughts go racing through your head, you jump from one subject to another, and you talk a lot.
_____ You're a non-stop party, constantly running around.
_____ You do too many wild or risky things—with driving, with spending money, with sex, and so on.
_____ You're so up that you don't need much sleep.
_____ You're rebellious or irritable and can't get along at home or school or with your friends.

If you are concerned about depression in yourself or a friend, or if you are thinking about hurting or killing yourself, talk to someone about it and get help immediately.

In major depression, symptoms are often severe; a diagnosis of *dysthymic disorder* may be applied to people who experience persistent symptoms of mild or moderate depression for two years or longer. In some cases, depression is a clear-cut reaction to specific events, such as the loss of a loved one or failing in school or work. In other cases, no trigger event is obvious.

RECOGNIZING THE WARNING SIGNS OF SUICIDE   One of the principal dangers of severe depression is suicide. Although a suicide attempt can occur unpredictably and unaccompanied by depression, the chances are greater if symptoms are numerous and severe. Additional warning signs of suicide include the following:
- the expression of the wish to be dead or the revealing of contemplated methods
- increasing social withdrawal and isolation
- a sudden, inexplicable lightening of mood (which can mean the person has decided to commit suicide)

Certain risk factors increase the likelihood of suicide:
- a history of previous attempts
- a suicide by a family member or friend
- readily available means, such as guns or pills
- a history of substance abuse or eating disorders
- serious medical problems

In Canada, men have much higher suicide rates than women; men aged 85 and older have the highest suicide rate, and men between the ages of 50 and 54 have the next highest rate (see Figure 2.2). Canadian Aboriginal peoples, and especially Canadian Aboriginal youth, have much higher rates than most other groups, with estimates ranging from five to seven times the national average. Suicide rates for Inuit youth are among the highest in the world, at 11 times the national average. It is important that culturally sensitive suicide prevention programs be offered. Women attempt suicide three to four times as often as men, yet men succeed at more than three times the rate of women (see the Gender Matters box). Suicide rates among adolescents and young adults and among adults over 70 have been falling for the last one to two decades.

Sometimes mistaken for suicide attempts are acts of *self-injury*, including cutting, burning, hitting, and other forms of self-inflicted harm. In a 2013 study, almost 20 percent of post-secondary students surveyed said they had injured themselves intentionally. A maladaptive coping strategy, self-injury is believed to provide relief from unbearable psychological distress or pain, perhaps through the release of endorphins. A variety of psychotherapeutic interventions can help people who injure themselves. Whatever the reason behind it,

FIGURE 2.2

Rates of Suicide, by Sex and Age, per 100 000 Population

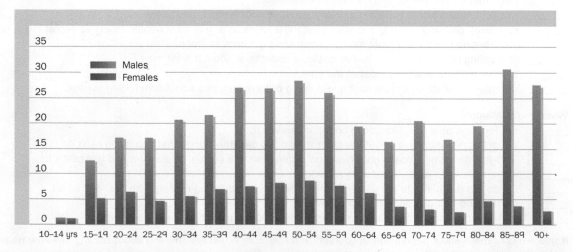

Source: Adapted from Statistics Canada, CANSIM, table 102-0551, last modified: 2012-05-31, http://www.statcan.gc.ca/tables-tableaux/sum-som/l01/cst01/hlth66f-eng.htm (retrieved January 20, 2015).

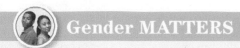

Gender MATTERS

Depression, Anxiety, and Gender

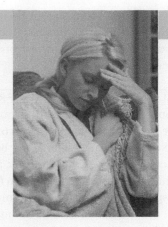

It is evident that gender is a determinant of many aspects of health, including aspects of psychological well-being. The common belief that females are more emotional than males has both a positive and a negative side. On the one hand, women are thought to express positive emotions more clearly than men, especially those related to sympathy and caring. On the other hand, women are more prone to negative emotions, such as depression and worry.

One of the defining characteristics of a psychiatric disorder is that it interferes with daily activities and the ability to live a happy life. Thus, the higher incidence of anxiety and mood disorders in women is convincing evidence that they are more likely to experience psychological distress than are men.

Anxiety Disorders

Panic disorder is almost twice as common in women as in men, whereas obsessive-compulsive disorder occurs in men and women at about the same rate. In population surveys, social anxiety disorder is more common in women than in men, but men are more likely to seek treatment for it—perhaps because men are more likely to find it a barrier to success in white-collar jobs. In some surveys, PTSD is more common in women, but the incidence of PTSD depends on the incidence of traumatic events, which varies in different environments. Men are more often exposed to military combat, and women are more often exposed to rape. Trauma from motor vehicle crashes is a fairly common cause of PTSD in both sexes.

Depression and Suicide

When women are depressed, they are more likely than men to experience guilt, anxiety, increased appetite and weight gain, and increased sleep. When women take antidepressants, they may need a lower dose than men; at the same dosage, blood levels of medication tend to be higher in women. An issue for women who may become pregnant is whether antidepressants can harm a fetus or newborn. The best evidence indicates that the most frequently prescribed types of antidepressants do not cause birth defects, although several studies have reported withdrawal symptoms in some newborns whose mothers used certain antidepressants.

Although suicidal behaviour is strongly associated with depression, and depression is more prevalent in women, many more men than women commit suicide. Overall, about three times as many women as men attempt suicide, but women's attempts are less likely to be lethal.

Underlying Factors

Why women have more anxiety and depression than men is a matter of debate. Some experts think much of the difference is due to reporting bias: Women are more willing to admit to experiencing negative emotions, being stressed, or having difficulty coping. Women may also be more likely to seek treatment.

Other experts point to biologically-based sex differences, particularly in the level and action of hormones. Greater anxiety and depression in women compared with men is most pronounced between puberty and menopause, when female hormones are most active. However, this period of life is also the time in which women's social roles and expectations may be the most different from those of men. Women may put more emphasis on relationships in determining self-esteem, and so the deterioration of a relationship is a cause of depression that can hit women harder than men. In addition, culturally-determined gender roles are more likely to place women in situations in which they have less control over key life decisions, and lack of autonomy is associated with depression.

The higher suicide rate among young men may relate to gender norms and expectations that men assert independence and physical prowess—sometimes expressed in risky, dangerous, and potentially self-destructive behaviour. Such behaviour, often involving drugs and alcohol and resulting in motor vehicle crashes, occurs more often in young people who later commit suicide. Even when suicidal intention is never expressed, suicidal impulses are often suspected of contributing to sudden deaths in this age group.

Sources: Sanz, E. J., et al. 2005. Selective serotonin reuptake inhibitors in pregnant women and neonatal withdrawal syndrome. *Lancet* 365(9458): 482–487; Kessler, R. C. 2003. Epidemiology of women and depression. *Journal of Affective Disorders* 74: 5–13; World Health Organization. 2002. *Gender and Mental Health*. Geneva: World Health Organization; Pigott, T. A. 1999. Gender differences in the epidemiology and treatment of anxiety disorders. *Journal of Clinical Psychiatry* 60(18 Suppl.): 4–15; and Seedat, S. et al. 2009. Cross-national associations between gender and mental disorders in the WHO World Mental Health Surveys. *Archives of General Psychiatry* 66(7): 785–795.

however, self-harm should be taken very seriously because it indicates that a person is struggling to cope with life, and may signal an increased risk for suicide, sometimes by accident. According to a 2007 British study, young people who purposely hurt themselves were much more likely to commit suicide than were the general population.

HELPING YOURSELF OR A FRIEND   If you are severely depressed or know someone who is, expert help from a mental health professional is essential. Don't be afraid to discuss the possibility of suicide with some-one you fear is suicidal. You won't give them an idea they haven't already thought of (see the In Focus box). Asking direct questions is the best way to determine whether someone seriously intends to commit suicide. Encourage your friend to talk and to take positive steps to improve his situation (e.g., talk with a mental health professional). If you are feeling unsure about how to help a depressed friend, it may be helpful for you to speak with a mental health professional for support and guidance.

Most communities have emergency help available, often in the form of a hotline telephone counselling service run by a suicide prevention agency (check online). If you feel the danger of suicide is immediate, do not leave the person alone. Call for help or take her to an emergency room.

TREATING DEPRESSION   Although more than 80 percent of Canadians with depression respond very well to treatment, only about 10 percent of Canadians with depression seek treatment. Treatment for depression depends on its severity and on whether the depressed person is suicidal. The best initial treatment for

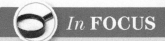 *In* **FOCUS**

Myths About Suicide

Myth People who really intend to kill themselves do not let anyone know about it.

Fact This belief can be an excuse for doing nothing when someone says he or she might commit suicide. In fact, most people who eventually commit suicide have talked about doing it.

Myth People who made a suicide attempt but survived did not really intend to die.

Fact This may be true for certain people, but people who seriously want to end their life may fail because they misjudge what it takes. Even a pharmacist may misjudge the lethal dose of a drug.

Myth People who succeed in suicide really wanted to die.

Fact We cannot be sure of that either. Some people are only trying to make a dramatic gesture or plea for help but miscalculate.

Myth People who really want to kill themselves will do it regardless of any attempts to prevent them.

Fact Few people are single-minded about suicide even at the moment of attempting it. People who are quite determined to take their life today may change their mind completely tomorrow.

Myth Suicide is proof of mental health problems.

Fact Many suicides are committed by people who do not meet ordinary criteria for a mental illness, although people with depression, schizophrenia, and other psychological disorders have a much higher than average suicide rate.

Myth People inherit suicidal tendencies.

Fact Certain kinds of depression that lead to suicide do have a genetic component. But many examples of suicide running in a family can be explained by other factors, such as psychologically identifying with a family member, often a parent, who committed suicide.

Myth All suicides are irrational.

Fact By some standards all suicides may seem irrational. But many people find it at least understandable that someone might want to commit suicide, for example, when approaching the end of a terminal illness or when facing a long prison term.

moderate to severe depression is usually a combination of drug therapy and psychotherapy. Newer prescription antidepressants work well, although they may take several weeks to take effect, and patients may need to try multiple medications before finding one that works well. Therefore, when suicidal impulses are strong, hospitalization may be necessary.

Antidepressants work by affecting key neurotransmitters in the brain, including serotonin (see Figure 2.3). The herbal supplement St. John's wort may also affect serotonin levels, but it has not been subject to the same testing and regulation as prescription medications, and recent evidence suggests it is not as effective as previously hoped. Anyone who may be experiencing depression should seek a medical evaluation rather than self-treating with supplements.

Electroconvulsive therapy (ECT) is effective for severe depression when other approaches, including medications and other electronic therapies, such as magnetic stimulation, have failed. In ECT, an epileptic-like seizure is induced by an electrical impulse transmitted through electrodes placed on the head. Patients are given an anaesthetic and a muscle relaxant to reduce anxiety and prevent injuries associated with seizures. A typical course of ECT includes three treatments per week for two to four weeks.

electroconvulsive therapy (ECT)
The use of electric shock to induce brief, generalized seizures; used in the treatment of selected psychological disorders.

One type of depression is treated by having people sit with their eyes open in front of a bright light source every morning. These people have **seasonal affective disorder (SAD)**; their depression worsens during

FIGURE 2.3

Nerve Cell Communication

Nerve cells (neurons) communicate through a combination of electrical impulses and chemical messages. Neurotransmitters, such as serotonin and norepinephrine, alter the overall responsiveness of the brain and are responsible for mood, level of attentiveness, and other psychological states. Many psychological disorders are related to problems with neurotransmitters and their receptors, and drug treatments frequently target them. For example, the antidepressant drug Prozac increases levels of serotonin by slowing the resorption (reuptake) of serotonin.

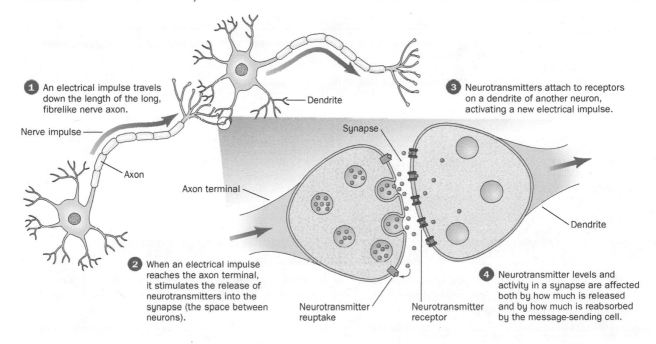

1 An electrical impulse travels down the length of the long, fibrelike nerve axon.

Nerve impulse

Axon

2 When an electrical impulse reaches the axon terminal, it stimulates the release of neurotransmitters into the synapse (the space between neurons).

Dendrite

Synapse

Axon terminal

Neurotransmitter reuptake

Neurotransmitter receptor

Dendrite

3 Neurotransmitters attach to receptors on a dendrite of another neuron, activating a new electrical impulse.

4 Neurotransmitter levels and activity in a synapse are affected both by how much is released and by how much is reabsorbed by the message-sending cell.

winter months as the number of hours of daylight diminishes, and then improves with the spring and summer. The Mood Disorders Society of Canada estimates that 15 percent of Canadians experience the winter blues, and 2–3 percent experience symptoms severe enough to be diagnosed as SAD. SAD is more common among people who live at higher latitudes, which receive fewer hours of light in winter. Light therapy may work by extending the perceived length of the day and thus convincing the brain that it is summertime even during the winter months.

seasonal affective disorder (SAD)
A mood disorder characterized by seasonal depression, usually occurring in winter, when there is less daylight.

THINKING ABOUT THE ENVIRONMENT

Some depressive disorders, such as SAD, are triggered by environmental factors, such as the long nights and grey skies of winter or job schedules that require people to work at night and sleep during the day. Anxiety disorders, such as social phobia, can be greatly compounded by living or working in a crowded area where the person with the disorder must deal with many other people.

If an environmental factor adds to your depression or anxiety, look for resources in your community that can help. For example, counselling can help with social anxiety, and inexpensive light treatments can relieve seasonal depression for some people. For more information on the environment and environmental health, see Chapter 21.

Mania and Bipolar Disorder

People who experience **mania**, a less common feature of mood disorders, are restless, have a lot of energy, need little sleep, and often talk non-stop. They may devote themselves to fantastic projects and spend more money than they can afford. Many manic people swing between manic and depressive states, a syndrome called **bipolar disorder**, because of the two opposite poles of mood. Bipolar disorder affects men and women equally. Tranquilizers are used to treat individual manic episodes, while special drugs taken daily, such as the salt lithium carbonate, can prevent future mood swings. Anticonvulsants (drugs used to prevent epileptic seizures) are also prescribed to stabilize moods; examples are Tegretol (carbamazepine) and Lamictal (lamotrigine).

mania
A mood disorder characterized by excessive elation, irritability, talkativeness, inflated self-esteem, and expansiveness.

bipolar disorder
A mood disorder characterized by alternating periods of depression and mania.

QUICK STATS

1% of Canadians (ages 15+) have bipolar disorder.
—Statistics Canada, 2012

QUESTIONS FOR CRITICAL THINKING AND REFLECTION

Have you ever wondered if you were depressed? Try to recall your situation at the time. How did you feel, and what do you think brought about those feelings? What, if anything, did you do to bring about change and to feel better?

Schizophrenia

Schizophrenia can be severe and debilitating or quite mild and hardly noticeable. Although people are capable of diagnosing their own depression, they usually don't diagnose their own schizophrenia, because they often can't see that anything is wrong. This disorder is not rare; in fact, 1.3 percent of Canadians (15 years+) have a diagnosed schizophrenic episode in their lifetime, most commonly starting in adolescence.

> **schizophrenia**
> A psychological disorder that involves a disturbance in thinking and in perceiving reality.

Scientists are uncertain about the exact causes of schizophrenia. Researchers have identified possible chemical and structural differences in the brains of people with the disorder, as well as several genes that appear to increase the risk. Schizophrenia is likely caused by a combination of genes and environmental factors that occur during pregnancy and development. For example, children born to a parent with schizophrenia have higher rates of schizophrenia, as do children with prenatal exposure to certain infections or medications.

Some general characteristics of schizophrenia include the following:

- *Disorganized thoughts:* Thoughts may be expressed in a vague or confusing way.
- *Inappropriate emotions:* Emotions may be either absent or strong but inappropriate.
- *Delusions:* People with delusions—firmly held false beliefs—may think that their minds are controlled by outside forces, that people can read their minds, that they are great personages, such as Jesus Christ or the prime minister of Canada, or that they are being persecuted by a group, such as the RCMP.
- *Auditory hallucinations:* People with schizophrenia may hear voices when no one is present.
- *Deteriorating social and work functioning:* Social withdrawal and increasingly poor performance at school or work may be so gradual that they are hardly noticed at first.

None of these characteristics is invariably present. Some people with schizophrenia are quite logical, except on the subject of their delusions. Others show disorganized thoughts but no delusions or hallucinations.

A person with schizophrenia needs help from a mental health professional. Suicide is a risk in schizophrenia, and expert treatment can reduce that risk and minimize the social consequences of the illness by shortening the period when symptoms are active. The key element in treatment is regular medication. At times, medication is like insulin for diabetes—it makes the difference between being able to function or not. Sometimes hospitalization is temporarily required.

Models of Human Nature and Therapeutic Change

At least four different perspectives—biological, behavioural, cognitive, and psychodynamic—can be applied to human problems, such as the psychological disorders discussed in this chapter. Each perspective has a distinct view of human nature, and from those views of human nature come distinct therapeutic approaches.

The Biological Model

The *biological model* emphasizes that the mind's activity depends entirely on an organic structure, the brain, whose composition is genetically determined. The activity of neurons, mediated by complex chemical reactions, gives rise to our most complex thoughts, our most ardent desires, and our most pathological behaviour.

Pharmacological Therapy

The most important kind of therapy inspired by the biological model is pharmacological therapy. A list of some of the popular medications currently used for treating psychological disorders follows. All require a prescription from a psychiatrist or other medical doctor. All have been evaluated as being safe and more effective than a **placebo**. Those included in this chapter have received approval from Health Canada but may not necessarily be available in other countries. See the Critical Consumer box for more information on Health Canada's approval process. As with all pharmacological therapies, these drugs may cause side effects. For example, the side effects of widely-used antidepressants range from diminished appetite to loss of sexual

Critical CONSUMER

Psychiatric Drug Use and the Medication Approval Process in Canada

Per capita, Canadians use more psychiatric medication than anyone else in the world. In 2012, more than 74 million psychiatric prescriptions worth $2.6 billion were dispensed. We are also the second highest users of sedatives and the fourth highest users of prescription narcotics worldwide. But the frequent use of these drugs has caused the Mood Disorders Society of Canada to voice some concerns about how drugs are approved in our country.

In *Quick Facts: Mental Illness and Addiction in Canada* (3rd ed.), the Society notes that 90 percent of drug trials are created and funded by the same pharmaceutical companies that intend to market the drugs. This fact draws into question the accuracy of the findings being reported, as these companies want favourable results. The duration of the studies is also of concern because most end before any adverse reactions can appear; many longer-term negative side effects may go unreported.

The Society also points out that some physicians prescribe the drugs for purposes other than that approved by Health Canada. That practice may be putting Canadians' health at risk, but the problems arising from these off-label uses have never been studied.

Several organizations, such as the Canadian Agency of Drugs and Technologies in Health (CADTH), can help Canadians make good choices when it comes to taking medications. According to its website, the CADTH is "an independent, not-for-profit agency funded by Canadian federal, provincial, and territorial governments to provide credible, impartial advice and evidence-based information about the effectiveness of drugs and other health technologies to Canadian health care decision makers." When you receive a prescription for a medication, be sure to ask your health care provider or pharmacist about the evidence supporting the drug's effectiveness and the conditions for which it has received Health Canada approval.

Sources: Mood Disorders Society of Canada, *Quick Facts: Mental Illness and Addiction in Canada*, 3rd ed., 2009, http://www.mooddisorderscanada.ca/documents/Media%20Room/Quick%20Facts%203rd%20Edition%20Eng%20Nov%2012%2009.pdf (retrieved January 25, 2015); and Canadian Agency of Drugs and Technologies in Health, *Media Centre*, 2011, http://www.cadth.ca/index.php/en/media-centre/2011/01/25/238 (retrieved January 25, 2015).

pleasure. In addition, a person may have to try several drugs before finding one that is effective and has acceptable side effects.

placebo

A chemically inactive substance that a patient believes is an effective medical therapy for his or her condition. To help evaluate a therapy, medical researchers compare the effects of a particular therapy with the effects of a placebo. The placebo effect occurs when a patient responds to a placebo as if it were an active drug.

1. *Antidepressants:* One group is called the selective serotonin reuptake inhibitors (SSRIs) because of one of their actions. This group includes Prozac (fluoxetine), Paxil (paroxetine), Zoloft (sertraline), Luvox (fluvoxamine), Celexa (citalopram), and Lexapro (escitalopram). Another group is called the tricyclics after their chemical structure; it includes Aventyl (nortriptyline) and Elavil (amitriptyline). Nardil (phenelzine) is a monoamine oxidase inhibitor (MAOI). Antidepressants that do not fit into these groups include Effexor (venlafaxine), Wellbutrin (buproprion), Remeron (mirtazapine), and Cymbalta (duloxetine). Surprisingly, these antidepressants are as effective in treating panic disorder and certain kinds of chronic anxiety as they are in treating depression. They may also alleviate the symptoms of OCD.

QUICK STATS

Canadians spend about $1.7 billion each year on antidepressant medications.

—O'Shea et al., 2013

2. *Mood stabilizers:* Lithium carbonate, Depakene (valproic acid), Lamictal (lamotrigine), and Topamax (topiramate) are prescribed as mood stabilizers. They are taken to prevent mood swings that occur in bipolar disorder and certain kinds of schizophrenia.

3. *Antipsychotics:* Older antipsychotics include haloperidol and fluphenazine; newer antipsychotics (sometimes called atypical) are Clozaril (clozapine), Zyprexa (olanzapine), Risperdal (risperidone), Seroquel (quetiapine), Zeldox (ziprasidone), Abilify (aripiprazole), and Invega (paliperidone). These drugs reduce hallucinations and disordered thinking in people with schizophrenia, bipolar disorder, and delirium, and they have a calming effect on agitated patients.

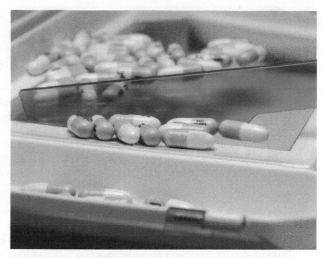

Pharmacological therapy (medication) is a common form of treatment for many psychological disorders. Medications can be very effective, but they do have risks and side effects, and they do not work for everyone.

4. *Anxiolytics (antianxiety agents) and hypnotics (sleeping pills):* One of the largest and most prescribed classes of anxiolytics is the benzodiazepines, a group of drugs that includes Valium (diazepam), Librax (chlordiazepoxide), Xanax (alprazolam), and Ativan (lorazepam); Dalmane (flurazepam), Restoril (temazepam), and triazolam are benzodiazepines marketed as sleeping aids. Newer hypnotics include Imovane (zopiclone).

5. *Stimulants:* Ritalin (methylphenidate) and Dexedrine (dextroamphetamine) are most commonly used for **attention deficit hyperactivity disorder (ADHD)** in children and less often in adults. Drugs of this type are also marketed under the names Adderall (amphetamine aspartate monohydrate), Strattera (atomoxetine), and Concerta (methylphenidate hydrochloride). They are also used for daytime sleepiness in adults, as is Alertec (modafinil).

attention deficit hyperactivity disorder (ADHD)
A disorder characterized by persistent, pervasive problems with inattention or hyperactivity, or both, to a degree that is considered inappropriate for a person's developmental stage and that causes significant difficulties in school, work, or relationships.

6. *Anti-dementia drugs:* Dementia is an impairment in memory and thinking that occurs almost exclusively in older adults. The most common type is Alzheimer's disease (see Chapter 17). Many people with this problem are now prescribed Aricept (donepezil) or Ebixa (memantine). Other anti-dementia drugs are Exelon (rivastigmine) and Reminyl (galantamine).

Issues in the Use of Pharmacological Therapy

The discovery that many psychological disorders have a biological basis in disordered brain chemistry has led to a revolution in the treatment of many disorders, particularly depression. The new view of depression as based in brain chemistry has also lessened the stigma attached to the condition, leading more people to seek treatment. Antidepressants are now among the most widely prescribed drugs in Canada. The development of effective drugs has provided relief for many people, but the widespread use of antidepressants has also raised many questions (see the In the News box).

Research indicates that for mild cases of depression, psychotherapy and antidepressants are about equally effective. For major depression, combined therapy is significantly more effective than either type of treatment alone. Therapy can help provide insight into factors that precipitated the depression, such as high levels of stress or a history of abuse. A therapist can also provide guidance in changing patterns of thinking and behaviour that contribute to the problem.

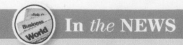

In *the* NEWS

Antidepressant Use in Young People

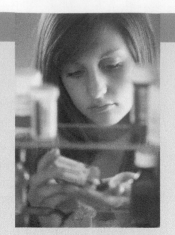

People have become increasingly concerned about the use of antidepressants by youth. On September 14, 2004, a U.S. Food and Drug Administration (FDA) advisory committee recommended a warning label be added to antidepressant drugs based on evidence that their use increases the risk of suicidal thinking and behaviour in children and adolescents. On February 3 of the same year, Health Canada issued a public warning and asked drug manufacturers to provide a review of all (worldwide) safety data pertaining to their drug when used by youth.

Effectiveness

Drug treatment for depression is part of a success story in which people take seriously symptoms of depression and hints of suicidal thinking in children and teens. Over the past decade, the suicide rate among adolescents has fallen. Drug treatment has been considered a key factor in the decline in suicide rates.

A 2005 review of reported childhood depression cases showed that between 1995 and 2002, the number of pediatric psychotherapy sessions declined significantly while prescriptions for antidepressants rose. Most of those prescriptions were for drugs that have not been approved for use in children. In North America, one drug—fluoxetine (Prozac)—has been prescribed regularly for use in children and teens. Studies have found that fluoxetine causes a greater improvement than a placebo, but the combination of drug therapy and cognitive behavioural therapy is more beneficial than either treatment alone. The placebo effect, in which people improve while taking pills containing inactive compounds, is significant in studies of depression and can exceed 30 percent—meaning about one-third of people receiving a placebo experience an improvement in their symptoms. In fact, in a 2011 study exploring the benefits of antidepressant medication for children and adolescents over and above that created by the placebo effect, only 16 percent of the medication impact could be attributed to the medication itself (i.e., 84 percent of the response to the pharmaceutical medication was replicated by the placebo effect).

Many antidepressants other than fluoxetine, especially other SSRIs, are also prescribed to young people, but these other drugs haven't been shown to be effective for that age group. Unpublished research data indicate that some SSRIs are not effective in children and teens or are only slightly more effective than a placebo.

Safety

The problem associated with SSRIs is the possibility that they increase the risk of suicide in some young people, particularly in the period immediately following the start of medication use. When study results were pooled, researchers found that in the short term, about 2–3 percent of users have an increased risk of suicidal thoughts and actions beyond the risk inherent in depression itself.

Researchers aren't exactly sure what causes this effect. One theory is that SSRIs reverse the lethargy associated with depression more quickly than they relieve the depression itself, giving users the energy to contemplate suicide in the interim. Antidepressants may also work differently on the brains of young people than on the brains of adults, so as yet unidentified effects may occur.

In February 2004, Health Canada advised that pediatric patients not discontinue their antidepressant medications without consulting their physician. Doctors would make sure the benefits outweighed the potential risks. Depression is a serious illness that can increase the risk of suicide, and mental health professionals and patients must balance the risks of doing nothing against the potential risks and benefits of different types of treatments.

The result of the Health Canada advisory was a 14 percent reduction in the number of antidepressant prescriptions for this age group. Along with this reduction in prescriptions was a 25 percent increase in the group's suicide rate. An advisory about antidepressants in children and adolescents was issued in the Netherlands at about the same time, with the same result: SSRI prescriptions dropped, but the suicide rate increased. These statistics do not prove a cause-and-effect relationship, but certainly are a reason for concern. For some young people, psychological treatment for depression may not have been a practical alternative to medication, because it was not available or not accepted.

Sources: Gibbons, R. D. 2007. Early evidence on the effects of regulators' suicidality warnings on SSRI prescriptions and suicide in children and adolescents. *American Journal of Psychiatry* 164(9): 1356–1363; Newman, T. B. 2004. Treating depression in children: A black-box warning for antidepressants in children? *New England Journal of Medicine* 351(16): 1595–1598; Brent, D. A. 2004. Treating depression in children: Antidepressants and pediatric depression—the risk of doing nothing. *New England Journal of Medicine* 351(16): 1598–1601; Treatment for Adolescents with Depression Study (TADS) Team. 2004. Fluoxetine, cognitive behavioral therapy, and their combination for adolescents with depression. *Journal of the American Medical Association* 292(7): 807–820; Stafford, R. S., et al. 2005. Depression treatment during outpatient visits by U.S. children and adolescents. *Journal of Adolescent Health* 37(6): 434–442; Katz, L. Y., et al. 2008. Effect of regulatory warnings on antidepressant prescription rates, use of health services and outcomes among children, adolescents and young adults. *Canadian Medical Association Journal* 178(8): 1005–1011; and Drews, A.D., Antonuccio, D.O. and Kirsch, I. 2011. A meta-analysis of randomized placebo controlled trials of anti-depressant medications in depressed children: do the benefits justify the risks? *The Journal of Mind-Body Regulation* 1(2): 85-95.

The Behavioural Model

The *behavioural model* focuses on what people do—their overt behaviour—rather than on brain structures and chemistry or on thoughts and consciousness. This model regards psychological problems as maladaptive behaviours or bad habits. When and how a person learned the maladaptive behaviour is less important than what makes it continue.

Behaviourists analyze behaviour in terms of **stimulus**, **response**, and **reinforcement**. The essence of behaviour therapy is to discover what reinforcements keep an undesirable behaviour going and then to try to alter those reinforcements. For example, if people who fear speaking in class (the stimulus) remove themselves from that situation (the response), they experience immediate relief, which acts as reinforcement for future avoidance and escape.

stimulus
Anything that causes a response.

response
A reaction to a stimulus.

reinforcement
Increasing the future probability of a response by following it with a reward.

To change their behaviour, fearful people are taught to practise **exposure**—to deliberately and repeatedly enter the feared situation and remain in it until their fear begins to abate. A student who is afraid to speak in class might begin his behavioural therapy program by keeping a diary listing each time he makes a contribution to a classroom discussion, how long he speaks, and his anxiety levels before, during, and after speaking. He would then develop concrete but realistic goals for increasing his speaking frequency and contract with himself to reward his successes by spending more time in activities he finds enjoyable. This approach is much like the general behaviour change strategy described in Chapter 1.

exposure
A therapeutic technique for treating fear in which the subject learns to come into direct contact with a feared situation.

Although exposure to the real situation works best, exposure in the imagination or through the virtual reality of computer simulation can also be effective. For example, in the case of someone afraid of flying, an imagined scenario would likely be vivid enough to elicit the fear necessary to practise exposure techniques.

The Cognitive Model

The *cognitive model* emphasizes the effect of ideas on behaviour and feeling. According to this model, behaviour results from complicated attitudes, expectations, and motives rather than from simple, immediate reinforcements. When behavioural therapies, such as exposure, work, it is because they change the way a person thinks about the feared situation and his or her ability to cope with it.

Cognitive therapy tries to expose and identify false ideas that produce negative feelings, such as anxiety and depression. For example, a student afraid of speaking in class may harbour such thoughts as "If I begin to speak, I'll say something stupid; if I say something stupid, the

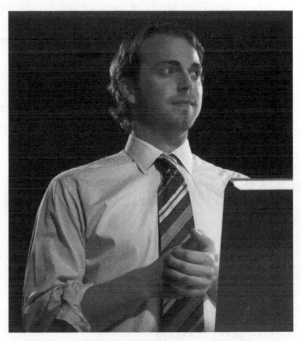

Behavioural therapy can help people overcome many kinds of fears, improving their quality of life.

teacher and my classmates will lose respect for me; then I'll get a low grade, my classmates will avoid me, and life will be hell." In cognitive therapy, these ideas will be examined critically. If the student prepares, will she really sound stupid? Does every sentence said have to be exactly correct and beautifully delivered, or is that an unrealistic expectation? Will classmates' opinions be completely transformed by one presentation? Do classmates even care that much? And why does the student care so much about what they think? People in cognitive therapy are taught to notice their unrealistic thoughts and to substitute more realistic ones, and they are advised to repeatedly test their assumptions.

The Psychodynamic Model

The *psychodynamic model* also emphasizes thoughts. Proponents of this model, however, do not believe thoughts can be changed directly because they are fed by other unconscious ideas and impulses. Symptoms are not isolated pieces of behaviour, but rather are the result of a complex set of desires and emotions hidden by active defence mechanisms (see Table 2.2). In psychodynamic therapy, patients speak as freely as possible in front of the therapist and try to understand the basis of their feelings toward the therapist and others. Through this process, patients gain insights that allow them to overcome their maladaptive behaviour. Current therapies of this type tend to focus more on the present (the here and now) than on the past, and the therapist tries to facilitate self-exploration rather than providing explanations.

Evaluating the Models

Ignoring theoretical conflicts among psychological models, therapists have recently developed pragmatic *cognitive behavioural therapies* that combine effective elements of both models in a single package. For example, the package for treating social anxiety emphasizes exposure as well as changing problematic patterns of thinking. Combined therapies have also been developed for panic disorder, obsessive-compulsive disorder, generalized anxiety disorder, and depression. These packages, involving ten or more individual or group sessions with a therapist and homework between sessions, have been shown to produce significant improvement.

Drug therapy and cognitive behavioural therapies are also sometimes combined, especially in the case of depression. Both kinds of therapy are equally effective for anxiety disorders, but the effects of drug therapy last only as long as the drug is being taken, while cognitive behavioural therapies produce longer-term improvement. For schizophrenia, drug therapy is necessary, but a continuing relationship with therapists who give support and advice is also indispensable.

Psychodynamic therapies have been criticized as ineffective and endless. Of course, effectiveness is hard to demonstrate for therapies that do not focus on specific symptoms. But common sense tells us that being able to open yourself up and discuss your problems with a supportive but objective person who focuses on you and lets you speak freely can enhance your sense of self and reduce feelings of confusion and despair.

QUESTIONS FOR CRITICAL THINKING AND REFLECTION

Are you open to discussing the intimate details of your life, your emotions, your fears, your deepest thoughts? Have you ever truly opened up to another person in this manner? Would you be more open to this kind of sharing if it meant getting help for a psychological disorder?

Getting Help

Knowing when self-help or professional help is required for mental health problems is usually not as difficult as knowing how to start or which professional to choose.

Self-Help

If you have a personal problem to solve, a smart way to begin is by finding out what you can do on your own. Some problems are specifically addressed in this text. Behavioural and some cognitive approaches are especially useful for helping yourself. They all involve becoming more aware of self-defeating actions and ideas and combating them in some way: by being more assertive; by communicating honestly; by raising your self-esteem by counteracting negative thoughts, people, and actions that undermine it; and by confronting, rather than avoiding, the things you fear. You can get more information from books in the psychology or self-help sections of libraries and bookstores, but be selective. Watch out for self-help books making fantastic claims that deviate from mainstream approaches.

Some people find it helpful to express their feelings in a journal. Grappling with a painful experience in this way provides an emotional release and can help you develop more constructive ways of dealing with similar situations in the future. Research indicates that using a journal this way can improve physical and emotional wellness.

For some people, religious belief and practice may promote psychological health. Religious organizations provide a social network and a supportive community, and religious practices, such as prayer and meditation, offer a path for personal change and transformation.

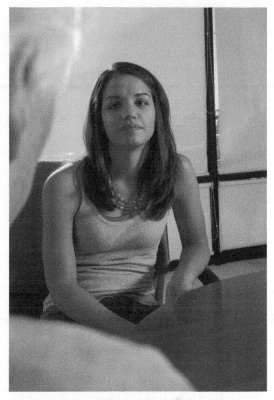

Individual therapy is just one of many different approaches to psychological counselling.

Peer Counselling and Support Groups

Sharing your concerns with others is another helpful way of dealing with psychological health challenges. Just being able to share what's troubling you with an accepting, empathetic person can bring relief. Comparing notes with people who have problems similar to yours can give you new ideas about coping.

QUICK STATS

4100 psychiatrists practise in Canada, but the demand for their services far outweighs the supply.

—Canadian Psychiatric Association, 2009

Many colleges and universities offer peer counselling through a health centre or through the psychology or education department. Peer counselling is usually done by volunteer students who have received special training that emphasizes confidentiality. Peer counsellors may steer you toward an appropriate campus or community resource, or may simply offer a sympathetic ear.

Many self-help groups work on the principle of bringing together people with similar problems to share their experiences and support one another. Support groups are typically organized around a specific problem, such as eating disorders or substance abuse. Self-help groups may be listed online or in the campus newspaper.

QUESTIONS FOR CRITICAL THINKING AND REFLECTION

Have you ever thought professional psychological counselling or therapy might be appropriate for you or a loved one? What circumstances made you think this? Did you or your loved one seek professional help? What was the outcome?

Professional Help

Sometimes self-help or talking to non-professionals is not enough. More objective, more expert, or more discreet help is needed. Many people have trouble accepting the need for professional help, and often those who most need help are the most unwilling to get it. You may someday find yourself having to overcome your own reluctance, or that of a friend, about seeking help.

Determining the Need for Professional Help

In some cases, professional help is optional. Some people are interested in improving their psychological health in a general way by going into individual or group therapy to learn more about themselves and how to interact with others. Clearly, seeking professional help for these reasons is a matter of individual choice. In some situations, such as friction among family members or between partners, professional help can mean the difference between a painful split and a satisfying relationship.

The following are some strong indications that you or someone you know needs professional help:

- Depression, anxiety, or other emotional problems begin to interfere seriously with school or work performance or in getting along with others.
- Suicide is attempted or is seriously considered (refer to the warning signs earlier in the chapter).
- Such symptoms as hallucinations, delusions, incoherent speech, or loss of memory occur.
- Alcohol or drugs are used to the extent that they impair normal functioning during much of the week, finding or taking drugs occupies much of the week, or reducing the dosage leads to psychological or physiological withdrawal symptoms.

Choosing a Mental Health Professional

Mental health workers belong to several different professions and have different roles. Psychiatrists are medical doctors. They are experts in deciding whether a medical disease lies behind psychological symptoms, and they are usually involved in treatment if medication or hospitalization is required. Clinical psychologists typically hold a PhD degree; they are often experts in behavioural and cognitive therapies. Other mental health workers include social workers, licensed counsellors, and clergy with special training in pastoral counselling. In hospitals and clinics, various mental health professionals may join together in treatment teams.

For more on finding appropriate help, see "Choosing and Evaluating Mental Health Professionals" in connect.

Take CHARGE

Dealing with Social Anxiety

Shyness is often the result of both high anxiety levels and lack of key social skills. To help overcome shyness, you need to learn to manage your fear of social situations and to develop social skills, such as making appropriate eye contact, initiating topics in conversations, and maintaining the flow of conversations by asking questions and making appropriate responses.

As described in the chapter, repeated exposure to the source of the fear—in this case, social situations—is the best method for reducing anxiety. When you practise new behaviours, they gradually become easier and you experience less anxiety.

A counterproductive strategy is avoiding situations that make you anxious. Although this approach works in the short term—you eliminate your anxiety because you escape the situation—it keeps you from meeting new people and having new experiences. Another counterproductive strategy is self-medicating with alcohol or drugs. Being under their influence actually prevents you from learning new social skills and new ways to handle your anxiety.

To reduce your anxiety in social situations, try some of the following strategies:

- Remember that physical stress reactions are short-term responses to fear. Don't dwell on them—remind yourself that they will pass, and they will.
- Refocus your attention away from the stress reaction you're experiencing and toward the social task at hand. Your nervousness is much less visible than you think.

- Allow a warm-up period for new situations. Realize that you will feel more nervous at first, and take steps to relax and become more comfortable. Refer to the suggestions for deep breathing and other relaxation techniques in Chapter 3.
- If possible, take breaks during anxiety-producing situations. For example, if you're at a party, take a moment to visit the restroom or step outside. Alternate between speaking with good friends and striking up conversations with new acquaintances.
- Watch your interpretations; having a stress reaction doesn't mean that you don't belong in the group, that you're unattractive or unworthy, or that the situation is too much for you. Try thinking of yourself as excited or highly alert instead of anxious.
- Avoid cognitive distortions and practise realistic self-talk. Replace your self-critical thoughts with more supportive ones: "No one else is perfect, and I don't have to be either"; "It would have been good if I had a funny story to tell, but the conversation was interesting anyway."
- Give yourself a reality check: Ask if you're really in a life-threatening situation (or just at a party), if the outcome you're imagining is really likely (or the worst thing that could possibly happen), or if you're the only one who feels nervous (or if many other people might feel the same way).
- Don't think of conversations as evaluations; remind yourself that you don't have to prove yourself with every social interaction. And remember that most people are thinking more about themselves than they are about you.

Starting and maintaining conversations can be difficult for shy people, who may feel overwhelmed by their physical stress reaction. If small talk is a problem for you, try the following strategies:

- Introduce yourself early in the conversation. If you tend to forget names, repeat your new acquaintance's name to help fix it in your mind ("Nice to meet you, Amelia").
- Ask questions and look for shared topics of interest. Simple, open-ended questions, such as "How's your presentation coming along?" or "How do you know our host?" encourage others to carry the conversation for a while and help bring forth a variety of subjects.
- Take turns talking, and elaborate on your answers. Simple yes and no answers don't move the conversation along. Try to relate something in your life—a course you're taking or a hobby you have—to something in the other person's life. Match self-disclosure with self-disclosure.
- Have something to say. Expand your mind and become knowledgeable about current events and local or campus news. If you have specialized knowledge about a topic, practise discussing it in ways that both beginners and experts can understand and appreciate.
- If you are stuck for something to say, try giving a compliment ("Great presentation!" or "I love your earrings.") or performing a social grace (pass the chips or get someone a drink).
- Be an active listener. Reward the other person with your full attention and with regular responses. Make frequent eye contact and maintain a relaxed but alert posture. (See Chapter 10 for more on being an active listener.)

At first, your new behaviours will likely make you anxious. Don't give up—things *will* get easier. Create many opportunities to practise your new behaviours; your goal is to make them routine activities. For example, striking up a conversation with someone in a registration or movie line can help you practise your skills at small talk in a non-threatening setting. Once you are comfortable doing that, you might try initiating brief conversations with classmates about academic topics—the upcoming exams, for example, or an assignment. Following that, you might try something more challenging, such as discussing a more personal topic or meeting new people in a social setting.

Regular practice and stress-management skills are critical. Using these techniques, you can increase your social skills and confidence level at the same time as you decrease your anxiety. Eventually, you'll be able to sustain social interactions with comfort and enjoyment. If you find that social anxiety is a major problem for you and self-help techniques don't work, consider looking into a shyness clinic or treatment program on your campus.

Sources: University of Texas at Dallas, Student Counseling Center. 2008. *Self-Help: Overcoming Social Anxiety,* http://www.utdallas.edu/counseling/selfhelp/social-anxiety.html (retrieved January 25, 2015); and Carducci, B. J. 2000. *Shyness: A Bold New Approach.* New York: Harper Paperbacks.

SUMMARY

- Psychological health encompasses more than a single particular state of normality. Psychological diversity is valuable among groups of people.
- Defining psychological health as the presence of wellness means that to be healthy you must strive to fulfill your potential.

- Maslow's definition of psychological health centred on self-actualization, the highest level in his hierarchy of needs. Self-actualized people have high self-esteem and are realistic, inner-directed, authentic, capable of emotional intimacy, and creative.
- Crucial parts of psychological wellness include developing an adult identity, establishing intimate relationships, and developing values and purpose in life.
- A sense of self-esteem develops during childhood as a result of giving and receiving love and learning to accomplish goals. Self-concept is challenged every day; healthy people adjust their goals to their abilities.
- Using defence mechanisms to cope with problems can make finding solutions harder. Analyzing thoughts and behaviour can help people develop less defensive and more effective ways of coping.
- A pessimistic outlook can be damaging; it can be overcome by developing more realistic self-talk.
- Honest communication requires recognizing what needs to be said and saying it clearly. Assertiveness enables people to insist on their rights and to participate in the give-and-take of good communication.
- People may be lonely if they haven't developed ways to be happy on their own or if they interpret being alone as a sign of rejection. Lonely people can take action to expand their social contacts.
- Dealing successfully with anger involves distinguishing between a reasonable level of assertiveness and gratuitous expressions of anger, heading off rage by reframing thoughts and distracting yourself, and responding to the anger of others with an asymmetrical, problem-solving orientation.
- People with psychological disorders have symptoms severe enough to interfere with daily living.
- Anxiety is a fear that is not directed toward any definite threat. Anxiety disorders include simple phobias, social phobias, panic disorder, generalized anxiety disorder, obsessive-compulsive disorder, and post-traumatic stress disorder.
- Depression is a common mood disorder; loss of interest or pleasure in things seems to be a universal symptom. Severe depression carries a high risk of suicide, and suicidally depressed people need professional help.
- Symptoms of mania include exalted moods with unrealistically high self-esteem, little need for sleep, and rapid speech. Mood swings between mania and depression characterize bipolar disorder.
- Schizophrenia is characterized by disorganized thoughts, inappropriate emotions, delusions, auditory hallucinations, and deteriorating social and work performance.
- The biological model emphasizes that the mind's activity depends on the brain, whose composition is genetically determined. Therapy based on the biological model is primarily pharmacological.
- The behavioural model focuses on overt behaviour and treats psychological problems as bad habits. Behaviour change is the focus of therapy.
- The cognitive model considers how ideas affect behaviour and feelings; behaviour results from complicated attitudes, expectations, and motives, not just from simple reinforcements. Cognitive therapy focuses on changing a person's thinking.
- The psychodynamic model asserts that false ideas are fed by unconscious ideas and cannot be addressed directly. Treatment is based on psychotherapy.
- Help is available in a variety of forms, including self-help, peer counselling, support groups, and therapy with a mental health professional. For serious problems, professional help may be the most appropriate.

FOR MORE INFORMATION

BOOKS

Antony, M. M. 2008. *The Shyness & Social Anxiety Workbook: Proven, Step-by-Step Techniques for Overcoming Your Fear*, 2nd ed. Oakland, Calif.: New Harbinger. Practical suggestions for fears of interacting with people you don't know.

Grieco, R. and L. Edwards. 2009. *The Other Depression: Bipolar Disorder.* New York: Routledge. A complete introduction to bipolar disorder, its symptoms, and its current treatments.

Hayden, J. 2009. *Introduction to Health Behavior Theory.* Sudbury, Mass.: Jones and Bartlett. An introduction to the ways theories are developed and the factors that influence health behaviour theory.

Jenkins, J., D. Keltner, and K. Oatley. 2006. *Understanding Emotions,* 2nd ed. Oxford: Blackwell. A comprehensive guide to emotions, including current research on the neuroscience of emotions, evolutionary and cultural approaches to emotion, and the expression and communication of emotions.

Leahy, R. L. 2010. *Beating the Blues Before They Beat You: How to Overcome Depression.* New York: Hay House. Describes strategies from cognitive behavioral therapy for changing thinking patterns that contribute to low self-esteem and depression; outlines symptoms, causes, and treatments, including therapy and medication.

Nathan, P. E., and J. M. Gorman. 2007. *A Guide to Treatments That Work,* 3rd ed. New York: Oxford University Press. A balanced and comprehensive report on various treatments for psychological disorders.

Nutbeam, D., and E. Harris. 1999. *Theory in a Nutshell: A Guide to Health Promotion Theory,* 2nd ed. Sydney, Australia: McGraw-Hill. An overview of some of the central theoretical approaches informing health-related behaviour changes.

Seligman, M.E. 2012. *Flourish: A Visionary New Understanding of Happiness and Well-Being.* New York: Free Press. The author refines his ideas about learned optimism and happiness, identifying factors that contribute to a satisfying life: positive emotion, engagement, relationships, meaning, and accomplishment.

Thase, M. E., and S. S. Lang. 2006. *Beating the Blues: New Approaches to Overcoming Dysthymia and Chronic Mild Depression.* New York: Oxford University Press. Describes strategies for changing negative thinking patterns that lead to discouragement and pessimism; also discusses newer medications and alternative therapies.

ORGANIZATIONS, HOTLINES, AND WEBSITES

Canadian Agency for Drugs and Technologies in Health. A national body that provides Canada's health care decision makers with credible, impartial advice and evidence-based information about the effectiveness and efficiency of drugs and other health technologies.
http://www.cadth.ca

Canadian Centre for Addiction and Mental Health. Provides information to help Canadians affected by mental health and addiction issues.
http://www.camh.net

Canada Suicide Support Groups. Provides information about suicide support groups throughout Canada.
http://www.suicide.org

Canadian Mental Health Association. Provides information and resources on many aspects of mental health for Canadians.
http://www.cmha.ca

Cope, Care, Deal. Offers information on mental health issues specifically for teens.
http://www.annenbergpublicpolicycenter.org/aci/copecaredeal-org/

Centre for Suicide Prevention. Provides knowledge and training in the prevention of suicide.
http://www.suicideinfo.ca

Internet Mental Health. Includes an encyclopedia of mental health information with medical diagnostic criteria.
http://www.mentalhealth.com

Organization for Bipolar Affective Disorder. Provides information to help people affected directly or indirectly by bipolar disorder, depression, or anxiety live better lives.
http://www.obad.ca

U.S. National Institute of Mental Health. Provides helpful information about anxiety, depression, eating disorders, and other challenges to psychological health.
http://www.nimh.nih.gov

SELECTED BIBLIOGRAPHY

Adams, R. E., and J. A. Boscarino. 2006. Predictors of PTSD and delayed PTSD after disaster: The impact of exposure and psychosocial resources. *Journal of Nervous and Mental Disease* 194(7): 485–493.

Agency for Healthcare Research and Quality. 2007. *Newer Class of Antidepressants Similar in Effectiveness, but Side Effects Differ,* http://www.ahrq.gov/news/press/pr2007/antideppr.htm (retrieved December 29, 2015).

Allard, Y. E., R. Wilkins, and J-M. Berthelot. 2004. Premature mortality in health regions with high Aboriginal populations. *Health Reports* 15(1): 51–60, http://www.statcan.gc.ca/studies-etudes/82-003/archive/2004/6765-eng.pdf (retrieved March 11, 2015).

American College Health Association. 2013. *American College Health Association-National College Health Assessment II: Canadian Reference Group Data Reporting Spring 2013.* Hanover, MD: American College Health Association.

American Psychiatric Association. 2000. *Diagnostic and Statistical Manual of Mental Disorders,* 4th ed., Text Revision *(DSM-IV-TR).* Washington, D.C.: American Psychiatric Association Press.

Antidepressants for children and adolescents: An update. 2006. *Harvard Mental Health Letter* 22(12): 4–5.

Avagianou, P. A., and M. Zafiropoulou. 2008. Parental bonding and depression: Personality as a mediating factor. *International Journal of Adolescent Medicine & Health* 20(3): 261–269.

Brenes, G. A. 2006. Age differences in the presentation of anxiety. *Aging and Mental Health* 10(3): 298–302.

Canadian Institutes of Health Research. 2012. Fact Sheet – Suicide Prevention, http://www.cihr-irsc.gc.ca/e/44716.html (retrieved January 21, 2015).

Coryell, W. H. 2006. Clinical assessment of suicide risk in depressive disorder. *CNS Spectrums* 11(6): 455–461.

Drews, A.D., Antonuccio, D.O. and Kirsch, I. 2011. A meta-analysis of randomized placebo controlled trials of antidepressant medications in depressed children: do the benefits justify the risks? *The Journal of Mind-Body Regulation* 1(2): 85–95.

Eranti, S., et al. 2007. A randomized, controlled trial with 6-month follow-up of repetitive transcranial magnetic stimulation and electroconvulsive therapy for severe depression. *American Journal of Psychiatry* 164(1): 73–81.

Favaro, A., et al. 2007. Self-injurious behavior in a community sample of young women: Relationship with childhood abuse and other types of self-damaging behaviors. *Journal of Clinical Psychiatry* 68(1): 122–131.

Fazel, S., and M. Grann. 2006. The population impact of severe mental illness on violent crime. *American Journal of Psychiatry* 163(8): 1397–1403.

Forty, L., et al. 2009. Polarity at illness onset in bipolar I disorder and clinical course of illness. *Bipolar Disorders* 11(1): 82–88.

Gunnell, D., P. K. Magnusson, and F. Rasmussen. 2005. Low intelligence test scores in 18-year-old men and risk of suicide: Cohort study. *British Medical Journal* 330(7484): 167.

Hamilton, B. E., et al. 2007. Annual summary of vital statistics: 2005. *Pediatrics* 119(2): 345–360.

Hettema, J. M., et al. 2006. A population-based twin study of the relationship between neuroticism and internalizing disorders. *American Journal of Psychiatry* 163(5): 857–864.

Jones, S. H., and G. Burrell-Hodgson. 2008. Cognitive-behavioral treatment of first diagnosis bipolar disorder. *Clinical Psychology & Psychotherapy* 15(6): 367–377.

Kasper, S., et al. 2006. Superior efficacy of St. John's wort extract WS(R) 5570 compared to placebo in patients with major depression: A randomized, double-blind, placebo-controlled, multi-center trial. *BMC Medicine* 4(1): 14.

Katz, L. Y. et al. 2008. Effects of regulatory warnings on antidepressant prescription rates, use of health services and outcomes among children, adolescents and young adults. *Canadian Medical Association Journal* 178(8): 1005–1011.

Kendler, K. S., J. Myers, and C. A. Prescott. 2005. Sex differences in the relationship between social support and risk for major depression: A longitudinal study of opposite-sex twin pairs. *American Journal of Psychiatry* 162(2): 250–256.

Kurlansik, S.L., and A. Ibay. 2012. Seasonal Affective Disorder. *American Family Physician* 86(11): 1037-1041.

Licinio, J., and M. L. Wong. 2005. Opinion: Depression, antidepressants and suicidality: A critical appraisal. *Nature Reviews: Drug Discovery* 4(2): 165–171.

Lin, Y. R., et al. 2008. Evaluation of assertiveness training for psychiatric patients. *Journal of Clinical Nursing* 17(21): 2875–2883.

McGirr, A., et al. 2007. An examination of *DSM-IV* depressive symptoms and risk for suicide completion in major depressive disorder: A psychological autopsy study. *Journal of Affective Disorders* 97(1–3): 203–209.

Mental Health Commission of Canada. 2013. Making the Case for Investing in Mental Health in Canada, http://www.mentalhealthcommission.ca/English/system/files/private/document/Investing_in_Mental_Health_FINAL_Version_ENG.pdf (retrieved January 21, 2015).

Mood Disorders Society of Canada. 2009. *Quick Facts: Mental Illness and Addiction in Canada*, 3rd ed., http://www.mooddisorderscanada.ca/page/quick-facts (retrieved January 17, 2015).

Nemeroff, C. B. 2007. The burden of severe depression: A review of diagnostic challenges and treatment alternatives. *Journal of Psychiatric Research* 41(3–4): 189–206.

Ozer, D. J., and V. Benet-Martinez. 2006. Personality and prediction of consequential outcomes. *Annual Review of Psychology* 57: 401–421.

Rados, C. 2005. Safeguards for children taking antidepressants strengthened. *FDA Consumer* 39 (1): 18–19.

Rothwell, J. D. 2009. *In the Company of Others: An Introduction to Communication*, 3rd ed. New York: McGraw-Hill.

Saewyc, E. M., and R. Tonkin. 2008. Surveying adolescents: Focusing on positive development. *Pediatrics & Child Health* 13(1): 43–47.

Schatzberg, A. F., J. O. Cole, and C. DeBattista. 2007. *Manual of Clinical Psychopharmacology*, 6th ed. Washington, D.C.: American Psychiatric Publishing.

Seedat, S. et al. 2009. Cross-national associations between gender and mental disorders in the WHO World Mental Health Surveys. *Archives of General Psychiatry* 66(7): 785–795 .

Simon, G. E., and J. Savarino. 2007. Suicide attempts among patients starting depression treatment with medications or psychotherapy. *American Journal of Psychiatry* 164(7): 1029–1034.

Simon, G. 2009. Collaborative care for mood disorders. *Current Opinion in Psychiatry* 22(1): 37–41.

Singh, N. N., et al. 2007. Individuals with mental illness can control their aggressive behavior through mindfulness training. *Behavior Modification* 31(3): 313–328.

Statistics Canada. 2010. *Suicides and Suicide Rate, by Sex and by Age Group*, http://www.statcan.gc.ca/tables-tableaux/sum-som/l01/cst01/hlth66a-eng.htm (retrieved March 11, 2015).

Statistics Canada. 2013. Table105-1101 *Mental Health Profile, Canadian Community Health Survey - Mental Health (CCHS), by age group and sex, Canada and provinces, occasional*, http://www5.statcan.gc.ca/cansim/a26?lang=eng&retrLang=eng&id=1051101&paSer=&pattern=&stByVal=1&p1=1&p2=31&tabMode=dataTable&csid=#F4 (retrieved January 20, 2015)

Statistics Canada. 2015. Table105-0503 *Health indicator profile, age-standardized rate, annual estimates, by sex, Canada, provinces and territories, occasional*, http://www5.statcan.gc.ca/cansim/a26?lang=eng&retrLang=eng&id=1050503&paSer=&pattern=&stByVal=1&p1=1&p2=-1&tabMode=dataTable&csid (retrieved January 21, 2015).

Verhaak, P. F., et al. 2009. Receiving treatment for common mental disorders. *General Hospital Psychiatry* 31(1): 46–55.

Williams, D., et al. 2007. Prevalence and distribution of major depressive disorder in African Americans, Caribbean blacks, and non-Hispanic whites. *Archives of General Psychiatry* 64: 305–315.

Wong, F.K and Edmond H. P. 2012. Ethnopsychopharmacology considerations for Asians and Asian Americans, *Asian Journal of Psychiatry* 5: 18–23..

World Health Organization. 2013. *Mental health action plan 2013 – 2020*, http://www.who.int/mental_health/publications/action_plan/en/index.html (retrieved January 25, 2015)

Zarit, S. H., and J. M. Zarit. 2006. *Mental Disorders in Older Adults: Fundamentals of Assessment and Treatment*, 2nd ed. New York: Guilford Press.

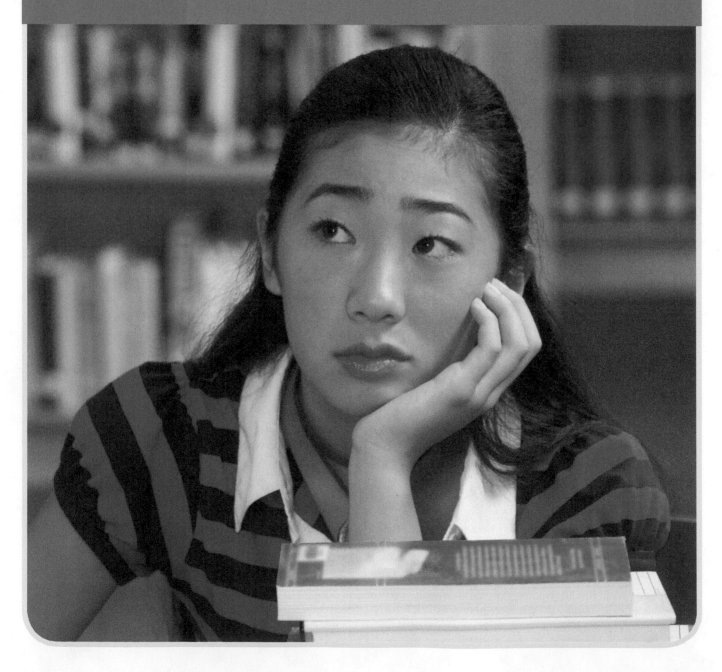

CHAPTER 3

Stress: The Constant Challenge

LOOKING AHEAD

After you have read and studied this chapter, you should be able to:

LO1 Explain what stress is and how people react to it—physically, emotionally, and behaviourally

LO2 Describe the relationship between stress and disease

LO3 List common sources of stress

LO4 Describe techniques for preventing and managing stress

LO5 Create a plan for successfully managing the stress in your life

TEST YOUR KNOWLEDGE

1. Which of the following events can cause stress?
a. taking out a loan b. failing a test c. graduating from university or college

2. Exercise stimulates which of the following?
a. analgesia (pain relief) b. birth of new brain cells c. relaxation

3. High levels of stress can impair memory and cause physical changes in the brain.
True or false?

4. Which of the following can result from chronic stress?
a. violence b. heart attack c. stroke

5. Because eating induces relaxation, it is an excellent means of coping with stress.
True or false?

ANSWERS

1. ALL THREE.   Stress-producing factors can be pleasant or unpleasant and can include physical challenges and goal achievement, as well as events that are perceived as negative.

2. ALL THREE.   Regular exercise is linked to improvements in many dimensions of wellness.

3. TRUE.   Low levels of stress may improve memory, but high stress levels impair learning and memory and, over the long term, may shrink an area of the brain called the hippocampus.

4. ALL THREE.   Chronic—or ongoing—stress can last for years. People who suffer from long-term stress may ultimately become violent toward themselves or others. They also run a greater than normal risk for certain ailments, especially cardiovascular disease.

5. FALSE.   Eating as a means of coping with stress may lead to weight gain and to binge eating, a risky behaviour associated with eating disorders.

Like the term *wellness*, *stress* is a word many people use without really understanding its precise meaning. Stress is popularly viewed as an uncomfortable response to a negative event, which probably describes *nervous tension* more than the cluster of physical and psychological responses that actually constitute stress. In fact, stress is not limited to negative situations; it is also a response to pleasurable physical challenges and the achievement of personal goals. Whether stress is experienced as pleasant or unpleasant depends largely on the situation and the individual. Because learning effective responses to stress can enhance psychological health and help prevent a number of serious diseases, stress management can be an important part of daily life.

As a post-secondary student, you may be in one of the most stressful times of your life (see the Assess Yourself box). This chapter explains the physiological and psychological reactions that make up the stress response and describes how these reactions can be risks to good health. The chapter also provides methods for managing stress.

What is Stress?

In common usage, the term *stress* refers to two different things: situations that trigger physical and emotional reactions, *and* the reactions themselves. This text uses the more precise term **stressor** for a situation or event that triggers physical and emotional reactions and the term **stress response** for those reactions. A first date and a final exam are examples of stressors; sweaty palms and a pounding heart are symptoms of the stress response. We will use the term **stress** to describe the general physical and emotional state that accompanies the stress response. So, a person taking a final exam experiences stress.

stressor
Any physical or psychological event or condition that produces stress.

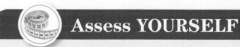

Assess YOURSELF

How High Is Your Stress Level?

Many symptoms of excess stress are easy to self-diagnose. To help determine how much stress you experience on a daily basis, answer the following questions:

1. How many of the symptoms of excess stress listed in Table 3.1 do you experience frequently?
2. Are you easily startled or irritated?
3. Are you increasingly forgetful?
4. Do you have trouble falling or staying asleep?
5. Do you continually worry about events in your future?
6. Do you feel as if you are constantly under pressure to produce?
7. Do you often use tobacco, alcohol, or other drugs to help you relax?
8. Do you often feel as if you have less energy than you need to finish the day?
9. Do you have recurrent stomach aches or headaches?
10. Is it difficult for you to find satisfaction in simple life pleasures?
11. Are you often disappointed in yourself and others?
12. Are you overly concerned with being liked or accepted by others?
13. Have you lost interest in intimacy or sex?
14. Are you concerned that you do not have enough money?

Experiencing some of the stress-related symptoms or answering yes to a few questions is normal. However, if you experience a large number of stress symptoms or you answered yes to a majority of the questions, you are likely experiencing a high level of stress. Take time out to develop effective stress-management techniques. This chapter describes many coping strategies that can aid you in dealing with your stressors. Additionally, your school's counselling centre can provide valuable support.

stress response
The physical and emotional changes associated with stress.

stress
The general physiological and emotional state that accompanies the stress response.

Physical Responses to Stressors

Imagine a near miss: As you step off the curb, a car swerves toward you. With just a fraction of a second to spare, you leap safely out of harm's way. In that split second of danger and in the moments following it, you experience a predictable series of physical reactions. Your body goes from a relaxed state to one prepared for physical action to cope with a threat to your life.

Two systems in your body control for your physical response to stressors: the nervous system and the endocrine system. Through rapid chemical reactions affecting almost every part of your body, you are primed to act quickly and appropriately in times of danger.

Actions of the Nervous System

The nervous system consists of the brain, spinal cord, and nerves. Part of the nervous system is under voluntary control, as seen when you tell your arm to reach for a banana. The part that is not under conscious supervision—for example, the part that controls the digestion of the banana—is the **autonomic nervous system**. In addition to digestion, it controls your heart rate, breathing, blood pressure, and hundreds of other involuntary functions.

autonomic nervous system
The branch of the nervous system that controls basic body processes; consists of the sympathetic and parasympathetic divisions.

The autonomic nervous system consists of two divisions:
- The **parasympathetic division** is in control when you are relaxed; it aids in digesting food, storing energy, and promoting growth.
- The **sympathetic division** is activated during times of arousal, including exercise, and when there is an emergency, such as severe pain, anger, or fear.

parasympathetic division
A division of the autonomic nervous system that moderates the excitatory effect of the sympathetic division, slowing metabolism and restoring energy supplies.

sympathetic division
A division of the autonomic nervous system that reacts to danger or other challenges by almost instantly accelerating body processes.

Sympathetic nerves use the neurotransmitter **norepinephrine** to exert their actions on nearly every organ, sweat gland, blood vessel, and muscle to enable your body to handle an emergency. In general, the sympathetic division commands your body to stop storing energy and to use it in response to a crisis.

norepinephrine
A neurotransmitter released by the sympathetic nervous system onto specific tissues to increase their function during increased activity; when released by the brain, causes arousal (increased attention, awareness, and alertness); also called *noradrenaline*.

Actions of the Endocrine System

During stress, the sympathetic nervous system triggers the **endocrine system**. This system of glands, tissues, and cells helps control body functions by releasing **hormones** and other chemical messengers into the bloodstream to influence metabolism and other body processes. These chemicals act on a variety of targets throughout the body. Along with the nervous system, the endocrine system prepares the body to respond to a stressor.

> **endocrine system**
> The system of glands, tissues, and cells that secrete hormones into the bloodstream to influence metabolism and other body processes.
>
> **hormones**
> Chemical messengers produced in the body and transported in the bloodstream to target cells or organs for specific regulation of their activities.

The Two Systems Together

How do both systems work together in an emergency? Let's go back to your near-collision with a car. Both reflexes and higher cognitive areas in your brain quickly make the decision that you are facing a threat—and your body prepares to meet the danger. Chemical messages and actions of sympathetic nerves cause the release of key hormones, including **cortisol** and **epinephrine**. These hormones trigger the physiological changes shown in Figure 3.1, including these:

- Heart and respiration rates accelerate to speed oxygen through the body.
- Hearing and vision become more acute.
- The liver releases extra sugar into the bloodstream to boost energy.
- Perspiration increases to cool the skin.
- The brain releases **endorphins**—chemicals that can inhibit or block sensations of pain—in case you are injured.

> **cortisol**
> A steroid hormone secreted by the cortex (outer layer) of the adrenal gland; also called *hydrocortisone*.
>
> **epinephrine**
> A hormone secreted by the medulla (inner core) of the adrenal gland that affects the functioning of organs involved in responding to a stressor; also called *adrenaline*.
>
> **endorphins**
> Brain secretions that have pain-inhibiting effects.

Taken together, these almost-instantaneous physical changes are called the **fight-or-flight reaction**. They give you the heightened reflexes and strength you need to dodge the car or deal with other stressors. Although these physical changes vary in intensity, the same basic set of physical reactions occurs in response to any type of stressor: positive or negative, physical or psychological.

> **fight-or-flight reaction**
> A defence reaction that prepares an individual for conflict or escape by triggering hormonal, cardiovascular, metabolic, and other changes.

The Return to Homeostasis

Once a stressful situation ends, the parasympathetic division of your autonomic nervous system takes command and halts the stress response. It restores **homeostasis**, a state in which blood pressure, heart rate, hormone levels, and other vital functions are maintained within a narrow range of normal. Your parasympathetic nervous system calms your body, slowing a rapid heartbeat, drying sweaty palms, and returning breathing to normal. Gradually, your body resumes its normal functions, such as digestion and temperature regulation. Damage that may have been sustained during the fight-or-flight reaction is repaired. The day after you narrowly dodge the car, you wake up feeling fine. In this way, your body can grow, repair itself, and acquire reserves of energy. When the next crisis comes, you will be ready to respond—instantly—again.

> **homeostasis**
> A state of stability and consistency in an individual's physiological functioning.

FIGURE 3.1

The Fight-or-Flight Reaction

In response to a stressor, the autonomic nervous system and the endocrine system prepare the body to deal with an emergency.

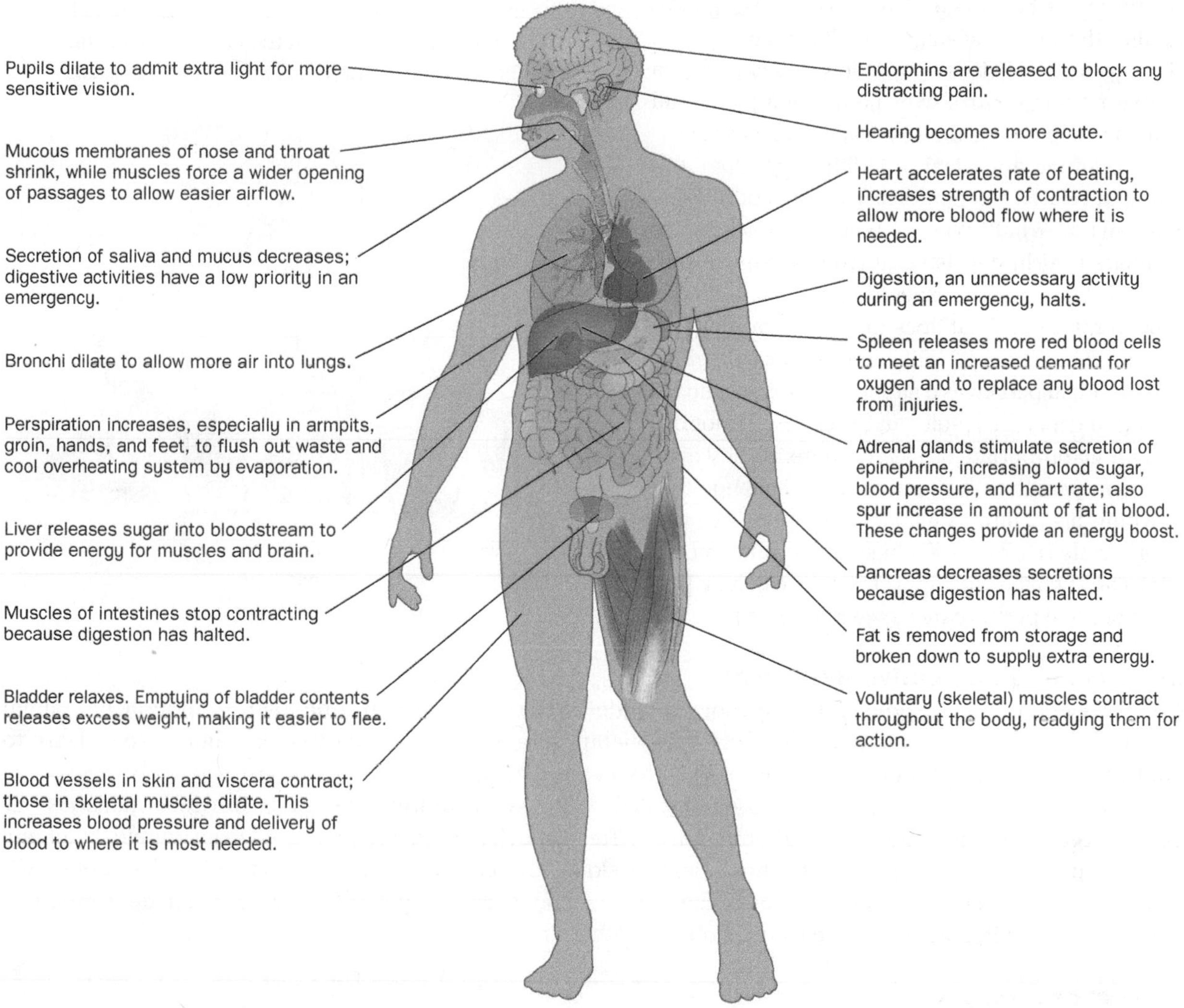

Pupils dilate to admit extra light for more sensitive vision.

Mucous membranes of nose and throat shrink, while muscles force a wider opening of passages to allow easier airflow.

Secretion of saliva and mucus decreases; digestive activities have a low priority in an emergency.

Bronchi dilate to allow more air into lungs.

Perspiration increases, especially in armpits, groin, hands, and feet, to flush out waste and cool overheating system by evaporation.

Liver releases sugar into bloodstream to provide energy for muscles and brain.

Muscles of intestines stop contracting because digestion has halted.

Bladder relaxes. Emptying of bladder contents releases excess weight, making it easier to flee.

Blood vessels in skin and viscera contract; those in skeletal muscles dilate. This increases blood pressure and delivery of blood to where it is most needed.

Endorphins are released to block any distracting pain.

Hearing becomes more acute.

Heart accelerates rate of beating, increases strength of contraction to allow more blood flow where it is needed.

Digestion, an unnecessary activity during an emergency, halts.

Spleen releases more red blood cells to meet an increased demand for oxygen and to replace any blood lost from injuries.

Adrenal glands stimulate secretion of epinephrine, increasing blood sugar, blood pressure, and heart rate; also spur increase in amount of fat in blood. These changes provide an energy boost.

Pancreas decreases secretions because digestion has halted.

Fat is removed from storage and broken down to supply extra energy.

Voluntary (skeletal) muscles contract throughout the body, readying them for action.

The Fight-or-Flight Reaction in Modern Life

The fight-or-flight reaction is a part of our biological heritage, and it's a survival mechanism that has served humans well. In modern life, however, it is often absurdly inappropriate. Many of the stressors we face in everyday life do not require a physical response—for example, an exam, a mess left by a roommate, or a stop light. The fight-or-flight reaction prepares the body for physical action regardless of whether such action is a necessary or appropriate response to a particular stressor.

Emotional and Behavioural Responses to Stressors

We all experience a similar set of physical responses to stressors, which make up the fight-or-flight reaction. These responses, however, vary from person to person and from one situation to another. People's perceptions of potential stressors—and of their reactions to such stressors—also vary greatly. For example, you may feel confident about taking exams but be nervous about talking to people you don't know, while your roommate may love challenging social situations but may be very nervous about taking tests. Many factors, some external and some internal, help explain these differences.

Your cognitive (mental) appraisal of a potential stressor strongly influences how you view it. Two factors that can reduce the magnitude of the stress response are successful prediction and the perception of control. For instance, receiving course syllabi at the beginning of the term allows you to predict the timing of major deadlines and exams. Having this predictive knowledge also allows you to exert some control over your study plans and can thus help reduce the stress caused by exams.

Cognitive appraisal is highly individual and strongly related to emotions. The facts of a situation—Who? What? Where? When?—typically are evaluated fairly consistently from person to person. Evaluation with respect to personal outcome, however, varies: What does this mean for me? Can I do anything about it? Will it improve or worsen? If an individual perceives a situation as exceeding his ability to cope, the result can be negative emotions and an inappropriate stress response. If, however, a person perceives a situation as a challenge that is within his ability to manage, more positive and appropriate responses are likely. A certain amount of stress, if coped with appropriately, can help promote optimal performance (see Figure 3.2).

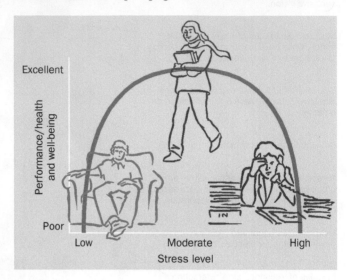

FIGURE 3.2

Stress Level, Performance, and Well-being

A moderate level of stress challenges individuals in a way that promotes optimal performance and well-being. Too little stress, and people are not challenged enough to improve; too much stress, and the challenges become stressors that can impair physical and emotional health.

Effective and Ineffective Responses

Common emotional responses to stressors include anxiety, depression, and fear. Although emotional responses are determined in part by inborn personality or temperament, we often can moderate or learn to control them. Coping techniques are discussed later in the chapter.

Behavioural responses to stressors—controlled by the **somatic nervous system**, which manages our conscious actions—are entirely under our control. Effective behavioural responses, such as talking, laughing, exercising, meditating, learning time-management skills, and becoming more assertive, can promote wellness and enable us to function at our best. Ineffective behavioural responses to stressors include overeating, expressing hostility, and using tobacco, alcohol, or other drugs.

> **somatic nervous system**
> The branch of the peripheral nervous system that governs motor functions and sensory information, largely under conscious control.

Let's consider the individual variations demonstrated by two students, David and Amelia, responding to the same stressor—the first exam of the term. David enters the exam with a feeling of dread, and as he reads the exam questions, he responds to his initial anxiety with more anxiety. The more upset he gets, the less he can remember and the more anxious he becomes. Soon he is staring into space, imagining what will happen if he fails the course. Amelia, conversely, takes a deep breath to relax before she reads the questions, wills herself to focus on the answers she knows, and then goes back over the exam to deal with those questions she's unsure of. She leaves the room feeling calm, relaxed, and confident that she has done well.

As this simple example shows, avoiding destructive responses to stress and adopting effective and appropriate ones can have a direct effect on well-being.

Personality and Stress

Some people seem to be nervous, irritable, and easily upset by minor annoyances; others are calm and composed even in difficult situations. Scientists remain unsure just why this is or how the brain's complex emotional mechanisms work. But **personality**, the sum of cognitive, behavioural, and emotional tendencies, clearly affects how people perceive and react to stressors. To investigate the links among personality, stress, and overall wellness, researchers have looked at different constellations of characteristics, or *personality types*.

> **personality**
> The sum of behavioural, cognitive, and emotional tendencies.

QUICK STATS

57.6% of Canadian university and college students feel *more than average* or *tremendous* stress.
—*National College Health Assessment II: Canadian Reference Group Data Report*, 2013

- *Type A:* People with type A personality are described as ultracompetitive, controlling, impatient, aggressive, and even hostile. Type A people have a higher perceived stress level and more problems coping with stress. They react explosively to stressors and are upset by events that others would consider only annoyances. Studies indicate that certain characteristics of the type A pattern—anger, cynicism, and hostility—increase the risk of heart disease.
- *Type B:* The type B personality is relaxed and contemplative. Type B people are less frustrated by daily events and more tolerant of the behaviour of others.
- *Type C:* The type C personality is characterized by anger suppression, difficulty expressing emotions, feelings of hopelessness and despair, and an exaggerated response to minor stressors. This heightened response may impair immune functions.
- *Type D:* The type D, or distressed personality is a new personality construct. People with this pattern have a joint tendency to feel (but not express) negative emotions and avoid social contact with others. They tend to be gloomy, socially inept, and anxious worriers, a combination that puts them at risk for heart problems.

Studies of type A, C, and D personalities suggest that expressing your emotions is beneficial, not expressing them is problematic, but habitually expressing exaggerated stress responses or hostility is unhealthy.

Researchers have also looked for personality traits that enable people to deal more successfully with stress. One such trait is *hardiness*, a particular form of optimism. People with a hardy personality view potential stressors as challenges and opportunities for growth and learning—not as burdens. They see fewer situations as stressful and react less intensely to stress than nonhardy people might. Hardy people are committed to their activities, have a sense of inner purpose and an inner locus of control, and feel at least partly in control of their lives.

The term *resilience* refers to personality traits associated with social and academic success in at-risk populations, such as people from low-income families and those with mental or physical disabilities. Resilience is associated with emotional intelligence and violence prevention. Resilient people tend to set goals and face adversity through individual effort. There are three basic types of resilience, and each one determines how a person responds to stress:

- *non-reactive resilience*, in which a person does not react to a stressor
- *homeostatic resilience*, in which a person may react strongly but returns to baseline functioning quickly
- *positive growth resilience*, in which a person learns and grows from the stress experience

Can you do anything to change your personality traits and become more stress resistant? It isn't likely. You can, however, change some of your typical behaviours and patterns of thinking and develop positive techniques for coping with stressors. Strategies for successful stress management are described later in this chapter.

Cultural Background

Young adults from around the world come to Canada for a higher education; most students finish university or college with a greater appreciation for other cultures and worldviews. The clashing of cultures, however, can be a big source of stress for many students—especially when it leads to disrespectful treatment, harassment, or violence. It is important to remember that reaction to stress is influenced by family and cultural background. Learning to accept and appreciate the cultural backgrounds of other people is both a mind-opening experience and a way to avoid stress over cultural differences.

Gender

Our **gender role**—the activities, abilities, and behaviours our culture expects of us based on our sex—can affect our experience of stress. Some behaviour responses to stressors, such as crying or openly expressing anger, may be deemed more appropriate for one gender than for the other.

> **gender role**
> A culturally expected pattern of behaviour and attitudes determined by a person's sex.

Strict adherence to gender roles, however, can limit a person's response to stress and can itself become a source of stress. Gender roles can also affect our perception of a stressor. If a man derives most of his self-worth from his work, for example, retirement may be more stressful for him than for a woman whose self-image is based on several different roles. See the Gender Matters box for more on gender and stress.

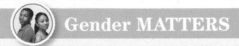 **Gender MATTERS**

How Women and Men Experience Stress

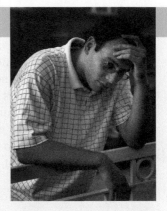

Men and women experience stress, but they experience it differently.

Women and Stress

Research has found that women are more likely than men to find themselves balancing multiple roles, such as those of student, spouse, and parent. Women who work outside the home still do most of the housework—although today's husbands are helping more than previous generations did—and housework isn't limited to cleaning or doing laundry. For example, more than 64 percent of women make all decisions about their family's health care, including decisions about aging parents. The combined pressures of home, workplace, and school can create very high stress levels. Recent reports suggest these findings apply to people in both Canada and the United States.

Men and Stress

Men who fit a traditional male gender role may feel compelled to be in charge at all times. This may create tension in interpersonal situations and limit men's ability to build a support network. Such men may keenly feel the responsibility to support a family, which can compound existing pressures at home and work.

Perceptions of Stress

The Canadian Heart and Stroke Foundation's *Annual Report Card on Canadians' Health* found that when it comes to stress, many Canadians feel overwhelmed. Specifically, Canadians received fairly mediocre grades in several areas, as shown in the table.

Proportion of Canadians Who	Percentage	Grade
Are not frequently stressed	57	D
Have enough quality time	47	F
Feel supported in the workplace	77	B
Cope well with stress	26	F

In Canada, employed women are more likely than their male counterparts to report high work stress, although both sexes feel the stress of having too little time in the day to accomplish everything. When it comes to coping, women are more likely than men to cope with stress through unhealthy behaviours, such as overeating or taking prescription medications.

Physiological Differences

Levels of testosterone (the primary male hormone, responsible for many masculine traits) increase from puberty onward, and so men tend to have higher blood pressure than women of the same age. This factor contributes to greater wear on the male circulatory system, sometimes increasing a man's risk for cardiovascular disease. A part of the brain that regulates emotions, the amygdala, is sensitive to testosterone. This may be one reason that men are more likely than women to find certain situations (such as social interactions) to be stressful.

Conversely, women have higher levels of oxytocin (a hormone involved in social interaction and mood regulation) and are more likely to respond to stressors by seeking social support. This coping response may give women a longevity advantage over men by decreasing the risk of some stress-related disorders. It does not, however, free women from stress-related ailments, and women are more likely than men to suffer stress-related hypertensions, depression, and obesity.

Experience

Past experiences can profoundly influence the evaluation of a potential stressor. Consider someone who has had a bad experience giving a speech in the past. The individual is much more likely to perceive an upcoming speech as stressful than is someone who has had positive public speaking experiences.

The Stress Experience as a Whole

As Table 3.1 shows, the physical, emotional, and behavioural symptoms of excess negative stress are distinct. Even so, they are also intimately interrelated. The more intense the emotional response, for example, the stronger the physical response will be.

Effective behavioural responses can lessen stress, while ineffective ones make it worse. Sometimes, people have such intense responses to stressors or such ineffective coping techniques that they need professional help to overcome the stress in their lives. This chapter also discusses a variety of ineffective coping behaviours and describes the destructiveness of relying on such habits to deal with stress.

TABLE 3.1

Symptoms of Excess Stress

Physical Symptoms	Emotional Symptoms	Behavioural Symptoms
Dry mouth	Anxiety	Crying
Excessive perspiration	Depression	Disrupted eating habits
Frequent illnesses	Edginess	Disrupted sleeping habits
Gastrointestinal problems	Fatigue	Harsh treatment of others
Grinding of teeth	Hypervigilance	Problems communicating
Headaches	Impulsiveness	Sexual problems
High blood pressure	Inability to concentrate	Social isolation
Pounding heart	Irritability	Increased use of tobacco, alcohol, or other drugs
Stiff neck or aching lower back	Trouble remembering things	

QUESTIONS FOR CRITICAL THINKING AND REFLECTION

Think of the last time you faced a significant stressor. How did you respond? List the physical, emotional, and behavioural reactions you experienced. Did these responses help you deal with the stress, or did they interfere with your efforts to handle it? What do you know about what works best for you in dealing with stress?

THINKING ABOUT THE ENVIRONMENT

Environmental problems—whether natural or caused by people—can compound other sources of stress, such as working, commuting, or taking care of a family. Consider the environment where you live, attend school, or work. Do you live with any of the following?

- smog or other pollutants, which make the air hard to breathe
- crowding, which makes it difficult to move around
- poverty, which limits your choices in many aspects of life
- crime, which can make you feel unsafe or hypervigilant

If one or more environmental factors make life more stressful for you, look for resources in your community that can help. For example, public transportation may ease your commute while helping to reduce pollution in your city or town. For more information on the environment and environmental health, see Chapter 21.

More often, however, people can learn to handle stressors on their own. Strategies for successful stress management are described throughout this chapter. For starters, review the following list of basic stress-management strategies and consider whether any of them has ever worked for you:

- building greater social support through meaningful relationships
- participating in and contributing to your family and community in productive ways
- setting higher expectations for yourself but with clear boundaries and fair, consistent expectations
- building life skills, such as decision making, effective communication, and conflict management
- avoiding the urge to control the outcome of every situation
- knowing your own limits and limitations
- trusting others

Stress and Health

According to Statistics Canada, about 23 percent of Canadians (ages 15 and older) report that most days feel "quite a bit" or "extremely" stressful. The burden of stress, both in terms of human suffering and medical costs, are staggering for Canadians. The role of stress in health is complex, but evidence suggests that stress can increase vulnerability to many ailments. For instance, many post-secondary students (and instructors) notice an increase in the cases of colds and other illnesses following exam periods. Several theories have been proposed to explain the relationship between stress and disease.

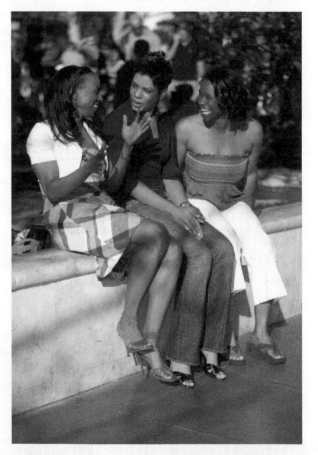

A person's emotional and behavioural responses to stressors depend on many different factors, including personality, gender, and cultural background. Research suggests that women are more likely than men to respond to stressors by seeking social support, a pattern referred to as tend and befriend.

The General Adaptation Syndrome

The term **general adaptation syndrome (GAS)**, coined by Canadian researcher Hans Seyle, describes what many believe is a universal and predictable response pattern to all stressors. As mentioned earlier, some stressors are pleasant (such as attending a party), but others are unpleasant (such as getting a bad grade). In the GAS theory, the stress triggered by a pleasant stressor is called **eustress**; stress brought on by an unpleasant stressor is called **distress**. The sequence of physical responses associated with GAS is the same for eustress and distress and occurs in three stages (see Figure 3.3):

- *Alarm:* The alarm stage includes the complex sequence of events brought on by the fight-or-flight reaction. At this stage, the body is more susceptible to disease or injury because it is geared up to deal with a crisis. Someone in this stage may experience headaches, indigestion, anxiety, and disrupted eating or sleep patterns.
- *Resistance:* With continued stress, the body develops a new level of homeostasis in which it is more resistant to disease and injury than usual. In this stage, a person can cope with normal life and added stress.
- *Exhaustion:* The first two stages of GAS require a great deal of energy. If a stressor persists, or if several stressors occur in succession, general exhaustion sets in. This is not the sort of exhaustion you feel after a long, busy day; rather, it's a life-threatening physiological state.

FIGURE 3.3

The General Adaptation Syndrome

During the alarm phase, a lower resistance to injury is evident. With continued stress, resistance to injury is enhanced. With prolonged exposure to repeated stressors, exhaustion sets in, with a return of low resistance levels seen during acute stress.

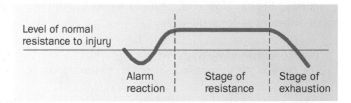

---

general adaptation syndrome (GAS)
A pattern of stress responses consisting of three stages: alarm, resistance, and exhaustion.

eustress
Stress resulting from a pleasant stressor.

distress
Stress resulting from an unpleasant stressor.

Allostatic Load

Although the GAS model is still viewed as a key conceptual contribution to the understanding of stress, some aspects of it are outdated. For example, increased susceptibility to disease after repeated or prolonged stress is now thought to be due to the effects of the stress response itself rather than to a depletion of resources (exhaustion state). In particular, long-term overexposure to stress hormones, such as cortisol, has been linked with health problems. Further, although physical stress reactions promote homeostasis (resistance stage), they also have negative effects on the body.

The long-term wear and tear of the stress response is called the **allostatic load**. An individual's allostatic load is dependent on many factors, including genetics, life experiences, and emotional and behavioural responses to stressors. A high allostatic load may be due to frequent stressors, poor adaptation to common stressors, an inability to shut down the stress response, or imbalances in the stress response of different body systems. A high allostatic load is linked with heart disease, hypertension, obesity, and reduced brain and immune system functioning. In other words, when your allostatic load exceeds your ability to cope, you are more likely to get sick.

---

allostatic load
The long-term negative impact of the stress response on the body.

Psychoneuroimmunology

One of the most fruitful areas of current research into the relationship between stress and disease is **psychoneuroimmunology (PNI)**. PNI is the study of the interactions among the nervous system, the endocrine system, and the immune system. The underlying premise of PNI is that stress, through the actions of the nervous and endocrine systems, impairs the immune system and thereby affects health. It is important to note, however, that even large stress-induced immune changes can have small clinical (medical) consequences because they are short term or because the immune system has redundant components and compensates for changes. In short, the immune system is remarkably flexible and capable of substantial change without compromising health. However, chronic stress in individuals predisposed to or experiencing disease may have more substantial consequences.

> **psychoneuroimmunology (PNI)**
> The study of the interactions among the nervous, endocrine, and immune systems.

A complex network of nerve and chemical connections exists between the nervous and endocrine systems and the immune system. In general, increased levels of cortisol are linked to a decreased number of immune system cells called lymphocytes (see Chapter 9 for more on the immune system). Epinephrine appears to promote the release of lymphocytes but at the same time reduces their efficiency. Scientists have identified hormonelike substances called *neuropeptides* that appear to translate stressful emotions into biochemical events, some of which affect the immune system, providing a physical link between emotions and immune function.

Different types of stress may affect immunity in different ways. For instance, during acute stress (typically lasting between 5 and 100 minutes), white blood cells move into the skin, where they enhance the immune response. During a stressful event sequence, such as a personal trauma and the events that follow, however, there are typically no overall significant immune changes. Chronic (ongoing) stressors, such as unemployment, have negative effects on almost all functional measures of immunity. Chronic stress may cause prolonged secretion of cortisol and may accelerate the course of diseases that involve inflammation, including multiple sclerosis, heart disease, and type 2 diabetes.

Mood, personality, behaviour, and immune functioning are intertwined. For example, people who are generally pessimistic may neglect the basics of health care, become passive when ill, and fail to engage in health-promoting behaviours. People who are depressed may reduce physical activity and social interaction, which may in turn affect the immune system and the cognitive appraisal of a stressor. Optimism, successful coping, and positive problem solving, conversely, may positively influence immunity.

Links Between Stress and Specific Conditions

Although much remains to be learned, it is clear that people who have unresolved chronic stress in their lives or who handle stressors poorly are at risk for a wide range of health problems. In the short term, the problem might be just a cold, a stiff neck, or a stomach ache. Over the long term, the problems can be more severe: cardiovascular disease (CVD), high blood pressure, impaired immune function, or accelerated aging.

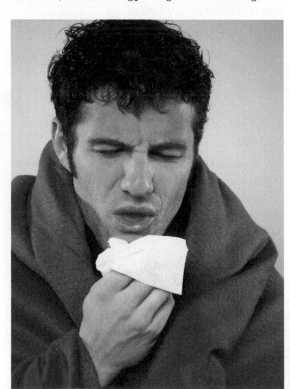

Ongoing stress has been shown to make people more vulnerable to everyday ailments, such as colds and allergies.

QUICK STATS

Although 80% of Canadians know that prolonged stress increases the risk for CVD, only one in four knows that lifestyle changes can reduce the risk of CVD by 80%.

—Canadian Heart and Stroke Foundation, 2000; 2013

Cardiovascular Disease

During the stress response, heart rate increases and blood vessels constrict, causing blood pressure to rise. Chronic high blood pressure is a major cause of atherosclerosis, a disease in which blood vessels become damaged and caked with fatty deposits. These deposits can block arteries, causing heart attacks and strokes. The stress response can precipitate a heart attack in someone with atherosclerosis. The stress response can also cause stress cardiomyopathy ("broken heart syndrome"), a condition that mimics a heart attack but doesn't damage the heart.

Certain types of emotional responses may increase a person's risk of CVD. As described earlier, people who tend to react to situations with anger and hostility are more likely to have heart attacks than are people with a less explosive, more trusting personality.

Stress has also been linked to some of the more recently identified risk factors for CVD, including elevated cholesterol. For example, inflammation is a key component of the damage to blood vessels that leads to heart attacks. Stress increases inflammation throughout the body. Stress-induced increases in inflammatory messenger molecules are also linked to elevated levels of homocysteine and C-reactive protein (CRP), two compounds that appear to be markers for CVD risk. Stress-related depression and anger are associated with elevated homocysteine levels, and job-related exhaustion is linked to high CRP levels in some people. Elevated CRP levels have also been implicated in insulin resistance and the development of diabetes, which is in turn a risk factor for CVD. Clearly, stress reduction can improve cardiovascular health. See Chapter 7 for more on CVD.

Psychological Problems

The hormones and other chemicals released during the stress response cause emotional as well as physical changes (see the Mind Body Spirit box). Stress also activates the enzyme PKC, which influences the brain's prefrontal cortex. Excess PKC can negatively affect focus, judgment, and the ability to think clearly. Moreover, many stressors are inherently anxiety producing, depressing, or both. Stress has been found to contribute to psychological problems, such as depression, panic attacks, anxiety, eating disorders, and post-traumatic stress disorder (PTSD). PTSD, which affects war veterans, rape and child abuse survivors, and others who have suffered or witnessed severe trauma, is characterized by nightmares, flashbacks, and a diminished capacity to experience or express emotion. Recent research suggests that PTSD symptoms may occur in some individuals who have not experienced a major trauma. (For more information, see Chapter 2.)

 Mind *Body* **SPIRIT**

Stress and Your Brain

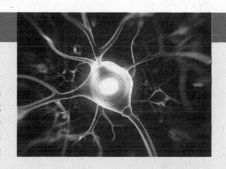

Like a computer that registers information in response to typing on a keyboard, your brain is able to respond to and store information about changes in your environment. Unlike a computer, your brain has the attribute of *plasticity*—it physically changes its structure and function in response to experience. Plasticity allows your brain to be altered by psychological stress.

Moderate stress enhances the ability to acquire and remember information, while high levels of acute stress can impair learning. For example, people can often remember minute details following a fender bender but can't recall the events surrounding a major car crash. Thus, it is good to be a little nervous before an exam—but not too nervous.

The effects of stress on brain form and function are apparent in a structure called the *hippocampus*, which is involved in learning and memory. High levels of chronic stress cause brain cells (neurons) in the hippocampus to shrink in size or die, thus impairing learning and memory. New research in neuroscience has revealed that the hippocampus actually grows new neurons during adulthood. However, stress acts to reduce new cell birth in the hippocampus, reducing the replacement of lost neurons. Together, these effects of stress result in fewer neurons and fewer connections between neurons in the hippocampus, thus decreasing the capacity for information processing.

People who are depressed or who experience PTSD have higher levels of stress hormones in their bloodstream and smaller hippocampi than others. Even in the absence of a serious disorder, it is thought that the accumulation of stress effects across the lifespan can contribute to brain aging. Thus, the way you cope with stress can affect the way your brain works both immediately and over the long term.

Altered Functioning of the Immune System

PNI research helps explain how stress affects the immune system. Some of the health problems linked to stress-related changes in immune function include vulnerability to colds and other infections, asthma and allergy attacks, susceptibility to cancer, and flare-ups of chronic diseases, such as genital herpes and HIV infection.

Other Health Problems

Many other health problems may be caused or worsened by excessive stress, including the following:

- digestive problems, such as stomach aches, diarrhea, constipation, irritable bowel syndrome, and ulcers
- tension headaches and migraines (see the In Focus box)
- insomnia and fatigue
- injuries, including on-the-job injuries caused by repetitive strain
- menstrual irregularities, impotence, and pregnancy complications
- loss of interest in previously enjoyable activities

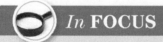 *In* FOCUS

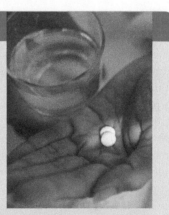

Headaches: A Common Symptom of Stress

Many Canadians have chronic, recurrent headaches. Headaches come in various types but are often grouped into three major categories: tension headaches, migraines, and cluster headaches. Other types of headaches have underlying organic causes, such as sinus congestion or infection.

Tension Headaches

Almost 60 percent of Canadian adults experience headaches, and approximately 90 percent of all headaches are *tension headaches*, characterized by a dull, steady pain, usually on both sides of the head. It may feel as though a band of pressure is tightening around your head, and the pain may extend to your neck and shoulders. Acute tension headaches can last from hours to days, while chronic tension headaches may occur almost every day for months or even years.

Psychological stress, poor posture, and immobility are the leading causes of tension headaches. They have no cure, but the pain can sometimes be relieved with over-the-counter painkillers and with therapies, such as massage, acupuncture, relaxation, hot or cold showers, and rest.

If your headaches are frequent, keep a diary with details about the events surrounding each one. If you can identify the stressors that are consistently associated with your headaches, you can begin to gain more control over the situation. If you have persistent tension headaches, you should consult your physician.

Migraines

About 17 percent of Canadians have *migraines*, which typically progress through a series of stages lasting from several minutes to several days. There are two categories of migraine: those with aura (called classical migraine) and those without aura (called common migraine). Sometimes, prior to the aura, the migraine sufferer experiences challenging mood changes that can interfere with normal activities. The aura itself usually lasts about 20 minutes and comes immediately before the onset of the other symptoms. Whether with or without an aura, migraines can produce a variety of symptoms, including throbbing pain that starts on one side of the head and may spread; heightened sensitivity to light; visual disturbances, such as flashing lights; nausea; and fatigue. About 70 percent of migraine sufferers are women, with the highest rates among 25- to 54-year-olds, and migraine headaches may have a genetic component.

Research suggests that people who get migraines may have abnormally excitable nerve cells in their brains. When triggered, these nerve cells send a wave of electrical activity throughout the brain, which in turn causes migraine symptoms. Potential triggers include menstruation, stress, fatigue, atmospheric changes, specific sounds or odours, and certain foods. The frequency of attacks varies from a few in a lifetime to several per week.

Keeping a headache journal can help a person with migraines identify headache triggers—the first step to avoiding them. In addition, many new treatments can help reduce the frequency, severity, and duration of migraines.

Cluster Headaches

Cluster headaches are extremely severe headaches that cause intense pain in and around one eye. They usually occur in clusters of one to three headaches each day over weeks or months, alternating with periods of remission in which no headaches occur. About 80 percent of people with cluster headaches are male.

There is no known cause or cure for cluster headaches, but a number of treatments are available. During cluster periods, it is important to refrain from smoking cigarettes and drinking alcohol because these activities can trigger attacks.

QUESTIONS FOR CRITICAL THINKING AND REFLECTION

Have you ever been so stressed that you felt ill in some way? If so, what were your symptoms? How did you handle them? Did the experience affect the way you reacted to other stressful events? What is one lifestyle change you can make to positively impact your daily experience of stress?

Common Sources of Stress

Being able to recognize potential sources of stress is an important step in successfully managing the stress in your life.

Major Life Changes

Any major change in your life that requires adjustment and accommodation can be a source of stress. Early adulthood and the post-secondary years are associated with many significant changes, such as moving out of the family home, changes in financial circumstances, and relationship changes. Even changes typically thought of as positive—graduation, job promotion, marriage—can be stressful.

Clusters of life changes, particularly those that are perceived negatively, may be linked to health problems in some people. Personality and coping skills, however, are important moderating influences. People with a strong support network and a stress-resistant personality are less likely to become ill in response to life changes than people with fewer resources.

Daily Hassles

Although major life changes are undoubtedly stressful, they seldom occur regularly. Researchers have proposed that minor problems—life's daily hassles, such as losing your keys or wallet—can be an even greater source of stress because they occur much more often.

People who perceive hassles negatively are likely to experience a moderate stress response every time they are faced with one. Over time, this can take a significant toll on health. Studies indicate that for some people, daily hassles contribute to a general decrease in overall wellness.

Post-Secondary Stressors

University or college is a time of major changes and minor hassles. For many students, post-secondary education means being away from home and family for the first time. Nearly all students share similar stresses, such as the following:

- *Academic stress:* Exams, grades, and an endless workload await every post-secondary student, but can be especially troublesome for young students just out of high school. Test anxiety is a source of stress for many students. To help yourself take control and learn some proven techniques for overcoming test anxiety, see the Take Charge box at the end of this chapter.
- *Interpersonal stress:* Most students are more than just students; they are also friends, children, employees, spouses, parents, and so on. Managing relationships while juggling the rigours of university or college life can be daunting, especially if some friends or family are less than supportive.
- *Time pressures:* Class schedules, assignments, and deadlines are an inescapable part of post-secondary life. But these time pressures can be drastically compounded for students who also have a job and family responsibilities.
- *Financial concerns:* The majority of post-secondary students need financial aid not just to cover the cost of tuition, but also to survive from day to day while in school. For many, this isn't possible without a job, and the pressure to stay afloat financially competes with academic and other stressors.
- *Worries about the future:* As school life comes to an end, students face the reality of life after university or college. This means thinking about a career, choosing a place to live, and leaving the friends and routines of school behind.

Job-Related Stressors

Canadians rate their jobs as a key source of stress in their lives, and the World Health Organization has deemed job-related stress a worldwide epidemic. The Canadian Mental Health Association recently identified the rise in unemployment and job instability as key stressors. And for those who are employed, tight schedules and overtime leave less time to exercise, socialize, and engage in other stress-proofing activities. More than three-quarters of Canadians report that they regularly feel rushed and that they do not have enough time, and more than one-third of Canadians report feeling constantly under stress trying to accomplish more than they can handle. Worries about job performance, salary, and job security, and interactions with bosses, co-workers, and customers can contribute to this experience. High levels of job stress are also common for people who are left out of important decisions relating to their jobs. When workers are given the opportunity to shape how their jobs are performed, job satisfaction goes up and stress levels go down.

If job-related (or school-related) stress is severe or chronic, the result can be **burnout**, a state of physical, mental, and emotional exhaustion. Burnout occurs most often in highly motivated and driven individuals who come to feel that their work is not recognized or that they are not accomplishing their goals. People in the helping professions—teachers, social workers, caregivers, police officers, and so on—are also prone to burnout. For some people who suffer from burnout, a vacation or leave of absence may be appropriate. For others, a reduced work schedule, better communication with superiors, or a change in job goals may be necessary. Improving time-management skills can also help.

burnout
A state of physical, mental, and emotional exhaustion.

Millions of workdays are lost annually because of illness. Stress-related sleep disturbances, headaches, and damaged relationships are quick to arise and easy to identify, but the effects of job stress on chronic diseases are harder to see because they take longer to develop. It's telling, however, that health care costs are nearly 50 percent greater for workers with high levels of stress. (For some recent statistics on job-related stress, see the In Focus box.)

Social Stressors

Social networks can be real or virtual. Both types can help improve your ability to deal with stress, but any social network can also become a stressor in itself.

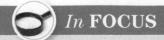

In FOCUS

What Stresses Us Out?

The Canadian Mental Health Association conducted a survey to determine the leading sources of stress in Canadians' lives, their perceptions of stress, and the ways in which stress affects them. The top ten key sources of serious stress for Canadians are shown in the table.

Work-related stress affects a large number of Canadians, so much so that more than a quarter of Canadian workers find their daily lives to be highly stressful. That being said, Canadian employers are actually receiving fairly positive reviews; 60 percent of employed Canadians reported that their bosses are effective or somewhat effective in dealing with employee stress.

Work	51%
Money	48%
Parenting/children	33%
Health problems	27%
Spousal/partner problems	21%
Unemployment	20%
Aging	19%
Housework/maintenance	18%
Elder care	12%
School	2%

Real Social Networks

Although social support is a key buffer against stress, your interactions with others can themselves be a source of stress. The post-secondary years, in particular, can be a time of great change in interpersonal relationships. The larger community where you live can also act as a stressor.

Social stressors include prejudice and discrimination. You may feel stress as you try to relate to people of other ethnic or socioeconomic groups. If you are a member of a minority ethnic group, you may feel pressure to assimilate into mainstream society, or to spend as much time as possible with others who share your ethnicity or background. If English is not your first language, you may face the added burden of conducting daily activities in a language with which you are not comfortable. All these pressures can become significant sources of stress. (See the Dimensions of Diversity box for more information.)

Dimensions *of* DIVERSITY

Diverse Populations, Discrimination, and Stress

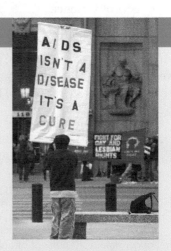

Stress is universal, but in diverse multiethnic and multicultural nations such as Canada, some groups face special stressors and have higher-than-average rates of stress-related physical and emotional problems. These groups include members of ethnic minority groups, the poor, those with disabilities, and gays, lesbians, and transgender people. As you read the information in this box, notice how a variety of the determinants of health introduced in Chapter 1 (particularly the determinants related to cultural background, gender, and social conditions) come together to affect the stress levels of some Canadians.

Discrimination occurs when people act according to their prejudices—biased, negative attitudes toward some group. Blatant examples are painting a swastika on a Jewish studies house or defacing a sculpture depicting a same-sex couple holding hands. More subtle examples include a black Canadian student noticing that white shopkeepers in a mostly white university town tend to keep a close eye on him; a male-to-female transgender individual being treated with less respect by her professors and peers; a student using a wheelchair finding no accessible bathrooms; or an obese woman overhearing remarks about eating and self-control.

Recent immigrants to Canada have to learn to live in a new society. This requires a balance between assimilating and changing to be like the majority, and maintaining a connection to their own culture, language, and religion. The process of acculturation is generally stressful, especially when their background is radically different from that of the people they are now living among. Parental expectations generate stress if they are too high or too low. When they are too high, the child may work too hard in an attempt to succeed at everything; when they are too low, the child may not work hard enough to succeed at anything.

Both immigrants and members of minority groups that have lived for generations in Canada can face job-related and school-related stressors because of stereotypes and discrimination. They may make less money in comparable jobs with comparable levels of education and may find it more difficult to achieve leadership positions. However, on a positive note, many who experience hardship, disability, or prejudice develop effective, goal-directed coping skills and are successful at overcoming obstacles and managing the stress they face.

Virtual Social Networks

New technologies can potentially be time-savers because we don't have to go home or to the office to check our email or phone messages, and we can make a call on a cellphone instead of jotting down notes to pass on at a later time. Telecommuting can ease the time pressures on people who find it necessary to work from home, such as parents with young children or people with disabilities. Increased electronic interactivity, however, can also impinge on our personal space, facilitate cyber-bullying, waste time, and cause stress. On a typical day, for example, you may check for email or voice mail several times, only to find no messages waiting for you. When you do have messages, you may find that some are of little or no value. If you are "always on" (that is, always available by voice or text messaging), some friends or colleagues may think it's all right to contact you any time, even if you're in class or trying to work. The convenience of staying electronically connected, therefore, comes at a price. It is important to create boundaries for daily interactions with technology, otherwise it can become an obsessions or even addiction and can feel like the technologies are in charge of us, rather than us using the devices to enhance the quality of our lives.

Environmental Stressors

Have you ever tried to eat at a restaurant where the food was great, but the atmosphere was so noisy that it put you on edge? This is an example of a mild environmental stress—a condition or an event in the physical environment that causes stress. Examples of more severe environmental stressors include the following:

- natural disasters
- acts of violence
- industrial accidents

Like the noisy atmosphere of some restaurants, many environmental stressors are mere inconveniences that are easy to avoid. Others, such as pollen or construction noise, may be an unavoidable daily source of stress. For those who live in poor or violent neighbourhoods or in a war-torn country, environmental stressors can be major stressors (see the In the News box).

 In *the* NEWS

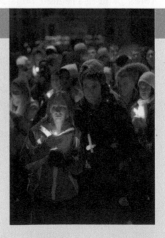

Coping After Violence on Campus

Stories of violence on North American campuses have become all-too familiar. A University of British Columbia researcher (Elizabeth Saewyc) led a study that found almost 20 percent of university students in Canada and the United States had experienced violence within the last six months, with men and women being equally likely to be victims of physical or emotional violence. The authors found links between violence and alcohol use, and noted that nearly half of the emotional violence and 20 percent of the physical violence reported by both sexes came from intimate partners. Violence on university and college campuses has become a terrible reality for many students, and at times, that violence turns deadly, as the following incidents depict:

- On April 2, 2012, One Goh, a 43-year-old former student at Oikos University, a Christian school populated by mostly Korean and Korean-Americans, opened fire on the campus, killing seven people and wounding several others.
- On December 8, 2011, a Virginia Tech police officer was shot and killed by a 22-year old student of Radford University. The shooting took place in a parking lot on Virginia Tech's campus in Blacksburg, Virginia.
- In March 2008, an Auburn University student died from gunshot wounds sustained during a robbery. One day later, a University of North Carolina student was killed while being robbed in Chapel Hill, North Carolina.
- On February 14, 2008, a former Northern Illinois University student walked into one of the school's lecture halls and fatally shot five students before killing himself. Gunfire injured at least 16 other people.
- Just a few days earlier, a student at Louisiana Technical College in Baton Rouge, Louisiana shot two other students to death, then killed herself as classmates watched in horror.
- On April 16, 2007, a student killed 28 students and 5 teachers and injured 29 others during two attacks at Virginia Polytechnic Institute and State University (Virginia Tech). Four Canadian students were among the survivors. The attacker was acting out fantasies of revenge in a drama that held the nation's attention for weeks.
- On September 13, 2006, a young man started shooting people at Dawson College in Montreal, killing 1 woman and injuring 19 others before taking his own life.
- On December 6, 1989, a 25-year-old man killed 13 female students, wounded 13 more, and then killed himself at L'École Polytechnique in Montreal.

People react to news of school violence in different ways, depending on their proximity to the event and its recency. In the case of school massacres, people far from the site may suffer emotional reactions simply from watching endless coverage online or on television. Responses to violence or reports of violence include disbelief, shock, fear, anger, resentment, anxiety, mood swings, irritability, sadness, depression, panic, guilt, apathy, feelings of isolation or powerlessness, and many of the symptoms of excess stress. Most of those affected return to normal after a few weeks or months, but a few go on to develop PTSD, a more serious condition.

In the case of the Virginia Tech shootings, the school and community mobilized quickly to respond to the expected surge in behavioural health needs generated by the attack. Hotline calls and emergency room visits increased dramatically, especially during the second and third weeks following the shootings. Information sources and support groups were established for people grieving the loss of friends, family, neighbours, or colleagues. Volunteers contacted each family that was directly affected by the shootings to offer help in making arrangements and other services.

If you are affected by a disastrous event, such as a school shooting or terrorist attack, take these steps:

- Be sure that you have the best information about what happened, whether a continuing risk is present, and what you can do to avoid it. That information may be posted online or on local radio or TV stations.
- Don't expose yourself to so much media coverage that you begin to feel overwhelmed by it.
- Take care of yourself. Use the stress-relief techniques discussed in this chapter.
- Share your feelings and concerns with others. Be a supportive listener.
- If you feel able, help others in any way you can, such as by volunteering to work with victims.
- If you feel emotionally distressed days or weeks after the event, consider asking for professional help.

Internal Stressors

Some stressors are found not in our environment, but within ourselves. We pressure ourselves to reach goals and continually evaluate our progress and performance. Setting goals and striving to reach them can enhance self-esteem if the goals are reasonable. Unrealistic expectations, however, can be a significant source of stress and can damage self-esteem (for example, expecting to earn 100 percent on every test or assignment, or being the top performer at work every week). Other internal stressors are physical and emotional states, such as illness and exhaustion (e.g., fighting cancer, having the flu, or even experiencing relationship upsets); these can be both a cause and an effect of unmanaged stress.

 QUESTIONS FOR CRITICAL THINKING AND REFLECTION

What are the top two or three stressors in your life right now? Are they new to your life—as part of your post-secondary experience—or are they stressors you have experienced in the past? Do they include both positive and negative experiences (eustress and distress)? What might you do differently to manage your difficult stressors?

Managing Stress

You can control the stress in your life by taking the following steps:

- Shore up your support system.
- Improve your communication skills.
- Develop healthy exercise, eating, and sleeping habits.
- Learn to identify and moderate individual stressors.

The effort required is well worth the time. People who manage stress effectively not only are healthier, but also have more time to enjoy life and accomplish goals.

Social Support

The ability to share fears, frustrations, and joys makes life richer. Having the support of friends and family members seems to contribute to the well-being of body and mind. Research supports this conclusion, as the following examples demonstrate:

- Among university students living in overcrowded apartments, a study revealed that those students with a strong social support system were less distressed by their cramped quarters than were the loners who navigated life's challenges on their own.
- Young adults who have strong relationships with their parents tend to cope with stress better than peers with poor parental relationships.
- Many studies have shown that married people live longer than single people (including those who are divorced, widowed, or never married) and have lower mortality rates from practically all causes of death.

Social support can provide a critical counterbalance to the stress in our lives. Give yourself time to develop and maintain a network of people you can count on for emotional support, feedback, and nurturing. If you believe you don't have enough social support, consider becoming a volunteer to help build your network of friends and to enhance your spiritual wellness.

Communication

How do you communicate your wants and needs to others? Communicating in an assertive way that respects the rights of others—while protecting your own rights—can prevent potentially stressful situations from getting out of control.

Some people have trouble either telling others what they need or saying no to the needs of others. They may suppress their feelings of anger, frustration, and resentment, and they may end up feeling taken advantage of or suffering in unhealthy relationships. At the other extreme are people who express anger openly and directly by being verbally or physically aggressive, or indirectly by making critical, hurtful comments to others. Their abusive behaviour pushes other people away, and so they also have problems with relationships.

QUICK STATS

More than 63% of Canadian college and university students are interested in receiving information from their schools about how to help others in distress.

—*National College Health Assessment II: Canadian Reference Group Data Report*, 2013

Better communication skills can help everyone form and maintain healthy relationships. If you typically suppress your feelings, you might want to take an assertiveness training course that can help you identify and change your patterns of communication. If you have trouble controlling your anger, you may benefit from learning anger-management strategies.

Chapter 2 includes a detailed discussion of anger and its impact on health and relationships. Chapter 10 discusses strategies for building healthy relationships, including positive communication techniques.

Exercise

Exercise helps maintain a healthy body and mind and even stimulates the birth of new brain cells. Regular physical activity can also reduce many of the negative effects of stress. Consider the following examples:

- Taking a long walk can help decrease anxiety and blood pressure.
- A brisk ten-minute walk can leave you feeling more relaxed and energetic for up to two hours.
- People who exercise regularly react with milder physical stress responses before, during, and after exposure to stressors.
- In a study, people who took three brisk 45-minute walks each week for three months reported that they perceived fewer daily hassles. Their sense of wellness also increased.

These findings should not be surprising, because the stress response mobilizes energy resources and readies the body for physical emergencies. If you experience stress and do not physically exert yourself, you are not completing the energy cycle. You may not be able to exercise while your daily stressors occur—during class, for example, or while sitting in a traffic jam—but you can be active at other times of the day. Physical activity allows you to expend

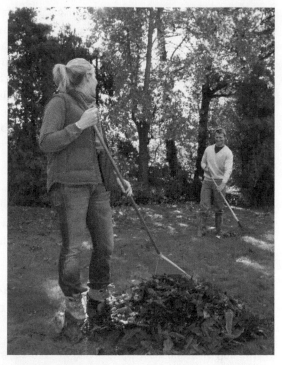

Exercise—even light activity—can be an effective antidote to stress.

the nervous energy you have built up and trains your body to more readily achieve homeostasis following stressful situations.

It isn't hard to incorporate light to moderate exercise into your day. For example, you may be able to walk to class or ride your bike to the store instead of driving, or plan occasional activities with a friend, such as playing tennis or going for a walk. The important thing is to find an activity that you enjoy so that it can become a habit and a regular stress reducer.

One warning: For some people, exercise can become just one more stressor in a highly stressed life. People who exercise compulsively risk overtraining, a condition characterized by fatigue, irritability, depression, and diminished athletic performance. An overly strenuous exercise program can even make you sick by compromising your immune function. (For details on creating a safe and effective exercise program, see Chapter 6.)

Nutrition

A healthy diet gives you an energy bank to draw from whenever you experience stress. Eating wisely also can enhance your feelings of self-control and self-esteem. Learning the principles of sound nutrition is easy, and sensible eating habits rapidly become second nature when practised regularly. (For information on nutrition and healthy eating habits, see Chapter 5.)

For the purposes of managing stress, you may find it especially helpful to limit or avoid caffeine. Although one or two cups of coffee a day probably won't hurt you, caffeine is a mildly addictive stimulant that leaves some people jittery, irritable, and unable to sleep. Consuming caffeine during stressful situations can raise blood pressure and increase levels of cortisol. The following items can contain caffeine, sometimes in high doses:

- tea
- cola and some other soft drinks
- chocolate
- cold remedies
- aspirin products
- weight-loss preparations

If you are concerned about your caffeine intake, read the labels of products you consume daily. You may be surprised at the amount of caffeine you are ingesting, from a variety of sources.

Although your diet has an effect on the way your body handles stress, the reverse is also true. Excess stress can negatively affect the way you eat. Many people, for example, respond to stress by overeating; other people skip meals or stop eating altogether during stressful periods. Both responses are not only ineffective (they don't address the causes of stress) but also potentially unhealthy. It can be helpful for busy students who are on-the-go to invest a few minutes each day to prepare healthy snacks to have on-hand between classes. Some alternatives to the easily accessible coffee/donut combination could be a small bag of carrots, celery, cheese, or sunflower seeds.

Sleep

Most adults need seven to nine hours of sleep every night to stay healthy and perform their best. Getting enough sleep isn't just good for you physically; adequate sleep also improves mood, fosters feelings of competence and self-worth, enhances mental functioning, and supports emotional functioning.

How Sleep Works

Sleep occurs in two phases: **rapid eye movement (REM) sleep** and **non-rapid eye movement (NREM) sleep**. A sleeper goes through several cycles of non-REM and REM sleep each night.

> **rapid eye movement (REM) sleep**
> The portion of the sleep cycle during which dreaming occurs.
>
> **non-rapid eye movement (non-REM) sleep**
> The portion of the sleep cycle that involves deep sleep; non-REM sleep includes four states of successively deeper sleep.

NREM sleep actually includes four stages of successively deeper sleep. As you move through these stages of sleep, a variety of physiological changes occur, including the following:

- Blood pressure drops.
- Respiration and heart rates slow.
- Body temperature declines.
- Growth hormone is released.
- Brain wave patterns become slow and even.

During REM sleep, dreams occur. REM sleep is characterized by the rapid movement of the eyes under closed eyelids. Heart rate, blood pressure, and breathing rate rise, and brain activity increases to levels equal to or greater than those during waking hours. Muscles in the limbs relax completely, resulting in a temporary paralysis. (This total relaxation may prevent you from acting out your dreams while you're asleep.)

Sleep and Stress

Stress hormone levels in the bloodstream vary throughout the day and are related to sleep patterns. Peak concentrations occur in the early morning, followed by a slow decline during the day and evening (see Figure 3.4). Concentrations return to peak levels during the final stages of sleep and in the early morning hours. Stress

FIGURE 3.4

Changing Levels of Stress Hormones in the Bloodstream

Stress hormones, such as cortisol, fluctuate throughout the day and night and reach a high level during the last stages of sleep.

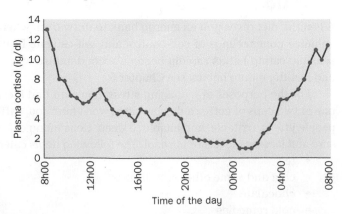

Source: Palma B. D., et al. 2008. Immune outcomes of sleep disorders: The hypothalamic-pituitary adrenal axis as a modulatory factor. *Revista Brasileiro de Psiquiatria*, Vol. 29 Suppl., Figure 3.l, São Paulo, May 2007.

hormone levels are low during non-REM sleep and increase during REM sleep. With each successive sleep cycle during the night, REM sleep lasts a little longer. This increase in REM sleep duration with each sleep cycle may underlie the progressive increase in circulating stress hormones during the final stages of sleep.

Even though stress hormones are released during sleep, it is the *lack* of sleep that has the greatest impact on stress. In someone who experiences **sleep deprivation** (not getting enough sleep over time), mental and physical processes steadily deteriorate. A sleep-deprived person has headaches, feels irritable, is unable to concentrate, and is more prone to forgetfulness. Poor-quality sleep has long been associated with stress and depression. A small 2008 study of female university students further associated sleep deprivation with an increased risk of suicide, and in 2012, similar findings were reported among young adults in the military.

sleep deprivation
A lack of sleep over time.

Acute sleep deprivation slows the daytime decline in stress hormones, and so evening levels are higher than normal. A decrease in total sleep time also causes an increase in the level of stress hormones. Together, these changes may cause an increase in stress hormone levels throughout the day and may contribute to physical and mental exhaustion. Extreme sleep deprivation can lead to hallucinations and other psychotic symptoms, as well as to a significant increase in heart attack risk.

QUICK STATS

Canadians spend nearly $340 million a year on alcohol to help promote sleep.
—Daley and colleagues, 2009

Sleep Problems

According to a study by Statistics Canada, Canadians sleep about eight hours per night, with men sleeping about 11 minutes more than women and women having a harder time falling asleep and staying asleep. Post-secondary students often cite sleep problems, or rather, not enough sleep, as part of the challenge of university or college life. Although many of us can attribute the lack of sleep to long (school and employment) workdays and family responsibilities, many Canadians have chronic sleep disorders—medical conditions that prevent them from sleeping well.

Researchers from the University of Laval in Quebec found that more than one-third of Canadian adults (about 35 percent of women and 25 percent of men) have trouble falling asleep or staying asleep—a condition called **insomnia**. The Canadian Sleep Society notes that when a person experiences sleep difficulty for at least three nights per week for one month or longer, and distress and/or functional impairment are present as a result, the condition is considered **insomnia syndrome**. Similar to bouts of insomnia, women are more likely than men to meet the criteria for insomnia syndrome (at about 16 percent compared to 11 percent, respectively). The most common causes of insomnia are lifestyle factors, such as high caffeine or alcohol intake before bedtime (which can actually cause disturbances in sleep quality and duration, even though it can help reduce the time needed to fall asleep); medical problems, such as a breathing disorder; and stress. About 75 percent of people who suffer from chronic insomnia report some stressful life event at the onset of their sleeping problems. (For more information, see the Take Charge box.)

Insomnia
A sleep problem involving the inability to fall or stay asleep.

insomnia syndrome
Experiencing insomnia for at least three nights per week for a minimum of one month, and experiencing associated impairment or distress

Take CHARGE

Overcoming Insomnia

Most people can resolve their insomnia by discovering the cause of their poor sleep and taking steps to remedy it. Insomnia that lasts for more than six months and interferes with daytime functioning requires consultation with a physician. Sleeping pills are not recommended for chronic insomnia because they can be habit forming; they also lose their effectiveness over time.

If you are bothered by insomnia, try the following:

- Determine how much sleep you need to feel refreshed the next day, and don't sleep longer than that.
- Go to bed at the same time every night and, more important, get up at the same time every morning, seven days a week, regardless of how much sleep you got. Don't nap for more than 30 minutes per day.
- Exercise every day, but not too close to bedtime. Your metabolism takes up to six hours to slow down after exercise.
- Avoid tobacco and caffeine late in the day, and avoid alcohol before bedtime (it causes disturbed, fragmented sleep).
- If you take any medications (prescription or not), ask your doctor or pharmacist if they are known to interfere with sleep.
- Use your bed only for sleep. Don't eat, read, study, or watch television in bed.
- Relax before bedtime with a warm bath (again, not too close to bedtime—allow about two hours for your metabolism to slow down afterward), a book, music, or relaxation exercises. Don't lie down in bed until you're sleepy.
- If you don't fall asleep in 15–20 minutes, or if you wake up and can't fall asleep again, get out of bed, leave the room if possible, and do something monotonous until you feel sleepy. Try distracting yourself with imagery instead of counting sheep; imagine yourself on a pleasant vacation or enjoying some beautiful scenery.
- If sleep problems persist, ask your physician for a referral to a sleep specialist in your area. You may be a candidate for a sleep study—an overnight evaluation of your sleep pattern that can uncover many sleep-related disorders.

Another type of chronic sleep problem, called **sleep apnea**, occurs when a person stops breathing while asleep. Apnea can be caused by a number of factors, but it typically results when the soft tissue at the back of the mouth (such as the tongue or soft palate) collapses during sleep, blocking the airway. When breathing is interrupted, so is sleep, as the sleeper awakens repeatedly throughout the night to begin breathing again. In most cases, this occurs without the sleeper even being aware of it. However, the disruption to sleep can be significant, and over time acute sleep deprivation can result from apnea. Apnea has several treatments, including medications, the use of a special apparatus that helps keep the airway open during sleep, and surgery.

sleep apnea
The interruption of normal breathing during sleep.

Time Management

Learning to manage your time can be crucial to coping with everyday stressors. Overcommitment, procrastination, and even boredom are significant stressors for many people. Along with gaining control of nutrition and exercise to maintain a healthy energy balance, time management is an important element in a wellness program. Try these strategies for improving your time-management skills:

- *Set priorities.* Divide your tasks into three groups: essential, important, and trivial. Focus on the first two, and ignore the third.
- *Schedule tasks for peak efficiency.* You have undoubtedly noticed you are most productive at certain times of the day (or night). Schedule as many of your tasks for those hours as you can, and stick to your schedule.
- *Set realistic goals and write them down.* Attainable goals spur you on. Impossible goals, by definition, cause frustration and failure. Fully commit yourself to achieving your goals by putting them in writing.

- *Budget your time.* For each project you undertake, calculate how long it will take to complete. Then tack on another 10–15 percent, or even 25 percent, as a buffer.
- *Break up long-term goals into short-term ones.* Instead of waiting for or relying on large blocks of time, use short amounts of time to start a project or keep it moving.
- *Visualize the achievement of your goals.* By mentally rehearsing your performance of a task, you will be able to reach your goal more smoothly.
- *Keep track of the tasks you put off.* Analyze the reasons you procrastinate. If the task is difficult or unpleasant, look for ways to make it easier or more fun. For example, if you find the readings for one of your classes particularly difficult, choose an especially nice setting for your reading, and then reward yourself each time you complete a section or chapter.
- *Consider doing your least-favourite tasks first.* Once you have the most unpleasant ones out of the way, work on the tasks you enjoy more.
- *Consolidate tasks when possible.* For example, try walking to the store so that you run your errands and exercise in the same block of time.

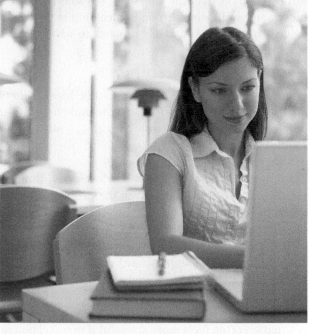

Managing the many commitments of adult life—including work, school, and parenthood—can sometimes feel overwhelming and produce a great deal of stress. Time-management and problem-solving skills, including careful scheduling with a date book or handheld computer, can help you cope with busy days.

- *Identify quick transitional tasks.* Keep a list of five-minute to ten-minute tasks, such as watering your plants, doing the dishes, or checking a homework assignment, that you can do while waiting or between other tasks.
- *Delegate responsibility.* Asking for help when you have too much to do is not a cop-out; it's good time management. Just don't delegate the jobs you know you should do yourself.
- *Say no when necessary.* If the demands made on you don't seem reasonable, say no—tactfully, but without guilt or apology.
- *Give yourself a break.* Allow time for play—free, unstructured time when you can ignore the clock. Don't consider this a waste of time. Play renews you and enables you to work more efficiently.
- *Avoid your personal time sinks.* You can probably identify your own time sinks—activities such as watching television, surfing the Internet, texting for the sake of texting, or talking on the phone that consistently use up more time than you anticipate and put you behind schedule. Some days, it may be best to avoid problematic activities altogether; for example, if you have a big paper due, don't sit down for a five-minute TV break if it is likely to turn into a two-hour break. Try a five-minute walk if you need to clear your head.
- *Stop thinking or talking about what you're going to do, and just do it!* Sometimes the best solution for procrastination is to stop waiting for the right moment and just get started. You will probably find that things are not as bad as you feared, and your momentum will keep you going.

Confiding in Yourself Through Writing

Keeping a diary is analogous to confiding in others, except that you are confiding in yourself. This form of coping with severe stress may be especially helpful for those who are shy or introverted and find it difficult to open up to others. Although writing about traumatic and stressful events may have a short-term negative effect on mood, over the long term, stress is reduced and positive changes in health occur. A key to promoting health and well-being through journaling is to write about your emotional responses to stressful events. Set aside a special time each day or week to write down your feelings about stressful events in your life.

Cognitive Techniques

Some stressors arise in our own minds. Ideas, beliefs, perceptions, and patterns of thinking can add to our stress level. Each of the following techniques can help you change unhealthy thought patterns to ones that will help you cope with stress. As with any skill, mastering these techniques takes practice and patience.

Think and Act Constructively

Think back to the worries you had last week. How many of them were needless? Think about things you *can* control. Try to stand aside from the problem, consider the positive steps you can take to solve it, and then carry them out. Remember, if you can successfully predict that a stressor will occur, you can better control your response to it. In the evening, try to predict stressful events you might encounter the following day. Then decide how to handle them constructively. This may mean dealing positively with an unpleasant person or figuring out how to stay focused during a boring class. By taking a constructive approach, you can prevent stressors from becoming negative events, and perhaps even turn them into positive experiences.

Take Control

A situation often feels more stressful if you feel you're not in control of it. Time may seem to be slipping away before a big exam, for example. Unexpected obstacles may appear in your path, throwing you off course. When you feel your environment is controlling you instead of the other way around, take charge! Concentrate on what is possible to control, and set realistic goals. Be confident of your ability to succeed.

Problem Solve

Students with greater problem-solving abilities report easier adjustment to university or college life, higher motivation levels, lower stress levels, and higher grades. When you find yourself stewing over a problem, sit down and do some problem solving on paper or at your computer. Try this approach:

1. Define the problem in one or two sentences.
2. Identify the causes of the problem.
3. Consider all solutions; don't just stop with the most obvious one.
4. Weigh positive and negative consequences for each solution.
5. Make a decision—choose a solution.
6. List what you will need to do to act on your decision.
7. Begin to carry out your list; if you're unable to do that, temporarily turn to other things.
8. Evaluate the outcome and revise your approach if necessary.

Modify Your Expectations

Expectations are exhausting and restricting. The fewer expectations you have, the more you can live spontaneously and joyfully. The more you expect from others, the more often you will feel let down. And trying to meet the expectations others have of you is often futile.

Stay Positive

If you beat up on yourself—"Late for class again! You can't even cope with university! How do you expect to ever hold down a professional job?"—change your inner dialogue. Talk to yourself as you would to a child you love: "You're a smart, capable person. You've solved other problems; you'll handle this one. Tomorrow you'll simply schedule things so you get to class with a few minutes to spare." (Chapter 2 has more information on self-talk.)

Cultivate Your Sense of Humour

When it comes to stress, laughter may be the best medicine. Even a fleeting smile produces changes in your autonomic nervous system that can lift your spirits. And a few minutes of belly laughing can be as invigorating as brisk exercise. Hearty laughter elevates your heart rate, aids digestion, eases pain, and triggers the release of endorphins and other pleasurable and stimulating chemicals in the brain. After a good laugh, your muscles go slack; your pulse and blood pressure dip below normal. You are relaxed. Cultivate the ability to laugh at yourself, and you will have a handy and instantly effective stress reliever.

Focus on What's Important

A major source of stress is trying to store too much data. Forget unimportant details (they will usually be self-evident) and organize important information. One technique you can try is to chunk the important material into categories. If your next exam covers three chapters from your text, consider each chapter a chunk of information. Then break down each chunk into its three or four most important features. Create a mental outline that allows you to trace your way from the most general category down to the most specific details. This technique can be applied to managing daily responsibilities as well.

Relaxation Techniques

The **relaxation response** is a physiological state characterized by a feeling of warmth and quiet mental alertness. This is the opposite of the fight-or-flight reaction. When the relaxation response is triggered by a relaxation technique, heart rate, breathing, and metabolism slow down. Blood pressure and oxygen consumption decrease. At the same time, blood flow to the brain and skin increases, and brain waves shift from an alert beta rhythm to a relaxed alpha rhythm. Practised regularly, relaxation techniques can counteract the debilitating effects of stress.

> **relaxation response**
> A physiological state characterized by a feeling of warmth and quiet mental alertness.

If you decide to try a relaxation technique, practise it daily until it becomes natural to you, and then use it whenever you feel the need. You may feel calmer and more refreshed after each session. You will know you have mastered a deep relaxation technique when you start to see subtle changes in other areas of your life: You may notice you have been encountering fewer hassles, working more efficiently, or enjoying more free time. None of the techniques takes long to do.

Progressive Relaxation

Unlike most of the others, this simple method requires no imagination, willpower, or self-suggestion. You simply tense, and then relax, the muscles in your body, group by group. The technique, also known as deep muscle relaxation, helps you become aware of the muscle tension that occurs when you are under stress. When you consciously relax those muscles, other systems of the body get the message and ease up on the stress response.

Start, for example, with your right fist. Inhale as you tense it. Exhale as you relax it. Repeat. Next, contract and relax your right upper arm. Repeat. Do the same with your left arm. Then, beginning at your forehead and ending at your feet, contract and relax your other muscle groups. Repeat each contraction at least once, breathing in as you tense, breathing out as you relax. To speed up the process, tense and relax more muscles at one time—both arms simultaneously, for instance. With practice, you will be able to relax very quickly and effectively by clenching and releasing only your fists.

Visualization

Also known as *imagery*, **visualization** lets you daydream without guilt. Athletes find that the technique enhances sports performance, and visualization is reportedly used by 99 percent of Canadian Olympic athletes. You can use visualization to help you relax, change your habits, or perform well—whether on an exam, a stage, or a playing field.

> **visualization**
> A technique for promoting relaxation or improving performance that involves creating or re-creating vivid mental pictures of a place or an experience; also called *imagery*.

Next time you feel stressed, close your eyes. Imagine yourself floating on a cloud, sitting on a mountain-top, or lying in a meadow. Involve all your senses; imagine the sounds, the smells, and the other sensations that would be part of the scene. Your body will respond as if your imagery were real. As an alternative, close your eyes and imagine a deep-purple light filling your body. Now change the colour into a soothing gold. As the colour lightens, so should your distress.

Visualization can also be used to rehearse for an upcoming event and enhance performance. By experiencing an event ahead of time in your mind, you can practise coping with any difficulties that may arise. Think positively, and you can psych yourself up for a successful experience.

Meditation

The need to periodically stop our incessant mental chatter is so great that, since ancient times, hundreds of forms of **meditation** have developed in cultures all over the world. Meditation is a way of telling the mind to be quiet for a while. Because meditation has been at the core of many Eastern religions and philosophies, it has acquired a mystique that has caused some people to shy away from it. Yet meditation requires no special knowledge or background. Whatever the philosophical, religious, or emotional reasons may be given for meditation, it is potentially useful for reducing stress. According to a recent study, post-secondary students who learned how to use meditation for stress management were able to significantly reduce their daily stress levels. Further, those students found it easier to forgive others for perceived wrongdoings and spent less time focusing on negative thoughts.

> **meditation**
> A technique for quieting the mind by focusing on a particular word, object (such as a candle flame), or process (such as breathing).

Meditation helps you tune out the world temporarily, removing you from both internal and external sources of stress. The thinker takes time out to become the observer—calmly attentive, without analyzing, judging, comparing, or rationalizing. Regular practice of this quiet awareness will subtly carry over into your daily life, encouraging physical and emotional balance no matter what confronts you. For a step-by-step description of a basic meditation technique, see "Meditation and the Relaxation Response" on connect.

Another form of meditation, known as *mindfulness meditation*, involves paying attention to physical sensations, perceptions, thoughts, and imagery. Instead of focusing on a word or an object to quiet the mind, you observe any thoughts that occur without evaluating or judging them. Development of this ability requires regular practice but may eventually result in a more objective view of your perceptions. It is believed that a greater understanding of moment-to-moment thought processes (mindful awareness) provides a richer and more vital sense of life and improves coping. Studies also suggest that people who rate high in mindfulness are less anxious and better able to deal with stress; among people with specific health problems, mindfulness can provide substantial benefits.

Deep Breathing

Your breathing pattern is closely tied to your stress level. Deep, slow breathing is associated with relaxation. Rapid, shallow, irregular breathing occurs during the stress response. With practice, you can learn to slow and quiet your breathing pattern, thereby also quieting your mind and relaxing your body. Breathing techniques can be used for on-the-spot tension relief as well as for long-term stress reduction.

The primary goal of many breathing exercises is to change your breathing pattern from chest breathing to diaphragmatic (stomach) breathing. During the day, most adults breathe by expanding their chest and raising their shoulders rather than by expanding their abdomen. Diaphragmatic breathing, which involves free expansion of the diaphragm and lower abdomen, is the pattern of breathing characteristic of children and sleeping adults. (The diaphragm is a sheet of muscle and connective tissue that divides the chest and abdominal cavities.) Diaphragmatic breathing is slower and deeper than chest breathing. For instructions on how to perform diaphragmatic breathing, refer to "Breathing for Relaxation" on connect.

Yoga

Hatha yoga, the yoga style most commonly practised in Canada, emphasizes physical balance and breath control. It integrates components of flexibility, muscular strength and endurance, and muscle relaxation; it also sometimes serves as a preliminary to meditation. A session of yoga typically involves a series of postures, each held for a few seconds to several minutes, which involve stretching and balance and coordinated breathing. Yoga can induce the relaxation response and promote body awareness and flexibility. If you are interested in trying yoga, it's best to take a class from an experienced instructor.

Tai Chi

This martial art (in Chinese, *taijiquan*) is a system of self-defence that incorporates philosophical concepts from Taoism and Confucianism. In addition to self-defence, tai chi aims to bring the body into balance and harmony to promote health and spiritual growth. It teaches practitioners to remain calm and centred, to conserve and concentrate energy, and to manipulate force by becoming part of it—by going with the flow. Tai chi is considered the gentlest of the martial arts. Instead of quick and powerful movements, tai chi consists of a series of slow, fluid, elegant movements, which reinforce the idea of moving *with* rather than *against* the stressors of everyday life. As with yoga, it's best to start tai chi with a class from an experienced instructor.

QUICK STATS

Physically active people are 25–30% less likely to feel distressed than inactive people.

—U.S. Dept. of Health and Human Service, Physical Activity Guidelines Advisory Committee, 2008

Listening to Music

Listening to music is another method of inducing relaxation. It can influence pulse, blood pressure, and the electrical activity of muscles. Studies of newborns and people hospitalized with a stroke have shown that listening to soothing, lyrical music can lessen depression, anxiety, and stress levels. Researchers have found that exposure to soothing music leads to reduced levels of the stress hormone cortisol and causes changes in the electrical activity in the brain.

To experience the stress-management benefits of music yourself, set aside a time to listen. Choose music that you enjoy and that makes you feel relaxed.

Biofeedback

Biofeedback helps people reduce the stress response by enabling them to become more aware of their level of physiological arousal. It involves electrical monitoring of some measure of the physiological stress response, such as perspiration, heart rate, skin temperature, or muscle tension. People receive feedback about their condition through the use of sound (a tone or music), light, or a meter or dial. For example, as heart rate increases, the tone becomes louder; as it decreases, the tone becomes softer. In this way, people can learn to reduce their physiological stress response through conscious control even without biofeedback.

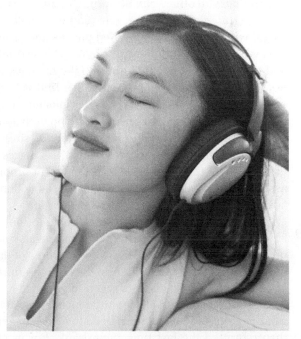

> **biofeedback**
> A technique in which monitoring devices help a person become conscious of unconscious body processes, such as body temperature or blood pressure, to exert some control over them.

Listening to soothing music leads to reduced levels of stress hormones and can induce the relaxation response.

The point of biofeedback training is to learn how relaxation feels, how to induce relaxation, and how to transfer this skill to daily life (without the use of electronic equipment). In addition to monitoring equipment, biofeedback usually also requires the initial help of a therapist, stress counsellor, or technician.

Other relaxation techniques include massage, hypnosis and self-hypnosis, and autogenic training. To learn more about these and other techniques for inducing the relaxation response, refer to the For More Information section at the end of the chapter.

Counterproductive Coping Strategies

University or college is a time when you will learn to adapt to new and challenging situations and gain skills that will last a lifetime. It is also a time when many people develop habits, in response to stress, that are counterproductive and unhealthy. Such habits can last well beyond graduation.

Tobacco Use

Many young adults who never smoked in high school smoke their first cigarette in university or college, usually at a party or a bar or in a dorm with friends. Many smokers report that smoking helps them to cope with stress by providing a feeling of relaxation, giving them something to do with their hands in social situations, or breaking up monotony and routine.

Cigarettes and other tobacco products contain nicotine, a chemical that enhances the actions of neurotransmitters. Nicotine can make you feel relaxed and even increase your ability to concentrate, but it is highly addictive, and nicotine dependence itself is considered a psychological disorder. Current research has found that smokers are actually more likely to experience frequent stress than non-smokers or ex-smokers. Cigarette smoke also contains substances that cause heart disease, stroke, lung cancer, and emphysema. These negative consequences far outweigh any beneficial effects, and tobacco use should be avoided. The easiest thing to do is to not start.

See Chapter 16 for more on the health effects of tobacco use and for tips on how to quit.

Use of Alcohol and Other Drugs

No post-secondary experience is complete without a party or two. Letting loose, dancing, laughing, and interacting with others can be very effective short-term coping strategies. However, partying is usually associated with drinking alcohol. Keg parties and drinking games can be fun, but they contribute to binge drinking and other forms of alcohol abuse. Like nicotine, alcohol is addictive, and many alcoholics find it hard to relax without a drink. Having a few drinks might make you feel temporarily at ease, and drinking until you are intoxicated may help you forget your current stressors. However, using alcohol to deal with stress places you at risk for all the short-term and long-term problems associated with alcohol abuse. It also does nothing to address the actual causes of stress in your life.

Although moderate alcohol consumption may have potential health benefits for some people, many university and college students have patterns of drinking that detract from wellness. Nearly one-third of Canadian university students recently reported having *at least* one indicator of alcohol dependence and the same percent (about one-third) said they did something they regretted the last time they drank. For more on the responsible use of alcohol, refer to Chapter 15.

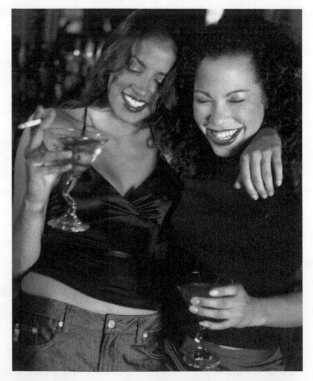

Tobacco and alcohol use may help you relax for a little while, but long-term use is unhealthy and an ineffective way to cope with stress.

Using other psychoactive drugs to cope with stress is also counterproductive:

- *Caffeine* raises cortisol levels and blood pressure and can make you feel more stressed; caffeine also disrupts sleep. Other stimulants, such as amphetamine, can activate the stress response, and they affect the same areas of the brain that are involved in regulating the stress response.
- *Marijuana* use is relatively common among post-secondary students, who report that they smoke marijuana in an effort to induce relaxation and for "mind expansion." Use of marijuana causes a brief period of euphoria and decreased short-term memory and attentional abilities. Physiological effects clearly show that marijuana use doesn't cause relaxation; in fact, some neurochemicals in marijuana act to enhance the stress response, and getting high on a regular basis can elicit panic attacks. To compound this, withdrawal from marijuana may also be associated with an increase in circulating stress hormones.
- *Opioids*, such as morphine and heroin, can mimic the effects of your body's natural painkillers and act to reduce anxiety. However, tolerance to opioids develops quickly, and many users become dependent.

For more information on the use of psychoactive drugs, see Chapter 14.

Unhealthy Eating Habits

The nutrients in the food you eat provide energy and the substances needed to maintain your body. Eating is also psychologically rewarding. The feelings of satiation and sedation that follow eating produce a relaxed state. However, regular use of eating as a means of coping with stress may lead to unhealthy eating habits. In fact, the recent *Report Card on Canadians' Health* revealed that about 75 percent of Canadians use television, alcohol, cigarettes, and comfort food as a means of coping with stress or anxiety. Comfort eaters are twice as likely as other people to be obese.

Certain foods and supplements are sometimes thought to fight stress. Carbohydrates may reduce the stress response by promoting activity of the parasympathetic nervous system; however, a high-carbohydrate diet can lead to excessive weight gain in sedentary people and is not recommended as a strategy for coping with stressors. In addition, some evidence suggests that greater ingestion of carbohydrates, simple sugars, and fatty foods may be a predisposing factor for psychological distress. Many dietary supplements are marketed for stress reduction, but supplements are not required to meet the same standards as medications in terms of safety, effectiveness, and manufacturing (see Chapters 5 and 19).

Creating a Personal Plan for Managing Stress

What are the most important sources of stress in your life? Are you coping successfully with these stressors? No single strategy or program for managing stress will work for everyone, but you can use the principles of behaviour management described in Chapter 1 to tailor a plan specifically to your needs. The most important starting point for a successful stress-management plan is to learn to listen to your body. When you learn to recognize the stress response and the emotions and thoughts that accompany it, you will be in a position to take charge of that crucial moment and handle it in a healthy way.

Identifying Stressors

Before you can learn to manage the stressors in your life, you have to identify them. Many experts recommend keeping a stress journal for a week or two (see Figure 3.5). Each time you feel or express a stress response, record the time and the circumstances in your journal. Note what you were doing at the time, what you were thinking or feeling, and the outcome of your response.

After keeping your journal for a few weeks, you should be able to identify your key stressors and spot patterns in how you respond to them. Take note of the people, places, events, and patterns of thought and behaviour that cause you the most stress. You may notice, for example, that mornings are usually the most stressful part of your day. Or you may discover that when you're angry at your roommate, you tend to respond with behaviours that only make matters worse. Keeping a journal allows you to be analytical about what produces the most stress in your life and fills in where your conscious memory fails you.

Designing Your Plan

Once you have identified the key stressors in your life, choose the stress reduction techniques that will work best for you and create an action plan for change. Finding a friend to work with you can make the process more fun and increase your chances of success. Some experts recommend drawing up a formal contract with yourself.

Whether or not you complete a contract, it's important to design rewards into your plan, such as treating yourself to a concert or a movie. It's also important to evaluate your plan regularly and redesign it as your needs change. Under times of increased stress, for example, you might want to focus on good eating, exercise, and relaxation habits. Over time, your new stress-management skills will become almost automatic. You will feel better, accomplish more, and reduce your risk of disease.

Getting Help

If the techniques discussed so far don't provide you with enough relief from the stress in your life, you might want to learn more about specific areas you want to work on. Excellent self-help guides can be found in bookstores or the library. Additional resources are listed in the For More Information section at the end of the chapter.

Your student health centre or student affairs office can tell you whether your campus has a peer counselling program. Such programs are usually staffed by volunteer students with special training that emphasizes maintaining confidentiality. Peer counsellors can guide you to other campus or community resources, or can simply provide understanding.

Support groups are typically organized around a particular issue or problem. In your area, you might find a support group for first-year students; for older students; for single parents; for students of your ethnicity, religion, or national origin; for people with eating disorders; or for rape survivors. The number of such groups has increased in recent years as more people discover how therapeutic it can be to talk with others who share the same situation.

Short-term psychotherapy can also be tremendously helpful in dealing with stress-related problems. Your student health centre may offer psychotherapy on a sliding-fee scale; the local mental health centre in your area may do the same. If you belong to any type of religious organization, check to see whether pastoral counselling is available. Your physician can refer you to psychotherapists in your community. Not all therapists are right for all people, so be prepared to have initial sessions with several. Choose the one you feel most comfortable with.

FIGURE 3.5

A Sample Stress Journal

Tracking stressful events and reactions can help you understand how you normally cope with stress.

Stress Journal		Date 9-18-15
Time	Stressor	Reaction/Coping Strategy
7:45 a.m.	Tara wouldn't get out of the shower	Yelled at her, started an argument
8:35 a.m.	Late for class	Slouched in back of room; chewed my nails
11:55 a.m.	Dad called to discuss credit card debt	Cried, skipped lunch, and went out to smoke with Greg
5:30 p.m.	Power outage at dorm, couldn't study	Took a walk with Tara, made up for arguing this morning, then went to library to study
7:45 p.m.	Ed called, asked to borrow money	Stayed calm, put down phone, and counted to 10, then explained that he already owes me $50
8:30 p.m.	Ed called, angry, said he wanted to break up	Argued on phone, then went out with Tara for a drink

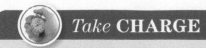 *Take* **CHARGE**

Dealing with Test Anxiety

Do you not perform as well as you should on tests? Do you find that anxiety interferes with your ability to study effectively before the test and to think clearly in the test situation? If so, you may be experiencing test anxiety. Two methods that have proven effective in helping people deal with test anxiety are systematic desensitization and success rehearsal.

Systematic Desensitization

Systematic desensitization is based on the premise that you can't feel anxiety and be relaxed at the same time.

- *Phase I – Constructing an anxiety hierarchy:* Begin the first phase by thinking of ten or more situations related to your fear, such as hearing the announcement of the test date in class, studying for the test, sitting in the classroom waiting for the test to begin, reading the test questions, and so on. Write each situation on an index card, using a brief phrase to describe it on one side of the card. On the other side, list several realistic details or prompts that will help you vividly imagine yourself actually experiencing the situation. For example, if the situation is "hearing that 50 percent of the final grade will be based on the two exams," the prompts might include specific details, such as "sitting in the big lecture auditorium in Baily Hall," "taking notes in my blue notebook," and "listening to Professor Lee's voice." Next, arrange your cards in order, from least-tense to most-tense situation. Rate each situation to reflect the amount of anxiety you feel when you encounter it in real life, to confirm your anxiety hierarchy. Assign ratings on a scale of 0–100, and make sure the distances between items are fairly small and about equal. When your anxiety hierarchy is a true reflection of your feelings, number the cards.
- *Phase II – Learning and practising muscle relaxation:* The second phase of the program involves learning to relax your muscles and to recognize when they are relaxed (see the description of progressive relaxation in this chapter). As you become proficient at this technique, you will be able to go to a deeply relaxed state within just a few minutes. When you can do this, go on to the next phase of the program.
- *Phase III – Implementing the desensitization program:* Use the quiet place where you practised your relaxation exercises. Sit comfortably and place your stack of numbered cards within reach. Take several minutes to relax completely, and then look at the first card, reading both the brief phrase and the descriptive prompts. Close your eyes and imagine yourself in that situation for about 10 seconds. Then put the card down and relax completely for about 30 seconds. Look at the card again, imagine the situation for 10 seconds, and relax again for 30 seconds.

    At this point, evaluate your level of anxiety about the situation on the card in terms of the rating scale you devised earlier. If your anxiety level is 10 or lower, relax for 2 minutes and go on to the second card. If it's higher than 10, repeat the routine with the same card until the anxiety decreases.

    If you have difficulty with a particular item, go back to the previous item and try it again. If you still can't visualize it without anxiety, try to construct three new items with smaller steps between them and insert them before the troublesome item. You should be able to move through one to four items per session.

    Sessions can be conducted from twice a day to twice a week and should last no longer than 20 minutes. It's helpful to graph your progress in a way that has meaning for you.

    After you have successfully completed your program, you should be desensitized to the real-life situations that previously caused anxiety. If you find that you do experience some anxiety in the real situations, take 30 seconds or a minute to relax completely, just as you did when you were practising.

Success Rehearsal

To practise this variation on systematic desensitization, take your hierarchy of anxiety-producing situations and vividly imagine yourself successfully dealing with each one. Create a detailed scenario for each situation, and use your imagination to experience genuine feelings of confidence. Recognize your negative thoughts ("I'll be so nervous I won't be able to think straight") and replace them with positive ones ("Anxiety will keep me alert so I can do a good job").

Proceed one step at a time, thinking as you go of strategies for success that you can later implement. These might include the following:

- Before the test, find out everything you can about it: its format, the material to be covered, the grading criteria. Ask the instructor for practice materials. Study in advance—don't just cram the night before. Avoid all-nighters.
- Devise a study plan. This might include forming a study group with one or more classmates or outlining what you will study, when, where, and for how long. Generate your own questions and answer them.
- In the actual test situation, sit away from possible distractions, listen carefully to instructions, and ask for clarification if you don't understand a direction.

- During the test, answer the easiest questions first. If you don't know an answer and there is no penalty for incorrect answers, guess. If you have difficulty answering several questions, review the ones you have already handled. Figure out approximately how much time you have to cover each remaining question.
- For math problems, try to estimate the answer before doing the precise calculations.
- For true-false questions, look for qualifiers, such as *always* and *never*. Such questions are likely to be false.
- For essay questions, look for key words in the question that indicate what the instructor is looking for in the answer. Develop a brief outline of your answer, sketching out what you will cover. Stick to your outline, and keep track of the time you're spending on your answer. Don't get caught with unanswered questions when time is up.
- Remain calm and focused throughout the test. Don't let negative thoughts rattle you. Avoid worrying about past performance, how others are doing, or the negative consequences of a poor test grade. If you start to become nervous, take some deep breaths and relax your muscles completely for a minute or so.

The best way to counter test anxiety is with successful test-taking experiences. The more times you succeed, the more your test anxiety will recede. If you find that these methods aren't sufficient to get your anxiety under control, you may want to seek professional help.

SUMMARY

- When confronted with a stressor, the body undergoes a set of physical changes known as the fight-or-flight reaction. The sympathetic nervous system and endocrine system act on many targets in the body to prepare it for action.
- Emotional and behavioural responses to stressors vary among individuals. Ineffective responses increase stress but can be moderated or changed.
- Factors that influence emotional and behavioural responses to stressors include personality, cultural background, gender, and past experiences.
- The general adaptation syndrome (GAS) has three stages: alarm, resistance, and exhaustion.
- A high allostatic load characterized by prolonged or repeated exposure to stress hormones can increase a person's risk of health problems.
- Psychoneuroimmunology (PNI) looks at how the physiological changes of the stress response affect the immune system and thereby increase the risk of illness.
- Health problems linked to stress include cardiovascular disease (CVD), colds and other infections, asthma and allergies, cancer, flare-ups of chronic diseases, psychological problems, digestive problems, headaches, insomnia, and injuries.
- A cluster of major life events that require adjustment and accommodation can lead to increased stress and an increased risk of health problems. Minor daily hassles increase stress if they are perceived negatively.
- Sources of stress associated with post-secondary education may be academic, interpersonal, time-related, or financial pressures.
- Job-related stress is common, particularly for employees who have little control over decisions relating to their jobs. If stress is severe or prolonged, burnout may occur.
- New and changing relationships, prejudice, and discrimination are examples of interpersonal and social stressors.
- Social support systems help buffer people against the effects of stress and make illness less likely. Good communication skills foster healthy relationships.
- Exercise, nutrition, sleep, and time management are wellness behaviours that reduce stress and increase energy.
- Cognitive techniques for managing stress involve developing new and healthy patterns of thinking, such as practising problem solving, monitoring self-talk, and cultivating a sense of humour.
- The relaxation response is the opposite of the fight-or-flight reaction. Techniques that trigger it, including progressive relaxation, imagery, meditation, and deep breathing, counteract the

effects of chronic stress. Counterproductive coping strategies include smoking, drinking, and unhealthy eating.

- A successful individualized plan for coping with stress begins with the use of a stress journal or log to identify and study stressors and inappropriate behavioural responses. Completing a contract and recruiting a friend can help your stress-management plan succeed.

- Additional help in dealing with stress is available from self-help books, peer counselling, support groups, and psychotherapy.

FOR MORE INFORMATION

BOOKS

Goelitz, J., and R. A. Rees. 2011. *The College De-Stress Handbook: Keeping Cool Under Pressure from the Inside Out.* Boulder Creek, CA: Institute of HeartMath. A brief guide to managing college stress, with tips on recognizing stressors, reducing their intensity, and learning new ways to respond.

Greenberg, J. 2010. *Comprehensive Stress Management.* 12th ed. New York: McGraw-Hill. A clear explanation of the physical, psychological, sociological, and spiritual aspects of stress, with numerous stress management techniques.

Kabat-Zinn, J. 2011. *Mindfulness for Beginners: Reclaiming the Present Moment—and Your Life.* Louisville, CO: Sounds True. A distillation of the ideas, attitudes, and practices that constitute the basics of mindfulness and mindful living.

Maté, G. 2004. *When the Body Says No: The Cost of Hidden Stress.* Toronto: Vintage Canada. An examination of the connections among emotion, stress, and disease.

Pennebaker, J. W. 2004. *Writing to Heal: A Guided Journal for Recovering from Trauma and Emotional Upheaval.* Oakland, Calif.: New Harbinger Press. Information about using journaling to cope with stress.

ORGANIZATIONS, HOTLINES, AND WEBSITES

The Internet addresses listed here were accurate at the time of publication.

American Psychological Association. Provides information on stress management and psychological disorders.
   http://www.apa.org/helpcenter/ and http://www.apa.org

Association for Applied Psychophysiology and Biofeedback. Provides information about biofeedback and referrals to certified biofeedback practitioners.
   http://www.aapb.org

Benson-Henry Institute for Mind Body Medicine. Provides information about stress-management and relaxation techniques.
   http://www.massgeneral.org/bhi/

Canadian Centre for Occupational Health and Safety. Provides information and links on job stress.
   http://www.ccohs.ca/oshanswers/psychosocial/stress.html

Canadian Mental Health Association. Provides information about mental health issues and offers related services and resources for Canadians.
   http://www.cmha.ca

Canadian Psychiatric Association. Advocates for the professional needs of its members and promotes excellence in education, research, and clinical practice.
   http://www.cpa-apc.org

Canadian Sleep Society. A professional association of clinicians, scientists, and technologists formed to further the advancement and understanding of sleep and its disorders through scientific study and public awareness.
   http://www.css-scs.ca/

National Network for Mental Health. Provides a national voice on decisions that affect people with mental illnesses.
   http://nnmh.ca/

Medical Basis for Stress. Includes information on recognizing stress and on the physiological basis of stress, self-assessments for stress levels, and techniques for managing stress.

> http://www.teachhealth.com

Public Health Agency of Canada: Mental Health Promotion Unit. Addresses mental health promotion from a population health perspective that takes into account the broad range of determinants of mental health.

> http://www.phac-aspc.gc.ca/mh-sm/mhp-psm/index-eng.php

Student Counseling Virtual Pamphlet Collection. Links to online pamphlets from student counselling centres; topics include stress, sleep, and time management.

> http://counseling.uchicago.edu/page/about-us

U.S. National Institute of Mental Health (NIMH). Publishes informative brochures about stress and stress management as well as other aspects of mental health.

> http://www.nimh.nih.gov

U.S. National Sleep Foundation. Provides information about sleep and how to deal with sleep problems, such as insomnia and jet lag.

> http://www.sleepfoundation.org

SELECTED BIBLIOGRAPHY

Adlaf, E. M., Demers, A., and Gliksman, L. (eds.). 2005. *Canadian Campus Survey 2004.* Toronto: Centre for Addiction and Mental Health.

American College Health Association. *American College Health Association-National College Health Assessment II: Canadian Reference Group Data Reporting Spring 2013.* Hanover, MD: American College Health Association, 2013

American Psychological Association. 2005. *The Different Kinds of Stress,* http://www.apa.org/helpcenter/stress-kinds.aspx (retrieved February 3, 2015).

American Psychological Association. 2005. *Learning to Deal with Stress,* http://www.apa.org/helpcenter/stress-learning.aspx (retrieved February 3, 2015).

Ano, G. G., and E. B. Vasconcelles. 2005. Religious coping and psychological adjustment to stress: A meta-analysis. *Journal of Clinical Psychology* 61(4): 461–480.

Canadian Institute for Health Information. 2008. *Improving the Health of Canadians: Mental Health, Delinquency and Criminal Activity.* Ottawa: Canadian Institute for Health Information.

Canadian Mental Health Association. 2004. Your Education – Your Future; A Guide to College and University for Students with Psychiatric Disabilities, http://www.cmha.ca/youreducation (retrieved February 3, 2015).

Centers for Disease Control. 2005. *Coping with a Traumatic Event: Information for the Public,* http://www.bt.cdc.gov/masscasualties/copingpub.asp (retrieved March 13, 2011).

Cohen, S., W. J. Doyle, and A. Baum. 2006. Socioeconomic status is associated with stress hormones. *Psychosomatic Medicine* 68(3): 414–420.

Constantine, M. G, S. Okazaki, and S. O. Utsey. 2004. Self-concealment, social self-efficacy, acculturative stress, and depression in African, Asian, and Latin American international college students. *American Journal of Orthopsychiatry* 74(3): 230–241.

Crompton, S. Statistics Canada. 2011. What's stressing the stressed? Main sources of stress among workers. *Canadian Social Trends.* Catalogue No. 11-008, http://www.statcan.gc.ca/pub/11-008-x/2011002/article/11562-eng.pdf (retrieved February 3, 2015).

Daley, M., et al. 2009. The economic burden of insomnia: Direct and indirect costs for individuals with insomnia syndrome, insomnia symptoms, and good sleepers. *Sleep* 32(1): 1–10.

Driver, H. Canadian Sleep Society. 2012. Insomnia Rounds – Sleepless Women: Insomnia from the Female Perspective, http://www.canadiansleepsociety.ca/images/150-006_Eng.pdf (retrieved February 2, 2014).

Gilmour, H., and K. Wilkins. 2001. Migraine. *Health Reports* 12(2): 23–40.

Grossman, P., et al. 2004. Mindfulness-based stress reduction and health benefits: A meta analysis. *Journal of Psychosomatic Research* 57(1): 35–43.

Harkins, D. and M. Ronayne. 2010. Challenging the Balancing Act: Women, postmodernism, and the demand to "Have it All". *American Journal of Psychological Research*, 6(10):103–133.

Harvard Health Publications Harvard Medical School. 2012. Why Stress Causes People to Overeat, http://www.health.harvard.edu/newsletters/Harvard_Mental_Health_Letter/2012/February/why-stress-causes-people-to-overeat (retrieved February 3, 2015).

Health Canada. 2008. *Mental Health: Coping with Stress,* http://www.hc-sc.gc.ca/hl-vs/alt_formats/pacrb-dgapcr/pdf/iyh-vsv/life-vie/stress-eng.pdf (retrieved February 3, 2015).

Heart and Stroke Foundation. 2013. Canadians Face a Decade of Sickness in Later Years, http://www.heartandstroke.com/site/c.ikIQLcMWJtE/b.8543059/k.5536/2013_Report_on_health__Canadians_face_decade_of_sickness_in_later_years.htm (retrieved February 3, 2015).

Higgins, C., L. Duxbury, and S. Lyons, S. 2008. *Report 5: Reducing Work-Life Conflict: What Works? What Doesn't?* http://www.hc-sc.gc.ca/ewh-semt/pubs/occup-travail/balancing-equilibre/index-eng.php (retrieved March 13, 2015).

Hurst, M. 2008. *Who Gets Any Sleep These Days? Sleep Patterns of Canadians,* http://www.statcan.gc.ca/pub/11-008-x/2008001/article/10553-eng.htm (retrieved February 3, 2015).

Institute of Medicine Committee on Sleep Medicine and Research. 2006. *Sleep Disorders and Sleep Deprivation: An Unmet Public Health Problem,* ed. H. R. Colton and B. M. Altevogt. Washington, D.C. National Academies Press.

Lauderdale, D. S., et al. 2006. Objectively measured sleep characteristics among early-middle-aged adults: The CARDIA study. *American Journal of Epidemiology* 164(1): 17–18.

MacGeorge, E. L., et al. 2004. Stress, social support, and health among college students after September 11, 2001. *Journal of College Student Development* 45(6): 655–670.

Mayo Foundation for Medical Education and Research. 2010. *Stress: Constant Stress Puts Your Health at Risk,* http://www.mayoclinic.com/health/stress/SR00001 (retrieved December 27, 2015).

Meier-Ewert, H. K., et al. 2004. Effect of sleep loss on C-reactive protein, an inflammatory marker of cardiovascular risk. *Journal of the American College of Cardiology* 43: 678–683.

Melamed, S., et al. 2004. Association of fear of terror with low-grade inflammation among apparently healthy employed adults. *Psychosomatic Medicine* 66(4): 484–491.

National Mental Health Association. 2006. *Coping with Disaster: Tips for College Students,* http://www.nmha.org/go/information/get-info/coping-with-disaster/coping-with-the-war-and-terrorism-tips-for-college-students (retrieved March 13, 2015).

Nordboe, D. J., et al. 2007. Immediate behavioural health response to the Virginia Tech shootings. *Disaster Medicine and Public Health Preparedness* 1(1 Suppl.): S31–S32.

Park, J. 2007. Work stress and job performance. *Perspectives on Labour and Income* 8(12): 5–17.

Parmet, S. Headaches. 2006. *Journal of the American Medical Association* 295(19): 2320.

Saewyc, E. M., et al. 2009. Gender differences in violence exposure among university students attending campus health clinics in the United States and Canada. *Journal of Adolescent Health* 45(6): 587–594.

Segerstrom, S. C., and G. E. Miller. 2004. Psychological stress and the human immune system: A meta-analytic study of 30 years of inquiry. *Psychological Bulletin* 130(4): 601–630.

Sher, L. 2005. Type D personality: the heart, stress, and cortisol. *QJM: An International Journal of Medicine* 98: 323–329.

Stambor, Z. 2006. Stressed out nation. *Monitor on Psychology* 37(4), http://www.apa.org/monitor/apr06/nation.html (retrieved December 27, 2015).

Statistics Canada. 2013. Perceived life stress, 2012, http://www.statcan.gc.ca/pub/82-625-x/2013001/article/11842-eng.htm (retrieved February 3, 2015).

Transport Canada. 2010. Headaches, http://www.tc.gc.ca/eng/civilaviation/publications/tp13312-2-neurology-headaches-2159.htm (retrieved February 3, 2015).

Wittstein, I. S., et al. 2005. Neurohumoral features of myocardial stunning due to sudden emotional stress. *New England Journal of Medicine* 352(6): 539–548.

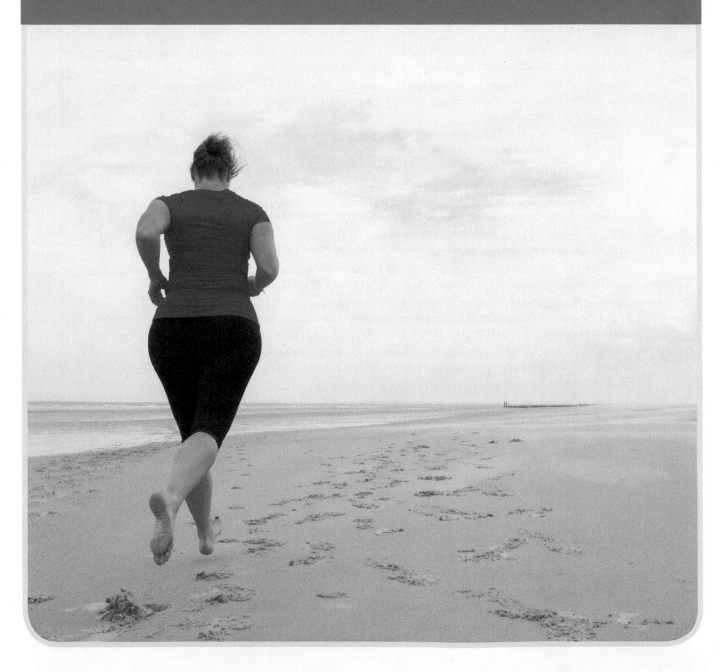

CHAPTER 4

Weight Management

LOOKING AHEAD

After you have read and studied this chapter, you should be able to:

LO1 Discuss different methods of assessing body weight and body composition

LO2 Explain the health risks associated with overweight and obesity

LO3 Explain factors that may contribute to a weight problem, including genetic, physiological, lifestyle, environmental, and psychosocial factors

LO4 Describe lifestyle factors that contribute to weight gain and loss, including the roles of diet, exercise, and emotional factors

LO5 Identify and describe the symptoms of eating disorders and the health risks associated with them

LO6 Design a personal plan for managing body weight successfully

TEST YOUR KNOWLEDGE

1. **About what percentage of Canadian adults have a healthy body weight?**
   a. 58% b. 48% c. 38%

2. **Genetic factors explain most cases of obesity.**
   True or false?

3. **The consumption of low-calorie sweeteners has helped Canadians control their weight.**
   True or false?

4. **Which eating disorder is considered most common across all age groups?**
   a. anorexia nervosa b. bulimia nervosa c. binge-eating disorder

5. **Which of the following is the most significant risk factor for type 2 diabetes (the most common type of diabetes)?**
   a. smoking b. overweight or obesity c. inactivity

ANSWERS

1. c.   Only 38 percent of Canadian adults have a healthy body weight according to their body mass index (BMI); 60 percent are either overweight or obese, and 2 percent are underweight.

2. FALSE.   Genetic factors may increase an individual's tendency to gain weight, but lifestyle is the key contributing factor.

3. FALSE.   Since the introduction of low-calorie sweeteners, both total calorie intake and total sugar intake have increased, as has the proportion of Canadians who are overweight.

4. c.   Binge-eating disorder is considered more common in all age groups; however, anorexia and bulimia nervosa often receive significant medical attention due to the high risk they pose to health.

5. b.   All are risk factors for type 2 diabetes, but overweight or obesity is the most significant. It is estimated that 80–90 percent of those with type 2 diabetes can be classified as overweight or obese; approximately 90 percent of cases could be prevented through the adoption of healthy lifestyle behaviours.

Achieving and maintaining a healthy body weight is a serious public health challenge and a source of distress for many Canadians. Under standards developed by Health Canada, about 54 percent of Canadian adults self-report that they are overweight, including 18 percent who identify themselves as obese (see Figure 4.1). In Canada, the number of adults with obesity tripled between 1985 and 2010. Experts say that by 2021, 70 percent of males and nearly 50 percent of females in Canada will be either overweight or obese. And while millions struggle to lose weight, others fall into dangerous eating patterns, such as binge eating or self-starvation.

Although not completely understood, management of body weight is not a mysterious process. In large part, it is a matter of balancing calories consumed with calories expended in daily activities—in other words, eating a moderate diet and exercising regularly. Unfortunately, this is not as exciting as the latest fad diet or "scientific breakthrough" that promises rapid weight loss without effort. Many people fail in their efforts to manage their weight because they focus on short-term weight loss rather than permanent changes in lifestyle. Successful weight management requires the long-term coordination of many aspects of a wellness lifestyle, including proper nutrition, adequate physical activity, and stress management.

This chapter explores the factors that contribute to the development of overweight/obesity and to eating disorders. It also takes a closer look at weight management through lifestyle behaviours and suggests specific strategies for reaching and maintaining a healthy weight.

QUICK STATS

Direct physical measurements have found that about 34% of adult Canadians are overweight and 26% are obese.

—*Canadian Health Measures Survey*, 2009–2011

FIGURE 4.1

Prevalence of Self-reported Obesity Among People 18 years and Older, by Age and Sex, 2013

The self-report nature of this information may mean that actual values are higher than reported here; research suggests that people tend to under-report rather than over-report their obesity-related attributes.

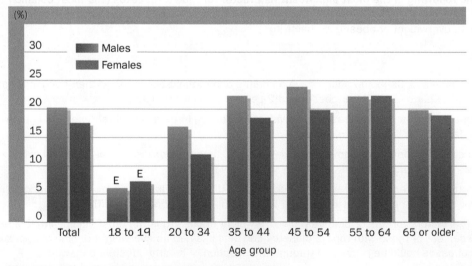

Note: E Use with caution (coefficient of variation 16.6% to 33.3%)

Source: Statistics Canada. (2014). *Overweight and Obese Adults (self-reported)*. Retrieved from http://www.statcan.gc.ca/pub/82-625-x/2014001/article/14021-eng.htm.

Basic Concepts of Weight Management

If you are like most people, you are concerned about your weight. But how do you decide if you are overweight? At what point does being overweight present a health risk? And how thin is too thin?

Body Composition

The human body can be divided into fat-free mass and body fat. Fat-free mass is composed of all the body's non-fat tissues: bone, water, muscle, connective tissue, organ tissues, and teeth. There are three types of body fat:

- **Subcutaneous fat** is the fat located just beneath the skin. Research has found subcutaneous fat to be protective for a variety of diseases. Subcutaneous fat accumulation represents the normal physiological buffer for excess energy intake. When its storage capacity is exceeded, fat starts to accumulate in other places of the body. About 80 percent of all body fat is in the subcutaneous area.
- **Visceral fat** is the fat embedded within the mesentery (which is tissue that connects the intestines to the back of the abdominal wall) surrounding the abdominal organs. Excess visceral fat has been linked to cardiovascular and a host of other diseases. Visceral fat accounts for 10–20 percent of total fat in men and 5–8 percent in women, and this amount increases with age for both sexes.
- **Ectopic fat** is the fat located on or within organs, such as the liver, heart, and brain. Ectopic fat increases the risk for metabolic syndrome (discussed more fully in Chapter 7), heart disease, and stroke.

subcutaneous fat
The fat just beneath the skin; critical for normal body functioning.

visceral fat
The fat inside the abdominal wall and around the internal organs; an excess leads to a greater risk of heart disease, insulin resistance, and metabolic syndrome.

ectopic fat
The fat located on or within organs, such as the liver, heart, and brain; increases the risk for metabolic syndrome, heart disease, and stroke.

One kilogram of body fat is equal to 7000 calories. This means that having only an extra 22 calories each day will cause a 1-kilogram weight gain over the course of a year. In 10 years, that is 10 kilograms gained. But what is most important for health is not total weight, but rather the proportion of the body's total weight that is fat—the **percent body fat**.

percent body fat
The percentage of total body weight that is composed of fat.

For example, two women may both be 1.7 metres tall and weigh 60 kilograms. But one woman, an endurance runner, may have only 15 percent of her body weight as fat, whereas the other woman, who is sedentary, may have 34 percent body fat. Although 60 kilograms is not considered overweight for women of this height, the sedentary woman may be overfat. (Methods for measuring and evaluating percent body fat are presented later in this chapter.) Most people use the word *overweight* to describe the condition of having too much body fat, although *overfat* is actually a more accurate term.

QUICK STATS

In Canada, the direct and indirect costs associated with overweight and obesity are estimated to reach $11 billion dollars annually.

—Quebec Government, INSPQ Public Health Expertise and Reference Centre, 2014

Energy Balance

The key to keeping a healthy ratio of fat-to-fat-free mass is maintaining an energy balance (see Figure 4.2). You take in energy (calories) from the food you eat. Your body uses energy (calories) to maintain vital body functions (resting metabolism), to digest food, and to fuel physical activity. When energy-in equals energy-out, you maintain your current weight. To change your weight and body composition, you must tip the energy balance equation in a particular direction. If you take in more calories daily than your body burns (a *positive* energy balance), the excess calories will be stored as fat and you will gain weight over time. If you eat fewer calories than you burn each day (a *negative* energy balance), you will lose some of the stored fat and probably lose weight.

If we look at the energy balance equation today as expressed for the general Canadian population, the equation is tipped heavily toward the energy-in side. Our environment is rich in large portion sizes, high-fat, high-calorie foods and palatable, easily available, and inexpensive foods. Unfortunately, the energy-out side of the equation has not compensated for increased energy intake; instead, we have decreased work-related physical activity, decreased activity associated with daily living, and increased time spent in sedentary pastimes, such as TV viewing and computer use.

The good news, however, is that you control both parts of the energy balance equation. Specific strategies for altering energy balance are discussed later in the chapter.

FIGURE 4.2

The Energy Balance Equation

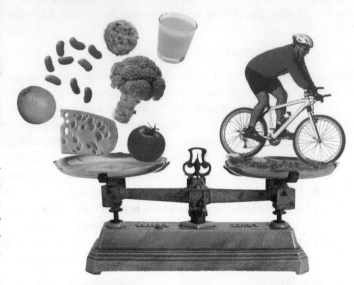

ENERGY IN
Food calories

ENERGY OUT
Physical activity 20–30%
Food digestion ±10%
Resting metabolism 65–70%

Evaluating Body Weight and Body Composition

Overweight is usually defined as total body weight above the recommended range for good health (as determined by large-scale population surveys). **Obesity** is defined as a more serious degree of overweight. Many methods are available for measuring and evaluating body weight and percent body fat; the cut-off points for defining overweight and obesity vary with the method chosen.

> **overweight**
> Body weight that falls above the recommended range for good health.
>
> **obesity**
> The condition of having an excess of non-essential body fat; having a body mass index (BMI) of 30 or greater or having a percent body fat greater than about 25 percent for men and 33 percent for women.

Height–Weight Charts

In the past, many people relied on height–weight charts to evaluate body weight. Based on insurance company statistics, these charts list a range of ideal or recommended body weights associated with the lowest mortality for people of a particular sex, age, and height. Although easy to use, height–weight charts can be highly inaccurate for some people, and they provide only an indirect measure of body fat.

Body Mass Index

Body mass index (BMI) is a measure that is useful for classifying the health risks of body weight if you don't have access to more sophisticated methods. Though more accurate than height–weight charts, BMI is also based on the concept that weight should be proportional to height. Easy to calculate and rate, BMI is a fairly accurate measure of the health risks of body weight for average people. Researchers frequently use BMI in conjunction with waist circumference in studies that examine the health risks associated with body weight.

> **body mass index (BMI)**
> A measure of relative body weight that takes height into account and is highly correlated with more direct measures of body fat; calculated by dividing total body weight (in kilograms) by the square of height (in metres).

However, because BMI does not distinguish between fat weight and fat-free weight, it can be very inaccurate for some groups, including short people (under 1.5 metres tall), muscular athletes, and older adults with little muscle mass because of inactivity or an underlying disease. If you fall into one of these groups, use one of the methods described in the next section for estimating percent body fat to assess whether your current weight and body composition are healthy. BMI is also not particularly useful for tracking changes in body composition—gains in muscle mass and losses of fat. Women are likely to have more body fat for a given BMI than men.

You can calculate your BMI by dividing your body weight (expressed in kilograms) by the square of your height (expressed in metres). You can look up your BMI by using the chart in Figure 4.3.

FIGURE 4.3

Body Mass Index (BMI)

To determine your BMI, find your height in the left column. Move across the appropriate row until you find the weight closest to your own. The number at the top of the column is the BMI at that height and weight.

Legend: Obese (>30)   Overweight (25–30)   Normal (18.5–25)   Underweight (<18.5)

Height in feet/inches and centimetres

lb	(kg)	4'8" 142 cm	4'9"	4'10" 147	4'11" 150	5'0" 152	5'1" 155	5'2" 157	5'3" 160	5'4" 163	5'5" 165	5'6" 168	5'7" 170	5'8" 173	5'9" 175	5'10" 178	5'11" 180	6'0" 183	6'1" 185	6'2" 188	6'3" 191	6'4" 193	6'5" 196
260	(117.9)	58	56	54	53	51	49	48	46	45	43	42	41	40	38	37	36	35	34	33	32	32	31
255	(115.7)	57	55	53	51	50	48	47	45	44	42	41	40	39	38	37	36	35	34	33	32	31	30
250	(113.4)	56	54	52	50	49	47	46	44	43	42	40	39	38	37	36	35	34	33	32	31	30	30
245	(111.1)	55	53	51	49	48	46	45	43	42	41	40	38	37	36	35	34	33	32	31	31	30	29
240	(108.9)	54	52	50	48	47	45	44	43	41	40	39	38	36	35	34	33	33	32	31	30	29	28
235	(106.6)	53	51	49	47	46	44	43	42	40	39	38	37	36	35	34	33	32	31	30	29	29	28
230	(104.3)	52	50	48	46	45	43	42	41	39	38	37	36	35	34	33	32	31	30	30	29	28	27
225	(102.1)	50	49	47	45	44	43	41	40	39	37	36	35	34	33	32	31	31	30	29	28	27	27
220	(99.8)	49	48	46	44	43	42	40	39	38	37	36	34	33	32	32	31	30	29	28	27	27	26
215	(97.5)	48	47	45	43	42	41	39	38	37	36	35	34	33	32	31	30	29	28	28	27	26	25
210	(95.3)	47	45	44	42	41	40	38	37	36	35	34	33	32	31	30	29	28	28	27	26	26	25
205	(93.0)	46	44	43	41	40	39	37	36	35	34	33	32	31	30	29	28	27	26	26	25	25	24
200	(90.7)	45	43	42	40	39	38	37	35	34	33	32	31	30	30	29	28	27	26	26	25	24	24
195	(88.5)	44	42	41	39	38	37	36	35	33	32	31	31	30	29	28	27	26	26	25	24	24	23
190	(86.2)	43	41	40	38	37	36	35	34	33	32	31	30	29	28	27	26	26	25	24	24	23	23
185	(83.9)	41	40	39	37	36	35	34	33	32	31	30	29	28	27	27	26	25	24	24	23	23	22
180	(81.6)	40	39	38	36	35	34	33	32	31	30	29	28	27	27	26	25	24	24	23	22	22	21
175	(79.4)	39	38	37	35	34	33	32	31	30	29	28	27	27	26	25	24	24	23	22	22	21	21
170	(77.1)	38	37	36	34	33	32	31	30	29	28	27	26	25	24	24	23	22	22	21	21	20	20
165	(74.8)	37	36	34	33	32	31	30	29	28	27	27	26	25	24	24	23	22	22	21	21	20	20
160	(72.6)	36	35	33	32	31	30	29	28	27	27	26	25	24	24	23	22	22	21	21	20	19	19
155	(70.3)	35	34	32	31	30	29	28	27	27	26	25	24	24	23	22	22	21	20	20	19	19	18
150	(68.0)	34	32	31	30	29	28	27	27	26	25	24	23	23	22	22	21	20	20	19	19	18	18
145	(65.8)	33	31	30	29	28	27	27	26	25	24	23	23	22	21	21	20	20	19	19	18	18	17
140	(63.5)	31	30	29	28	27	26	26	25	24	23	23	22	21	21	20	20	19	18	18	17	17	17
135	(61.2)	30	29	28	27	26	26	25	24	23	22	22	21	21	20	19	19	18	18	17	17	16	16
130	(59.0)	29	28	27	26	25	25	24	23	22	22	21	20	20	19	19	18	18	17	17	16	16	15
125	(56.7)	28	27	26	25	24	24	23	22	21	21	20	20	19	18	18	17	17	16	16	15	15	14
120	(54.4)	27	26	25	24	23	23	22	21	21	20	19	19	18	18	17	17	16	16	15	15	15	14
115	(52.2)	26	25	24	23	22	22	21	20	20	19	19	18	17	17	16	16	15	15	14	14	14	14
110	(49.9)	25	24	23	22	21	21	20	19	19	18	18	17	17	16	16	15	15	15	14	14	13	13
105	(47.6)	24	23	22	21	21	20	19	19	18	17	17	16	16	15	15	14	14	14	13	13	13	12
100	(45.4)	22	22	21	20	20	19	18	18	17	17	16	16	15	15	14	14	14	13	13	12	12	12
95	(43.1)	21	21	20	19	19	18	17	17	16	16	15	15	14	14	14	13	13	13	12	12	12	11
90	(40.8)	20	19	19	18	18	17	16	16	15	15	15	14	14	13	13	13	12	12	12	11	11	11
85	(38.6)	19	18	18	17	17	16	16	15	15	14	14	13	13	13	12	12	12	11	11	11	10	10
80	(36.3)	18	17	17	16	16	15	15	14	14	13	13	13	12	12	11	11	11	11	10	10	10	9

Note: BMI values rounded to the nearest whole number. BMI categories based on CDC (Centers for Disease Control and Prevention) criteria.

Source: © 2009 Vertex42 LLC. BMI chart created by Vertex42.com. Used with permission (http://www.vertex42.com/ExcelTemplates/bmi-chart.html; retrieved March 16, 2015).

Under standards issued by the World Health Organization (WHO), a BMI between 18.5 and 24.9 is considered average, a person with a BMI above 25 is overweight, 25–29.99 is considered pre-obese, 30–34.99 is considered obese class I, 35–39.99 is obese class II, and 40 or higher is obese class III. As obesity classes increase, the risk of associated health problems also increases. A person with a BMI below 18.5 is classified as underweight, although low BMI values may be healthy in some cases if they are not the result of smoking, an eating disorder, or an underlying disease. A BMI of 17.5 or lower is sometimes used as a diagnostic criterion for the eating disorder anorexia nervosa.

Body Composition Analysis

The most accurate and direct way to evaluate body composition is to determine percent body fat, but it is worth noting that the WHO has not established specific guidelines for body composition assessment. A variety of methods are available and range in terms of their complexity, reproducibility, cost, and the skills required by those taking the measurement. Not only is it important to be mindful of these factors when selecting the measure, the comfort of the individual being assessed should also be considered. Table 4.1 shows body composition ratings based on percent body fat. As with BMI, the percent body fat ratings indicate cut-off points for health risks associated with underweight and obesity.

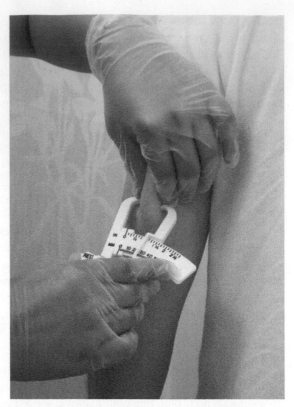

Calipers are used to perform skinfold measurements, which is a simple and inexpensive way to determine body fat levels. To ensure accuracy, skinfold measurements must be done by someone with appropriate training.

HYDROSTATIC (UNDERWATER) WEIGHING AND BOD POD One of the most accurate techniques for analyzing body composition is hydrostatic weighing. In this method, a person is submerged and weighed under water. Percent body fat can be calculated from body density. Muscle has a higher density and fat a lower density than water, so people with more fat tend to float and weigh less under water, while lean people tend to sink and weigh more under water.

A specialized body composition analysis device called the Bod Pod uses air instead of water. A person sits in a chamber and computerized pressure sensors determine the amount of air displaced by the person's body. This provides the needed information to calculate body composition density (i.e., lean and fat body mass).

SKINFOLD MEASUREMENTS The skinfold-thickness technique measures the thickness of fat under the skin. Measurements are taken at several sites and plugged into formulas that calculate body fat percentages.

CIRCUMFERENCE MEASURES Waist circumference and waist-to-hip ratio can be used to measure abdominal obesity and predict health risk. Waist circumference can be taken in between the top

TABLE 4.1

Body Fat Percentages for Males and Females and their Classification

Males	Females	Rating
5–10	8–15	Athletic
11–14	16–23	Good
15–20	24–30	Acceptable
21–24	31–36	Overweight
>24	>37	Obese

Keep in mind that these are only rough estimates. The term athletic in this context refers to sports where low body fat is an advantage.

Source: Jeukendrup, A., and M. Gleeson. (2010). *Sport nutrition: An introduction to energy production and performance (2nd ed.).* Windsor, ON: Human Kinetics (http://www.humankinetics.com/excerpts/excerpts/normal-ranges-of-body-weight-and-body-fat).

of the hip bone and the lowest rib, at the umbilicus (navel), or at the midsection's narrowest point. Waist-to-hip ratio involves measuring the waist and hip diameters, and then dividing the waist value by the hip value.

ELECTRICAL IMPEDANCE ANALYSIS In this method, electrodes are attached to the body and a harmless electrical current is transmitted from electrode to electrode. The electrical conduction through the body favours the path of the fat-free tissues over fat tissues. A computer can calculate fat percentages from measurements of current.

SCANNING PROCEDURES High-tech scanning procedures are highly accurate means of assessing body composition, but they require expensive equipment. These procedures include computed tomography (CT), magnetic resonance imaging (MRI), dual-energy X-ray absorptiometry (DEXA), and dual-photon absorptiometry. Other procedures include infrared reactance (Futrex 1100) and total body electrical conductivity (TOBEC).

Excess Body Fat and Wellness

The amount of fat in the body—and its location—can have profound effects on health.

The Health Risks of Excess Body Fat

Obesity significantly increases mortality rates and can reduce life expectancy by 10–20 years. In fact, if the current trends in overweight and obesity (and their related health problems) continue, scientists believe that the average North American's life expectancy will soon decline by five years. According to the Canadian House of Commons Health Committee, obesity is the reason that, for the first time in history, the current generation of children is at risk for shorter life expectancies than their parents.

People with obesity have a 50–100 percent increased risk of early death from all causes, compared with healthy weight people. Obesity is associated with unhealthy cholesterol and triglyceride levels, impaired heart function, and death from cardiovascular disease. Other health risks include hypertension, many kinds of cancer, impaired immune function, gallbladder and kidney diseases, skin problems, impotence, sleep and breathing disorders, back pain, arthritis, and other bone and joint disorders. Obesity is also associated with complications of pregnancy, menstrual irregularities, urine leakage (stress incontinence), increased surgical risk, and psychological disorders and problems (such as depression, low self-esteem, and body dissatisfaction).

A strong association exists between excess body fat and diabetes mellitus, a disease that causes a disruption of normal metabolism. The pancreas normally secretes the hormone insulin, which stimulates cells to take up blood sugar (glucose) to produce energy (see Figure 4.4). In diabetes, this process is disrupted, causing a buildup of glucose in the bloodstream. Diabetes is associated with kidney failure; nerve damage; circulation problems and amputations; retinal damage and blindness; and increased rates of heart attack, stroke, and hypertension. Excess body fat is a major risk factor for type 2 diabetes (the most common form of diabetes). Obese people are more than three times as likely to develop type 2 diabetes when compared to their healthy weight counterparts, and the incidence of type 2 diabetes among Canadians has increased dramatically as the rate of obesity has climbed. Diabetes is currently the sixth leading cause of death in the Canada. (See the In Focus box for more information.)

QUICK STATS

Approximately 347 million adults worldwide have diabetes.
—World Health Organization, 2013

The health risks from obesity increase with its severity, and they are much more likely to occur in people who are more than twice their desirable body weight. Controversy exists about the precise degree of risk at lower levels of overweight, particularly among overweight individuals who are physically active. The health risks associated with overweight depend in part on an individual's overall health and other risk factors, such as high blood pressure, unhealthy cholesterol levels, body fat distribution, and tobacco use. Weight loss is

FIGURE 4.4

Diabetes Mellitus

During digestion, carbohydrates are broken down in the small intestine into glucose, a simple sugar that enters the bloodstream. The presence of glucose signals the pancreas to release insulin, a hormone that helps cells take up glucose; once inside a cell, glucose can be converted to energy. In diabetes, this process is disrupted, resulting in a buildup of glucose in the bloodstream.

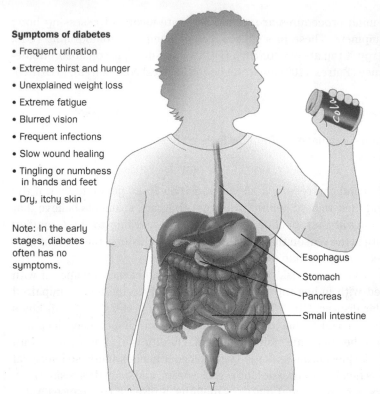

Symptoms of diabetes

- Frequent urination
- Extreme thirst and hunger
- Unexplained weight loss
- Extreme fatigue
- Blurred vision
- Frequent infections
- Slow wound healing
- Tingling or numbness in hands and feet
- Dry, itchy skin

Note: In the early stages, diabetes often has no symptoms.

Esophagus
Stomach
Pancreas
Small intestine

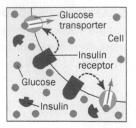

Normal
Insulin binds to receptors on the surface of a cell and signals special transporters in the cell to transport glucose inside.

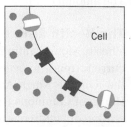

Type 1 diabetes
The pancreas produces little or no insulin. Thus, no signal is sent instructing the cell to transport glucose, and glucose builds up in the bloodstream.

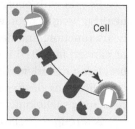

Type 2 diabetes
The pancreas produces too little insulin or the body's cells are resistant to it. Some insulin binds to receptors on the cell's surface, but the signal to transport glucose is blocked. Glucose builds up in the bloodstream.

recommended for people whose BMI places them in the obese category and for those who are overweight *and* have two or more major risk factors for disease. If your BMI is 25 or higher, consult a physician for help in determining a healthy BMI for you.

Many people who are overweight have some of the risk factors associated with obesity. The Nurses' Health Study, in which Harvard researchers have followed more than 120 000 women since 1976, has found that even mildly to moderately overweight women have an 80 percent increased risk of developing coronary heart disease compared with leaner women. This study also confirmed that to reduce the risk of dying prematurely of any cause, maintaining a desirable body weight is important. This conclusion was supported by a 10-year study that ended in 2006 after following 500 000 people in their fifties. Researchers concluded that subjects who were even slightly overweight were up to 40 percent more likely to die within the next decade, compared with age-matched people who had a desirable weight. But it is also important to realize that small weight losses—5–10 percent of total body weight—can lead to significant health improvements.

QUICK STATS

Among First Nations adults in Canada, nearly 34% can be classified as overweight, while 35% fall within the obese class I/II categories, and 5% fall in the obese class III category.

—*First Nations Regional Health Survey, 2012*

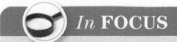 *In* FOCUS

Diabetes

Types of Diabetes

In 2013, 6 percent of female Canadians aged 12 and older, and 7.2 percent of male Canadians aged 12 and older (almost 2 million people or 1 in 17) had diabetes. The prevalence was lowest in British Columbia and Alberta, and highest in Newfoundland and Labrador, Nova Scotia, and New Brunswick.

More than 300 000 Canadians live with *type 1 diabetes*. In this type of diabetes, the pancreas produces little or no insulin so that daily doses of insulin are required. Type 1 diabetes occurs when the body's immune system, triggered by a viral infection or some other environmental factor, mistakenly destroys the insulin-producing cells in the pancreas. It usually strikes before age 30. The incidence rate of type 1 diabetes is rising by 3–5 percent yearly in Canada. While the onset can occur in children in young as one, the most common onset is between 10 and 14 years of age.

The remaining people have *type 2 diabetes*, and its prevalence is also rising dramatically. This condition can develop slowly, and about 33 percent of affected individuals are unaware of their condition. In type 2 diabetes, the pancreas doesn't produce enough insulin, or cells are resistant to insulin, or both. This condition is usually diagnosed in people over age 40, although a significant increase in type 2 diabetes in children has occurred in the past two decades. About one-third of people with type 2 diabetes must take insulin; others take medications that increase insulin production or stimulate cells to take up glucose.

A third type of diabetes occurs in some women during pregnancy. *Gestational diabetes* usually disappears after pregnancy, but approximately 30 percent of women who experience it eventually develop type 2 diabetes within 15 years. In Canada, the prevalence of gestational diabetes is higher than previously thought, with rates varying from 3.7 percent in non-Aboriginal women to 8–18 percent in Aboriginal women. The number of people with diabetes continues to grow; as of 2009, 2.4 million Canadians were diagnosed, a 230 percent increase from 1998 estimates. It is projected that this number will rise to 3.7 million by 2019.

Older Canadians are more likely to have diabetes. In 2013, 17.4 percent of people who were 65 years and older had been diagnosed with diabetes. This was almost 20 times the proportion seen in Canadian adults aged 20–34 (prevalence = .9 percent), and six times the proportion seen among 35–44 year olds (prevalence = 2.9 percent).

Overall, those with diabetes in every age group are at least twice as likely to die prematurely compared to those without the condition. Among 20–39-year-olds, individuals with diabetes die at a rate 4.2–5.8 times higher than the general population, while those who are 40–70 years old experience rates two to three times as high.

Research has shown that Aboriginal peoples and certain populations, such as Asians, Hispanics, and Africans, have a significantly higher risk of developing diabetes. Estimates of the prevalence of diabetes in Aboriginal peoples have been found to be as much as three to five times that seen among non-Aboriginal populations.

Prevention

It is estimated that as many as 90 percent of type 2 diabetes cases could be prevented if people adopted healthy lifestyle behaviours, including regular physical activity, a moderate diet, and modest weight loss. For people with pre-diabetes, lifestyle measures are more effective than medication for delaying or preventing the development of diabetes. Studies of people with pre-diabetes show that just a 5–7 percent weight loss can lower diabetes onset by up to 69 percent. Exercise (endurance and strength training) makes cells more sensitive to insulin and helps stabilize blood glucose levels; it also helps keep body fat at healthy levels.

A moderate diet to control body fat is perhaps the most important dietary recommendation for the prevention of diabetes. However, the composition of the diet may also be important. Studies have linked diets low in fibre and high in sugar, refined carbohydrates, saturated fat, red meat, and high-fat dairy products to increased risk of diabetes; diets rich in whole grains, fruits, vegetables, legumes, fish, and poultry may be protective. Specific foods linked to higher risk of diabetes include soft drinks, white bread, white rice, french fries, processed meats, and sugary desserts.

Treatment

Diabetes has no cure, but it can be successfully managed by keeping blood glucose levels within safe limits through diet, exercise, and, if necessary, medication. Blood glucose levels can be monitored by using a home test; close monitoring and control of glucose levels can significantly reduce the rate of serious complications. New drug therapies include inhibitors known as DDP-4, which lower blood glucose without causing weight gain.

About 85 percent of people with type 2 diabetes are struggling with overweight or obesity when diagnosed. An important step in treatment is weight loss; even a small amount lost can be beneficial. People with diabetes should get their carbohydrates from whole grains, fruits, vegetables, and low-fat dairy products; carbohydrate and monounsaturated fat together should provide 60–70 percent of total daily calories. Regular exercise and a healthy diet are often sufficient to control type 2 diabetes.

Warning Signs and Testing
Be alert for the warning signs of diabetes, which include frequent urination and infections, extreme hunger or thirst and fatigue, unexplained weight loss, blurred vision, cuts and bruises that are slow to heal, tingling or numbness in hands or feet, and generalized itching with no rash.

The best way to avoid complications is to recognize these symptoms and get early diagnosis and treatment. Type 2 diabetes is often asymptomatic in the early stages, so routine screening is recommended for people over age 45 and anyone younger who is at high risk. Screening involves a blood test to check glucose levels after either fasting or the administration of a set dose of glucose. A fasting glucose level of 7 mmol/L or higher indicates diabetes; a level of 6.1–6.9 mmol/L indicates pre-diabetes.

Sources: Statistics Canada. 2014. *Diabetes by sex, provinces, and territories 2013,* http://www.statcan.gc.ca/tables-tableaux/sum-som/l01/cst01/health54a-eng.htm (retrieved July 25, 2015); Juvenile Diabetes Research Foundation of Canada. 2014. *Fact Sheets,* http://www.jdrf.ca/news-and-media/fact-sheets/type-1-diabetes/ (retrieved July 25, 2015); Public Health Agency of Canada. 2011. *Diabetes in Canada: Facts and figures from a public health perspective,* http://www.phac-aspc.gc.ca/cd-mc/publications/diabetes-diabete/facts-figures-faits-chiffres-2011/pdf/facts-figures-faits-chiffres-eng.pdf (retrieved July 25, 2015); Government of Canada. 2013. *Type 2 diabetes,* http://www.healthycanadians.gc.ca/health-sante/disease-maladie/diabete-eng.php (retrieved July 25, 2015); and Canadian Diabetes Association. 2014. *Risk factors: Mothers at risk,* http://www.diabetes.ca/about-diabetes/risk-factors/mothers-at-risk (retrieved July 25, 2015).

Body Fat Distribution and Health

The distribution of body fat (that is, the locations of fat on the body) is also an important indicator of health. Men and postmenopausal women tend to store fat in the upper regions of their bodies, particularly in the abdominal area (the apple shape). Premenopausal women usually store fat in hips, buttocks, and thighs (the pear shape). Excess fat in the abdominal area increases the risk of high blood pressure, type 2 diabetes, early-onset heart disease, stroke, certain types of cancer, and mortality. This risk is independent of a person's BMI. The reason for this increase in risk is not entirely clear, but it appears that abdominal fat is more easily mobilized and sent into the bloodstream, increasing disease-related blood fat levels.

The risks from body fat distribution are usually assessed by measuring waist circumference (the distance around the abdomen at the level of the hip bone, known as the iliac crest). Waist circumference can be used as a measure of abdominal obesity, as an indicator of disease risk, and to monitor changes in body composition over time. More research is needed to determine the precise degree of risk associated with specific values of waist measurement. However, a total waist measurement of more than 102 centimetres for men and 88 centimetres for women is associated with a significantly increased risk of disease.

A person doesn't have to be technically overfat to have fat distribution be a risk factor, nor do all overfat people face this increased risk. The Health Canada guidelines state that large waist circumference can be a marker for increased risk of type 2 diabetes, high blood pressure, and cardiovascular disease even in people with a BMI in the normal range. Health Canada recommends measuring waist circumference among people with BMIs between 18.5 and 34.9; for BMIs equal to or great than 35, waist circumference does not seem to provide additional information on health risks. That being said, at any given level of overweight, people with a large waist circumference or additional disease risk factors are considered at greater risk for health problems. For example, a man with a BMI of 27, a waist circumference of more than 102 centimetres, and type 2 diabetes is at greater risk for health problems than another man who has a BMI of 27 but has a smaller waist and no other risk factors. Abdominal obesity and any two other risk factors associated with cardiovascular health put an individual at risk for metabolic syndrome. Abdominal obesity (as measured by waist circumference) is a primary component of metabolic syndrome and a forewarning of type 2 diabetes and heart disease.

Body Image

The collective picture of the body as seen through the mind's eye, body image consists of perceptions, images, thoughts, attitudes, and emotions. A negative **body image** is characterized by dissatisfaction with the body in general or some part of the body in particular. Recent surveys indicate that the majority of North Americans, many of whom are not actually overweight, are unhappy with their body weight or with some aspect of their appearance.

> **body image**
> The mental representation a person holds about his or her body at any given moment in time, consisting of perceptions, images, thoughts, attitudes, and emotions about the body.

Losing weight or getting cosmetic surgery does not necessarily improve body image. However, improvements in body image may occur in the absence of changes in weight or appearance. Many experts now believe that body image issues must be dealt with as part of treating obesity and eating disorders. See the Eating Disorders section later in the chapter for more information on body image and eating disorders.

Problems Associated with Very Low Levels of Body Fat

Health experts have generally viewed very low levels of body fat—less than 8–12 percent for women and 3–5 percent for men—as a threat to wellness. Extreme leanness has been linked with reproductive, circulatory, and immune system disorders. Extremely lean people may experience muscle wasting and fatigue; they are also more likely to have dangerous eating disorders.

In physically active women and girls, particularly those involved in sports where weight and appearance are important (ballet, gymnastics, skating, and distance running, for example), a condition called the **female athlete triad** may develop. The triad consists of three interrelated disorders: abnormal eating patterns (see the Eating Disorders section later in this chapter) and excessive exercising, followed by **amenorrhea** (absence of menstruation), followed by decreased bone density (premature osteoporosis). Prolonged amenorrhea can cause bone density to erode to a point that a woman in her twenties will have the bone density of a woman in her sixties. Left untreated, the triad can lead to decreased physical performance, increased incidence of bone fractures, disturbances of heart rhythm and metabolism, and even death.

> **female athlete triad**
> A condition consisting of three interrelated disorders: abnormal eating patterns and excessive exercising, followed by lack of menstrual periods (amenorrhea) and decreased bone density (premature osteoporosis).
>
> **amenorrhea**
> The absence of menstruation.

What Is the Right Weight for You?

BMI, percent body fat, and waist circumference measurement can best serve as general guides or estimates for body weight (see Table 4.2).

To answer the question of what you should weigh, let your lifestyle be your guide. Don't focus on a particular weight as your goal. Instead, focus on living a lifestyle that includes eating moderate amounts of healthful foods, getting plenty of exercise and adequate sleep, thinking positively, and learning to cope with stress. Then let the kilograms fall where they may. For most people, the result will be close to the recommended weight ranges discussed earlier. For some, their weight will be somewhat higher than societal standards—but right for them. By letting a healthy lifestyle determine your weight, you can avoid developing unhealthy patterns of eating and a negative body image.

TABLE 4.2

Body Mass Index (BMI) and Waist Circumference Classification and Disease Risk

Classification	BMI (kg/m²)	Obesity Class	Disease Risk Relative to Normal Weight and Waist Circumference[a]	
			Men ≤ 102 cm Women ≤ 88 cm	Men > 102 cm Women > 88 cm
Underweight[b]	< 18.5		—	—
Normal[c]	18.5–24.9		—	—
Overweight	25.0–29.9		Increased	High
Obesity	30.0–34.9	I	High	Very high
	35.0–39.9	II	Very high	Very high
Extreme obesity	40.0+	III	Extremely high	Extremely high

Sources: Adapted from National Heart, Lung, and Blood Institute. 1998. *Clinical Guidelines on the Identification, Evaluation, and Treatment of Overweight and Obesity in Adults: The Evidence Report.* Bethesda, Md.: National Institutes of Health; *Canadian Guidelines for Body Weight Classification in Adults,* http://www.hc-sc.gc.ca/fn-an/ nutrition/weights-poids/guide-ld-adult/index-eng.php. Health Canada. Reproduced with the permission of the Minister of Public Works and Government Services Canada, 2011.

[a] Disease risk for type 2 diabetes, hypertension, and cardiovascular disease. The waist circumference cut-offs for increased risk are 102 centimetres for men and 88 centimetres for women.

[b] Research suggests that a low BMI can be healthy in some cases, as long as it is not the result of smoking, an eating disorder, or an underlying disease process. A BMI of 17.5 or lower is sometimes used as a diagnostic criterion for the eating disorder anorexia nervosa.

[c] Increased waist circumference can also be a marker for increased risk, even in people of normal weight.

Factors Contributing to Excess Body Fat

Body weight and body composition are determined by multiple factors that vary with each individual. These factors can be grouped into genetic, physiological, lifestyle, and psychosocial factors.

Genetic Factors

Nutrigenomics is the study of how nutrients and genes interact and how genetic variations can cause people to respond differently to nutrients in food. Estimates of the genetic contribution to obesity vary widely, ranging from 40 percent to 70 percent heritability in children and adults for measures such as body mass index and regional fat distribution. Scientists have so far identified more than 600 genes associated with obesity. Genes influence body size and shape, body fat distribution, and metabolic rate. Genetic factors also affect the ease in which weight is gained as a result of overeating and where extra body weight is added. Researchers have suggested a link between a mother's level of obesity and her baby's body-weight-regulating mechanisms while in the womb.

QUESTIONS FOR CRITICAL THINKING AND REFLECTION

What is important to you about having a healthy body weight? How does your use of food, drink, and physical activity reflect your level of respect for yourself? What does it mean to you to be kind to your body?

If both parents are obese, their children have an 80 percent risk of being obese; children with only one obese parent face a 40 percent risk of becoming obese. In studies that compared adoptees and their biological parents, the weights of the adoptees were found to be more like those of the biological parents than the adoptive parents, again indicating a strong genetic link.

However, hereditary influences must be balanced against the contribution of environmental factors. Not all children of obese parents become obese, and non-obese parents may have obese children. Environmental factors, such as diet and exercise, are probably responsible for such differences. Thus, the *tendency* to develop obesity may be inherited, but the expression of this tendency is affected by environmental influences.

The message you should take from this research is that genes are not destiny. It is true that some people have a harder time losing weight and maintaining weight loss than others. However, with increased exercise and attention to diet, even those with a genetic tendency toward obesity can maintain a healthy body weight. And regardless of genetic factors, lifestyle choices remain the cornerstone of successful weight management.

Physiological Factors

Metabolism is a key physiological factor in the regulation of body fat and body weight; hormones and fat cell types also play a role.

Metabolism

Metabolism is the sum of all the vital processes by which food energy and nutrients are made available to and used by the body. The largest component of metabolism, **resting metabolic rate (RMR)**, is the energy required to maintain vital body functions, including respiration, heart rate, body temperature, and blood pressure, while the body is at rest. As was shown in Figure 4.2, RMR accounts for about 65–70 percent of daily energy expenditure. The energy required to digest food accounts for an additional ±10 percent of daily energy expenditure. The remaining 20–30 percent is expended during physical activity.

> **resting metabolic rate (RMR)**
> The energy required to maintain vital body functions, including respiration, heart rate, body temperature, and blood pressure, while the body is at rest.

Both heredity and behaviour affect metabolic rate. Men, who have a higher proportion of muscle mass than women, have a higher RMR because muscle tissue is more metabolically active than fat. Also, some individuals inherit a higher or lower RMR than others. A higher RMR means that a person burns more calories while at rest and can therefore take in more calories without gaining weight.

Weight loss or gain also affects metabolic rate. When a person loses weight, both RMR and the energy required to perform physical tasks decrease. The reverse occurs when weight is gained. One of the reasons exercise is so important during a weight-loss program is that exercise, especially resistance training, helps maintain muscle mass and metabolic rate.

Exercise has a positive effect on metabolism. When people exercise, they slightly increase their RMR— the number of calories their bodies burn at rest. They also increase their muscle mass, which is associated with a higher metabolic rate. The exercise itself also burns calories, raising total energy expenditure. The higher the energy expenditure, the more the person can eat without gaining weight. (The role of exercise in weight management is discussed in greater detail later in the chapter.)

Hormones

Hormones clearly play a role in the accumulation of body fat, especially for females. Hormonal changes at puberty, during pregnancy, and at menopause contribute to the amount and location of fat accumulation. For example, during puberty, hormones cause the development of secondary sex characteristics, including larger breasts, wider hips, and a fatty layer under the skin.

One hormone thought to be linked to obesity is leptin. Secreted by the body's fat cells, leptin is carried to the brain, where it appears to let the brain know how big or small the body's fat stores are. With this information, the brain can regulate appetite and metabolic rate accordingly. Several other hormones may be involved in the regulation of appetite. Researchers hope to use these hormones to develop treatments for obesity based on appetite control; however, as most of us will admit, hunger is often not the primary reason we overeat. Cases of obesity based solely or primarily on hormone abnormalities do exist, but they are rare. Lifestyle choices still account for the largest proportion of the differences in body weight and body composition among individuals.

Fat Cells

The amount of fat (adipose tissue) the body can store is a function of the number and size of fat (adipose) cells. These fat cells are like little compartments that can inflate to hold body fat; when existing fat cells are filled, the body makes more, thereby increasing its ability to store fat.

Some people are born with an above-average number of fat cells and thus have the potential for storing more energy as body fat. Overeating at critical times, such as in childhood and adolescence, can cause the body to create more fat cells. If a person loses weight, fat cell content is depleted, but it is unclear whether the number of fat cells can be decreased.

Further, it appears that all fat cells are not created equal. As mentioned earlier, visceral adipose tissue is located at waist level, inside the abdominal wall and surrounding the organs. This type of fat contains many biologically active substances, such as inflammatory chemicals and growth factors, which can adhere to the lining of blood vessels, cause insulin resistance, and have a negative influence on cardiovascular health. The more visceral fat and ectopic fat you have, the greater your chances of developing insulin resistance, metabolic syndrome, type 2 diabetes, and heart disease. Researchers consider visceral fat to be an active endocrine organ (like the pancreas), responsible for many of the pathological conditions of obesity. Visceral fat may also be the reason waist circumference is such a critical indicator of obesity risk.

In contrast, subcutaneous fat carries little or no health risk. Subcutaneous fat lies just under your skin, outside the abdominal wall. This fat tends to be soft and flabby (whereas visceral fat is hard) and is not metabolically active like visceral fat.

Found more often in women than men, subcutaneous fat appears on the lower body—the hips, upper thighs, and buttocks—a trait called *gynoid obesity* (see Figure 4.5). As a result of their body shape, people with excess subcutaneous fat are described as "pears." People with excess visceral and ectopic fat tend to carry it on their upper body (*android obesity*) and are called "apples." In terms of health risk, apples are bad and pears are good.

Location of Fat Cells

Overweight men tend to have an apple (android) shape; overweight women tend to have a pear (gynoid) shape.

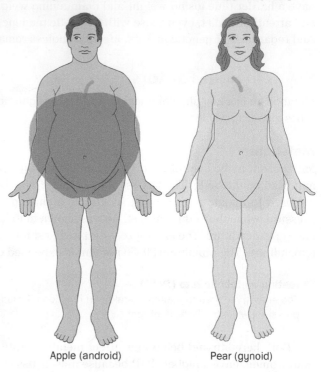

Apple (android)   Pear (gynoid)

Lifestyle Factors

Although genetic and physiological factors may increase the risk for excess body fat, they are not sufficient to explain the increasingly high rate of obesity seen in Canada (see Figure 4.6). The gene pool has not changed in the past 40 years, but the rate of obesity among Canadians has increased dramatically (see Table 4.2 and the Dimensions of Diversity box). Clearly, other factors are at work—particularly lifestyle factors, such as increased eating and decreased physical activity.

QUICK STATS

Obesity among children and youth increased from 2% in 1981 to 9% in 2011. This means that the prevalence of childhood obesity has tripled in one generation.

—*Canadian Health Measures Survey*, 2009–2011; Janssen, 2013

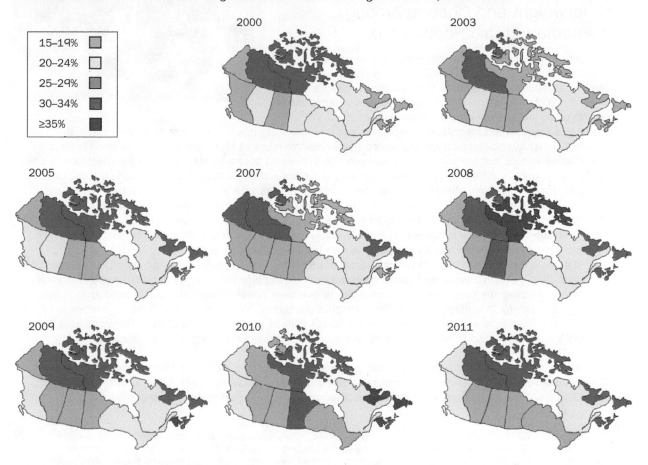

FIGURE 4.6

Estimated Prevalence of Obesity in Canadian Adults by Province, 2000–2011

15–19%	☐
20–24%	☐
25–29%	☐
30–34%	☐
≥35%	■

2000   2003

2005   2007   2008

2009   2010   2011

Source: Gotay, C. C., et al. 2013. "Updating the Canadian Obesity Maps: An Epidemic in Progress", Figure I. *Canadian Journal of Public Health* 104(1): e64-68; retrieved August 8, 2015.

QUICK STATS

According to their measured body mass index (BMI), the proportion of Canadian children and youth who were classified as overweight or obese in 2009–2011 was 32%.

—*Canadian Health Measures Survey*, 2009–2011

Eating

Canadians have access to plenty of calorie-dense foods, and many have eating habits that contribute to weight gain. Most overweight adults admit to eating more than they should of high-fat, high-sugar, high-calorie foods. Canadians eat out more frequently now than in the past, and we rely more heavily on fast food and packaged convenience foods. Restaurant and convenience food portion sizes tend to be large, and the foods themselves are likely to be high in fat, sugar, and calories, and low in essential nutrients.

Canadians' average calorie intake has been climbing since 1995. Studies have consistently found that people underestimate calories consumed by an average of 30 percent. Many of our extra calories come from carbohydrates, such as refined sugars. The popularity of sugar-free soft drinks does not appear to be helping

Dimensions *of* DIVERSITY

Overweight and Obesity Among Canadian Ethnic Populations

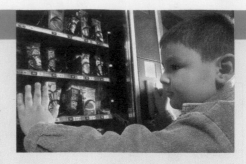

Culture, gender, income, and environment are among the determinants of obesity. The impact of culture is particularly interesting. Among all population groups in Canada, the prevalence of overweight and obesity is growing. However, rates and trends vary by ethnic group and other population characteristics.

- Certain groups, including Aboriginal peoples and Canadians of Chinese and South Asian descent, may have higher-than-average rates of obesity-related chronic disease (such as heart disease and high blood pressure).
- Cultural factors that influence dietary and exercise behaviours appear to play a role in the development of obesity. Cultural differences also exist regarding acceptance of larger body size and in body image perception. For example, one study found that black North Americans were more likely to think they were thinner than they really were and whites were more likely to think they were fatter than they really were.
- Rates of overweight and obesity tend to be higher among Canadian men than women; however, women experience larger socioeconomic disparities. For example, women with less education are approximately 1.6 times more likely to experience obesity compared to their more educated counterparts.
- In general, low socioeconomic status is associated with higher rates of overweight and obesity. Researchers theorize that people living in poor communities are more greatly affected by a toxic food and exercise environment—meaning they have fewer opportunities to purchase healthy foods and safely engage in regular physical activity. In addition, many foods low in price are high in calorie density (fast food, for example).
- Although overweight and obesity are a problem across Canada, provincial and territorial differences exist with the lowest rates found in British Columbia, and the highest rates found in both rural areas and in the Atlantic provinces.
- For Asian Canadians or people of Asian descent, waist circumference is a better indicator of relative disease risk than is BMI. According to the WHO, observed disease risk goes up at a lower level of BMI (22–25 kg/m^2) than it does for individuals of other groups, while high disease risk ranges from 26 kg/m^2 to 31 kg/m^2.

Sources: *World Health Organization BMI Classification,* http://apps.who.int/bmi/index.jsp?introPage= intro_3.html& (retrieved August 6, 2015); Targeting interventions for ethnic minority and low-income populations. *The Future of Children* 16(1): 187–207; Whitaker, R. C., and S. M. Orzol. 2006. Obesity among US urban preschool children: Relationships to race, ethnicity, and socioeconomic status. *Archives of Pediatric and Adolescent Medicine* 160(6): 578–584; Goel, M. S., et al. 2004. Obesity among U.S. immigrant subgroups by duration of residence. *Journal of the American Medical Association* 292(23): 2860–2867; and Heart and Stroke Foundation of Canada. 2008. *Overweight, Obesity and Heart Disease and Stroke,* http://www.heartandstroke.com/site/c.iklQLcMWJtE/b.3799193/k.C2EF/ Overweight_obesity_and_heart_disease_and_stroke.htm (retrieved March 17, 2015).

people lose weight (see the In the News box). Levels of physical activity have also been declining. The result has been a substantial increase in the number of overweight and obese Canadians. Eating for weight management is discussed later in this chapter.

Physical Activity

Research has shown that activity levels among Canadians are declining, beginning in childhood and continuing throughout life (see Chapter 6). Many schools have cut back on physical education classes and recess. Recent data show that only 7 percent of Canadian children and youth are meeting the national guidelines of 60 minutes of moderate to vigorous physical activity each day. Most adults drive to work, sit all day, and then relax in front of the TV at night. One study found that 60 percent of the incidence of overweight can be linked to excessive television viewing. Modern conveniences, such as remote controls, elevators, and power mowers, have also reduced daily physical activity. On average, Canadian adults spend 580 minutes (9.7 hours) each day in sedentary pursuits.

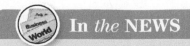

In *the* NEWS

Are Diet Soft Drinks Bad for You?

Soft drink consumption has grown significantly in Canada among children, adolescents, and adults in the past 30 years. Regular soft drinks, in fact, are now among the leading source of calories in the Canadian diet.

A can of regular pop contains about 150 calories. High consumption of sugary pop has previously been linked with obesity and type 2 diabetes in children and adolescents and with high blood pressure in adults. Further, some studies have shown that the added sweeteners in soft drinks are linked to increased triglycerides in the blood, leading to a greater risk of heart disease.

Why does drinking more pop lead to obesity and insulin resistance? Researchers have attributed this effect to the following factors:

- the consumption of more calories in general
- the high-fructose corn syrup content in soft drinks
- lower feelings of satiety (satisfaction)
- the general effect of eating a diet that is high in refined carbohydrates, including sugar

Many weight-conscious people have changed to diet pop in the hope that this is a sugar-free, calorie-free alternative to regular pop. But is it? Recent research indicates that drinking more than one soft drink a day, even if it is diet pop, may be associated with an increased incidence of metabolic syndrome. As described elsewhere in this text, metabolic syndrome is a cluster of risk factors linked to the development of type 2 diabetes, heart disease, and stroke. The syndrome includes high blood pressure, elevated triglyceride levels, low levels of HDL ("good" cholesterol), high fasting blood glucose levels, and excessive waist circumference.

The news about diet pop came from the Framingham Heart Study, which examined more than 6000 middle-aged people who were initially free of metabolic syndrome. The link between diet soft drink consumption and metabolic syndrome was clear even when the researchers accounted for other factors, such as saturated fat and fibre in the diet, total calories, physical activity, and smoking.

Compared with people who did not drink pop frequently, researchers found that people who consumed more than one soft drink per day—regular or diet—were:

- 44 percent as likely to develop metabolic syndrome
- 37 percent as likely to be obese
- 22 percent as likely to have hypertension

What is the possible explanation for the association? Some research has suggested that the artificial sweeteners in diet drinks make a person more prone to eating sweet, higher-calorie foods. Another theory is that the caramel content in both regular and diet pops may play a role in insulin resistance.

Conversely, some contradictory studies show the benefit of diet pop consumption in overweight individuals and suggest that other factors could explain the development of risk factors for heart disease. Regardless, everyone agrees that more research should be done before a final verdict on diet pop consumption is reached.

Meanwhile, nutritionists say that this is a wake-up call for some diet soft drink drinkers, suggesting that a zero-calorie beverage cannot undo the damage of an otherwise unhealthy diet.

An "Obesogenic" Environment

An increasing amount of research is focusing on the "obesogenic" environment where most North Americans live. This environment promotes overconsumption of calories while at the same time discouraging physical activity. Food and activity choices are influenced by socioeconomic status, religion, culture, and geographic location. People living in areas with limited access to supermarkets, an abundance of fast-food outlets, and few opportunities for physical activity do not have the same options for choosing a healthy lifestyle as do people living in more enriched environments.

While lifestyle choices remain the primary focus of weight management, an area of study that has seen recent growth involves endocrine disrupting chemicals (EDCs) and their relationship to weight gain. Diethylstilbestrol (DES), bisphenol A (BPA), phthalates, and organotins are examples of EDCs, or "obesogens," which can be found in a variety of man-made products including cosmetics, plastics, lubricants, shampoos, pesticides, and paints. EDCs are thought to disrupt the body's control over fat production and energy balance, and may increase one's susceptibility to diseases such as obesity and diabetes later in life.

THINKING ABOUT THE ENVIRONMENT

Environmental factors are determinants of obesity and can make weight management even more difficult for many people. In this case, it is the human-made environment (sometimes referred to as the "built environment"), and not the natural one, that creates obstacles to a healthy lifestyle. For example:

- A noisy environment can make it difficult to sleep, and poor sleep quality has been associated with weight gain, difficulty in losing weight, and other conditions, such as depression and high blood pressure.
- In some urban and high-poverty areas, it is not always easy to make ideal food choices because fresh, healthy foods may be more expensive or harder to obtain than cheaper, less healthy fast food or junk food.
- People who live in unsafe environments, such as some inner-city areas, may not get as much physical activity as they need, simply because there are not enough safe places to walk or exercise.

As you create your own weight-management program, remember to account for environmental factors that may interfere with your efforts. You may need creative solutions to keep your program on track.

For more information on health and the environment, see Chapter 21.

Psychosocial Factors

Many people have learned to use food as a means of coping with stress and negative emotions. Eating can provide a powerful distraction from difficult feelings: loneliness, anger, boredom, anxiety, shame, sadness, and inadequacy. It can be used to combat low moods, low energy levels, and low self-esteem (see the Assess Yourself box). When food and eating become the primary means of regulating emotions, binge eating or other disturbed eating patterns can develop.

Obesity is strongly associated with socioeconomic status. In general, the prevalence of obesity goes down as income level goes up. More women than men are obese at lower income levels, but men are somewhat more obese at higher levels. These differences may reflect the greater sensitivity and concern for a slim physical appearance among upper-income women, as well as greater access to information about nutrition, to low-fat and low-calorie foods, and to opportunities for physical activity. It may also reflect the greater acceptance of obesity among certain ethnic groups, as well as different cultural values related to food choices.

In some families and cultures, food is used as a symbol of love and caring. It is an integral part of social gatherings and celebrations. In such cases, it may be difficult to change established eating patterns because they are linked to cultural and family values.

QUESTIONS FOR CRITICAL THINKING AND REFLECTION

How do you view your own body composition? Where do you think you have gotten your ideas about how your body should look and perform? In light of what you have read in this chapter, do the ideals and images promoted in our culture seem reasonable? Do they seem healthy?

Assess YOURSELF

What Triggers Your Eating?

Hunger isn't the only reason people eat. Efforts to maintain a healthy body weight can be sabotaged by eating related to other factors, including emotions, environment, and patterns of thinking. This quiz is designed to provide you with a score for five factors that describe many people's eating habits. This information will put you in a better position to manage your eating behaviour and control your weight. Circle the number that indicates to what degree each situation is likely to make you start eating.

Social	Very Unlikely					Very Likely				
1. Arguing or having a conflict with someone	1	2	3	4	5	6	7	8	9	10
2. Being with others when they are eating	1	2	3	4	5	6	7	8	9	10
3. Being urged to eat by someone else	1	2	3	4	5	6	7	8	9	10
4. Feeling inadequate around others	1	2	3	4	5	6	7	8	9	10
Emotional										
5. Feeling bad, such as being anxious or depressed	1	2	3	4	5	6	7	8	9	10
6. Feeling good, happy, or relaxed	1	2	3	4	5	6	7	8	9	10
7. Feeling bored or having time on my hands	1	2	3	4	5	6	7	8	9	10
8. Feeling stressed or excited	1	2	3	4	5	6	7	8	9	10
Situational										
9. Seeing an advertisement for food or eating	1	2	3	4	5	6	7	8	9	10
10. Passing by a bakery, cookie shop, or other enticement to eat	1	2	3	4	5	6	7	8	9	10
11. Being involved in a party, celebration, or special occasion	1	2	3	4	5	6	7	8	9	10
12. Eating out	1	2	3	4	5	6	7	8	9	10
Thinking										
13. Making excuses to myself about why it's OK to eat	1	2	3	4	5	6	7	8	9	10
14. Berating myself for being fat or unable to control my eating	1	2	3	4	5	6	7	8	9	10
15. Worrying about others or about difficulties I'm having	1	2	3	4	5	6	7	8	9	10
16. Thinking about how things should or shouldn't be	1	2	3	4	5	6	7	8	9	10
Physiological										
17. Experiencing pain or physical discomfort	1	2	3	4	5	6	7	8	9	10
18. Experiencing trembling, headache, or light-headedness associated with not eating or consuming too much caffeine	1	2	3	4	5	6	7	8	9	10
19. Experiencing fatigue or feeling overtired	1	2	3	4	5	6	7	8	9	10
20. Experiencing hunger pangs or urges to eat, even though I have eaten recently	1	2	3	4	5	6	7	8	9	10

Scoring

Total your scores for each category, and enter them below. Then rank the scores by marking the highest score 1, next highest score 2, and so on. Focus on the highest-ranked categories first, but any score above 24 is high and indicates that you need to work on that category.

Category	Total Score	Rank Order
Social (Items 1–4)	_____	_____
Emotional (Items 5–8)	_____	_____
Situational (Items 9–12)	_____	_____
Thinking (Items 13–16)	_____	_____
Physiological (Items 17–20)	_____	_____

What Your Score Means

Social A high score here means you are very susceptible to the influence of others. Work on better ways to communicate more assertively, handle conflict, and manage anger. Challenge your beliefs about the need to be polite and the obligations you feel you must fulfil.

Emotional A high score here means you need to develop effective ways to cope with emotions. Work on developing skills in stress management, time management, and communication. Practising positive but realistic self-talk can help you handle small daily upsets.

Situational A high score here means you are especially susceptible to external influences. Try to avoid external cues and respond differently to those you cannot avoid. Control your environment by changing the way you buy, store, cook, and serve food. Anticipate potential problems, and have a plan for handling them.

Thinking A high score here means that the way you think—how you talk to yourself, the beliefs you hold, your memories, and your expectations—have a powerful influence on your eating habits. Try to be less self-critical, less perfectionistic, and more flexible in your ideas about the way things ought to be. Recognize when you are making excuses or rationalizations that allow you to eat.

Physiological A high score here means that the way you eat, what you eat, or medications you are taking may be affecting your eating behaviour. You may be eating to reduce physical arousal or deal with physical discomfort. Try eating three meals a day, supplemented with regular snacks if needed. Avoid too much caffeine. If any medication you are taking produces adverse physical reactions, switch to an alternative, if possible. If your medications may be affecting your hormone levels, discuss possible alternatives with your physician.

Source: Adapted from Nash, J. D. 1997. *The New Maximize Your Body Potential*. Boulder, Colorado: Bull. Reprinted with permission from Bull Publishing Company.

Adopting a Healthy Lifestyle for Successful Weight Management

The Canadian Medical Association's *Canadian Clinical Practice Guidelines on the Management and Prevention of Obesity in Adults and Children* stress the importance of a lifestyle geared toward healthy bodies. This recommendation is logical, given that when all the research has been assessed, it is clear that most weight problems are lifestyle problems. Even though more and more young people are developing weight problems, most arrive at early adulthood with the advantage of having a normal body weight—neither too fat nor too thin. In fact, many young adults have less than desirable eating and exercise habits and don't develop a weight problem. But as the rapid growth that occurs during adolescence slows, and family and career obligations increase, maintaining a healthy weight becomes a greater challenge. Slow weight gain is a major cause of overweight and obesity, and so weight management is important for everyone, not just for people who are currently overweight. A good time to develop a lifestyle for successful weight management is during early adulthood, when healthy behaviour patterns have a better chance of taking a firm hold.

Permanent weight loss is not something people can start and stop. They need to adopt healthy behaviours that they can maintain throughout life, including eating habits, level of physical activity, an ability to think positively and manage emotions effectively, and the coping strategies they use to deal with the stresses and challenges.

Diet and Eating Habits

In contrast to dieting, which involves some form of food restriction, the term *diet* refers to your daily food choices. Everyone has a diet, but not everyone is dieting. You need to develop a diet that you enjoy and that enables you to maintain a healthy body composition. Use Health Canada's *Eating Well with Canada's Food Guide* as the basis for a healthy diet (see Chapter 5). For weight management, pay special attention to total calories, portion sizes, energy density, and eating habits.

Total Calories

Chapter 5 includes suggestions for approximate daily energy intakes based on gender, age, and activity level. However, energy balance may be a more important consideration for weight management than total calories consumed (refer back to Figure 4.2). To maintain your current weight, the total number of calories you eat must equal the number you burn. To lose weight, you must decrease your calorie intake or increase the number of calories you burn (or both); to gain weight, the reverse is true (1 kilogram of body fat represents 7000 calories).

The best approach for weight loss is combining an increase in physical activity with moderate calorie restriction. Don't go on a crash diet. To maintain weight loss, you will probably have to maintain some degree of the calorie restriction you used to lose the weight. Therefore, you need to adopt a level of food intake that provides all the essential nutrients and that you can live with over the long term. For most people, maintaining weight loss is more difficult than losing the weight.

Portion Sizes

Overconsumption of total calories is closely tied to portion sizes. Many Canadians are unaware that the portions of packaged foods and of foods served at restaurants have increased in size, and most of us significantly underestimate the amount of food we eat. Studies have found that the larger the meal, the greater the underestimation of calories. People also commonly eat much more of the foods that they perceive as being healthy, but in the process consume far more calories than they need. Limiting portion sizes is critical for maintaining good health. For many people, concentrating on portion sizes is easier than counting calories.

QUICK STATS

Canadians obtain more than 20% of their total daily calories from "other foods," which are not found in the four food groups.

—Heart and Stroke Foundation, 2014; Statistics Canada, 2006

To counteract portion distortion, weigh and measure your food at home for a few days every now and then. In addition, check the serving sizes listed on packaged foods. With practice, you will learn to judge portion sizes more accurately. When eating out, try to order the smallest-sized items on the menu. It is especially important to limit serving sizes of foods that are high in calories and low in nutrients. Don't supersize your meals and snacks; although huge servings may seem like the best deal, it is more important to order just what you need. Refer to Chapter 5 for more information on choosing appropriate portion sizes.

Energy (Calorie) Density

Experts also recommend that you pay attention to *energy density*—the number of calories per gram of food. Studies suggest that it isn't consumption of a certain amount of fat or calories in food that reduces hunger and leads to feelings of fullness and satisfaction; rather, it is consumption of a certain weight of food. Foods that are low in energy density have more volume and bulk—that is, they are relatively heavy but have few calories (see Table 4.3). For example, for the same 100 calories, you could eat 21 baby carrots or 4 pretzel twists; you are more likely to feel full after eating the serving of carrots because it weighs 10 times as much as the serving of pretzels (280 grams versus 28 grams).

Fresh fruits and vegetables, with their high water and fibre content, are low in energy density, as are whole-grain foods. Fresh fruits contain fewer calories and more fibre than fruit juices or drinks. Meat, ice cream, potato chips, croissants, crackers, cakes, and cookies are examples of foods high in energy density. Strategies for lowering the energy density of your diet include the following:

- Eat fruit with breakfast and for dessert.
- Add extra vegetables to sandwiches, casseroles, stir-fry dishes, pizza, pasta dishes, and fajitas.
- Start meals with a bowl of broth-based soup; include a green salad or fruit salad.
- Snack on fresh fruits and vegetables rather than crackers, chips, or other energy-dense snack foods.

TABLE 4.3

Examples of Foods Low in Energy Density

Food	Amount	Calories
Egg whites	2 large	35
Plain instant oatmeal	85 g (½ cup)	80
Fresh blueberries	130 g (1 cup)	80
Corn on the cob (plain)	1 ear	80
Cantaloupe	½ melon	95
Unsweetened apple sauce	250 mL (1 cup)	100
Pear	1 medium	100
Mixed vegetables	130 g (1 cup)	110
Sweet potato	1 medium	120

Limit serving sizes of energy-dense foods, such as butter, mayonnaise, cheese, chocolate, fatty meats, croissants, and snack foods that are fried, high in added sugars (including sugar substitutes and reduced-fat products), or contain trans fats. It is also important to watch out for processed foods, which can be high in fat and sodium. Even processed foods labelled "fat free" or "reduced fat" may be high in calories; such products may contain sugar or fat substitutes. And although a number of sugar substitutes (such as Aspartame and Sorbitol) have been approved for use in Canada, controversy about potential long-term side effects continues. Many of the foods containing fat and sugar substitutes are low-nutrient snack foods. Although substituting a lower-fat or lower-sugar version of the same food may be beneficial, fruits, vegetables, and whole grains are healthier snack choices. Otherwise, stick to the calorie and nutrient recommendations offered in *Eating Well with Canada's Food Guide*. These guidelines are described in detail in Chapter 5.

Eating Habits

Equally important to weight management is the habit of eating several small meals—four to five meals per day, including breakfast and snacks—on a regular schedule. Skipping meals leads to excessive hunger, feelings of deprivation, and increased vulnerability to binge eating or snacking. In addition to establishing a regular pattern of eating, set some rules to govern your food choices. Rules for breakfast might include choosing a (naturally) sugar-free, high-fibre cereal with fat-free milk on most days; having a hard-boiled egg (no more than three per week); and saving pancakes and waffles for special occasions, unless they are whole grain. For effective weight management, it is better to consume the majority of calories during the day rather than in the evening.

Decreeing some foods off limits generally sets up a rule to be broken. A more sensible principle is "everything in moderation." If a particular food becomes troublesome, place it off limits until you gain control over it. The ultimate goal is to eat in moderation; no foods need to be entirely off limits, though some should be eaten judiciously.

Physical Activity and Exercise

Regular physical activity is a very important lifestyle factor in weight management. Physical activity, which includes activity that is part of your daily life such as walking to school or "active transportation," and exercise, a more structured form of physical activity that is planned and structured such as lifting weights or doing a yoga class, burn calories and keep the metabolism geared to using food for energy instead of storing it as fat. Making *significant* cuts in food intake to lose weight can be a difficult strategy to maintain; increasing your physical activity tends to be a more easily tolerated approach for the long term. Additional good news about physical activity and weight management is that researchers have found that exercise does not automatically prompt increases in feelings of hunger (to replace the energy used from activity). And, in some situations, exercise can suppress appetite. Regular physical activity protects against weight gain, is essential for maintaining weight loss, and improves quality of life (see the Mind Body Spirit box). The sooner you establish good habits, the better. The key to success is making physical activity and exercise an integral part of the lifestyle you can enjoy now and in the future. Chapter 6 contains many suggestions for becoming a more active, physically fit person.

 Mind *Body* **SPIRIT**

Exercise, Body Image, and Self-Esteem

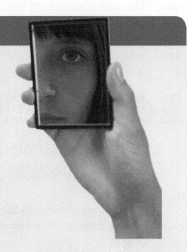

If you gaze into the mirror and wish you could change the way your body looks, consider getting some exercise—not to reshape your contours, but to firm up your body image and enhance your self-esteem. In a recent study, 82 adults completed a 12-week aerobic exercise program and had 12 months of follow-up. Compared with the control group, these participants improved their fitness and also benefited psychologically in tests of mood, anxiety, and self-concept. These same physical and psychological benefits were still significant at the one-year follow-up.

One reason for the findings may be that people who exercise regularly often gain a sense of mastery and competence that enhances their self-esteem and body image. In addition, exercise contributes to a more toned look, which many adults prefer.

Research suggests that physically active people are more comfortable with their body and their image than sedentary people are. In one workplace study, 60 employees were asked to complete a 36-session stretching program whose main purpose was to prevent muscle strains at work. At the end of the program, besides the significant increase by all participants in measurements of flexibility, their perceptions of their bodies improved, and so did their overall sense of self-worth.

Similar results were obtained in a Norwegian study, in which 219 middle-aged people at risk for heart disease were randomly assigned to one of four groups: (1) diet, (2) diet plus exercise, (3) exercise, and (4) no intervention. The greater the participation of individuals in the exercise component of the program, the higher their scores in perceived competence and self-esteem and coping.

Thinking and Emotions

The way you think about yourself and your world influences, and is influenced by, how you feel and how you act. In fact, research on people who have a weight problem indicates that low self-esteem and the negative emotions that accompany it are significant problems. Often, people with low self-esteem mentally compare the actual self to an internally held picture of an ideal self, an image based on perfectionistic goals and beliefs about how they and others should be. The more these two pictures differ, the larger the impact on self-esteem and the more likely the presence of negative emotions.

Along with the internal picture we carry of ourselves, we all carry on an internal dialogue about events happening to us and around us. This *self-talk* can be either self-deprecating or positively motivating, depending on our beliefs and attitudes. Having realistic beliefs and goals, and practising positive self-talk and problem solving, support a healthy lifestyle.

 QUESTIONS FOR CRITICAL THINKING AND REFLECTION

Have you ever used food as an escape when you were stressed out or distraught? Were you aware of what you were doing at the time? How can you avoid using food as a coping mechanism in the future?

Coping Strategies

Appropriate coping strategies help you deal with the stresses of life (see Chapter 3); they are also an important lifestyle factor in weight management. Many people use eating as a way to cope; others may cope by turning to drugs, alcohol, smoking, or gambling. Those who overeat might use food to alleviate loneliness or to serve as a pickup for fatigue, as an antidote to boredom, or as a distraction from problems. Some people even overeat to punish themselves for real or imagined transgressions.

Those who recognize that they are misusing food in such ways can analyze their eating habits with fresh eyes. They can consciously attempt to find new coping strategies (e.g., developing a support system, setting realistic goals, being kind to oneself) and begin to use food appropriately—to fuel life's activities, to foster growth, and to bring pleasure, but *not* as a way to manage stress. For a summary of the components of weight management through healthy lifestyle choices, see the Take Charge box.

Take CHARGE

Lifestyle Strategies for Successful Weight Management

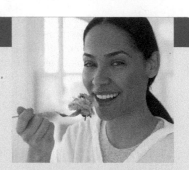

Food Choices

- Follow the recommendations in *Eating Well with Canada's Food Guide* for eating a moderate, varied diet. Focus on making good choices from each food group.
- Favour foods with a low energy density and a high nutrient density.
- Check food labels for serving sizes, calories, and nutrient levels.
- Watch for hidden calories. Reduced-fat foods often have as many calories as their full-fat versions. Fat-based condiments, such as butter, margarine, mayonnaise, and salad dressings, provide about 100 calories per tablespoon; added sugars, such as jams, jellies, and syrup, are also packed with calories.
- Drink fewer calories in the form of pop, fruit drinks, sports drinks, alcohol, and specialty coffees and teas.
- For problem foods, try eating small amounts under controlled conditions. Go out for a scoop of ice cream, for example, rather than buying a couple of litres for your freezer.

Planning and Serving

- Keep a log of what you eat. Before you begin your program, your log will provide a realistic picture of your current diet and what changes you can make. Once you start your program, a log will keep you focused on your food choices and portion sizes. Track the food eaten, your hunger level, the circumstances (location, other activities), outside influences (environment, other people), and your thoughts and emotions.
- Eat four to five meals and snacks daily, *including breakfast*, to distribute calories throughout your day. In studies, people who eat breakfast consume fewer calories overall over the course of the day. Make more meals yourself and eat out less often. Keep low-calorie snacks on hand to combat the munchies: baby carrots, popcorn, and fresh fruits and vegetables are good choices.
- When shopping, make a list and stick to it. Don't shop when you are hungry. Avoid aisles that contain problem foods. Generally, the perimeter of the grocery store contains the healthier choices.
- Consume the majority of your daily calories during the day, not in the evening.
- Pay special attention to portion sizes. Use measuring cups and spoons and a food scale to become more familiar with appropriate portion sizes.
- Serve meals on small plates and in small bowls to help you eat smaller portions without feeling deprived.
- Eat only in specifically designated spots. Remove food from other areas of your home.
- When you eat, just eat—don't do anything else, such as reading or watching TV.
- Avoid late-night eating, a behaviour specifically associated with weight gain among university and college students.
- Eat slowly. It takes time for your brain to get the message that your stomach is full. Take small bites and chew food thoroughly. Pay attention to every bite, and enjoy your food. Between bites, try putting your fork or spoon down and taking sips of a beverage.
- When you are done eating, remove your plate. Cue yourself that the meal is over; drink a glass of water, suck on a mint, chew gum, or brush your teeth.

Special Occasions

- When you eat out, choose a restaurant where you can make healthy food choices. Ask the server not to put bread and butter on the table before the meal, and request that sauces and salad dressings be served on the side. If portion sizes are large, take half your food home for a meal later in the week. Don't choose supersized meals.
- If you cook a large meal for friends, send leftovers home with your guests.
- If you are eating at a friend's, eat a little and leave the rest. Don't eat to be polite; if someone offers you food you don't want, thank the person and decline firmly.
- Take care during the winter holidays. Research indicates that people gain less than they think during the winter holidays (about a half kilogram) but that the weight isn't lost during the rest of the year, leading to slow, steady weight gain.

Physical Activity and Stress Management

- Increase your level of daily physical activity. If you have been sedentary for a long time or are seriously overweight, increase your level of activity slowly. Start by walking 10 minutes at a time, and work toward 30–60 minutes or more of moderate physical activity per day.
- Begin a formal exercise program that includes cardiorespiratory endurance exercise, strength training, and stretching.
- Develop techniques for handling stress. Try walking, or use a relaxation technique. Practise positive self-talk. Get adequate sleep. (See Chapter 3 for more on stress management.)
- Develop strategies for coping with non-hunger cues to eat, such as boredom, sleepiness, or anxiety. Try calling a friend, taking a shower, or reading a magazine.
- Tell family members and friends that you are changing your eating and exercise habits. Ask them to be supportive.

Approaches to Overcoming a Weight Problem

What should you do if you are overweight? You have several options.

Doing It Yourself

If you need to lose weight, decide what is important about doing so: Is this a way to be kinder to yourself? Treat yourself with more respect? Reduce potential health risks? All of the above? Once you have decided for yourself why it is important for you to lose weight, focus on adopting the healthy lifestyle described throughout this book. The right weight for you will naturally evolve, and you won't have to diet. Combine modest cuts in energy intake with exercise, and avoid very-low-calorie diets. (In general, a low-calorie diet should have 1500–1800 calories per day.) By producing a negative energy balance of 250–1000 calories per day, you will produce the recommended weight loss of 0.25 to 1 kilogram per week.

Don't try to lose weight more rapidly. Most low-calorie diets cause a rapid loss of body water at first. When this phase passes, weight loss slows. As a result, dieters are often misled into believing that their efforts are not working. They then give up, not realizing that smaller, mostly fat, losses later in the diet are actually better than the initial larger, mostly fluid losses. Reasonable weight loss is 8–10 percent of body weight over six months.

For many Canadians, maintaining weight loss is a bigger challenge than losing weight. Most weight lost during dieting is regained. When planning a weight-management program, it is extremely important to include

QUICK STATS

In 2012, the North American weight loss management market (e.g., fitness equipment; weight loss/diet supplements, foods, and beverages; surgery-related devices) was worth $120 billion dollars.

—*North America Weight Loss/Obesity Management Market Report*, 2012

strategies that you can maintain over the long term, both for food choices and for physical activity. Weight management is a lifelong project. A registered dietitian or nutritionist can recommend an appropriate plan for you when you want to lose weight on your own. For more tips, refer to the Take Charge box at the end of the chapter.

Diet Books and Fad Diets

Many people who try to lose weight by themselves try using one or more of the dozens of diet books on the market or following a fad diet. Although some contain useful advice and motivational tips, most make empty promises. Fad diets are frequently promoted in the media as offering quick and easy weight loss, but weight that is lost quickly is often regained. In many cases, the person gains even more weight back. Typically based on unsound nutrition or the elimination of certain foods or even entire food groups, fad diets may not meet a person's nutrient and calorie requirements. Simply stated, if a dietary change is not something you can see yourself maintaining in the long-term, it's not going to provide you with sustainable results. Here are some guidelines for evaluating and choosing a diet book and recognizing a fad diet book:

- Reject books that advocate an unbalanced way of eating, such as a carbohydrate-only diet or a low-carbohydrate, high-protein diet. Also reject books that promote a single food, such as cabbage or grapefruit.
- Reject books that claim to be based on a "scientific breakthrough" or to have the "secret to success."
- Reject books that use gimmicks, such as matching eating to blood type, hyping insulin resistance as the single cause of obesity, combining foods in special ways to achieve weight loss, rotating levels of calories, or purporting that a weight problem is due to food allergies, food sensitivities, yeast infections, or hormone imbalances.
- Reject books that promise quick weight loss, that limit the selection of foods, or that promise more than one kilogram of weight loss each week.
- Reject books that require you to meet your nutritional needs with supplements instead of food.
- Reject books that advocate diets for men with fewer than 1800 calories a day and for women with fewer than 1500 calories a day.
- Reject books that promote the idea that it is healthy to lose more than one kilogram a week.
- Accept books that advocate a balanced approach to diet along with exercise and sound nutrition advice.

Many diets can cause weight loss if maintained; the real difficulty is finding a safe and healthy pattern of food choices and physical activity that results in long-term maintenance of a healthy body weight and reduced risk of chronic disease (see the Critical Consumer box).

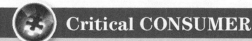

Critical CONSUMER

Is Any Diet Best for Weight Loss?

Experts agree that reducing calorie intake promotes weight loss. However, many popular weight-loss plans include a special hook and promote specific food choices and macronutrient (protein, fat, carbohydrate) combinations as best for weight loss. Research findings have been mixed, but two points are clear. Total calorie intake matters, and the best diet is probably the one you can stick with. It stands to reason that if you go on a diet, you will eventually go off it; you are better off choosing a healthy dietary lifestyle that you can live with over the long term.

Low-Carbohydrate Diets
Some low-carbohydrate diets advocate fewer than 10 percent of total calories from carbohydrates, compared with the 45–65 percent recommended by nutrition experts. Some suggest daily carbohydrate intake below the 130 grams needed to provide essential carbohydrates in the diet. Small studies have found that low-carbohydrate diets can help with short-term weight loss and be safe for relatively short periods of time—although unpleasant effects, such as bad breath, constipation, and headache, are fairly common.

Some low-carbohydrate diets tend to be very high in protein and saturated fat and low in fibre, whole grains, vegetables, and fruits (and thus lack some essential nutrients). Diets high in protein and saturated fat have been linked to an increased risk of heart disease, high blood pressure, and cancer. Other low-carbohydrate diets, though still emphasizing protein, limit saturated fats, allow most vegetables after an initial period, and advocate switching to "healthy carbs." These diets are healthier than the more extreme versions.

Low-Fat Diets

Many experts advocate diets that are relatively low in fat, high in carbohydrates, and moderate in protein. Critics of these diets blame them for rising rates of obesity and note that very-low-fat, very-high-carbohydrate diets can increase triglyceride levels and reduce levels of good (HDL) cholesterol in some people. However, these negative effects can be counteracted with moderate intensity exercise, and low-fat diets combined with physical activity can be safe and effective for many people.

Few experts take the position that low-fat, high-carbohydrate diets, apart from overall diet and activity patterns, are responsible for the increase in obesity among North Americans. However, the debate has highlighted the importance of total calorie intake and the quality of carbohydrate choices. A low-fat diet is not a licence to consume excess calories, even in low-fat foods.

How Do Popular Diets Measure Up?

In one recent study, people with obesity on a very-low-carbohydrate, high-fat diet lost more weight over six months than did people following a moderate-fat diet. After a year, however, the difference in weight loss between the two groups was no longer significant, and the dropout rate from both groups was high.

A 2005 study followed participants in four popular diets that emphasize different strategies—Weight Watchers (restricted portion sizes and calories), Atkins (low carbohydrate, high fat), the Zone (relatively high protein, moderate fat and carbohydrate), and Ornish (very low fat). Each of these diets modestly reduced body weight and heart disease risk factors. No significant difference in weight loss was found at one year among the diets, and the more closely people adhered to each diet, the more weight they lost. Dropout rates were high—about 50 percent for Atkins and Ornish and 35 percent for Weight Watchers and the Zone. According to a recent article in the *New England Journal of Medicine*, while diets have been shown to reduce weight effectively, maintaining a diet in the long-term generally does not work well. Identifying realistic healthy practices (e.g., eating more fruits and vegetables and eating breakfast daily), in combination with reduced energy intake, are important considerations for lasting change.

Energy Balance Counts: The National Weight Control Registry

Future research may determine that certain macronutrient patterns are somewhat more helpful for disease reduction in people with particular risk profiles. In terms of weight loss, however, such differences among diets are likely overshadowed by the importance of total calorie intake and physical activity. Important lessons about energy balance can be drawn from The National Weight Control Registry, an ongoing study of people who have lost significant amounts of weight and kept it off. Although the Registry is based in the United States, it accepts members from anywhere in the world. Participants have lost an average of 32 kilograms and kept the weight off for more than five years. Nearly all participants use a combination of diet and exercise to manage their weight. Most consume diets moderate in calories and relatively low in fat and fried foods; they monitor their body weight and their food intake frequently. Participants engage in an average of 60 minutes of moderate physical activity daily. The National Weight Control Registry study illustrates that to lose weight and keep it off, you must decrease daily calorie intake or increase daily physical activity—and continue to do so over your lifetime.

Sources: Battle of the diet books II. 2006. *Nutrition Action Healthletter*, July/August; Dansinger, M. L., et al. 2005. Comparison of the Atkins, Ornish, Weight Watchers, and Zone diets for weight loss and heart disease risk reduction. *Journal of the American Medical Association* 293(1): 43–53; Hays, N. P., et al. 2004. Effects of an ad libitum low-fat, high-carbohydrate diet on body weight, body composition, and fat distribution in older men and women. *Archives of Internal Medicine* 164(2): 210–217. Hill, J., and R. Wing. 2003. The National Weight Control Registry. *Permanente Journal* 7(3): 34–37; Bravata, D. M., et al. 2003. Efficacy and safety of low-carbohydrate diets. *Journal of the American Medical Association* 289: 1837–1850; Foster, G. D., et al. 2003. A randomized trial of low-carbohydrate diet for obesity. *New England Journal of Medicine* 348: 2082–2090; and Casazza, K. et al. 2013. Myths, presumptions, and facts about obesity. *New England Journal of Medicine* 368(5) 446–454. Screenshot from The National Weight Control Registry reprinted with permission.

Dietary Supplements and Diet Aids

The number of dietary supplements and other weight-loss aids on the market has also increased in recent years. Promoted in advertisements, magazines, social media, direct mail campaigns, infomercials, and websites, these products typically promise a quick and easy path to weight loss. Most of these products are marketed as dietary supplements and so are subject to fewer regulations than over-the-counter (OTC) medications. A 2002 report stated that more than half of advertisements for weight-loss products made representations that are likely to be false. In 2011, the number one type of fraud claim submitted to the Federal Trade Commission pertained to weight-loss products: more than double any other category. In addition, use of OTC products doesn't assist with the adoption of lifestyle behaviours that can help people achieve and maintain a healthy weight over the long term.

The bottom line on non-prescription diet aids is caveat emptor—let the buyer beware. There is no quick and easy way to lose weight. The most effective approach is to develop healthy diet and exercise habits and make them a permanent part of your life. The following sections describe some commonly marketed OTC products for weight loss.

Formula Drinks and Food Bars

Canned diet drinks, powders used to make shakes, and diet food bars and snacks are designed to achieve weight loss by substituting for some or all of a person's daily food intake. However, most people find it difficult to use these products for long periods, and muscle loss and other serious health problems may result if they are used as the sole source of nutrition for an extended period. Use of such products sometimes results in rapid short-term weight loss, but the weight is typically regained because users don't learn to change their eating and lifestyle behaviours.

Herbal Supplements

As described in Chapter 5, herbs are marketed as dietary supplements (natural health products), and so little information is available about effectiveness, proper dosage, drug interactions, and side effects. In addition, labels may not accurately list the ingredients and dosages, and safe manufacturing practices are not guaranteed. For example, the substitution of a toxic herb for another compound during the manufacture of a Chinese herbal weight-loss preparation caused more than 100 cases of kidney damage and cancer among users in Europe.

In 2002 and 2008, Health Canada issued a health advisory about the sale of ephedra (*ma huang*), stating that it presents a significant and unreasonable risk to human health. Ephedrine, the active ingredient in ephedra, is structurally similar to amphetamine and was widely used in weight-loss supplements. It may suppress appetite, but adverse and possibly fatal effects have included elevated blood pressure, panic attacks, seizures, insomnia, and increased risk of heart attack or stroke, particularly when combined with another stimulant, such as caffeine. Products containing ephedra for sale in Canada must be caffeine free and must not have more than 8 milligrams of ephedrine per dose. Other herbal stimulants are described in Table 4.4.

Other Supplements

Fibre is another common ingredient in OTC diet aids, promoted for appetite control. However, dietary fibre acts as a bulking agent in the large intestine, not the stomach, and so it doesn't have a pronounced effect on

TABLE 4.4

Ingredients Commonly Found in Weight-Loss Products

Common Name	Use/Claim	Evidence/Efficacy	Safety Issues
Bitter orange extract (Citrus aurantium)	Central nervous system (CNS) stimulant	Limited evidence	Highly concentrated extracts may increase blood pressure; should not be used by people with cardiac problems
Caffeine	CNS stimulant; increases fat metabolism	Amplifies effects of ephedra	Generally considered safe; caution advised in caffeine-sensitive individuals
Garcinia cambogia	May interfere with fat metabolism or suppress appetite	Inconclusive evidence	Short-term use (< 12 weeks) generally considered safe when used as directed
Green tea extract	Diuretic; increases metabolism	Limited evidence	Generally considered safe
Guarana	CNS stimulant; diuretic	Few clinical trials	Same as for caffeine; overdose can cause painful urination, abdominal spasms, and vomiting
Senna, cascara, aloe, buckthorn berries	Stimulant, laxative	Not effective for weight loss	Chronic use decreases muscle tone in large intestine, causes electrolyte imbalances, and leads to dependence on laxatives
Tea, kola, dandelion, bucho, uva-ursi, damiana, juniper	Diuretic	Not effective for weight loss	Chronic use can cause electrolyte imbalance in some people
Yerba mate	Stimulant, laxative, diuretic	Limited evidence	Long-term use as a beverage may increase risk of oral cancer

Source: Adapted from Leslie, K. K. 2003. Herbal weight-loss products: Effective and appropriate? *Today's Dietician* 5(8): 12.

appetite. In addition, many diet aids contain only 3 grams of fibre or fewer, which does not contribute much toward the recommended daily intake of 25–38 grams. Other popular dietary supplements include conjugated linoleic acid, carnitine, chromium, pyruvate, calcium, B vitamins, chitosan, and a number of products labelled "fat absorbers," "fat blockers," and "starch blockers." Research has not found these products to be effective, and many have potentially adverse side effects.

Weight-Loss Programs

Weight-loss programs come in a variety of types, including non-commercial support organizations, commercial programs, websites, and clinical programs.

Non-commercial Weight-Loss Programs

Non-commercial programs, such as TOPS (Take Off Pounds Sensibly) and Overeaters Anonymous (OA), mainly provide group support. They do not advocate any particular diet, but do recommend seeking professional advice for creating an individualized plan. Like Alcoholics Anonymous, OA is a 12-step program with a spiritual orientation that promotes abstinence from compulsive overeating. These types of programs are generally free. Your physician or a registered dietitian can also provide information and support for weight loss.

Commercial Weight-Loss Programs

Commercial weight-loss programs typically provide group support, nutrition education, physical activity recommendations, and behaviour modification advice. Some also make available packaged foods to assist in following dietary advice.

One study evaluated major commercial weight-loss programs, including Weight Watchers, NutriSystem, Jenny Craig, and LA Weight Loss, for 12 weeks or more with a one-year follow-up assessment. Results showed Weight Watchers to be the only moderately priced commercial program with a mean loss of 5 percent of initial weight.

A responsible and safe weight-loss program should have the following features:

- The recommended diet should be safe and balanced, include all the food groups, and meet the Daily Recommended Intakes (DRIs) for all nutrients. Regular physical activity and exercise should be strongly encouraged.
- The program should promote slow, steady weight loss averaging 0.25–1.0 kilogram per week. Some greater weight loss may occur initially through fluid loss.
- If a participant plans to lose more than 10 kilograms, has any health problems, or is taking medication on a regular basis, physician evaluation and monitoring should be recommended. The program staff should include qualified counsellors and health professionals.
- The program should include plans for weight maintenance after the weight-loss phase is over.
- The program should provide information on all fees and costs, including those of supplements and prepackaged foods, as well as data on risks and expected outcomes of participating in the program.

In addition, you should consider whether a program fits your lifestyle and whether you are truly ready to make a commitment to it. A strong commitment and a plan for maintenance are especially important because only about 10–15 percent of program participants maintain their weight loss—the rest gain back all or more than they had lost. One study of participants found that regular exercise was the best predictor of maintaining weight loss, whereas frequent television viewing was the best predictor of weight gain.

Online Weight-Loss Programs

A recent addition to the weight-loss program scene is the Internet-based program. Most such websites provide a cross between self-help and group support through chat rooms, bulletin boards, and e-newsletters. Many sites offer online self-assessment for diet, physical activity habits, and meal plans; some provide access to a staff professional for individualized help. Many are free, but some charge a small weekly or monthly fee.

Preliminary research suggests that this type of program provides an alternative to in-person diet counselling and can lead to weight loss for some people. Studies found that people who logged on to Internet programs more frequently tended to lose more weight; weekly online contact proved most successful for weight loss. The criteria used to evaluate commercial programs can also be applied to Internet-based programs. In addition, the program should offer member-to-member support and access to staff professionals.

Clinical Weight-Loss Programs

Medically supervised clinical programs are usually located in a hospital or other medical setting. Designed to help those who are severely obese, these programs typically involve a closely monitored very-low-calorie diet.

Prescription Drugs

For a medicine to cause weight loss, it must reduce energy consumption, increase energy expenditure, or interfere with energy absorption. The medications most often prescribed for weight loss are appetite suppressants that reduce feelings of hunger or increase feelings of fullness. Appetite suppressants usually work by increasing levels of catecholamine or serotonin, two brain chemicals that affect mood and appetite.

All prescription weight-loss drugs have potential side effects, and some are very dangerous. Most approved by Health Canada are only for short-term use, but a few are approved for longer-term use, such as orlistat (Xenical). Orlistat is not an appetite suppressant but rather is considered an anti-obesity drug because it lowers calorie consumption by blocking fat absorption in the intestines; it prevents about 30 percent of the fat in food from being digested. Because orlistat reduces the absorption of fat-soluble vitamins and antioxidants, taking a vitamin supplement is highly recommended when taking it. Its side effects include diarrhea, cramping, and other gastrointestinal problems if users do not follow a low-fat diet.

All medications work best in conjunction with behaviour modification. Studies have generally found that appetite suppressants produce modest weight loss—about 2–10 kilograms above the loss expected with non-drug obesity treatments. Individuals respond very differently, however, and some experience more weight loss than others. Unfortunately, weight loss tends to level off or reverse after four to six months on a medication, and many people regain the weight they have lost when they stop taking the drug.

Prescription weight-loss drugs are recommended only in certain cases: for people who have been unable to lose weight with non-drug options and who have a BMI higher than 30 (or higher than 27 if two or more additional risk factors, such as diabetes and high blood pressure, are present). For severely obese people who have been unable to lose weight by other methods, prescription drugs may provide a good option.

Surgery

According to the *2009-2011 Canadian Health Measures Survey*, about 26 percent (or 7 million) Canadian adults have a BMI greater than 30 (obese). About 4 percent (or about 1 million) of the adult population falls into the class III obesity category, and nearly two-thirds of these individuals are women. Because severe obesity is a serious medical condition that is often complicated by other health problems such as diabetes, sleep disorders, heart disease, and arthritis, it important to look at obesity by category, rather than as a whole. Surgical intervention may be necessary as a treatment of last resort. According to the U.S. National Institutes of Health, gastric bypass surgery is recommended for patients with a BMI greater than 40, or greater than 35 with obesity-related illnesses. A 2010 article in *Canadian Family Physician* noted that several Canadian provinces are working to improve access to obesity surgery in our country.

QUICK STATS

In 2007–2009, approximately 1.5 million Canadian adults were considered eligible for bariatric surgery with a mean BMI of 40.1 kg/m^2.

—*Canadian Health Measures Survey*, 2007–2009; Padwal et al., 2012

Because of the increasing prevalence of severe obesity, surgical treatment of obesity is growing worldwide. Obesity-related health conditions, as well as risk of premature death, generally improve after surgical weight loss. However, lifestyle changes coupled with the surgery are essential for long-term success, and surgery is not without risks. A recent study found that patients with poor cardiorespiratory fitness before surgery experienced more post-operative complications, including stroke, kidney failure, and even death, than patients with higher fitness levels.

Gastric bypass surgery modifies the gastrointestinal tract by changing either the size of the stomach or how the intestine drains, thereby reducing food intake. Two of the most common surgeries are the Roux-en-Y gastric bypass and the vertical banded gastroplasty.

Roux-en-Y Gastric Bypass

In the *Roux-en-Y gastric bypass* procedure, the stomach is separated into two pouches, one large and one small. A Y segment of the small intestine is attached to the smaller pouch. The small stomach pouch restricts food intake, and the bypass of the lower stomach and part of the small intestine results in the absorption of fewer calories (and nutrients). Side effects include fat intolerance, nutritional deficiencies, and dumping syndrome, which involves gastrointestinal distress.

Vertical Banded Gastroplasty

In *vertical banded gastroplasty (VBG)*, a small gastric pouch is created in the upper part of the stomach by applying a double row of staples that essentially elongates the esophagus. This small pouch empties into the remaining stomach through an outlet that is restricted with a band. The procedure controls the gastric emptying of food and the volume of foods eaten. Common complications associated with this kind of surgery are nausea, vomiting, band slippage, gastroesophageal reflux, and stenosis (constriction of the outlet). When compared with Roux-en-Y gastric bypass, VBG has a lower initial weight loss and a greater weight regain.

In a variation of VGB, called Lap-Band, an adjustable band is placed around the stomach. The band is implanted laparoscopically via a tube inserted through a small incision in the abdomen. The band ties off a portion of the stomach, creating a small pouch similar to that created in VGB surgery. The band is filled with saline and can be tightened or loosened by adding or removing saline through a small tube that exits through the patient's abdomen. The Lap-Band procedure has about the same success rate as VGB and is generally considered to be safe.

Weight loss from surgery generally ranges between 40–70 percent of total body weight in a year. In a 2006 study that included mild to moderately obese (BMI 30–35) adults, gastric banding surgery was significantly more effective in reducing weight and improving quality of life than non-surgical methods, even after two years. For surgical procedures, the key to success is to have adequate follow-up and to stay motivated so that lifestyle behaviours and eating patterns are changed permanently. Behavioural counselling should be done in conjunction with surgery—the surgery physically reduces a person's ability to eat large amounts of food, but it doesn't change that person's eating behaviours and food choices or identify psychosocial reasons for overeating or not exercising.

QUESTIONS FOR CRITICAL THINKING AND REFLECTION

Why do you think people continue to buy into fad diets and weight-loss gimmicks, even though they are constantly reminded that the key to weight management is lifestyle change? Have you ever tried a fad diet or dietary supplement? If so, what were your reasons for trying it? What were the results?

Liposuction

Another procedure, *liposuction*, involves the removal of localized fat deposits. According to the American Society for Aesthetic Plastic Surgery, liposuction was the most popular surgical procedure performed in 2013, with more than 360 000 individuals electing to take part. This cosmetic procedure does not improve health the way weight loss does, and it involves considerable pain and discomfort.

Professional Help

Some obesity experts argue that how we eat and whether we exercise can be symptoms of how we feel about ourselves; if we help people deal with other challenges in their lives, weight loss may follow. A number of recent Canadian studies have evaluated the effect of one-on-one life coaching, with a certified coach, on the waist circumference, BMI, self-esteem, physical activity, and functional health status of adults with obesity. The studies found that after as few as six sessions, participants experienced significant decreases in their waist circumference and weight, and increases in self-esteem and functional health status. Qualitatively, participants reported an increase in daily physical activity and healthier dietary choices, feelings of optimism, and greater self-acceptance. The researchers concluded that the particular form of life coaching used shows promise as an intervention for obesity, and that more research should be conducted.

When concern about body weight develops into an eating disorder, the help of a professional is recommended. In choosing a therapist, be sure to ask about credentials and experience (see Chapter 2). The therapist should have experience working with weight management, body image issues, eating disorders, addictions, and abuse issues.

Body Image

As described earlier in the chapter, body image consists of perceptions, images, thoughts, attitudes, and emotions. Developing a positive body image is an important aspect of psychological wellness and an important component of successful weight management.

Severe Body Image Problems

Poor body image can cause significant psychological distress. A person can become preoccupied with a perceived defect in appearance, thereby damaging self-esteem and interfering with relationships. Adolescents and adults who have a negative body image are more likely to diet restrictively, eat compulsively, or develop some other form of disordered eating.

When dissatisfaction becomes extreme, the condition is called *body dysmorphic disorder (BDD)*. It is estimated that BDD affects about 350 000 Canadians, males and females in equal numbers. Rates are particularly high in certain groups such as students (2–13.1 percent compared to 0.7–2.4 percent in the general population). BDD usually begins before age 18, but can begin in adulthood. People with BDD are overly concerned with physical appearance, often focusing on slight flaws that are not obvious to others. Low self-esteem is common. People with BDD may spend hours every day thinking about their flaws and looking at themselves in mirrors; they may desire and seek repeated cosmetic surgeries. BDD is related to obsessive-compulsive disorder and can lead to depression, social phobia, and suicide if left untreated. A person with BDD needs professional evaluation and treatment; medication and therapy can help.

QUESTIONS FOR CRITICAL THINKING AND REFLECTION

Describe your body image in the fewest words possible. What satisfies you most and least about your body? Do you think your self-image is in line with the way others see you?

In some cases, body image may bear little resemblance to fact. People who have the eating disorder anorexia nervosa typically have a severely distorted body image—they believe themselves to be fat even when they have become emaciated (see the next section for more on anorexia nervosa). Distorted body image is also a hallmark of *muscle dysmorphia*, a disorder experienced by some bodybuilders and other active people in which they see themselves as small and out of shape despite being very muscular. Those who suffer from muscle dysmorphia may let obsessive bodybuilding interfere with their work and relationships. They may also use steroids and other potentially dangerous muscle-building drugs.

Acceptance and Change

There are limits to the changes that can be made to body weight and body shape, both of which are influenced by heredity. The changes that can and should be made are lifestyle changes, as described throughout this chapter.

Knowing when the limits to healthy change have been reached—and learning to accept those limits—is crucial for overall wellness. Women in particular tend to measure self-worth in terms of their appearance; when they don't measure up to an unrealistic cultural ideal, they see themselves as defective and their self-esteem falls (see the Gender Matters box). The result can be negative body image, disordered eating, or even a full-blown eating disorder. Women who view their bodies positively tend to be more intuitive eaters, relying on internal hunger and fullness cues to regulate what and how much they eat. They think more about how their bodies feel and function than how they appear to others.

Weight management needs to take place in a positive and realistic atmosphere. For a person with obesity, losing as few as five kilograms can

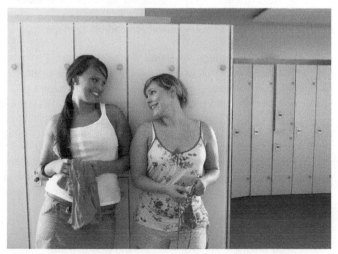

A balanced, realistic attitude toward weight management is part of overall wellness. Many healthy people do not fit society's image of ideal body size and shape.

Gender MATTERS

Gender, Ethnicity, and Body Image

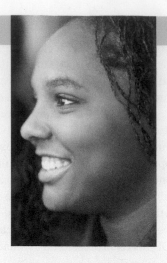

Body Image and Gender

Women are much more likely than men to be dissatisfied with their bodies, often wanting to be thinner than they are. In one study, only 30 percent of girls in Grade 8 reported being content with their bodies, while 70 percent of their male classmates expressed satisfaction with theirs. Girls and women are much more likely than boys and men to diet and develop eating disorders.

One reason that girls and women are dissatisfied with their bodies is that they are influenced by the media—particularly advertisements, women's fashion magazines, and more recently, social networking sites (SNS) such as Facebook. Most teen girls report that the media influence their idea of the perfect body and their decision to diet. Correlations have been shown between elevated appearance exposure and weight dissatisfaction among adolescent female SNS users. In a study of adult women, viewing pictures of thin models in magazines had an immediate negative effect on their mood. In another study, 68 percent of female university students felt worse about their own appearance after looking through women's magazines. Some 75 percent of normal-weight women think they are overweight, and 90 percent overestimate their body size.

It is important to note that the image of the ideal woman presented in the media is often unrealistic and even unhealthy. In a review of BMI data for Miss America pageant winners since 1922, researchers noted a significant decline in BMI over time, with an increasing number of recent winners having BMIs in the underweight category. The average fashion model is 10–18 centimetres taller and almost 23 kilograms lighter than the average North American woman. Most fashion models are thinner than 98 percent of North American women.

Our culture may be promoting an unattainable masculine ideal as well. Researchers have found that media consumption is positively associated with a desire for thinness and muscularity. Researchers studying male action figures, such as GI Joe, from the past 40 years noted that they have become increasingly muscular. A recent Batman action figure, if projected onto a man of average height, would result in someone with a 76-centimetre waist, 145-centimetre chest, and 70-centimetre biceps. Such media messages can be demoralizing; although not as common, boys and men also develop body image problems.

Body Image and Ethnicity

Although some groups espouse thinness as an ideal body type, others do not. In many traditional African societies, for example, full-figured women's bodies are seen as symbols of health, prosperity, and fertility. Black Canadian teenage girls typically have a much more positive body image than do white girls; in one survey, two-thirds of them defined beauty as "the right attitude," whereas white girls were more preoccupied with weight and body shape.

Nevertheless, recent evidence indicates that black women are as likely to engage in disordered eating behaviour, especially binge eating and vomiting, as other ethnic counterparts. These findings underscore the complex nature of eating disorders and body image.

Avoiding Body Image Problems

To minimize your risk of developing a body image problem, keep the following strategies in mind:

- Focus on healthy habits and good physical health.
- Focus on good psychological health and put concerns about physical appearance in perspective. Your worth as a human being does not depend on how you look.
- Practise body acceptance. You can influence your body size and type to some degree through lifestyle, but the basic fact is that some people are genetically designed to be bigger or heavier than others.
- Find things to appreciate in yourself besides an idealized body image. Men and women whose self-esteem is based primarily on standards of physical attractiveness can find it difficult to age gracefully. Those who can learn to value other aspects of themselves are more accepting of the physical changes that occur naturally with age.
- View food choices as morally neutral—eating dessert isn't "bad" and doesn't make you a bad person. Healthy eating habits are an important part of a wellness lifestyle, but the things you really care about and do are more important in defining who you are.
- See the beauty and fitness industries for what they are. Realize that one of their goals is to prompt dissatisfaction with yourself so that you will buy their products.

reduce blood pressure and improve mood. The hazards of excessive dieting and overconcern about body weight need to be countered by a change in attitude. A reasonable weight must take into account a person's weight history, social circumstances, metabolic profile, and psychological well-being.

Eating Disorders

Problems with body weight and weight control are not limited to excessive body fat. A growing number of people, especially adolescent girls and young women, experience an **eating disorder**, characterized by severe disturbances in body image, eating patterns, and eating-related behaviours. The major eating disorders are anorexia nervosa, bulimia nervosa, and binge-eating disorder. Disordered eating affects an estimated 1.1 percent of Canadian females and not as many males (approximately 0.15 percent); acquiring accurate statistics is difficult as only those hospitalized are included. Many more people have abnormal eating habits and attitudes about food that, although not meeting the criteria for a major eating disorder, do disrupt their lives.

> **eating disorder**
> A serious disturbance in eating patterns or eating-related behaviour, characterized by a negative body image and concerns about body weight or body fat.

Many factors are probably involved in the development of an eating disorder. Although many different explanations have been proposed, they share one central feature: dissatisfaction with body image and body weight. Such dissatisfaction is created by distorted thinking, including perfectionistic beliefs, unreasonable demands for self-control, and excessive self-criticism. Dissatisfaction with body weight leads to dysfunctional attitudes about eating, such as fear of fat and preoccupation with food, and problematic eating behaviours, including excessive dieting, constant calorie counting, and frequent weighing.

Heredity appears to play a role in the development of eating disorders, accounting for more than 50 percent of the risk. But as with other conditions, only the tendency to develop an eating disorder is explained by heredity; the expression of this tendency is affected by other factors. The home environment is one factor. Families in which there is hostility, abuse, or lack of cohesion provide fertile ground for the development of an eating disorder; a rigid or overprotective parent can also increase risk. Cultural messages, as well as family, friends, and peers, shape attitudes toward the self and others. Comparing yourself negatively with others can damage self-esteem and increase vulnerability. Young people who see themselves as lacking control over their lives are also at high risk for eating orders. About 90 percent of eating disorders begin during adolescence. A 25-year life span reduction can result when the onset occurs between 10 and 15 years of age. In recent years, eating disorder cases have increased among children as young as eight.

QUICK STATS

Nearly 2% of surveyed students felt their academic performance was affected negatively by an eating disorder.

—American College Health Association: Canadian Reference Group, 2013

Certain turning points in life, such as leaving home for university or college, often trigger an eating disorder. How a person copes with such stresses can influence risk, particularly in individuals who have few stress-management skills. An eating disorder may become a means of coping: The abnormal eating behaviour reduces anxiety by producing numbness and alleviating emotional pain. Restrictive dieting is another possible trigger for the development of eating disorders.

Anorexia Nervosa

A person with **anorexia nervosa** does not eat enough food to maintain an adequate, healthy body weight. Anorexia nervosa affects 1 percent of North Americans, 95 percent of whom are female. Because men tend to be more reluctant when it comes to seeking medical assistance or participating in research studies, the rates among males are likely higher than reported. Although it can occur later, anorexia typically develops between the ages of 12 and 18.

> **anorexia nervosa**
> An eating disorder characterized by a refusal to maintain body weight at a minimally healthy level and an intense fear of gaining weight or becoming fat; self-starvation.

Characteristics of Anorexia Nervosa

People with anorexia have an intense fear of gaining weight or becoming fat. Their body image is so distorted that even when emaciated, they think they are fat. People with anorexia may engage in compulsive behaviours or rituals that help keep them from eating, though some may also binge and **purge**. They often use vigorous and prolonged exercise to reduce body weight as well. Although they may express a great interest in food, even taking over the cooking responsibilities for the rest of the family, their own diet becomes more and more extreme. People with anorexia often hide or hoard food without eating it.

> **purge**
> The use of vomiting, laxatives, excessive exercise, restrictive dieting, enemas, diuretics, or diet pills to compensate for food that has been eaten and that the person fears will produce weight gain.

Anorexic people are typically introverted, emotionally reserved, and socially insecure. They are often model children who rarely complain and are anxious to please others and win their approval. Although school performance is typically above average, they are often critical of themselves and not satisfied with their accomplishments. For people with anorexia nervosa, their entire sense of self-esteem may be tied up in their evaluation of their body shape and weight.

Health Risks of Anorexia Nervosa

Because of extreme weight loss, females with anorexia often stop menstruating, become intolerant of cold, and develop low blood pressure and heart rate. They also develop dry skin that is often covered by fine body hair like that of an infant. Their hands and feet may swell and take on a blue tinge.

Anorexia nervosa has been linked to a variety of medical complications, including disorders of the cardiovascular, gastrointestinal, endocrine, and skeletal systems. When body fat is virtually gone and muscles are severely wasted, the body turns to its own organs in a desperate search for protein. Death can occur from heart failure caused by electrolyte imbalances. About one in ten people with anorexia dies of starvation, cardiac arrest, or other medical complications—the highest death rate for any psychiatric disorder. Depression is also a serious risk, and about 20 percent of the fatalities related to anorexia are suicides.

Bulimia Nervosa

A person with **bulimia nervosa** engages in recurrent episodes of binge eating followed by purging. Bulimia is often difficult to recognize because sufferers conceal their eating habits and usually maintain a normal weight, although they may experience weight fluctuations of 5–10 kilograms. Although bulimia usually begins in adolescence or young adulthood, it has begun to emerge at increasingly younger (11–12 years) and older (40–60 years) ages. About 90 percent of bulimia cases are among women.

> **bulimia nervosa**
> An eating disorder characterized by recurrent episodes of binge eating and purging—overeating and then using compensatory behaviours, such as vomiting, laxatives, and excessive exercise, to prevent weight gain.

Characteristics of Bulimia Nervosa

During a binge, a bulimic person may rapidly consume thousands of calories. This is followed by an attempt to get rid of the food by purging, usually by vomiting or using laxatives or diuretics. During a binge, bulimics feel as though they have lost control and cannot stop or limit how much they eat. Some binge and purge only occasionally; others do so many times every day.

People with bulimia may appear to eat normally, but they are rarely comfortable around food. Binges usually occur in secret and can become nightmarish—raiding the kitchen for food, going from one grocery store to another to buy food, or even stealing food. During the binge, food acts as an anaesthetic, and all feelings are blocked out. Afterward, bulimics feel physically drained and emotionally spent. They usually feel deeply ashamed and disgusted with both themselves and their behaviour and terrified that they will gain weight from the binge.

Major life changes, such as leaving for college or university, getting married, having a baby, or losing a job, can trigger a binge-purge cycle. At such times, stress is high and the person may have no good outlet for emotional conflict or tension. As with people with anorexia, people with bulimia are often insecure and depend on others for approval and self-esteem. They may hide difficult emotions, such as anger and disappointment, from themselves and others. Binge eating and purging become a way of dealing with feelings.

Health Risks of Bulimia Nervosa

The binge-purge cycle of bulimia places a tremendous strain on the body and can have serious health effects. Contact with vomited stomach acids erodes tooth enamel. Bulimic people often develop tooth decay because they binge on foods that are high in simple sugars. Repeated vomiting or the use of laxatives, in combination with deficient calorie intake, can damage the liver and kidneys and cause cardiac arrhythmia. Chronic hoarseness and esophageal tearing with bleeding may also result from vomiting. More rarely, binge eating can lead to rupture of the stomach. Although many bulimic women maintain normal weight, even a small weight loss to lower-than-normal weight can cause menstrual problems. And although less often associated with suicide or premature death than anorexia, bulimia is associated with increased depression, excessive preoccupation with food and body image, and sometimes disturbances in cognitive functioning.

Binge-Eating Disorder

Health Canada estimates that **binge-eating disorder** affects about 2 percent of Canadians. It is characterized by uncontrollable eating, usually followed by feelings of guilt and shame with weight gain. Common eating patterns are eating more rapidly than normal, eating until uncomfortably full, eating when not hungry, and preferring to eat alone. Binge eaters may eat large amounts of food throughout the day, with no planned mealtimes. Many people with binge-eating disorder mistakenly see rigid dieting as the only solution to their problem. However, rigid dieting usually causes feelings of deprivation and a return to overeating.

> **binge-eating disorder**
> An eating disorder characterized by binge eating and a lack of control over eating behaviour in general.

Compulsive overeaters rarely eat because of hunger. Instead, food is used as a means of coping with stress, conflict, and other difficult emotions or to provide solace and entertainment. People who do not have the resources to deal effectively with stress may be more vulnerable to binge-eating disorder. Inappropriate overeating often begins during childhood. In some families, eating may be used as an activity to fill otherwise empty time. Parents may reward children with food for good behaviour or withhold food as a means of punishment, thereby creating distorted feelings about the use of food.

Binge eaters are almost always obese, and so they face all the health risks associated with obesity. In addition, binge eaters may have higher rates of depression and anxiety. To overcome binge eating, a person must learn to put food and eating into proper perspective and develop other ways of coping with stress and painful emotions.

Borderline Disordered Eating

Eating habits and body image can fall anywhere on the continuum from healthy to seriously disordered. Where each of us falls can change depending on life stresses, illnesses, and many other factors. People with borderline disordered eating (otherwise referred to as Eating Disorder Not Otherwise Specified or EDNOS) have some or many symptoms of eating disorders but do not meet the full diagnostic criteria for anorexia or bulimia. Such behaviours as excessive dieting, occasional bingeing or purging, or the inability to control eating turn food into the enemy and create havoc in the lives of thousands of Canadians. EDNOS can pose serious health risks to those affected.

How do you know if you have disordered eating habits? When thoughts about food and weight dominate your life, you have a problem. If you are convinced that your worth as a person hinges on how you look and how much you weigh, it's time to get help. Other danger signs include frequent feelings of guilt after a meal or snack, any use of vomiting or laxatives after meals, or over-exercising or severely restricting your food intake to compensate for what you have already eaten.

QUESTIONS FOR CRITICAL THINKING AND REFLECTION

Do you suspect someone you know has an eating disorder? Does the advice in this chapter seem helpful to you? Do you think you could follow it? Why or why not? Have you ever experienced disordered eating patterns yourself? If so, can you identify the reasons for it?

If you suspect you have an eating problem, don't go it alone or delay getting help: Disordered eating habits can develop into a full-blown eating disorder. Check with your student health or counselling centre—nearly all universities and colleges have counsellors and medical personnel who can help you in confidence, or refer you to a specialist if needed. If you are concerned about the eating habits of a family member or friend, refer to the suggestions in the Take Charge box.

Take CHARGE

Does Someone You Know Have an Eating Disorder?

Secrecy and denial are two hallmarks of eating disorders, and so it can be hard to know if someone has anorexia or bulimia. Signs that someone may have anorexia include sudden weight loss, excessive dieting or exercise, guilt or preoccupation with food or eating, frequent weighing, fear of becoming fat despite being thin, and the wearing of baggy or layered clothes to conceal weight loss. Signs that someone may have bulimia include excessive eating without weight gain, secretiveness about food (stealing, hiding, or hoarding food), self-induced vomiting (bathroom visits during or after a meal), swollen glands or a puffy face, erosion of tooth enamel, and use of laxatives, diuretics, or diet pills to control weight.

   If you decide to approach a friend with your concerns, here are some tips to follow:

- Find out about treatment resources in your community (see the For More Information section for suggestions). You may want to consult a professional at your school clinic or counselling centre about the best way to approach the situation.
- Arrange to speak with your friend in a private place, and allow enough time to talk.
- Express your concerns, with specific observations of your friend's behaviour. Expect him or her to deny or minimize the problem and possibly to become angry with you. Stay calm and non-judgmental, and continue to express your concern.
- Avoid giving simplistic advice about eating habits. Listen if your friend wants to talk, and offer your support and understanding. Give your friend the information you found about where he or she can get help, and offer to go along.
- If the situation is an emergency—if your friend has fainted, for example, or attempted suicide—call 911 for help immediately.
- If you are upset about the situation, consider talking to someone yourself. The professionals at the clinic or counselling centre can help you, too. Remember, you are not to blame for another person's eating disorder.

Treating Eating Disorders

The treatment of eating disorders must address both problematic eating behaviours and the misuse of food to manage stress and emotions. Treatment for anorexia nervosa first involves averting a medical crisis by restoring adequate body weight, and then the psychological aspects of the disorder can be addressed. The treatment of bulimia nervosa or binge-eating disorder involves first stabilizing the eating patterns, then identifying and changing the patterns of thinking that led to disordered eating, and then improving coping skills. Concurrent problems, such as depression or anxiety, must also be addressed.

In 2006, a study published in the *Journal of the American Medical Association* showed that the antidepressant Prozac, which is widely used to treat anorexia, worked no better than a placebo in preventing recurrence in women recovering from the disorder. However, the anti-seizure drug topiramate has shown promise in the treatment of bulimia by reducing the urges to binge and purge.

QUICK STATS

15–20% of Canadian women have many of the symptoms of an eating disorder.

—Government of Saskatchewan, 2012

Treatment of eating disorders usually involves a combination of psychotherapy and medical management. The therapy may be carried out individually or in a group; sessions involving the entire family may be recommended. A support or self-help group can be a useful adjunct to such treatment. Medical professionals, including physicians, dentists, gynecologists, and registered dietitians, can evaluate and manage the physical damage caused by the disorder. If a patient is severely depressed or emaciated, hospitalization may be necessary.

 Take **CHARGE**

A Weight-Management Program

The behaviour-management plan described in Chapter 1 provides an excellent framework for a weight-management program. The following are some suggestions about specific ways you can adapt that general plan to controlling your weight.

Motivation and Commitment
Make sure you are motivated and committed before you begin. Failure at weight loss is a frustrating experience that can make it more difficult to lose weight in the future. Think about why you want to lose weight. Self-focused reasons, such as to feel good about yourself or to have a greater sense of well-being, are often associated with success. Trying to lose weight for others or out of concern for how others view you is a poor foundation for a weight-loss program. Make a list of your reasons for wanting to lose weight, and post it in a prominent place.

Setting Goals
Choose a reasonable weight you think you would like to reach over the long term, and be willing to renegotiate it as you get further along. Break down your long-term weight and behavioural goals into a series of short-term goals. Develop a new way of behaving by designing small, manageable steps that will get you to where you want to go.

Creating a Negative Energy Balance
When your weight is constant, you are burning approximately the same number of calories as you are taking in. To tip the energy balance toward weight loss, you must either consume fewer calories or burn more calories through

physical activity or both. One kilogram of body fat represents 7000 calories. To lose weight at the recommended rate of 0.25–1.0 kilogram per week, you must create a negative energy balance of 1750–7000 calories per week or 250–1000 calories per day. To generate a negative energy balance, it's important to consider increasing your activity level and evaluating your calorie consumption.

Physical Activity

Consider how you can increase your energy output simply by increasing routine physical activity, such as walking or taking the stairs. (Chapter 6 lists some activities that use about 150 calories.) If you are not already involved in a regular exercise routine aimed at increasing endurance and building or maintaining muscle mass, seek help from someone who is competent to help you plan and start an appropriate exercise routine. If you are already doing regular physical exercise, evaluate your program according to the guidelines in Chapter 6.

Don't try to use exercise to spot reduce. Leg lifts, for example, contribute to fat loss only to the extent that they burn calories; they don't burn fat just from your legs. You can make parts of your body appear more fit by exercising them, but the only way you can reduce fat in any specific part of your body is to create an overall negative energy balance.

Diet and Eating Habits

If you can't generate a large enough negative energy balance solely by increasing physical activity, you may want to supplement exercise with modest cuts in your calorie intake. Don't think of this as going on a diet; your goal is to make small changes in your diet that you can maintain for a lifetime. Focus on cutting your intake of saturated and trans fats and added sugars and on eating a variety of nutritious foods in moderation. Don't skip meals, fast, or go on a very-low-calorie diet or a diet that is unbalanced.

Making changes in eating habits is another important strategy for weight management. If your program centres on a conscious restriction of certain food items, you are likely to spend all your time thinking about the forbidden foods. Focus on *how* to eat rather than *what* to eat.

Self-Monitoring

Keep a record of your weight and behaviour change progress. Try keeping a record of everything you eat. Write down what you plan to eat, in what quantity, *before* you eat. You will find that just having to record something that is not OK to eat right now is likely to stop you from eating it. If you also note what seems to be triggering your urges to eat (for example, you feel bored, or someone offered you something), you will become more aware of your triggers and be better able to take corrective action. Also, keep track of your daily activities and your formal exercise program so you can monitor increases in physical activity.

Putting Your Plan into Action

- Examine the environmental cues that trigger poor eating and exercise habits, and devise strategies for dealing with them. For example, you may need to remove problem foods from your house temporarily or put a sign on the refrigerator reminding you to go for a walk instead of having a snack. Anticipate problem situations, and plan ways to handle them more effectively. Create new environmental cues that will support your new healthy behaviours. Put your walking shoes by the front door. Move fruits and vegetables to the front of the refrigerator.
- Get others to help. Talk to friends and family members about what they can do to support your efforts. Find a buddy to join you in your exercise program.
- Give yourself lots of praise and rewards. Think about your accomplishments and achievements and congratulate yourself. Plan special non-food treats for yourself, such as a walk or a movie. Reward yourself often and for anything that counts toward success.
- If you slip, tell yourself to get back on track immediately, and don't waste time on self-criticism. Think positively instead of getting into a cycle of guilt and self-blame. Don't demand too much of yourself.
- Don't get discouraged. Be aware that although weight loss is bound to slow down after the first loss of body fluid, the weight loss at this slower rate is more permanent than earlier, more dramatic, losses.
- Remember that weight management is a lifelong project. You need to adopt reasonable goals and strategies that you can maintain over the long term.

SUMMARY

- Body composition is the relative amounts of fat-free mass and fat in the body. *Overweight* and *obesity* refer to body weight or the percentage of body fat that exceeds what is associated with good health.
- The key to weight management is maintaining a balance of calories in (food) and calories out (resting metabolism, food digestion, and physical activity).
- Standards for assessing body weight and body composition include the body mass index (BMI) and percent body fat.
- Too much or too little body fat is linked to health problems; the distribution of body fat can also be a significant risk factor.
- An inaccurate or negative body image is common and can lead to psychological distress.
- Genetic factors help determine a person's weight, but the influence of heredity can be overcome with attention to lifestyle factors.
- Physiological factors involved in the regulation of body weight and body fat include metabolic rate, hormonal influences, and the size and number of fat cells.
- Nutritional guidelines for weight management include consuming a moderate number of calories; limiting portion sizes, energy density, and the intake of fat, simple sugars, refined carbohydrates, and protein to recommended levels; and developing an eating schedule and rules for food choices.
- Activity guidelines for weight management emphasize daily physical activity and regular sessions of cardiorespiratory endurance exercise and strength training.
- Weight management requires developing positive, realistic self-talk and self-esteem and a repertoire of appropriate techniques for handling stress and other emotional and physical challenges.
- Many people are successful at long-term weight loss on their own by combining diet and exercise.
- Diet books, fad diets, OTC diet aids and supplements, and formal weight-loss programs should be assessed for safety and efficacy.
- Professional help is needed in cases of severe or morbid obesity; medical treatments include prescription drugs, surgery, and psychological therapy.
- Dissatisfaction with weight and shape are common to all eating disorders. Anorexia nervosa is characterized by self-starvation, distorted body image, and an intense fear of gaining weight. Bulimia nervosa is characterized by recurrent episodes of uncontrolled binge eating and frequent purging. Binge-eating disorder involves binge eating without regular use of compensatory purging.

FOR MORE INFORMATION

BOOKS

Akabas, S. R., S. A. Lederman, and B. J. Moore. 2012. *Textbook of Obesity*. Sussex, UK: Wiley-Blackwell. A discussion of the biological, psychological, and cultural influences of obesity.

Brownell, K. D. 2004. *The LEARN Program for Weight Management (10th ed.)*. Dallas, Tx: American Health Publishing. An approach to weight management that considers lifestyle, exercise, attitudes, relationships, and nutrition.

Freedhoff, Y. 2014. *The Diet Fix: Why Diets Fail and How to Make Yours Work*. USA: Random House Canada. An approach to weight-management that considers physical and mental realms.

Gaesser, G. A., and K. Kratina. 2006. *It's the Calories, Not the Carbs*. Victoria, B.C.: Trafford. A detailed look at the facts behind successful weight loss that shuns fad diets and encourages sound energy balance.

Hensrud, D. D. 2005. *Mayo Clinic Healthy Weight for Everyone*. Rochester, Minn.: Mayo Clinic. Guidelines for successful weight management.

Hu, F. B. 2008. *Obesity Epidemiology*. New York: Oxford University Press. An in-depth look at the latest research on all facets of obesity.

Ihde, G. M. 2006. *Considering Weight-Loss Surgery: The Facts You Need to Know for a Healthy Recovery.* Victoria, BC: Trafford. An easy-to-read guide to the benefits and risks of weight-loss surgery.

Milchovich, S. K., and B. Dunn-Long. 2011. *Diabetes Mellitus: A Practical Handbook,* 10th. ed. Boulder, Colo.: Bull. A user-friendly guide to diabetes.

ORGANIZATIONS, HOTLINES, AND WEBSITES

The Internet addresses listed here were accurate at the time of publication.

Canadian Diabetes Association. Provides information, literature, and guidance for living with and managing diabetes.
http://www.diabetes.ca

Canadian Fitness and Lifestyle Research Institute. Provides research findings and recommendations to increase population levels of physical activity and improve the health of all Canadians.
http://www.cflri.ca

Canadian Obesity Network. Provides Canadian obesity-related research, guidelines, and resources for everyone interested in reducing obesity rates.
http://www.obesitynetwork.ca

Calorie Control Council. Provides a variety of interactive calculators, including an Exercise Calculator that estimates the calories burned from various forms of physical activity.
http://www.caloriecontrol.org

Directory of Canada Eating Disorder Treatment Programs. Provides a comprehensive list of links to resources on eating disorders throughout Canada.
http://www.canadadrugrehab.ca/Eating-Disorder-Treatment.html

MedlinePlus: Eating Disorders. Includes information from the U.S. National Library of Medicine.
http://www.nlm.nih.gov/medlineplus/eatingdisorders.html

National Eating Disorders Information Centre. Provides information and resources on eating disorders and food and weight preoccupation.
http://www.nedic.ca

U.S. National Heart, Lung, and Blood Institute: What is a Healthy Weight? Provides information and tips on diet and physical activity, as well as a BMI calculator.
http://www.nhlbi.nih.gov/health/educational/wecan/healthy-weight-basics/healthy-weight.htm

See also the listings in Chapters 5 and 6.

SELECTED BIBLIOGRAPHY

Adams, K. F., et al. 2006. Overweight, obesity, and mortality in a large prospective cohort of persons 50 to 71 years old. *New England Journal of Medicine* 355(8): 763–778.

American Heart Association. *Policy statement on environmental endocrine disrupting chemicals and the impact on obesity and cardiovascular disease,* http://www.heart.org/idc/groups/heart-public/@ wcm/@adv/documents/downloadable/ucm_467655.pdf (retrieved June 6, 2015).

Baker, B. 2006. Weight loss and diet plans. *American Journal of Nursing* 106(6): 52–59.

Behn, A., and E. Ur. 2006. The obesity epidemic and its cardiovascular consequences. *Current Opinions in Cardiology* 21(4): 353–360.

Bowman, S. A., et al. 2004. Effects of fast-food consumption on energy intake and diet quality among children in a national household survey. *Pediatrics* 113(1 Pt 1): 112–118.

Buchwald, H., et al. 2004. Bariatric surgery: A systematic review and meta-analysis. *Journal of the American Medical Association* 292(14): 1724–1737.

Canada. House of Commons Health Committee. 2007. *Healthy Weights for Healthy Kids,* http://www. parl.gc.ca/content/hoc/Committee/391/HESA/Reports/RP2795145/hesarp07/hesarp07-e.pdf (retrieved March 17, 2015).

Canadian Medical Association. 2007. 2006 Canadian clinical practice guidelines on the management and prevention of obesity in adults and children, *CMAJ* 176 (8 Suppl.): 1–120, http://www.cmaj.ca/cgi/content/full/176/8/S1/DC1 (retrieved March 20, 2015).

Casazza, K. et al. 2013. Myths, presumptions, and facts and obesity. *New England Journal of Medicine* 368(5): 446–454.

Chandon, P., and B. Wansink. 2007. The biasing health halos of fast-food restaurant health claims: Lower calorie estimates and higher side-dish consumption intentions. *Journal of Consumer Research* 34(3): 301–314.

Dahlman, I., and P. Arner. Obesity and polymorphisms in genes regulating human adipose tissue. *International Journal of Obesity* 31(11): 1629–1641.

Dhingra, R., et al. 2007. Soft drink consumption and risk of developing cardiometabolic risk factors and the metabolic syndrome in middle-aged adults in the community. *Circulation* 116(5): 480–488.

Dietz, W. H. 1994. Critical periods in childhood for the development of obesity. *American Journal of Clinical Nutrition* 59: 955–959.

Dong, L., G. Block, and S. Mandel. 2004. Activities contributing to total energy expenditure in the United States: Results from the NHAPS Study. *International Journal of Behavioral Nutrition and Physical Activity* 1(4): 1–11.

Drewnowski, A., and F. Bellisle. 2007. Liquid calories, sugar and body weight. *American Journal of Clinical Nutrition* 85(3): 651–661.

Farshchi, H. R., M. A. Taylor, and I. A. Macdonald. 2005. Deleterious effects of omitting breakfast on insulin sensitivity and fasting lipid profiles in healthy lean women. *American Journal of Clinical Nutrition* 81(2): 388–396.

Fenicchia, L. M., et al. 2004. Influence of resistance exercise training on glucose control in women with type 2 diabetes. *Metabolism* 53(3): 284–289.

Flegal, K. M., et al. 2005. Excess deaths associated with underweight, overweight, and obesity. *Journal of the American Medical Association* 293(15): 1861–1867.

Fung, T. T., et al. 2004. Dietary patterns, meat intake, and the risk of type 2 diabetes in women. *Archives of Internal Medicine* 64(20): 2235–2240.

Graves, B. S., and R. L. Welsh. 2004. Recognizing the signs of body dysmorphic disorder and muscle dysmorphia. *ACSM's Health and Fitness Journal* 8(1): 11–13.

Hamilton, M., et al. 2007. Role of low energy expenditure and sitting in obesity, metabolic syndrome, type 2 diabetes, and cardiovascular disease. *Diabetes* 56(11): 2655–2667.

Harvard T. H. Chan School of Public Health. 2015. *Measuring Obesity,* http://www.hsph.harvard.edu/obesity-prevention-source/obesity-definition/how-to-measure-body-fatness/ (retrieved June 6, 2015).

He, M., et al. 2012. Obesogenic neighbourhoods: The impact of neighbourhood restaurants and convenience stores on adolecents' food consumption behaviours. *Public Health Nutrition* 15(12): 2331–2339.

Health Canada. 2002. *A Report on Mental Illnesses in Canada,* http://www.phac-aspc.gc.ca/publicat/miic-mmac/index-eng.php (retrieved March 20, 2015).

Herrera, B. M. 2011. Genetics and epigenetics of obesity. *Maturitas* 69: 41–49.

Hu, F. B., et al. 2004. Adiposity as compared with physical activity in predicting mortality among women. *New England Journal of Medicine* 351(26): 2694–2703.

Ibrahim, M. M. 2010. Etiology and pathophysiology: Subcutaneous and visceral adipose tissue: Structural and functional differences. *Obesity Reviews* 11: 11–18.

INSPQ Public Health Expertise and Reference Centre. 2014. The economic impact of obesity and overweight, http://www.inspq.qc.ca/pdf/publications/1799_Topo_9_VA.pdf (retrieved July 23, 2015).

Janssen, I. 2013. The public health burden of obesity in Canada. *Canadian Journal of Diabetes* 37:90–96.

Kaiser Family Foundation. 2004. The role of media in childhood obesity. *Issue Brief,* February, http://kff.org/other/issue-brief/the-role-of-media-in-childhood-obesity-2/ (retrieved March 20, 2015).

Karmali, S., et al. 2010. Bariatric surgery: A primer. *Canadian Family Physician* 56(9): 873–879.

Kumanyika, S. K, et al. 2008. Population-based prevention of obesity: The need for comprehensive promotion of healthful eating, physical activity, and energy balance: A scientific statement from American Heart Association Council on Epidemiology and Prevention, Interdisciplinary Committee for Prevention (formerly the Expert Panel on Population and Prevention Science). *Circulation* 118(4): 428–464.

Lau, D. C. W., et al. 2007. 2006 Canadian clinical practice guidelines on the management and prevention of obesity in adults and Children. *Canadian Medical Association Journal* 176(8): S1–13.

Le Petit, C. 2005. *How many obese Canadians can we expect by 2010 and 2020?* Presented at the 96th Annual Canadian Public Health Association Conference. Ottawa, Ontario, September 18–21.

Ma, Y., et al. 2005. Association between dietary carbohydrates and body weight. *American Journal of Epidemiology* 161(4): 359–367.

McBride, B. F., et al. 2004. Electrocardiographic and hemodynamic effects of a multicomponent dietary supplement containing ephedra and caffeine. *Journal of the American Medical Association* 291(4): 216–221.

McCullough, P. A., et al. 2006. Cardiorespiratory fitness and short-term complications after bariatric surgery. *CHEST* 130: 517–525.

Meier, E. P., and J. Gray. 2014. Facebook photo activity associated with body image disturbance in adolescent girls. *Cyberpsychology, Behavior, and Social Networking* 17(4): 199–206.

Muenning, P., et al. 2006. Gender and the burden of disease attributable to obesity. *American Journal of Public Health* 96(9): 1662–1668.

Newnham-Kanas, C., J. D. Irwin, and D. Morrow. 2008. Life coaching as an intervention for individual with obesity. *International Journal of Evidence-Based Coaching and Mentoring* 6(2): 1–12.

Nicklas, B. J., et al. 2004. Association of visceral adipose tissue with incident myocardial infarction in older men and women: "The Health, Aging and Body Composition Study." *American Journal of Epidemiology* 160(8): 741–749.

O'Brien, P., et al. 2006. Treatment of mild to moderate obesity with laparoscopic adjustable gastric banding or an intensive medical program. *Annals of Internal Medicine* 144(9): 625–633.

Ogden, C. L., et al. 2007. Obesity among adults in the United States: No change since 2003–2004. *National Center for Health Statistics Data Brief* 1: 1–8.

Olshansky, S. J., et al. 2005. A potential decline in life expectancy in the United States in the 21st century. *New England Journal of Medicine* 352(11): 1138–1145.

Padwal, R. S., et al. 2012. Characteristics of the population eligible for and receiving publicly funded bariatric surgery in Canada. *International Journal for Equity in Health* 11: 54.

Pearson, E. S., et al. 2013. The CHANGE Program: Comparing an interactive versus prescriptive approach to self-management among university students with obesity. *Canadian Journal of Diabetes* 37: 4–11.

Rubin, C. T., et al. 2007. Adipogenesis is inhibited by brief, daily exposure to high-frequency, extremely low-magnitude mechanical signals. *Proceedings of the National Academy of Sciences* 104(45): 17879–17884.

Saaristo, T., et al. 2010. Lifestyle intervention for prevention of type 2 diabetes in primary health care: One-year follow-up of the Finnish National Diabetes Prevention Program (FIN-D2D). *Diabetes Care* 33 (10): 2146–2151.

Schulze, M. B., et al. 2004. Sugar-sweetened beverages, weight gain, and incidence of type 2 diabetes in young and middle-aged women. *Journal of the American Medical Association* 292(8): 927–934.

Shankar, K., et al. 2008. Maternal obesity at conception programs obesity in the offspring. *American Journal of Physiology: Regulatory, Integrative and Comparative Physiology* 294: R528–R523.

Statistics Canada. 2010. *Canadian Health Measures Survey: Cycle 1 Data Tables, 2007–2009,* http://www.statcan.gc.ca/pub/82-623-x/82-623-x2010002-eng.pdf (retrieved March 20, 2015).

Taillon, A., et al. 2013. Inference-based therapy for body dysmorphic disorder. *Clinical Psychology and Psychotherapy* 20: 67–76.

Taylor, E. N., et al. 2005. Obesity, weight gain, and risk of kidney stones. *Journal of the American Medical Association* 293(4): 455–462.

Tsai, A. G., and T. A. Wadden. 2005. Systematic review: An evaluation of major commercial weight loss programs in the United States. *Annals of Internal Medicine* 142(1): 56–66.

University of Montreal. 2010. New therapy to overcome body dysmorphic disorder. *U de M Nouvelles,* http://www.nouvelles.umontreal.ca/udem-news/news/20100628-new-therapy-to-overcome-body-dysmorphic-disorder.html (retrieved March 20, 2015).

van Dam, R. M., et al. 2006. The relationship between overweight in adolescence and premature death in women. *Annals of Internal Medicine* 145(2): 91–97.

Vorona, R. D., et al. 2005. Overweight and obese patients in a primary care population report less sleep than patients with a normal body mass index. *Archives of Internal Medicine* 165: 25–30.

Walsh, T. B., et al. 2006. Fluoxetine after weight restoration in anorexia nervosa. *Journal of the American Medical Association* 295(22): 2605–2612.

Wang, Y., and M. A. Beydoun. 2007. The obesity epidemic in the United States—gender, age, socioeconomic, racial/ethnic and geographical characteristics: A systematic review and meta-regression analysis. *Epidemiologic Reviews* 29: 6–28.

Wansink, B., and P. Chandon. 2006. Meal size, not body size, explains errors in estimating calorie content of meals. *Annals of Internal Medicine* 145: 326–332.

Weinstein, A. R., et al. 2004. Relationship of physical activity vs. body mass index with type 2 diabetes in women. *Journal of the American Medical Association* 292(10): 1188–1194.

Weinstein, P. K. 2006. A review of weight loss programs delivered via the Internet. *Journal of Cardiovascular Nursing* 21(4): 251–258.

Wong, S. L., et al. 2004. Cardiorespiratory fitness is associated with lower abdominal fat independent of body mass index. *Medicine and Science in Sports and Exercise* 36(2): 286–291.

World Health Organization. 1998. *Obesity: Preventing and Managing the Global Epidemic: Report of a WHO Consultation on Obesity.* Geneva, Switzerland: WHO.

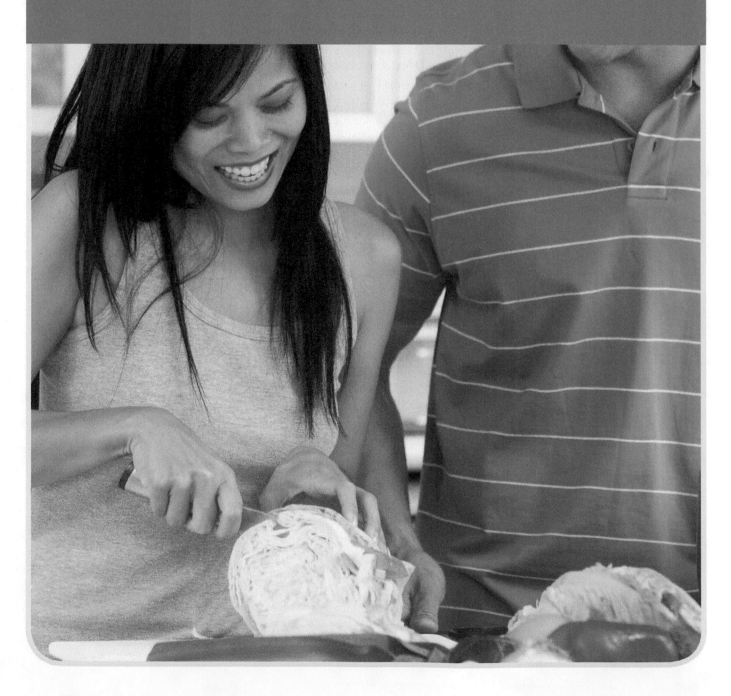

CHAPTER 5

Nutrition Basics

LOOKING AHEAD

After you have read and studied this chapter, you should be able to:

LO1 List the essential nutrients, and describe the functions they perform in the body

LO2 Describe the guidelines that have been developed to help people choose a healthy diet, avoid nutritional deficiencies, and reduce their risk of diet-related chronic diseases

LO3 Discuss nutritional guidelines for vegetarians and for special population groups

LO4 Explain how to use food labels and other consumer tools to make informed choices about foods

LO5 Put together a personal nutrition plan based on affordable foods that you enjoy and that will promote wellness, today as well as in the future

TEST YOUR KNOWLEDGE

1. **It is recommended that all adults consume one to two servings of fruits and vegetables every day.**
   True or false?

2. **How many French fries are in one small serving?**
   a. 10 b. 15 c. 25

3. **Which of the following is not a whole grain?**
   a. brown rice b. wheat flour c. popcorn

4. **Registered dietitians advise reduced intake of saturated and trans fats for which of the following reasons?**
   a. They increase the levels of low-density lipoproteins (LDL), or "bad" cholesterol.
   b. They provide more calories than other types of fat.
   c. They increase the risk of heart disease.

ANSWERS

1. FALSE.   Adult females should consume seven to eight servings of vegetables and fruit daily; adult males should consume eight to ten servings of vegetables and fruit daily.

2. c.   Many people underestimate the size of the portions they eat, leading to overconsumption of calories and fat. A small serving of French fries (about 75 grams) contains between 20 and 25 fries.

3. b.   Unless labelled as whole wheat, wheat flour is processed to remove the bran and the germ and is not a whole grain.

4. a and c.   High intake of saturated and trans fats raises LDL levels and the risk of heart disease. Saturated and trans fats provide the same number of calories as other types of fat: 9 calories per gram (compared with 4 calories per gram for protein and carbohydrate).

In the course of your lifetime, you will spend about six years eating—about 70 000 meals and 54 metric tons of food. What you eat can have profound effects on your health and well-being. Your nutritional habits help determine your risk of major chronic diseases, including heart disease, cancer, stroke, and diabetes. Choosing foods that provide the nutrients you need while limiting the substances linked to disease should be an important part of your daily life.

Choosing a healthy diet is a two-part process. First, you have to know which nutrients you need and in what amounts. Second, you have to translate those requirements into a diet consisting of foods you like that are both available and affordable. Once you know what constitutes a healthy diet for you, you can adjust your current diet to bring it into line with your goals.

This chapter explains the basic principles of **nutrition**. It introduces the six classes of essential nutrients and explains their roles in the functioning of the body. It also provides guidelines that you can use to design a healthy diet plan. Finally, it offers practical tools and advice to help you apply the guidelines to your own life.

nutrition
The science of food and how the body uses it in health and disease.

Nutritional Requirements: Components of a Healthy Diet

You probably think about your diet in terms of the foods you like to eat. What's important for your health, though, are the nutrients contained in those foods. Your body requires proteins, fats, carbohydrates, vitamins, minerals, and water—about 50 **essential nutrients**. In this context, the word *essential* means that you must get these substances from food because your body is unable to manufacture them, or at least not fast enough to meet your physiological needs. The six classes of nutrients, along with their functions and major sources, are listed in Table 5.1. The body needs some essential nutrients in relatively large amounts; these **macronutrients** include protein, fat, and carbohydrate. **Micronutrients**, such as vitamins and minerals, are required in much smaller amounts. Your body obtains these nutrients through the process of **digestion**, in which the foods you eat are broken down into compounds your gastrointestinal tract can absorb and your body can

TABLE 5.1

The Six Classes of Essential Nutrients

Nutrient	Function	Major Sources
Proteins (4 calories/gram)	Form important parts of muscles, bone, blood, enzymes, some hormones, and cell membranes; repair tissue; regulate water and acid-base balance; help in growth; supply energy	Meat, fish, poultry, eggs, milk products, legumes, nuts
Carbohydrates (4 calories/gram)	Supply energy to cells in brain, nervous system, and blood; supply energy to muscles during exercise	Grains (breads and cereals), fruits, vegetables, milk
Fats (9 calories/gram)	Supply energy; insulate, support, and cushion organs; provide medium for absorption of fat-soluble vitamins	Animal foods, grains, nuts, seeds, fish, vegetables
Vitamins	Promote (initiate or speed up) specific chemical reactions within cells	Abundant in fruits, vegetables, and grains; also found in meat and dairy products
Minerals	Help regulate body functions; aid in growth and maintenance of body tissues; act as catalysts for release of energy	Found in most food groups
Water	Makes up approximately 60 percent of body weight; provides medium for chemical reactions; transports chemicals; regulates temperature; removes waste products	Fruits, vegetables, liquids

use (see Figure 5.1). A diet that provides enough essential nutrients is vital because various nutrients provide energy, help build and maintain body tissues, and help regulate body functions (see the Mind Body Spirit box).

essential nutrients
Substances the body must get from foods because it cannot manufacture them at all or fast enough to meet its needs; include proteins, fats, carbohydrates, vitamins, minerals, and water.

macronutrients
Essential nutrients required by the body in relatively large amounts.

micronutrients
Essential nutrients required by the body in minute amounts.

digestion
The process of breaking down foods in the gastrointestinal tract into compounds the body can absorb.

Calories

The energy in foods is expressed as **kilocalories**. One kilocalorie represents the amount of heat it takes to raise the temperature of 1 litre of water by 1 degree Celsius. A person needs about 2000 kilocalories per day to meet his or her energy needs. In common usage, people usually refer to kilocalories as *calories*, which is technically a much smaller energy unit: 1 kilocalorie contains 1000 calories. This text uses the familiar word *calorie* to stand for the larger energy unit; you will also find the word *calorie* used on food labels.

kilocalorie
A measure of energy content in food; 1 kilocalorie represents the amount of heat needed to raise the temperature of 1 litre of water by 1 degree Celsius; commonly referred to as a *calorie*.

Of the six classes of essential nutrients, three supply energy:
- Fat = 9 calories per gram
- Protein = 4 calories per gram
- Carbohydrate = 4 calories per gram

Alcohol, though not an essential nutrient, also supplies energy, providing 7 calories per gram. The high caloric content of fat is one reason experts often advise against high fat consumption; most of us do not need the extra calories to meet energy needs. Regardless of their source, calories consumed in excess of energy needs are converted to fat and stored in the body.

But just meeting energy needs is not enough; our bodies need enough of the essential nutrients to grow and function properly. Practically all

FIGURE 5.1

The Digestive System

Food is partially broken down by being chewed and mixed with saliva in the mouth. After travelling to the stomach via the esophagus, food is broken down further by stomach acids and other secretions. As food moves through the digestive tract, it is mixed by muscular contractions and broken down by chemicals. Most absorption of nutrients occurs in the small intestine, aided by secretions from the pancreas, gallbladder, and intestinal lining. The large intestine reabsorbs excess water; the remaining solid wastes are collected in the rectum and excreted through the anus.

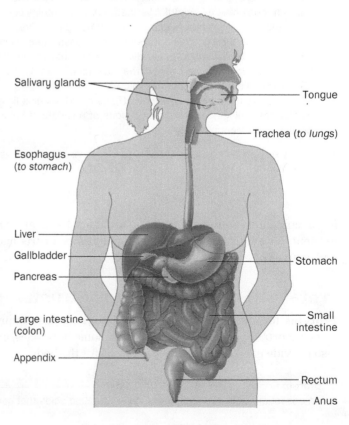

Salivary glands
Tongue
Trachea (*to lungs*)
Esophagus (*to stomach*)
Liver
Gallbladder
Pancreas
Stomach
Large intestine (colon)
Small intestine
Appendix
Rectum
Anus

Mind *Body* SPIRIT

Eating Habits and Total Wellness

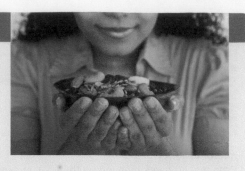

Healthy eating does more than nourish your body; it enhances your ability to enjoy life to the fullest by improving overall wellness, both physical and mental. One study examined a group of adults who followed a healthy eating plan for four years. At the end of this period, the study subjects were more confident with their food choices and more satisfied with their lives in general than their peers who did not make any dietary changes. The reverse is also true: when people overeat, they often have feelings of guilt, anger, discouragement, and even self-loathing. Out-of-control eating can erode self-confidence and lead to depression.

Can individual foods affect the way we feel? Limited scientific evidence points to some correlation between certain foods and our mood. Many people, especially women, seem to crave chocolate when they feel slightly depressed. Studies show that chocolate, in small quantities, may indeed give you a lift. Sugary foods tend to temporarily raise serotonin levels in the brain, which can improve mood (serotonin is a neurotransmitter associated with a calm, relaxed state). The fat found in chocolate acts to increase endorphins, brain chemicals that reduce pain and increase feelings of well-being. Chocolate also contains a variety of other less studied chemicals that may have a positive impact on mood.

A commonly held belief about the connection between food and the mind is that eating sugary foods makes people (especially children) hyperactive. Parents often comment on the wild behaviour observed at parties and festive events where many sweets are consumed. However, several carefully controlled studies showed no correlation between behaviour and the consumption of sugary foods. Researchers speculate that high-sugar foods tend to be eaten at birthday parties and other exciting occasions when children tend to be highly stimulated regardless of what they eat.

Some recent research shows that eating certain carbohydrate-rich foods, such as a plain baked potato or a bagel with jelly, can have a temporary calming effect. This effect is most pronounced when rapidly digestible carbohydrates are consumed alone, with no fats or proteins in the meal. The practical implications of this research are uncertain.

If you are looking for a mental boost, some scientists think that eating a meal consisting primarily of protein-rich foods may be helpful. The theory is that proteins contain the amino acid tyrosine, which the body uses to make the neurotransmitters dopamine and norepinephrine. Some researchers think that eating protein-rich foods could increase the synthesis of these neurotransmitters, which can speed reaction time and increase alertness. Whether this really works, especially in well-nourished individuals who have not been lacking these nutrients to begin with, remains to be seen. In the meantime, it wouldn't hurt, and might even help, to include some protein in the meal you eat before your next big exam.

What we know about how food affects mood remains limited. But evidence points to the common-sense conclusion that enjoying reasonable portions of a variety of healthy and tasty foods is a great way to optimize your physical and mental health.

Source: Fahey, T. D., P. M. Insel, and W. T. Roth. 2007. *Fit and Well*, 8th ed. New York: McGraw-Hill. Copyright © 2007 The McGraw-Hill Companies, Inc.

foods contain mixtures of nutrients, although foods are commonly classified according to the predominant nutrient; for example, spaghetti is thought of as a carbohydrate. The following sections discuss the function and sources of each class of nutrients.

Proteins: The Basis of Body Structure

Proteins form important parts of the body's main structural components: muscles and bones. Proteins also form important parts of blood, enzymes, some hormones, and cell membranes. As mentioned earlier, proteins also provide energy (4 calories per gram) for the body.

> **protein**
> An essential nutrient; a compound made of amino acids that contains carbon, hydrogen, oxygen, and nitrogen.

Amino Acids

The building blocks of proteins are called **amino acids**. Twenty common amino acids are found in food; nine of these are essential: histidine, isoleucine, leucine, lysine, methionine, phenylalanine, threonine, tryptophan, and valine. The other eleven amino acids can be produced by the body, given the presence of the needed components supplied by foods.

amino acids
The building blocks of proteins.

Complete and Incomplete Proteins

Individual protein sources are considered *complete* if they supply all the essential amino acids in adequate amounts and are *incomplete* if they do not. Meat, fish, poultry, eggs, milk, cheese, and soy provide complete proteins. Incomplete proteins, which come from other plant sources, such as **legumes** and nuts, are good sources of most essential amino acids but are usually low in one or two.

legumes
Vegetables, such as peas and beans, that are high in fibre and are also important sources of protein.

Certain combinations of vegetable proteins, such as wheat and peanuts in a peanut butter sandwich, allow each vegetable protein to make up for the amino acids missing in the other protein. The combination yields a complete protein. Many traditional Aboriginal food pairings, such as wild turkey, wild rice, potatoes, bannock or cornbread, squash, and beans, emerged as dietary staples because they are complementary proteins.

QUICK STATS

Worldwide, 45% of childhood deaths and 11% of diseases are attributable to undernutrition.
—*Lancet*, 2013; United Nations, 2012

It was once believed that vegetarians had to complement their proteins at each meal to receive the benefit of a complete protein. It is now known, however, that proteins consumed throughout the day can complement one another and form a pool of amino acids the body can draw from to produce the necessary proteins. Vegetarians should include a variety of vegetable protein sources in their diets to make sure they get all the essential amino acids in adequate amounts. (Healthy vegetarian diets are discussed later in the chapter.) The majority of the protein in the Canadian comes from animal sources (meat and dairy), making our diet rich in essential amino acids.

Hemp, chia seeds, and quinoa are other popular sources of protein. These foods do not have as much protein as legumes, meats, fish, or poultry but can contribute to your overall intake of protein in a moderate way. For example, quinoa is a nutritious grain that happens to be higher in protein and iron compared to other grain products. It is also a good source of fibre in the diet. There is 2 grams of protein in ½ cup (125 mL) of cooked quinoa.

Recommended Protein Intake

Adequate daily intake of protein for adults is 0.8 gram per kilogram of body weight, corresponding to about 50 grams of protein per day for someone who weighs 63 kilograms and 65 grams of protein for someone who weighs 81 kilograms. Table 5.2 lists some popular food items and the amount of protein each provides.

TABLE 5.2

Protein Content of Common Food Items

Item	Protein (grams)
90 g lean meat, poultry, or fish	20–25
125 mL (½ cup) tofu	20–25
250 mL (1 cup) dried beans	15–20
250 mL (1 cup) milk, yogourt	8–12
45 g cheese	8–12
1 serving of cereals, grains, nuts, vegetables	2–4

Most Canadians meet or exceed the protein intake needed for adequate nutrition. If you consume more protein than your body needs, the extra protein is synthesized into fat for energy storage or burned for energy requirements. A little extra protein is not harmful, but it can contribute fat to the diet because protein-rich foods are often fat-rich as well.

A very high protein intake can also strain the kidneys. A fairly broad range of protein intakes is associated with good health, and Health Canada's Expert Advisory Committee on Dietary Reference Intakes (DRIs) recommends that protein intake should be 10–35 percent of total daily caloric intake, depending on the individual's age. The average Canadian diet for adult men and women includes about 17 percent of total daily calories as protein.

Fats: Essential in Small Amounts

Fats, also known as *lipids*, are the most concentrated source of energy, at 9 calories per gram. The fats stored in your body represent usable energy, they help insulate your body, and they support and cushion your organs. Fats in the diet help your body absorb fat-soluble vitamins and add important flavour and texture to foods. Fats are the major fuel for the body during rest and light activity.

Two fats, linoleic acid and alpha-linolenic acid, are essential components of the diet. They are used to make compounds that are key regulators of many body functions, such as the maintenance of blood pressure and the progress of a healthy pregnancy.

Types and Sources of Fats

Most of the fats in foods are fairly similar in composition, generally including a molecule of glycerol (an alcohol) with three fatty acid chains attached to it. The resulting structure is called a *triglyceride* (see Figure 5.2). Animal fat, for example, is made primarily of triglycerides.

Within a triglyceride, differences in the fatty acid structure result in different types of fats. Depending on this structure, a fat may be unsaturated, monounsaturated, polyunsaturated, or saturated. (The essential fatty acids—linoleic and alpha-linolenic acids—are both polyunsaturated.) The different types of fatty acids have different characteristics and different effects on your health.

Food fats are usually composed of both saturated and unsaturated fatty acids; the dominant type of fatty acid determines the fat's characteristics. Food fats containing large amounts of saturated fatty acids are usually solid at room temperature; they are generally found naturally in animal products. The leading sources of saturated fat in the Canadian diet are red meats (hamburger, steak, roasts), homogenized milk, cheese, hot dogs, and lunchmeats. Food fats containing large amounts of monounsaturated and polyunsaturated fatty acids usually come from plant sources and are liquid at room temperature. Olive, canola, safflower, and peanut oils contain mostly monounsaturated fatty acids. Soybean, corn, and cottonseed oils contain mostly polyunsaturated fatty acids.

FIGURE 5.2

A Triglyceride

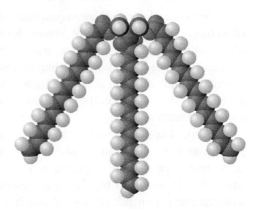

QUICK STATS

Canadians, on average, consume 8.4 grams of trans fatty acids each day.

—Trans Fat Task Force, 2006

Hydrogenation

Notable exceptions to these generalizations exist. When unsaturated vegetable oils undergo the process of **hydrogenation**, a mixture of saturated and unsaturated fatty acids is produced, creating a more solid fat from a liquid oil. Hydrogenation also changes some unsaturated fatty acids to **trans fatty acids,** unsaturated fatty acids with an atypical shape that affects their behaviour in the body. Food manufacturers use hydrogenation to increase the stability of an oil so it can be reused for deep frying, to improve the texture of certain foods (to make pastries and pie crusts flakier, for example), and to extend the shelf life of foods made with oil. Hydrogenation is also used to transform a liquid oil into margarine or vegetable shortening.

> **hydrogenation**
> A process by which hydrogens are addedto unsaturated fats, increasing the degree of saturation and turning liquid oils into solid fats. Hydrogenation produces a mixture of saturated fatty acids and standard and trans forms of unsaturated fatty acids.
>
> **trans fatty acid**
> A type of unsaturated fatty acid produced during the process of hydrogenation; trans fats have an atypical shape that affects their chemical activity.

Many baked and fried foods are prepared with hydrogenated vegetable oils, so they can be relatively high in saturated and trans fatty acids. Leading sources of trans fats in the Canadian diet are processed foods, such as crackers, cookies, doughnuts, cakes, pastries, muffins, croissants, snack foods, fried foods (such as French fries), and breaded foods. In general, the more solid a hydrogenated oil is, the more saturated and trans fats it contains; for example, hard margarines typically contain more saturated and trans fats than do soft margarines. Small amounts of trans fatty acids are also found naturally in meat and milk.

Hydrogenated vegetable oils are not the only plant fats that contain saturated fats. Palm and coconut oils, although derived from plants, are also highly saturated. However, fish oils, derived from an animal source, are rich in polyunsaturated fats.

Fats and Health

Different types of fats have very different effects on health. Many studies have examined the effects of dietary fat intake on blood **cholesterol** levels and the risk of heart disease. Saturated and trans fatty acids raise blood levels of **low-density lipoprotein (LDL),** or "bad" cholesterol, thereby increasing a person's risk of heart disease. Unsaturated fatty acids lower LDL. Monounsaturated fatty acids, such as those found in olive and canola oils, may also increase levels of **high-density lipoprotein (HDL),** or "good" cholesterol, providing even greater benefits for heart health. In large amounts, trans fatty acids may lower HDL. Saturated fats have been found to impair the ability of HDLs to prevent inflammation of the blood vessels, one of the key factors in vascular disease; they have also been found to reduce the ability of the blood vessels to react normally to stress. Thus, to reduce the risk of heart disease, it is important to choose unsaturated fats instead of saturated and trans fats. (See Chapter 7 for more on cholesterol.)

> **cholesterol**
> A waxy substance found in the blood and cells and needed for synthesis of cell membranes, vitamin D, and hormones.
>
> **low-density lipoprotein (LDL)**
> Blood fat that transports cholesterol to organs and tissues; excess amounts result in the accumulation of deposits on artery walls.
>
> **high-density lipoprotein (HDL)**
> Blood fat that helps transport cholesterol out of the arteries, thereby protecting against heart disease.

Health experts are particularly concerned about Canadians' consumption of trans fats because of their triple negative effects on heart health—they raise LDL, lower HDL, and produce inflammation—and because the public is less aware of trans fats than of saturated fats. Since September 2005, food labels have included the trans fat content. Consumers can also check for the presence of trans fats by reading the ingredient list of a food, looking for *partially hydrogenated oil* or *vegetable shortening.*

For heart health, it's important to have a moderate intake of your consumption of saturated and minimize your intake of trans fats. The best way to reduce saturated fat in your diet is to lower your intake of meat and full-fat dairy products (homogenized milk, cream, butter, cheese, yogourt, ice cream). To lower trans fats, decrease your intake of deep-fried foods and processed foods, such as crackers, cookies, and other baked goods made with hydrogenated vegetable oils; use liquid oils for cooking; and favour soft margarines over hard margarines. Remember, the softer or more liquid a fat is, the less saturated and trans fat it is likely to contain.

Although saturated and trans fats pose health hazards, other fats can be beneficial. When used in place of saturated fats, monounsaturated fatty acids, found in avocados, most nuts, and olive, canola, peanut, and safflower oils, improve blood cholesterol levels and may help protect against some cancers. Remember that fats can quickly add up in your diet. Whatever the source of fat in your diet, enjoy it in moderation.

Omega-3 fatty acids, a form of polyunsaturated fat found primarily in fish, may be even more healthful. Foods rich in omega-3s are important because they contain the essential nutrient alpha-linolenic acid. Omega-3s and the compounds the body makes from them have a number of heart-healthy effects: They reduce the tendency of blood to clot, inhibit inflammation and abnormal heart rhythms, and reduce blood pressure and risk of heart attack and stroke in some people. Because of these benefits, dietitians recommend that Canadians increase the proportion of omega-3s in their diet by eating at least two servings of fish each week. Serving sizes are based on *Eating Well with Canada's Food Guide*. Salmon, tuna, trout, mackerel, herring, sardines, and anchovies are all good sources of omega-3s; lesser amounts are found in plant foods, including dark-green leafy vegetables; walnuts; flaxseeds; and canola, walnut, and flaxseed oils.

omega-3 fatty acids
Polyunsaturated fatty acids commonly found in fish oils that are beneficial to cardiovascular health.

Most of the polyunsaturated fats currently consumed by Canadians are omega-6 fatty acids, primarily from corn oil and soybean oil. Foods rich in omega-6s are important because they contain the essential nutrient linoleic acid. However, some nutritionists recommend that people reduce the proportion of omega-6s they consume in favour of omega-3s. To make this adjustment, use canola oil rather than corn oil in cooking, and check for corn, soybean, or cottonseed oil in such products as mayonnaise, margarine, and salad dressing.

In addition to its effects on heart disease risk, dietary fat can affect health in other ways. Diets high in fatty red meat are associated with an increased risk of certain forms of cancer, especially colon cancer. A high-fat diet can also make weight management more difficult. Because fat is a concentrated source of calories (9 calories per gram versus 4 calories per gram for protein and carbohydrate), a high-fat diet is often a high-calorie diet that can lead to weight gain. In addition, some evidence shows that calories from fat are more easily converted to body fat than calories from protein or carbohydrate.

Although more research is needed on the precise effects of different types and amounts of fat on overall health, a great deal of evidence points to the fact that most people benefit from keeping their overall fat intake at recommended levels and choosing unsaturated fats instead of saturated and trans fats. The types of fatty acids and their effects on health are summarized in Figure 5.3.

Recommended Fat Intake

To meet the body's demand for essential fats, adult men need about 17 grams per day of linoleic acid and 1.6 grams per day of alpha-linolenic acid; adult women need 12 grams of linoleic acid and 1.1 grams of alpha-linolenic acid. It takes only 30–45 mL (2–3 tablespoons) of unsaturated fat per day incorporated into your diet to supply the essential fats. This includes oil used for cooking, salad dressings, margarine, and mayonnaise. Most Canadians consume sufficient amounts of the essential fats; limiting unhealthy fats is a much greater health concern.

Limits for total fat, saturated fat, and trans fat intake have been set by a number of government and research organizations. In 2002, Health Canada adopted recommendations for the balance of energy sources in a healthful diet from the Institute of Medicine. These new recommendations, called Acceptable Macronutrient Distribution Ranges (AMDRs), are based on ensuring adequate intake of essential nutrients while also reducing the risk of chronic diseases, such as heart disease and cancer. As with protein, a range of levels of fat consumption is associated with good health; the AMDR for total fat is 20–35 percent of total calories. Although more difficult for consumers to monitor, AMDRs have also been set for omega-6 fatty acids (5–10 percent)

FIGURE 5.3

Types of Fatty Acids and their Possible Effects on Health

Type of Fatty Acid	Found In[a]	Possible Effects on Health
SATURATED 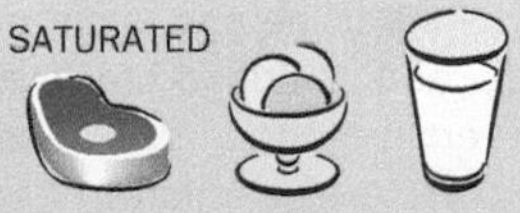	Animal fats (especially fatty meats and poultry fat and skin) Butter, cheese, and other high-fat dairy products Palm and coconut oils	Raises total cholesterol and LDL cholesterol levels Increases risk of heart disease May increase risk of colon and prostate cancers
TRANS 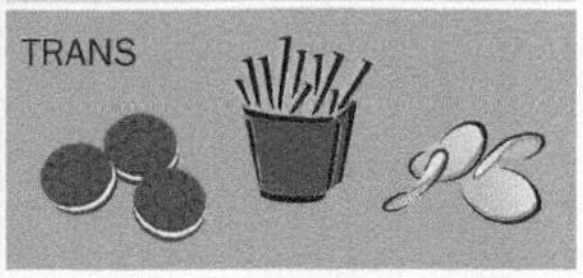	French fries and other deep-fried fast foods Stick margarines, shortening Packaged cookies and crackers Processed snacks and sweets	Raises total cholesterol and LDL cholesterol levels Lowers HDL cholesterol levels May increase risk of heart disease and breast cancer
MONOUNSATURATED 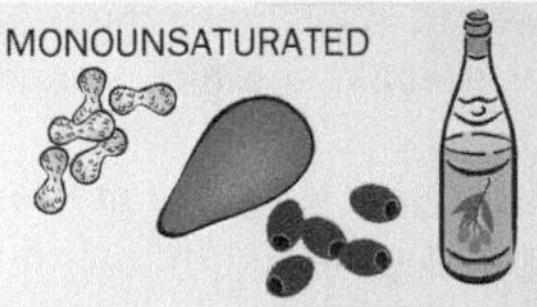	Olive, canola, and safflower oils Avocados, olives Peanut butter (without added fat) Many nuts, including almonds, cashews, pecans, and pistachios	Lowers total cholesterol and LDL cholesterol levels May reduce blood pressure and lower triglyceride levels (a risk factor for CVD) May reduce risk of heart disease, stroke, and some cancers
POLYUNSATURATED (two groups)[b]		
Omega-3 fatty acids 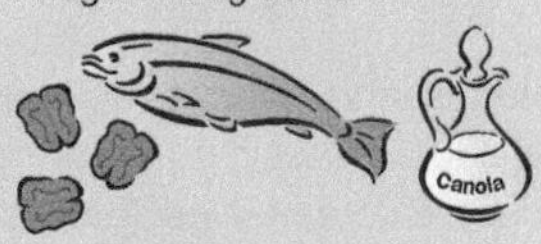	Fatty fish, including salmon, white albacore tuna, mackerel, anchovies, and sardines Lesser amounts in walnut, flaxseed, canola, and soybean oils; tofu; walnuts; flaxseeds; and dark-green leafy vegetables	Reduces blood clotting and inflammation and inhibits abnormal heart rhythms Lowers triglyceride levels (a risk factor for CVD) May lower blood pressure in some people May reduce risk of fatal heart attack, stroke, and some cancers
Omega-6 fatty acids 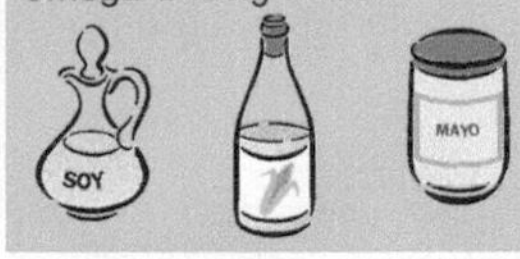	Corn, soybean, and cottonseed oils (often used in margarine, mayonnaise, and salad dressing)	Lowers total cholesterol and LDL cholesterol levels May lower HDL cholesterol levels May reduce risk of heart disease May slightly increase risk of cancer if omega-6 intake is high and omega-3 intake is low

Keep Intake Low — Choose Moderate Amounts

[a] Food fats contain a combination of types of fatty acids in various proportions; for example, canola oil is composed mainly of monounsaturated fatty acids (62 percent) but also contains polyunsaturated (32 percent) and saturated (6 percent) fatty acids. Food fats are categorized here according to their predominant fatty acid.

[b] The essential fatty acids are polyunsaturated: Linoleic acid is an omega-6 fatty acid and alpha-linolenic acid is an omega-3 fatty acid.

and omega-3 fatty acids (0.6–1.2 percent) as part of total energy intake. Because any amount of saturated and trans fats increases the risk of heart disease, the Food and Nutrition Board, a committee of the Institute of Medicine, recommends that saturated fat and trans fat intake be kept as low as possible; most fat in a healthy diet should be unsaturated. In Canada, 25 percent of males and 23 percent of females, ages 19 years and older, have fat intakes above the AMDR of 25–35 percent. The best way to minimize the risk of adverse health effects related to trans fat is to reduce your intake of foods that contain trans fatty acids.

QUICK STATS

100 grams of Atlantic salmon provides 2 grams of omega-3 fatty acids, while 1 teaspoon of flaxseed oil provides 2.6 grams of omega-3 fatty acids.

—Marine Harvest Canada, 2010; Dietitians of Canada, 2012

For advice on setting individual intake goals, see the Take Charge box. To determine how close you are to meeting your personal intake goals for fat, keep a running total over the course of the day. For prepared foods, food labels list the number of grams of fat, protein, and carbohydrate. The breakdown of some popular fast-food items can be found on the website for the fast-food restaurant for which you have interest. Look for their nutrition information of menu items. Nutrition information is also available in many grocery stores, in

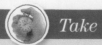 *Take* **CHARGE**

Setting Intake Goals for Protein, Fat, and Carbohydrate

The Acceptable Macronutrient Distribution Ranges (AMDRs), established by the Institute of Medicine and adopted by Health Canada, help ensure adequate intake of the essential amino acids, fatty acids, and carbohydrate. The ranges can help you balance your intake of the energy-providing nutrients in ways that ensure adequate intake while reducing the risk of chronic disease. The AMDRs for protein, total fat, and carbohydrate are as follows:

Protein   10–35% of total daily calories

Total fat   20–35% of total daily calories

Carbohydrate   45–65% of total daily calories

Protein intake goals can be calculated more specifically by multiplying your body weight in kilograms by 0.8. (Refer to the Nutrition Resources section at the end of the chapter for information for specific age groups and life stages.)

To set individual goals, begin by estimating your total daily energy (calorie) needs; if your weight is stable, your current energy intake is the number of calories you need to maintain your weight at your current activity level. Next, select percentage goals for protein, fat, and carbohydrate. You can allocate your total daily calories among the three classes of macronutrients to suit your preferences; just make sure that the three percentages you select total 100 percent and that you meet the minimum intake AMDR for each macronutrient. Two samples showing different total energy intake and nutrient intake goals are included below.

To translate your own percentage goals into daily intake goals expressed in calories and grams, multiply the appropriate percentages by total calorie intake and then divide the results by the corresponding calories per gram. For example, a fat limit of 35 percent applied to a 2200-calorie diet would be calculated as follows: 0.35 x 2200 = 770 calories of total fat; 770 ÷ 9 calories per gram = 86 grams of total fat.

(Remember that fat has 9 calories per gram and that protein and carbohydrate have 4 calories per gram.)

Two Sample Macronutrient Distributions

Nutrient	AMDR	Sample 1		Sample 2	
		Individual Goals	Amounts for a 1600-Calorie Diet	Individual Goals	Amounts for a 2800-Calorie Diet
Protein	10–35%	15%	240 calories = 60 g	30%	840 calories = 210 g
Fat	20–35%	30%	480 calories = 53 g	25%	700 calories = 78 g
Carbohydrate	45–65%	55%	880 calories = 220 g	45%	1260 calories = 315 g

Source: Food and Nutrition Board, Institute of Medicine, National Academies. 2002. *Dietary Reference Intakes: Applications in Dietary Planning,* Washington, D.C.: National Academies Press. Reprinted with permission from the National Academies Press, Washington, D.C.

inexpensive published nutrition guides, and online (see the For More Information section at the end of the chapter). By checking these resources, you can keep track of the total grams of fat, protein, and carbohydrate you eat and assess your current diet.

You can still eat high-fat foods, but it makes sense to limit the size of your portions and to balance your intake with low-fat foods. For example, peanut butter is high in fat: 15 millilitres (1 tablespoon) has 90 calories, with 72 of those calories (8 grams) coming from fat. A full serving of peanut butter is 30 millilitres. This amount spread on whole wheat bread and served with a banana, carrot sticks, and a glass of skim milk makes a nutritious lunch, high in protein and carbohydrate, and relatively low in fat (500 calories, 18 grams of total fat, 4 grams of saturated fat). Sixty millilitres (4 tablespoons) of peanut butter on high-fat crackers, eaten with potato chips, cookies, and homogenized milk is a far less healthy combination (1000 calories, 62 grams of total fat, 15 grams of saturated fat). So although it's important to evaluate individual food items for their fat content, it is more important to look at them in the context of your overall diet.

Carbohydrates: An Ideal Source of Energy

Carbohydrates are needed in the diet primarily to supply energy for body cells. Some cells, such as those found in the brain and other parts of the nervous system and in blood, use only carbohydrates for fuel. During high-intensity exercise, muscles also use primarily carbohydrates for fuel.

> **carbohydrate**
> An essential nutrient; sugars, starches, and dietary fibre are all carbohydrates.

When we don't eat enough carbohydrates to satisfy the needs of the brain and red blood cells, our bodies synthesize carbohydrates from proteins. In situations of extreme deprivation, when the diet lacks a sufficient amount of both carbohydrates and proteins, the body turns to its own organs and tissues, breaking down proteins in muscles, the heart, kidneys, and other vital organs to supply carbohydrate needs. This rarely occurs, however, because consuming the equivalent of just three or four slices of bread supplies the body's daily minimum need for carbohydrates.

Simple and Complex Carbohydrates

Carbohydrates are classified into two groups: simple and complex. Simple carbohydrates include sucrose (table sugar), fructose (fruit sugar, honey), maltose (malt sugar), and lactose (milk sugar). Simple carbohydrates provide much of the sweetness in foods and are found naturally in fruits and milk and are added to soft drinks, fruit drinks, candy, and sweet desserts. No evidence suggests that any type of simple carbohydrate is more nutritious than the others.

Complex carbohydrates include starches and most types of dietary fibre. Starches are found in a variety of plants, especially grains (wheat, rye, rice, oats, barley, millet), legumes (dry beans, peas, and lentils), and tubers (potatoes and yams). Most other vegetables contain a mixture of complex and simple carbohydrates. Fibre, discussed in the next section, is found in grains, fruits, and vegetables.

During digestion in the mouth and small intestine, your body breaks down carbohydrates into simple sugar molecules, such as **glucose**, for absorption. Once glucose is in the bloodstream, the pancreas releases the hormone insulin, which allows cells to take up glucose and use it for energy. The liver and muscles also take up glucose to provide carbohydrate storage in the form of **glycogen**. Some people have problems controlling blood glucose levels, a disorder called *diabetes mellitus* (see Chapter 4 for more on diabetes).

> **glucose**
> A simple sugar that is the body's basic fuel.
>
> **glycogen**
> An animal starch stored in the liver and muscles.

Refined Carbohydrates Versus Whole Grains

Complex carbohydrates can be further divided between refined, or processed, carbohydrates and unrefined carbohydrates, or **whole grains**. Before they are processed, all grains are whole grains, consisting of an inner layer, the germ; a middle layer, the endosperm; and an outer layer, called bran (see Figure 5.4). During processing, the germ and bran are often removed, leaving just the starchy endosperm. The refinement of whole grains transforms whole wheat flour to white flour, brown rice to white rice, and so on.

> **whole grain**
> The entire edible portion of a grain, such as wheat, rice, or oats, consisting of the germ, endosperm, and bran. During milling or processing, parts of the grain are removed, often leaving just the endosperm.

Refined carbohydrates usually retain all the calories of their unrefined counterparts, but they tend to be much lower in fibre, vitamins, minerals, and other beneficial compounds. Many refined grain products are enriched or fortified with vitamins and minerals, but often the nutrients lost in processing are not replaced.

FIGURE 5.4

The Parts of a Whole-grain Kernel

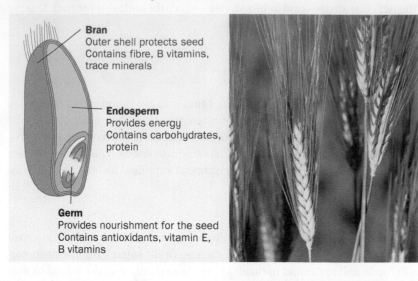

Bran
Outer shell protects seed
Contains fibre, B vitamins,
trace minerals

Endosperm
Provides energy
Contains carbohydrates,
protein

Germ
Provides nourishment for the seed
Contains antioxidants, vitamin E,
B vitamins

Added sugar in foods is problematic. Consuming too much sugar increases your risk for heart disease, stroke, obesity, diabetes, high blood cholesterol, cancer, and dental cavities. Canadians are consuming too much added sugar, which can be found mostly in foods that have minimal or no nutritional value. The Heart and Stroke Foundation recently recommended that Canadians decrease their consumption of added sugar (excluding naturally occurring sugar in fruit, vegetables, milk, grains, and other nutrient-dense foods) to no more than 10 percent of their total daily calories. For an average 2000 calories per day diet, 10 percent of added sugars translates to approximately 48 grams or about 12 teaspoons of sugar. To put this into context, one 355mL can of pop contains about 85 percent of the daily sugar limit.

Unrefined carbohydrates tend to take longer to chew and digest than refined ones; they also enter the bloodstream more slowly. This slower digestive pace tends to make people feel full sooner and for longer. The slower rise in blood glucose levels following consumption of complex carbohydrates may help in the management of diabetes. Whole grains are also high in dietary fibre and so have all the benefits of fibre (discussed later). Consumption of whole grains has been linked to a reduced risk of heart disease, diabetes, high blood pressure, stroke, and certain forms of cancer. For all these reasons, whole grains are recommended over those that have been refined. This does not mean that you should never eat refined carbohydrates, such as white bread or white rice; it simply means that whole wheat bread, brown rice, and other whole grains are healthier choices. See the Take Charge box for tips on increasing your intake of whole grains.

QUICK STATS

A healthy adult needs 21 to 38 grams of fibre a day, but Canadian nutrition surveillance surveys show that the average daily Canadian intake is only about 14 grams.

—Heart and Stroke Foundation, 2011

Glycemic Index and Glycemic Response

Insulin and glucose levels rise and fall following a meal or snack containing any type of carbohydrate. Some foods cause a quick and dramatic rise in glucose and insulin levels; others have a slower, more moderate effect. A food that has a rapid effect on blood glucose levels is said to have a high **glycemic index**. Research findings have been mixed, but some studies have found that a meal containing high glycemic index foods may increase appetite and that over the long term, diets rich in these foods may increase the risk of diabetes and heart disease for some people. High glycemic index foods do not, as some popular diets claim, directly cause weight gain beyond the calories they contain.

glycemic index
A measure of how the ingestion of a particular food affects blood glucose levels.

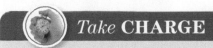

Take CHARGE

Choosing More Whole-Grain Foods

Whole-grain foods are good weapons against heart disease, diabetes, high blood pressure, stroke, and certain cancers. They are also low in fat and so can be a good choice for managing weight. Health Canada recommends that half of your grain products every day should be whole grains.

What Are Whole Grains?
The first step in increasing your intake of whole grains is to correctly identify them. The following are whole grains:

- whole wheat
- whole rye
- whole oats
- oatmeal

- whole-grain corn
- popcorn
- brown rice
- whole-grain barley

More unusual choices include bulgur (cracked wheat), millet, kasha (roasted buckwheat kernels), quinoa, wheat and rye berries, amaranth, wild rice, graham flour, whole-grain kamut, whole-grain spelt, and whole-grain triticale.

Wheat flour, unbleached flour, enriched flour, and degerminated corn meal are not whole grains. Wheat germ and wheat bran are also not whole grains, but they are the constituents of wheat typically left out when wheat is processed and so are healthier choices than regular wheat flour, which typically contains just the endosperm.

Reading Food Packages to Find Whole Grains
To find packaged foods rich in whole grains, read the list of ingredients and check for special health claims related to whole grains. The *first* item on the list of ingredients should be one of the whole grains listed above. Product names and colours used on food packaging can be misleading. When in doubt, always check the list of ingredients, looking for *whole* as the first word on the list.

Incorporating Whole Grains into Your Daily Diet
Small changes can make a big difference in your fibre intake:
- *Bread:* Look for sandwich breads, bagels, English muffins, buns, and pita breads with a whole grain listed as the first ingredient.
- *Breakfast cereals:* Check the ingredient list for whole grains. Whole-grain choices include oatmeal, muesli, shredded wheat, and some types of raisin bran, bran flakes, wheat flakes, toasted oats, and granola.
- *Rice:* Choose brown rice or rice blends that include brown rice.
- *Pasta:* Look for whole wheat, whole-grain kamut, or whole-grain spelt pasta.
- *Tortillas:* Choose whole wheat or whole-corn tortillas.
- *Crackers and snacks:* Some varieties of crackers are made from whole grains, including some flatbreads or crispbreads, woven wheat crackers, and rye crackers. Other whole-grain snack possibilities include popcorn, popcorn cakes, brown rice cakes, whole-corn tortilla chips, and whole wheat fig cookies. Be sure to check food labels for fat content, as many popular snacks are high in fat.
- *Mixed-grain dishes:* Combine whole grains with other foods to create healthy mixed dishes. Possibilities include tabouli; soups made with hulled barley or wheat berries; and pilafs, casseroles, and salads made with brown rice, whole wheat couscous, kasha, millet, wheat bulgur, or quinoa.
  If your grocery store doesn't carry all of these items, try your local health food store.

Attempting to base food choices on the glycemic index is a difficult task, however. Although unrefined complex carbohydrates and high-fibre foods generally tend to have a low glycemic index, patterns are less clear for other types of foods and do not follow an easy distinction, such as that of simple versus complex carbohydrates. For example, some fruits with fairly high levels of simple carbohydrates have only a moderate effect on blood glucose levels, whereas white rice, potatoes, and white bread, which are rich in complex carbohydrates, have a high glycemic index. Watermelon has a glycemic index more than twice that of strawberries, and the glycemic index of a banana changes dramatically as it ripens. The acid and fat content of a food also affect its glycemic index; the more acidic and higher in fat a food is, the lower its effect on glucose levels. The body's response to carbohydrates also depends on many other factors, such as how foods are combined and prepared and the fitness status of the individual.

This complexity is one reason major health organizations have not issued specific guidelines for the glycemic index of foods. For people with particular health concerns, a food's glycemic index may be an important consideration; however, it should not be the sole criterion for food choices. For example, ice cream has a much lower glycemic index than brown rice or carrots—but that doesn't make it a healthier choice overall. Remember that most unrefined grains, fruits, vegetables, and legumes are rich in nutrients, have a relatively low energy density, and have a low to moderate glycemic index. Choose a variety of vegetables daily. Limit foods that are high in added sugars but provide few other nutrients. Some studies have specifically linked soft drinks, with their large dose of rapidly absorbable sugar, to increased risk for diabetes and obesity.

Recommended Carbohydrate Intak

Experts recommend that adults consume 45–65 percent of their total daily calories as carbohydrate, about 225–325 grams of carbohydrate for someone consuming 2000 calories per day. The focus should be on consuming a variety of foods rich in complex carbohydrates, especially whole grains.

Canada has no specific recommendations for added sugar consumption. That said, foods high in added sugar are generally high in calories and low in nutrients and fibre, thus providing empty calories. Although the Institute of Medicine has set an AMDR for added sugars of no more than 25 percent of total daily calories, many health experts recommend an even lower intake.

The 2014 WHO sugar draft guideline suggests that a reduction to below 5 percent of total energy intake per day would have additional health benefits, which is equivalent to around 25 grams (around 6 teaspoons) of sugar per day for an adult of healthy body weight. To reduce your intake of added sugars, limit soft drinks, candy, sweet desserts, and sweetened fruit drinks. The simple carbohydrates in your diet should come mainly from fruits, which are excellent sources of vitamins and minerals, and from low-fat or skim milk and other dairy products, which are high in protein and calcium.

Athletes in training can benefit from high-carbohydrate diets (60–70 percent of total daily calories), which enhance the amount of carbohydrates stored in their muscles (as glycogen) and therefore provide more carbohydrate fuel for use during endurance events or long workouts (more than 60 minutes). In addition, carbohydrates consumed during prolonged athletic events can help fuel muscles and extend the availability of the glycogen stored in muscles. Caution is in order, however, because overconsumption of carbohydrates can lead to fatigue and under-consumption of other nutrients. Athletes should focus on complex carbohydrates, such as whole-grain breads, cereals, brown rice, whole wheat pastas, and starchy vegetables, such as sweet potatoes, corn, and peas.

QUICK STATS

Breakfast foods typically contain mostly carbohydrate-rich foods, and about 18% of daily calories are consumed at breakfast.

—*Canadian Community Health Survey*, 2004

Fibre: A Closer Look

Fibre is the term given to non-digestible carbohydrates provided by plants. Instead of being digested, like starch, fibre passes through the intestinal tract and provides bulk for feces in the large intestine, which in turn facilitates elimination. In the large intestine, some types of fibre are broken down by bacteria into acids and gases, which explains why consuming too much fibre can lead to intestinal gas. Because humans cannot digest fibre, it is not a source of carbohydrate in the diet; however, the consumption of fibre is necessary for good health.

Types of Fibre

Fibre comes in two types: dietary fibre and functional fibre. **Dietary fibre** refers to the non-digestible carbohydrates (and the non-carbohydrate substance lignin) that are present naturally in plants, such as grains, legumes, and vegetables. **Functional fibre** refers to non-digestible carbohydrates that have been either isolated from natural sources or synthesized in a lab and then added to a food product or dietary supplement. **Total fibre** is the sum of dietary and functional fibre.

dietary fibre
Non-digestible carbohydrates and lignin that are intact in plants.

functional fibre
Non-digestible carbohydrates either isolated from natural sources or synthesized; may be added to foods and dietary supplements.

total fibre
The total amount of dietary fibre and functional fibre in the diet.

Fibres have different properties that lead to different physiological effects in the body. For example, **soluble (viscous) fibre**, such as that found in oat bran or legumes, can delay stomach emptying, slow the movement of glucose into the blood after eating, and reduce absorption of cholesterol. **Insoluble fibre**, such as that found in wheat bran or psyllium seed, increases fecal bulk and helps prevent constipation, hemorrhoids, and other digestive disorders. A diet high in fibre can help reduce the risk of type 2 diabetes and heart disease and improve gastrointestinal health. Some studies have linked high-fibre diets with reduced risk of colon and rectal cancer; other studies have suggested that other characteristics of diets rich in fruits, vegetables, and whole grains may be responsible for this reduction in risk (see Chapter 8 for more on cancer and diet).

soluble (viscous) fibre
Fibre that dissolves in water or is broken down by bacteria in the large intestine.

insoluble fibre
Fibre that does not dissolve in water and is not broken down by bacteria in the large intestine.

Sources of Fibre
All plant foods contain some dietary fibre. Fruits, legumes, oats (especially oat bran), and barley all contain the viscous type of fibre that help lower blood glucose and cholesterol levels. Wheat (especially wheat bran), other grains and cereals, and vegetables are good sources of cellulose and other fibres that help prevent constipation. Psyllium, which is often added to cereals or used in fibre supplements and laxatives, improves intestinal health and also helps control glucose and cholesterol levels. The processing of packaged foods can remove fibre, so it is important to rely on fresh fruits and vegetables and foods made from whole grains as your main sources of fibre.

Recommended Fibre Intake
To reduce the risk of chronic disease and maintain intestinal health, Health Canada suggests a daily fibre intake of 38 grams for adult men (ages 19–50; 30 g/day for men 51 and older) and 25 grams for adult women (ages 19–50; 30 g/day for women 51 and older). Canadians, on average, consume about half this amount. Fibre should come from foods, not supplements, which should be used only under medical supervision.

QUESTIONS FOR CRITICAL THINKING AND REFLECTION

Experts say that two of the most important factors in a healthy diet are eating the right kinds of carbohydrates and the right kinds of fats. Based on what you have read so far in this chapter, which are the right carbohydrates and fats? How would you say your own diet stacks up when it comes to carbs and fats?

Vitamins: Organic Micronutrients

Vitamins are organic (carbon-containing) substances required in small amounts to regulate various processes within living cells (see Table 5.3). Humans need 13 vitamins; four are fat soluble (A, D, E, and K), and nine are water soluble (C and the eight B-complex vitamins: thiamine, riboflavin, niacin, vitamin B6, folate, vitamin B12, biotin, and pantothenic acid).

> **vitamins**
> Carbon-containing substances needed in small amounts to help promote and regulate chemical reactions and processes in the body.

Solubility affects how a vitamin is absorbed, transported, and stored in the body. The water-soluble vitamins are absorbed directly into the bloodstream, where they travel freely; excess water-soluble vitamins are detected and removed by the kidneys and excreted in urine. Fat-soluble vitamins require a more complex absorptive process; they are usually carried in the blood by special proteins and are stored in the liver and in fat tissues rather than excreted.

Functions of Vitamins

Many vitamins help chemical reactions take place. They provide no energy to the body directly, but help unleash the energy stored in carbohydrates, proteins, and fats. Vitamins are critical in the production of red blood cells and the maintenance of the nervous, skeletal, and immune systems. Some vitamins act as **antioxidants**, which help preserve healthy cells in the body. Key vitamin antioxidants include vitamin E, vitamin C, and the vitamin A precursor beta-carotene. (Antioxidants are described later in the chapter.)

> **antioxidants**
> Substances that can lessen the breakdown of food or body constituents by free radicals; actions include binding oxygen, donating electrons to free radicals, and repairing damage to molecules.

Sources of Vitamins

The human body does not manufacture most of the vitamins it requires and must obtain them from foods. Vitamins are abundant in fruits, vegetables, and grains. In addition, many processed foods, such as flour and breakfast cereals, contain added vitamins. A few vitamins are made in certain parts of the body: The skin makes vitamin D when it is exposed to sunlight, and intestinal bacteria make vitamin K. Nonetheless, you still need to obtain vitamin D and vitamin K from foods. Table 5.3 lists good food sources of vitamins.

Vitamin Deficiencies

If your diet lacks a particular vitamin, characteristic symptoms of deficiency can develop. Table 5.3 lists the signs of certain vitamin deficiencies. Physicians have known about some common deficiency-related ailments for generations. For example, *scurvy* is a potentially fatal illness caused by a long-term lack of vitamin C. Children who do not get enough vitamin D can develop *rickets*, which leads to potentially disabling bone deformations. Vitamin A deficiency may cause blindness, and seizures can develop in people whose diet lacks vitamin B6. Low intake of folate and vitamins B6 and B12 has been linked to an increased risk of heart disease.

New research is tying vitamin deficiencies with other health risks, as well. For example, two recent studies showed that a lack of vitamin K may contribute to bone brittleness and contribute to bone fractures. A great deal of recent research has focused on vitamin D, with surprising results. Several studies have associated vitamin D deficiency with an increased risk of cardiovascular disease in adults, and show that the vitamin plays an important role in arterial health and blood clotting. A 2008 study also raised the possibility that women with certain types of breast cancer may be more likely to die from their cancer if they do not get enough vitamin D.

Vitamin deficiency diseases are most often seen in developing countries, and they are relatively rare in Canada because vitamins are readily available from our food supply. Still, many Canadians consume less-than-recommended amounts of several vitamins, including vitamins A, C, and E. At the request of Health

TABLE 5.3

Facts About Vitamins

Vitamin	Important Dietary Sources	Major Functions	Signs of Prolonged Deficiency	Toxic Effects of Megadoses
Fat Soluble				
Vitamin A	Liver, milk, butter, cheese, and fortified margarine; carrots, spinach, and other orange and deep-green vegetables and fruits	Maintenance of vision, skin, linings of the nose, mouth, digestive and urinary tracts, immune function	Night blindness; dry, scaling skin; increased susceptibility to infection; loss of appetite; anemia; kidney stones	Liver damage, miscarriage and birth defects, headache, vomiting and diarrhea, vertigo, double vision, bone abnormalities
Vitamin D	Fortified milk and margarine, fish oils, butter, egg yolks (sunlight on skin also produces vitamin D)	Development and maintenance of bones and teeth, promotion of calcium absorption	Rickets (bone deformities) in children; bone softening, loss, and fractures in adults	Kidney damage, calcium deposits in soft tissues, depression, death
Vitamin E	Vegetable oils, whole grains, nuts and seeds, green leafy vegetables, asparagus, peaches	Protection and maintenance of cellular membranes	Red blood cell breakage and anemia, weakness, neurological problems, muscle cramps	Relatively nontoxic, but may cause excess bleeding or formation of blood clots
Vitamin K	Green leafy vegetables; smaller amounts widespread in other foods	Production of factors essential for blood clotting and bone metabolism	Hemorrhaging	None reported
Water Soluble				
Biotin	Cereals, yeast, egg yolks, soy flour, liver; widespread in foods	Synthesis of fat, glycogen, and amino acids	Rash, nausea, vomiting, weight loss, depression, fatigue, hair loss	None reported
Folate	Green leafy vegetables, yeast, oranges, whole grains, legumes, liver	Amino acid metabolism, synthesis of RNA and DNA, new cell synthesis	Anemia, weakness, fatigue, irritability, shortness of breath, swollen tongue	Masking of vitamin B12 deficiency
Niacin	Eggs, poultry, fish, milk, whole grains, nuts, enriched breads and cereals, meats, legumes	Conversion of carbohydrates, fats, and protein into usable forms of energy	Pellagra (symptoms include diarrhea, dermatitis, inflammation of mucous membranes, dementia)	Flushing of the skin, nausea, vomiting, diarrhea, liver dysfunction, glucose intolerance
Pantothenic acid	Animal foods, whole grains, broccoli, potatoes; widespread in foods	Metabolism of fats, carbohydrates, and proteins	Fatigue, numbness and tingling of hands and feet, gastrointestinal disturbances	None reported
Riboflavin	Dairy products, enriched breads and cereals, lean meats, poultry, fish, green vegetables	Energy metabolism; maintenance of skin, mucous membranes, and nervous system structures	Cracks at corners of mouth, sore throat, skin rash, hypersensitivity to light, purple tongue	None reported
Thiamine	Whole-grain and enriched breads and cereals, organ meats, lean pork, nuts, legumes	Conversion of carbohydrates into usable forms of energy, maintenance of appetite and nervous system function	Beriberi (symptoms include muscle wasting, mental confusion, anorexia, enlarged heart, nerve changes)	None reported
Vitamin B6	Eggs, poultry, fish, whole grains, nuts, soybeans, liver, kidney, pork	Metabolism of amino acids and glycogen	Anemia, convulsions, cracks at corners of mouth, dermatitis, nausea, confusion	Neurological abnormalities and damage
Vitamin B12	Meat, fish, poultry, fortified cereals	Synthesis of blood cells; other metabolic reactions	Anemia, fatigue, nervous system damage, sore tongue	None reported
Vitamin C	Peppers, broccoli, spinach, Brussels sprouts, citrus fruits, strawberries, tomatoes, potatoes, cabbage, other fruits and vegetables	Maintenance and repair of connective tissue, bones, teeth, and cartilage; promotion of healing; aid in iron absorption	Scurvy, anemia, reduced resistance to infection, loosened teeth, joint pain, poor wound healing, hair loss, poor iron absorption	Urinary stones in some people, acid stomach from ingesting supplements in pill form, nausea, diarrhea, headache, fatigue

Sources: Food and Nutrition Board, Institute of Medicine. 2006. *Dietary Reference Intakes: The Essential Guide to Nutrient Requirements*. Washington, D.C.: The National Academies Press. The complete Dietary Reference Intake reports are available from the National Academy Press (http://www.nap.edu); and Shils, M. E., et al., eds. 2005. *Modern Nutrition in Health and Disease*, 10th ed. Baltimore: Lippincott Williams & Wilkins.

Canada and several federal agencies in the United States, the Institute of Medicine undertook a study to assess all available data and review the DRIs for vitamin D and calcium. These two essential nutrients have long been known for their important role in bone health, and new research has indicated that they may also play a role in cancer, cardiovascular disease, hypertension, diabetes, metabolic syndrome, falls, immune response, neuropsychological functions, physical performance, preeclampsia, and reproductive outcomes. The Institute of Medicine's report was released at the end of 2010, and although the DRIs were updated for both calcium and vitamin D, additional research is required to determine the benefit of vitamin D and calcium for conditions other than bone health.

Vitamin Excesses

Extra vitamins in the diet can also be harmful, especially when taken as supplements. Megadoses of fat-soluble vitamins are particularly dangerous because the excess is stored in the body rather than excreted, increasing the risk of toxicity. Even when vitamins are not taken in excess, relying on supplements for an adequate intake of vitamins can be a problem. Foods have many substances other than vitamins and minerals, and some of these compounds may have important health effects.

As Canadians consume more supplements and eat more foods that have been fortified with vitamin D, they must do so cautiously. Very high levels of vitamin D (more than 10 000 IU per day) are known to cause kidney and tissue damage. High levels have not been shown to provide greater benefits, and in fact have been linked to other health issues. More is not always better, especially in the case of vitamin D.

Later in the chapter we discuss specific recommendations for vitamin intake and when a vitamin supplement is advisable. For now, keep in mind that it's best to get most of your vitamins from foods rather than from supplements.

QUICK STATS

At least 80% of fractures in people 50 years of age and older are related to osteoporosis.

—Osteoporosis Canada, 2013

Keeping the Nutrient Value in Food

Vitamins and minerals can be lost or destroyed during the storage and cooking of foods. To retain nutrients, consume or process vegetables as soon as possible after purchasing. Store fruits and vegetables in the refrigerator in covered containers or plastic bags to minimize moisture loss; freeze foods that won't be eaten within a few days. Frozen and canned vegetables are usually as high in nutrients as fresh vegetables because nutrients are locked in when produce is frozen or canned. Canned vegetables may have high amounts of sodium added during the processing of the vegetables, so be sure to read the labels. To reduce nutrient losses during food preparation, minimize the amount of water used and the total cooking time. Develop a taste for a crunchier texture in cooked vegetables. Baking, steaming, broiling, grilling, and microwaving are all healthy methods of preparing vegetables.

Minerals: Inorganic Micronutrients

Minerals are inorganic (non-carbon-containing) elements you need in relatively small amounts to help regulate body functions, aid in the growth and maintenance of body tissues, and help release energy (see Table 5.4). There are about 17 essential minerals. The major minerals, those that the body needs in amounts exceeding 100 milligrams per day, include calcium, phosphorus, magnesium, sodium, potassium, and chloride. The essential trace minerals, those that you need in minute amounts, include copper, fluoride, iodide, iron, selenium, and zinc.

minerals
Inorganic compounds needed in relatively small amounts for regulation, growth, and maintenance of body tissues and functions.

TABLE 5.4

Facts About Selected Minerals

Mineral	Important Dietary Sources	Major Functions	Signs of Prolonged Deficiency	Toxic Effects of Megadoses
Calcium	Milk and milk products, tofu, fortified orange juice and bread, green leafy vegetables, bones in fish	Formation of bones and teeth, control of nerve impulses, muscle contraction, blood clotting	Stunted growth in children, bone mineral loss in adults; urinary stones	Kidney stones, calcium deposits in soft tissues, inhibition of mineral absorption, constipation
Fluoride	Fluoridated water, tea, marine fish eaten with bones	Maintenance of tooth and bone structure	Higher frequency of tooth decay	Increased bone density, mottling of teeth, impaired kidney function
Iodine	Iodized salt, seafood, processed foods	Essential part of thyroid hormones, regulation of body metabolism	Goitre (enlarged thyroid), cretinism (birth defect)	Depression of thyroid activity, hyperthyroidism in susceptible people
Iron	Meat and poultry, fortified grain products, dark-green vegetables, dried fruit	Component of hemoglobin, myoglobin, and enzymes	Iron-deficiency anemia, weakness, impaired immune function, gastrointestinal distress	Nausea, diarrhea, liver and kidney damage, joint pains, sterility, disruption of cardiac function, death
Magnesium	Widespread in foods and water (except soft water); especially found in grains, legumes, nuts, seeds, green vegetables, milk	Transmission of nerve impulses, energy transfer, activation of many enzymes	Neurological disturbances, cardiovascular problems, kidney disorders, nausea, growth failure in children	Nausea, vomiting, diarrhea, central nervous system depression, coma; death in people with impaired kidney function
Phosphorus	Present in nearly all foods, especially milk, cereal, peas, eggs, meat	Bone growth and maintenance, energy transfer in cells	Impaired growth, weakness, kidney disorders, cardio-respiratory and nervous system dysfunction	Drop in blood calcium levels, calcium deposits in soft tissues, bone loss
Potassium	Meats, milk, fruits, vegetables, grains, legumes	Nerve function and body water balance	Muscular weakness, nausea, drowsiness, paralysis, confusion, disruption of cardiac rhythm	Cardiac arrest
Selenium	Seafood, meat, eggs, whole grains	Defence against oxidative stress, regulation of thyroid hormone action	Muscle pain and weakness, heart disorders	Hair and nail loss, nausea and vomiting, weakness, irritability
Sodium	Salt, soy sauce, salted foods, tomato juice	Body water balance, acid-base balance, nerve function	Muscle weakness, loss of appetite, nausea, vomiting; deficiency is rarely seen	Edema, hypertension in sensitive people
Zinc	Whole grains, meat, eggs, liver, seafood (especially oysters)	Synthesis of proteins, RNA, and DNA; wound healing; immune response; ability to taste	Growth failure, loss of appetite, impaired taste acuity, skin rash, impaired immune function, poor wound healing	Vomiting, impaired immune function, decline in blood HDL levels, impaired copper absorption

Sources: Food and Nutrition Board, Institute of Medicine. 2006. *Dietary Reference Intakes: The Essential Guide to Nutrient Requirements.* Washington, D.C.: The National Academies Press. The complete Dietary Reference Intake reports are available from the National Academy Press (http://www.nap.edu); and Shils, M. E., et al., eds. 2005. *Modern Nutrition in Health and Disease,* 10th ed. Baltimore: Lippincott Williams & Wilkins.

Characteristic symptoms develop if an essential mineral is consumed in a quantity too small or too large for good health. The minerals commonly lacking in the Canadian diet are calcium, magnesium, potassium, iron, and folate. Iron-deficiency **anemia** is a problem in many age groups, and researchers fear poor calcium intake in childhood is sowing the seeds for future **osteoporosis**, especially in women. See Chapter 21 for more information on osteoporosis; the Take Charge box has tips for building and maintaining bone density.

anemia
A deficiency in the oxygen-carrying material in the red blood cells.

osteoporosis
A condition in which the bones become extremely thin and brittle and break easily.

Take **CHARGE**

Eating for Healthy Bones

Osteoporosis is a condition in which the bones become dangerously thin and fragile over time. An estimated 1.4 million Canadians are living with osteoporosis. In 2009, approximately 19 percent of women and 3 percent of men aged 50 or older reported that they had been diagnosed with osteoporosis. Most bone mass is built by age 18. After bone density peaks between ages 25 and 35, bone mass is lost over time. To prevent osteoporosis, the best strategy is to build as much bone as possible during your youth and do everything you can to maintain it as you age. Genetic factors may determine as much as 50–90 percent of bone mass, and environmental factors make up for the remaining 10–50 percent. Key nutrients for bone health include the following:

- *Calcium:* Consuming an adequate amount of calcium is important throughout life to build and maintain bone mass. Milk, yogourt, and calcium-fortified orange juice, bread, and cereals are all good sources.
- *Vitamin D:* Vitamin D is necessary for bones to absorb calcium; a daily intake of 15 micrograms is recommended for adults ages 19–50. Vitamin D can be obtained from foods and is manufactured by the skin when exposed to sunlight. Candidates for vitamin D supplements include people who don't eat many foods rich in vitamin D; those who don't have incidental exposure to UV radiation from the sun on their face, arms, and hands (without sunscreen) for 5–15 minutes a few times each week; and people who live in northern latitudes throughout Canada where the sun is weaker. Remember that ultraviolet light from the sun can cause skin cancer. Limit your exposure to the sunshine when you are not wearing sunscreen, and do not use tanning beds. Most skin cancers are largely preventable. Regardless of where the melanoma shows up on the body, it is typically a result of ultraviolet radiation exposure, either from natural sunlight or artificial tanning.
- *Vitamin K:* Vitamin K promotes the synthesis of proteins that help keep bones strong. Broccoli and leafy green vegetables are rich in vitamin K.
- *Other nutrients:* Other nutrients that may play an important role in bone health include vitamin C, magnesium, potassium, manganese, zinc, copper, and boron.

On the other side, several dietary substances may have a *negative* effect on bone health, especially if consumed in excess, including alcohol, sodium, caffeine, and retinol (a form of vitamin A). Drinking lots of soft drinks, which often replace milk in the diet and which are high in phosphorus (a mineral that may interfere with calcium absorption), has been shown to increase the risk of bone fracture in teenage girls.

The effect of protein intake on bone mass depends on other nutrients: Protein helps build bone as long as calcium and vitamin D intake are adequate. If intake of calcium and vitamin D is low, high protein intake can lead to bone loss.

Weight-bearing aerobic exercise helps maintain bone mass throughout life, and strength training improves bone density, muscle mass, strength, and balance. Drinking alcohol only in moderation, refraining from smoking, and managing depression and stress are also important for maintaining strong bones. For people who develop osteoporosis, a variety of medications are available to treat the condition.

Water: Vital but Often Ignored

Water is the major component in both foods and the human body: You are composed of about 60 percent water. Your need for other nutrients, in terms of weight, is much less than your need for water. You can live up to 50 days without food, but only a few days without water.

Water is distributed all over the body, among lean and other tissues and in blood and other body fluids. Water is used in the digestion and absorption of food and is the medium in which most of the chemical reactions take place within the body. Some water-based fluids, such as blood, transport substances around the body, whereas other fluids serve as lubricants or cushions. Water also helps regulate body temperature.

Water is contained in almost all foods, particularly in liquids, fruits, and vegetables. The foods and fluids you consume provide 80–90 percent of your daily water intake; the remainder is generated through metabolism. You lose water each day in urine, feces, and sweat and through evaporation from your lungs.

Most people can maintain a healthy water balance by consuming beverages at meals and drinking fluids in response to thirst. Health Canada has set levels of adequate water intake to maintain hydration; all fluids, including those containing caffeine, can count toward your total daily fluid intake. Under these guidelines and those set by the Institute of Medicine, men need to consume about 3.7 litres of water, while women need 2.7

litres. (See Table 1 in the Nutrition Resources section at the end of the chapter for information on specific age groups.) If you exercise vigorously or live in a hot climate, you need to consume additional fluids to maintain a balance between water consumed and water lost. Severe dehydration causes weakness and can lead to death.

Other Substances in Food

Many substances in food are not essential nutrients, but they may influence health.

Antioxidants

When the body uses oxygen or breaks down certain fats or proteins as a normal part of metabolism, it gives rise to substances called **free radicals**. Environmental factors, such as cigarette smoke, exhaust fumes, radiation, excessive sunlight, certain drugs, and stress, can increase free radical production. A free radical is a chemically unstable molecule that reacts with fats, proteins, and DNA, damaging cell membranes and mutating genes. Free radicals have been implicated in aging, cancer, cardiovascular disease, and other degenerative diseases, such as arthritis.

> **free radical**
> An electron-seeking compound that can react with fats, proteins, and DNA, damaging cell membranes and mutating genes in its search for electrons; produced through chemical reactions in the body and by exposure to environmental factors, such as sunlight and tobacco smoke.

Antioxidants found in foods can help protect the body from damage by free radicals in several ways. Some prevent or reduce the formation of free radicals; others remove free radicals from the body; still others repair some types of free radical damage after it occurs. Some antioxidants, such as vitamin C, vitamin E, and selenium, are also essential nutrients. Others—such as the carotenoids found in yellow, orange, and deep-green vegetables—are not. Researchers have identified the top antioxidant-containing foods and beverages as blackberries, walnuts, strawberries, artichokes, cranberries, brewed coffee, raspberries, pecans, blueberries, cloves, grape juice, unsweetened baking chocolate, sour cherries, and red wine. Also high in antioxidants are Brussels sprouts, kale, cauliflower, and pomegranates.

Phytochemicals

Antioxidants fall into the broader category of **phytochemicals**, substances found in plant foods that may help prevent chronic disease. Researchers have just begun to identify and study all the different compounds found in foods, and many preliminary findings are promising. For example, certain substances found in soy foods may help lower cholesterol levels. Sulphoraphane, a compound isolated from broccoli and other **cruciferous vegetables**, may render some carcinogenic compounds harmless. Allyl sulphides, a group of chemicals found in garlic and onions, appear to boost the activity of cancer-fighting immune cells. Further research on phytochemicals may extend the role of nutrition to the prevention and treatment of many chronic diseases.

> **phytochemicals**
> Naturally occurring substances found in plant foods that may help prevent and treat chronic diseases, such as cancer and heart disease; *phyto* means "plant."
>
> **cruciferous vegetables**
> Vegetables of the cabbage family, including cabbage, broccoli, Brussels sprouts, kale, and cauliflower; the flower petals of these plants form the shape of a cross, hence the name.

If you want to increase your intake of phytochemicals, it is best to eat a variety of fruits,

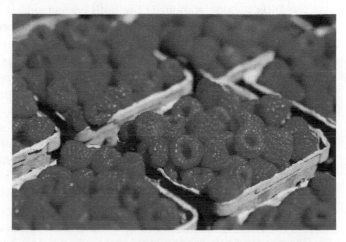

Berries are rich in antioxidants, vitamins, and dietary fibre.

vegetables, and grains rather than relying on supplements. Like many vitamins and minerals, isolated phytochemicals may be harmful if taken in high doses. In addition, it is likely that their health benefits are the result of chemical substances working in combination. The role of phytochemicals in disease prevention is discussed further in Chapters 7 and 8.

Nutritional Guidelines: Planning Your Diet

Scientific and government groups have created various tools to help people design healthy diets. As noted earlier, the **Dietary Reference Intakes (DRIs)** are standards for nutrient intake designed to prevent nutritional deficiencies and reduce the risk of chronic disease. Health Canada has established **Guidelines for Healthy Eating** to promote health and reduce the risk for major chronic diseases through diet and physical activity. *Eating Well with Canada's Food Guide* provides further guidance on daily food intake patterns that meet the DRIs and are consistent with the dietary guidelines.

Dietary Reference Intakes (DRIs)
An umbrella term for four types of nutrient standards. Estimated Average Requirement (EAR) is the amount estimated to meet the nutrient needs of half the individuals in a population group; Adequate Intake (AI) and Recommended Dietary Allowance (RDA) are levels of intake considered adequate to prevent nutrient deficiencies and reduce the risk of chronic disease for most individuals in a population group; Tolerable Upper Intake Level (UL) is the maximum daily intake that is unlikely to cause health problems.

Guidelines for Healthy Eating
General principles of good nutrition presented as practical ways that Canadians can follow a healthy diet and reduce their risk for chronic diseases.

Eating Well with Canada's Food Guide
A food-group plan that provides practical advice to ensure a balanced intake of the essential nutrients.

Dietary Reference Intakes (DRIs)

The Food and Nutrition Board of the Institute of Medicine, in partnership with Health Canada, establishes dietary standards, or recommended intake levels, for Canadians of all ages. The current set of standards, called Dietary Reference Intakes (DRIs), was introduced in 1997. The DRIs are frequently reviewed and updated as new nutrition-related information becomes available. The DRIs present different categories of nutrients in an easy-to-read table format. An earlier set of standards, called the Recommended Nutrient Intakes (RNIs) in Canada, focused on preventing nutritional deficiency diseases, such as anemia. The DRIs have a broader focus because research looked not just at the prevention of nutrient deficiencies, but also at the role of nutrients in promoting health and preventing chronic diseases such as cancer, osteoporosis, and heart disease.

The DRIs include standards for both recommended intakes and maximum safe intakes. The recommended intake of each nutrient is expressed as either a *Recommended Dietary Allowance (RDA)* or *Adequate Intake (AI)*. An AI is set when not enough information is available to set an RDA value; regardless of the type of standard used, however, the DRI represents the best available estimate of intake for optimal health. The *Tolerable Upper Intake Level (UL)* is the maximum daily intake that is unlikely to cause health problems in a healthy person. For example, the AI for calcium for an 18-year-old female is 1300 milligrams per day; the UL is 3000 milligrams per day.

Because of lack of data, ULs have not been set for all nutrients. This does not mean that people can tolerate chronic intakes of these vitamins and minerals above recommended levels (see the In Focus box). Like all chemical agents, nutrients can produce adverse effects if intakes are excessive. No benefit from consuming nutrients at levels above the RDA or AI has been established. The DRIs can be found in the Nutrition Resources section at the end of the chapter.

The Estimated Average Requirement (EAR) is also part of the DRIs. It is the amount estimated to meet the nutrient needs of half the individuals in a population group. EARs are used to calculate the RDA.

Because the DRIs are too cumbersome to use as a basis for food labels, Health Canada has introduced another set of dietary standards on food labels, the **Daily Values**. The Daily Values are based on several

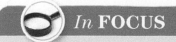

Should You Take Supplements?

The aim of the Dietary Reference Intakes (DRIs) is to guide you in meeting your nutritional needs primarily with food, rather than with vitamin and mineral supplements. Supplements lack potentially beneficial phytochemicals and fibres that are found only in whole foods. Most Canadians can get the vitamins and minerals they need by eating a nutritionally balanced diet of various foods. The use of supplements to reduce heart disease or cancer risk remains controversial, so experts suggest that you avoid taking any nutrient at a level exceeding the Tolerable Upper Intake Level (UL).

The question of whether to take supplements is a serious one. Some vitamins and minerals are dangerous when taken in excess. Large doses of particular nutrients can also cause health problems by affecting the absorption of certain vitamins or minerals. For this reason, ask your doctor or a dietitian before taking any high-dosage supplement.

In setting the DRIs, Health Canada and the Institute of Medicine recommended supplements of particular nutrients for specific groups:

- Women who are capable of getting pregnant should get 400 micrograms per day of folic acid (the synthetic form of the vitamin folate) from fortified foods and supplements in addition to folate from a varied diet. This level of folate can reduce the risk of neural tube defects in a developing fetus. Enriched breads, flours, cornmeal, rice, noodles, and other grain products are fortified with folic acid. Folate is found naturally in leafy green vegetables, legumes, oranges, and strawberries.
- Because of the oxidative stress caused by smoking, smokers should get 35 milligrams more vitamin C per day than the RDA set for their age and sex. Supplements are not usually necessary, however, because this extra vitamin C can easily be found in foods. For example, 250 millilitres (1 cup) of orange juice has about 100 milligrams of vitamin C.
- Vitamin D and calcium are important for bone strength and to reduce the risk of osteoporosis and fractures in older adults. Canadians under the age of 71 need 600 IU (IU is the symbol for international units, which vitamin D is measured in) of vitamin D a day, and those 71 and older need 800 IU. Five hundred millilitres (2 cups) of milk provide about 200 IU of vitamin D. Because the skin's ability to produce vitamin D decreases with age, men and women 50 and older need a daily vitamin D supplement of 400 IU, in addition to following *Eating Well with Canada's Food Guide*. People with dark skin and people who are exposed to little sunlight (such as nightshift workers and those living in institutions) may need vitamin D supplements as well.

Supplements may be recommended in other cases. Women with heavy menstrual flows, for example, may need extra iron. Some vegetarians may need supplemental calcium, iron, zinc, and B12, depending on their food choices. Other people may benefit from supplementation based on their physical conditions, the medicines they take, or their dietary habits.

Before deciding whether to take a vitamin or mineral supplement, consider whether you already consume a fortified breakfast cereal every day. Many breakfast cereals contain almost as many nutrients as a multivitamin pill. If you elect to take a supplement, choose one that contains 50–100 percent of the Daily Value for vitamins and minerals. Avoid supplements containing large doses of particular nutrients. To determine which supplement may be best for you, consult your doctor or pharmacist.

different sets of guidelines and include standards for fat, cholesterol, carbohydrate, dietary fibre, and selected vitamins and minerals. The Daily Values represent appropriate intake levels for a 2000-calorie diet. The percent Daily Value shown on a food label shows how well that food contributes to your recommended daily intake. Food labels are described in detail later in the chapter.

Daily Values
A simplified version of the RDAs used on food labels; includes values for nutrients with no RDA.

Guidelines for Healthy Eating

To provide general guidance for choosing a healthy diet, Health Canada has issued Guidelines for Healthy Eating. Most people look for more than just additional information on nutrition to help them decipher the scientific concepts used to establish the Dietary Reference Intakes. The Guidelines for Healthy Eating provide practical, concrete actions that Canadians can take to ensure they follow a healthy diet, such as:

- Enjoy a variety of foods.
- Emphasize cereals, breads, grain products, vegetables, and fruit.
- Choose lower-fat dairy products, leaner meats, and foods prepared with little or no fats.
- Achieve and maintain a healthy weight by enjoying regular physical activity and healthy eating.
- Limit salt, alcohol, and caffeine.

Following these guidelines promotes health and reduces the risk for chronic diseases, including heart disease, cancer, diabetes, stroke, osteoporosis, and obesity. Each of the Guidelines for Healthy Eating recommendations is supported by an extensive review of scientific and medical evidence.

Adequate Nutrients Within Calorie Needs

Many people consume more calories than they need while failing to meet recommended intakes for all nutrients. The DRIs provide a foundation not only for current health, but also for reducing chronic disease risk.

Following *Eating Well with Canada's Food Guide* can help you to obtain all the nutrients you need by choosing the recommended number of daily servings from basic food groups and following the advice about selecting nutrient-dense foods within the groups.

People's food choices can be affected by individual and cultural preferences, moral beliefs, the cost and availability of food, and food intolerances and allergies. But healthy eating is possible no matter how foods are prepared or combined (see the Dimensions of Diversity box). If you avoid most or all foods from any of the major food groups, be sure to get enough nutrients from the other groups. *Eating Well with Canada's Food Guide* can also be applied to vegetarian diets.

Weight Management

Overweight and obesity are a major public health problem in Canada. Calorie intake and physical activity work together to influence body weight. Most Canadians need to reduce the number of calories they consume, increase their level of physical activity, and make wiser food choices. Many adults gain weight slowly over time, but even small changes in behaviour can help avoid weight gain. For more information on weight management, see Chapter 4.

Physical Activity

Regular physical activity improves fitness, helps manage weight, promotes psychological well-being, and reduces the risk of heart disease, high blood pressure, cancer, and diabetes. Become active if you are inactive, and maintain or increase physical activity if you are already active. It is important to balance a healthy diet with regular physical activity to maintain optimal health. The amount of daily physical activity recommended for you depends on your current health status and goals. See Chapter 6 for information on exercise and physical fitness.

THINKING ABOUT THE ENVIRONMENT

Environmental issues—including booming populations and changing weather patterns—have coupled with fuel shortages to create a potential global food crisis. In 2008, evidence of such a crisis began to mount, even as worldwide production of many food staples reached all-time highs.

- The growing demand for corn to create ethanol (an alternative to gasoline) has driven up corn prices and greatly reduced the amount of grain used for human and animal consumption.
- Driven by fears of future shortages, the price of rice rose by more than 75 percent between December 2007 and April 2008. Some rice-producing countries began restricting rice exports to meet their own needs for the staple.
- Riots erupted in Haiti, Egypt, Bangladesh, and other countries in the spring of 2008, as residents protested food shortages and high prices. Many experts warned that if the current trend continues, the world's poorest people soon will not be able to feed themselves.

For more information on the environment and health, see Chapter 21.

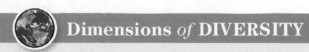

Dimensions *of* DIVERSITY

Ethnic Foods

No single ethnic diet clearly surpasses all others in providing people with healthful foods. However, every diet has its advantages and disadvantages and, within each cuisine, some foods are better choices. The dietary guidelines described in this chapter can be applied to any ethnic cuisine. For additional guidance, refer to the table below.

	Choose More Often	Choose Less Often
Chinese	• Dishes that are steamed, poached (jum), boiled (chu), roasted (kow), barbecued (shu), or lightly stir-fried • Hoisin sauce, oyster sauce, wine sauce, plum sauce, velvet sauce, or hot mustard • Fresh fish and seafood, skinless chicken, tofu • Mixed vegetables, Chinese greens • Steamed rice, steamed spring rolls, soft noodles	• Fried wontons or egg rolls • Crab rangoon • Crispy (Peking) duck or chicken • Sweet-and-sour dishes made with breaded and deep-fried meat, poultry, or fish • Fried rice • Fried or crispy noodles
French	• Dishes prepared *au vapeur* (steamed), *en brochette* (skewered and broiled), or *grillé* (grilled) • Fresh fish, shrimp, scallops, mussels, or skinless chicken, without sauces • Clear soups	• Dishes prepared *à gratinée* (baked with cream and cheese), or *en croûte* (in pastry crust) • Drawn butter, hollandaise sauce, and remoulade (mayonnaise-based sauce)
Greek	• Dishes that are stewed, broiled, or grilled, including souvlaki • Dolmas (grape leaves) stuffed with rice • Tzatziki (yogourt, cucumbers, and garlic) • Pita bread, especially whole wheat	• Moussaka, saganaki (fried cheese) • Vegetable pies, such as spanakopita and tyropita • Gyros stuffed with ground meat • Baklava
Indian	• Dishes prepared *masala* (curry), *tandoori* (roasted in a clay oven), or *tikke* (pan roasted); kebabs • Raita (yogourt and cucumber salad) and other yogourt-based dishes and sauces • Dal (lentils), pullao or pilau (basmati rice) • Chapati (baked bread)	• Ghee (clarified butter) • Korma (meat in cream sauce) • Samosas, pakoras (fried dishes) • Molee and other coconut milk–based dishes • Poori, bhatura, or paratha (fried breads)
Italian	• Pasta primavera or pasta, polenta, risotto, or gnocchi with marinara, red or white wine, white or red clam, or light mushroom sauce • Dishes that are grilled or prepared *cacciatore* (tomato-based sauce), *marsala* (broth and wine sauce), or *piccata* (lemon sauce) • Cioppino (seafood stew) • Vegetable soup, minestrone or fagioli (beans)	• Antipasto (cheese, smoked meats) • Dishes that are prepared *alfredo*, *frito* (fried), *crema* (creamed), *alla panna* (with cream), or *carbonara* • Veal scaloppini • Chicken, veal, or eggplant parmigiana • Italian sausage, salami, and prosciutto • Buttered garlic bread • Cannoli
Japanese	• Dishes prepared *nabemono* (boiled), *shabu-shabu* (in boiling broth), *mushimono* (steamed), *nimono* (simmered), *yaki* (broiled), or *yakimono* (grilled) • Sushi or domburi (mixed rice dish) • Steamed rice or soba (buckwheat), udon (wheat), or rice noodles	• Tempura (battered and fried) • Agemono (deep fried) • Katsu (fried pork cutlet) • Sukiyaki • Fried tofu
Mexican	• Soft corn or wheat tortillas • Burritos, fajitas, enchiladas, soft tacos, and tamales filled with beans, vegetables, or lean meats • Refried beans, nonfat or low-fat; rice and beans • Ceviche (fish marinated in lime juice) • Salsa, enchilada sauce, and *picante* sauce • Gazpacho, menudo, or black bean soup • Fruit or flan for dessert	• Crispy, fried tortillas • Dishes that are fried, such as chile flautas, and tostadas • Nachos and cheese, chili con queso, and other dishes made with cheese or cheese sauce • Guacamole, sour cream, and extra cheese • Refried beans made with lard • Fried ice cream
Middle Eastern	• Dishes that are stewed, broiled, or grilled, including shish kebabs • Tabouli (bulgur-based salad) • Pita bread, especially whole wheat	• Moussaka • Baba ghanoush (eggplant and olive oil) • Deep-fried falafel (chickpea patties)
Thai	• Dishes that are barbecued, sautéed, broiled, boiled, steamed, braised, or marinated • Sâté (skewered and grilled meats) • Fish sauce, basil sauce, chili or hot sauces • Bean thread noodles, Thai salad	• Coconut milk soup • Peanut sauce or dishes topped with nuts • Mee-krob (crispy noodles) • Red, green, and yellow curries, which typically contain coconut milk

Sources: National Heart, Lung, and Blood Institute. 2006. *Guidelines on Overweight and Obesity: Electronic Textbook,* http://www.nhlbi.nih.gov/health-pro/guidelines/current/obesity-guidelines/e_textbook/ (retrieved February 9, 2015); and Duyff, R. L. 2006. *The American Dietetic Association's Complete Food and Nutrition Guide,* 2nd ed. Hoboken, N.J.: Wiley.

Food Groups to Encourage

The Guidelines for Healthy Eating and *Eating Well with Canada's Food Guide* both emphasize eating a wide range of foods. Central to these plans are fruits, vegetables, whole grains, and low-fat and fat-free milk and alternatives. Each of these food groups offers a nearly endless array of choices. The discussion of *Eating Well with Canada's Food Guide* later in this chapter provides detailed information on choices and serving sizes.

Fats

The type and amount of fats consumed can make a difference for health. A diet low in saturated fat, trans fat, and cholesterol helps keep blood cholesterol low and reduces the risk for heart disease. Goals for fat intake for most adults are as follows:

- Total fat: 20–35 percent of total daily calories
- Saturated fat: Less than 7 percent of total daily calories
- Trans fat: Less than 2 percent of total caloric intake
- Cholesterol: Less than 300 milligrams per day

Most fats in the diet should come from sources of unsaturated fats, such as fish, nuts, and vegetable oils. When selecting and preparing meat, poultry, dry beans, and milk or milk products, make choices that are lean, low fat, or fat free. To reduce trans fat intake, limit intake of foods made with hydrogenated vegetable oils. (See the In the News box.)

Cholesterol is found only in animal foods. If you need to reduce your cholesterol intake, limit your intake of foods that are particularly high in cholesterol, including egg yolks, dairy fats, certain shellfish, and liver and other organ meats, and watch your serving sizes of animal foods. Food labels list the fat and cholesterol content of foods.

Two servings per week of fish rich in heart-healthy omega-3 fatty acids are also recommended for people at high risk for heart disease. However, for certain groups, intake limits are set for varieties of fish that may contain mercury; see the section "Guidelines for Fish Consumption" later in the chapter for more information. Fish rich in omega-3 fatty acids include salmon, mackerel, and trout.

Carbohydrates

Carbohydrates are an important energy source in a healthy diet. Foods rich in carbohydrates may also be rich in dietary fibre, which promotes healthy digestion and helps reduce the risk of type 2 diabetes and heart disease. Fruits, vegetables, whole grains, and fat-free or low-fat milk can provide the recommended amount of carbohydrate. Choose fibre-rich foods often—for example, whole fruits, whole grains, and legumes.

People who consume foods and beverages high in added sugars tend to consume more calories but smaller amounts of vitamins and minerals than those who limit their intake of added sugars. A food is likely high in sugar if one of the following appears first or second in the list of ingredients or if several are listed: sugar (any type, including beet, brown, invert, raw, and cane), corn syrup or sweetener, fruit juice concentrate, honey, malt syrup, molasses, syrup, cane juice, dextrose, fructose, glucose, lactose, maltose, or sucrose.

To reduce added sugar consumption, cut back on soft drinks, candies, sweet desserts, fruit drinks, and other foods high in added sugars. Watch out for specialty drinks,

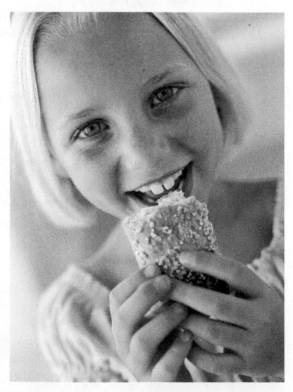

Half of your daily grain servings should come from whole grains. To check whether a food contains whole grains, read the ingredient list on the food label.

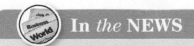
In *the* NEWS

Going Trans Fat Free

In 2005, Health Canada commissioned the Trans Fat Task Force to study ways to reduce or eliminate the trans fats added to our food supply, and in 2006, *TRANS forming the Food Supply*, the Task Force's final report, was released. In 2007, the minister of health endorsed the trans fat levels recommended by the Task Force (2 percent of the total fat content in vegetable oils and soft margarines; and 5 percent of the total fat in all other foods, including those sold to restaurants) and gave the food industry two years to voluntarily meet those levels. If the levels were not met, the minister promised regulation of the industry to achieve that goal. Some food companies achieved or bettered these levels, but others have not. Unfortunately, many foods often consumed by children as treats, such as cakes, doughnuts, and brownies, still contain trans fats.

Denmark, Switzerland, California, and many cities in the United States have trans fat regulations. In Canada, British Columbia implemented trans fat regulations in September 2009.

What Are Trans Fats?

Trans fats are unsaturated fatty acids that have at least one double bond in the *trans* configuration. This refers to the way the hydrogen atoms are arranged on either side of the double bond. Normally, these hydrogen atoms are on the same side of the double bond, but in a trans fatty acid, they are on opposite sides. This gives the fatty acid a physical structure more like a saturated fatty acid. Although trans fats are found in small amounts naturally in milk, beef, and lamb, most trans fats are formed through the process of hydrogenation. Many popular food items contain trans fat (see the table below).

Hydrogenation makes liquid oils into solid or semi-solid fats and is the process used to make margarine and shortening. These partially hydrogenated oils have a longer shelf life and ideal physical properties for use in baked goods, such as pastries, pie crusts, pizza dough, biscuits, cookies, and crackers. Partially hydrogenated oils are used for deep-fat frying because they are more stable, don't break down quickly, and therefore are more cost effective than non-hydrogenated oils.

The use of partially hydrogenated oils in restaurant and commercially prepared foods grew throughout the 1960s, 1970s, and 1980s in response to public health recommendations to reduce saturated fat intake from animal fats and tropical oils (such as palm and coconut oil).

Trans Fat Content of Common Food Items

Product	Common Serving Size	Total Fat (g)	Trans Fat (g)
French fries	Medium pkg (147 g)	27	8
Hard margarine	1 tbsp	11	3
Soft margarine	1 tbsp	7	0.5
Shortening	1 tbsp	13	4
Potato chips	Small bag (42.5 g)	11	3
Doughnut	1	18	5
Candy bar	1 (40 g)	10	3
Pound cake	1 slice (80 g)	16	4.5

Why Worry About Trans Fats?

In the 1990s, studies began to show that trans fats had similar effects in the body as saturated fat. Further research found that trans fats were actually worse for heart health because not only do they raise LDL cholesterol, but they also lower HDL cholesterol. Trans fats are at least five times more harmful, on a gram by gram basis, than saturated fats. Other studies suggest that trans fats may promote obesity and diabetes.

Can Trans Fats Be Eliminated?

Trans fats are not a dietary essential. Health organizations recommend that trans fat intake be as low as possible. Because some trans fats are naturally occurring, unless you are a strict vegetarian, your diet has no room for trans fats from partially hydrogenated oils. More and more products in the grocery store are available without trans fat, and as interest in trans-fat-free restaurants grows, it will be easier for consumers to limit trans fats when eating out.

Denmark has made it illegal for any food to contain more than 2 percent trans fat, and Canada is considering a nationwide ban on trans fats in restaurants. In the United States in 2004, the Center for Science in the Public Interest petitioned the Food and Drug Administration to ban trans fat as a food ingredient.

Reducing Your Trans Fat Intake

To reduce your intake of trans fat, start by reading food labels; trans fat content is required to be listed. A word of caution, however: A serving of a food can contain up to 0.5 grams of trans fat and still show zero grams on the Nutrition Fact label and the words "trans fat free" on the label. So check the ingredient list. If partially hydrogenated oil is included in the list, then the product contains trans fat.

Next, check the product's calorie and saturated fat content. Foods without trans fat are not healthier if they contain more saturated fat or more calories from added sugars. Ask at restaurants whether trans-fat-free oils are used in cooking. Proposals being considered could require national chain restaurants to include information about the calorie content of their foods, which could also help consumers make smart choices.

Sources: Mozaffarian, D., et al. 2006. Trans fatty acids and cardiovascular disease. *New England Journal of Medicine* 354(15): 1601–1613; Eckel, R. H., et al. 2006. Understanding the complexity of trans fatty acid reduction in the American diet. American Heart Association Trans Fat Conference 2006. Report of the *Trans Fat* Conference Planning Group. *Circulation* 115(16): 2231–2246; American Heart Association. 2009. *Trans Fats,* http://www.americanheart.org/presenter.jhtml?identifier=3045792 (retrieved February 9, 2015); Center for Science in the Public Interest. 2009. *Trans Fat,* http://www.cspinet.org/transfat (retrieved February 9, 2015); U.S. Food and Drug Administration, Center for Food Safety and Applied Nutrition. 2006 Update. *Questions and Answers about Trans Fat Nutrition Labeling,* http://vm.cfsan.fda.gov/~dms/qatrans2.html (retrieved February 9, 2015); U.S. Food and Drug Administration. 2003. *Revealing Trans Fats,* http://www.fda.gov/FDAC/features/2003/503_fats.html (retrieved February 9, 2015); Trans Fat Task Force. 2006. *TRANS forming the Food Supply,* http://www.hc-sc.gc.ca/fn-an/alt_formats/hpfb-dgpsa/pdf/nutrition/tf-gt_rep-rap-eng.pdf (retrieved April 2, 2015).

such as café mochas, chai tea, smoothies, and sports drinks, which can contain hundreds of extra calories from sugar. Drink water rather than sweetened drinks, and don't let soft drinks and other sweets crowd out more nutritious foods, such as low-fat milk. Regular soft drinks are the leading source of both added sugars and calories in the Canadian diet, but they provide little in the way of nutrients except sugar (see Figure 5.5).

Sodium and Potassium

Many people can reduce their chance of developing high blood pressure or lower already-elevated blood pressure by consuming less salt; reducing blood pressure lowers the risk for stroke, heart disease, and kidney disease. Salt is made up of the minerals sodium and chloride, and although both of these minerals are essential for normal body function, we need only small amounts (1500 milligrams per day for adults). Most Canadians consume much more salt than they need. The goal is to reduce sodium intake to less than 2300 milligrams per day, the equivalent of about one teaspoon of salt. Certain groups, including people with hypertension, blacks, those of South Asian descent, and older adults, benefit from an even lower sodium intake (no more than 1500 milligrams per day).

Salt is found mainly in processed and prepared foods; smaller amounts may also be added during cooking or at the table. To lower your intake of salt, choose fresh or plain frozen meat, poultry, seafood, and vegetables most often, which are lower in salt than processed forms are. Check and compare the sodium content in processed foods, including frozen dinners, cheeses, soups, salad dressings, sauces, and canned mixed dishes. Add less salt during cooking and at the table, and limit your use of high-sodium condiments, such as soy sauce, ketchup, mustard, pickles, and olives. Use lemon juice, herbs, and spices instead of salt to enhance the flavour of foods.

Along with lowering salt intake, increasing potassium intake helps lower blood pressure. Fruits, vegetables, and most milk products are available in forms that contain no salt, and many of these are sources of potassium. Potassium-rich foods include leafy green vegetables, sweet and white potatoes, winter squash, soybeans, tomato sauce, bananas, peaches, apricots, cantaloupes, and orange juice.

FIGURE 5.5

Nutrient Density of 355-millilitre Portions of Selected Beverages

The coloured bars represent percentage of recommended daily intake or limit for each nutrient.

Nutrient	Recommended Daily Intake*	Orange Juice		Low-Fat (1%) Milk		Regular Cola		Bottled Iced Tea	
Calories	2000 calories	168 calories		150 calories		152 calories		150 calories	
Carbohydrate	300 g		40.5 g		18 g		38 g		37.5 g
Added sugars	32 g						38 g		34.5 g
Fat	65 g				3.9 g				
Protein	55 g				12 g				
Calcium	1000 mg		33 mg		450 mg		11 mg		
Potassium	4700 mg	15%	710 mg	12%	570 mg		4 mg		
Vitamin A	700 µg	4%	30 µg	31%	216 µg				
Vitamin C	75 mg		145.5 mg		3.6 mg				
Vitamin D	5 µg				3.7 µg				
Folate	400 µg		160 µg		20 µg				

*Recommended intakes and limits appropriate for a 20-year-old woman consuming 2000 calories per day.

Alcoholic Beverages

Alcoholic beverages supply calories but few nutrients. Drinking in moderation—that is, no more than two drinks per day for women and no more than three drinks per day for men—is associated with mortality reduction among some groups, primarily males age 45 and older and women age 55 and older. Among younger people, alcohol use provides little if any health benefit, and heavy drinking is associated with motor vehicle injuries and deaths, liver disease, stroke, violence, and other health problems (see Chapter 15 for more on the health risks and potential benefits of alcohol use). If you drink alcohol, follow the low-risk drinking guidelines at all times.

QUICK STATS

In 2011–2012, 8.3% of households, or almost 1.1 million households, experienced food insecurity. Of those households, 5.8% experienced a moderate rate food insecurity and 2.5% experienced a severe rate.

—Canadian Community Health Survey, 2004

Eating Well with Canada's Food Guide

When the Canada's first food guide was published in 1942, it acknowledged the difficulties of coping with wartime food rationing while still trying to prevent nutritional deficiencies and improve health. Since then, scientists have updated both nutrient recommendations (the DRIs) and the Guidelines for Healthy Eating. The food guide has had several different names, different looks, and even different messages, but it's core purpose has remained the same: "guiding food selection to promote the nutritional health of Canadians." In 2002, Health Canada began a revision of the food guide that was evidence based. In 2007, it released *Eating Well with Canada's Food Guide* (see Figure 5.6).

More than half of Canadians are consuming more than double the recommended daily amount of sodium. Most Canadians take in more than twice the amount of sodium they need in a day. It is estimated that Canadians 1 year of age and older eat an average of about 3400 mg/day of sodium.

—Health Canada, 2012

Another food plan that has received attention in recent years is the Mediterranean diet, which emphasizes vegetables, fruits, and whole grains; daily servings of beans, legumes, and nuts; moderate consumption of fish, poultry, and dairy products; and the use of olive oil over other types of fat, especially saturated fat. The Mediterranean diet has been associated with lower rates of heart disease and cancer, and recent studies have found a link between the diet and a greatly reduced risk of Alzheimer's disease.

Key Messages of *Eating Well with Canada's Food Guide*

The most recent version of the food guide was developed to remind consumers to make healthy food choices and to be active every day. Consuming a balance of servings from each food group will not only meet nutrient needs, but will also help to reduce chronic disease risk. The key messages include the following:

- *Variety* is represented by the wide range of foods graphically represented in the guide. Many foods, including those typically consumed by different ethic groups living in Canada, are given as examples. Foods from all groups are needed daily for good health.

- *Food guide serving sizes and quantities* are given in both pictures and specific measurements, showing serving sizes of a variety of foods and amounts required by consumers of different ages and sexes.

- *Make each food guide serving count* is represented by directional statements that give consumers ways to ensure they are choosing food with high nutritional quality more often.

- *Advice for different ages and stages* ensures optimal growth, development, and maintenance of health are achieved.

Eating Well with Canada's Food Guide

Health Canada's food guidance system, called *Eating Well with Canada's Food Guide*, can be personalized based on your sex, age, and activity level; visit http://www.myfoodguide.ca to obtain a food plan appropriate for you. *Eating Well with Canada's Food Guide* contains four main food groups. Directional statements, examples of food guide servings, and recommended numbers of servings guide consumers to choose a variety of healthy foods. The guide is available in English, French, Arabic, Chinese (simple), Farsi (Persian), Korean, Punjabi, Russian, Spanish, Tagalog, Urdu, and Tamil.

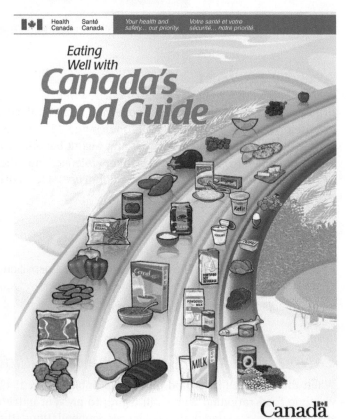

Source: © Health Canada, 2011. *Eating Well with Canada's Food Guide*, Health Canada, 2011. Adapted and reproduced with permission from the Minister of Health, 2015. All rights reserved.

- *Promotion of physical activity* includes recommendations about building physical activity into daily life.

To determine how much and what foods you should be consuming every day, create a personalized version of *Eating Well with Canada's Food Guide* at http://www.myfoodguide.ca. Each food group is described briefly below. Past experiences have shown that many Canadians have trouble identifying serving sizes, so recommended daily intakes from each group are now given; see the Take Charge box for additional advice.

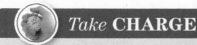 Take **CHARGE**

Judging Portion Sizes

Studies have shown that most people underestimate the size of their food portions. Consequently they underestimate their true calorie intake by at least 30 percent, with a range of 10–45 percent. If you need to retrain your eye, try using measuring cups and spoons and an inexpensive kitchen scale when you eat at home. With a little practice, you will learn the difference between 90 and 225 grams of chicken or meat, and what 125 millilitres of rice really looks like. For quick estimates, use the following equivalents:
- 5 millilitres (1 teaspoon) of margarine = the tip of your thumb
- 30 grams of cheese = two thumbs, four dice stacked together
- 90 grams of chicken or meat = a deck of cards
- 250 millilitres (1 cup) of pasta = a small fist or a baseball
- 125 millilitres (½ cup) of rice or cooked vegetables = a tennis ball
- 30 millilitres (2 tablespoons) of peanut butter = a golf ball
- 1 medium potato = a computer mouse
- 1 small bagel = a hockey puck
- 1 medium fruit (apple or orange) = a baseball or light bulb
- 50 millilitres (¼ cup) of nuts = a golf ball

Grains

Foods from this group are usually low in fat and rich in complex carbohydrates, dietary fibre (if the grains are unrefined), and many vitamins and minerals, including thiamine, riboflavin, iron, niacin, folic acid (if enriched or fortified), and zinc. An adult between the ages of 19 and 50 should include six to eight servings each day, depending on their sex, with half of those servings from whole grains, such as whole-grain bread, whole wheat pasta, high-fibre cereal, and brown rice. The following count as one serving:
- 1 slice of bread
- 1 small (6-centimetre diameter) muffin
- 250 millilitres (1 cup) of ready-to-eat cereal flakes
- 125 millilitres (½ cup) cooked cereal, rice, grains, or pasta
- 1 15-centimetre tortilla

Choose foods that are typically made with little fat or sugar (bread, rice, pasta) over those that are high in fat and sugar (croissants, chips, cookies, doughnuts).

Vegetables and Fruit

Vegetables contain carbohydrates, dietary fibre, vitamin A, vitamin C, folate, potassium, and other nutrients. They are also naturally low in fat. Each of the following counts as one serving of vegetables:
- 125 millilitres (½ cup) of raw or cooked vegetables
- 250 millilitres (1 cup) of raw leafy salad greens
- 125 millilitres (½ cup) vegetable juice

Because vegetables vary in the nutrients they provide, it is important to consume a variety of types of vegetables to obtain maximum nutrition. Many Canadians consume only a few types of vegetables, with white potatoes (baked or served as French fries) being the most popular. You should eat at least one dark-green and one orange vegetable each day; choose vegetables and fruit prepared with little or no added fat, sugar, or salt; and have vegetables and fruit more often than juice. The following examples will give you ideas to help boost your vegetable intake:

- Dark-green vegetables include spinach, chard, collards, bok choy, broccoli, kale, romaine, turnip greens, and mustard greens.
- Orange and deep-yellow vegetables include carrots, winter squash, sweet potatoes, and pumpkin.
- Starchy vegetables include corn, green peas, and white potatoes.
- Other vegetables, such as tomatoes, bell peppers (red, orange, yellow, or green), green beans, and cruciferous vegetables, such as cauliflower, are also good choices.

Fruits are rich in carbohydrates, dietary fibre, and many vitamins, especially vitamin C. The following each count as one serving of fruit:

- 125 millilitres (½ cup) fresh, canned, or frozen fruit
- 125 millilitres (½ cup) fruit juice (100 percent juice)
- 1 small whole fruit
- 50 millilitres (½ cup) dried fruit

Good choices from this group are citrus fruits and juices, melons, pears, apples, bananas, and berries. Choose whole fruits often—they are higher in fibre and often lower in calories than fruit juices. Fruit *juices* typically contain more nutrients and less added sugar than fruit *drinks*. For canned fruits, choose those packed in 100 percent fruit juice or water rather than in syrup.

QUICK STATS

47% of Canadian females and 34.6% of males report consuming five or more servings of fruits and vegetables each day.

—*Canadian Community Health Survey*, 2012

Milk and Alternatives

This group includes all milk, milk products, and milk alternatives, such as yogourt and cheeses (except cream cheese), lactose-free and lactose-reduced products, and soy and rice beverages. Foods from this group are high in protein, carbohydrate, calcium, riboflavin, and vitamin D (if fortified). Each of the following counts as one serving:

- 250 millilitres (1 cup) of milk or fortified soy beverage
- 50 grams of natural cheese
- 175 millilitres (¾ cup) of kefir or yogourt

Meat and Alternatives

This group includes meat, poultry, fish, dry beans and peas, eggs, nuts, and seeds. These foods provide protein, niacin, iron, vitamin B6, zinc, and thiamine; the animal foods in the group also provide vitamin B12. Each of the following counts as one serving:

- 75 grams of cooked lean meat, poultry, or fish
- 175 millilitres (¾ cup) of cooked dry beans (legumes) or tofu
- 2 eggs
- 30 millilitres (1 tablespoon) of peanut butter
- 60 millilitres (¼ cup) of nuts or seeds

One egg at breakfast, 175 millilitres of cooked pinto beans at lunch, and a 75-gram (cooked weight) hamburger at dinner would give you 170 grams of lean meat for the day. To limit your intake of fat and saturated fat, choose lean cuts of meat and skinless poultry, and watch your serving sizes carefully. Choose at least one serving of plant proteins, such as black beans, lentils, or tofu, every day.

Discretionary Calories, Solid Fats, and Added Sugars

The suggested intakes from the basic food groups in *Eating Well with Canada's Food Guide* assume that nutrient-dense forms are selected from each group; nutrient-dense forms are those that are low in fat, sodium, and sugar. If this pattern is followed, then a small amount of additional calories can be consumed—the *discretionary calorie allowance.*

People who are trying to lose weight may choose not to use discretionary calories. For those wanting to maintain weight, discretionary calories may be used to increase the amount of food from a food group; to consume foods that are not in the lowest-fat form or that contain added sugars; to add oil, fat, or sugars to foods; or to consume alcohol.

The values for additional fat suggest no more than 30 percent of total calories from fat and less than 7 percent of calories from saturated fat. Examples of discretionary solid fat calories include choosing higher-fat meats, such as sausage or chicken with the skin, drinking whole milk instead of fat-free milk, and topping foods with butter. For example, 250 millilitres (1 cup) of whole milk has 60 calories more than 250 millilitres (1 cup) of skim milk; these 60 calories would be counted as discretionary calories.

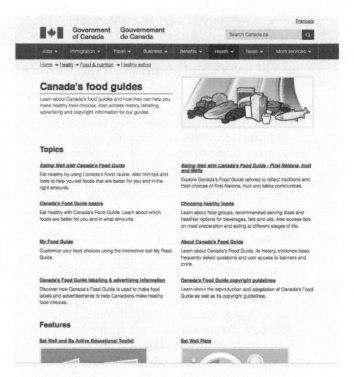

You can track your diet and physical activity and create a personal diet plan by using the online tools at http://www.MyFoodGuide.ca.

As described earlier in the chapter, added sugars are the sugars added to foods and beverages in processing or preparation, not the naturally occurring sugars in fruits or milk. The suggested amounts of added sugars may be helpful limits for including some sweetened foods or beverages in your daily diet without exceeding your energy needs or underconsuming other nutrients. In the Canadian diet, added sugars are often found in sweetened beverages (regular soft drinks, sweetened teas, fruit drinks), dairy products (ice cream, some yogurts), and grain products (bakery goods). For example, a 591-millilitre bottle of a regular soft drink has 260 calories from added sugars that would be counted as discretionary calories. Remember, to control weight and get enough essential nutrients, it is important to choose nutrient-dense forms of foods for most of your daily servings.

For an evaluation of your diet, complete the activity in the Assess Yourself box.

The Vegetarian Alternative

Some people choose a diet with one essential difference from the diets we have already described—foods of animal origin (meat, poultry, fish, eggs, milk) are eliminated or restricted. Many do so for health reasons; vegetarian diets tend to be lower in saturated fat and cholesterol and higher in complex carbohydrates, dietary fibre, folate, vitamins C and E, carotenoids, and phytochemicals. Some people adopt a vegetarian diet out of concern for the environment, for financial considerations, or for reasons related to ethics or religion.

Assess YOURSELF

Your Diet Versus the *Eating Well with Canada's Food Guide* Recommendations

1. *Keep a food record.* To evaluate your daily diet, begin by keeping a record of everything you eat on a typical day. To help with your analysis, break down each food item into its component parts and note your portion sizes; for example, a turkey sandwich might be listed as 2 slices sourdough bread, 90 grams turkey, 1 tomato, 15 millilitres mayonnaise, and so on.
2. *Compare your servings with the recommendations* of Eating Well with Canada's Food Guide. Complete the chart below to compare your daily diet with *Eating Well with Canada's Food Guide.* It may be difficult to track values for added sugars and, especially, oils and fats, but be as accurate as you can. Check food labels for information on fat and sugar. For a more complete and accurate analysis of your diet, keep food records for three days and then average the results. MyFoodGuide.ca has additional guidelines for counting discretionary calories.
3. *Further evaluate your food choices within the groups.* Based on the data you collected and what you learned in the chapter, what were the especially healthy choices you made (for example, whole grains and citrus fruits) and what were your less healthy choices? Identify and list foods in the latter category, as these are areas where you can make changes to improve your diet. In particular, you may want to limit your intake of the following: processed, sweetened grains; high-fat meats and poultry skin; deep-fried fast foods; homogenized milk products; regular soft drinks, sweetened teas, fruit drinks; alcoholic beverages; and other foods that primarily provide sugar and fat and few other nutrients.
4. *Make healthy changes.* Bring your diet in line with *Eating Well with Canada's Food Guide* by adding servings from food groups for which you fall short of the recommendations. To maintain a healthy weight, you may need to balance these additions by reductions in other areas—by eliminating some of the fats, oils, sweets, and alcohol you consume; by cutting extra servings from food groups for which your intake is more than adequate; or by making healthier choices within the food groups. Make a list of foods to add and a list of foods to eliminate; post your lists in a prominent location.

For a more detailed analysis of your current diet, including intakes of specific nutrients, use the online tools for *Eating Well with Canada's Food Guide* available at MyFoodGuide.ca.

Food Group	Recommended Daily, Amounts/Servings for Your Energy Intake	Your Actual Daily Intake (Amounts/Servings)	Serving Sizes and Equivalents
Grain Products (total)			1 serving = 1 slice of bread; 1 small muffin; 250 mL ready-to-eat cereal flakes; or 125 mL cooked cereal, rice, grains, or pasta
Whole grains			
Other grains			
Vegetables and Fruit (total)			1 serving = 125 mL raw or cooked vegetables; 250 mL raw leafy salad greens; 125 mL vegetable juice; 125 mL fresh, canned, or frozen fruit; 125 mL fruit juice; 1 small whole fruit; or 50 mL dried fruit
Dark green*			
Deep yellow*			
Starchy*			
Other*			
Milk and Alternatives			1 serving = 250 mL milk or 175 mL yogourt; 50 g natural cheese
Meat and Alternatives			1 serving = 75 g lean meat, poultry, or fish; 175 mL cooked dry beans or tofu; 2 eggs; 30 mL peanut butter; or 60 mL nuts or seeds
Oils			
Solid Fats			
Added Sugars			

Types of Vegetarian Diets

There are various vegetarian styles; the wider the variety of the diet eaten, the easier it is to meet nutritional needs.

- **Vegans** eat only plant foods.
- **Lacto-vegetarians** eat plant foods and dairy products.
- **Lacto-ovo-vegetarians** eat plant foods, dairy products, and eggs.

vegans
Vegetarians who eat no animal products at all.

lacto-vegetarians
Vegetarians who include milk and cheese products in the diet.

lacto-ovo-vegetarians
Vegetarians who eat no meat, poultry, or fish but do eat eggs and milk products.

Others can be categorized as **partial vegetarians**, **semivegetarians**, or **pescovegetarians**; these individuals eat plant foods, dairy products, eggs, and usually a small selection of poultry, fish, and other seafood. Many other people choose vegetarian meals frequently but are not strictly vegetarian. Including some animal protein (such as dairy products) in a vegetarian diet makes planning easier, but it is not necessary.

partial vegetarians, semivegetarians, or pescovegetarians
Vegetarians who include eggs, dairy products, and small amounts of poultry and seafood in the diet.

Strong evidence links vegetarian diets to the reduction in risk of many chronic diseases. Vegetarian diets often include more potassium, fibre, and antioxidant-rich nutrients, which may play a role in reducing disease risk. Additionally, many people choosing vegetarian diets also choose a healthier lifestyle overall, which includes not smoking, being more physically active, and consuming alcohol in moderation, if at all. This healthy lifestyle also reduces the risk for chronic diseases, such as diabetes, heart disease, cancers, and obesity.

A Food Plan for Vegetarians

Eating Well with Canada's Food Guide can be adapted for use by vegetarians with only a few key modifications. For the meat and alternatives group, vegetarians can focus on the non-meat choices of dry beans (legumes), nuts, seeds, eggs, and soy foods, such as tofu (soybean curd) and tempeh (a cultured soy product). Vegans and other vegetarians who do not consume any dairy products must find other rich sources of calcium. Fruits, vegetables, and whole grains are healthy choices for people following all types of vegetarian diets.

QUICK STATS

4% of Canadians describe their typical diet as vegetarian.
—Government of Alberta, 2011

A healthy vegetarian diet emphasizes a wide variety of plant foods. Although plant proteins are generally of lower quality than animal proteins, choosing a variety of plant foods will supply all of the essential amino acids. Choosing minimally processed and unrefined foods will maximize nutrient value and provide ample dietary fibre. Daily consumption of a variety of plant foods in amounts that meet total energy needs can provide all needed nutrients, except vitamin B12 and possibly vitamin D. Strategies for obtaining nutrients of concern include the following:

- *Vitamin B12* is found naturally only in animal foods; if dairy products and eggs are limited or avoided, B12 can be obtained from fortified foods, such as ready-to-eat cereals, soy beverages, meat substitutes, and special yeast products, or from supplements.
- *Vitamin D* can be obtained by consuming vitamin D–fortified products like ready-to-eat cereals and soy or rice milk, or by taking a supplement. Although unprotected exposure to the sun can manufacture vitamin

D in your body, it can also increase your risk for skin cancer. It is recommended that people get their vitamin D from fortified foods and supplements rather than by spending time in the sun or in tanning beds.

- *Calcium* is found in legumes, tofu processed with calcium, dark-green leafy vegetables, nuts, and fortified orange juice, soy milk, bread, and other foods.
- *Iron* can be obtained from whole grains, fortified bread and breakfast cereals, dried fruits, green leafy vegetables, nuts and seeds, legumes, and soy foods. The iron in plant foods is more difficult for the body to absorb than is the iron from animal sources; consuming a good source of vitamin C with most meals is helpful because vitamin C improves iron absorption.
- *Zinc* is found in whole grains, nuts, legumes, and soy foods.

If you are a vegetarian or considering becoming one, devote some extra time and thought to your diet. It's especially important to eat as wide a variety of foods as possible to ensure that all your nutritional needs are satisfied. Consulting with a registered dietitian will make your planning even easier. Vegetarian diets for children, teens, and pregnant and lactating women warrant guidance from a health professional.

Dietary Challenges for Special Population Groups

The Guidelines for Healthy Eating and *Eating Well with Canada's Food Guide* provide a basis that everyone can use to create a healthy diet. However, some population groups face special dietary challenges (see the Gender Matters box).

 Gender MATTERS

How Different Are the Nutritional Needs of Women and Men?

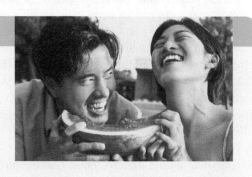

When it comes to nutrition, men and women have a lot in common. Both sexes need the same essential nutrients, and the Guidelines for Healthy Eating apply equally to both. But beyond the basics, men and women need different amounts of essential nutrients and have different nutritional concerns.

Women tend to be smaller and weigh less than men, and thus have lower energy requirements and need to consume fewer calories than men to maintain a healthy weight. For most nutrients, women need the same or slightly lower amounts than men. But because women consume fewer calories, they may have more difficulty getting adequate amounts of all essential nutrients and need to focus on nutrient-dense foods.

Two nutrients of special concern to women are calcium and iron. Low calcium intake may be linked to the development of osteoporosis in later life. Low-fat milk and alternatives and fortified cereal, bread, and orange juice are good choices for calcium-rich foods. Menstruating women also have higher iron needs than other groups, and low iron intake can lead to iron-deficiency anemia. Lean red meat, green leafy vegetables, and fortified breakfast cereals are good sources of iron. As discussed earlier, all women capable of becoming pregnant should consume adequate folic acid from fortified foods and supplements.

Men are seldom thought of as having nutritional deficiencies because they generally have high-calorie diets. However, many men have a diet that does not follow recommended food intake patterns and includes more red meat and fewer fruits, vegetables, and whole grains than recommended. This dietary pattern is linked to heart disease and some types of cancer. A high intake of calories can lead to weight gain over time if a man's activity level decreases as he ages. To reduce chronic disease risk, men should focus on increasing their consumption of fruits, vegetables, and whole grains to obtain vitamins, minerals, fibre, and phytochemicals.

The Northern Fruit and Vegetable Program is a provincial initiative that aims to increase fruit and vegetable consumption and increase awareness of the importance of fruits and vegetables among elementary school children in communities in Northern Ontario. It also hopes to educate elementary-school-age children and their families about the importance of eating fruit and vegetables, and the associated benefits of healthy eating and physical activity to overall health. In 2012, only 40.9 percent of Canadians reported consuming five or more servings of fruits and vegetables each day.

Children and Teenagers

Young people often simply need to be encouraged to eat. Perhaps the best thing a parent can do for younger children is to provide them with a variety of foods. Add vegetables to casseroles and fruit to cereal; offer fruit and vegetable juices or homemade yogourt or fruit shakes instead of sugary drinks. Allowing children to help prepare meals is another good way to increase overall food consumption and variety. Many children and teenagers enjoy eating at fast-food restaurants; they should be encouraged to select the healthiest choices from fast-food menus and to complete the day's diet with low-fat, nutrient-rich foods.

College and University Students

Foods that are convenient for post-secondary students are not always the healthiest choices. It is easy for students who eat in buffet-style dining halls or food courts to overeat, and the foods offered are not necessarily high in essential nutrients and low in fat. The same is true of meals at fast-food restaurants, another convenient source of quick and inexpensive meals for busy students. Although no food is entirely bad, consuming a wide variety of foods is critical for a healthy diet. See the Take Charge box for tips on making healthy eating convenient and affordable.

Take **CHARGE**

Eating Strategies for Post-secondary Students

General Guidelines
- Eat slowly, and enjoy your food. Set aside a separate time to eat, and don't eat while you study.
- Eat a colourful, varied diet. The more colourful your diet is, the more varied and rich in fruits and vegetables it will be. Many Canadians eat few servings of fruits and vegetables, despite the fact that these foods are typically inexpensive, delicious, rich in nutrients, and low in fat and calories.
- Eat breakfast. You will have more energy in the morning and be less likely to grab an unhealthy snack later on.
- Choose healthy snacks, such as fruits, vegetables, grains, and cereals.
- Drink water more often than soft drinks or other sweetened beverages. Rent a mini-refrigerator for your dorm room and stock up on healthy beverages, such as milk, water, and 100 percent fruit juice.
- Pay attention to portion sizes.
- Combine physical activity with healthy eating. You will feel better and have a much lower risk of many chronic diseases. Even a little exercise is better than none.

Eating in the Dining Hall or Cafeteria
- Choose a meal plan that includes breakfast, and don't skip it.
- Accept that dining hall food is not going to taste the same as home cooking. Find healthy dishes that you like.
- If menus are posted or distributed, decide what you want to eat before you get in line, and stick to your choices. Consider what you plan to do and eat for the rest of the day before making your choices.
- Ask for large servings of vegetables and small servings of meat and other high-fat main dishes. Build your meals around grains and vegetables.
- Try whole grains like brown rice, whole wheat bread, and whole-grain cereals.
- Choose leaner poultry, fish, or bean dishes rather than high-fat meats and fried entrees.
- Ask that gravies and sauces be served on the side; limit your intake.
- Choose broth-based or vegetable soups rather than cream soups.
- At the salad bar, load up on leafy greens, beans, and fresh vegetables. Avoid mayonnaise-coated salads, bacon, croutons, and high-fat dressings. Put dressing on the side, and dip your fork into it rather than pouring it over the salad.
- Drink low-fat milk, water, mineral water, or 100 percent fruit juice rather than heavily sweetened fruit drinks, whole milk, or soft drinks.
- Choose fruit for dessert rather than pastries, cookies, or cakes.
- Do some research about the foods and preparation methods used in your dining hall or cafeteria. Discuss any suggestions you have with your food-service manager. Students have the ability to advocate for healthy food choices. Make your voice heard if you have concerns.

Eating in Fast-Food Restaurants
- Most fast-food chains can provide a brochure with a nutritional breakdown of the foods on the menu. Ask for it or visit their website to find nutrition information posted about their products.
- Order small single burgers with no cheese instead of double burgers with many toppings. If possible, ask for them broiled instead of fried.
- Ask for items to be prepared without mayonnaise, tartar sauce, sour cream, or other high-fat sauces. Ketchup, mustard, and low-fat mayonnaise or sour cream are better choices and are available at many fast-food restaurants.
- Choose whole-grain buns or bread for burgers and sandwiches.
- Choose chicken items made from chicken breast, not processed chicken.
- Order vegetarian pizzas without extra cheese.
- If you order french fries or onion rings, get the smallest size, or share them with a friend. Better yet, get a salad or fruit cup instead.

Eating on the Run
Are you chronically short of time? Pack these items for a quick snack or meal: fresh or dried fruit, fruit juices, raw fresh vegetables, plain bagels, bread sticks, whole wheat fig bars, low-fat cheese sticks or cubes, low-fat crackers or granola bars, fat-free or low-fat yogourt, snack-size cereal boxes, pretzels, rice or corn cakes, plain popcorn, soup (if you have access to a microwave), or water.

Older Adults

Nutrient needs do not change much as people age, but because older adults tend to become less active, they require fewer calories to maintain body weight. At the same time, the absorption of nutrients tends to be lower in older adults because of age-related changes in the digestive tract. Thus, they must consume nutrient-dense foods to meet their nutritional requirements. Because constipation is a common problem, consuming foods high in fibre and getting adequate fluids are important goals.

Athletes

Key dietary concerns for athletes are meeting their increased energy requirements and drinking enough fluids during practice and throughout the day to remain fully hydrated. Endurance athletes may also benefit from increasing the amount of carbohydrate in the diet to 60–70 percent of total daily calories; this increase should come in the form of complex, rather than simple, carbohydrates. Athletes for whom maintaining low body weight and body fat is important—such as skaters, gymnasts, and wrestlers—should consume adequate nutrients and avoid falling into unhealthy patterns of eating. Eating for exercise is discussed in more detail in Chapter 6; refer to Chapter 4 for information on eating disorders.

Low-Income Families

Families surviving on low or fixed incomes may have difficulty meeting their nutritional needs. Often, they do not have enough income to support a healthy diet. If they have to use emergency food supports, such as food banks and soup kitchens, their challenge in consistently finding healthy foods is even greater.

First Nations, Inuit, and Metis

Aboriginal peoples, especially First Nations living on-reserve, face challenges in maintaining traditional food preparation and eating practices while trying to improve their health. They are also at risk for a variety of chronic diseases (predominantly obesity and diabetes), mental health issues, and addictions. The First Nations, Inuit, and Aboriginal Health Program established by Health Canada supports community-based and community delivered programs, initiatives, and strategies that aim to improve the health of mothers, infants, and families and to support the development of children in an effort to address the gap in life chances between Aboriginal and non-Aboriginal children.

Health Canada has also, for the first time, produced a food guide that specifically addresses the values, traditions, and food choices of Canada's First Nations, Inuit, and Metis. *Eating Well with Canada's Food Guide: First Nations, Inuit and Métis* meshes traditional food choices with those available in stores, especially the sometimes-limited selection available in rural and remote areas. The food guide is available in English, Inuktitut, Ojibwe, Plains Cree, and Woods Cree.

People with Special Health Concerns

Many Canadians have special health concerns that affect their dietary needs. For example, women who are pregnant or breastfeeding require extra calories, vitamins, and minerals (see Chapter 12). People with diabetes benefit from a well-balanced diet that is low in simple sugars, high in complex carbohydrates, and relatively rich in monounsaturated fats. People with high blood pressure need to control their weight and limit their sodium consumption. If you have a health problem or concern that may require a special diet, discuss your situation with a physician or registered dietitian.

QUESTIONS FOR CRITICAL THINKING AND REFLECTION

What factors influence your food choices: convenience, cost, availability, habit? Do you ever consider nutritional content or nutritional recommendations like those found in *Eating Well with Canada's Food Guide*? If not, how big a change would it be for you to think of nutritional content first when choosing food? Is it something you could do easily?

A Personal Plan: Making Informed Choices about Food

Now that you understand the basis of good nutrition and a healthy diet, you can put together a diet that works for you. Focus on the likely causes of any health problems in your life, and make specific dietary changes to address them. You may also have some specific areas of concern, such as interpreting food labels and dietary supplement or natural health product labels, avoiding food-borne illnesses and environmental contaminants, and understanding food additives. We turn to these and other topics next.

Reading Food Labels

All processed foods regulated by Health Canada and the Canadian Food Inspection Agency (CFIA) include standardized nutrition information on their labels. Every food label shows serving sizes and the amount of fat, saturated fat, trans fat, cholesterol, sodium, total carbohydrate, dietary fibre, sugars, and protein in each serving. To make intelligent choices about food, learn to read and *understand* food labels (see the Critical Consumer box).

Fresh meat, poultry, fish, fruits, vegetables, herbs, spices, and alcoholic beverages are not required to have food labels, and many of these products are not packaged. You can find information on the nutrient content of these items from basic nutrition books, registered dietitians, nutrient analysis computer software, websites, and the companies that produce or distribute these foods. Supermarkets often have large posters or pamphlets listing the nutrient contents of these foods.

Natural Health Products

In Canada, vitamins and minerals, herbal remedies, homeopathic medicines, traditional medicines, such as traditional Chinese medicines, probiotics, and other products, such as amino acids and essential fatty acids, are called natural health products. They may come in the form of tablets, capsules, liquids, or powders. Although many consumers often consider the use of natural health products to be safe, the products do contain powerful bioactive chemicals that have the potential for harm. Botanicals continue to serve as a beneficial source of therapeutic preparations: morphine from poppies and digoxin from foxglove, for example. And, as described earlier, even essential vitamins and minerals can have toxic effects if consumed in excess.

QUICK STATS

73% of Canadians take natural health products.
—Health Canada, 2010

Critical CONSUMER

Using Food Labels

Food labels are designed to help consumers make food choices based on the nutrients that are most important to good health. In addition to listing nutrient content by weight, the label puts the information in the context of a daily diet of 2000 calories that includes no more than 65 grams of fat (approximately 30 percent of total calories). For example, if a serving of a particular product has 13 grams of fat, the label will show that the serving represents 20 percent of the daily fat allowance. If your daily diet contains fewer or more than 2000 calories, you need to adjust these calculations accordingly.

Food labels contain uniform serving sizes. This means that if you look at different brands of salad dressing, for example, you can compare calories and fat content based on the serving amount. (Food label serving sizes may be larger or smaller than *Eating Well with Canada's Food Guide* serving size equivalents, however.) Regulations also require that foods meet strict definitions if their packaging includes the terms *light*, *low fat*, or *high fibre* (see below). Health claims, such as "good source of dietary fibre" or "low in saturated fat," on packages are signals

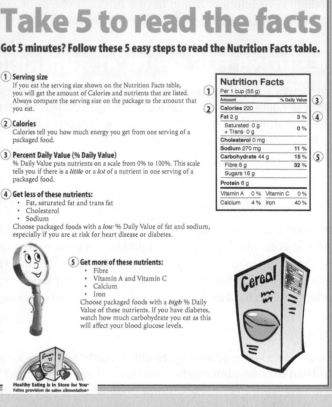

that those products can wisely be included in your diet. Overall, the food label is an important tool to help you choose a diet that conforms to *Eating Well with Canada's Food Guide* recommendations.

Selected Nutrient Claims and What They Mean

- *Light:* Reduced in energy or reduced in fat (criteria for "reduced" or "lower in" claims are based on the reference amount of the food)
- *Reduced or fewer:* At least 25 percent less of a nutrient than a similar product; can be applied to fat ("reduced fat"), saturated fat, cholesterol, sodium, and calories
- *Low in calories:* 40 calories or less per serving
- *High source of fibre:* 4 grams or more of fibre or of each identified fibre
- *Good source of fibre:* 2 grams or more of fibre or of each identified fibre
- *Fat free:* Less than 0.5 grams of fat per serving
- *Reduced fat or low in fat:* 3 grams of fat or less per serving
- *Saturated fatty acid free:* Less than 0.2 grams of saturated fat and 0.2 grams of trans fatty acids per serving
- *Low in saturated fatty acids:* 2 grams or less of saturated fat per serving and no more than 15 percent of total calories
- *Cholesterol free:* Less than 2 milligrams of cholesterol per serving and "low in saturated fatty acids"
- *Low in cholesterol:* 20 milligrams or less of cholesterol per serving and "low in saturated fatty acids"
- *Low in sodium or salt:* 140 milligrams or less of sodium or salt per serving
- *Sodium free or salt free:* Less than 5 milligrams of sodium or salt per serving
- *Lean:* Cooked seafood, meat, or poultry no more than 17 percent fat
- *Extra lean:* Cooked seafood, meat, or poultry with no more than 10 percent fat

Note: Health Canada has not yet defined nutrient claims relating to carbohydrate, so foods labelled low- or reduced-carbohydrate do not conform to any approved standard.

Source: Based on information from Health Canada. 2010. *Nutrition Labelling*, http://www.hc-sc.gc.ca/fn-an/label-etiquet/nutrition/index-eng.php (retrieved May 20, 2015).

The Natural Health Products Directorate, part of Health Canada, is the regulating authority for natural health products for sale in Canada. The role of this directorate is to ensure that Canadians have ready access to natural health products that are safe, effective, and of high quality. Before they are approved by Health Canada and put on the market, all drugs undergo clinical studies to determine safety, effectiveness, side effects and risks, possible interactions with other substances, and appropriate dosages. Although dosage guidelines exist for some of the compounds in natural health products, dosages for many are not well established.

Key differences also exist in how drugs and supplements are manufactured. The potency of herbal natural health products tends to vary widely because of differences in growing and harvesting conditions, preparation methods, and storage. Some manufacturers attempt to standardize their products by isolating the compounds believed to be responsible for a herb's action. However, potency is often still highly variable, and when several compounds are thought to be responsible for a herb's effect, often only one is standardized. In addition, herbs can be contaminated or misidentified at any stage from harvest to packaging. (See Chapter 19 for more on herbal remedies.) Health Canada has recalled several products because of the presence of dangerous contaminants, including heavy metals and pharmaceutical drugs.

To be sold in Canada, a natural health product must have a product licence from Health Canada, and applicants have to provide detailed information about the product, including the medicinal ingredients, source, dose, potency, non-medicinal ingredients, and recommended uses. If a product is granted a licence, it is also assigned an eight-digit Natural Product Number (NPN) or Homeopathic Medicine Number (DIN-HM). The number, which must appear on the label, tells you that the product has been reviewed and approved by Health Canada.

In some cases, exceptions are given for products that have had an initial assessment but have not been fully evaluated. The exemption number (EN) will be listed on the product label.

Finally, it is important to remember that natural health products, including dietary supplements, are no substitute for a healthy diet. Supplements do not provide all the known—or yet-to-be-discovered—benefits of whole foods. Supplements should also not be used as a replacement for medical treatment for serious illnesses.

Protecting Yourself Against Food-Borne Illness

Many people worry about additives or pesticide residues in their food, but a greater threat comes from microorganisms that cause food-borne illnesses. Raw or undercooked animal products, such as chicken, hamburger, and oysters, pose the greatest threat, although in recent years contaminated fruits and vegetables have been catching up.

The Public Health Agency of Canada estimates that 11 million to 13 million illnesses are attributed to food-borne illnesses annually. Although most people fully recover, food-borne illnesses can result in chronic health problems in up to 3 percent of cases, including chronic arthritis and kidney failure. Some illnesses have long-term consequences for people and for the economy and society as a whole. Health Canada also estimates that the annual cost related to these illnesses is between $12 billion and $14 billion. Symptoms of food-borne illness include diarrhea, vomiting, fever, and weakness. Although the effects of food-borne illnesses are usually not serious, some groups, such as children, pregnant women, older adults, and people with suppressed or weakened immune systems, are more at risk for severe complications, such as rheumatic diseases, seizures, blood poisoning, other ailments, and death.

Causes of Food-Borne Illnesses

Most cases of food-borne illness are caused by **pathogens**, disease-causing microorganisms. Food can be contaminated with pathogens through improper handling; pathogens can grow if food is prepared or stored improperly. Causes of food-borne illness in Canada include the following pathogens:

pathogens
Microorganisms that cause disease.

- *Campylobacter jejuni* causes more cases of food-borne illness than any other bacteria. It is most commonly found in contaminated water, raw milk, and raw or undercooked poultry, meat, or shellfish; the majority of chickens sold in Canada test positive for the presence of *C. jejuni*. Symptoms of infection include diarrhea, fever, abdominal and muscle pain, and headache, which resolve in 7–10 days. However, in about 1 in 1690 cases, *Campylobacter* infection triggers Guillain-Barré syndrome, a neurological disease that can cause numbness, weakness, and (usually temporary) paralysis.

- *Salmonella* bacteria are most often found in raw or undercooked eggs, poultry, and meat; milk and dairy products; seafood; fruits and vegetables, including sprouts; and inadequately refrigerated and reheated leftovers. The recent identification of an antibiotic-resistant strain of *Salmonella* has raised concerns about a potential increase in serious illness from *Salmonella*.

QUICK STATS

About 87 510 cases of *Salmonella* infection occur annually in Canada.

—Health Canada, 2010

- *Shigella* bacteria are found in the human intestinal tract and usually transmitted via fecal contamination of food and water. Outbreaks are typically traced to foods, especially salads, that have been handled by people with poor personal hygiene. Contaminated water, milk, and dairy products are other possible sources of infection.
- *Escherichia coli* bacteria, found in the intestinal tracts of humans and animals, most commonly contaminate water, raw milk, raw to rare ground beef, unpasteurized juices, and fruits and vegetables. A certain strain, known as *E. coli* O157:H7, is of particular concern because it produces a toxin that causes serious illness and sometimes death. Children are particularly at risk for developing hemolytic uremic syndrome, which causes kidney failure.
- *Listeria monocytogenes* causes listeriosis, which is reported to affect about 100–140 Canadians a year, causing death in about 20–30 percent of cases. It is found in soft cheeses, raw milk, improperly processed ice cream, raw leafy vegetables, hot dogs and lunchmeats, and other meat, poultry, and processed foods. For the most part, healthy people who come into contact with *Listeria* are rarely affected by the bacteria. However, *Listeria* is particularly dangerous for pregnant women and their fetuses, babies and children, older adults, and people with weakened immune systems.
- *Staphylococcus aureus* lives mainly in nasal passages and skin sores; it is transferred to food when people handle food or sneeze or cough over food. Foods contaminated with *S. aureus* may include cooked hams, egg and potato salads, cheese, seafood, whipped cream, and milk. *S. aureus* multiplies rapidly at room temperature to produce a toxin that causes illness.
- *Clostridium botulinum* is widely distributed in nature, but it grows only in environments with little or no oxygen; it produces a toxin that causes illness. Potential sources of *C. botulinum* include improperly canned foods, garlic in oil, sausages and other meat products, and vacuum-packed and tightly wrapped foods. Although rare, botulism is potentially fatal if untreated because the toxin affects the nervous system.
- *Noroviruses*, are a group of viruses that cause gastroenteritis, an illness that usually includes vomiting, diarrhea, and abdominal pain, lasting one to three days. Gastroenteritis is often called the *stomach flu*, although it is not related to the flu (or influenza), which is a respiratory illness caused by the influenza virus. *Novovirus* is the most common viral cause of food-borne illness and may be found in contaminated water, raw or insufficiently cooked shellfish, and salads contaminated by food handlers.

Other causes of food-borne illness include the bacteria *Clostridium perfringens*, *Vibrio vulnificus*, and *Yersinia enterocolitica*; the hepatitis A virus; the parasites *Trichinella spiralis* (found in pork and wild game), *Anisakis* (found in raw fish), *Giardia lamblia*, *Cyclospora cayetanensis*, and tapeworms; and certain moulds.

A potential new threat from food is bovine spongiform encephalopathy (BSE), or mad cow disease, a fatal degenerative neurological disease caused by an abnormal protein (called a prion) that forms deposits in the brain. A variant form that appears in people, known as Creutzfeldt-Jakob disease (CJD), is believed to be caused by eating beef contaminated with central nervous system tissue from BSE-infected cows. To date, there have been about 200 confirmed cases of this variant CJD worldwide, most of them in Great

Britain. In 1993, the first case of BSE diagnosed in Canada was in a cow that had been imported from the United Kingdom in 1987, when it was six months old. The animal was destroyed and the Canadian government attempted to trace and destroy all cattle imported from the United Kingdom between 1982 and 1990 (in 1990, cattle imports from the United Kingdom were banned because of BSE). According to Health Canada and the Canadian Food Inspection Agency, the risk to Canadians from BSE is extremely low, but steps are being taken to prevent the BSE protein from entering the food supply.

Preventing and Treating Food-Borne Illnesses

Because every teaspoon of the soil that our food grows in contains about 2 billion bacteria (only some of which are pathogenic), we are always exposed to the possibility of a food-borne illness. You can't tell by taste, smell, or sight whether a food is contaminated. Some studies have revealed high levels of contamination. In 2003, for example, *Consumer Reports* tested 484 chickens purchased in grocery stores and found that half were contaminated with *Campylobacter* or *Salmonella* or both; many of the strains of bacteria found were resistant to antibiotics.

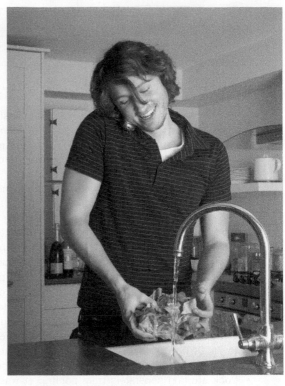

Careful food handling greatly reduces the risk of food-borne illness.

Although pathogens are usually destroyed during cooking, Health Canada is trying to bring down levels of contamination. In addition to new microbiological testing methods for inspection of meat and poultry processing plants, raw meat and poultry products are now sold with safe handling and cooking instructions, and all packaged, unpasteurized fresh fruit and vegetable juices carry warnings about potential contamination. Food-borne illness outbreaks associated with food-processing plants make headlines, but most cases of illness trace back to poor food handling in the home or in food-service establishments. To decrease your risk of food-borne illness, follow the guidelines in the Take Charge box.

If you think you may be have a food-borne illness, drink plenty of clear fluids to prevent dehydration and rest to speed recovery. To prevent further contamination, wash your hands often and always before handling food. A fever higher than 38.9 degrees Celsius, blood in the stool, or dehydration deserves a physician's evaluation, especially if the symptoms persist for more than two to three days. In cases of suspected botulism—characterized by such symptoms as double vision, paralysis, dizziness, and vomiting—consult a physician immediately to receive an antitoxin.

Environmental Contaminants and Organic Foods

Contaminants are also present in the food-growing environment, but few of them ever enter the food and water supply in amounts sufficient to cause health problems. Environmental contaminants include various minerals, antibiotics, hormones, pesticides, the industrial chemicals known as **PCBs (polychlorinated biphenyls)**, and naturally occurring substances, such as cyanogenic glycosides (found in lima beans and the pits of some fruits) and certain moulds. Their effects depend on many factors, including concentration, length of exposure, and the age and health status of the person involved. Safety regulations attempt to keep our exposure to contaminants at safe levels, but monitoring is difficult and many substances (such as pesticides) persist in the environment long after being banned from use.

PCB (polychlorinated biphenyl)
An industrial chemical used as an insulator in electrical transformers and linked to certain human cancers.

Safe Food Handling

- Don't buy food in containers that leak, bulge, or are severely dented. Refrigerated foods should be cold, and frozen foods should be solid.
- Refrigerate perishable items as soon as possible after purchase. Use or freeze fresh meats within three to five days and fresh poultry, fish, and ground meat within one to two days.
- Store raw meat, poultry, fish, and shellfish in containers in the refrigerator so that the juices don't drip onto other foods. Keep these items away from other foods, surfaces, utensils, or serving dishes to prevent cross-contamination.
- Thaw frozen food in the refrigerator or in the microwave oven, not on the kitchen counter. Cook foods immediately after thawing.
- Thoroughly wash your hands with warm soapy water for a minimum of 20 seconds before and after handling food, especially raw meat, fish, shellfish, poultry, or eggs.
- Make sure counters, cutting boards, dishes, utensils, and other equipment are thoroughly cleaned in hot soapy water before and after use. Wash dishcloths and kitchen towels frequently.
- Use separate cutting boards for meat, poultry, and seafood and for foods that will be eaten raw, such as fruits and vegetables. Replace cutting boards once they become worn or develop hard-to-clean grooves.
- Thoroughly rinse and scrub fruits and vegetables with a brush, if possible, or peel off the skin.
- Cook foods thoroughly, especially beef, poultry, fish, pork, and eggs; cooking kills most microorganisms. Use a foodthermometer to ensure that foods are cooked to a safe temperature. Hamburgers should be cooked to 71°C. Turn or stir microwaved food to make sure it is heated evenly throughout. When eating out, order hamburger cooked well done and make sure foods are served piping hot.
- Cook stuffing separately from poultry; or wash poultry thoroughly, stuff immediately before cooking, and transfer the stuffing to a clean bowl immediately after cooking. The temperature of cooked stuffing should reach 74°C.
- Keep hot foods hot (60°C or above) and cold foods cold (4°C or below); harmful bacteria can grow rapidly between these two temperatures. Refrigerate foods within two hours of purchase or preparation, and within one hour if the air temperature is above 32°C. Refrigerate foods at or below 4°C and freeze at or below −17°C. Use refrigerated leftovers within three to four days.
- Even for experienced cooks, improper heating and preparation of food means bacteria can survive. Use a food thermometer: You can't tell if food is cooked safely by how it looks. Refer to a temperature chart to see if your food is cooked completely.
- Don't eat raw animal products, including raw eggs in homemade hollandaise sauce or eggnog. Use only pasteurized milk and juice.
- Cook eggs until they are firm, and fully cook foods containing eggs. Store eggs in the coldest part of the refrigerator, not in the door, and use them within three to five weeks.
- Because of possible contamination with *E. coli* O157:H7 and *Salmonella*, avoid raw sprouts. Even sprouts grown under clean conditions in the home can be risky because bacteria may be present in the seeds. Cook sprouts before eating them.
- Read the food label and package information, and follow safety instructions, such as "Keep Refrigerated" and the "Safe Handling Instructions."
- According to the Canadian Food Inspection Agency, "When in doubt, throw it out." Even if a food looks and smells fine, it may not be safe. If you aren't sure that a food has been prepared, served, and stored safely, don't eat it.

Additional precautions are recommended for people at particularly high risk for food-borne illness: pregnant women, young children, older persons, and people with weakened immune systems or certain chronic illnesses. If you are a member of one of these groups, don't eat or drink any of the following products: unpasteurized juices; raw sprouts; unpasteurized (raw) milk and products made from unpasteurized milk; raw or undercooked meat, poultry, eggs, fish, and shellfish; and soft cheeses, such as feta, Brie, Camembert, or blue-veined cheeses. To protect against *Listeria*, it's also important to avoid ready-to-eat foods, such as hot dogs, lunchmeats, and cold cuts, unless they are reheated until they are steaming hot.

Organic Foods

Some people who are concerned about pesticides and other environmental contaminants choose to buy foods that are **organic**. To be certified as organic by Canadian Food Inspection Agency, foods must meet strict production, processing, handling, and labelling criteria. Organic crops must meet limits on pesticide residues; for meat, milk, eggs, and other animal products to be certified organic, animals must be given organic feed and access to the outdoors and may not be given antibiotics or growth hormones. The use of genetic engineering, ionizing radiation, and sewage sludge is prohibited. General principles of organic production include protection of the environment; maintenance of long-term soil fertility; maintenance of biological diversity; recycling and maintenance of resources to the greatest extent possible; and provision of attentive care to livestock.

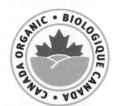

> **organic**
> A designation applied to foods grown and produced according to strict guidelines limiting the use of pesticides, non-organic ingredients, hormones, antibiotics, irradiation, genetic engineering, and other practices.

Organic foods are not necessarily chemical-free, however. Synthetic pesticides are not permitted for use in organic production. Some organic or naturally-based pesticides are permitted for use as long as they are included on an approved list by Canadian Organic Standards. The practices allowed by the Canadian Organic Standards are developed to ensure the least possible amount of residues at the lowest possible levels. It should be noted, though, that it can be possible that products produced in accordance with organic standards could have come into contact with pesticides—for example, drift from neighbouring fields—during transport. However, organically produced foods do tend to have lower levels of pesticide residues than conventionally grown crops. Some experts recommend that consumers who want to buy organic fruits and vegetables spend their money on those that carry lower pesticide residues than their conventional counterparts (the "dirty dozen"): apples, bell peppers, celery, cherries, imported grapes, nectarines, peaches, pears, potatoes, red raspberries, spinach, and strawberries. Experts also recommend buying organic beef, poultry, eggs, dairy products, and baby food. Fruits and vegetables that carry little pesticide residue whether grown conventionally or organically include asparagus, avocadoes, bananas, broccoli, cauliflower, corn, kiwi, mangoes, onions, papaya, pineapples, and peas. Although all foods are subject to strict pesticide limits, the debate about the health effects of small amounts of residue is ongoing.

Whether organic foods are better for your health or not, organic farming is better for the environment. It helps maintain biodiversity of crops and replenish Earth's resources; and it is less likely to degrade soil, contaminate water, or expose farm workers to toxic chemicals. As multinational food companies get into the organic food business, however, consumers who want to support environmentally friendly farming methods should look for foods that are not only organic, but also locally grown.

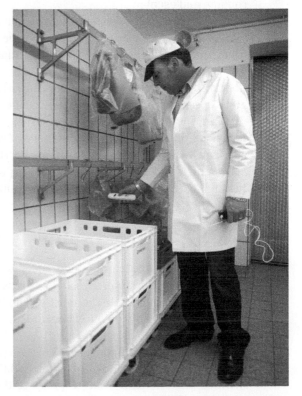

Government inspectors regularly check Canada's food supply to ensure its safety.

Local Foods and Slow Food

New food movements are taking place across Canada, including eating locally and the slow food movement. Eating locally promotes the benefits of buying agricultural products grown close to our backyards. Some marketing agencies and companies promoting their local foods identify how far food travels to reach the consumer; others choose to promote the economic and health benefits of purchasing food grown closer to home.

Eating locally-grown food supports local agriculture, which in turn supports the local economy while protecting farmland. This benefits both consumers and producers. In addition, local food purchased from nearby farms is often as affordable as non-local food, but is of higher quality. Price is often the main reason that shoppers purchase imported food, but some consumers in favour of local foods are willing to pay more for foods produced closer to home. Consumers committed to purchasing locally grown food cite the peace of mind that comes with knowing where their food comes from and with making a contribution to the economic stability of the local agricultural industry as their main reasons for purchasing local foods. It should be noted, however, that cost and access to foods, especially in the vast rural locations across Canada, can influence food choice and may impact on one's ability to ensure healthy options are always available in the home. This context is important for consideration.

The slow food movement is a global, grassroots movement with supporters in 150 countries. According to Slow Food Canada, it is "a national eco-gastronomic organization founded to counteract fast food and fast life and the disappearance of local food traditions."

Guidelines for Fish Consumption

A specific area of concern is possible mercury contamination in fish. Overall, fish and shellfish are healthy sources of protein, omega-3 fats, and other nutrients. Prudent choices can minimize the risk of any possible negative health effects. High mercury concentrations are most likely to be found in predator fish—large fish that eat smaller fish. Mercury can cause brain damage to fetuses and young children.

Health Canada has released an advisory with guidelines for certain groups. To reduce exposure to mercury, women who are or who may become pregnant and breastfeeding mothers should follow these guidelines:

- Some fish contain higher amounts of methylmercury and should be limited to no more than 150 grams per month (that's two servings). These fish include fresh/frozen tuna, shark, swordfish, marlin, orange roughy, and escolar.
- For other varieties of fish and shellfish that are lower in methylmercury, eat up to two servings a week (150 grams total). These varieties include shrimp, canned light tuna, salmon, pollock, and catfish. Albacore tuna (sometimes called white tuna) contains more mercury than light tuna, so you need to watch how much you are eating.
- Check advisories about the safety of recreationally caught fish from local lakes, rivers, and coastal areas; if no information is available, limit consumption to two servings (150 grams total) per month.
- Children should consume only one serving (75 grams) of fish lower in methylmercury per week.

The levels of mercury in the muscle tissue of salmon are very low. Separate studies have identified other chemicals, such as polychlorinated biphenyls (PCBs), in the fat of both wild-caught and farmed salmon. These chemicals can be found in most fish and in many other foods, but at low levels that do not cause concern for human health. Fish should be labelled with its country of origin and whether it is wild or farmed; most canned salmon is wild.

Additives in Food

Today, some 2800 substances are intentionally added to foods to maintain or improve nutritional quality, to maintain freshness, to help in processing or preparation, or to alter taste or appearance. Additives make up less than 1 percent of our food. The most widely used are sugar, salt, and corn syrup; these three and citric acid, baking soda, vegetable colours, mustard, and pepper account for 98 percent by weight of all food additives used in Canada.

Some additives may be of concern for certain people, either because they are consumed in large quantities or because they cause some type of reaction. Additives having potential health concerns include the following:

- *Nitrates and nitrites:* Used to preserve the colour of meats, to enhance their flavour by inhibiting rancidity (in cured meats), and to protect against bacterial growth, specifically from contamination with botulism. Consumption of nitrates and nitrites is associated with the synthesis of cancer-causing agents in the stomach, but the cancer risk appears to be low, except for people with low stomach acid output (such as some older adults). That said, a person's overall exposure to nitrosamine-related compounds comes from other substances, such as tobacco smoke, beer and bacon consumption, and exhaust from vehicles.

- *BHA and BHT:* Used to help maintain the freshness of foods. BHT has been shown to reduce the risk of cancer by providing an antioxidant effect similar to that of vitamin E. However, other studies indicate a potential link between BHT and an increased risk of certain cancers when BHT is consumed in very large amounts, but any risk from these agents is considered to be low. Some manufacturers have stopped using BHT and BHA.
- *Sulphites:* Used to keep vegetables from turning brown. They can cause severe allergic reactions in some people. Health Canada severely limits the use of sulphites and requires any foods containing sulphites to be clearly labelled.
- *Monosodium glutamate (MSG):* Typically used as a flavour enhancer. MSG may cause some people to experience episodes of increased blood pressure and sweating. If you are sensitive to MSG, check food labels when shopping, and ask to have it left out of dishes you order at restaurants.

Food additives pose no significant health hazard to most people because the levels used are well below any that could produce toxic effects. To avoid potential problems, eat a variety of foods in moderation. If you are sensitive to an additive, check food labels when you shop, and ask questions when you eat out.

Food Irradiation

Food irradiation is the treatment of foods with gamma rays, X-rays, or high-voltage electrons to kill potentially harmful pathogens, including bacteria, parasites, insects, and fungi that cause food-borne illness. It also reduces spoilage and extends shelf life. For example, irradiated strawberries stay unspoiled in the refrigerator up to three weeks, versus only three to five days for untreated berries. The same irradiation process has also been used for decades on many items, such as plastic wrap, milk cartons, teething rings, contact lenses, and medical supplies.

> **food irradiation**
> The treatment of foods with gamma rays, X-rays, or high-voltage electrons to kill potentially harmful pathogens and increase shelf life.

Even though irradiation has been generally endorsed by such agencies as the World Health Organization, the Centers for Disease Control and Prevention, and the American Medical Association, few irradiated foods are on the market because of consumer resistance and skepticism. Currently, onions, potatoes, wheat, flour, whole wheat flour, and whole or ground spices and dehydrated seasonings are approved for irradiation and sale in Canada.

Studies haven't conclusively identified any harmful effects of food irradiation, and the newer methods of irradiation involving electricity and X-rays do not require the use of any radioactive materials. However, studies do indicate that when consumers are given information about the process of irradiation and the benefits of irradiated foods, most want to purchase them. Without such information, many remain skeptical. Irradiated foods are labelled with the flowerlike radura symbol and a brief information label; spices and foods that are merely ingredients do not have to be labelled. It is important to remember that although irradiation kills most pathogens, it does not completely sterilize foods. Proper handling of irradiated foods is still critical for preventing food-borne illness.

Genetically Modified Foods

Genetic engineering involves altering the characteristics of a plant, an animal, or a microorganism by adding, rearranging, or replacing genes in its DNA; the result is a **genetically modified (GM) organism**. New DNA may come from related species or from entirely different types of organisms. In Canada, 95 percent of the canola, 90 percent of the corn, and 80 percent of the soybeans farmers plant is genetically modified. Products

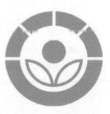

made with GM organisms include juice, soft drinks, nuts, tuna, frozen pizza, spaghetti sauce, canola oil, chips, salad dressings, and soup.

---

genetically modified (GM) organism
A plant, an animal, or a microorganism in which genes have been added, rearranged, or replaced through genetic engineering.

The potential benefits of GM foods cited by supporters include improved yields overall and in difficult growing conditions, increased disease resistance, improved nutritional content, lower prices, and less pesticide use. Critics of biotechnology argue that unexpected effects may occur: Gene manipulation could elevate levels of naturally occurring toxins or allergens, permanently change the gene pool and reduce biodiversity, and produce pesticide-resistant insects through the transfer of genes. Experience has shown that GM products are difficult to keep separate from non-GM products; animal escapes, cross-pollination, and contamination during processing are just a few ways GM organisms could potentially appear unexpectedly in the food supply or the environment.

According to the National Academy of Sciences, there is currently no proof that the GM food already on the market is unsafe. However, experts have recommended regulatory changes and further study of key issues, particularly the environmental effects of the escape of GM animals.

Animal Cloning

Cloning allows producers to create animals with highly desirable characteristics, such as disease resistance and more predictable fat-to-lean meat ratios. Cloned animals are similar to identical twins. For example, scientists can produce a cloned cow by taking an egg from a female cow, removing the egg's gene-containing nucleus, and inserting genes from another cow that the scientists want to copy. The egg is then urged to create an embryo, and the embryo is implanted into the uterus of another female cow, which carries it to term and delivers it. (This surrogate cow's DNA does not affect the clone's DNA.)

The recently developed method of animal cloning called somatic cell nuclear transfer (SCNT) has raised potential food safety concerns. At this time, it is unclear if this cloning technique would have an impact on the safety and nutritional quality of foods derived from animals generated by SCNT. SCNT technology is still at the research and development stage, and as a result, very limited data are available to provide answers to these questions. The fact that significant health problems are observed in some animals cloned by using this technology reinforces the fact that questions need to be asked about food products derived from them.

Until more is known about the products of this technology, Health Canada considers foods produced from livestock developed by using SCNT and the progeny of such livestock to be what is termed "novel food" in the Food and Drug Regulations. At this time, Health Canada does not allow food producers to have cloned animals in the food supply.

Labelling of GM Foods

Labelling has been another major concern, with surveys indicating that most Canadians want to know if their food contains GM ingredients. Health Canada does not require special labelling for foods from genetically modified or cloned sources. Under current rules, Health Canada requires special labelling only when a food's composition or nutrition profile is changed significantly or when a known allergen, such as a peanut gene, is introduced into a food. Health Canada needs to determine what type of information is required on the label to inform Canadians about these changes in the food. The only foods guaranteed not to contain GM ingredients are those certified as organic.

Food Allergies and Food Intolerances

For some people, consuming a particular food causes uncomfortable symptoms, such as itchiness, swollen lips, or abdominal pain. Adverse reactions, such as these, may be due to a food allergy or a food intolerance, and symptoms may range from annoying to life threatening. If you have had an adverse reaction to a food, it's important to determine whether your symptoms are due to an allergy or an intolerance so that you can take appropriate action.

Food Allergies

A true **food allergy** is a reaction of the body's immune system to a food or food ingredient, usually a protein. The immune system perceives the reaction-provoking substance, or allergen, as foreign and acts to destroy it. This immune reaction can occur within minutes of ingesting the food, resulting in symptoms that affect the skin (hives), gastrointestinal tract (cramps or diarrhea), respiratory tract (asthma), or mouth (swelling of the lips or tongue). The most severe response is a systemic reaction called *anaphylaxis*, which involves a potentially life-threatening drop in blood pressure.

> **food allergy**
> An adverse reaction to a food or food ingredient in which the immune system perceives a particular substance (allergen) as foreign and acts to destroy it.

Food allergies affect only about 1.8 million Canadians, and 5–6 percent of young children have a physician-diagnosed food allergy. Although numerous food allergens have been identified, just eight foods account for more than 90 percent of the food allergies in Canada: cow's milk, eggs, peanuts, tree nuts (e.g., walnuts, cashews), soy, wheat, fish, and shellfish. Food labels are now required to state the presence of the eight most common allergens in plain language in the ingredient list. People with food allergies, especially those prone to anaphylaxis, must diligently avoid trigger foods. This involves carefully reading food labels and asking questions about ingredients when eating out. People at risk are usually advised to carry medications to treat anaphylaxis, such as injectable epinephrine. Refer to Chapter 9 for more on allergies.

QUICK STATS

About 2% of children ages 5 to nine 9 have a peanut allergy. For 80% of people with a peanut allergy, this allergy will be lifelong.

—Allergy Asthma Information Association, 2008

Food Intolerances

Many people who believe they have food allergies may actually have a much more common source of adverse food reactions: a food intolerance. In the case of a **food intolerance**, the problem usually lies with metabolism rather than with the immune system. Typically, the body cannot adequately digest a food or food component, often because of some type of chemical deficiency; in other cases, the body reacts to a particular compound in a food. Lactose intolerance is a fairly common food intolerance. A more serious condition is intolerance of gluten, a protein component of some grains; in affected individuals, consumption of gluten damages the lining of the true small intestine. Sulphite, a common food additive, can produce severe asthmatic reactions in sensitive individuals. Food intolerances have also been attributed to tartrazine (a yellow food colouring), MSG, and the sweetener aspartame.

> **food intolerance**
> An adverse reaction to a food or food ingredient that doesn't involve the immune system; intolerances are often caused by a problem with metabolism.

A "popular" food intolerance lately has been gluten-free dieting. Celiac disease is a medical condition the results in damage of the surface of the small intestine caused by gluten, a protein found in wheat, rye, triticale, barley. As a result of the damage to the absorptive surface of the small intestine, the body is unable to absorb protein, fat, carbohydrates, vitamins, and minerals. It is estimated that 1 in 133 people in Canada are affected by celiac disease. However, many more people without a confirmed diagnosis of celiac disease are choosing to follow a gluten-free diet. The challenge with removing all sources of gluten from your diet without carefully replacing the nutrients those foods would have provided is the potential for not achieving a dietary intake containing the full complement of nutrients required for health. If you think you need to remove the gluten from your diet, it is recommended that you speak to a registered dietitian or regulated health care provider to determine whether or not this is a safe and practical dietary change to make.

QUESTIONS FOR CRITICAL THINKING AND REFLECTION

What is the least healthy food you eat every day (either during meals or as a snack)? Identify at least one substitute that would be healthier but just as satisfying.

Food intolerance reactions often produce symptoms similar to food allergies, such as diarrhea or abdominal cramps, but reactions are typically localized and not life threatening. Many people with food intolerances can consume small amounts of the food that affects them; exceptions are gluten and sulphites, which must be avoided by sensitive individuals. Through trial and error, most people with food intolerances can adjust their intake of the trigger food to an appropriate level.

If you suspect that you have a food allergy or intolerance, a good first step is to keep a food diary. Note everything you eat or drink, any symptoms you develop, and how long after eating the symptoms appear. Then make an appointment with your physician to go over your diary and determine if any additional tests are needed.

 Take **CHARGE**

Improving Your Diet by Choosing Healthy Beverages

After reading this chapter and completing the dietary assessment in the Assess Yourself box, you can probably identify several changes you could make to improve your diet. Here, we focus on choosing healthy beverages to increase intake of nutrients and decrease intake of empty calories from added sugars and fat. However, this model of dietary change can be applied to any modification you'd like to make to your diet. Additional specific plans for improving diet can be found in the Behaviour Change Strategy in Chapter 7 (decreasing saturated and trans fat intake) and Chapter 8 (increasing intake of fruits and vegetables).

Gather Data and Establish a Baseline

Begin by tracking your beverage consumption in your health journal. Write down the types and amounts of beverages you drink, including water. Also note where you were at the time and whether you obtained the beverage there or brought it with you. At the same time, investigate your options. Find out what other beverages you can easily obtain during your daily routine. For example, what drinks are available in the dining hall where you eat lunch or at the food court where you often grab snacks? How many drinking fountains do you walk by over the course of the day? This information will help you put together a successful plan for change.

Analyze Your Data and Set Goals

Evaluate your beverage consumption by dividing your typical daily consumption between healthy and less healthy choices. Use the following guide as a basis, and add other beverages to the lists as needed.

Choose less often:
- Regular soft drinks
- Sweetened iced tea
- Fruit beverages made with little fruit juice (usually labelled fruit drinks, punches, beverages, blends, or ades)
- Homogenized milk

Choose more often:
- Water
- Low-fat or skim milk

- Fruit juice (100 percent juice)
- Unsweetened herbal tea

How many beverages do you consume daily from each category? What would be a healthy and realistic goal for change? For example, if your beverage consumption is currently evenly divided between the "choose more often" and "choose less often" categories (four from each list), you might set a final goal for your behaviour change program of increasing your healthy choices by two (to six from the "more often" list and two from the "less often" list).

Develop a Plan for Change

Once you have set your goal, you need to develop strategies that will help you choose healthy beverages more often. Consider the following possibilities:

- Keep healthy beverages on hand; if you live in a student dorm, rent a small refrigerator or keep bottled water, juice, low-fat or skim milk, and other healthy choices in the dorm kitchen's refrigerator.
- Plan ahead, and put a bottle of water or 100 percent juice in your backpack every day.
- Check food labels on beverages for serving sizes, calories, and nutrients; comparison shop to find the healthiest choices, and watch your serving sizes. Use this information to make your "choose more often" list longer and more specific.
- If you eat out frequently, examine all the beverages available at the places you typically eat your meals. You will probably find that healthy choices are available; if not, bring along your own drink or find somewhere else to eat.
- For a snack, try water and a piece of fruit rather than a heavily sweetened beverage.
- Create healthy beverages that appeal to you; for example, try adding slices of citrus fruit to water or mixing 100 percent fruit juice with sparkling water.

You may also need to make some changes in your routine to decrease the likelihood that you will make unhealthy choices. For example, you might discover from your health journal that you always buy a soft drink after class when you pass a particular vending machine. If this is the case, try another route that allows you to avoid the machine. And try to guard against impulse buying by carrying water or a healthy snack with you every day.

To complete your plan, try some of the other behaviour change strategies described in Chapter 1: Develop and sign a contract, set up a system of rewards, involve other people in your program, and develop strategies for challenging situations. Once your plan is complete, take action. Keep track of your progress in your health journal by continuing to monitor and evaluate your beverage consumption.

SUMMARY

- To function at its best, the human body requires about 50 essential nutrients in specific proportions. People get the nutrients needed to fuel their bodies and maintain tissues and organ systems from foods; the body cannot synthesize most of them.
- Proteins, made up of amino acids, form muscles and bones and help make up blood, enzymes, hormones, and cell membranes. Foods from animal sources provide complete proteins; plants provide incomplete proteins.
- Fats, a concentrated source of energy, also help insulate the body and cushion the organs; 15 mL of vegetable oil per day supplies the essential fats. Dietary fat intake should be 20–35 percent of total daily calories. Unsaturated fats should be favoured over saturated and trans fats.
- Carbohydrates supply energy to the brain and other parts of the nervous system as well as to red blood cells.
- Fibre includes non-digestible carbohydrates provided mainly by plants. Adequate intake of fibre (38 grams per day for men and 25 grams per day for women) can help people manage diabetes and high cholesterol levels and improve intestinal health.
- The 13 vitamins needed in the diet are organic substances that promote specific chemical and cell processes within living tissue. Deficiencies or excesses can cause serious illnesses and even death.

- The approximately 17 minerals needed in the diet are inorganic substances that regulate body functions, aid in the growth and maintenance of body tissues, and help in the release of energy from foods.
- Water is used to digest and absorb food, transport substances around the body, lubricate joints and organs, and regulate body temperature.
- Foods contain other substances, such as phytochemicals, which may not be essential nutrients but which reduce chronic disease risk.
- Dietary Reference Intakes (DRIs) are recommended intakes for essential nutrients that meet the needs of healthy people.
- The Guidelines for Healthy Eating address the prevention of diet-related diseases such as heart disease, cancer, and diabetes. The guidelines advise us to consume a variety of foods while staying within calorie needs; manage body weight through calorie control and regular physical activity; eat more fruits, vegetables, whole grains, and reduced-fat dairy products; choose fats and carbohydrates wisely; consume less salt and caffeine; be moderate with alcohol intake; and handle foods safely.
- Choosing foods from each group in *Eating Well with Canada's Food Guide* every day helps ensure the appropriate amounts of necessary nutrients.
- A vegetarian diet can meet our nutritional needs.
- Almost all foods have labels that show how much fat, cholesterol, protein, fibre, and sodium they contain. Serving sizes are standardized, and health claims are carefully regulated.
- Food-borne illnesses are a greater threat to health than additives and environmental contaminants. Other dietary issues of concern to some people include organic foods, food irradiation, genetic modification of foods, and food allergies and intolerances.

FOR MORE INFORMATION

BOOKS

Nestle, M. 2007. *What to Eat*. New York: North Point Press. Examines the marketing of food and how to interpret food-related information while shopping.

NEWSLETTERS

Nutrition Action Health Letter (613-244-7337; http://www.cspinet.org/nah/canada.htm)

Tufts University Health & Nutrition Letter (800-274-7581;http://www.tuftshealthletter.com)

ORGANIZATIONS, HOTLINES, AND WEBSITES

The Internet addresses listed here were accurate at the time of publication.

Beyond the Basics: Meal Planning for Healthy Eating, Diabetes Management and Prevention. Provides resources for choosing foods and portions sizes to manage diabetes and maintain a healthy body weight.
  http://orders.diabetes.ca/products/beyond-the-basics-resource

Canadian Food Inspection Agency. Offers information about many topics, such as food labelling, food additives, dietary supplements, and food-borne illness.
  http://www.inspection.gc.ca

Canadian Foundation for Dietetic Research. Provides links to reliable food and nutrition information.
  http://www.cfdr.ca/sharing/CCFNLibrary.aspx

Dietitians of Canada. Provides a wide variety of nutrition-related educational materials, including information related to healthy eating, body image, self-esteem, physical activity. Includes a tool called EATracker, which allows you to track your day's food and activity choices and compare them with Health Canada guidelines.
  http://www.dietitians.ca

Eat Right Ontario. Offers nutrition information for consumers on a wide range of topics, in more than 100 languages. Staffed by registered dietitians throughout the weekdays and with extended hours into the evenings.

http://www.Ontario.ca/EatRight or call toll free 1-877-510-5102

Eating Well with Canada's Food Guide. Provides personalized dietary plans and interactive food and activity tracking tools.

http://www.myfoodguide.ca

Food Safety Network. Provides information on safe purchase, handling, cooking, and storage of food.

1-866-50-FSNET (1-866-503-7638) or e-mail queries to fsnrsn@uoguelph.ca

Health Canada. Provides access to government resources relating to food safety and nutrition.

http://www.hc-sc.gc.ca/fn-an/index-eng.php

Health Canada: Nutrient Value of Some Common Foods. Provides nutrient breakdowns of individual foods.

http://www.hc-sc.gc.ca/fn-an/nutrition/fiche-nutri-data/nutrient_value-valeurs_nutritives-eng.php

Health Nexus. Offers health-promotion resources to help organizations and individuals develop and implement prevention and health-promotion strategies to enhance well-being and reduce demand on the health care and social service systems.

http://www.healthnexus.ca

Heart and Stroke Foundation of Canada. Provides basic information about nutrition, tips for shopping and eating out, and heart-healthy recipes.

http://www.heartandstroke.ca

International Food Information Council. Provides information for consumers, journalists, and educators about food safety and nutrition.

http://www.foodinsight.org

Institute of Medicine: Food and Nutrition Board. Provides information about the Dietary Reference Intakes and related guidelines.

http://iom.nationalacademies.org/Activities/Nutrition/SummaryDRIs/~/media/Files/Activity%20Files/Nutrition/DRIs/New%20Material/5DRI%20Values%20SummaryTables%2014.pdf

Public Health Agency of Canada. Includes information on promoting health; preventing and controlling chronic diseases and injuries; preventing and controlling infectious diseases; preparing for and responding to public health emergencies, and strengthening Canada's public health capacity.

http://www.publichealth.gc.ca

Vegetarian Diets. Provides information for vegetarians and people interested in learning more about vegetarian diets.

http://www.dietitians.ca/Your-Health/Nutrition-A-Z/Vegetarian-Diets.aspx?categoryID=54

See also the listings for Chapters 4, 6–8, and 17.

SELECTED BIBLIOGRAPHY

Aboriginal Canada Portal. 2010. *Food and Recipes,* http://www.aboriginalcanada.gc.ca/acp/site.nsf/eng/ao35296.html (retrieved January 13, 2015).

Benardot, D. 2005. *Advanced Sports Nutrition: Carbohydrate Requirements,* http://www.healthline.com/hlbook/nut-carbohydrate-requirements (retrieved April 15, 2015).

Bush, M. A., et al. 2007. *Eating Well with Canada's Food Guide*: A tool for the times. *Canadian Journal of Dietetic Practice and Research* 68(2): 92–96.

Canadian Food Inspection Agency. 2007. *Food,* http://www.inspection.gc.ca/english/fssa/fssae.shtml; (retrieved April 15, 2015).

Canadian Food Inspection Agency. 2010. *Causes of Foodborne Illness,* http://www.inspection.gc.ca/english/fssa/concen/causee.shtml (retrieved June 15, 2015).

Canadian Food Inspection Agency. 2010. *Food Allergens,* http://www.inspection.gc.ca/english/fssa/labeti/allerg/allerge.shtml (retrieved June 15, 2015).

Canadian Food Inspection Agency. 2010. *Organic Products,* http://www.inspection.gc.ca/english/fssa/orgbio/orgbioe.shtml (retrieved June 15, 2015).

Capital Health. 2007. *Sugar Shocker: An Activity Kit to Help Teach Students About Healthy Drink Choices,* http://www.capitalhealth.ca/nr/rdonlyres/e6nstouxulgpkbvzot7as7dhtyvv6storxwnl57sbz4gl6o2im2rgwio4tthag2r5vag2aoqodp7fst6zyagrafdccb/sugar+shocker+kit_nov07.pdf (retrieved December 12, 2015).

Capital Health, Regional Nutrition and Food Service. 2005. *Canada's Food Guide: Serving size handout,* http://www.capitalhealth.ca/NR/rdonlyres/etgansnparwmjhldsvhl4nmhp6bvkynxnoao2bm3qrcounb6nzu5jcpqhocw4wk576apdb7v4dmaeywfqk7rdjx6cec/Portion+size+Handout.pdf (retrieved December 12, 2015).

Cheung, A. M., et al. 2004. Prevention of osteoporosis and osteoporotic fractures in postmenopausal women: Recommendation statement from the Canadian Task Force on Preventive Health Care. *Canadian Medical Association Journal* 170(11): 1665–1667.

Dairy Nutrition. 2010. *Trans Fats in the Canadian Diet,* http://www.dairynutrition.ca/nutrients-in-milk-products/fat/trans-fats-in-the-canadian-diet (retrieved April 10, 2015).

Egg Farmers of Canada. 2008. *Omega-3 Fatty Acids,* http://www.eggs.ca/AllAboutEggs/FAQ_Omega3FattyAcids.aspx (retrieved February 15, 2015).

Garriguet, D. 2004. *Nutrition: Findings from the Canadian Community Health Survey: Overview of Canadians' Eating Habits,* http://www.statcan.gc.ca/pub/82-620-m/82-620-m2006002-eng.pdf (retrieved May 14, 2015).

Government of Alberta. 2004. *Vegetarianism: A Meatless Eating Experience,* http://www1.agric.gov.ab.ca/$department/deptdocs.nsf/all/sis8739 (retrieved April 4, 2015).

Hanley, D. M., and K. S. Davison. 2005. Vitamin D insufficiency in North America: A significant risk factor in chronic diseases and potential disease-specific biomarkers of Vitamin D sufficiency. *Journal of Nutrition,* 135: 332–337.

Health Canada. 2003. *Guiding Canadians Towards Healthy Eating: National Nutrition Leadership,* http://www.hc-sc.gc.ca/fn-an/res-rech/res-prog/eat-aliment/guiding_cdn_lead-lead_cdn_inciter-eng.php (retrieved March 5, 2015).

Health Canada. 2003. *Using the Dietary Reference Intakes,* http://www.hc-sc.gc.ca/fn-an/nutrition/reference/dri_using-util_anref-eng.php (retrieved December 9, 2015).

Health Canada. 2006. *Dietary Reference Intakes: Questions and Answers,* http://www.hc-sc.gc.ca/fn-an/nutrition/reference/dri_ques-ques_anref-eng.php (retrieved April 3, 2015).

Health Canada. 2006. *Salmonella Prevention,* http://www.hc-sc.gc.ca/hl-vs/iyh-vsv/food-aliment/salmonella-eng.php (retrieved April 4, 2015).

Health Canada. 2007. *Canada's Food Guide: Questions and Answers for Educators,* http://www.hc-sc.gc.ca/fn-an/food-guide-aliment/educ-comm/faq_educat-eng.php#14 (retrieved December 12, 2015).

Health Canada. 2007. *It's Your Health: Trans Fats,* http://www.hc-sc.gc.ca/hl-vs/alt_formats/pacrb-dgapcr/pdf/iyh-vsv/food-aliment/trans-eng.pdf (retrieved March 24, 2015).

Health Canada. 2008. *Eating Well with Canada's Food Guide,* http://www.hc-sc.gc.ca/fn-an/food-guide-aliment/order-commander/eating_well_bien_manger-eng.php (retrieved February 21, 2015).

Health Canada. 2008. *Human Health Risk Assessment of Mercury in Fish and Health Benefits of Fish Consumption,* http://www.hc-sc.gc.ca/fn-an/pubs/mercur/merc_fish_poisson-eng.php (retrieved January 15, 2015).

Health Canada. 2008. *It's Your Health: Sodium,* http://www.hc-sc.gc.ca/hl-vs/alt_formats/pacrb-dgapcr/pdf/iyh-vsv/food-aliment/sodium_eng.pdf (retrieved March 5, 2015).

Health Canada. 2008. *My Food Guide,* http://www.hc-sc.gc.ca/fn-an/food-guide-aliment/myguide-monguide/index-eng.php (retrieved March 5, 2015).

Health Canada. 2010. *Eating Well with Canada's Food Guide: First Nations, Inuit and Métis,* http://www.hc-sc.gc.ca/fn-an/pubs/fnim-pnim/index-eng.php (retrieved April 5, 2015).

Health Canada. 2010. *Food and Nutrition,* http://www.hc-sc.gc.ca/fn-an/index-eng.php (retrieved April 5, 2015).

Health Canada. 2011. *Natural Health Products,* http://www.hc-sc.gc.ca/dhp-mps/prodnatur/index-eng.php (retrieved April 4, 2015).

Health Canada and Statistics Canada. 2004. *Canadian Community Health Survey Cycle 2.2, Nutrition. Nutrient Intakes from Food. Provincial, Regional and National Summary Data Tables: Volume 1.* Ottawa: Health Canada.

Institute of Medicine. 2010. *Dietary Reference Intakes for Calcium and Vitamin D: Report at a Glance,* http://www.iom.edu/Reports/2010/Dietary-Reference-Intakes-for-Calcium-and-Vitamin-D/Report-Brief. aspx (retrieved April 3, 2015).

Katamay, S. W., et al. 2007. *Eating Well with Canada's Food Guide* 2007: Development of the Food Intake Pattern. *Nutrition Reviews* 65(4): 155–166.

L'Abbé, M. R., S. J. Whiting, and D. A. Hanley. 2004. The Canadian health claim for calcium, vitamin D and osteoporosis. *Journal of the American College of Nutrition* 23(4): 303–308.

Lambton Community Health Services Department (n.d.) *New Nutrition Labels,* http://www. lambtonhealth.on.ca/nutrition/readlabels.asp (retrieved February 15, 2015).

Marine Harvest Canada. 2010. *Salmon Nutrition Facts,* http://www.marineharvestcanada.com/pdf/mics/ Nutrition_Facts.pdf (retrieved April 2, 2015).

McDonald, B. E. 2004. The Canadian experience: Why Canada decided against an upper limit for cholesterol. *Journal of the American College of Nutrition* 23(90006): 616S–620S.

National Research Council of Canada. 2006. *Highlights: Missing Ingredients Can Be a Recipe for Disaster,* http://www.nrc-cnrc.gc.ca/eng/news/nrc/2006/12/06/low-folate.html (retrieved February 21, 2015).

Norris, S. 2007. *Trans Fats: The Health Burden,* http://www2.parl.gc.ca/content/LOP/ ResearchPublications/prb0521-e.pdf (retrieved February 15, 2015).

Peng, Y. 2004. *Canadian Consumer Trends in Obesity and Food Consumption,* http://www1.agric.gov. ab.ca/$department/deptdocs.nsf/all/sis8438/$file/obesityandnutrition.pdf?OpenElement (retrieved May 14, 2015).

Public Health Agency of Canada. 2009. *Healthy Eating and Healthy Aging,* http://www.phac-aspc.gc.ca/ seniors-aines/publications/pro/healthy-sante/haging_newvision/vison-rpt/eating-alimentation-eng.php (retrieved March 5, 2015).

Samra, R. A., and G. H. Anderson. 2007. Insoluble cereal fiber reduces appetite and short-term food intake and glycemic response to food consumed 75 min later by healthy men. *American Journal of Clinical Nutrition* 86(4): 972–979.

Trans Fat Task Force. 2006. *TRANSforming the Food Supply,* http://www.hc-sc.gc.ca/fn-an/alt_formats/ hpfb-dgpsa/pdf/nutrition/tf-gt_rep-rap-eng.pdf (retrieved April 2, 2015).

Wolever, T. M., and D. J. Jenkins. 1997. What is a high fiber diet? *Advances in Experimental Medicine and Biology* 427: 35–42.

Nutrition Resources

TABLE 1

Dietary Reference Intakes (DRIs): Recommended Levels for Individual Intake

Life Stage	Group	Biotin (µg/day)	Choline (mg/day)[a]	Folate (µg/day)[b]	Niacin (mg/day)	Pantothenic Acid (mg/day)	Riboflavin (mg/day)
Infants	0–6 months	5	125	65	2	1.7	0.3
	7–12 months	6	150	80	4	1.8	0.4
Children	1–3 years	8	200	150	6	2	0.5
	4–8 years	12	250	200	8	3	0.6
Males	9–13 years	20	375	300	12	4	0.9
	14–18 years	25	550	400	16	5	1.3
	19–30 years	30	550	400	16	5	1.3
	31–50 years	30	550	400	16	5	1.3
	51–70 years	30	550	400	16	5	1.3
	>70 years	30	550	400	16	5	1.3
Females	9–13 years	20	375	300	12	4	0.9
	14–18 years	25	400	400i	14	5	1.0
	19–30 years	30	425	400i	14	5	1.1
	31–50 years	30	425	400i	14	5	1.1
	51–70 years	30	425	400i	14	5	1.1
	>70 years	30	425	400	14	5	1.1
Pregnancy	≤18 years	30	450	600i	18	6	1.4
	19–30 years	30	450	600j	18	6	1.4
	31–50 years	30	450	600j	18	6	1.4
Lactation	≤18 years	35	550	500	17	7	1.6
	19–30 years	35	550	500	17	7	1.6
	31–50 years	35	550	500	17	7	1.6
Tolerable Upper Intake Levels for Adults (19–70)			3500	1000k	35k		

Life Stage	Group	Thiamine (mg/day)	Vitamin A (µg/day)^d	Vitamin B-6 (mg/day)	Vitamin B-12 (µg/day)	Vitamin C (mg/day)^e	Vitamin D (µg/day)^f	Vitamin E (mg/day)^g
Infants	0–6 months	0.2	400	0.1	0.4	40	5	4
	7–12 months	0.3	500	0.3	0.5	50	5	5
Children	1–3 years	**0.5**	**300**	**0.5**	**0.9**	**15**	5	**6**
	4–8 years	**0.6**	**400**	**0.6**	**1.2**	**25**	5	**7**
Males	9–13 years	**0.9**	**600**	**1.0**	**1.8**	**45**	5	**11**
	14–18 years	**1.2**	**900**	**1.3**	**2.4**	**75**	5	**15**
	19–30 years	**1.2**	**900**	**1.3**	**2.4**	**90**	5	**15**
	31–50 years	**1.2**	**900**	**1.3**	**2.4**	**90**	5	**15**
	51–70 years	**1.2**	**900**	**1.7**	**2.4h**	**90**	10	**15**
	>70 years	**1.2**	**900**	**1.7**	**2.4h**	**90**	15	**15**
Females	9–13 years	**0.9**	**600**	**1.0**	**1.8**	**45**	5	**11**
	14–18 years	**1.0**	**700**	**1.2**	**2.4**	**65**	5	**15**
	19–30 years	**1.1**	**700**	**1.3**	**2.4**	**75**	5	**15**
	31–50 years	**1.1**	**700**	**1.3**	**2.4**	**75**	5	**15**
	51–70 years	**1.1**	**700**	**1.5**	**2.4h**	**75**	10	**15**
	>70 years	**1.1**	**700**	**1.5**	**2.4h**	**75**	15	**15**
Pregnancy	≤18 years	**1.4**	**750**	**1.9**	**2.6**	**80**	5	**15**
	19–30 years	**1.4**	**770**	**1.9**	**2.6**	**85**	5	**15**
	31–50 years	**1.4**	**770**	**1.9**	**2.6**	**85**	5	**15**
Lactation	≤18 years	**1.4**	**1200**	**2.0**	**2.8**	**115**	5	**19**
	19–30 years	**1.4**	**1300**	**2.0**	**2.8**	**120**	5	**19**
	31–50 years	**1.4**	**1300**	**2.0**	**2.8**	**120**	5	**19**
Tolerable Upper Intake Levels for Adults (19–70)			3000	100		2000	50	1000k

Note: The table includes values for the type of DRI standard—Adequate Intake (AI) or Recommended Dietary Allowance (RDA)—that has bee n established for that particular nutrient and life stage; RDAs are shown in **bold type**. The final row of the table shows the Tolerable Upper Intake Levels (ULs) for adults; refer to the full DRI report for information on other ages and life stages. A UL is the maximum level of daily nutrient intake that is likely to pose no risk of adverse effects. There is insufficient data to set ULs for all nutrients, but this does not mean that there is no potential for adverse effects; source of intake should be from food only to prevent high levels of intake of nutrients without established ULs. In healthy individuals, there is no established benefit from nutrient intakes above the RDA or AI.

µg is the symbol for micrograms.

^{a} Although AIs have been set for choline, there are few data to assess whether a dietary supply of choline is needed at all stages of the life cycle, and it may be that the choline requirement can be met by endogenous synthesis at some of these stages.

^{b} As dietary folate equivalents (DFE): I DFE = I µg food folate = 0.6 µg folate from fortified food or as a supplement consumed with food = 0.5 µg of a supplement taken on an empty stomach.

^{c} As niacin equivalents (NE): I mg niacin = 60 mg tryptophan.

^{d} As retinol activity equivalents (RAEs): I RAE = I µg retinol, 12 µg b-carotene, or 24 µg a-carotene or b-cryptoxanthin. Preformed vitamin A (retinol) is abundant in animal-derived foods; provitamin A carotenoids are abundant in some dark-yellow, orange, red, and deep-green fruits and vegetables. For preformed vitamin A and for provitamin A carotenoids in supplements, I RE = I RAE; for provitamin A carotenoids in foods, divide the REs by 2 to obtain RAEs. The UL applies only to preformed vitamin A.

TABLE 1

Dietary Reference Intakes (DRIs): Recommended Levels for Individual Intake (*continued*)

Life Stage	Group	Vitamin K (µg/day)	Calcium (mg/day)	Chromium (µg/day)	Copper (µg/day)	Fluoride (mg/day)	Iodine (µg/day)
Infants	0–6 months	2.0	210	0.2	200	0.01	110
	7–12 months	2.5	270	5.5	220	0.5	130
Children	1–3 years	30	500	11	**340**	0.7	**90**
	4–8 years	55	800	15	**440**	1	**90**
Males	9–13 years	60	1300	25	**700**	2	**120**
	14–18 years	75	1300	35	**890**	3	**150**
	19–30 years	120	1000	35	**900**	4	**150**
	31–50 years	120	1000	35	**900**	4	**150**
	51–70 years	120	1200	30	**900**	4	**150**
	>70 years	120	1200	30	**900**	4	**150**
Females	9–13 years	60	1300	21	**700**	2	**120**
	14–18 years	75	1300	24	**890**	3	**150**
	19–30 years	90	1000	25	**900**	3	**150**
	31–50 years	90	1000	25	**900**	3	**150**
	51–70 years	90	1200	20	**900**	3	**150**
	>70 years	90	1200	20	**900**	3	**150**
Pregnancy	≤18 years	75	1300	29	**1000**	3	**220**
	19–30 years	90	1000	30	**1000**	3	**220**
	31–50 years	90	1000	30	**1000**	3	**220**
Lactation	≤18 years	75	1300	44	**1300**	3	**290**
	19–30 years	90	1000	45	**1300**	3	**290**
	31–50 years	90	1000	45	**1300**	3	**290**
Tolerable Upper Intake Levels for Adults (19–70)			2500		10,000	10	1100

Life Stage	Group	Iron (mg/day)[i]	Magnesium (mg/day)	Manganese (mg/day)	Molybdenum (µg/day)	Phosphorus (mg/day)	Selenium (µg/day)	Zinc (mg/day)[m]
Infants	0–6 months	0.27	30	0.003	2	100	15	2
	7–12 months	11	75	0.6	3	275	20	3
Children	1–3 years	7	80	1.2	17	460	20	3
	4–8 years	10	130	1.5	22	500	30	5
Males	9–13 years	8	240	1.9	34	1250	40	8
	14–18 years	11	410	2.2	43	1250	55	11
	19–30 years	8	400	2.3	45	700	55	11
	31–50 years	8	420	2.3	45	700	55	11
	51–70 years	8	420	2.3	45	700	55	11
	>70 years	8	420	2.3	45	700	55	11
Females	9–13 years	8	240	1.6	34	1250	40	8
	14–18 years	15	360	1.6	43	1250	55	9
	19–30 years	18	310	1.8	45	700	55	8
	31–50 years	18	320	1.8	45	700	55	8
	51–70 years	8	320	1.8	45	700	55	8
	>70 years	8	320	1.8	45	700	55	8
Pregnancy	≤18 years	27	400	2.0	50	1250	60	13
	19–30 years	27	350	2.0	50	700	60	11
	31–50 years	27	360	2.0	50	700	60	11
Lactation	≤18 years	10	360	2.6	50	1250	70	14
	19–30 years	9	310	2.6	50	700	70	12
	31–50 years	9	320	2.6	50	700	70	12
Tolerable Upper Intake Levels for Adults (19-70)		45	350k	11	2000	4000	400	40

e Individuals who smoke require an additional 35 mg/day of vitamin C over that needed by nonsmokers; nonsmokers regularly exposed to tobacco smoke should ensure they meet the RDA for vitamin C.

f As cholecalciferol: I µg cholecalciferol = 40 IU vitamin D. DRI values are based on the absence of adequate exposure to sunlight.

g As a-tocopherol. Includes naturally occurring RRR-a-tocopherol and the 2R-stereoisomeric forms from supplements; does not include the 2S-stereoisomeric forms from supplements.

h Because 10 –30 percent of older people may malabsorb food-bound B12, those over age 50 should meet their RDA mainly with supplements or foods fortified with B12.

i In view of evidence linking folate intake with neural tube defects in the fetus. It is recommended that all women capable of becoming pregnant consume 400 µg from supplements or fortified foods in addition to consuming folate from a varied diet.

j It is assumed that women will continue consuming 400 µg from supplements or fortified food until their pregnancy is confirmed and they enter prenatal care, which ordinarily occurs after the end of the periconceptional period—the critical time for formation of the neural tube.

k The UL applies only to intake from supplements, fortified foods, and/or pharmacological agents and not to intake from foods.

l Because the absorption of iron from plant foods is low compared with that from animal foods, the RDA for strict vegetarians is approximately 1.8 times as high as the values established for omnivores (14 mg/day for adult male vegetarians; 33 mg/day for premenopausal female vegetarians). Oral contraceptives (OCs) reduce menstrual blood losses, so women taking them need less daily iron; the RDA for premenopausal women taking OCs is 10.9 mg/day. For more on iron requirements for other special situations, refer to *Dietary Reference Intakes for Vitamin A, Vitamin K, Arsenic, Boron, Chromium, Copper, Iodine, Iron, Manganese, Molybdenum, Nickel, Silicon, Vanadium, and Zinc* (visit http://www.nap.edu for the complete report).

m Zinc absorption is lower for those consuming vegetarian diets so the zinc requirement for vegetarians is approximately twofold greater than for those consuming a nonvegetarian diet.

TABLE 1

Dietary Reference Intakes (DRIs): Recommended Levels for Individual Intake (*continued*)

Life Stage	Group	Potassium (g/day)	Sodium (g/day)	Chloride (g/day)	Carbohydrate RDA/AI (g/day)	Carbohydrate AMDR (%)	Total Fibre RDA/AI (g/day)	Total Fat AMDR (%)
Infants	0–6 months	0.4	0.12	0.18	60	NDq	ND	r
	7–12 months	0.7	0.37	0.57	95	NDq	ND	r
Children	1–3 years	3.0	1.0	1.5	**130**	45–65	19	30–40
	4–8 years	3.8	1.2	1.9	**130**	45–65	25	25–35
Males	9–13 years	4.5	1.5	2.3	**130**	45–65	31	25–35
	14–18 years	4.7	1.5	2.3	**130**	45–65	38	25–35
	19–30 years	4.7	1.5	2.3	**130**	45–65	38	20–35
	31–50 years	4.7	1.5	2.3	**130**	45–65	38	20–35
	51–70 years	4.7	1.3	2.0	**130**	45–65	30	20–35
	>70 years	4.7	1.2	1.8	**130**	45–65	30	20–35
Females	9–13 years	4.5	1.5	2.3	**130**	45–65	26	25–35
	14–18 years	4.7	1.5	2.3	**130**	45–65	26	25–35
	19–30 years	4.7	1.5	2.3	**130**	45–65	25	20–35
	31–50 years	4.7	1.5	2.3	**130**	45–65	25	20–35
	51–70 years	4.7	1.3	2.0	**130**	45–65	21	20–35
	>70 years	4.7	1.2	1.8	**130**	45–65	21	20–35
Pregnancy	≤18 years	4.7	1.5	2.3	**175**	45–65	28	20–35
	19–30 years	4.7	1.5	2.3	**175**	45–65	28	20–35
	31–50 years	4.7	1.5	2.3	**175**	45–65	28	20–35
Lactation	≤18 years	5.1	1.5	2.3	**210**	45–65	29	20–35
	19–30 years	5.1	1.5	2.3	**210**	45–65	29	20–35
	31–50 years	5.1	1.5	2.3	**210**	45–65	29	20–35
Tolerable Upper Intake Levels for Adults (19–70)			2.3	3.6				

Life Stage	Group	Linoleic Acid		Alpha-linolenic Acid		Protein[n]		Water[p] (L/day)
		RDA/AI (g/day)	AMDR[o] (%)	RDA/AI (g/day)	AMDR[o] (%)	RDA/AI (g/day)	AMDR[o] (%)	
Infants	0–6 months	4.4	ND[q]	0.5	ND[q]	9.1	ND[q]	0.7
	7–12 months	4.6	ND[q]	0.5	ND[q]	13.5	ND[q]	0.8
Children	1–3 years	7	5–10	0.7	0.6–1.2	13	5–20	1.3
	4–8 years	10	5–10	0.9	0.6–1.2	19	10–30	1.7
Males	9–13 years	12	5–10	1.2	0.6–1.2	34	10–30	2.4
	14–18 years	16	5–10	1.6	0.6–1.2	52	10–30	3.3
	19–30 years	17	5–10	1.6	0.6–1.2	56	10–35	3.7
	31–50 years	17	5–10	1.6	0.6–1.2	56	10–35	3.7
	51–70 years	14	5–10	1.6	0.6–1.2	56	10–35	3.7
	>70 years	14	5–10	1.6	0.6–1.2	56	10–35	3.7
Females	9–13 years	10	5–10	1.0	0.6–1.2	34	10–30	2.1
	14–18 years	11	5–10	1.1	0.6–1.2	46	10–30	2.3
	19–30 years	12	5–10	1.1	0.6–1.2	46	10–35	2.7
	31–50 years	12	5–10	1.1	0.6–1.2	46	10–35	2.7
	51–70 years	11	5–10	1.1	0.6–1.2	46	10–35	2.7
	>70 years	11	5–10	1.1	0.6–1.2	46	10–35	2.7
Pregnancy	≤18 years	13	5–10	1.4	0.6–1.2	71	10–35	3.0
	19–30 years	13	5–10	1.4	0.6–1.2	71	10–35	3.0
	31–50 years	13	5–10	1.4	0.6–1.2	71	10–35	3.0
Lactation	≤18 years	13	5–10	1.3	0.6–1.2	71	10–35	3.8
	19–30 years	13	5–10	1.3	0.6–1.2	71	10–35	3.8
	31–50 years	13	5–10	1.3	0.6–1.2	71	10–35	3.8

[n] Daily protein recommendations are based on body weight for reference body weights. To calculate for a specific body weight, use the following values: 1.5 g/kg for infants, 1.1 g/kg for 1-3 years, 0.95 g/kg for 4-13 years, 0.85 g/kg for 14-18 years, 0.8 g/kg for adults, and 1.1 g/kg for pregnant (using prepregnancy weight) and lactating women.

[o] Acceptable Macronutrient Distribution Range (AMDR), expressed as a percent of total daily calories, is the range of intake for a particular energy source that is associated with reduced risk of chronic disease while providing intakes of essential nutrients. If an individual consumes in excess of the AMDR, there is a potential for increasing the risk of chronic diseases and/or insufficient intakes of essential nutrients.

[p] Total water intake from fluids and food.

[q] Not determinable because of lack of data of adverse effects in this age group and concern with regard to lack of ability to handle excess amounts. Source of intake should be from food only to prevent high levels of intake.

[r] For infants, Adequate Intake of total fat is 31 grams/day (0-6 months) and 30 grams per day (7-12 months) from breast milk and, for infants 7-12 months, complementary food and beverages.

Source: Reprinted with permission from *Dietary Reference Intakes: Applications in Dietary Planning*, copyright © 2003 by the National Academy of Sciences. Reprinted with permission from the National Academies Press, Washington, D.C.

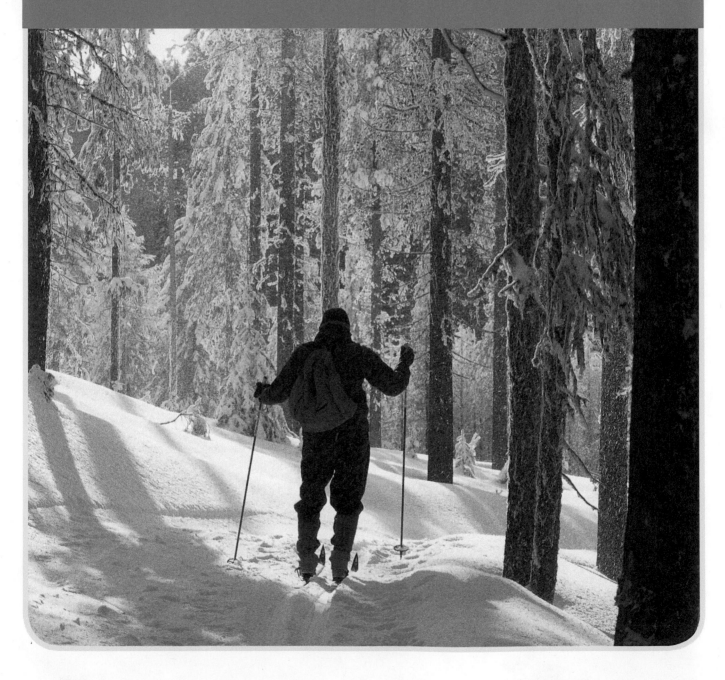

CHAPTER 6

Exercise for Health
and Fitness

LOOKING AHEAD

After you have read and studied this chapter, you should be able to:

LO1 Define physical fitness, and list the health-related components of fitness

LO2 Explain the wellness benefits of physical activity and exercise

LO3 Describe how to develop each of the health-related components of fitness

LO4 Discuss how to choose appropriate exercise equipment, how to eat and drink for exercise, how to assess fitness, and how to prevent and manage injuries

LO5 Put together a personalized exercise program that you enjoy and that will enable you to achieve your fitness goals

TEST YOUR KNOWLEDGE

1. **To improve your health, you must exercise vigorously for at least 30 minutes straight, five or more days per week.**
   True or false?

2. **Which of the following is considered a form of cardiorespiratory endurance exercise?**
   a. walking b. swimming c. aerobic dancing

3. **Developing strength in the trunk muscles is the most important way to prevent low-back pain.**
   True or false?

4. **The terms *physical activity* and *exercise* mean the same thing.**
   True or false?

5. **Which principle of fitness states that when you stop exercising, you can lose up to 50 percent of fitness improvements in two months?**
   a. FITT b. reversibility c. progressive overload

ANSWERS

1. FALSE.   Experts recommend 150 minutes of moderate physical activity per week, and activity can be done in short bouts—10-minute sessions, for example.

2. ALL THREE.   You can develop cardiorespiratory endurance through activities that involve continuous, rhythmic movements of large-muscle groups, such as the legs. Many kinds of activities count as cardiorespiratory endurance exercise.

3. FALSE.   Although muscular strength is an important factor in low-back health, muscular endurance in the trunk is actually more important to preventing low-back pain.

4. FALSE.   Physical activity is any body movement carried out by the skeletal muscles that requires energy. Exercise is planned, structured, repetitive movement performed specifically to improve or maintain physical fitness.

5. b.   The body adapts to any level of physical activity. The harder you exercise, the greater the improvements in fitness you will make. The reverse is also true; as you work less, your fitness drops to lower levels.

Your body is a wonderful moving machine made to work best when it is physically active. It readily adapts to practically any level of activity and exercise: The more you ask of your body—your muscles, bones, heart, lungs—the stronger and fitter it becomes. The opposite is also true. Left unchallenged, bones lose their density, joints stiffen, muscles become weak, and cellular energy systems begin to degenerate. To be truly healthy, human beings must be active.

This chapter gives you the basic information you need to put together a physical fitness program that will work for you. If approached correctly, physical activity and exercise can contribute immeasurably to overall wellness, add fun and joy to life, and provide the foundation for a lifetime of fitness.

What is Physical Fitness?

Physical fitness is the body's ability to respond or adapt to the demands and stress of physical effort—that is, to perform moderate to vigorous levels of physical activity without becoming overly tired.

> **physical fitness**
> The body's ability to respond or adapt to the demands and stress of physical effort.

Some components of fitness are related to specific activities or sports; others relate to general health. **Health-related fitness** includes the following components:
- cardiorespiratory endurance
- muscular strength
- muscular endurance
- flexibility
- body composition

> **health-related fitness**
> Physical capabilities that contribute to health, including cardiorespiratory endurance, muscular strength, muscular endurance, flexibility, and body composition.

Health-related fitness helps you withstand physical challenges and protects you from diseases.

Cardiorespiratory Endurance

Cardiorespiratory endurance is the ability to perform prolonged, large-muscle, dynamic exercise at moderate to high intensity. It depends on such factors as the lungs' ability to deliver oxygen to the bloodstream, the heart's capacity to pump blood, the ability of the nervous system and blood vessels to regulate blood flow, and the body's ability to use oxygen and process fuels for exercise.

> **cardiorespiratory endurance**
> The ability of the body to perform prolonged, large-muscle, dynamic exercise at moderate to high levels of intensity.

QUICK STATS

Physical inactivity is one of the top five global risk factors for mortality and is estimated to cause 2 million deaths per year.
—World Health Organization, 2009

When cardiorespiratory fitness is low, the heart has to work hard during normal daily activities and may not be able to work hard enough to sustain high-intensity physical activity in an emergency. Poor cardiorespiratory fitness is linked with heart disease, diabetes, colon cancer, stroke, depression, and anxiety.

Regular cardiorespiratory **endurance training**, however, conditions the heart. Endurance training makes the heart stronger and improves the function of the entire cardiorespiratory system. As cardiorespiratory fitness improves, related physical functions also improve:

- The heart pumps more blood per heartbeat.
- Resting heart rate slows and resting blood pressure decreases.
- Blood volume increases.
- Blood supply to tissues improves.
- The body can cool itself better.

endurance training
Exercise intended specifically to improve cardiorespiratory endurance; usually involves prolonged, large-muscle, dynamic exercises.

A healthy heart can better withstand the strains of daily life, the stress of occasional emergencies, and the wear and tear of time.

Endurance training also improves the function of the body's chemical systems, particularly in the muscles and liver, enhancing the body's ability to use energy from food and to do more exercise with less effort.

You can develop cardiorespiratory endurance through activities that involve continuous, rhythmic movements of large-muscle groups, such as the legs. Such activities include walking, jogging, cycling, and aerobic dancing.

Muscular Strength

Muscular strength is the amount of force a muscle can produce with a single maximum effort. It depends on such factors as the size of muscle cells and the ability of nerves to activate muscle cells. Strong muscles are important for everyday activities, such as climbing stairs, as well as for emergencies. They help keep the skeleton in proper alignment, preventing back and leg pain and providing the support necessary for good posture. Muscular strength has obvious importance in recreational activities. Strong people can hit a tennis ball harder, kick a soccer ball farther, and ride a bicycle uphill more easily.

muscular strength
The amount of force a muscle can produce with a single maximum effort.

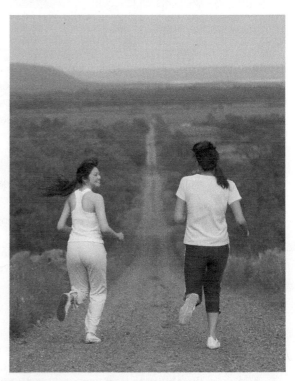

Muscle tissue is an important element of overall body composition. Greater muscle mass makes possible a higher rate of metabolism and faster energy use, which help to maintain a healthy body weight.

Maintaining strength and muscle mass is vital for healthy aging. Older people tend to lose muscle cells (a condition called *sarcopenia*), and many of the remaining muscle cells become non-functional because they lose their attachment to the nervous system. Strength training helps maintain muscle mass, function, and balance in older people, which greatly enhances their quality of life and prevents life-threatening injuries. Strength training has also been shown to benefit cardiovascular health and reduce the risk of osteoporosis (bone loss).

Muscular strength can be developed by training with weights or by using the weight of the body for resistance during callisthenic exercises, such as push-ups and curl-ups.

Cardiorespiratory endurance is a critical component of health-related fitness.

Muscular Endurance

Muscular endurance is the ability to resist fatigue and sustain a given level of muscle tension—that is, to hold a muscle contraction for a long time or to contract a muscle over and over again. It depends on such factors as the size of muscle cells, the ability of muscles to store fuel, and the blood supply to muscles.

> **muscular endurance**
> The ability of a muscle or group of muscles to remain contracted or to contract repeatedly for a long time.

Muscular endurance is important for good posture and for injury prevention. For example, if abdominal and back muscles cannot hold the spine correctly, the chances of low-back pain and back injury are increased. In fact, good muscular endurance in the trunk muscles is more important than muscular strength for preventing back pain. Muscular endurance helps people cope with the physical demands of everyday life and enhances performance in sports and work.

Like muscular strength, muscular endurance is developed by stressing the muscles with a greater load (weight) than they are used to. The degree to which strength or endurance develops depends on the type and amount of stress that is applied.

Flexibility

Flexibility is the ability to move joints through their full range of motion. It depends on joint structure, the length and elasticity of connective tissue, and nervous system activity. Flexible, pain-free joints are important for good health and well-being. Inactivity causes the joints to become stiffer with age. Stiffness, in turn, can cause people (of any age) to assume unnatural body postures that can stress joints and muscles. Stretching exercises can help ensure a healthy range of motion for all major joints.

> **flexibility**
> The ability to move joints through their full range of motion.

Body Composition

Body composition refers to the proportion of fat and **fat-free mass** (muscle, bone, and water) in the body. Healthy body composition involves a high proportion of fat-free mass and an acceptably low level of body fat, for a given age and sex. A person with excessive body fat—especially in the abdomen—is more likely to experience health problems, including heart disease, high blood pressure, stroke, joint problems, diabetes, gallbladder disease, cancer, and back pain.

> **body composition**
> The proportion of fat and fat-free mass (muscle, bone, and water) in the body.
>
> **fat-free mass**
> The non-fat component of the human body, consisting of skeletal muscle, bone, and water.

The best way to lose fat is through a lifestyle that includes a sensible diet and exercise. The best way to add muscle mass is through resistance training, such as weight training. (Body composition is discussed in detail in Chapter 4.)

Skill-Related Components of Fitness

In addition to the five health-related components of physical fitness, the ability to perform a particular sport or activity may depend on **skill-related fitness** components, such as the following:
- *Speed:* the ability to perform a movement in a short time
- *Power:* the ability to exert force rapidly, based on a combination of strength and speed
- *Agility:* the ability to change the body's position quickly and accurately

- *Balance:* the ability to maintain equilibrium while either moving or stationary
- *Coordination:* the ability to perform motor tasks accurately and smoothly by using body movements and the senses
- *Reaction time:* the ability to respond quickly to a stimulus

skill-related fitness
Physical abilities that contribute to performance in a sport or activity, including speed, power, agility, balance, coordination, and reaction time.

Skill-related fitness tends to be sport-specific and is best developed through practice. For example, the speed, coordination, and agility needed to play basketball are best developed by playing basketball. Some fitness experts contend that certain sports don't contribute to all the health-related components of physical fitness. Nevertheless, playing a sport can be fun, can help you build fitness, and may contribute to other areas of wellness.

QUICK STATS

Physical inactivity contributes to more than 21 000 premature deaths in Canada each year and about $2.4 billion in direct and $4.3 billion in indirect costs.

—Public Health Agency of Canada, 2007; Janssen, 2012

Physical Activity and Exercise for Health and Fitness

Despite the many benefits of an active lifestyle, levels of physical activity remain low for all populations of Canadians. Canadian males are more active than females at all ages, with the exception of 35–54 year olds where males and females are roughly the same. However, less than half of the population is active enough to trigger health gains. According to the most recent Canadian Health Measures Survey, the fitness levels of all Canadians have declined significantly over the last three decades.

Although studies have shown that physical activity helps to boost concentration, memory, and learning in school, a startling 95 percent of children and youth (ages 5–17 years) do not get the recommended amount of physical activity every day. One contributor to children and youth's reduction in physical activity over the years is their mode of transportation to and from school. Between the years 2000 and 2010, there was more than a 10 percent increase in the percentage of Canadian children and youth who use *only* inactive modes (such as taking the bus or getting a ride) every day. As illustrated in Figure 6.1, while children and youth across the country are not getting enough physical activity overall, the percentage who engage in active and inactive modes of transportation to and from school each day differs by province.

Differences also exist among different ethnic groups when it comes to meeting guidelines for moderate to vigorous physical activity (MVPA): White and Aboriginal people are most likely to be moderately active, while black, West Asian and South Asian, and Arab people are least likely to be sufficiently active. Evidence is growing that for many Canadians, becoming more physically active may be the single most important lifestyle change they can make to improve their health and well-being (see the Mind Body Spirit box).

Canadian adults are also struggling to get in enough active minutes each week, with about 15 percent meeting the guideline. As depicted in Figure 6.2, Canadian men and women at a healthy weight accumulate significantly more minutes of MVPA than their overweight and obese counterparts.

QUESTIONS FOR CRITICAL THINKING AND REFLECTION

When you think about exercise, do you think of only one or two of the five components of health-related fitness, such as muscular strength or body composition? If so, where do you think your ideas come from? What role do the media play in shaping your ideas about fitness?

FIGURE 6.1

Transportation Behaviours to/from School, by Province/Territory

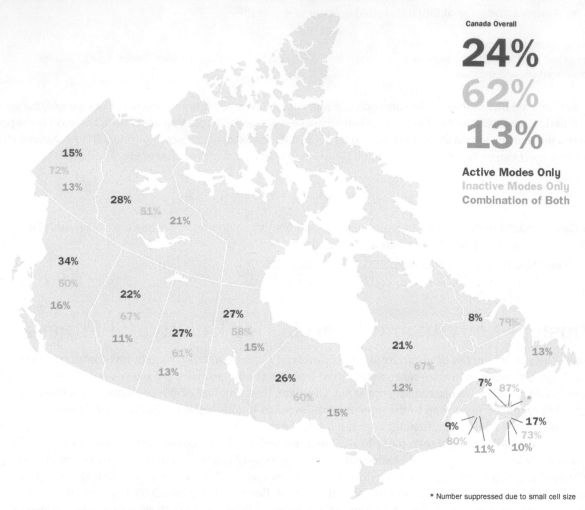

Canada Overall

24%

62%

13%

Active Modes Only
Inactive Modes Only
Combination of Both

* Number suppressed due to small cell size

Source: Active Healthy KidsCanada, *Are We Driving Our Kids to Unhealthy Habits?* 2013 Active Healthy Kids Canada Report Card on Physical Activity for Children and Youth, http://dvqdas9jty7g6.cloudfront.net/reportcard2013/AHKC2013ReportCardENG.pdf, p. 10.

 Mind *Body* SPIRIT

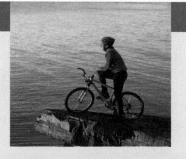

Exercise and Total Wellness

As you will see throughout this chapter, an active lifestyle provides a multitude of benefits. For example, physically active adults live from about two to four and a half years longer, on average, than do sedentary adults. The benefits of regular physical activity, however, go beyond longevity—they affect quality of life across multiple dimensions of wellness.

Physical Wellness

In terms of general health, exercise increases your physical capacity so that you are better able to meet the challenges of daily life with energy and vigour. Physical activity can help you do the following:
- Generate more energy.
- Increase your stamina.

- Control your weight.
- Manage stress.
- Boost your immune system.

Over the long term, even moderate physical activity can help you avoid illnesses, such as heart disease, diabetes, high blood pressure, depression, osteoporosis, and some cancers. Evidence shows that exercise can even prevent premature death from several causes.

Emotional Wellness

Exercise provides psychological and emotional benefits, contributing to your sense of competence and well-being. People who focus on staying active can also enjoy an improved self-image and a higher level of self-confidence. Such healthy self-esteem can positively affect other aspects of your life. For example, a good self-image can be helpful when dealing with others or when competing.

Intellectual Wellness

Recent studies indicate that regular exercise is good for the brain—literally. One study shows that brain volume actually increases in adults who exercise regularly. Other studies show that exercise helps to reduce mental declines seen with aging. Such valuable impacts in brain mass (growth or replenishment of brain matter) can improve cognitive functions and the overall health of the nervous system. Additionally, the process of mastering physical challenges—such as learning a proper golf swing—can boost intellectual fitness in the same manner as solving puzzles or engaging in other learning experiences.

Interpersonal Wellness

Joining in physical activity with a friend or a group can be a boon to your interpersonal or social wellness, too. By sharing physical challenges with others, you can make new friends, deepen your existing relationships, and build a stronger overall network of support.

Physical Activity on a Continuum

Physical activity is any body movement carried out by the skeletal muscles and requiring energy. Different types of physical activity can be arranged on a continuum based on the amount of energy they require. Quick, easy movements, such as standing up or walking down a hallway, require little energy or effort; more intense, sustained activities, such as cycling 10 kilometres or running in a race, require considerably more.

> **physical activity**
> Any body movement carried out by the skeletal muscles and requiring energy.

Exercise refers to a subset of physical activity—planned, structured, repetitive movement of the body intended specifically to improve or maintain physical fitness. Levels of fitness depend on such physiological factors as the heart's ability to pump blood and the size of muscle fibres. These factors are a function both of genetics—a person's inborn potential for physical fitness—and of behaviour—the amount of exercise a person does to improve fitness. To develop fitness, a person must perform enough physical activity to stress the body and cause long-term physiological changes.

FIGURE 6.2

Average Daily Minutes of Moderate to Vigorous Physical Activity by Body Mass Index Category

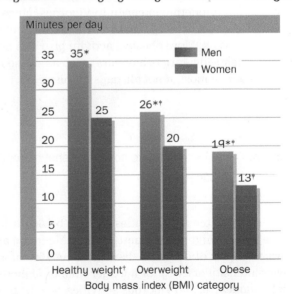

† reference category
* significantly different from estimate for women (p < 0.05)
‡ significantly different from estimate for reference category (p < 0.05)

Source: Statistics Canada, *Canadian Health Measures Survey, 2007 to 2009*. Chart 2, "Average daily minutes of moderate-to-vigorous physical activity by BMI category". http://www.statcan.gc.ca/pub/82-625-x/2011001/article/11552-eng.htm (accessed: August 25, 2015)

exercise
Planned, structured, repetitive movement of the body intended to improve or maintain physical fitness.

Physical activity is essential to health and confers wide-ranging health benefits, but exercise is necessary to significantly improve physical fitness. This important distinction between physical activity and exercise is a key concept in understanding the guidelines discussed in this chapter.

Increasing Physical Activity to Improve Health and Wellness

In 1998, Health Canada and the Canadian Society for Exercise Physiology (CSEP) worked in partnership to launch *Canada's Physical Activity Guide to Healthy Active Living*. At that time, research indicated that Canadians were unaware that physical inactivity is a serious risk factor for premature death, chronic disease, and disability, with a magnitude of risk comparable with that of smoking. Further, two-thirds of Canadians were inactive, a serious threat to their health and a burden on the public health care system. Canadians were confused by all the data and information available about physical activity and fitness and wanted a valid and practical guide, similar to what is now called *Eating Well with Canada's Food Guide* (discussed in Chapter 5), that would help them judge how much physical activity they needed to achieve better health.

QUICK STATS

Only 13% of Canadians ages 60–79 get enough physical activity in a week to meet Canadian guidelines.
—Colley et al., 2011

In 2011, CSEP released new guidelines with the support of the Public Health Agency of Canada. The new guidelines for Canadian adults (18–64 years old) recommend strength-training activities at least two days per week, and moderate-intensity to vigorous-intensity aerobic physical activity most days per week. Each session of aerobic activity must be at least 10 minutes, and adults should accumulate a total of at least 150 minutes per week. More physical activity provides greater health benefits. Canadians are also encouraged to minimize their sedentary behaviours (such as sitting for long periods) as much as possible. Ideally, Canadians should be active most, if not all, days of the week.

QUICK STATS

85% of Canadian adults are not active enough for health benefits.
—Statistics Canada, 2013

Moderate-intensity activities include brisk walking and bike riding, while vigorous-intensity activities include jogging and cross-country skiing. Moderate activity for 30 minutes uses about 150 calories. Figure 6.3 shows examples of activities that use about 150 calories. You can burn the same number of calories by doing a lower-intensity activity for a longer time or higher-intensity activity for a shorter time. For more examples of light, moderate, and vigorous activities, see the In Focus box. Research shows that being active for at least 150 minutes every week promotes health and wellness by lowering the risk of high blood pressure, stroke, heart disease, type 2 diabetes, colon cancer, and osteoporosis and by reducing feelings of mild to moderate depression and anxiety.

It's easy to fit in the required amount of physical activity because the activities can be done all at once or in 10-minute intervals throughout the week; for example, 10-minute bike rides to and from class and a brisk

10-minute walk to the store each day add up to 150 minutes in a week. In this lifestyle approach to physical activity, people can choose activities that they find enjoyable and that fit into their daily routine. Everyday tasks at school, work, and home can be structured to contribute to the daily activity total (see "Making Time for Physical Activity" on connect). Public health and individual well-being would receive an enormous benefit if all sedentary Canadians were to increase their lifestyle physical activity to 30 minutes per day.

In addition to the activity guide for adults 18 to 64, CSEP has produced guides for adults 65 and older, for children 5–11 years old, and for youth between the ages of 12 and 17 (see Figure 6.4). Not only is it important for all Canadians to get sufficient physical activity, researchers are finding that *also* reducing sedentary time is essential for our health. In fact, in addition to the recommendation for everyone to reduce time spent being sedentary, CSEP recently released specific sedentary guides for children and youth. The guides encourage children up to 4 years of age to have minimal time being sedentary during waking hours, including reducing prolonged sitting or being restrained (e.g., stroller, high chair) to

FIGURE 6.3

Examples of Moderate Amounts of Physical Activity

Each example uses about 150 calories.

Activity	Duration (min)	
Washing a car	45–60	***Less Vigorous, More Time***
Washing windows or floors	45–60	
Playing volleyball	45	
Playing touch football	30–45	
Gardening	30–45	
Wheeling self in wheelchair	30–40	
Walking 1.75 miles (2.75 km)	35 (20 min/mile)	
Shooting a basketball	30	
Bicycling 5 miles	30 (6 min/mile)	
Dancing fast	30	
Pushing a stroller 1.5 miles (2.5 km)	30	
Raking leaves	30	
Walking 2 miles (3.25 km)	30 (15 min/mile)	
Doing water aerobics	30	
Swimming laps	20	
Wheelchair basketball	20	
Playing a game of basketball	15–20	
Bicycling 4 miles (6.5 km)	15 (3$^3/_4$ min/mile)	
Jumping rope	15	
Running 1.5 miles (2.5 km)	15 (10 min/mile)	
Shovelling snow	15	***More Vigorous, Less Time***
Stairwalking	15	

Source: Department of Health and Human Services. 1996. *Physical Activity and Health: A Report of the Surgeon General.* Atlanta: DHHS.

FIGURE 6.4

Canadian Physical Activity Guidelines

For children 5–11 years

For health benefits, children aged 5–11 years should accumulate at least 60 minutes of moderate- to vigorous-intensity physical activity daily.
This should include:

- Vigorous-intensity activities at least 3 days per week.
- Activities that strengthen muscle and bone at least 3 days per week.
- More daily physical activity provides greater health benefits.

For youth 12–17 years

For health benefits, youth aged 12–17 years should accumulate at least 60 minutes of moderate- to vigorous-intensity physical activity daily.
This should include:

- Vigorous-intensity activities at least 3 days per week.
- Activities that strengthen muscle and bone at least 3 days per week.
- More daily physical activity provides greater health benefits.

For adults 18–64 years

To achieve health benefits, adults aged 18–64 years should accumulate at least 150 minutes of moderate- to vigorous-intensity aerobic physical activity per week, in bouts of 10 minutes or more.

- It is also beneficial to add muscle and bone strengthening activities using major muscle groups, at least 2 days per week.
- More physical activity provides greater health benefits.

For older adults 65 years and older

To achieve health benefits, and improve functional abilities, adults aged 65 and older should accumulate at least 150 minutes of moderate- to vigorous-intensity aerobic physical activity per week, in bouts of 10 minutes or more.

- It is also beneficial to add muscle and bone strengthening activities using major muscle groups, at least 2 days per week.
- Those with poor mobility should perform physical activities to enhance balance and prevent falls.
- More physical activity provides greater health benefits.

Source: Reprinted with permission from the Canadian Society for Exercise Physiology, http://www.csep.ca/guidelines (retrieved May 19, 2015).

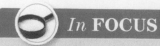 *In* FOCUS

Classifying Activity Levels

Assessing your physical activity level is easier if you know how to classify different kinds of activities. Fitness experts categorize activities into the following three levels:

- *Light activity* includes the routine tasks associated with typical day-to-day life, such as vacuuming or walking to class. You probably perform dozens of light activities every day without even thinking about it. You can gain significant health benefits by turning light activities into moderate activities—by walking briskly instead of slowly, for example.
- *Moderate activity* causes your breathing and heart rate to accelerate but still allows for comfortable conversation. An example is walking at 4 to 5 kilometres per hour. It is sometimes described as activity that can be performed comfortably for about 45 minutes. Raking leaves is an example of moderate physical activity, as are most occupational tasks that involve extended periods of moderate effort.
- *Vigorous activity* elevates your heart rate considerably and has other physical effects that improve your fitness level. During vigorous activity you are breathing too heavily to hold a conversation very easily. An example is walking faster than 6 kilometres per hour.

Here are some examples:

Light	Moderate	Vigorous
Walking slowly	Walking briskly	Walking briskly uphill
Routine tasks: • Cooking • Shopping	Cycling moderately on level terrain Social dancing	Cycling on steep uphill terrain Heavy housework: • Moving furniture • Carrying heavy objects upstairs
Light housework: • Ironing • Dusting • Washing dishes	Moderate housework: • Scrubbing floors • Washing windows	Vigorous yardwork or home activities: • Shovelling snow • Trimming trees • Doing construction work • Digging
Light yardwork or home activities: • Pruning • Weeding • Plumbing	Moderate yardwork or home activities: • Planting • Raking • Painting • Washing car	
Light fitness activities: • Light stretching or warm-up • Swimming, slow treading	Fitness activities requiring moderate effort: • Low-impact aerobics • Frisbee • Swimming • Tennis, doubles	Fitness activities requiring vigorous effort: • Running • High-impact aerobics • Circuit weight training • Swimming laps • Most competitive sports

no more than an hour at a time. They also recommend children under 2 years of age have no screen time (e.g., watching TV, computer), and that children ages 2–4 years have less than an hour per day of screen time. For children and youth ages 5–17 years, the sedentary guidelines recommend limiting recreational screen time to no more than 2 hours per day and limiting the amount of time spent in sedentary motorized transport, extended sitting, and time spent indoors throughout the day. You can order or download free copies of the guides from the CSEP website listed in the "For More Information" section at the end of the chapter.

Increasing Physical Activity to Manage Weight

Because more than half of Canadians are overweight or obese, various agencies and health organizations have created physical activity guidelines focusing on weight management. These guidelines call for more daily physical activity than the guidelines designed for general health promotion. These guidelines do not conflict with those from CSEP, but they do have a different emphasis. They recognize that for people who need to prevent weight gain, lose weight, or maintain weight loss, 150 minutes of physical activity each week may not be enough. Instead, they recommend 45–90 or more minutes of physical activity each day. The different recommendations may seem confusing, but all major international health organizations have the same message: People can improve their health by becoming more active.

Exercising to Improve Physical Fitness

As mentioned earlier, moderate physical activity confers significant health and wellness benefits, especially for those who are currently sedentary and become moderately active. The leading international physical activity authorities all conclude that people can obtain even greater health and wellness benefits by increasing the duration and intensity of physical activity. With increased activity, they will see more improvements in quality of life and greater reductions in disease and mortality risk.

More vigorous activity, as occurs in a structured, systematic exercise program, is also needed to improve physical fitness; moderate physical activity alone is not enough. Physical fitness requires more intense movement that poses a substantially greater challenge to the body. The Canadian Society for Exercise Physiology (CSEP), along with researchers with the American College of Sports Medicine (ACSM), world leaders in exercise science, have issued specific recommendations for creating a formal exercise program that will develop physical fitness. These guidelines are described in detail later in the chapter.

How Much Physical Activity Is Enough?

Some experts feel that people get most of the health benefits of an exercise program simply by becoming more active during the day; the amount of activity needed depends on an individual's health status and goals. Other experts feel that the activity goal set by the lifestyle approach is too low; they argue that people should exercise long enough and intensely enough to improve their body's capacity for exercise—that is, to improve physical fitness. More research is needed to clarify the health effects of different amounts of lifestyle physical activity, of moderate-intensity versus high-intensity exercise, and of continuous versus intermittent exercise. However, there is probably some truth in both of these positions.

Where does this leave you? Most experts agree that some physical activity is better than none, but that more—as long as it does not result in injury—is better than some. To set a personal goal for physical activity and exercise, consider your current activity level, your health status, and your overall goals. At the very least, strive to become more active and meet the goal set by CSEP of 150 minutes of MVPA each week. Choose to be active whenever you can. If weight management is a concern for you, you may need to start slowly, depending on how long you have been inactive, and raise your activity level gradually to 45–90 minutes per day or more. For even better health and well-being, participate in a structured exercise program that develops physical fitness. This is important for all Canadians—the profile of the typical Canadian has changed (and not necessarily for the better) over the last 30 years. Figure 6.5 illustrates the differences between a typical Canadian 12-year-old boy and girl from 1981 to 2007–2009. The bottom line is that any increase in physical activity will contribute to your health and well-being, now and in the future.

QUESTIONS FOR CRITICAL THINKING AND REFLECTION

Does your current lifestyle include enough physical activity—150 minutes of moderate to vigorous activity each week—to support health and wellness? Does your lifestyle go beyond this level to include enough vigorous physical activity and exercise to build physical fitness? What would be the impact on your life if you were more active? How would you feel? What is one change you could make in your lifestyle to start developing physical fitness?

FIGURE 6.5

Portrait of a Typical 12-year-old Boy and Girl, 1981 and 2007–2009

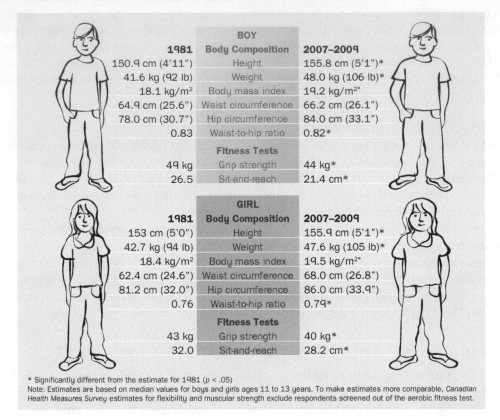

	BOY	
1981	**Body Composition**	**2007–2009**
150.9 cm (4'11")	Height	155.8 cm (5'1")*
41.6 kg (92 lb)	Weight	48.0 kg (106 lb)*
18.1 kg/m²	Body mass index	19.2 kg/m²*
64.9 cm (25.6")	Waist circumference	66.2 cm (26.1")
78.0 cm (30.7")	Hip circumference	84.0 cm (33.1")
0.83	Waist-to-hip ratio	0.82*
	Fitness Tests	
49 kg	Grip strength	44 kg*
26.5	Sit-and-reach	21.4 cm*

	GIRL	
1981	**Body Composition**	**2007–2009**
153 cm (5'0")	Height	155.9 cm (5'1")*
42.7 kg (94 lb)	Weight	47.6 kg (105 lb)*
18.4 kg/m²	Body mass index	19.5 kg/m²*
62.4 cm (24.6")	Waist circumference	68.0 cm (26.8")
81.2 cm (32.0")	Hip circumference	86.0 cm (33.9")
0.76	Waist-to-hip ratio	0.79*
	Fitness Tests	
43 kg	Grip strength	40 kg*
32.0	Sit-and-reach	28.2 cm*

* Significantly different from the estimate for 1981 ($p < .05$)
Note: Estimates are based on median values for boys and girls ages 11 to 13 years. To make estimates more comparable, *Canadian Health Measures Survey* estimates for flexibility and muscular strength exclude respondents screened out of the aerobic fitness test.

Source: M. S. Tremblay, M. Shields, M. Laviolette, et al. 2010. Fitness of Canadian children and youth: Results from the 2007–2009 Canadian Health Measures Survey, *Health Reports* 21(1). Statistics Canada, Catalogue 82-003.

The Benefits of Exercise

As mentioned earlier, the human body is very adaptable. The greater the demands made on it, the more it adjusts to meet the demands—it becomes fit. Over time, immediate, short-term adjustments translate into long-term changes and improvements (see Figure 6.6). The goal of regular physical activity is to bring about these kinds of long-term changes and improvements in the body's functioning.

Improved Cardiorespiratory Functioning

Every time you take a breath, oxygen in the air enters your lungs and is picked up by red blood cells and transported to your heart. From there, the heart pumps oxygenated blood throughout the body to organs and tissues that use it. During exercise, the cardiorespiratory system (heart, lungs, and circulatory system) must work harder to meet the body's increased demand for oxygen. Regular endurance exercise improves the functioning of the heart and the ability of the cardiorespiratory system to carry oxygen to body tissues. Exercise directly affects the health of your arteries, keeping them from stiffening or clogging with plaque and reducing the risk of cardiovascular disease. Exercise also improves sexual function and general vitality.

More Efficient Metabolism

Endurance exercise improves metabolism, the process that converts food to energy and builds tissue. This process involves oxygen, nutrients, hormones, and enzymes. A physically fit person can more efficiently

FIGURE 6.6

Immediate and Long-term Effects of Regular Exercise

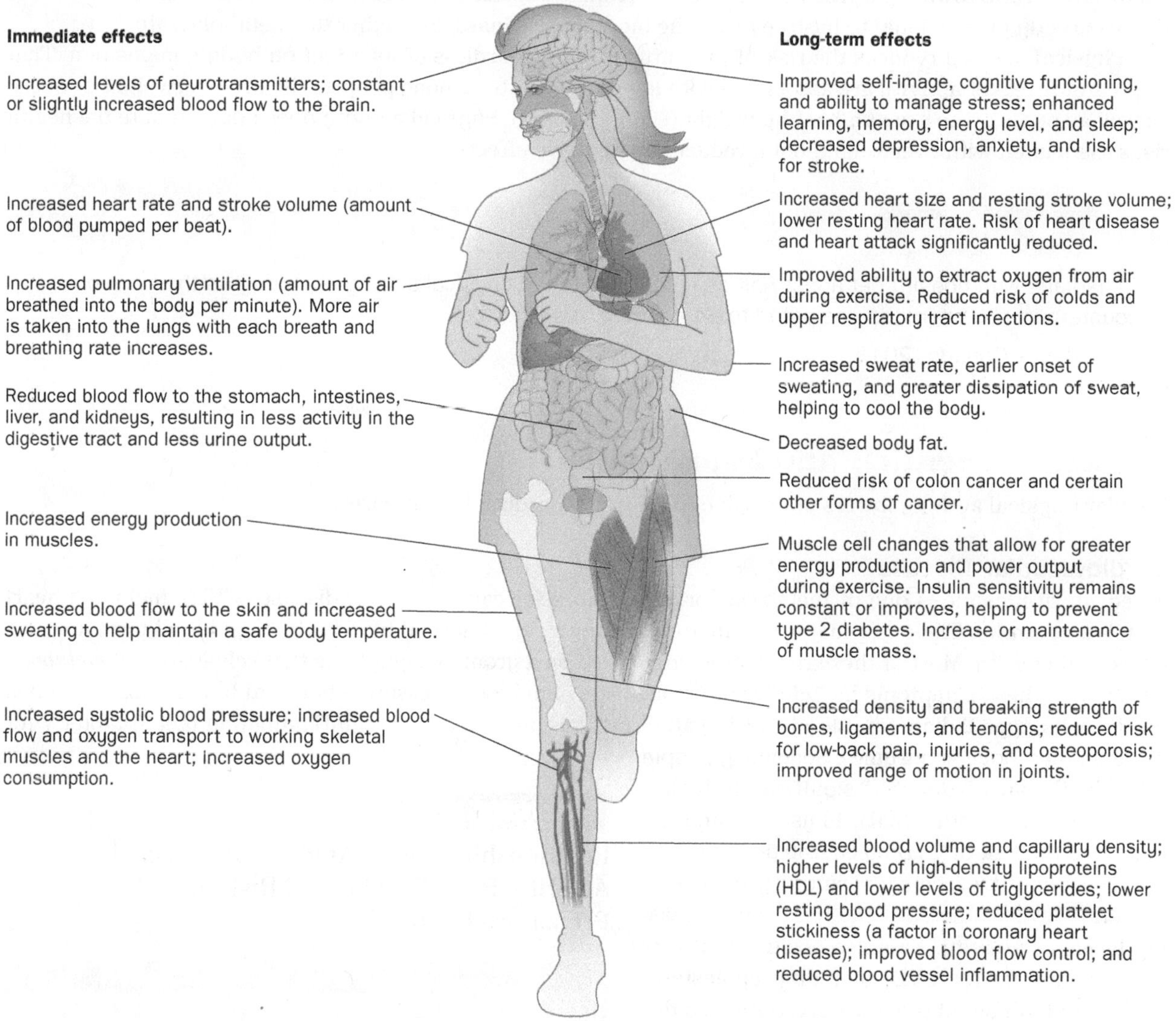

Immediate effects

Increased levels of neurotransmitters; constant or slightly increased blood flow to the brain.

Increased heart rate and stroke volume (amount of blood pumped per beat).

Increased pulmonary ventilation (amount of air breathed into the body per minute). More air is taken into the lungs with each breath and breathing rate increases.

Reduced blood flow to the stomach, intestines, liver, and kidneys, resulting in less activity in the digestive tract and less urine output.

Increased energy production in muscles.

Increased blood flow to the skin and increased sweating to help maintain a safe body temperature.

Increased systolic blood pressure; increased blood flow and oxygen transport to working skeletal muscles and the heart; increased oxygen consumption.

Long-term effects

Improved self-image, cognitive functioning, and ability to manage stress; enhanced learning, memory, energy level, and sleep; decreased depression, anxiety, and risk for stroke.

Increased heart size and resting stroke volume; lower resting heart rate. Risk of heart disease and heart attack significantly reduced.

Improved ability to extract oxygen from air during exercise. Reduced risk of colds and upper respiratory tract infections.

Increased sweat rate, earlier onset of sweating, and greater dissipation of sweat, helping to cool the body.

Decreased body fat.

Reduced risk of colon cancer and certain other forms of cancer.

Muscle cell changes that allow for greater energy production and power output during exercise. Insulin sensitivity remains constant or improves, helping to prevent type 2 diabetes. Increase or maintenance of muscle mass.

Increased density and breaking strength of bones, ligaments, and tendons; reduced risk for low-back pain, injuries, and osteoporosis; improved range of motion in joints.

Increased blood volume and capillary density; higher levels of high-density lipoproteins (HDL) and lower levels of triglycerides; lower resting blood pressure; reduced platelet stickiness (a factor in coronary heart disease); improved blood flow control; and reduced blood vessel inflammation.

generate energy, use carbohydrates and fats for energy, and regulate hormones. Exercise may also protect cells from damage by free radicals, which are destructive chemicals produced during normal metabolism (see Chapter 5), and from inflammation caused by high blood pressure or cholesterol, nicotine, and over-eating. Training activates antioxidant enzymes that prevent free radical damage and maintain the health of the body's cells.

Improved Body Composition

Healthy body composition means that the body has a high proportion of fat-free mass and a relatively small proportion of fat. Too much body fat, particularly abdominal fat, is linked to a variety of health problems, including heart disease, cancer, and diabetes. Healthy body composition can be difficult to achieve and maintain because a diet that contains all essential nutrients can be relatively high in calories, especially for someone who is sedentary. Excess calories are stored in the body as fat.

Exercise can improve body composition in several ways. Endurance exercise significantly increases daily calorie expenditure; it can also slightly raise *metabolic rate*, the rate at which the body burns calories, for several hours after an exercise session. Strength training increases muscle mass, thereby tipping the body composition ratio toward fat-free mass and away from fat. It can also help with losing fat because metabolic rate is directly proportional to fat-free mass: the more muscle mass, the higher the metabolic rate.

Physical activity reduces the risk of premature death regardless of its effect on body composition. That is, greater levels of activity are associated with lower death rates among people who are overweight or obese as well as people who are at a healthy weight (see Figure 6.7). Physical activity does not eliminate the health risks associated with overweight, but it reduces its negative effects.

QUICK STATS

Canadians with obesity get about half as many minutes of physical activity each day as their non-obese counterparts (19 minutes compared to 34 minutes, respectively).

—Statistics Canada, 2013

Disease Prevention and Management

Regular physical activity lowers your risk of many chronic, disabling diseases.

Cardiovascular Disease

A sedentary lifestyle is one of the six major risk factors for cardiovascular disease (CVD), including heart attack and stroke. The other major risk factors are smoking, abnormal blood fats, high blood pressure, diabetes, and obesity. Most of these risk factors are linked by a group of symptoms that scientists call *metabolic syndrome*. These symptoms include insulin resistance, high blood pressure, abnormal blood fats, abdominal fat deposits, type 2 diabetes, blood clotting abnormalities, and blood vessel inflammation (see Chapter 7 for more on metabolic syndrome). Sedentary people have death rates from CVD significantly higher than those of fit individuals. Physical inactivity increases the risk of CVD by 50–240 percent.

The benefit of physical activity occurs at moderate levels of activity and rises with increasing levels of activity. Exercise positively affects the risk factors for CVD, including cholesterol levels and high blood pressure. Exercise also directly interferes with the disease process itself, directly lowering risk of heart disease and stroke.

BLOOD FAT LEVELS Endurance exercise and strength training have a positive effect on the balance of lipids (fats) that circulate in the blood. High concentrations of lipids, such as cholesterol and triglycerides, are linked to heart disease because they contribute to the formation of fatty deposits on the linings of arteries. When blood clots block a narrowed artery, a heart attack or stroke can occur.

Cholesterol is carried in the blood by lipoproteins, which are classified according to size

FIGURE 6.7

Relationship Among Amount of Physical Activity, Body Weight, and Risk of Premature Death

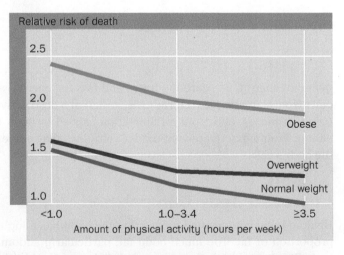

Source: Hu, F. B., et al. 2004. Adiposity compared with physical activity in predicting mortality among women. *New England Journal of Medicine* 351(26): 2694–2703.

and density. Cholesterol carried by low-density lipoproteins (LDLs) sticks to the walls of coronary arteries. High-density lipoproteins (HDLs) pick up excess cholesterol in the bloodstream and carry it back to the liver for excretion from the body. High LDL levels and low HDL levels increase the risk of cardiovascular disease. High levels of HDL and low levels of LDL are associated with lower risk.

Heart disease is covered in Chapter 7. For our purposes in this chapter, it is important to know only that endurance exercise and strength training influence blood lipids in a positive way, by increasing HDL levels and decreasing LDL levels and triglycerides—reducing the risk of CVD.

HIGH BLOOD PRESSURE   Regular endurance exercise tends to reduce high blood pressure (hypertension), a contributing factor in many diseases, such as coronary heart disease, stroke, heart failure, kidney failure, and blindness. Intense, long-duration exercise works best, but even moderate exercise can produce significant improvements. Strength training also reduces blood pressure.

CORONARY HEART DISEASE   Coronary heart disease (CHD), also called coronary artery disease (CAD), involves blockage of one of the coronary arteries. These blood vessels supply the heart with oxygenated blood, and an obstruction in one of them can cause a heart attack. Exercise directly interferes with the disease process that causes coronary artery blockage. It also enhances the function of cells lining the arteries that help regulate blood flow.

STROKE   A stroke occurs when a blood vessel leading to the brain is blocked or ruptures, often through the same disease process that leads to heart attacks. Regular exercise reduces the risk of stroke.

Cancer

Studies have shown a relationship between increased physical activity and a reduced risk of cancer, but these findings are not conclusive. Evidence suggests that exercise reduces the risk of colon cancer and some studies are showing promising data that it reduces the risk of cancer of the breast and reproductive organs in women and prostate cancer in men. Exercise may decrease the risk of colon cancer by speeding the movement of food through the gastro-intestinal tract (quickly eliminating potential carcinogens), lowering blood insulin levels, enhancing immune function, and reducing blood fats. The protective mechanism in the case of reproductive system cancers is less clear, but physical activity during the high school and the post-secondary years may be particularly important for preventing breast cancer later in life. Some studies have also found that regular physical activity reduces the risk of pancreatic cancer.

Osteoporosis

A special benefit of exercise, especially for women, is protection against osteoporosis, a disease that results in loss of bone density and poor bone strength. Weight-bearing exercise, which includes almost everything except swimming, helps build bone during childhood, the teens, and the twenties. Older people with denser bones can better endure the bone loss that occurs with aging. Strength training and impact exercises, such as jumping rope, can increase bone density throughout life. With stronger bones and muscles and better balance, fit people are less likely to experience debilitating falls and bone fractures. Along with exercise, a well-balanced diet containing adequate calcium and vitamin D and normal hormone function are also essential for strong bones. One caution: Too much exercise can depress levels of estrogen, which helps maintain bone density, thereby leading to bone loss, even in young women.

Type 2 Diabetes

People with diabetes are prone to heart disease, blindness, and severe problems of the nervous and circulatory systems. Exercise prevents the development of type 2 diabetes, the most common form of the disease. Exercise burns excess sugar and makes cells more sensitive to insulin. Exercise also helps keep body fat at healthy levels. (Obesity is a key risk factor for type 2 diabetes.) For people who have diabetes, physical activity is an important part of treatment. See Chapter 4 for more on diabetes.

Improved Psychological and Emotional Wellness

People who are physically active experience many social, psychological, and emotional benefits, including the following:

- *Reduced stress:* In response to stressors, physically fit people experience milder physical responses and less emotional distress than sedentary individuals. Physical activity also provides protection against the effects of stress that have been linked to poor cardiorespiratory health. Endurance exercise decreases the secretion of hormones and neurotransmitters triggered by emotional stress. It also can diffuse hostility and alleviate feelings of stress and anxiety by providing an emotional outlet and inducing feelings of relaxation. Regular exercise can also relieve sleeping problems.
- *Reduced anxiety and depression:* Sedentary adults are much more likely to feel fatigue and depression than those who are physically active. Exercise is an effective treatment for people with depression and improves mood in people who aren't experiencing depression.
- *Improved self-image:* Performing physical activities provides proof of skill and self-control, thus enhancing your self-concept. Sticking with an exercise program increases people's belief in their ability to be active, thereby boosting self-efficacy. Exercise also helps you look and feel better, boosting self-confidence and body image.
- *Learning and memory:* Exercise enhances the formation and survival of new nerve cells and the connections between nerves, which in turn improve memory and learning. Physical activity helps maintain mental functioning in older adults and may ward off dementia.
- *Enjoyment:* Exercise is fun. It offers a way to interact with other people, as well as opportunities to strive and excel. Physically fit people can perform everyday tasks with ease. They have plenty of energy and can lead lives that are full and varied.

Improved Immune Function

Exercise can have either positive or negative effects on the immune system, the physiological processes that protect us from disease. It appears that moderate endurance exercise boosts immune function, whereas excessive training depresses it. Physically fit people get fewer colds and upper respiratory tract infections than people who are not fit. The immune system—and ways to strengthen it—is discussed further in Chapter 9.

Prevention of Injuries and Low-Back Pain

Increased muscle strength provides protection against injury because it helps people maintain good posture and appropriate body mechanics when carrying out everyday activities, such as walking, lifting, and carrying. Good muscle endurance in the abdomen, hips, lower back, and legs supports the back in proper alignment and helps prevent low-back pain, which affects a significant majority of Canadians at some time in their lives.

Improved Wellness for Life

Although people differ in the maximum levels of fitness they can achieve through exercise, the wellness benefits of exercise are available to everyone (see the Dimensions of Diversity box). Exercising regularly may be the single most important thing you can do now to improve the quality of your life in the future. All the benefits of exercise continue to accrue but gain new importance as the resilience of youth begins to wane. Specific information about physical activity for older adults is discussed more in Chapter 17. Simply stated, exercising can help you live a longer and healthier life.

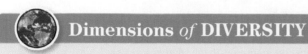

Dimensions *of* DIVERSITY

Exercise for People with Special Health Concerns

Regular, appropriate exercise is safe and beneficial for many people with chronic conditions or other special health concerns. For many people with special health concerns, in fact, the risks associated with not exercising are far greater than those associated with a moderate program of regular exercise.

If you have a special health concern and have hesitated becoming more active, one helpful strategy is to take a class or join an exercise group specifically designed for your condition. Many health centres and support groups sponsor specially tailored activity programs. Such a class or group activity can provide you with both expert advice and exercise partners who share your concerns and goals. If you prefer to exercise at home, exercise videos are available for people with a variety of conditions.

The fitness recommendations for the general population presented in this chapter can serve as general guidelines for any exercise program. However, for people with special health concerns, certain precautions and monitoring may be required. *Anyone with special health concerns should consult a physician before beginning an exercise program.* Guidelines and cautions for some common conditions are described below.

Most of the following conditions are influenced by many of the determinants of health noted in Chapter 1; as you read this section, see if you can identify which determinants affect each condition.

Asthma
- Carry medication during workouts and avoid exercising alone. Use your inhaler before exercise, if recommended by your physician.
- Exercise regularly, and warm up and cool down slowly to reduce the risk of acute attacks.
- When starting a fitness program, choose self-paced endurance activities, especially those involving interval training (short bouts of exercise followed by rest periods).
- When possible, avoid circumstances that may trigger an asthma attack, including cold, dry air, or pollen or dust. Drink water to keep your airways moist, and in cold weather, cover your mouth with a mask or scarf to warm and humidify the air you breathe. Swimming is a good activity choice for people with asthma.

Diabetes
- Don't exercise alone; wear a bracelet identifying you as having diabetes.
- If you are taking insulin or another medication, you may need to adjust the timing and amount of each dose as you learn to balance your energy intake and output and your medication dosage.
- To prevent abnormally rapid absorption of injected insulin, inject it over a muscle that won't be exercised and wait at least an hour before exercising.
- Check blood sugar levels before, during, and after exercise, and adjust your diet or insulin dosage if needed. Avoid exercise if your blood sugar level is above 13.5 mmol/L, and ingest carbohydrates before exercise if your blood sugar level is below 5.5 mmol/L. Have high-carbohydrate foods available during a workout.
- Check your skin regularly for blisters and abrasions, especially on your feet.

Obesity
- For maximum benefit and minimum risk, begin with low- to moderate-intensity activities and increase the intensity slowly as your fitness improves.
- To lose weight or maintain lost weight, exercise moderately 60 minutes or more every day; you can exercise all at once or divide your total activity time into sessions of 10 or more minutes.
- At first choose non- or low-weight-bearing activities, such as swimming, water exercises, cycling, or walking.
- Stay alert for symptoms of heat-related problems during exercise.
- Try to include as much lifestyle physical activity in your daily routine as possible.
- Include strength training in your program to build or maintain muscle mass.

Heart Disease and Hypertension
- Warm-up and cool-down sessions should be gradual and should last at least 10 minutes.
- Exercise at a moderate rather than a high intensity; monitor your heart rate during exercise, and stop if you experience dizziness or chest pain.
- Increase exercise frequency, intensity, and time very gradually.
- Don't hold your breath when exercising as this can cause a sudden, steep increase in blood pressure.

- Discuss the effects of your medication with your physician; for example, certain drugs for hypertension affect heart rate. If your physician has prescribed nitroglycerine, carry it with you during exercise.

Arthritis
- Begin an exercise program as early as possible in the course of the disease.
- Warm up thoroughly before each workout to loosen stiff muscles and lower the risk of injury.
- Avoid high-impact activities that may damage arthritic joints; consider swimming or water aerobics.
- In strength training, pay special attention to muscles that support and protect affected joints; add weight very gradually.
- Perform flexibility exercises regularly.

Osteoporosis
- If possible, choose low-impact, weight-bearing activities to help safely maintain bone density.
- To prevent fractures, avoid any activity or movement that stresses the back or carries a risk of falling.
- Weight train to improve strength and balance and reduce the risk of falls and fractures, but avoid lifting heavy weights.

QUESTIONS FOR CRITICAL THINKING AND REFLECTION

Which benefits of exercise are most important to you, and why? For example, is there a history of heart disease or diabetes in your family? Have you thought about how regular exercise could reduce your risks for specific diseases?

Designing Your Exercise Program

The best exercise program has two primary characteristics: It promotes your health, and it's fun for you to do. Exercise does not have to be a chore. On the contrary, it can provide some of the most pleasurable moments of your day, once you make it a habit. A little thought and planning will help you achieve these goals.

QUICK STATS

Only 22% of Canadian schools provide daily physical education.

—Canadian Heart and Stroke Foundation, 2012

For even greater benefits, consider integrating a formal exercise program into your life. Table 6.1 summarizes the current physical activity and exercise recommendations based on the various goals of promoting general health, fitness, and weight management. Leading physical activity and exercise scientists have established guidelines for an exercise program that includes cardiorespiratory endurance (aerobic) exercise, strength training, flexibility training, and neuromuscular training. Such a program will develop all the health-related components of physical fitness.

The sections of this chapter that follow will show you how to develop a personalized exercise program. For a summary of the health and fitness benefits of different levels of physical activity, see Figure 6.8.

TABLE 6.1

Physical Activity and Exercise Recommendations for Promoting General Health, Fitness, and Weight Management

Goal	Recommendation
General health	Perform moderate- to vigorous-intensity aerobic physical activity for at least 150 minutes per week. Also, be more active in your daily life: walk instead of drive, take the stairs instead of the elevator, and watch less television.
Increased health and fitness benefits	Exercise at a moderate intensity for 300 minutes per week or at a vigorous intensity for 150 minutes per week.
Achieve or maintain weight loss	Exercise at a moderate intensity for 60–90 minutes per day on most days of the week.
Muscle strength and endurance	Perform one or more sets of resistance exercises that work the major muscle groups for 8–12 repetitions (10–15 reps for older adults) on two or three non-consecutive days per week. Examples include weight training and exercises that use body weight as resistance (such as core-stabilizing exercises, pull-ups, push-ups, lunges, and squats).
Flexibility	Perform range-of-motion (stretching) exercises at least two days per week. Hold each stretch for 10–30 seconds.
Neuromuscular training	Older people should do balance training two or three days per week. Examples include yoga, tai chi, and balance exercises (standing on one foot, step-ups, and walking lunges). These exercises are probably beneficial for young and middle-aged adults.

Sources: Canadian Society of Exercise Physiology. Canadian Physical Activity Guidelines, http://www.csep.ca/CMFiles/Guidelines/CSEP-InfoSheetsComplete-Eng.pdf; Garber, C. E., et al. 2011. Quantity and quality of exercise for developing and maintaining cardiorespiratory, musculoskeletal, and neuromotor fitness in apparently healthy adults: guidance for prescribing exercise. *Medicine & Science in Sports & Exercise.* 43(7):1334–1359; Physical Activity Guidelines Advisory Committee. 2008. *Physical Activity Guidelines Advisory Committee Report, 2008.* Washington, DC: U.S. Department of Health and Human Services; and U.S. Department of Health and Human Services. 2010. *The Surgeon General's Vision for a Healthy and Fit Nation.* Rockville, MD: U.S. Department of Health and Human Services, Office of the Surgeon General.

FIGURE 6.8

Health and Fitness Benefits of Different Amounts of Physical Activity and Exercise

	Lifestyle physical activity 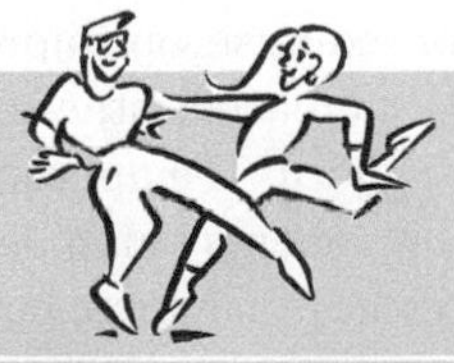	Moderate exercise program 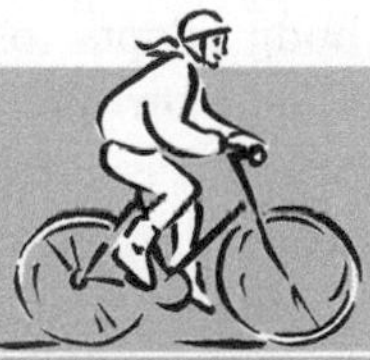	Vigorous exercise program 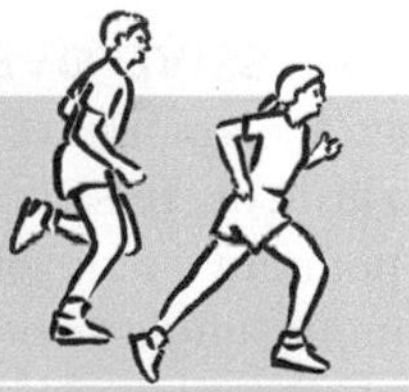
Description	Moderate physical activity—an amount of activity that uses about 150 calories per day Minimum of 150 minutes/week (about 5 days or more per week)	Cardiorespiratory endurance exercise (30 minutes, 5 days per week); strength training (at least 2 non-consecutive days per week) and stretching exercises (2 or more days per week)	Cardiorespiratory endurance exercise (20 minutes, 3 days per week); interval training; strength training (3–4 days per week); and stretching exercises (5–7 days per week)
Sample activities or program	One of the following: • Walking to and from work, 15 minutes each way • Cycling to and from class, 15 minutes each way • Yardwork for 30 minutes • Dancing (fast) for 30 minutes • Playing basketball for 20 minutes	• Walking for 30 minutes, 5 days per week • Weight training, 1 set of 8 exercises, 2 days per week • Stretching exercises, 3 days per week	• Jogging for 45 minutes, 3 days per week • Intervals: running 400 m at high effort, 4 sets, 2 days per week • Weight training, 3 sets of 10 exercises, 3 days per week • Stretching exercises, 6 days per week
Health and fitness benefits	Better blood cholesterol levels, reduced body fat, better control of blood pressure, improved metabolic health, and enhanced glucose metabolism; improved quality of life; reduced risk of some chronic diseases Greater amounts of activity can help prevent weight gain and promote weight loss	All the benefits of lifestyle physical activity, plus improved physical fitness (increased cardiorespiratory endurance, muscular strength and endurance, and flexibility) and even greater improvements in health and quality of life and reductions in chronic disease risk	All the benefits of lifestyle physical activity and a moderate exercise program, with greater increases in fitness and somewhat greater reductions in chronic disease risk Participating in a vigorous exercise program may increase risk of injury and overtraining

First Steps

Are you thinking about starting a formal exercise program? A little planning can help make it a success.

Medical Clearance

Some people are advised to check with their physicians before increasing their current level of activity or beginning an exercise program. You can use the Physical Activity Readiness Questionnaire (PAR-Q), a self-screening tool, originally designed by the British Columbia Ministry of Health and the Multidisciplinary Board on Exercise, to see whether you are in this group. You can take the updated questionnaire on the Public Health Agency of Canada's website listed in the "For More Information" section at the end of the chapter. In general, it is often recommended that previously inactive men over 40 and women over 50 get a medical examination before beginning an exercise program. Diabetes, asthma, heart disease, and extreme obesity are conditions that may call for a modified program. If you have an increased risk of heart disease because of smoking, high blood pressure, or obesity, get a complete physical checkup, including an **electrocardiogram (ECG or EKG)**, before beginning your program.

> **electrocardiogram (ECG or EKG)**
> A recording of the electrical activity of the heart.

Basic Principles of Physical Training

To put together an effective exercise program, you should first understand the basic principles of physical training.

SPECIFICITY To develop a fitness component, you must perform exercises that are specifically designed for that component. This is the principle of *specificity*. Weight training, for example, develops muscular strength but is less effective for developing flexibility. Specificity also applies to the skill-related fitness components and to the different parts of the body. A well-rounded exercise program includes exercises geared to each component of fitness, to different parts of the body, and to specific activities or sports.

PROGRESSIVE OVERLOAD Your body adapts to the demands of exercise by improving its functioning. When the amount of exercise, also called **overload**, is progressively increased, fitness continues to improve. Too little exercise will have no effect on fitness; too much may cause injury. The appropriate amount depends on your current level of fitness, your fitness goals, and the fitness components being developed. A novice, for example, might experience fitness benefits from jogging 2 kilometres in 15 minutes, but this level of exercise would cause no physical adaptations in a trained distance runner.

> **overload**
> The amount of stress placed on the body; a gradual increase in the amount of overload causes adaptations that improve fitness.

The amount of overload needed to maintain or improve a particular level of fitness is determined in four dimensions, represented by the acronym FITT: **F**requency, **I**ntensity, **T**ime, and **T**ype.

- *Frequency, or how often:* Optimum exercise frequency, expressed in number of days per week, varies with the component being developed, how vigorously you exercise, and your goals. A frequency of three to five days per week is recommended for cardiorespiratory endurance exercise, two or three days per week for strength training, and two to three days per week (ideally five to seven days per week) for stretching.
- *Intensity, or how hard:* Fitness benefits occur when you exercise harder than your normal level of activity. To develop cardiorespiratory endurance, you must raise your heart rate above normal; to develop muscular strength, you must lift a heavier weight than you normally do; to develop flexibility, you must stretch your muscles beyond their normal length. A gradual increase in intensity is recommended to avoid injury.

- *Time (duration), or how long:* If fitness benefits are to occur, exercise sessions must last for an extended time. Depending on the component being developed and your intensity level, a duration of 20–60 minutes is usually recommended.
- *Type or mode of activity:* The type of exercise in which you should engage varies with each fitness component and with your personal fitness goals. To develop cardiorespiratory endurance, you need to engage in continuous activities involving large-muscle groups—walking, cycling, or swimming, for example. Resistive exercises develop muscular strength and endurance; stretching exercises build flexibility. The frequency, intensity, and time of exercise will be different for each type of activity.

These dimensions of overload are described individually as they apply to the health-related components of fitness discussed in this chapter.

REST AND RECUPERATION Fitness gains occur following exercise as the body adapts to the stress of training. Adequate rest is as important to this process as training. Overtraining—an imbalance between training and recovery—leads to injury, illness, and excessive fatigue.

REVERSIBILITY The body adjusts to lower levels of physical activity in the same way it adjusts to higher levels—the principle of **reversibility**. When you stop exercising, you can lose up to 50 percent of fitness improvements within two months. Try to exercise consistently, and don't quit if you miss a few workouts. If you must temporarily curtail your training, you can maintain your fitness improvements by keeping the intensity of your workouts constant while reducing their frequency or duration.

> **reversibility**
> The training principle that fitness improvements are lost when demands on the body are lowered.

INDIVIDUAL DIFFERENCES There are limits to the potential for improvement and large individual differences in our ability to improve fitness, achieve a desirable body composition, and perform and learn sports skills. Scientists have identified specific genes that influence the capacity to alter body fat, strength, and endurance. In addition, men tend to have higher endurance capacity than women because of higher testosterone levels (which affect oxygen transport and cellular metabolism) and lower levels of body fat. However, men and women have the same capacity for improvement when gains are expressed as a percentage of initial fitness.

Selecting Activities

If you have been inactive, you should begin slowly by gradually increasing the amount of moderate physical activity in your life. Once your body adjusts to your new level of activity, you can choose additional activities for your exercise program.

Be sure the activities you choose contribute to your overall wellness and make sense for you. Are you competitive? If so, try racquetball, basketball, or squash. Do you prefer to exercise alone? Then consider cross-country skiing or road running. Have you been sedentary? A walking program may be a good place to start. If you think you may have trouble sticking with an exercise program, find a structured activity that you can do with a friend or a group.

Be realistic about the constraints presented by some sports, such as accessibility, expense, and time. For example, if you have to travel for hours to get to a ski area, skiing may not be a good choice for your regular exercise program. And if you have never played tennis, it will probably take some time to reach a reasonable skill level; you may be better off with a program of walking or jogging to get good workouts while you are improving your tennis game.

Cardiorespiratory Endurance Exercises

Exercises that condition your heart and lungs should have a central role in your fitness program. The best exercises for developing cardiorespiratory endurance stress a large portion of the body's muscle mass for a prolonged time. These include walking, jogging, running, swimming, bicycling, and aerobic dancing. Many popular sports and recreational activities, such as racquetball, tennis, basketball, and soccer, are also good if the skill level and intensity of the game are sufficient to provide a vigorous workout.

Frequency

The optimal workout schedule for endurance training is three to five days per week. Beginners should start with three and work up to five days. Training more than five days a week often leads to injury for recreational athletes. Although you do get health benefits from exercising very vigorously only one or two days per week, you risk injury because your body never gets a chance to adapt fully to regular exercise training.

Intensity

The most misunderstood aspect of conditioning, even among experienced athletes, is training intensity. Intensity is the crucial factor in attaining a significant training effect—that is, in increasing the body's cardiorespiratory capacity. A primary purpose of endurance training is to increase **maximal oxygen consumption** ($\dot{V}O_{2max}$) which represents the maximum ability of the cells to use oxygen and is considered the best measure of cardiorespiratory capacity. Intensity of training is the crucial factor in improving $\dot{V}O_{2max}$.

> **maximal oxygen consumption ($\dot{V}O_{2max}$)**
> The body's maximum ability to transport and use oxygen.

One of the easiest ways to determine exactly how intensely you should work involves measuring your heart rate. It is not necessary or desirable to exercise at your maximum heart rate—the fastest heart rate possible before exhaustion sets in—to improve your cardiorespiratory capacity. Beneficial effects occur at lower heart rates with a much lower risk of injury. **Target heart rate range** is the range of rates within which you should exercise to obtain cardiorespiratory benefits. To determine the intensity at which you should exercise, refer to the Take Charge box and Figure 6.9.

> **target heart rate range**
> The range of heart rates within which exercise yields cardiorespiratory benefits.

After you begin your fitness program, you may improve quickly because the body adapts readily to new exercises; the rate of improvement may slow after the first month or so. The more fit you become, the harder you will have to work to improve. By monitoring your heart rate, you will always know if you are working hard enough to improve, not hard enough, or too hard. For most people, a fitness program involves attaining an acceptable level of fitness and then maintaining that level. There is no need to keep working indefinitely to improve; doing so only increases the chance of injury. After you have reached the level you want, you can maintain fitness by exercising at the same intensity three to five days per week.

FIGURE 6.9

Checking your Pulse

The pulse can be taken at the carotid artery in the neck (top) or at the radial artery in the wrist (bottom). Be sure to not press too hard, particularly on the carotid artery.

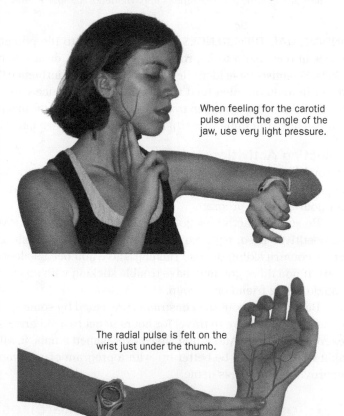

When feeling for the carotid pulse under the angle of the jaw, use very light pressure.

The radial pulse is felt on the wrist just under the thumb.

Take **CHARGE**

Determining Your Target Heart Rate Range

Your target heart rate is the range of rates at which you should exercise to experience cardiorespiratory benefits. Your target heart rate range is based on your maximum heart rate, which can be estimated from your age. (If you are a serious athlete or face possible cardiovascular risks from exercise, you may want to have your maximum heart rate determined more accurately through a treadmill test in a physician's office, hospital, or sports medicine laboratory.) Your target heart rate is a range: The lower value corresponds to moderate-intensity exercise, and the higher value is associated with high-intensity exercise. Target heart rate ranges are shown in the table.

You can monitor the intensity of your workouts by measuring your pulse either at your wrist or at one of your carotid arteries, located on either side of your Adam's apple. Your pulse rate drops rapidly after exercise, so begin counting immediately after you have finished exercising. You will obtain the most accurate results by counting beats for 10 seconds and then multiplying by 6 to get your heart rate in beats per minute (bpm). The 10-second counts corresponding to each target heart rate range are also shown in the table.

Age (years)	Target Heart Rate Range (bpm)*	10-Second Count (beats)*
20–24	127–180	21–30
25–29	124–176	20–29
30–34	121–171	20–28
35–39	118–167	19–27
40–44	114–162	19–27
45–49	111–158	18–26
50–54	108–153	18–25
55–59	105–149	17–24
60–64	101–144	16–24
65+	97–140	16–23

*Target heart rates lower than those shown here are appropriate for individuals with a very low initial level of fitness. Ranges are based on the following formula: Target heart rate = 0.65 to 0.90 of maximum heart rate, assuming maximum heart rate = 220 − age.

QUICK STATS

Throughout Canada, 51 YMCA/YWCAs serve 2 million Canadians in more than 1000 communities across the country.
—YMCA Canada, 2013

Time (Duration)
A total time of 20–60 minutes is recommended; exercise can take place in a single session or several sessions lasting 10 or more minutes. The total duration of exercise depends on its intensity. To improve cardiorespiratory endurance during a low-intensity to moderate-intensity activity, such as walking or slow swimming, you should exercise for 45–60 minutes. For high-intensity exercise performed at the top of your target heart rate zone, a duration of 20 minutes is sufficient. Start with less vigorous activities and gradually increase intensity.

You can use these three dimensions of cardiorespiratory endurance training—frequency, intensity, and time—to develop a fitness program that strengthens your heart and lungs and provides all the benefits described earlier in this chapter. Build your program around at least 20 minutes of endurance exercise at your target heart rate three to five days a week. Then add exercises that develop the other components of fitness.

The Warm-Up and Cool-Down
It is always important to warm up before you exercise and to cool down afterward. Warming up enhances your performance and decreases your chances of injury. Your muscles work better when their temperature is

elevated slightly above resting level. Warming up helps your body gradually progress from rest to exercise. Blood needs to be redirected to active muscles, and your heart needs time to adapt to the increased demands of exercise. A warm-up helps spread **synovial fluid** throughout the joints, which helps protect joint surfaces from wear and tear. (It's like warming up a car to spread oil through the engine parts before shifting into gear.)

> **synovial fluid**
> Fluid found within many joints that provides lubrication and nutrition to the cells of the joint surface.

A warm-up session should include low-intensity movements similar to those in the activity that will follow. For example, hit forehands and backhands before a tennis game or jog slowly for 400 metres before progressing to 1.6 kilometres in 8 minutes. Some people like to include stretching exercises in their warm-up. Experts recommend that you stretch *after* the active part of your warm-up, when your body temperature has been elevated. Studies have found that stretching before exercise can temporarily decrease muscle strength and power, so if a high-performance workout is your goal, it is best to stretch after a workout. See the section "Flexibility Exercises" later in this chapter for more on stretching.

Cooling down after exercise is important to restore the body's circulation to its normal resting condition. When you are at rest, a relatively small percentage of your total blood volume is directed to muscles, but during exercise, as much as 90 percent of the heart's output is directed to them. During recovery from exercise, it is important to continue exercising at a low level to provide a smooth transition to the resting state. Cooling down helps regulate the return of blood to your heart.

QUICK STATS

5–10 minutes of warming up and cooling down is adequate for a 30-minute workout of brisk walking.
—Mayo Clinic, 2011

Developing Muscular Strength and Endurance

Any program designed to promote health should include exercises that develop muscular strength and endurance (see the Gender Matters box). Your ability to maintain correct posture and move efficiently depends in part on adequate muscle fitness. Strengthening exercises also increase muscle tone, which improves the appearance of your body.

Types of Strength-training Exercises

Muscular strength and endurance can be developed in many ways, from weight training to calisthenics. Common exercises, such as curl-ups, push-ups, pull-ups, and wall-sitting (leaning against a wall in a seated position and supporting yourself with your leg muscles), maintain the muscular strength of most people if they practise them several times a week. To condition and tone your whole body, choose exercises that work the major muscles of the shoulders, chest, back, arms, abdomen, and legs.

To increase muscular strength and endurance, you must do **resistance exercise**—exercises in which your muscles must exert force against a significant amount of resistance. Resistance can be provided by weights, exercise machines, or your own body weight.

> **resistance exercise**
> Activities that force muscles to contract against increased resistance; also called *strength training*.

Isometric (static) exercises involve applying force without movement, such as when you contract your abdominal muscles. This static type of exercise is valuable for toning and strengthening muscles. Isometrics can be practised anywhere and do not require any equipment. For maximum strength gains, hold an isometric contraction maximally for six seconds; do five to ten repetitions. Don't hold your breath—that can restrict

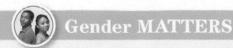

Gender MATTERS

Gender Differences in Muscular Strength

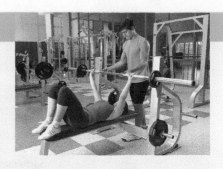

At this point in your reading of this text, it should be clear that gender often plays a role as a health determinant, and this is also the case when looking at building muscular strength. Men are generally stronger than women because they typically have larger bodies overall and a larger proportion of their total body mass is made up of muscle. But when strength is expressed per unit of muscle tissue, men are only 1–2 percent stronger than women in the upper body and about equal to women in the lower body. Individual muscle cells are larger in men, but the functioning of the cells is the same in both sexes.

Two factors that help explain these disparities are testosterone levels and the speed of nervous control of muscle. Testosterone promotes the growth of muscle tissue in both males and females, but testosterone levels are about 6–10 times as high in men as in women, so men develop larger muscles. Also, because the male nervous system can activate muscles faster, men tend to have more power.

Some women are concerned that they will develop large muscles from strength training. Because of hormonal differences, most women do not develop large muscles unless they train intensely over many years or take steroids. A study of average women who weight trained two to three days per week for eight weeks found that the women gained about 3.75 kilograms of muscle and lost about 7.7 kilograms of fat. Another study followed women who trained with weights for two years. Not only did the women reduce their overall body fat levels, but they ended up with less fat around their midsection.

Losing muscle over time is a much greater health concern for women than small gains in muscle weight in response to strength training, especially as any gains in muscle weight are typically more than balanced with loss of fat weight. Both men and women lose muscle mass and power as they age, but because men start out with more muscle when they are young and don't lose power as quickly as women, older women tend to have greater impairment of muscle function than older men. This may partially explain the higher incidence of life-threatening falls in older women.

Although world authorities recommend strength training two to four days per week, only 14 percent of Canadian women and 20 percent of men do so, underscoring the need for additional programs and campaigns that promote this form of exercise.

Sources: Fahey, T. D. 2013. Basic *Weight Training for Men and Women*, 8th ed. New York: McGraw-Hill; Centers for Disease Control and Prevention. 2006. Trends in strength training—United States, 1998–2004. *Morbidity and Mortality Weekly Report* 55(28): 769–772; and Canadian Fitness and Lifestyle Research Institute. 2005. *Physical Activity Levels Among Adults*, http://www.cflri.ca/eng/levels/popular_pa_adults.php (retrieved April 4, 2015).

blood flow to your heart and brain. Within a few weeks, you will notice the effect of this exercise. Isometrics are particularly useful when recovering from an injury.

isometric (static) exercise
The application of force without movement.

Isotonic (dynamic) exercises involve applying force with movement, as in weight training exercises such as the bench press. These are the most popular type of exercises for increasing muscle strength and seem to be most valuable for developing strength that can be transferred to other forms of physical activity. They include exercises using barbells, dumbbells, weight machines, and body weight, as in push-ups or curl-ups.

isotonic (dynamic) exercise
The application of force with movement.

Choosing Equipment

Many people prefer weight machines because they are safe, convenient, and easy to use (see the In Focus box). You just set the resistance, sit down at the machine, and start working. Machines make it easy to isolate and work

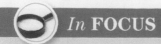 *In* FOCUS

Exercise Machines Versus Free Weights

Exercise Machines		Free Weights	
Advantages	**Disadvantages**	**Advantages**	**Disadvantages**
• Are safe and convenient • Don't require spotters	• Have limited availability • Are inappropriate for performing dynamic movements	• Allow dynamic movements • Allow user to develop control of weights	• Are not as safe • Require spotters
• Don't require lifter to balance bar • Provide variable resistance	• Allow limited number of exercises • Train muscles rather than movements	• Allow greater variety of exercises • Are widely available, inexpensive, and convenient for home use	• Require more skill • Cause more blisters and calluses
• Require less skill	• Place minimal stress on core-stabilizing muscles (those in torso)	• Train core-stabilizing muscles	
• Make it easy to move from one exercise to the next • Allow easy isolation of muscles and muscle groups • Support back (on many machines)		• Are better for building power • Are truer to real-life situations; strength transfers to daily activities	

specific muscles. Free weights require more care, balance, and coordination to use, but they strengthen your body in ways that are more adaptable to real life. When using free weights, you need to use a spotter, someone who stands by to assist in case you lose control over a weight (see "Safe Weight Training" on ▣ connect).

Choosing Exercises

A complete weight training program works all the major muscle groups: neck, upper back, shoulders, arms, chest, abdomen, lower back, thighs, buttocks, and calves. Different exercises work different muscles, so it usually takes about eight to ten exercises to get a complete workout for general fitness—for example, bench presses to develop the chest, shoulders, and upper arms; pull-ups to work the biceps and upper back; squats to develop the legs and buttocks; toe raises to work the calves; and so on. If you are also training for a particular sport, include exercises to strengthen the muscles important for optimal performance and those most likely to be injured.

Frequency

For general fitness, the American College of Sports Medicine recommends a frequency of at least two non-consecutive days per week. This allows your muscles one or more days of rest between workouts to avoid soreness and injury. If you enjoy weight training and would like to train more often, try working different muscle groups on alternate days.

Intensity and Time

The amount of weight (resistance) you lift in weight training exercises is equivalent to intensity in cardio-respiratory endurance training; the number of repetitions of each exercise is equivalent to time. To improve fitness, you must do enough repetitions of each exercise to temporarily fatigue your muscles. The number of repetitions needed to cause fatigue depends on the amount of resistance: the heavier the weight, the fewer repetitions to reach fatigue. In general, a heavy weight and a low number of repetitions (1–5) build strength, whereas a light weight and a high number of repetitions (20–25) build endurance. For a general fitness program to build both strength and endurance, try to do 8–12 repetitions of each exercise; a few exercises, such as abdominal crunches and calf raises, may require more. (For people who are 50–60 years of age and older, 10–15 repetitions of each exercise using a lighter weight is recommended.)

The first few sessions of weight training should be devoted to learning the exercises. To start, choose a weight that you can move easily through 8–12 repetitions. Add weight when you can do more than 12 repetitions of an exercise. If adding weight means you can do only seven or eight repetitions before your muscles fatigue, stay with that weight until you can again complete 12 repetitions. If you can do only four to six repetitions after adding weight, or if you can't maintain good form, you have added too much and should take some off. As a general guideline, try increases of approximately one kilogram of additional weight for each five kilograms you are currently lifting.

For developing strength and endurance for general fitness, a single set (group) of each exercise is sufficient, provided you use enough resistance (weight) to fatigue your muscles. Doing more than one set of each exercise may increase strength development, and most serious weight trainers do at least three sets of each exercise. If you do more than one set of an exercise, rest long enough between sets to allow your muscles to recover. More rapid strength gains occur with one, two, and three sets. If you do more than three sets, you will need to work much harder to get lower results (the law of diminishing returns).

You should warm up before every weight training session and cool down afterward. You can expect to improve rapidly during the first 6–10 weeks of training; gains will then come more slowly. Many factors, such as age, motivation, gender, and heredity, will affect your program. Your ultimate goal depends on you. After you have achieved the level of strength and muscularity that you want, you can maintain your gains by training two to three non-consecutive days per week.

A Caution About Supplements

No nutritional supplement or drug will change a weak person into a strong person. Those changes require regular training that stresses the body and causes physiological adaptations. Supplements or drugs that promise quick, large gains in strength usually don't work and are often either dangerous, expensive, or both (see the In the News box). Over-the-counter supplements are not carefully regulated, and their long-term effects have not been systematically studied.

 In *the* NEWS

Drugs and Supplements for Improved Athletic Performance

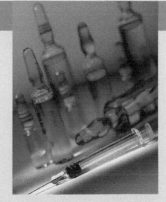

Doping scandals have snared athletes in sports as diverse as cycling, baseball, and track and field. After years of doping allegations that he vehemently denied, in 2012, Lance Armstrong was stripped of his seven Tour de France cycling titles. In 1988, Canadian sprinter Ben Johnson tested positive for anabolic steroids and was stripped of his gold medal in the 100-metre sprint. In 2007, cyclist Floyd Landis was stripped of his 2006 Tour de France title and banned from cycling for two years after testing positive for synthetic testosterone. Meantime, as baseball legends Barry Bonds and Roger Clemens fought to restore reputations damaged by allegations of steroid abuse, a special congressional report accused nearly 90 professional baseball players of using steroids and other performance-enhancing drugs. That same year, Olympic sprinter Marion Jones admitted to using banned substances before the 2000 Olympic Games. In the wake of these and other events, governments, professional sports leagues, and anti-doping agencies all sought ways to rid sports of banned substances.

Professional and Olympic athletes aren't the only ones using performance-enhancing drugs. About 2–6 percent of high school students report having used anabolic steroids. Interestingly, researchers recently found that although more than 50 percent of university students thought that the "typical student" had used them, less than 1 percent of university students reported actually doing so. Over-the-counter dietary supplements are much more popular. Many such substances are ineffective and expensive, and many are also dangerous. A few of the most widely used compounds are described below.

Anabolic Steroids

These synthetic derivatives of testosterone are taken to increase strength, power, speed, endurance, muscle size, and aggressiveness. Anabolic steroids have dangerous side effects, including disruption of the body's hormone system, liver disease, acne, breast development and testicular shrinkage in males, masculinization in women and children, and increased risk of heart disease and cancer. Evidence links steroid use and risk of heart attack, stroke, and sudden death.

In addition, steroid users who inject the drugs face the same health risks as other injection drug users, including increased risk of HIV infection. Steroids have been found to be a gateway to the use of other drugs.

Adrenal Androgens

This group of drugs, which includes dehydroepiandrosterone (DHEA) and androstenedione, are typically taken to stimulate muscle growth and aid in weight control. The few studies of these agents done on humans show that they are of very little value in improving athletic performance, and they have side effects similar to those of anabolic steroids, especially when taken in high doses.

Ephedra and Other Stimulants

These drugs may be taken to increase training intensity, suppress hunger, reduce fatigue, and promote weight loss. They raise heart rate and blood pressure and, at high doses, may increase the risk of heart attack, stroke, and heat-related illness. Several stimulants, including ephedra and phenylpropanolamine, have been banned by government authorities.

Erythropoietin (EPO)

A naturally occurring hormone that boosts the concentration of red blood cells, endurance athletes use EPO to improve performance. EPO can cause blood clots and death.

Creatine Monohydrate

Creatine is thought to improve performance in short-term, high-intensity, repetitive exercise and decrease the risk of injury. People vary in their responses to creatine. The long-term effects of creatine use, especially among young people, are not well established.

Protein, Amino Acid, and Polypeptide Supplements

Taking protein supplements after weight training may increase muscle strength and hypertrophy. Little research supports the use of such supplements, however, even in athletes on extremely heavy training regimens. The protein requirements of athletes are not much higher than those of sedentary individuals, and most people take in more than enough protein in their diets. By substituting supplements for food sources of protein, people may risk deficiencies in other key nutrients typically found in such foods, including iron and B vitamins.

Chromium Picolinate

Sold over the counter, chromium picolinate is a more easily digested form of the trace mineral chromium. Although often marketed as a means to build muscle and reduce fat, most studies have found no positive effects. Long-term use of high dosages may have serious health consequences.

Flexibility Exercises

Flexibility, or stretching, exercises are important for maintaining the normal range of motion in the major joints of the body. Some exercises, such as running, can actually decrease flexibility because they require only a partial range of motion. Like a good weight training program, a good stretching program includes exercises for all the major muscle groups and joints of the body: neck, shoulders, back, hips, thighs, hamstrings, and calves.

Proper Stretching Technique

Stretching should be performed statically. Ballistic stretching (known as *bouncing*) is dangerous and counterproductive. In active stretching, a muscle is stretched under a person's own power by contracting the opposing muscles. In passive stretching, an outside force or resistance provided by you, a partner, gravity, or a weight helps elongate the targeted muscle. You can achieve a greater range of motion and a more intense stretch by using passive stretching, but there is a greater risk of injury. The safest and most convenient technique may be active static stretching with a passive assist. For example, you might do a seated stretch of your calf muscles both by contracting the muscles on the top of your shin and by grabbing your feet and pulling them toward you.

QUICK STATS

As many as 25% of dietary supplements around the world contain substances that would cause an athlete to fail a drug test.

—Maughan, 2011

Frequency

Do stretching exercises at least two to three days per week, ideally five to seven days per week. If you stretch after cardiorespiratory endurance exercise or strength training, during your cool-down, you may develop more flexibility because your muscles are warmer then and can be stretched farther.

Intensity and Time

For each exercise, stretch to the point of tightness in the muscle, and hold the position for 15–30 seconds. Rest for 30–60 seconds, then repeat, trying to stretch a bit farther. Relax and breathe easily as you stretch. You should feel a pleasant, mild stretch as you let the muscles relax; stretching should not be painful. Do two to four repetitions of each exercise. A complete flexibility workout usually takes about 20–30 minutes.

Increase your intensity gradually over time. Improved flexibility takes many months to develop. There are large individual differences in joint flexibility. Don't feel you have to compete with others during stretching workouts.

Training in Specific Skills

The final component in your fitness program is learning the skills required for the sports or activities in which you choose to participate. By taking the time and effort to acquire competence, you can achieve a sense of mastery and add a new physical activity to your repertoire.

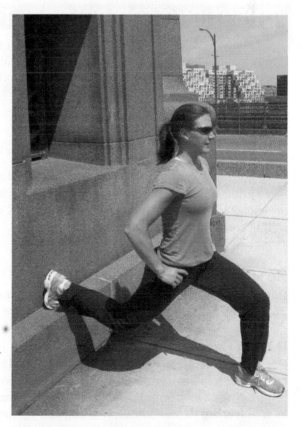

When performed regularly, stretching exercises help maintain or improve the range of motion in joints. For each exercise, stretch to the point of tightness in the muscle and hold the position for 15–30 seconds.

The first step in learning a new skill is getting help. Many sports, such as tennis, golf, sailing, and skiing, require mastery of basic movements and techniques, so instruction from a qualified teacher can save you hours of frustration and increase your enjoyment of the sport. Skill is also important in conditioning activities, such as jogging, swimming, and cycling. Even if you learned a sport as a child, additional instruction now can help you refine your technique, get over obstacles, and relearn skills that you may have learned incorrectly.

Putting It All Together

Now that you know the basic components of a fitness program, you can put them all together in a program that works for you. Remember to include the following:

- *Cardiorespiratory endurance exercise:* Do at least 20–60 minutes of aerobic exercise within your target heart rate range three to five days a week.
- *Muscular strength and endurance:* Work the major muscle groups (one or more sets of eight to ten exercises) at least two non-consecutive days a week.
- *Flexibility exercise:* Do stretches at least two or three days a week, ideally five to seven days a week, preferably after exercise, when your muscles are warm.
- *Skill training:* Incorporate some or all of your aerobic or strengthening exercise into an enjoyable sport or physical activity.

Refer to Figure 6.8 for a summary of the health benefits of different amounts of physical activity and exercise.

QUESTIONS FOR CRITICAL THINKING AND REFLECTION

Consider the different activities that have been suggested throughout this chapter. For which ones do you have the necessary fitness prerequisite? Given your current fitness and skill level, which ones could you incorporate into your exercise program?

Getting Started and Staying on Track

Once you have a program that fulfils your basic fitness needs and suits your personal tastes, adhering to a few basic principles will help you improve at the fastest rate, have more fun, and minimize the risk of injury. These principles include buying appropriate equipment, eating and drinking properly, and managing your program so it becomes an integral part of your life.

Selecting Instructors, Equipment, and Facilities

Once you have chosen the activities for your program, you may need to obtain appropriate information, instruction, and equipment, or find an appropriate facility.

Finding Help and Advice About Exercise

One of the best places to get help is an exercise class, where an expert instructor can help you learn the basics of training and answer your questions. A qualified personal trainer can also get you started on an exercise program or a new form of training. Make sure that your instructor or trainer has proper qualifications, such as a university degree in exercise physiology, kinesiology, or physical education and certification by such organizations as the Canadian Society for Exercise Physiology (CSEP), the American College of Sports Medicine (ACSM), Can-Fit-Pro, the YMCA, or another professional organization. Don't seek out advice from people simply because they look fit. You can further your knowledge by reading articles by experts in fitness magazines or online.

Many websites provide fitness programs, including ongoing support and feedback via email. Many of these sites charge a fee, so it is important to review the sites, decide which ones seem most appropriate, and if possible go through a free trial period before subscribing. Also remember to consider the reliability of the information at fitness websites, especially those that also advertise or sell products. A few popular sites are listed in the "For More Information" section at the end of the chapter.

Selecting Equipment

Try to purchase the best equipment you can afford. Good equipment will enhance your enjoyment and decrease your risk of injury. Appropriate safety equipment, such as pads and helmets for in-line skating, is particularly important. If you shop around, you can often find bargains online and through discount or used equipment stores.

Before you invest in a new piece of equipment, investigate it. Try it out at a local gym to make sure that you will use it regularly. Also check whether you have space to use and store it at home. Ask the experts (coaches, physical educators, and sports instructors) for their opinion. Better yet, educate yourself. Every sport, from running to volleyball, has its own magazine.

Footwear is an important piece of equipment for almost any activity; see "Choosing Exercise Footwear" in Connect for shopping strategies.

Choosing a Fitness Centre

Are you thinking of joining a health club or fitness centre? Be sure to choose one that has the right programs and equipment available at the times you will use them. You should feel comfortable with the classes and activities available; the age, fitness level, and dress of others in the club; and the types of music used in classes. The facility and equipment should be clean and well maintained, including the showers and lockers; the staff should be well trained, certified, and helpful.

Ask for a free trial workout, a one-day pass, or an inexpensive one-week to two-week trial membership before committing to a long-term contract. Be wary of promotional gimmicks and high-pressure sales tactics.

Eating and Drinking for Exercise

Most people do not need to change their eating habits when they begin a fitness program. Many athletes and other physically active people are lured into buying aggressively advertised vitamins, minerals, and protein supplements; but, in almost every case, a well-balanced diet contains all the energy and nutrients needed to sustain an exercise program (see Chapter 5).

A balanced diet is also the key to improving your body composition when you begin to exercise more. One of the promises of a fitness program is a decrease in body fat and an increase in muscular body mass. As mentioned earlier, the control of body fat is determined by the balance of energy in the body. If more calories are consumed than are expended through metabolism and exercise, then fat increases. If the reverse is true, fat is lost. The best way to control body fat is to follow a diet containing adequate but not excessive calories and to be physically active.

One of the most important principles to follow when exercising is to drink enough water. Your body depends on water to sustain many chemical reactions and to maintain correct body temperature. Sweating during exercise depletes the body's water supply and can lead to dehydration if fluids are not replaced. Serious dehydration can cause reduced blood volume, accelerated heart rate, elevated body temperature, muscle cramps, heat stroke, and other serious problems.

Drinking fluids before and during exercise is important to prevent dehydration and enhance performance. Thirst receptors in the brain make you want to drink fluids, but during heavy or prolonged exercise or exercise in hot weather, thirst alone isn't a good indication of how much fluid you need to drink. As a general rule, drink at least a half litre of fluid two hours before exercise and then drink enough during exercise to match fluid loss in sweat—at least 250 millilitres (1 cup) of fluid every 20–30 minutes of exercise, more in hot weather or if you sweat heavily. To determine if you are drinking the right amount of fluid, weigh yourself before and after an exercise session: Any weight loss is due to fluid loss and needs to be replaced. Any weight gain is due to overconsumption of fluid.

Bring a bottle of water when you exercise so you can replace your fluids when they are depleted. For exercise sessions lasting less than 60–90 minutes, cool water is an excellent fluid replacement. For longer workouts, a sports drink that contains water and small amounts of electrolytes (sodium, potassium, and magnesium) and simple carbohydrates (sugar, usually in the form of sucrose or glucose) is recommended.

THINKING ABOUT THE ENVIRONMENT

Wherever you see people exercising, you will see bottled water in abundance. For several years, however, a debate has been raging about the quality and safety of commercially bottled water. Recently, new evidence has emerged showing that most bottled waters are no better for you than regular tap water, and some bottled waters may actually be bad for you.

In a 2008 analysis, the Environmental Working Group (EWG) found 38 different contaminants in ten popular brands of bottled water. Contaminants included heavy metals, such as arsenic, pharmaceutical residues, and other pollutants commonly found in urban wastewater, and a variety of industrial chemicals.

In recent years, government and private agencies have revealed that many commercially-bottled water products are really just tap water drawn from municipal water systems. These products are priced many times higher than water from a residential tap. They also provide no benefit over standard tap water.

Further, plastic water bottles have become a huge solid waste problem, as millions of bottles end up in landfills each day. Once in a landfill, many kinds of plastic bottles will never decompose at all; at best, some types of plastic take years to biodegrade.

Experts say that when you are exercising, the cheapest and safest way to stay hydrated is to drink filtered tap water. If you need to carry water with you, buy a reusable container (preferably made of stainless steel) that can be cleaned and sterilized after each use. If you drink from plastic bottles, be sure they are recyclable and dispose of them by recycling.

For more information on the environment and environmental health, see Chapter 21.

Managing Your Fitness Program

How can you tell when you are in shape? When do you stop improving and start maintaining? How can you stay motivated? If your program is going to become an integral part of your life, and if the principles behind it are going to serve you well in the future, these are key questions.

Start Slowly, Get in Shape Gradually

As Figure 6.10 shows, an exercise program can be divided into three phases:
- *Beginning phase:* The body adjusts to the new type and level of activity.
- *Progress phase:* Fitness increases.
- *Maintenance phase:* The targeted level of fitness is sustained over the long term.

When beginning a program, start slowly to give your body time to adapt to the stress of exercise. Choose activities carefully, according to your fitness status; if you have been sedentary or are overweight, try an activity that won't jar the body or strain your joints, such as walking or swimming.

FIGURE 6.10

Progression of an Exercise Program

This figure shows how the amount of overload is increased gradually over time in a sample walking program. Regardless of the activity chosen, it is important that an exercise program begin slowly and progress gradually. Once you achieve the desired level of fitness, you can maintain it by exercising three to five days a week.

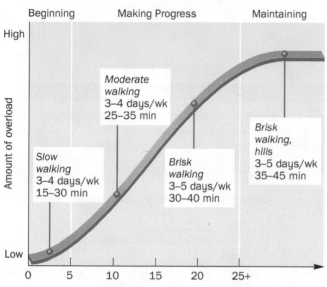

Source: Progression data from American College of Sports Medicine. 2006. *ACSM's Guidelines for Exercise Testing and Prescription*, 7th ed. Philadelphia: Lippincott Williams & Wilkins.

Exercising Consistently

Consistency is the key to getting into shape without injury. Steady fitness improvement comes when you overload your body consistently over a long time. The best way to ensure consistency is to keep a training journal in which you record the details of your workouts: how far you ran, how much weight you lifted, how many laps you swam, and so on. This record will help you evaluate your progress and plan your workout sessions intelligently. Don't increase your exercise volume by more than 5–10 percent per week.

Assessing Your Fitness

When are you in shape? It depends. One person may be out of shape running 1 to 2 kilometres in 5 minutes; another may be in shape running 1 to 2 kilometres in 12 minutes. As mentioned earlier, your ultimate level of fitness depends on your goals, your program, and your natural ability. The important thing is to set goals that make sense for you.

If you are interested in finding out exactly how fit you are before you begin a program, the best approach is to get an assessment from a sports medicine laboratory. Such laboratories can be found in university physical education departments and medical centres. Here you will receive an accurate profile of your capacity to exercise. Typically, your endurance will be measured on a treadmill or bicycle, your body fat will be estimated, and your strength and flexibility will be tested. This evaluation will reveal whether your physical condition is consistent with good health, and the staff members at the laboratory can suggest an exercise program that will be appropriate for your level of fitness. To assess your own approximate level of cardiorespiratory endurance, visit Connect and take "The 1.5-Mile Run–Walk Test").

Preventing and Managing Athletic Injuries

Although annoying, most injuries are neither serious nor permanent. However, an injury that is not cared for properly can escalate into a chronic problem. It is important to learn how to deal with injuries so they don't derail your fitness program (see Table 6.3).

Some injuries require medical attention. Consult a physician for head and eye injuries, possible ligament injuries, broken bones, and internal disorders, such as chest pain, fainting, and intolerance to heat. Also seek medical attention for apparently minor injuries that do not get better within a reasonable amount of time.

For minor cuts and scrapes, stop the bleeding and clean the wound with soap and water. Treat soft tissue injuries (muscles and joints) with the R-I-C-E principle:

- *Rest:* Stop using the injured area as soon as you experience pain, protect it from further injury, and avoid any activity that causes pain.
- *Ice:* Apply ice to the injured area to reduce swelling and alleviate pain. Apply ice immediately for 10–20 minutes, and repeat every few hours until the swelling disappears. Let the injured part return to normal

temperature between icings, and do not apply ice to one area for more than 20 minutes (10 minutes if you are using a cold gel pack).

- *Compression:* Wrap the injured area with an elastic bandage or a compression bandage between icings. If the area starts throbbing or begins to change colour, the bandage may be wrapped too tightly. Do not sleep with the bandage on.
- *Elevation:* Raise the injured area above heart level to decrease the blood supply and reduce swelling.

After about 36–48 hours, apply heat, if the swelling has completely disappeared, to help relieve pain, relax muscles, and reduce stiffness. Immerse the affected area in warm water or apply warm compresses, a hot water bottle, or a heating pad.

TABLE 6.2

Care of Common Exercise Injuries and Discomforts

Injury	Symptoms	Treatment
Blister	Accumulation of fluid in one spot under the skin	Don't pop or drain it unless it interferes too much with your daily activities. If it does pop, clean the area with antiseptic and cover with a bandage. Do not remove the skin covering the blister.
Bruise (contusion)	Pain, swelling, and discoloration	R-I-C-E: rest, ice, compression, elevation.
Fracture or dislocation	Pain, swelling, tenderness, loss of function, and deformity	Seek medical attention, immobilize the affected area, and apply cold.
Joint sprain	Pain, tenderness, swelling, discoloration, and loss of function	R-I-C-E; apply heat when swelling has disappeared. Stretch and strengthen affected area.
Muscle cramp	Painful, spasmodic muscle contractions	Gently stretch for 15–30 seconds at a time or massage the cramped area. Drink fluids and increase dietary salt intake if exercising in hot weather.
Muscle soreness or stiffness	Pain and tenderness in the affected muscle	Stretch the affected muscle gently; exercise at a low intensity; apply heat. Nonsteroidal anti-inflammatory drugs, such as ibuprofen, help some people.
Muscle strain	Pain, tenderness, swelling, and loss of strength in the affected muscle	R-I-C-E; apply heat when swelling has disappeared. Stretch and strengthen the affected area.
Plantar fasciitis	Pain and tenderness in the connective tissue on the bottom of your feet	Apply ice, take non-steroidal anti-inflammatory drugs, and stretch. Wear night splints when sleeping.
Shin splint	Pain and tenderness on the front of the lower leg; sometimes also pain in the calf muscle	Rest; apply ice to the affected area several times a day and before exercise; wrap with tape for support. Stretch and strengthen muscles in the lower legs. Purchase good-quality footwear and run on soft surfaces.
Side stitch	Pain on the side of the abdomen	Stretch the arm on the affected side as high as possible; if that doesn't help, try bending forward while tightening the abdominal muscles.
Tendinitis	Pain, swelling, and tenderness of the affected area	R-I-C-E; apply heat when swelling has disappeared. Stretch and strengthen the affected area.

Source: Fahey, T. D., P. M. Insel, and W. T. Roth. 2013. *Fit and Well: Core Concepts and Labs in Physical Fitness and Wellness,* 10th ed. New York: McGraw-Hill. Copyright © 2013 The McGraw-Hill Companies, Inc.

After a minor athletic injury, gradually reintroduce the stress of the activity until you are capable of returning to full intensity. Before returning to full exercise participation, you should have a full range of motion in your joints; normal strength and balance among your muscles; no injury-compensation movements, such as limping; and little or no pain.

To prevent injuries in the future, follow a few basic guidelines:

- Stay in condition; haphazard exercise programs invite injury.
- Warm up thoroughly before exercise.
- Use proper body mechanics when lifting objects or executing sports skills.
- Don't exercise when you are ill or over-trained (experiencing extreme fatigue because of over-exercising).
- Use the proper equipment.
- Don't return to your normal exercise program until athletic injuries have healed.

You can minimize the risk of injury by following safety guidelines, using proper technique and equipment, respecting signals from your body that something may be wrong, and treating any injuries that occur. Warm up, cool down, and drink plenty of fluids before, during, and after exercise. Use special caution in extreme heat or humidity (over 27°C or 60 percent humidity): Exercise slowly, rest frequently in the shade, wear clothing with ventilation, and drink plenty of fluids; slow down or stop if you begin to feel uncomfortable. During hot weather, it's best to exercise in the early morning or evening, when temperatures are lowest.

QUESTIONS FOR CRITICAL THINKING AND REFLECTION

Have you ever suffered an injury while exercising? If so, how did you treat the injury? Compare your treatment with the guidelines given in this chapter. Did you do the right things? What can you do to avoid such injuries in the future?

Staying with Your Program

Once you have attained your desired level of fitness, you can maintain it by exercising regularly at a consistent intensity, three to five days a week. You must work at the intensity that brought you to your desired fitness level. If you don't, your body will become less fit because less is expected of it. In general, if you exercise at the same intensity over a long period, your fitness will level out and can be maintained easily.

Adapt your program to changes in environment or schedule. Don't use wet weather or a new job as an excuse to give up your fitness program. If you walk in the summer, dress appropriately and walk in the winter as well. (Exercise is usually safe even in very cold temperatures as long as you dress warmly in layers and don't stay out too long.) If you can't walk outside because of darkness or an unsafe neighbourhood, walk in a local shopping mall or on campus or join a gym and walk on a treadmill.

What if you run out of steam? Although good health is an important *reason* to exercise, it's a poor *motivator* for consistent adherence to an exercise program. A variety of specific suggestions for staying with your program are given in "Maintaining Your Exercise Program" in Connect and in the Take Charge box at the end of the chapter. It's a good idea to have a meaningful goal, anything from fitting into the same-size jeans you used to wear to successfully skiing down a new slope.

Varying your program is another key strategy. Some people alternate two or more activities—swimming and jogging, for example—to improve a particular component of fitness. The practice, called **cross-training**, can help prevent boredom and overuse injuries. Explore many exercise options. (See the In Focus box for more information about high-intensity interval training.) Consider competitive sports at the recreational level: swimming, running, racquetball, volleyball, golf, and so on. Find out how you can participate in an activity you have never done before: canoeing, hang gliding, windsurfing, backpacking. Try new activities, especially ones that you will be able to do for the rest of your life.

cross-training
Participating in two or more activities to develop a particular component of fitness.

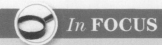

High-intensity Interval Training (HIIT)

High-intensity interval training (HIIT) has received increased attention recently as researchers have found it can help to improve both cardiorespiratory and metabolic function in athletes. HIIT involves alternating between brief bouts of intense exercise and lower-intensity activity or rest (e.g., 30 seconds of "all out" cycling followed by a few minutes of recovery, and repeating). Most sessions last less than 30 minutes and would include the warm-up, mix of intensive/non-intensive exercise, and the cool-down period, and are done a few times per week. While HITT provides a great workout, especially for those with time constraints, it is also more highly associated with injuries when compared to something like continuous jogging and as such, being cautious about starting this kind of program is wise, especially for beginning exercisers. In 2013, Canadian researchers out of McMaster University highlighted the promising findings of some early research that identifies alterations in the extreme nature of HIIT that may produce valuable fitness changes while being a safer and better tolerated alternative for the general population. The authors indicate that most research on HIIT has been done in laboratory settings, and more is needed to make a definitive recommendation in terms of its suitability for all.

 Take **CHARGE**

Planning a Personal Exercise Program

Although most people recognize the importance of incorporating exercise into their lives, many find it difficult to do. No single strategy will work for everyone, but the general steps outlined here should help you create an exercise program that fits your goals, preferences, and lifestyle. A carefully designed contract and program plan can help you convert your vague wishes into a detailed plan of action. And the strategies for program compliance outlined here and in Chapter 1 can help you enjoy and stick with your program for the rest of your life.

Step 1: Set Goals
Setting specific goals to accomplish by exercising is an important first step in a successful fitness program because it establishes the direction you want to take. Your goals might be specifically related to health, such as lowering your blood pressure and risk of heart disease, or they might relate to other aspects of your life, such as improving your tennis game or the fit of your clothes. If you can decide why you are starting to exercise, it can help you keep going.

Think carefully about your reasons for incorporating exercise into your life, and then fill in the goals portion of the Personal Fitness Contract.

Step 2: Select Activities
As discussed in the chapter, the success of your fitness program depends on the consistency of your involvement. Select activities that encourage your commitment: The right program will be its own incentive to continue; poor activity choices provide obstacles and can turn exercise into a chore. When choosing activities for your fitness program, consider the following:
- Is this activity fun? Will it hold my interest over time?
- Will this activity help me reach the goals I have set?
- Will my current fitness and skill level enable me to participate fully in this activity?
- Can I easily fit this activity into my daily schedule? Are there any special requirements (facilities, partners, equipment, etc.) that I must plan for?
- Can I afford any special costs required for equipment or facilities?
- If you have special exercise needs because of a particular health problem: Does this activity conform to those exercise needs? Will it enhance my ability to cope with my specific health problem?

Step 3: Make a Commitment
Complete your Fitness Contract and Program Plan by signing your contract and having it signed by someone who can help make you accountable for your progress. By completing a written contract, you will make a firm commitment and will be more likely to follow through until you meet your goals.

Step 4: Begin and Maintain Your Program

Start out slowly to allow your body time to adjust. Be realistic and patient—meeting your goals will take time. The following guidelines may help you start and stick with your program:

- Set aside regular periods for exercise. Choose times that fit in best with your schedule, and stick to them.
- Allow an adequate amount of time for warm-up, cool-down, and a shower.
- Take advantage of any opportunity for exercise that presents itself (for example, walk to class, take the stairs instead of the elevator).
- Do what you can to avoid boredom. Do stretching exercises or jumping jacks to music, or watch the evening news while riding your stationary bicycle.
- Exercise with a group that shares your goals and general level of competence.
- Vary the program. Change your activities periodically. Alter your route or distance if biking or jogging. Change racquetball partners, or find a new volleyball court.
- Establish mini-goals or a point system, and work rewards into your program. Until you reach your main goals, a series of small rewards will help you stick with your program. Rewards should be things you enjoy that are easily obtainable.

Step 5: Record and Assess Your Progress

Keeping a record that notes the daily results of your program will help remind you of your ongoing commitment to your program and give you a sense of accomplishment.

Create daily and weekly program logs that you can use to track your progress. Record the activity frequency, intensity, time, and type. Keep your log handy, and fill it in immediately after each exercise session. Post it in a visible place to remind you of your activity schedule and to provide incentive for improvement.

Personal Fitness Contract

I, _____, am contracting with myself to follow an exercise program to work at the following goals.

I will begin my program on _____.

Fitness Goals

1. _____   4. _____
2. _____   5. _____
3. _____   6. _____

Program Plan

Activities	Components (Check ✓)					Frequency (Check ✓)							Intensity	Time
	cre	MS	ME	F	BC	M	Tu	W	Th	F	Sa	Su		
1.														
2.														
3.														
4.														
5.														

Note: You should conduct activities for achieving CRE goals at your target heart rate.

I agree to maintain a record of my activity, assess my progress periodically, and, if necessary, revise my goals.

Signed _____   Date _____

Witness _____   Date _____

Source: Adapted from Kusinitz, I., and M. Fine. 1995. *Your Guide to Getting Fit*, 3rd ed. Mountain View, Calif.: Mayfield.

SUMMARY

- The five components of physical fitness most important to health are cardiorespiratory endurance, muscular strength, muscular endurance, flexibility, and body composition.
- Exercise improves the functioning of the heart and the ability of the cardiorespiratory system to carry oxygen to the body's tissues. It also increases the efficiency of the body's metabolism and improves body composition.
- Exercise lowers the risk of cardiovascular disease by improving blood fat levels, reducing high blood pressure, and interfering with the disease process that causes coronary artery blockage.
- Exercise reduces the risk of cancer, osteoporosis, and diabetes. It improves immune function and psychological health and helps prevent injuries and low-back pain.
- Everyone should accumulate at least 30–60 minutes per day of moderate endurance-type physical activity. Additional health and fitness benefits can be achieved through longer or more vigorous activity.
- Cardiorespiratory endurance exercises stress a large portion of the body's muscle mass. Endurance exercise should be performed three to five days per week for a total of 20–60 minutes per day. Intensity can be evaluated by measuring the heart rate.
- Warming up before exercising and cooling down afterward improve your performance and decrease your chances of injury.
- Exercises that develop muscular strength and endurance involve exerting force against a significant resistance. A strength-training program for general fitness typically involves one set of 8–12 repetitions of 8–10 exercises, at least two non-consecutive days per week.
- A good stretching program includes exercises for all the major muscle groups and joints of the body. Do a series of active, static stretches two to three days per week, ideally five to seven days per week. Hold each stretch for 15–30 seconds; do two to four repetitions. Stretch when muscles are warm.
- Choose nstructors, equipment, and facilities carefully to enhance enjoyment and prevent injuries.
- A well-balanced diet contains all the energy and nutrients needed to sustain a fitness program. When exercising, remember to drink enough fluids.
- Rest, ice, compression, and elevation (R-I-C-E) are treatments for muscle and joint injuries.
- A desired level of fitness can be maintained by exercising three to five days a week at a consistent intensity.
- Strategies for maintaining an exercise program over the long term include having meaningful goals, varying the program, and trying new activities.

FOR MORE INFORMATION

BOOKS

Fahey, T. 2013. *Basic Weight Training for Men and Women*, 8th ed. New York: McGraw-Hill. Weight training and plyometric exercises for fitness, weight control, and improved sports performance.

Fahey, T., P. Insel, and W. Roth. 2013. *Fit and Well: Core Concepts and Labs in Physical Fitness and Wellness*, 10th ed. New York: McGraw-Hill. A comprehensive guide to developing a complete fitness program.

Fenton, M. 2008. *The Complete Guide to Walking, New and Revised: For Health, Weight Loss, and Fitness.* Guildford, Conn.: Lyons Press. Discusses walking as a fitness method and a way to avoid diseases, such as diabetes.

Nieman, D. C. 2010. *Exercise Testing and Prescription: A Health-Related Approach*, 7th ed. New York: McGraw-Hill. A comprehensive discussion of the effect of exercise and exercise testing and prescription.

Richmond, M. 2011. *The Physiology Storybook: An Owner's Manual for the Human Body*. Monterey, CA: Healthy Learning. A discussion of human physiology and wellness written for the average person.

Rothman, J., and T. LaFontaine. 2011. *The Exercise Professional's Guide to Optimizing Health: Strategies for Pre-venting and Reducing Chronic Disease.* Baltimore: Lippincott Williams & Wilkins. Written for professionals in association with the American College of Sports Medicine, the book describes how exercise can help prevent and treat chronic disease.

Woods, R., and C. Jordon. 2010. *Energy Every Day.* Champaign, IL: Human Kinetics. A sensible guide to fitness and nutrition that will help you attain your fitness goals.

ORGANIZATIONS, HOTLINES, AND WEBSITES

The Internet addresses listed here were accurate at the time of publication.

American College of Sports Medicine. Provides brochures, publications, audiotapes, and videotapes on the positive effects of exercise.
http://www.acsm.org

Canadian Fitness and Lifestyle Research Institute. Provides research findings and recommendations to increase population levels of physical activity and improve the health of all Canadians.
http://www.cflri.ca

Canadian Centre for Activity and Aging. Provides information for, research about, and exercise programs tailored specifically for older adults.
http://www.uwo.ca/actage/index.html

Canadian Diabetes Association. Supports people affected by diabetes by providing information, diabetes research, education, service, and advocacy.
http://www.diabetes.ca

Canadian Society for Exercise Physiology. Provides information about the society, conferences, publications, press releases, and the physical activity guides.
http://www.csep.ca
http://www.csep.ca/guidelines

Can-Fit-Pro. Provides certification and continuing education of group fitness instructors, personal fitness trainers, and allied health professionals.
http://www.canfitpro.com

CDC Physical Activity Information. Provides information on the benefits of physical activity and suggestions for incorporating moderate physical activity into daily life.
http://www.cdc.gov/nccdphp/dnpa

Fitness Industry Council of Canada. Represents the Canadian fitness industry in pursuit of a more physically active and healthy country.
http://www.english.ficdn.ca

Heart and Stroke Foundation of Canada. Provides information about heart disease, stroke, and healthy living in Canada.
http://www.heartandstroke.ca

Mayo Clinic Healthy Living Centers: Fitness. Offers information on incorporating physical activity and exercise into your daily life.
http://www.mayoclinic.com/health/fitness/SM99999

MedlinePlus: Exercise and Physical Fitness. Provides links to news and reliable information about fitness and exercise from government agencies and professional associations.
http://www.nlm.nih.gov/medlineplus/exerciseandphysicalfitness.html

National Institute on Drug Abuse: Anabolic Steroid Abuse. Provides information and links about the dangers of anabolic steroids.
http://www.steroidabuse.org

Pace Canada—Counseling for Healthy, Active Living. Provides the Take the Physical Activity Readiness Questionnaire (PAR-Q).
http://www.pace-canada.org/products/pdfs/en/par-q-en.pdf

Public Health Agency of Canada. Provides physical activity information and tips for active living.
http://www.phac-aspc.gc.ca/hp-ps/hl-mvs/pa-ap/index-eng.php

U.S. Federal Trade Commission: Consumer Protection—Diet, Health, and Fitness. Provides several brochures with consumer advice about purchasing exercise equipment.
   http://www.consumer.ftc.gov/topics/weight-loss-fitness

World Health Organization (WHO): Move for Health. Provides information about the WHO initiative to promote increased physical activity.
   http://www.who.int/moveforhealth/en/

See also the listings for Chapters 4, 5, and 7.

SELECTED BIBLIOGRAPHY

Active Healthy Kids Canada (2013). *Are We Driving Our Kids to Unhealthy Habits? The 2013 Active Healthy Kids Canada Report Card on Physical Activity for Children and Youth.* Toronto: Active Healthy Kids Canada, http://dvqdas9jty7g6.cloudfront.net/reportcard2013/AHKC2013ReportCardENG.pdf (retrieved February 10, 2015).

American College of Sports Medicine. 2009. *ACSM's Guidelines for Exercise Testing and Prescription*, 8th ed. Philadelphia: Lippincott Williams & Wilkins.

American College of Sports Medicine. 2009. *ACSM's Resource Manual for Guidelines for Exercise Testing and Prescription*, 6th ed. Philadelphia: Lippincott Williams & Wilkins.

American College of Sports Medicine. 2011. "Quantity and quality of exercise for developing and maintaining cardiorespiratory, musculoskeletal, and neuromotor fitness in apparently healthy adults: guidance for prescribing exercise," Medecine & Science in Sports Exercise 43(7): 1334–1359.

American Heart Association. 2010. *Heart Disease and Stroke Statistics—2010 Update.* Dallas: American Heart Association..

Bertoli, S., et al. 2006. Nutritional status and dietary patterns in disabled people. *Nutrition Metabolism and Cardiovascular Diseases* 16(2): 100–112.

Blair, S. N., and J. N. Morris. 2009. Healthy hearts—and the universal benefits of being physically active: physical activity and health. *Annals of Epidemiology* 19(4): 253–256.

Brooks, G. A., et al. 2005. *Exercise Physiology: Human Bioenergetics and Its Applications,* 4th ed. New York: McGraw-Hill.

Bryan, S. N., et al. 2006. Physical activity and ethnicity: Evidence from the *Canadian Community Health Survey. Canadian Journal of Public Health* 97(4): 271–276.

Bryan, S., and P. Walsh. 2004. Physical activity and obesity in Canadian women. *BMC Women's Health* 4(1 Suppl.): S6.

Carnathon, M. R., M. Gulati, and P. Greenland. 2006. Prevalence and cardiovascular disease correlates of low cardiorespiratory fitness in adolescents and adults. *Journal of the American Medical Association* 294(23): 2981–2988.

Colley R.C., D. Garriguet, I. Janssen, C. Craig, J. Clarke, and M.S. Tremblay. 2011. Physical activity of Canadian children and youth: Accelerometer results from the 2007–2009 Canadian Health Measures Survey *Health Reports* 2(1): 12–20.

Cooper, C. B. 2006. Exercise testing does not have to be complicated. *Chronic Respiratory Disease* 3(2): 107–108.

Dal Maso, L., et al. 2006. Lifetime occupational and recreational physical activity and risk of benign prostatic hyperplasia. *International Journal of Cancer* 118(10): 2632–2635.

Dishman, R. K., et al. 2006. Neurobiology of exercise. *Obesity* (Silver Spring) 14(3): 345–356.

Fahey, T. 2013. *Basic Weight Training for Men and Women*, 8th ed. New York: McGraw-Hill.

Fahey, T., P. Insel, and W. Roth. 2013. *Fit and Well: Core Concepts and Labs in Physical Fitness and Wellness*, 10th ed. New York: McGraw-Hill.

Fenicchia, L. M., et al. 2004. Influence of resistance exercise training on glucose control in women with type 2 diabetes. *Metabolism* 53(3): 284–289.

Franco, O. H., et al. 2005. Effects of physical activity on life expectancy with cardiovascular disease. *Archives of Internal Medicine* 165(20): 2355–2360.

Gillen, J.B, and M.J. Gibala. 2014. Is high-intensity interval training a time-efficient exercise strategy to improve health and fitness? *Applied Physiology, Nutrition, and Metabolism* 39: 1–4 (2014) dx.doi. org/10.1139/apnm-2013-0187.

Gunter, M. J., and M. F. Leitzmann. 2006. Obesity and colorectal cancer: Epidemiology, mechanisms and candidate genes. *Journal of Nutritional Biochemistry* 17(3): 145–156.

Hambrecht, R., and S. Gielen. 2005. Essay: Hunter-gatherer to sedentary lifestyle. *Lancet* 366(1 Suppl.): S60–S61.

Hart, L. 2006. Exercise therapy for nonspecific low-back pain: A meta-analysis. *Clinical Journal of Sports Medicine* 16(2): 189–190.

Haskell, W. L., et al. 2007. Physical activity and public health: Updated recommendations for adults from the American College of Sports Medicine and the American Heart Association. *Circulation* 116(9): 1081–1093.

Janssen, I. 2012. Health care costs of physical inactivity in Canadian adults. *Applied Physiology, Nutrition, and Metabolism* 37(4): 803–806.

John, E. M., P. L. Horn-Ross, and J. Koo. 2004. Lifetime physical activity and breast cancer risk in a multiethnic population. *Cancer Epidemiology, Biomarkers & Prevention* 12(11 Pt. 1): 1143–1152.

Katzmarzyk, P. T., N. Gledhill, and R. J. Shephard. 2000. The economic burden of physical inactivity in Canada. *Canadian Medical Association Journal* 163(11): 1435–1440.

Kelly, C. W. 2005. Commitment to Health Scale. *Journal of Nursing Measurement* 13(3): 219–229.

Lakka, T. A., and C. Bouchard. 2005. Physical activity, obesity and cardiovascular diseases. *Handbook of Experimental Pharmacology* 2005(170): 137–163.

Larson, E. B., et al. 2006. Exercise is associated with reduced risk for incident dementia among persons 65 years of age and older. *Annals of Internal Medicine* 144(2): 73–81.

LaRoche, D. P., and D. A. Connolly. 2006. Effects of stretching on passive muscle tension and response to eccentric exercise. *American Journal of Sports Medicine* 34(6): 1000–1007.

Moore, SC. Et al. 2012. Leisure Time Physical Activity of Moderate to Vigorous Intensity and Mortality: A Large Pooled Cohort Analysis. *PLOS Medicine.* DOI : 10.1371/journal.pmed.1001335

Nattiv, A., et al. 2007. American College of Sports Medicine position stand: The female athlete triad. *Medicine and Science in Sports and Exercise* 39(10): 1867–1882.

Nelson, M. E., et al. 2007. Physical activity and public health in older adults: Recommendations from the American College of Sports Medicine and the American Heart Association. *Medicine and Science in Sports and Exercise* 39(8): 1435–1445.

Pescatello, L. S., et al. 2004. American College of Sports Medicine position stand: Exercise and hypertension. *Medicine and Science in Sports and Exercise* 36(3): 533–553.

Sawka, M. N., et al. 2005. Human water needs. *Nutritional Reviews* 63(6 Pt. 2): S30–S39.

Sawka, M. N., et al. 2007. American College of Sports Medicine position stand: Exercise and fluid replacement. *Medicine and Science in Sports and Exercise* 39(2): 377–390.

Shehab, R., et al. 2006. Pre-exercise stretching and sports-related injuries: Knowledge, attitudes and practices. *Clinical Journal of Sports Medicine* 16(3): 228–231.

Statistics Canada. 2013. *Directly measured physical activity of Canadian adults, 2007 to 2011.* Catalogue no.82-625-X Health Fact Sheets.

Statistics Canada. 2015. Table105-0503 - *Health indicator profile, age-standardized rate, annual estimates, by sex, Canada, provinces and territories, occasiona*l, CANSIM (database), http://www5.statcan.gc.ca/cansim/a26?lang=eng&retrLang=eng&id=1050503&paSer=&pattern=&stByVal=1&p1=1&p2=-1&tabMode=dataTable&csid (retrieved February 10, 2015).

Tremblay, M. S., et al. 2010. Fitness of Canadian children and youth: Results from the 2007–2009 Canadian Health Measures Survey. *Health Reports* 21(1), http://www.statcan.gc.ca/pub/82-003-x/2010001/article/11065-eng.pdf (retrieved February 10, 2015).

Wheeler, G. 2005. Active living and people with disabilities: The broader context of Access. *Wellspring* 16(4), http://www.centre4activeliving.ca/publications/wellspring/2005/aug-disabilities.pdf (retrieved February 10, 2015).

World Health Organization. 2009. *Global health risks: mortality and burden of disease attributable to selected major risks.* WHO Library Cataloguing-in-Publication Data. ISBN 978 92 156387 1, http://www.who.int/healthinfo/global_burden_disease/GlobalHealthRisks_report_full.pdf (retrieved February 10, 2015).

CHAPTER 7

Cardiovascular Health

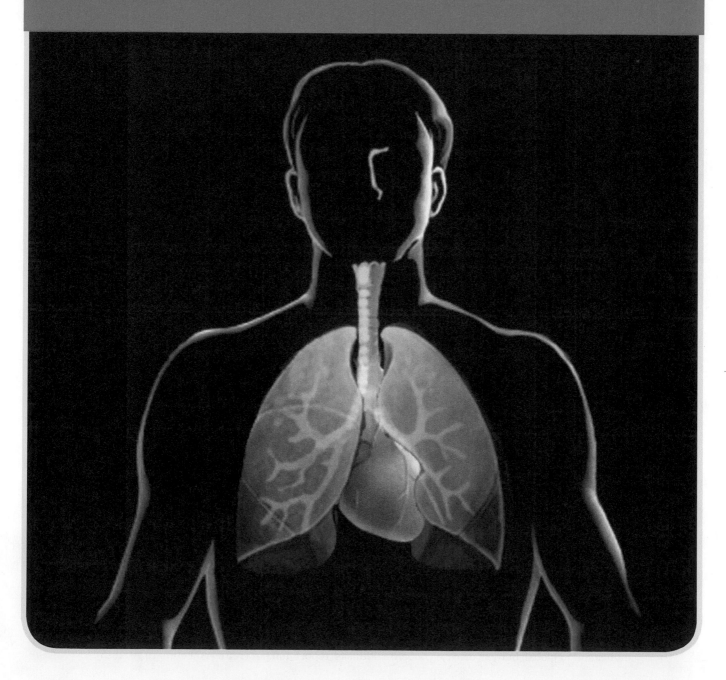

LOOKING AHEAD

After you have read and studied this chapter, you should be able to:

LO1 List the major components of the cardiovascular system and describe how blood is pumped and circulated throughout the body

LO2 Describe the controllable and uncontrollable risk factors associated with cardiovascular disease

LO3 Discuss the major forms of cardiovascular disease and how they develop

LO4 List the steps you can take to lower your personal risk of developing cardiovascular disease

TEST YOUR KNOWLEDGE

1. **Reducing the amount of cholesterol you eat is the most important dietary change you can make to improve your blood cholesterol levels.**
   True or false?

2. **Women are about as likely to die of cardiovascular disease as they are to die of breast cancer.**
   True or false?

3. **Which type of exercise improves cardiovascular health?**
   a. weight training b. aerobic activities c. both

4. **Healthy teenagers have no signs of cardiovascular disease.**
   True or false?

5. **Which of the following foods would be a good choice for promoting heart health?**
   a. whole grains b. salmon c. bananas

ANSWERS

1. FALSE.   Limiting your intake of saturated and trans fats, which promote the production of cholesterol by the liver, is the key dietary change for improving blood cholesterol levels; dietary cholesterol has much less of an effect on blood cholesterol.

2. FALSE.   Cardiovascular disease kills far more. Among Canadian women, nearly 1 in 3 deaths is due to cardiovascular disease, and about 1 in 29 is due to breast cancer.

3. c.   Both aerobic exercise and strength training significantly improve cardiovascular health.

4. FALSE.   Autopsy studies of young trauma victims show that narrowing of the arteries that supply the heart with blood begins in adolescence in many people.

5. ALL THREE.   Whole grains (such as whole wheat, oatmeal, rye, barley, and brown rice), foods with omega-3 fatty acids (salmon), and foods high in potassium and low in sodium (bananas) all improve cardiovascular health.

Cardiovascular disease (CVD) has been diagnosed in 1.3 million Canadians and together, heart disease and stroke claim one life every eight minutes. Heart attacks and strokes are the second and third leading causes of death in Canada, respectively, making them the most common life-threatening manifestations of CVD. Though we typically think of CVD as primarily affecting men and older adults, heart attack is the number-two killer of Canadian women (second to cancer), and an increasing number of fatal heart attacks occur in people ages 45–64.

> **cardiovascular disease (CVD)**
> The collective term for various diseases of the heart and blood vessels.

CVD is largely due to our way of life. Too many Canadians eat an unhealthy diet, are overweight and sedentary, smoke, manage stress ineffectively, have uncontrolled high blood pressure or high cholesterol levels, and don't know the signs of CVD. Not all the risk factors for CVD are controllable—for example, the older you are, the greater your risk for CVD. But many key risk factors can be treated or modified, and you can reduce your risk for CVD.

This chapter introduces the workings of the cardiovascular system, explains CVD and its risks, and shows you how to keep your heart healthy for life.

The Cardiovascular System

The **cardiovascular system** consists of the heart and blood vessels (see Figure 7.1); together, they move blood throughout the body.

> **cardiovascular system**
> The system that circulates blood through the body; consists of the heart and blood vessels.

The Heart

The heart is a four-chambered, fist-sized muscle located just beneath the sternum (breastbone). It pumps deoxygenated (oxygen-poor) blood to the lungs and delivers oxygenated (oxygen-rich) blood to the rest of the body. Blood actually travels through two separate circulatory systems: The right side of the heart pumps blood to the lungs in what is called **pulmonary circulation**, and the left side pumps blood through the rest of the body in **systemic circulation**.

FIGURE 7.1

The Cardiovascular System

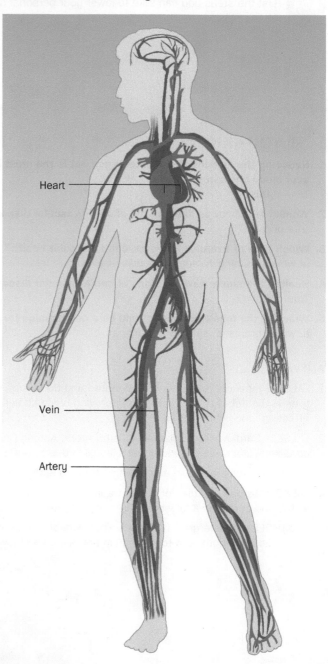

Heart

Vein

Artery

pulmonary circulation
The part of the circulatory system governed by the right side of the heart; the circulation of blood between the heart and the lungs.

systemic circulation
The part of the circulatory system governed by the left side of the heart; the circulation of blood between the heart and the rest of the body.

The following steps describe the path blood follows as it travels through the cardiovascular system (see Figure 7.2):

1. Waste-laden, oxygen-poor blood travels through large vessels, called **venae cavae**, into the heart's right upper chamber, called the **atrium**.
2. After the right atrium fills, it contracts and pumps blood into the heart's right lower chamber, called the **ventricle**.
3. When the right ventricle is full, it contracts and pumps blood through the pulmonary artery into the lungs.
4. In the lungs, blood picks up oxygen and discards carbon dioxide.
5. The cleaned, oxygenated blood flows from the lungs through the pulmonary veins into the heart's left atrium.
6. After the left atrium fills, it contracts and pumps blood into the left ventricle.
7. When the left ventricle is full, it pumps blood through the **aorta**—the body's largest artery—for distribution to the rest of the body's blood vessels.

FIGURE 7.2

Circulation in the Heart

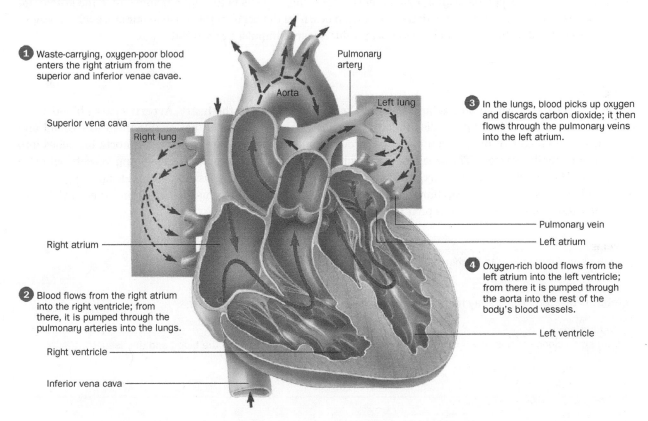

1 Waste-carrying, oxygen-poor blood enters the right atrium from the superior and inferior venae cavae.

Pulmonary artery

Aorta

Left lung

Superior vena cava

Right lung

3 In the lungs, blood picks up oxygen and discards carbon dioxide; it then flows through the pulmonary veins into the left atrium.

Pulmonary vein

Left atrium

Right atrium

4 Oxygen-rich blood flows from the left atrium into the left ventricle; from there it is pumped through the aorta into the rest of the body's blood vessels.

2 Blood flows from the right atrium into the right ventricle; from there, it is pumped through the pulmonary arteries into the lungs.

Right ventricle

Left ventricle

Inferior vena cava

vena cava
Either of two large veins through which blood is returned to the right atrium of the heart.

atrium
The two upper chambers of the heart in which blood collects before passing to the ventricles.

ventricle
The two lower chambers of the heart that pump blood through arteries to the lungs and other parts of the body.

aorta
The large artery that receives blood from the left ventricle and distributes it to the body.

The period of the heart's contraction is called **systole**; the period of relaxation is called **diastole**. During systole, the atria contract first, pumping blood into the ventricles. A fraction of a second later, the ventricles contract, pumping blood to the lungs and the body. During diastole, blood flows into the heart. **Blood pressure**, the force exerted by blood on the walls of the blood vessels, is created by the pumping action of the heart; blood pressure is greater during systole than during diastole.

systole
Contraction phase of the heart.

diastole
Relaxation phase of the heart.

blood pressure
The force exerted by the blood on the walls of the blood vessels; created by the pumping action of the heart.

The heartbeat—the split-second sequence of contractions of the heart's four chambers—is controlled by nerve impulses. These signals originate in a bundle of specialized cells in the right atrium called the *sinoatrial node*, or *pacemaker*. Unless it is speeded up or slowed down by the brain in response to stimuli, such as danger or the tissues' need for more oxygen, the heart produces nerve impulses at a steady rate.

The Blood Vessels

Blood vessels are classified by size and function. **Veins** carry blood to the heart. **Arteries** carry blood away from the heart. Veins have thin walls, but arteries have thick elastic walls that enable them to expand and relax with the volume of blood being pumped through them. After leaving the heart, the aorta branches into smaller and smaller vessels. The smallest arteries branch still further into **capillaries**, tiny vessels only one cell thick. The capillaries deliver oxygen and nutrient-rich blood to the tissues and pick up oxygen-poor, waste-laden blood. From the capillaries, this blood empties into small veins (*venules*) and then into larger veins that return it to the heart to repeat the cycle.

veins
Vessels that carry blood to the heart.

arteries
Vessels that carry blood away from the heart.

capillaries
Very small blood vessels that serve to exchange oxygen and nutrients between the blood and the tissues.

QUESTIONS FOR CRITICAL THINKING AND REFLECTION

How often do you think about the health of your heart? Are there certain situations, for example, that make you aware of your heart rate, or make you wonder how strong your heart is? What's one change you could make to support your heart's health?

Blood pumped through the heart does not reach the cells of the heart, so the organ has its own network of arteries, veins, and capillaries (see Figure 7.3). Two large vessels, the right and left **coronary arteries**, branch off the aorta and supply the heart muscle with oxygenated blood. Blockage of a coronary artery is a leading cause of heart attacks.

coronary arteries
A system of arteries branching from the aorta that provides blood to the heart muscle.

QUICK STATS

A 68-kilogram person has about 5 litres of blood, which circulates about once each minute.
—CDC, 2007

FIGURE 7.3

Blood Supply to the Heart

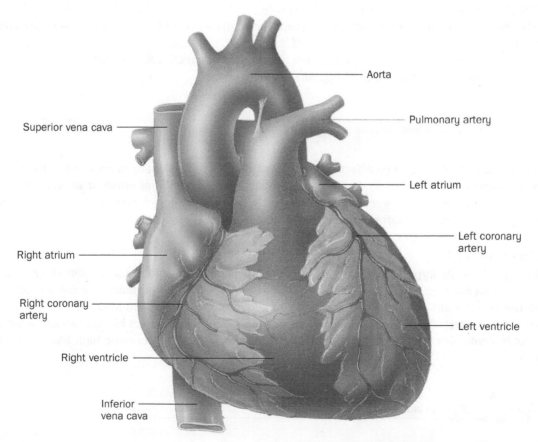

Risk Factors for Cardiovascular Disease

Researchers have identified a variety of factors associated with an increased risk of developing CVD. They are grouped into two categories: major risk factors and contributing risk factors. Some risk factors are linked to controllable aspects of lifestyle and can therefore be changed. Others are beyond your control.

Major Risk Factors that Can Be Changed

According to the Public Health Agency of Canada, about 90 percent of Canadians have at least one risk factor for heart disease or stroke. Therefore, all Canadians should be mindful of the six major risk factors for CVD that can be changed: tobacco use, high blood pressure, unhealthy blood cholesterol levels, physical inactivity, overweight and obesity, and diabetes.

Tobacco Use

About 1 in 7 (15 percent) deaths from CVD is attributable to smoking. In 2013, an estimated 4.4 million Canadians (aged 15+) were tobacco users, including almost 30 percent of university and college students who reported having used cigarettes. Smoking contributes to about 37 000 deaths annually in Canada, 11 000 of which are CVD related. People who smoke a pack of cigarettes a day have twice the risk of heart attack as non-smokers; smoking two or more packs a day triples the risk. When smokers have heart attacks, depending on how much they typically smoke, they are 60–80 percent more likely as non-smokers to die from them. Cigarette smoking also doubles the risk of stroke.

Smoking harms the cardiovascular system in several ways:
- It damages the lining of arteries.
- It reduces the level of high-density lipoproteins (HDL), or good cholesterol.
- It raises the levels of triglycerides and low-density lipoproteins (LDL), or bad cholesterol.
- Nicotine increases blood pressure and heart rate.
- The carbon monoxide in cigarette smoke displaces oxygen in the blood, reducing the oxygen available to the body.
- Smoking causes **platelets** to stick together in the blood stream, leading to clotting.
- It speeds the development of fatty deposits in the arteries.

platelets
Cell fragments in the blood that are necessary for the formation of blood clots.

You don't have to smoke to be affected. The risk of death from coronary heart disease increases up to 30 percent among those exposed to environmental tobacco smoke (ETS) at home or at work. Researchers estimate that about 800 non-smokers in Canada die from heart disease each year as a result of exposure to ETS. (See Chapter 16 for more information on smoking.)

High Blood Pressure

High blood pressure, or **hypertension**, is a risk factor for many forms of cardiovascular disease, including heart attacks and strokes, and is itself considered a form of CVD. Blood pressure, the force exerted by the blood on the vessel walls, is created by the pumping action of the heart. High blood pressure occurs when too much force is exerted against the walls of the arteries. Many factors affect blood pressure, such as exercise or excitement. Short periods of high blood pressure are normal, but chronic high blood pressure is a health risk.

hypertension
Sustained abnormally high blood pressure.

Blood pressure is measured with a stethoscope and an instrument called a *sphygmomanometer*. It is expressed as two numbers—for example, 120 over 80—and measured in millimetres of mercury (mm Hg). The first number is the systolic blood pressure; the second is the diastolic blood pressure. Research has found that CVD risk increases when blood pressure rises above 120 over 80. According to Hypertension Canada, although it is important for most people's blood pressure to be less than 140 over 90, people with diabetes or kidney disease should make sure their blood pressure is less than 130 over 80. See Table 7.1 for a more detailed breakdown of blood pressure categories in adults.

TABLE 7.1

Blood Pressure Classification for Healthy Adults

Category	Systolic/Diastolic
Normal	120–129 / 80–84
High-normal	130–139 / 85–89
High blood pressure (measured in a doctor's office)	140 / 90
High blood pressure (measured at home with home monitoring device)	135 / 85

Source: Adapted from The Canadian Heart and Stroke Foundation, *Getting your Blood Pressure In Check*, 2014, http://www.heartandstroke.com/site/c.ikIQLcMWJtE/b.3484023/ (retrieved March 10, 2015).

CAUSES High blood pressure results from an increased output of blood by the heart or from increased resistance to blood flow in the arteries. The latter condition can be caused by constriction of smooth muscle surrounding the arteries or by **atherosclerosis**, a disease process that causes arteries to become clogged and narrowed. (Atherosclerosis is discussed in detail later in this chapter.) High blood pressure also scars and hardens arteries, making them less elastic and further increasing blood pressure. When a person has high blood pressure, the heart must work harder than normal to force blood through the narrowed and stiffened arteries, straining both the heart and the arteries. Eventually, the strained heart weakens and tends to enlarge, which weakens it even more.

atherosclerosis
A form of CVD in which the inner layers of artery walls are made thick and irregular by plaque deposits; arteries become narrow, and blood supply is reduced.

HEALTH RISKS High blood pressure is often called a silent killer because it usually has no symptoms. A person may have high blood pressure for years without realizing it. But during that time, it damages vital organs and increases the risk of heart attack, congestive heart failure, stroke, kidney failure, and blindness. In about 90–95 percent of people with high blood pressure, the cause is unknown. This type of high blood pressure is called primary (or *essential*) hypertension and is probably due to a mixture of genetic and environmental factors, including obesity, stress, excessive alcohol intake, inactivity, and a high-fat, high-salt diet. In the remaining 5–10 percent of people, the condition is caused by an underlying illness and is referred to as *secondary* hypertension.

QUICK STATS

More than 90% of Canadians with hypertension have other cardiovascular risks as well.
—Canadian Hypertension Education Program, 2010

PREVALENCE Hypertension is common. About 20 percent of Canadian adults have hypertension, but only 66 percent of these individuals have it controlled. Another 20 percent of Canadians have prehypertension. The incidence of high blood pressure increases with age, however it can occur among children and young adults, and women sometimes develop hypertension during pregnancy (blood pressure usually returns to normal following the pregnancy). High blood pressure is more common in women taking oral contraceptives, especially in obese and older women; this risk increases with the duration of use. Following the start of menopause, women are more likely than men of the same age to have high blood pressure. The rate of hypertension is much higher among First Nations Canadian adults and those of African and South Asian descent, compared with the general population.

QUICK STATS

About 17% of Canadians with high blood pressure are not aware of their condition.

—Heart and Stroke Foundation of Canada, 2010

TREATMENT Primary hypertension cannot be cured, but it can be controlled. In 2010, a study by researchers with Statistics Canada found that hypertension control has improved considerably over the last two decades. Because hypertension has no early warning signs, it's crucial to have your blood pressure tested at least once every two years (more often if you have other CVD risk factors). In fact, experts now advise that anyone with hypertension or prehypertension monitor their own blood pressure several times each week. Self-monitoring is easy to do using a low-cost digital home blood pressure monitor. Follow your physician's advice about lifestyle changes and medication.

Lifestyle changes are recommended for everyone with prehypertension and hypertension. In fact, the Canadian Hypertension Education Program Recommendations stress lifestyle modification as the cornerstone for the prevention and control of hypertension. The specific changes they recommend include reaching a healthy weight, exercising regularly, eating a healthy diet, eating less salt, quitting smoking and avoiding second-hand smoke, and drinking alcohol only moderately. Nutrition experts recommend eating more fruits, vegetables, and whole grains, and increasing potassium and fibre intake (see Chapter 5). Even small increases in fruit and vegetable intake can create measurable drops in blood pressure.

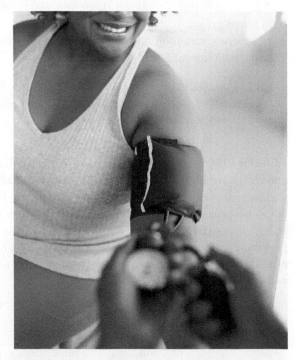

Sodium restriction is also helpful for most people with hypertension. People with or at risk for hypertension should aim to consume no more than 1500 milligrams of sodium per day. In fact, 1500 milligrams is the amount considered adequate for *all* adults. However, most Canadians consume about 3400 milligrams of sodium daily, which is well above Health Canada's recommended maximum of 2300 milligrams (about 5 millilitres or 1 teaspoon of salt) per day. Adequate potassium intake is also important. The recommended intake is 4.7 grams per day, which should be obtained through food. Supplements should be taken only when recommended by a physician; excessively high levels of potassium can be lethal.

For people whose blood pressure isn't adequately controlled with lifestyle changes, medication is prescribed. Many different types of antihypertensive drugs are available; the right one lowers blood pressure effectively with few side effects.

Monitoring blood pressure is a key strategy for the prevention of CVD. Blood pressure can be measured by a health care professional during a health care visit or at home with a home blood pressure monitor.

Recent research has shed new light on the importance of lowering blood pressure to improve cardiovascular health. Death rates from CVD begin to rise when blood pressure is above 115 over 75, well below the traditional 140 over 90 cut-off for hypertension. People with blood pressure in the prehypertension range are at increased risk of heart attack and stroke and at significant risk of developing full-blown hypertension.

High Cholesterol

Cholesterol is a fatty, wax-like substance that circulates through the bloodstream and is an important component of cell membranes, sex hormones, vitamin D, the fluid that coats the lungs, and the protective sheaths around nerves. Adequate cholesterol is essential for the proper functioning of the body. Excess cholesterol, however, can clog arteries and increase the risk of CVD. Your liver manufactures cholesterol, and you also get cholesterol from the foods you eat.

GOOD VERSUS BAD CHOLESTEROL   Cholesterol is carried in the blood in protein-lipid packages called **lipoproteins** (see Figure 7.4).

lipoproteins
Protein-and-lipid substances in the blood that carry fats and cholesterol; classified according to size, density, and chemical composition.

FIGURE 7.4

Cholesterol in the Body

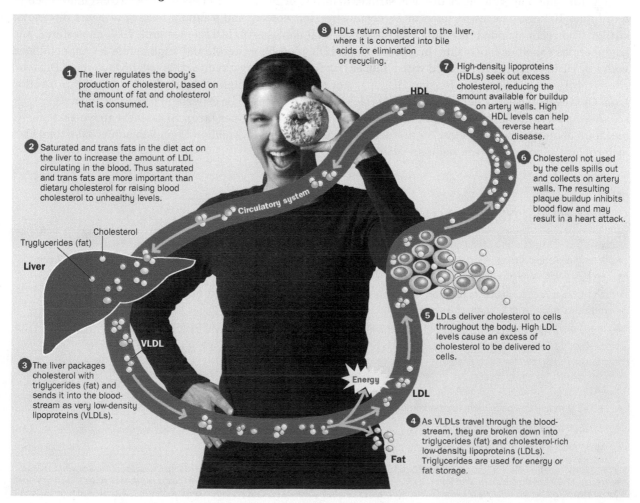

8 HDLs return cholesterol to the liver, where it is converted into bile acids for elimination or recycling.

1 The liver regulates the body's production of cholesterol, based on the amount of fat and cholesterol that is consumed.

7 High-density lipoproteins (HDLs) seek out excess cholesterol, reducing the amount available for buildup on artery walls. High HDL levels can help reverse heart disease.

HDL

2 Saturated and trans fats in the diet act on the liver to increase the amount of LDL circulating in the blood. Thus saturated and trans fats are more important than dietary cholesterol for raising blood cholesterol to unhealthy levels.

Circulatory system

6 Cholesterol not used by the cells spills out and collects on artery walls. The resulting plaque buildup inhibits blood flow and may result in a heart attack.

Cholesterol
Tryglycerides (fat)
Liver

VLDL

5 LDLs deliver cholesterol to cells throughout the body. High LDL levels cause an excess of cholesterol to be delivered to cells.

Energy

3 The liver packages cholesterol with triglycerides (fat) and sends it into the bloodstream as very low-density lipoproteins (VLDLs).

LDL

4 As VLDLs travel through the bloodstream, they are broken down into triglycerides (fat) and cholesterol-rich low-density lipoproteins (LDLs). Triglycerides are used for energy or fat storage.

Fat

Two types of lipoproteins influence the risk of heart disease:

- As discussed in Chapter 5, *low-density lipoproteins (LDLs)* shuttle cholesterol from the liver to the organs and tissues that require it. LDL is known as bad cholesterol because if there is more than the body can use, the excess is deposited in the blood vessels. LDL that accumulates and becomes trapped in artery walls may be oxidized by free radicals, speeding inflammation and damage to artery walls and increasing the likelihood of a blockage. If coronary arteries are blocked, the result may be a heart attack; if an artery carrying blood to the brain is blocked, a stroke may occur.
- *High-density lipoproteins (HDLs)*, or *good cholesterol*, shuttle unused cholesterol back to the liver for recycling. By removing cholesterol from blood vessels, HDL helps protect against atherosclerosis.

QUICK STATS

About 40% of Canadians have high blood cholesterol.

—Statistics Canada, 2012

RECOMMENDED BLOOD CHOLESTEROL LEVELS The risk for cardiovascular disease increases with higher blood cholesterol levels, especially LDL (see Table 7.2). The College of Family Physicians of Canada recommends that all adults over age 20 talk with their physician about whether cholesterol testing is appropriate for them. With no risk factors, routine screening typically begins at age 40 for men, and age 50 for women (earlier if they are postmenopausal). The Heart and Stroke Foundation of Canada also suggests cholesterol testing for anybody with heart disease, stroke, diabetes, or high blood pressure; a waist circumference of more than 102 centimetres for men or 88 centimetres for women; and a family history of heart disease or stroke. The recommended test typically measures total cholesterol, LDL cholesterol, HDL cholesterol, and triglycerides (another blood fat). In general, high LDL, total cholesterol, and triglyceride levels, combined with low HDL levels, are associated with a higher risk for CVD. You can reduce this risk by lowering LDL, total cholesterol, and triglycerides. Raising HDL is important because a high HDL level seems to offer protection from CVD even in cases where total cholesterol is high. This seems to be especially true for women.

As shown in Table 7.2, LDL levels below 3.4 mmol/L (millimoles per litre), HDL levels above 1.6 mmol/L, and total cholesterol levels below 5.2 are desirable. An estimated 13.9 million Canadian adults have total cholesterol levels higher than are recommended.

TABLE 7.2

Cholesterol and Triglyceride Guidelines

Cholesterol Guidelines
• A total cholesterol level below 5.2 mmol/L is desirable (5.2–6.2 mmol/L is considered borderline high, and above 6.2 is high).
• An LDL cholesterol level of 2.6–3.3 mmol/L is near ideal.
• An HDL above 1.6 mmol/L is best; an HDL cholesterol level of less than 1.0 mmol/L for men and 1.3 mmol/L for women indicates a higher risk for heart disease.
• *If you are at risk for heart disease*, your LDL cholesterol should be less than 2.6 mmol/L.
• *If your risk for heart disease is very high*, your LDL cholesterol should be less than 1.8 mmol/L .

Triglycerides Guidelines
• Less than 1.7 mmol/L is desirable.
• 1.7–2.2 mmol/L is considered borderline high.
• 2.3–5.6 mmol/L is considered high.
• More than 5.6 mmol/L is considered very high.

Sources: Adapted from The College of Family Physicians of Canada. 2007. *Cholesterol: What You Can Do to Lower Your Level*, http://www.cfpc.ca/ProjectAssets/Templates/Resource.aspx?id=1364&langType=4105 (retrieved March 10, 2015), used with permission of The College of Family Physicians of Canada; and Mayo Clinic. 2013. *Cholesterol Levels: What Numbers Should You Aim For?*, ⟨http://www.mayoclinic.org/diseases-conditions/high-blood-cholesterol/basics/tests-diagnosis/con-20020865; retrieved August 5, 2015).

The CVD risk associated with elevated cholesterol levels also depends on other factors. For example, an above-optimal level of LDL would be of more concern for an individual who also smokes and has high blood pressure than for someone without these additional CVD risk factors, and it is especially a concern for people with diabetes.

BENEFITS OF CONTROLLING CHOLESTEROL People can cut their heart attack risk by about 2 percent for every 1 percent that they reduce their total blood cholesterol levels. People who lower their total cholesterol from about 6.2 to 5.2 mmol/L, for example, reduce their risk of heart attack by 40 percent. Studies indicate that lowering LDL and raising HDL levels not only reduces the likelihood that arteries will become clogged, but may also reverse deposits on artery walls.

Your primary goal should be to reduce your LDL to healthy levels. Important dietary changes for reducing LDL levels include increasing fibre intake and substituting unsaturated for saturated and trans fats. Decreasing saturated and trans fats is particularly important because they promote the production of cholesterol by the liver. Exercising regularly and eating more fruits, vegetables, fish, and whole grains also help. Many experts believe cholesterol-lowering foods may be most effective when eaten in combination, rather than separately. You can raise your HDL levels by exercising regularly, losing weight if you are overweight, quitting smoking, and altering the amount and type of fat you consume.

See Chapter 5 for detailed information on nutrition and guidelines for heart-healthy eating.

Physical Inactivity

As discussed in Chapter 6, many Canadians are very sedentary, so much so that they are at high risk for developing CVD. Exercise is thought to be the closest thing we have to a magic bullet against heart disease. It lowers CVD risk by helping to decrease blood pressure and resting heart rate, increase HDL levels, maintain desirable weight, improve the condition of blood vessels, and prevent or control diabetes. One study found that women who accumulated at least three hours of brisk walking each week cut their risk of heart attack and stroke by more than 50 percent.

See Chapter 6 for detailed explanations of the benefits of physical activity and for help in creating your own exercise plan.

Obesity

As your weight increases, your risk of CVD increases. The risk of death from CVD is two to three times as likely in obese people (BMI ≥ 30) as it is in lean people (BMI 18.5–24.9), and for every five-unit increment of BMI, a person's risk of death from coronary heart disease increases by 30 percent. BMI at age 18 predicts mortality from CVD—the higher your BMI at age 18, the more likely you are to eventually die from CVD. Maintaining a healthy weight is also important. Researchers found that middle-aged women who had gained 10 kilograms or more since age 18 had a significantly higher risk of subsequent death from CVD than those who were able to maintain their weight over time.

As explained in Chapter 4, excess body fat is strongly associated with hypertension, high cholesterol levels, insulin resistance, diabetes, physical inactivity, and increasing age. It is also associated with endothelial cell dysfunction and increased inflammatory markers (discussed later in this chapter). **Endothelial cells** line the inside of arteries, including the coronary arteries, and they help regulate blood flow to the heart and keep platelets and other cells from sticking to artery walls. When the endothelial cells are healthy, the coronary arteries dilate (widen) when the heart needs more blood, but when the cells are dysfunctional, the coronary arteries instead constrict, limiting blood flow to the heart. With excess weight, there is also more blood to pump and the heart has to work harder. This causes chronically elevated pressures within the heart chambers that can lead to ventricular **hypertrophy** (enlargement), and eventually the heart muscle can start to fail.

endothelial cells
Cells lining the inside of arteries; they help regulate blood flow and prevent platelets from sticking.

hypertrophy
Abnormal enlargement of an organ secondary to an increase in cell size.

Physical activity and physical fitness have a strong positive influence on cardiovascular health in those who are overweight and obese. People who are obese but have at least moderate cardiorespiratory fitness may have lower rates of cardiovascular disease than their normal-weight but unfit peers. For someone who is overweight, even modest weight reduction—5–10 percent of body weight—can reduce CVD risk.

Diabetes

As described in Chapter 4, diabetes is a disorder characterized by elevated blood glucose levels because of an insufficient supply or inadequate action of insulin. Diabetes increases the risk of CVD by two to four times. The most common cause of death in adults with diabetes is CVD, and they usually die at younger ages than people without diabetes. There is an estimated loss of 5–10 years of life in those with diabetes.

People with diabetes have higher rates of other CVD risk factors, including hypertension, obesity, and unhealthy blood lipid levels (typically, high triglyceride levels and low HDL levels). The elevated blood glucose and insulin levels that occur in diabetes can damage the endothelial cells that line the arteries, making them more vulnerable to atherosclerosis. In addition, people with diabetes often have platelet and blood coagulation abnormalities that increase the risk of heart attacks and strokes. People with pre-diabetes also face a significantly increased risk of CVD.

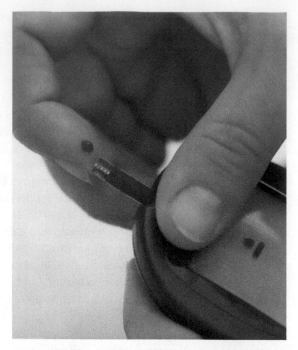

Blood glucose monitoring is important in managing diabetes and its associated risks.

The number of people with diabetes and pre-diabetes continues to climb and is closely linked to obesity. It is estimated that for every kilogram increase in weight, the risk of diabetes increases by approximately 9 percent. The increase in prevalence of type 2 diabetes over the past decade has been among Canadians of all age groups, and with a particularly alarming increase among children and adolescents. Children who are diagnosed with diabetes typically develop complications in their twenties or thirties.

Complications of diabetes mainly affect the arteries. When the larger arteries are affected, all forms of CVD result, including heart attacks, strokes, and peripheral vascular disease. Having diabetes is considered to be a heart disease risk equivalent, meaning that your CVD morbidity and mortality risk is the same as if you already had coronary artery disease (CAD). People with diabetes who also have CAD fare even worse; they have accelerated atherosclerosis and benefit less from common forms of treatment than people without diabetes.

In addition, evidence suggests that after a heart attack, the risk of diabetes steeply rises. A recent study demonstrated that within 3.5 years after a heart attack, one-third of patients without diabetes will develop diabetes or pre-diabetes. Thus, heart disease and elevated blood glucose are clearly linked, with each being a risk factor for the other.

QUICK STATS

First Nations adults with diabetes are 4 times as likely to have heart disease as their counterparts without diabetes.

—Heart and Stroke Foundation of Canada, 2009

Routine screening for diabetes is not currently recommended unless a person has symptoms of diabetes or other CVD risk factors. In people with pre-diabetes, a healthy diet and exercise are more effective than medication at preventing diabetes. For people with diabetes, a healthy diet, exercise, and careful control of glucose levels are recommended to decrease chances of developing complications. Even people whose diabetes is under control face a high risk of CVD, so control of other risk factors is critical.

Contributing Risk Factors that Can Be Changed

Other factors that can be changed have been identified as contributing to CVD risk, including triglyceride levels and psychological and social factors.

High Triglyceride Levels

Like cholesterol, **triglycerides** are blood fats that are obtained from food and manufactured by the body. High triglyceride levels are a reliable predictor of heart disease, especially if associated with other risk factors, such as low HDL levels, obesity, and diabetes. Factors contributing to elevated triglyceride levels include excess body fat, physical inactivity, cigarette smoking, type 2 diabetes, excess alcohol intake, very high carbohydrate diets, and certain diseases and medications. Much of the picture regarding triglycerides remains unclear, however. Studies have yet to show whether lowering triglyceride levels will actually decrease heart disease. Elevated triglyceride levels are most often seen in people with other lipid abnormalities; and the lifestyle modifications that help lower cholesterol also help decrease triglycerides, making it difficult to identify any potential independent benefit of lowering triglyceride levels.

> **triglyceride**
> A type of blood fat that can be a predictor of heart disease.

A full lipid profile should include testing and evaluation of triglyceride levels (see Table 7.2). For people with borderline high triglyceride levels, increased physical activity, reduced intake of added sugars, and weight reduction can help bring levels down into the healthy range. Drug therapy may be recommended for people with high triglyceride levels. Being moderate in the use of alcohol and quitting smoking are also important.

Psychological and Social Factors

Many of the psychological and social factors that influence other areas of wellness are also important risk factors for CVD. The cardiovascular system is affected by both sudden, acute episodes of mental stress and the more chronic, underlying emotions of anger, anxiety, and depression.

STRESS Excessive stress can strain the heart and blood vessels over time and contribute to CVD. When you experience stress, stress hormones activate the sympathetic nervous system. As described in Chapter 3, the sympathetic nervous system causes the fight-or-flight response; this response increases heart rate and blood pressure so that more blood is distributed to the heart and other muscles in anticipation of physical activity. Blood glucose concentrations and cholesterol also increase to provide a source of energy, and the platelets become activated so that they will be more likely to clot in case of injury. If you are healthy, you can tolerate the cardiovascular responses that take place during stress, but if you already have CVD, stress can lead to adverse outcomes, such as abnormal heart rhythms (arrhythmias), heart attacks, and sudden cardiac death.

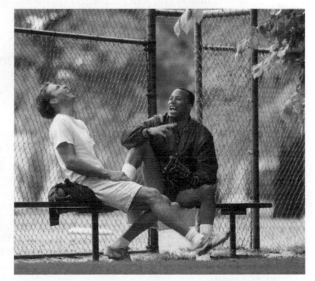

A strong social support network is a major antidote to stress and can help promote and support a healthy lifestyle, such as opportunities for exercise and relaxation.

Because avoiding all stress is impossible, having healthy mechanisms to cope with it is your best defence. Instead of adopting unhealthy habits, such as smoking or overeating, use healthier coping strategies, such as exercising, getting enough sleep, and talking to others.

CHRONIC HOSTILITY AND ANGER Certain traits in the hard-driving type A personality—hostility, cynicism, and anger—are associated with increased risk of heart disease. Men prone to anger have two to three times the heart attack risk of calmer men and are much more likely to develop CVD at young ages. In a 10-year study of young adults ages 18–30 years, those with high hostility levels were more than twice as likely to develop coronary artery calcification (a marker of early atherosclerosis) as those with low hostility levels. See the Mind Body Spirit box for more information.

Mind *Body* SPIRIT

Anger, Hostility, and Heart Disease

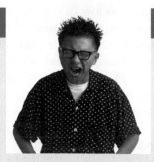

People with a quick temper, a persistently hostile outlook, and a cynical, mistrusting attitude toward life are more likely to develop heart disease than those with a calmer, more trusting attitude. People who are angry frequently, intensely, and for long periods experience the stress response much more often than more relaxed individuals. Over the long term, the effects of stress may damage arteries and promote CVD.

Are You Too Hostile?
To help answer that question, a short self-test has been devised. It's not a scientific evaluation, but it does offer a rough measure of hostility. Are the following statements true or false for you?
 1. I often get annoyed at checkout cashiers or the people in front of me when I'm waiting in line.
 2. I usually keep an eye on the people I work or live with to make sure they do what they should.
 3. I often wonder how homeless people can have so little respect for themselves.
 4. I believe that most people will take advantage of you if you let them.
 5. The habits of friends or family members often annoy me.
 6. When I'm stuck in traffic, I often start breathing faster and my heart pounds.
 7. When I'm annoyed with people, I really want to let them know it.
 8. If someone does me wrong, I want to get even.
 9. I like to have the last word in any argument.
 10. At least once a week, I have the urge to yell at or even hit someone.
    According to the survey creators, five or more "true" statements suggest that you are excessively hostile and should consider taking steps to learn to deal with it.

Managing Your Anger
Begin by monitoring your angry responses and looking for triggers—people or situations that typically make you angry. Familiarize yourself with the patterns of thinking that lead to angry or hostile feelings, and then try to head them off before they develop into full-blown anger. If you feel your anger starting to build, try reasoning with yourself by asking the following questions:
 1. Is this really important enough to get angry about?
 2. Am I really justified in getting angry?
 3. Is getting angry going to make a real and positive difference in this situation?
    If you answer yes to all three questions, then calm but assertive communication may be an appropriate response. If your anger isn't reasonable, try distracting yourself or removing yourself from the situation. Exercise, humour, social support, and other stress-management techniques can also help. (See Chapter 2 for additional anger-management tips.) Your heart—and the people around you—will benefit from your calmer, more positive outlook.

Sources: Virginia Williams and Redford Williams. 1999. *Lifeskills: Lifeskills: 8 Simple Ways to Build Stronger Relationships, Communicate More Clearly, and Improve Your Health.* New York: Times Books. Reprinted by permission.

SUPPRESSING PSYCHOLOGICAL DISTRESS   Consistently suppressing anger and other negative emotions may also be hazardous to a healthy heart. People who hide psychological distress appear to have higher rates of heart disease than people who experience similar distress but share it with others. People with such type D personalities tend to be pessimistic, negative, and unhappy, and to suppress these feelings. This type D trait may have physical effects, or it may lead to social isolation and poor communication with physicians.

DEPRESSION   Depression appears to increase the risk of CVD in healthy people, and it definitely increases the risk of adverse cardiac events in those who already have heart disease. You do not need to have a major depressive disorder to be affected: For each depressive symptom you have, the risk seems to increase in a linear fashion (see Chapter 2 for symptoms of depression).

Depression is common in people with coronary heart disease (CHD), and patients who are depressed tend to have worse outcomes than those who are not. Up to one-third of patients experience major depression within one year of having a heart attack, and those who are depressed after having a heart attack are more likely to have another heart attack or die of a cardiac cause. Even in those with CHD who have not had a recent cardiac event, up to 20 percent have depression, and this number may be even higher in women. Major depressive disorder at the time of treatment for coronary artery disease is associated with both short-term and long-term complications, including subsequent heart attack and death.

The relationship between depression and CHD is complex and not fully understood. Depressed people may be more likely to smoke or be sedentary. They may not consistently take prescribed medications, and they may not cope well with having an illness or undergoing a medical procedure. Depression also causes physiological changes; for example, it elevates basal levels of stress hormones, which, as described earlier, induce a variety of stress-related responses.

ANXIETY   There is evidence to suggest that chronic anxiety and anxiety disorders (such as phobias and panic disorder) are associated with up to a threefold increased risk of coronary heart disease, heart attack, and sudden cardiac death. There is also some evidence that, similar to people with depression, people with anxiety are more likely to have a subsequent adverse cardiac event after having a heart attack. At the same time, people with anxiety and depression often have medically unexplained chest pain, meaning that no evidence of coronary artery disease can be found. This can create difficulties in diagnosis and disease management, but it is important to always seek medical attention if you experience chest pain.

QUICK STATS

Heart disease patients who also have anxiety are 2 times as likely to die from any cause than are those who don't struggle with anxiety.
—Watkins et al., 2013

SOCIAL ISOLATION   Social isolation and low social support (living alone, or having few friends or family members) are associated with an increased incidence of CHD and poorer outcomes after the first diagnosis of CHD. Older men and women who report less emotional support from others before they have a heart attack are almost three times as likely to die in the first six months after the attack. A strong social support network is a major antidote to stress. Friends and family members can also promote and support a healthy lifestyle.

LOW SOCIOECONOMIC STATUS   Low socioeconomic status and low educational attainment also increase the risk for CVD. These associations are probably due to a variety of factors, including lifestyle and access to health care.

Alcohol and Other Drugs

Although moderate drinking (defined as no more than two drinks per day for men and no more than one drink per day for women) may have health benefits for some people, drinking too much alcohol raises blood pressure and can increase the risk of stroke and heart failure. Stimulant drugs, particularly cocaine, can also cause serious cardiac problems, including heart attack, stroke, and sudden cardiac death. Cocaine stimulates the nervous system, promotes platelet aggregation, and can cause spasm in the coronary arteries. Injection drug use can cause infection of the heart and stroke. See Chapters 14–16 for more information on the use of alcohol, tobacco, and other drugs.

Major Risk Factors that Can't Be Changed

A number of major risk factors, and consequent determinants, for CVD cannot be changed. They include heredity, aging, being male, and ethnicity.

Heredity

Multiple genes contribute to the development of CVD and its associated risk factors, such as high cholesterol, hypertension, diabetes, and obesity. Having a favourable set of genes decreases your risk of developing CVD, while having an unfavourable set of genes increases your risk. Risk, however, is modifiable by lifestyle factors, such as whether you smoke, exercise, or eat a healthy diet.

Because of the genetic complexity of CVD, genetic screening is usually recommended for only a few specific conditions (for example, certain cholesterol disorders), but you can learn more about your personal risk just by assessing your family history. If you have a first-degree relative (parent, sibling, child) with CAD, for example, you have a twofold increased risk of someday developing CAD yourself.

Don't forget the role of lifestyle factors, however. Coronary artery disease is usually the result of the interaction of several unfavourable genetic and lifestyle factors, and people with the greatest number of genetic and lifestyle risk factors will face the highest risks. People with favourable genes may not develop CAD despite having an unhealthy lifestyle, and people with many healthy habits may still develop CAD because they have an unfavourable genetic makeup. People who inherit a tendency for CVD are not destined to develop it. They may, however, have to work harder than other people to prevent CVD.

Aging

Nearly 85 percent of people who have a heart attack are 65 or older, and more than 16 000 Canadians die each year from heart attacks. For people over 55, the incidence of stroke more than doubles in each successive decade. However, even people in their thirties and forties, especially men, can have heart attacks. Figure 7.5 shows the percentage of deaths from CVD among Canadians by age and gender.

Being Male

Although CVD is the leading killer of both men and women in Canada, men face a greater risk of heart attack than women, especially earlier in life. Until age 55, men also have a greater risk of hypertension. The incidence of stroke is higher for males than females until age 65, and more Canadian women than men die of stroke each year. Estrogen production, which is highest during the childbearing years, may protect premenopausal women against CVD (see the Gender Matters box). By age 75, the gender gap nearly disappears.

Ethnicity

Rates of heart disease vary among ethnic groups in Canada, with Canadians of South Asian and African descent, as well as Aboriginal peoples, having much higher rates of hypertension, heart disease, and stroke than other groups.

Inflammation and C-Reactive Protein

Inflammation plays a key role in the development of CVD. When an artery is injured by smoking, cholesterol, hypertension, or other factors, the body's response is to produce inflammation. A substance called *C-reactive protein (CRP)* is released into the bloodstream during the inflammatory response, and high levels of CRP indicate a substantially elevated risk of heart attack and stroke. CRP may also be harmful to the coronary arteries themselves.

FIGURE 7.5

Percentage of Deaths from Cardiovascular Disease by Age Group and Sex

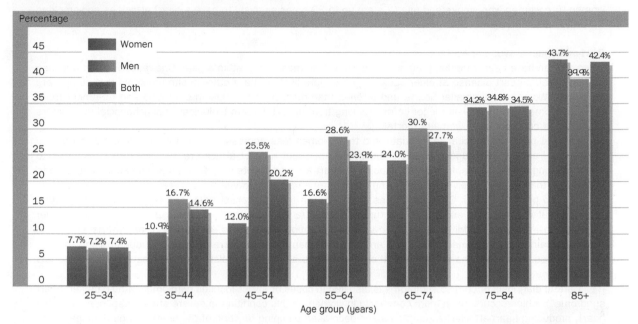

Percentage

Legend:
- Women
- Men
- Both

Values by age group:

- 25–34: 7.7%, 7.2%, 7.4%
- 35–44: 10.9%, 16.7%, 14.6%
- 45–54: 12.0%, 25.5%, 20.2%
- 55–64: 16.6%, 28.6%, 23.9%
- 65–74: 24.0%, 30.%, 27.7%
- 75–84: 34.2%, 34.8%, 34.5%
- 85+: 43.7%, 39.9%, 42.4%

Age group (years)

Source: Health Canada, using data from Mortality File, Statistics Canada. *The Growing Burden of Heart Disease and Stroke in Canada, 2003,* Figure 4.5. p. 54.

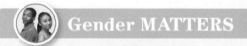

Gender MATTERS

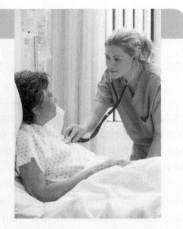

Women and CVD

CVD has traditionally been thought of as a man's disease, and until recently, this has been the justification for carrying out almost all CVD research on men. It is true that men have a higher incidence of cardiovascular problems than women, especially before age 50. On average, women live 10–15 more years free of coronary heart disease than men do. But heart disease is the leading cause of death among women.

Polls indicate that women vastly underestimate their risk of dying of a heart attack and, in turn, overestimate their risk of dying of breast cancer. In reality, CVD is responsible for seven times as many Canadian women's deaths as breast cancer. Women from minority groups face the highest risk of developing CVD, but their awareness of heart disease as a killer of women is lower than that of white women. Risk factors for CVD are similar for men and women and include age, family history, smoking, hypertension, high cholesterol, and diabetes. There are some gender differences, however. HDL appears to be an even more powerful predictor of CAD risk in women than it is in men. Also, women with diabetes have a greater risk of having CVD events, such as heart attack and stroke, than men with diabetes.

Estrogen: A Heart Protector?

The hormone estrogen, produced naturally by a woman's ovaries until menopause, improves blood lipid concentrations and other CVD risk factors. For the past several decades, many physicians encouraged menopausal women to take hormone replacement therapy (HT) to relieve menopause symptoms and presumably reduce the risk of CVD. However, studies found that HT may actually *increase* a woman's risk for heart disease and certain other health problems, including breast cancer. Some newer studies have found a reduced risk of CVD in women who start HT in the early stages of menopause (usually the mid-40s), suggesting that outcomes may depend on several factors, including the timing of hormone use. The Heart and Stroke Foundation of Canada currently recommends that HT not be used to protect against CVD.

For younger women, the most common form of hormonal medication is oral contraceptives (OCs). Typical OCs contain estrogen and progestin in relatively low doses and are generally considered safe for most non-smoking women. But women who smoke and use OCs are up to 32 times as likely to have a heart attack as non-smoking OC users.

Post-menopausal Women: At Risk

When women have heart attacks, they are more likely than men to die within a year. One reason is that because women develop heart disease at older ages, they are more likely to have other health problems that complicate treatment. Women have smaller hearts and arteries than men, possibly making diagnosis and treatment more difficult. Women may also wait longer before seeking treatment. Unknown biological or psychosocial risk factors may also be contributing to women's mortality.

Medical personnel appear to evaluate and treat women less aggressively than men. Women with positive stress tests and those whose evaluation raises concern about a heart attack are less likely to be referred to further testing than are men. In addition, studies of heart attack patients have found that women usually have to wait longer than men to receive clot-dissolving drugs in an emergency room.

Women presenting with CHD are just as likely as men to report chest pain, and a recent Canadian study revealed that women experience all of the typical heart attack symptoms that men experience, although other research has suggested additional symptoms, including fatigue, weakness, shortness of breath, nausea, vomiting, and pain in the abdomen, neck, jaw, and back. Women may also have pain at rest, during sleep, or with mental stress. A woman who experiences these symptoms should be persistent in seeking accurate diagnosis and appropriate treatment.

Careful diagnosis of cardiac symptoms is also key in cases of stress-induced cardiomyopathy ("broken heart syndrome"), which occurs much more commonly in women. In this condition, a severe stress response stuns the heart, producing heart-attack-like symptoms and decreased pumping function of the heart, but no damage to the heart muscle. Typically, the condition reverses quickly, and correct diagnosis is important to avoid unnecessary invasive procedures.

Experts recommend testing of CRP levels for people at intermediate risk for CVD because people in this risk category who are found to have high CRP levels may benefit from additional testing or treatment. (This guideline assumes that people at high risk for CVD are already receiving treatment.)

Lifestyle changes and certain drugs can reduce CRP levels. Statin drugs, widely prescribed to lower cholesterol, also decrease inflammation and reduce CRP levels; this may be one reason that statin drugs seem to lower CVD risk even in people with normal blood lipid levels. Patients who receive intensive statin treatment fare better than patients who receive less aggressive treatment that primarily targets LDL levels. The reduction in risk from decreased CRP levels is independent of changes in LDL.

The benefits of statins were underscored in 2008, when findings were released from a study involving 18 000 patients in 26 countries. Researchers found that volunteers who took statins reduced their risk of CVD by about 50 percent, even if they had normal cholesterol levels. The patients had undergone a simple blood test that checked for inflammation by measuring levels of CRP. Because statins lower CRP regardless of cholesterol levels, researchers concluded that CRP levels and inflammation are important markers of CVD risk. That said, statins have recently been the focus of controversy, with a 2013 report suggesting that prescribing statins for individuals at low risk of CVD may not produce benefits that outweigh the harms associated with potential side effects, which can include muscular problems known as myopathy, diabetes, kidney and liver damage, cataracts, and depression, among other challenges. Consequently, like any medication, it is important to discuss the possible benefits and dangers with a physician to help determine if statins are a suitable option for you.

QUICK STATS

CVD accounts for more than 15% of all hospitalizations in Canada each year.

—Heart and Stroke Foundation of Canada, 2009

Possible Risk Factors Currently Being Studied

In recent years, a number of other possible risk factors for cardiovascular disease have been identified.

Insulin Resistance and Metabolic Syndrome

When you consume carbohydrates, your blood glucose level increases. This stimulates the pancreas to secrete insulin, which allows body cells to pick up glucose to use for energy (see Chapter 4). The function of insulin is to maintain proper glucose levels in the body, which it does by affecting the uptake of glucose from the blood by muscle and fat tissue and by limiting the liver's production of glucose. As people gain weight and engage in less physical activity, their muscles, fat, and liver become less sensitive to the effect of insulin—a condition known as insulin resistance (or pre-diabetes). As the body becomes increasingly insulin resistant, the pancreas must secrete more and more insulin (hyperinsulinemia) to keep glucose levels within a normal range. Eventually, however, even high levels of insulin may become insufficient, and blood glucose levels will also start to rise (hyperglycemia), resulting in type 2 diabetes.

Those who have insulin resistance tend to have several other related risk factors. As a group, this cluster of abnormalities is called metabolic syndrome or insulin resistance syndrome (see Table 7.3). Metabolic syndrome significantly increases the risk of CVD—more so in women than in men. An estimated 19 percent of the Canadian population has metabolic syndrome, and even higher rates are estimated for Aboriginal peoples and Canadians of South Asian and African descent.

To reduce your risk for metabolic syndrome, choose a healthy diet and get plenty of exercise. Regular physical activity increases your body's sensitivity to insulin in addition to improving cholesterol levels and decreasing blood pressure. Reducing calorie intake to prevent weight gain or losing weight if needed will also reduce insulin resistance. The amount and type of carbohydrate intake is also important: Diets high in carbohydrates, especially high-glycemic-index foods, can raise levels of glucose and triglycerides and lower HDL, thus contributing to the development or worsening of metabolic syndrome and CVD, particularly in people who are already sedentary and overweight. For people prone to insulin resistance, eating more unsaturated fats, protein, vegetables, and fibre while limiting added sugars and starches may be beneficial.

Homocysteine

Elevated levels of homocysteine, an amino acid circulating in the blood, are associated with an increased risk of CVD. Homocysteine appears to damage the lining of blood vessels, resulting in inflammation and the development of fatty deposits in artery walls. These changes can lead to the formation of clots and blockages in arteries, which in turn can cause heart attacks and strokes. High homocysteine levels are also associated with cognitive impairment, such as memory loss.

Men generally have higher homocysteine levels than women, as do individuals with diets low in folic acid, vitamin B12, and vitamin B6. Many genes may cause elevated homocysteine levels, and some genes associated with small-to-moderate elevations are quite common in the general population. A recent study showed that taking folic acid will decrease homocysteine levels, but it does not lower the risk of CVD and may actually be harmful. Therefore, taking folic acid beyond the dose found in a multivitamin is not recommended. Instead, it may be more helpful to follow a diet rich in fruits,

TABLE 7.3

Defining Characteristics of Metabolic Syndrome*

Abdominal obesity (waist circumference)	
Men	> 102 cm
Women	> 88 cm
Triglycerides	≥ 1.69 mmol/L
HDL cholesterol	
Men	< 1.03 mmol/L
Women	< 1.29 mmol/L
Blood pressure	≥ 130/≥85 mm Hg
Fasting glucose	≥ 5.6 mmol/L

Sources: Grundy, S. M., B. J. Brewer, J. I. Cleeman, et al. 2004. Definition of metabolic syndrome: Report of the National Heart, Lung, and Blood Institute/American Heart Association conference on scientific issues related to definition. Circulation 109: 433–438; and National Cholesterol Education Program. 2001. *ATP III Guidelines At-A-Glance Quick Desk Reference*. Bethesda, Md.: National Heart, Lung, and Blood Institute. NIH Publication No. 01-3305.

*A person is diagnosed with metabolic syndrome if she or he has three or more of the risk factors listed here.

vegetables, and whole grains. Also, if your homocysteine level is high, aggressively controlling your other cardiac risk factors is that much more important.

Infectious Agents
Several infectious agents have been identified as possible culprits in the development of CVD. *Chlamydia pneumoniae*, a common cause of flulike respiratory infections, has been found in sections of clogged, damaged arteries but not in sections of healthy arteries. It does not appear that antibiotic treatment for *C. pneumoniae* reduces risk, but further research is needed. Other infectious agents may also play a role in CVD.

Lipoprotein(a)
A high level of a specific type of LDL called lipoprotein(a), or Lp(a), may be a risk factor for CHD, especially when associated with high LDL or low HDL levels. Lp(a) is thought to contribute to CVD by promoting clots and by delivering cholesterol to a site of vascular injury. Lp(a) levels have a strong genetic component and are difficult to treat, and they tend to increase with age and vary by race. Lifestyle modifications, such as diet, exercise, and weight loss, appear to have little effect in lowering Lp(a). High-dose niacin has been shown to decrease Lp(a), but studies are still needed to see if lower levels actually reduce the risk of CVD. In the meantime, if you have elevated Lp(a), any other cholesterol abnormalities—such as elevated LDL—should be treated even more aggressively.

LDL Particle Size
Research has shown that LDL particles differ in size and density, and that the concentrations of different particles vary among individuals. LDL cholesterol profiles can be divided into three general types: People with pattern A have mostly large, buoyant LDL particles; people with pattern B have mostly small, dense LDL particles; and people with pattern C have a mixture of particle types. Small, dense LDL particles pose a greater CVD risk than large particles; thus, people with LDL pattern B are at greater risk for CVD. Exercise, a low-fat diet, and certain lipid-lowering drugs may help lower CVD risk in people with LDL pattern B. In a recent study of men who walked or jogged 19–32 kilometres per week, total cholesterol and LDL levels were often unchanged, but the LDL particles became larger and less dense.

Blood Viscosity and Iron
High blood viscosity (thickness) may increase the risk of CVD; excess iron stores have also been linked to higher risk, especially for men and postmenopausal women (iron stores are usually lower in younger women because of menstrual blood loss). Regular blood donation, which reduces iron stores and blood viscosity, is associated with lower CVD risk in men. Drinking five or more glasses of water a day may also reduce risk by reducing blood viscosity. On the flip side, high consumption of heme iron—found in meat, fish, and poultry—is associated with an increased risk of heart attack. Men and post-menopausal women should consult a physician before taking iron supplements.

Uric Acid
Recent research suggests a link between high blood levels of uric acid and CVD mortality, particularly among those at elevated risk of CVD (i.e., based on diabetes and metabolic syndrome status, ethnicity, obesity). Uric acid may raise CVD risk by increasing inflammation and platelet aggregation or by influencing the development of hypertension; high uric acid levels also cause gout (a type of arthritis), kidney stones, and certain forms of kidney disease. Medications to lower uric acid levels are available, but it is not yet known if they will be useful in preventing CVD.

QUICK STATS

The estimated annual financial burden of CVD in Canada is about $21 billion in physician services, other hospital costs, lost wages, and reduced productivity.

— Conference Board of Canada, 2010

Time of Day and Time of Year

More heart attacks and sudden cardiac deaths occur between 6:00 a.m. and noon than during other times of the day. This trend may be explained by the natural increase in adrenaline and cortisol levels that occurs in the morning and by an increase in the sympathetic nervous system activity as people hurry around at the beginning of their day. Blood pressure is often lowest during sleep and highest in the morning, and endothelial function may be impaired in the early morning.

Heart attacks also follow a seasonal pattern, with up to 50 percent more occurring in winter months than in summer months. Heart attacks that occur in winter also tend to be more often fatal than those that occur during summer. Possible explanations include low temperature, which can constrict blood vessels; bursts of exertion, such as snow shovelling; increased rates of smoking; increased stress and depression, including seasonal affective disorder (see Chapter 2); holiday-related episodes of high-fat eating and binge drinking; and physiological factors, including levels of cholesterol and C-reactive protein, which appear to rise in winter. People who have symptoms of heart trouble may also be more reluctant to seek help during the holidays.

QUESTIONS FOR CRITICAL THINKING AND REFLECTION

What risk factors do you have for cardiovascular disease? Which ones are factors you have control over, and which are factors you can't change? If you have risk factors you cannot change (such as a family history of CVD), were you aware that you can make lifestyle adjustments to reduce your risk? Which lifestyle adjustments are important to help promote your cardiovascular health?

Major Forms of Cardiovascular Disease

Although deaths from CVD have declined drastically over the past 60 years, it remains the second leading cause of death in Canada (next to cancer). According to the Government of Canada, heart disease kills more than 49 000 Canadians each year. Figure 7.6 shows the life-altering limitations experienced by those who have CVD.

The main forms of CVD are atherosclerosis, heart disease and heart attack, stroke, peripheral arterial disease (PAD), congestive heart failure, congenital heart disease, rheumatic heart disease, and heart valve problems. Many forms are interrelated and have elements in common; we treat them separately here for the sake of clarity. Hypertension, which is both a major risk factor and a form of CVD, was described earlier in the chapter.

Atherosclerosis

Atherosclerosis is a form of arteriosclerosis, or thickening and hardening of the arteries. In atherosclerosis, arteries become narrowed by deposits of fat, cholesterol, and other substances. The process begins when the endothelial cells (cells that line the arteries) become damaged, most likely through a combination of factors, such as smoking, high blood pressure, high insulin or glucose levels, and deposits of oxidized LDL particles. The body's response to this damage

FIGURE 7.6

Limitations Experienced by Canadians Who Have and Have Not Had CVD

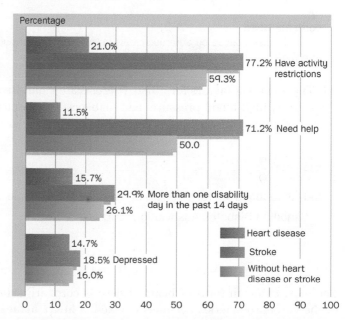

Source: Statistics Canada and Canadian Community Health Survey. *The Growing Burden of Heart Disease and Stroke in Canada, 2003,* Figure 4.3. p. 54.

results in inflammation and changes in the artery lining that create a sort of magnet for LDL, platelets, and other cells; these cells build up and cause a bulge in the wall of the artery. As these deposits, called **plaques**, accumulate on artery walls, the arteries lose their elasticity and their ability to expand and contract, restricting blood flow. Once narrowed by a plaque, an artery is vulnerable to blockage by blood clots (see Figure 7.7). The risk of life-threatening clots and heart attacks increases if the fibrous cap covering a plaque ruptures.

> **plaque**
> A deposit of fatty (and other) substances on the inner wall of the arteries.

FIGURE 7.7

Stages of Plaque Development

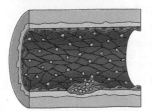 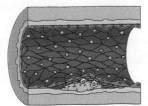 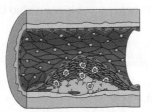 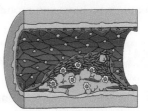

Plaque buildup begins when endothelial cells lining the arteries are damaged by smoking, high blood pressure, oxidized LDL, and other causes; excess cholesterol particles collect beneath these cells.

In response to the damage, platelets and other types of cells collect at the site; a fibrous cap forms, isolating the plaque within the artery wall. An early-stage plaque is called a fatty streak.

Chemicals released by cells in and around the plaque cause further inflammation and buildup; an advanced plaque contains LDL, white blood cells, connective tissue, smooth muscle cells, platelets, and other compounds.

The narrowed artery is vulnerable to blockage by clots. The risk of blockage and heart attack rises if the fibrous cap cracks (probably because of destructive enzymes released by white blood cells within the plaque).

If the heart, brain, or other organs are deprived of blood and the oxygen it carries, the effects of atherosclerosis can be deadly. Coronary arteries, which supply the heart with blood, are particularly susceptible to plaque buildup, a condition called **coronary heart disease (CHD)**, or *coronary artery disease (CAD)*. The blockage of a coronary artery causes a heart attack. If a cerebral artery (leading to the brain) is blocked, the result is a stroke. If an artery in a limb becomes narrowed or blocked, it causes *peripheral arterial disease*, a condition that causes pain and sometimes loss of the affected limb.

> **coronary heart disease (CHD)**
> Heart disease caused by atherosclerosis in the arteries that supply blood to the heart muscle; also called *coronary artery disease*.

The main risk factors for atherosclerosis are cigarette smoking, physical inactivity, high levels of blood cholesterol, high blood pressure, and diabetes. Atherosclerosis often begins in childhood; in fact, autopsy studies of young trauma victims have revealed atherosclerosis of the coronary arteries in adolescents.

QUICK STATS

CAD is responsible for 65–80% of deaths among people with diabetes.
—Canadian Diabetes Association, 2009

Heart Disease and Heart Attack

The most common form of heart disease is coronary artery disease caused by atherosclerosis. When one of the coronary arteries becomes blocked, a **heart attack**, or *myocardial infarction (MI)*, results. During a heart attack, the heart muscle (the myocardium) is damaged and part of it may die from lack of blood. Although a heart attack may come without warning, it is usually the end result of a long-term disease process.

> **heart attack**
> Damage to, or death of, heart muscle, resulting from a failure of the coronary arteries to deliver enough blood to the heart; also called *myocardial infarction (MI)*.

Myocardial infarctions are a significant issue in Canada, especially among people ages 65 and older. The average age for a first heart attack is 65 for men and 70 for women.

Heart attack symptoms may include the following:

- chest pain or pressure (even if it goes away with rest and comes on with exertion)
- arm, neck, shoulder, back, or jaw pain
- difficulty breathing or shortness of breath
- excessive sweating; cool, clammy skin
- nausea and vomiting
- loss of consciousness
- fear, anxiety, or denial

Most people having a heart attack have chest pain, but about one-third of men and 42 percent of women do not. In addition to women, ethnic minorities, older adults, and people with diabetes represent the groups most likely to experience heart attack without chest pain. Women may also experience other symptoms differently than men (see the Gender Matters box earlier in this chapter).

The Heart and Stroke Foundation of Canada estimates that 70 000 heart attacks occur each year in Canada, which is one every seven minutes. A Canadian Institute for Health Information report showed that deaths from first heart attacks dropped 2.5 percent across Canada between 2000 and 2005, which is a promising finding contributing to the hope that the Canadian Heart and Stroke Foundation can meet its goal of decreasing Canadians' rate of death from heart disease and stroke by 25 percent by 2020. Although there is still a long way to go toward reaching this goal, Canadians have introduced important initiatives over the years that are believed to have helped to create declines in CVD. See the In the News box for an overview of some of Canada's important milestones toward reducing CVD.

Angina

Arteries narrowed by disease may still be open enough to deliver blood to the heart. At times, however—during stress or exertion, for example—the heart needs more oxygen than can flow through narrowed arteries. When the need for oxygen exceeds the supply, chest pain, called **angina pectoris**, may occur.

> **angina pectoris**
> Pain in the chest, and often in the left arm and shoulder, caused by the heart muscle not receiving enough blood.

Angina pain is usually felt as an extreme tightness in the chest and heavy pressure behind the breastbone or in the shoulder, neck, arm, hand, or back. This pain, although not actually a heart attack, is a warning that the load on the heart must be reduced. The symptoms of angina are often very difficult to distinguish from a heart attack. Any severe chest pain that lasts more than a few minutes should be considered life threatening, and emergency medical help should be obtained immediately. About 2 percent of Canadians experience angina.

Angina may be controlled in a number of ways (with drugs and surgical or non-surgical procedures), but its course is unpredictable. Over a period ranging from hours to years, the narrowing may go on to full blockage and a heart attack.

Arrhythmias and Sudden Cardiac Death

The pumping of the heart is controlled by electrical impulses from the sinus node that maintain a regular heartbeat of 60–100 beats per minute. If this electrical conduction system is disrupted, the heart may beat too quickly, too slowly, or in an irregular fashion, a condition known as **arrhythmia**. Arrhythmia can cause symptoms ranging from imperceptible to severe, and it can even be fatal.

> **arrhythmia**
> A change in the normal pattern of the heartbeat.

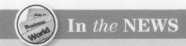

In *the* NEWS

Milestones: Decline in Deaths from Coronary Heart Disease and Stroke

The cardiovascular disease death rate has been declining steadily in Canada since the mid-1960s. The 1995 death rate for CVD was almost half that of 1969, and between 1994 and 2004 the death rate fell by 30 percent.

While the exact reason for this decrease is not known, it is likely the result of a combination of factors, including prevention, better diagnosis and treatment of high blood pressure and the level of lipids, and better management of those who have CVD. Some of the Canadian initiatives that may also have directly and indirectly contributed to the reduction in CVD are listed below.

1942 – Canada's first food guide was introduced, acknowledging wartime food rationing while endeavouring to prevent nutritional deficiencies and to improve the health of Canadians.

1945 – The Honourable Brooke Claxton, Minister of National Health and Welfare, announced a program to make the Canadian people the healthiest in the world. It included increased work in the fields of physical fitness, nutrition, child and maternal hygiene, industrial hygiene, and the like.

1961 – The Royal Canadian Air Force developed an 11-minute-a-day exercise program known as 5 Basic Exercises (5BX) to "give the nation twice as much energy"; it became famous worldwide.

1966 – The federal government introduced the Medical Care Act to provide publicly funded medical care insurance plans in provinces on a cost-shared basis. Between 1968 and 1972, the provinces and territories joined the nation's public medical care insurance, or Medicare, program.

1971 – ParticipACTION was launched and for 30 years nudged Canadians of all ages, sizes, and shapes to make physical activity a part of everyday life.

1974 – The landmark federal report, *New Perspectives on the Health of Canadians* (the Lalonde Report), showed that health care is just one factor in how health is created and set the stage for the modern movement in health promotion.

1977 – *Canada's Food Guide* got a dramatic new look, with colourful pictures of foods grouped in wheel-like fashion around a sun graphic. This Guide was supported by the premiere edition of *Canada's Food Guide Handbook*, considered by many to be a nutrition education milestone.

1986 – Health promotion became the guiding principle behind the further development of public health in Canada, driven by the federal report, *Achieving Health for All: A Framework for Health Promotion*. This report placed greater emphasis on the key determinants of health.

1986 – Canada hosted the first International Conference on Health Promotion, at which the Ottawa Charter for Health Promotion was presented. This Charter called on national governments to establish health promotion strategies and programs.

1999 – The Canadian Hypertension Education Program was introduced and significantly increased awareness that high blood pressure is a "silent killer" and needs to be regularly checked.

2003 – The Canadian Stroke Strategy was launched as a joint initiative of the Canadian Stroke Network and the Heart and Stroke Foundation of Canada. The goal of the strategy was to help support an integrated approach to stroke prevention, treatment, and rehabilitation in every province and territory by 2010.

2007 – Health Canada announced that it would adopt the Trans Fat Task Force's recommendation on trans fats in Canadian foods, by calling on Canada's food industry to limit the trans-fat content of vegetable oils and soft, spreadable margarines to 2 percent of the total fat content, and to limit the trans-fat content for all other foods to 5 percent, including ingredients sold to restaurants.

2007 – Nutrition labelling became mandatory for all pre-packaged foods.

2007 – The Minister of Health announced that the Government of Canada will establish an expert Sodium Working Group to explore options for reducing sodium intake and cardiovascular disease among Canadians.

Sources: Canadian Public Health Association, *Decline in Deaths from Coronary Heart Disease and Stroke,* http://www.cpha.ca/en/programs/history/achievements/03-hds.aspx; and Canadian Public Health Association, *Milestones: Decline in Deaths from Coronary Heart Disease and Stroke,* http://www.cpha.ca/en/programs/history/achievements/03-hds/milestones.aspx.

Sudden cardiac death, also called *cardiac arrest*, is most often caused by an arrhythmia called *ventricular fibrillation*, a kind of quivering of the ventricle that makes it ineffective in pumping blood. If ventricular fibrillation continues for more than a few minutes, it is generally fatal. Cardiac defibrillation, in which an electrical shock is delivered to the heart, can be effective in jolting the heart into a more efficient rhythm. Emergency personnel typically carry defibrillators, and automated external defibrillators (AEDs) are becoming increasingly available in public places for use by the general public. AEDs monitor the heart's rhythm and, if appropriate, deliver an electrical shock. Training in the use of AEDs is available from many organizations, such as St. John Ambulance Canada. Sudden cardiac death most often occurs in people with CHD. Serious arrhythmias frequently develop during or after a heart attack and are often the actual cause of death in cases of a fatal MI. In Canada, one cardiac arrest occurs every 12 minutes (about 40 000 a year).

> **sudden cardiac death**
> A non-traumatic, unexpected death from sudden cardiac arrest, most often from arrhythmia; in most instances, people have underlying heart disease.

Other potential causes of arrhythmia include congenital heart abnormalities, infections, drug use, chest trauma, and congestive heart failure. Some arrhythmias cause no problems and resolve without treatment. More serious arrhythmias are usually treated with medication or a surgically implanted pacemaker or defibrillator that delivers electrical stimulation to the heart to create a more normal rhythm.

Helping a Person Having a Heart Attack

Of those who die from heart attacks, about half die within an hour of the first symptom and before they reach the hospital, and most people who die from a heart attack do so within two hours from the time they experience the first symptoms. Unfortunately, half of all people having a heart attack wait more than two hours before getting help. If you or someone you are with has any of the warning signs of heart attack listed in the Take Charge box, take immediate action. Get help even if the person denies there is something wrong. Many experts also suggest that the person having the heart attack chew and swallow one adult Aspirin tablet (325 milligrams) as soon as possible after symptoms begin; Aspirin has an immediate anticlotting effect.

If the person loses consciousness, a qualified person should immediately start administering emergency **cardiopulmonary resuscitation (CPR)**. Damage to the heart muscle increases with time. If the person receives emergency care quickly enough, a clot-dissolving agent can be injected to break up a clot in the coronary artery.

> **cardiopulmonary resuscitation (CPR)**
> A technique involving mouth-to-mouth breathing and chest compression to keep oxygen flowing to the brain.

Detecting and Treating Heart Disease

Physicians have an expanding array of tools to evaluate the condition of the heart and its arteries. Currently, the most common initial screening tool for CAD is the stress, or exercise, test, in which a patient runs or walks on a treadmill or pedals a stationary cycle while being monitored for abnormalities with an electrocardiogram (ECG or EKG). Certain characteristic changes in the heart's electrical activity while under stress can reveal particular heart problems, such as restricted blood flow. Exercise testing can also be performed in conjunction with imaging techniques, such as nuclear medicine or echocardiography that provide pictures of the heart, which can help pinpoint problems.

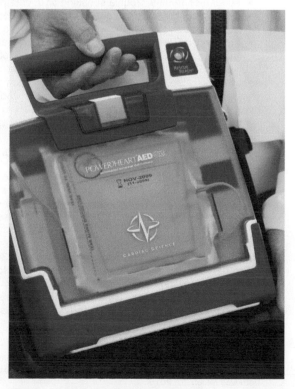

An automated external defibrillator.

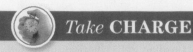 *Take* **CHARGE**

What to Do in Case of a Heart Attack, Stroke, or Cardiac Arrest

Heart Attack Warning Signs

Some heart attacks are sudden and intense—the "movie heart attack," where no one doubts what's happening. But most heart attacks start slowly, with mild pain or discomfort. Although chest pain is the most common symptom, some people experience no chest pain at all, while others will experience only mild chest pain or discomfort. Often people affected are not sure what's wrong and wait too long before getting help. Here are signs that can mean a heart attack is happening:

- *Chest discomfort:* Heart attacks often involve discomfort in the chest that feels like uncomfortable pressure, squeezing, burning, fullness, or pain.
- *Discomfort in other areas of the upper body:* Symptoms can include pain or discomfort in one or both arms, shoulders, the back, neck, jaw, or stomach.
- *Shortness of breath:* This may occur with or without chest discomfort.
- *Sweating*
- *Nausea*
- *Light-headedness*

If you or someone you are with experiences any of these signs, you should call 9-1-1 or your local emergency number immediately (or have someone call for you). Have the person stop all activity and sit or lie down. If the person takes nitroglycerin, he should be told to take their normal dose. If the 9-1-1 operator advises it, the person should chew and swallow one or two 80 mg tables of ASA (Aspirin). (Do not take other pain medication instead of Aspirin, and do not substitute Aspirin for medical care).

Calling 9-1-1 is almost always the fastest way to get lifesaving treatment. Emergency medical services staff can begin treatment when they arrive—up to an hour sooner than if someone gets to the hospital by car. The staff are also trained to revive someone whose heart has stopped. Patients with chest pain who arrive by ambulance usually receive faster treatment at the hospital, too.

If you can't access the emergency medical services, have someone drive you to the hospital right away. If you are the one having symptoms, don't drive yourself, unless you have absolutely no other option.

Stroke Warning Signs

The Heart and Stroke Foundation of Canada provides the following warning signs of stroke:

- sudden numbness or weakness of the face, arm, or leg, even if temporary
- sudden confusion, trouble speaking or understanding, even if temporary
- sudden trouble seeing in one or both eyes, even if temporary
- sudden, severe headache with no known cause
- sudden trouble walking, dizziness, or loss of balance or coordination, especially with any of the above signs

If you or someone with you has one or more of these signs (even temporarily), don't delay! Immediately call 9-1-1 or the emergency medical services number so an ambulance (ideally with advanced life support) can be sent for you. Also, check the time so you will know when the first symptoms appeared. It's very important to take immediate action. If given within three hours of the start of symptoms, a clot-busting drug can reduce long-term disability for the most common type of stroke.

Signs of Cardiac Arrest

Cardiac arrest strikes instantly and without warning. Here are the signs:

- Sudden loss of responsiveness. No response to being called or to gentle shaking. No movement or coughing.
- No normal breathing. The person does not take a normal breath for several seconds.
- No signs of circulation. No pulse or blood pressure.

If cardiac arrest occurs, call 9-1-1 and begin cardiopulmonary resuscitation (CPR) immediately. If an automated external defibrillator (AED) is available and someone trained to use it is nearby, involve the person.

Be Prepared

Research shows that heart attack victims have a 30 percent higher likelihood of survival if they are immediately given CPR (ideally after 9-1-1 has been called). More than 80 percent of cardiac arrest emergencies happen in the home. Knowing what to do in an emergency may help you to save the life of someone you love. The Heart and Stroke Foundation of Canada sets the guidelines for CPR and AED training and more than 1 million Canadians receive training each year. The Canadian Red Cross provides trainings for citizens all over the country.

Sources: The Heart and Stroke Foundation of Canada. 2013. *Health Information*, http://www.heartandstroke.com/site/c.iklQLcMWJtE/ b.3479403/k.BF78/Health_Information.htm, http://www.heartandstroke.com/site/apps/nlnet/content2.aspx?c=iklQLcMWJtE&b= 4016859&ct=13378863 and http://www.heartandstroke.on.ca/site/c.pvI3leNWJwE/b.3581655/k.9C4D/ResuscitationCPR.htm (retrieved March 13, 2015); and The Canadian Red Cross. 2014. First Aid and CPR, http://www.redcross.ca/what-we-do/first-aid-and-cpr (retrieved March 20, 2015).

Other tests for evaluating CHD include the following:

- Electron-beam computed tomography (EBCT) uses a sweeping electron beam to produce computerized cross-sectional images; it can detect calcium in the arteries, a marker for atherosclerosis.
- Echocardiography uses sound waves to examine the heart's pumping function and valves.
- Multi-slice computed tomography (MSCT) is another type of CT that produces very thinly sliced images of the heart, allowing physicians to see very small structures, such as the coronary arteries.
- **Magnetic resonance imaging (MRI)** uses powerful magnets to look inside the body and generate pictures of the heart and blood vessels.
- In nuclear myocardial perfusion imaging, radiotracers, such as thallium-201, are injected into the bloodstream. The radiotracers' location and density in the heart can be imaged and quantified; from this data, physicians can extrapolate the blow flow (perfusion) to various areas of the heart and diagnose coronary artery disease.
- Positron emission tomography (PET) involves the use of positron-emitting isotopes to image and quantify regional blood flow in the heart and diagnose coronary artery disease.

magnetic resonance imaging (MRI)
A computerized imaging technique that uses a strong magnetic field and radio frequency signals to examine a thin cross section of the body.

If symptoms or non-invasive tests suggest coronary artery disease, the next step is usually a coronary **angiogram**, performed in a cardiac catheterization lab. In this test, a catheter (a small plastic tube) is threaded into an artery, usually in the groin, and advanced through the aorta to the coronary arteries. The catheter is then placed into the opening of the coronary artery and a special dye is injected. The dye can be seen moving through the arteries under moving X-ray, and any narrowings or blockages can be identified. If a problem is found, it is commonly treated with **balloon angioplasty**, which is performed by specially trained cardiologists (see Figure 7.8). Surgeons in Canada performed more than 35 000 angioplasty procedures in 2009. This technique involves placing a small wire in the artery and feeding a deflated balloon over it. The balloon is advanced to the site of the narrowing and then inflated, flattening the fatty plaque and widening the arterial opening. This is generally followed by placement of a stent, a small metal tube that helps keep the artery open. Repeat clogging of the artery, known as restenosis, can occur, but the introduction of stents coated with medication, which is slowly released over a few months, significantly decreases the chance of restenosis.

FIGURE 7.8

Balloon Angioplasty and Stenting

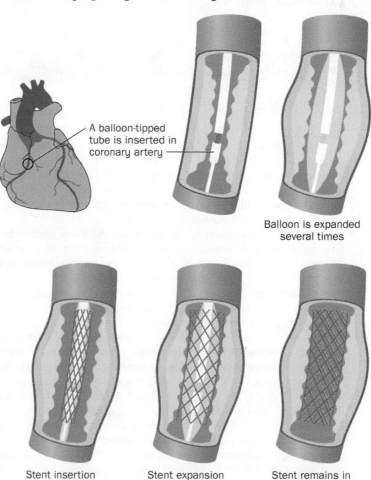

A balloon-tipped tube is inserted in coronary artery

Balloon is expanded several times

Stent insertion

Stent expansion

Stent remains in coronary artery

angiogram
A picture of the arterial system taken after injecting a dye that is opaque to X-rays; also called arteriogram.

balloon angioplasty
A technique in which a catheter with a deflated balloon on the tip is inserted into an artery; the balloon is then inflated at the point of obstruction in the artery, pressing the plaque against the artery wall to improve blood supply; also called *percutaneous coronary intervention (PCI)*.

Other treatments, ranging from medication to major surgery, are also available. Along with a low-fat diet, regular exercise, and smoking cessation, one frequent recommendation for people at high risk for CVD is to take a low-dose Aspirin tablet (81 milligrams) every day. Aspirin has an anticlotting effect, which discourages platelets in the blood from sticking to arterial plaques and forming clots; it also reduces inflammation. (Low-dose Aspirin therapy appears to help prevent first heart attacks in men, second heart attacks in men and women, and strokes in women over age 65. See the In the News box for more information.) Prescription drugs can help control heart rate, dilate arteries, lower blood pressure, and reduce the strain on the heart—raising both quality and length of life in heart patients. In patients with coronary artery disease, cholesterol-lowering statins are effective in preventing heart attacks; statins also have beneficial anti-inflammatory effects.

In **coronary bypass surgery** surgeons remove a healthy blood vessel, usually a vein from one of the patient's legs, and graft it from the aorta to one or more coronary arteries to bypass a blockage.

coronary bypass surgery
Surgery in which a vein is grafted from a point above to a point below an obstruction in a coronary artery, improving the blood supply to the heart.

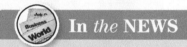 **In *the* NEWS**

Aspirin and CVD

There is significant evidence that Aspirin can help decrease the risk of CVD in a wide range of patients.

Aspirin functions by inactivating a clotting component of the blood called platelets. Platelets and their products play a role in virtually all events involving blocked blood vessels, including myocardial infarctions and ischemic strokes. It is believed that when atherosclerotic plaques in the blood vessels become dislodged, platelets begin accumulating at the site and ultimately form a blood clot (thrombus), which can lead to an acute cardiovascular event. Even in small amounts (as little as 75 milligram each day), Aspirin acts as a potent and irreversible inhibitor of platelet clotting function.

The strongest indications for Aspirin are for the acute treatment of thrombotic cardiovascular events and for the prevention of further such events after an initial episode, which is called secondary prevention. There is extremely strong evidence to show that Aspirin should be administered to virtually every patient with an acute MI. The benefits of Aspirin for reducing the risk of subsequent MI, stroke, or vascular death are substantial, and the risks of serious bleeding and other adverse reactions are very low and treatable in an acute care hospital setting. In some patients, prolonged Aspirin use carries side effects, such as gastrointestinal bleeding. Such people, however, are generally able to tolerate different formulations or lower doses of Aspirin.

The use of daily oral Aspirin is recommended in patients with prior MI, unstable angina, chronic stable angina, prior occlusive stroke, and certain other conditions. In addition all patients with chronic stable angina or other clinical or laboratory evidence of coronary artery disease should receive daily oral Aspirin indefinitely.

Aspirin can also be used to prevent an initial thrombotic cardiovascular event, which is called primary prevention. It is vital to remember that when Aspirin is used for primary prevention the benefit is much smaller than for secondary prevention, while the risk of major bleeding complication, such as gastrointestinal bleeding or hemorrhagic stroke, is the same. In one meta-analysis looking at multiple trials on this topic, the risk of a major gastrointestinal bleeding event in those treated with Aspirin was 2.30 percent versus 1.45 percent with placebo at an average of 28 months. Consequently, Aspirin is recommended along with efforts to use the lowest effective dose among both short- and long-term users to help minimize adverse effects.

Recent evidence has demonstrated that the use of Aspirin for the primary prevention of CVD events in women is more complicated. Low-dose Aspirin is often recommended for women 65 years or older who are at increased risk of CVD. For women under 65 years of age, Aspirin is recommended for the prevention of ischemic stroke in those at risk (for example, patients with TIAs), but not for the prevention of MI. There may be some instances when Aspirin use is not appropriate for some individuals; It Is Important to consult a physician for individualized recommendations and dosage.

Stroke

For brain cells to function as they should, they must have a continuous supply of oxygen-rich blood. If brain cells are deprived of blood for more than a few minutes, they die. A **stroke**, also called a *cerebrovascular accident (CVA)*, occurs when the blood supply to the brain is cut off. One study found that about 2 million brain cells die per minute during a stroke and the brain ages about 3.5 years each hour.

stroke
An impeded blood supply to some part of the brain resulting in the destruction of brain cells; also called *cerebrovascular accident.*

In the past, not much could be done for people having a stroke; today, however, prompt treatment of stroke can greatly decrease the risk of permanent disability. Everyone should know the warning signs of a stroke and seek immediate medical help, just as they would at the first sign of a heart attack.

QUICK STATS

50,000 Canadians have strokes each year—about 1 every 10 minutes.

—Heart and Stroke Foundation of Canada, 2012

Types of Strokes

There are two major types of strokes (see Figure 7.9), which are described in the following sections.

ISCHEMIC STROKE An **ischemic stroke** is caused by a blockage in a blood vessel. There are two types of ischemic strokes:

- A *thrombotic stroke* is caused by a **thrombus**, which is a blood clot that forms in a cerebral artery that has been narrowed or damaged by atherosclerosis.
- An *embolic stroke* is cause by an **embolus**, which is a wandering blood clot that is carried in the blood stream and may become wedged in a cerebral artery. Many embolic strokes are linked to a type of abnormal heart rhythm called *atrial fibrillation*; when this arrhythmia occurs, blood may pool in an atrium and form a clot.

ischemic stroke
Impeded blood supply to the brain caused by the obstruction of a blood vessel by a clot.

thrombus
A blood clot in a blood vessel that usually remains at the point of its formation.

embolus
A blood clot that breaks off from its place of origin in a blood vessel and travels through the bloodstream.

Ischemic strokes, which account for about 80 percent of all strokes, are potentially treatable with clot-busting drugs, so immediate medical help is critical to improving the chances of recovery.

FIGURE 7.9

Types of Stroke

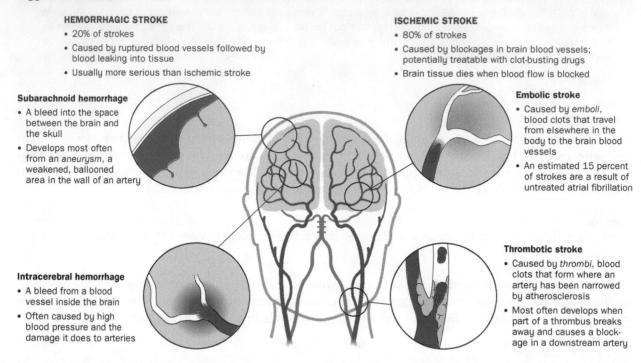

HEMORRHAGIC STROKE
- 20% of strokes
- Caused by ruptured blood vessels followed by blood leaking into tissue
- Usually more serious than ischemic stroke

ISCHEMIC STROKE
- 80% of strokes
- Caused by blockages in brain blood vessels; potentially treatable with clot-busting drugs
- Brain tissue dies when blood flow is blocked

Subarachnoid hemorrhage
- A bleed into the space between the brain and the skull
- Develops most often from an *aneurysm*, a weakened, ballooned area in the wall of an artery

Embolic stroke
- Caused by *emboli*, blood clots that travel from elsewhere in the body to the brain blood vessels
- An estimated 15 percent of strokes are a result of untreated atrial fibrillation

Intracerebral hemorrhage
- A bleed from a blood vessel inside the brain
- Often caused by high blood pressure and the damage it does to arteries

Thrombotic stroke
- Caused by *thrombi*, blood clots that form where an artery has been narrowed by atherosclerosis
- Most often develops when part of a thrombus breaks away and causes a blockage in a downstream artery

Sources: Excerpted from *Harvard Health Letter*, April 2000. Reprinted with permission obtained via The Copyright Clearance Center. Heart & Stroke Foundation; Statistics: http://www.heartandstroke.on.ca/site/c.pvI3IeNWJwE/b.358l729/; American Stroke Association. When the Beat is Off - Atrial Fibrillation: http://www.strokeassociation.org/STROKEORG/LifeAfterStroke/HealthyLivingAfterStroke/UnderstandingRiskyConditions/When-the-Beat-is-Off---Atrial-Fibrillation_UCM_3I0782_Article.jsp#.

HEMORRHAGIC STROKE   A **hemorrhagic stroke** occurs when a blood vessel in the brain bursts, spilling blood into the surrounding tissue. Cells normally nourished by the artery are deprived of blood and cannot function. In addition, accumulated blood from the burst vessel may put pressure on surrounding brain tissue, causing damage and even death. There are two types of hemorrhagic strokes:

- In an *intracerebral hemorrhage*, a blood vessel ruptures within the brain. About 10 percent of strokes are caused by intracerebral hemorrhages.
- In a *subarachnoid hemorrhage*, a blood vessel on the brain's surface ruptures and bleeds into the space between the brain and the skull. About 3 percent of strokes are of this type.

Hemorrhages can be caused by head injuries or the bursting of a malformed blood vessel called an **aneurysm**, which is a blood-filled pocket that bulges out from a weak spot in an artery wall. Aneurysms in the brain may remain stable and never break. But when they do, the result is a stroke. Aneurysms may be caused or worsened by hypertension.

hemorrhagic stroke
Impeded blood supply to the brain caused by the rupture of a blood vessel.

aneurysm
A sac formed by a distension or dilation of the artery wall.

The Effects of a Stroke

The interruption of the blood supply to any area of the brain prevents the nerve cells there from functioning—in some cases causing death. Stroke survivors usually have some lasting disability. Which parts of the body are affected depends on the area of the brain that has been damaged. Nerve cells control sensation and most of our body movements, and a stroke may cause paralysis, walking disability, speech impairment, memory loss, and changes in behaviour. The severity of the stroke and its long-term effects depend on which brain cells have been injured, how widespread the damage is, how effectively the body can restore the blood supply, and how rapidly other areas of the brain can take over. Early treatment can significantly reduce the severity of disability resulting from a stroke.

QUICK STATS

Alhough most Canadians recognize at least one sign of stroke, over 1/3 would not likely call 9-1-1 if they saw those signs in someone they know.
—Heart and Stroke Foundation of Canada, 2012

Detecting and Treating Stroke

Death rates from stroke have declined significantly in Canada over the past decades declining by 62 percent between 1969 and 1999. Effective treatment requires the prompt recognition of symptoms and correct diagnosis of the type of stroke. The signs of a stroke are listed in "Three Simple Ways to Recognize a Stroke" on ▣ connect.

Many people have strokes, however, without knowing it. These "silent strokes" do not cause any noticeable symptoms while they are occurring. Although they may be mild, having silent strokes leaves people at a higher risk for subsequent and more serious strokes later in life. They also contribute to loss of mental and cognitive skills. A recent study of MRI scans of 2000 older adults revealed that 11 percent of the subjects had brain damage from one or more strokes but did not realize they had ever had a stroke.

Some people experience a **transient ischemic attack (TIA)**, or mini-stroke, days, weeks, or months before they have a full-blown stroke. A TIA produces temporary stroke-like symptoms, such as weakness or numbness in an arm or a leg, speech difficulty, or dizziness. These symptoms are brief, often lasting just a few minutes, and do not cause permanent damage. TIAs should be taken as warning signs of a stroke, however, and anyone with a suspected TIA should get immediate medical help.

transient ischemic attack (TIA)
A small stroke; usually a temporary interruption of blood supply to the brain, causing numbness or difficulty with speech.

Strokes should be treated with the same urgency as heart attacks. A person with stroke symptoms should be rushed to the hospital. A **computed tomography (CT)** scan, which uses a computer to construct an image of the brain from X-rays, can assess brain damage and determine the type of stroke. Newer techniques using MRI and ultrasound are increasingly available and should improve the speed and accuracy of stroke diagnosis.

computed tomography (CT)
The use of computerized X-ray images to create a cross-sectional depiction (scan) of tissue density.

If tests reveal that a stroke is caused by a blood clot—and if help is sought within a few hours of the onset of symptoms—the person can be treated with the same kind of clot-dissolving drugs that are used to treat coronary artery blockages. If the clot is dissolved quickly enough, brain damage is minimized and symptoms may disappear. (The longer the brain goes without blood, the greater the risk of permanent damage.) People who have had TIAs or who are at high risk for stroke because of narrowing of the carotid arteries (large arteries on either side of the neck, which carry blood to the head) may undergo a surgical procedure called *carotid endarterectomy*, in which plaque is removed. There is also a non-surgical procedure, similar to coronary angioplasty and stenting, that can be done in the carotid arteries.

If tests reveal that a stroke was caused by a cerebral hemorrhage, drugs may be prescribed to lower the blood pressure, which will usually be high. Careful diagnosis is crucial, because administering clot-dissolving drugs to a person suffering a hemorrhagic stroke would cause more bleeding and potentially more brain damage.

If detection and treatment of stroke come too late, rehabilitation is the only treatment. Although damaged or destroyed brain tissue does not normally regenerate, nerve cells in the brain can make new pathways, and some functions can be taken over by other parts of the brain. Some spontaneous recovery starts immediately after a stroke and continues for a few months.

Rehabilitation consists of physical therapy, which helps strengthen muscles and improve balance and coordination; speech and language therapy, which helps those whose speech has been damaged; and occupational therapy, which helps improve hand–eye coordination and everyday living skills. Some people recover completely in a matter of days or weeks, but most people who have a stroke and survive must adapt to some disability.

Peripheral Arterial Disease

Peripheral arterial disease (PAD) refers to atherosclerosis in the leg (or arm) arteries, which can eventually limit or completely obstruct blood flow. The same process that occurs in the heart arteries can occur in any artery of the body. In fact, patients with PAD frequently also have coronary artery disease and cerebrovascular disease, and they have an increased risk of death from CVD. According to Canada's Vascular Disease Foundation, approximately 800 000 people in Canada have PAD, although a recent study published in the Canadian Journal of Cardiology indicated that only about one-quarter of Canadians are even aware of PAD.

> **peripheral arterial disease (PAD)**
> Atherosclerosis in arteries in the legs (or, less commonly, arms) that can impede blood flow and lead to pain, infection, and loss of the affected limb.

The risk factors associated with coronary atherosclerosis, such as smoking, diabetes, hypertension, and high cholesterol, also contribute to atherosclerosis in the peripheral circulation. The risk of PAD is significantly increased in people with diabetes and people who smoke. The likelihood of needing an amputation is increased in those who continue to smoke, and PAD in people with diabetes tends to be extensive and severe.

Symptoms of PAD include claudication and rest pain. *Claudication* is aching or fatigue in the affected leg with exertion, particularly walking, which resolves with rest. Claudication occurs when leg muscles do not get adequate blood and oxygen supply. *Rest pain* occurs when the limb artery is unable to supply adequate blood and oxygen, even when the body is not physically active. This occurs when the artery is significantly narrowed or completely blocked. If blood flow is not restored quickly, cells and tissues die; in severe cases, amputation may be needed. PAD is the leading cause of amputation in people over age 50.

Congestive Heart Failure

A number of conditions—high blood pressure, heart attack, atherosclerosis, alcoholism, viral infections, rheumatic fever, and birth defects—can damage the heart's pumping mechanism. When the heart cannot maintain its regular pumping rate and force, fluids begin to back up. When extra fluid seeps through capillary walls, edema (swelling) results, usually in the legs and ankles, but sometimes in other parts of the body as well. Fluid can collect in the lungs and interfere with breathing, particularly when a person is lying down. This condition is called **pulmonary edema**, and the entire process is known as **congestive heart failure**. According to The Heart and Stroke Foundation of Canada, about 500 000 Canadians are living with heart failure.

> **pulmonary edema**
> The accumulation of fluid in the lungs.
>
> **congestive heart failure**
> A condition resulting from the heart's inability to pump out all the blood that returns to it; blood backs up in the veins leading to the heart, causing an accumulation of fluid in various parts of the body.

Congestive heart failure can be controlled. Treatment includes reducing the workload on the heart, modifying salt intake, and using drugs that help the body eliminate excess fluid. Drugs used to treat congestive heart failure improve the pumping action of the heart, lower blood pressure so the heart doesn't have to work as hard, and help the body eliminate excess salt and water. When medical therapy is ineffective, heart transplant is a solution for some patients with severe heart failure, but the need greatly exceeds the number of hearts available.

The risk of heart failure increases with age, and being overweight is a significant independent risk factor. Experts fear that the incidence of heart failure will increase dramatically over the next few decades as our population ages and becomes increasingly obese.

QUICK STATS

165 heart transplants are performed in Canada annually.

—Canadian Institute for Health Information, 2010

Other Forms of Heart Disease

Other, less common, forms of heart disease include congenital heart disease, rheumatic heart disease, and heart valve disorders.

Congenital Heart Defects

About 1 percent of children born each year in Canada have a defect or malformation of the heart or major blood vessels. These conditions are collectively referred to as **congenital heart defects**. Most of the common congenital defects can now be accurately diagnosed and treated with medication or surgery. Early recognition of possible heart disease in a newborn is important in saving lives. The most common congenital defects are holes in the wall that divides the chambers of the heart. Such defects cause the heart to produce a distinctive sound, making diagnosis relatively simple. Another common defect is *coarctation of the aorta*, a narrowing, or constriction, of the aorta. Heart failure may result unless the constricted area is repaired by surgery.

> **congenital heart defects**
> Malformation of the heart or its major blood vessels, present at birth.

Hypertrophic cardiomyopathy (HCM) occurs in 1 out of every 500 people and is the most common cause of sudden death among athletes younger than age 35. It causes the heart muscle to become hypertrophic (enlarged), primarily in the septum, which is the area between the two ventricles. People with hypertrophic cardiomyopathy are at high risk for sudden death, mainly because of serious arrhythmias. Hypertrophic cardiomyopathy may be identified by a **murmur** and then diagnosed by using echocardiography. Possible treatments include medication and a pacemaker or internal defibrillator. If the hypertrophy is mainly in the septum, some of the septum can be surgically removed or a nonsurgical procedure can be done to kill off the extra muscle.

> **hypertrophic cardiomyopathy (HCM)**
> An inherited condition in which there is an enlargement of the heart muscle, especially between the two ventricles.
>
> **murmur**
> An abnormal heart sound indicating turbulent blood flow through a valve or hole in the heart.

Rheumatic Heart Disease

Rheumatic fever, a consequence of certain types of untreated streptococcal throat infections, is a leading cause of heart trouble worldwide. Rheumatic fever can permanently damage the heart muscle and heart valves, a condition called *rheumatic heart disease (RHD)*. Many operations on heart valves performed annually are related to RHD, and in 2011, 441 Canadians died from RHD. The incidence of rheumatic fever has declined significantly in Canada since the introduction of antibiotics.

> **rheumatic fever**
> A disease, mainly of children, characterized by fever, inflammation, and pain in the joints; often damages the heart valves and muscle, a condition called rheumatic heart disease.

Symptoms of strep throat include the sudden onset of a sore throat, painful swallowing, fever, swollen glands, headache, nausea, and vomiting. Careful laboratory diagnosis is important because strep throat is treated with antibiotics, which are not useful in the treatment of far more common viral sore throats. If left untreated, up to 3 percent of strep infections progress into rheumatic fever. Rheumatic fever primarily affects children between the ages of 5 and 15 years.

Heart Valve Disorders

Congenital defects and certain types of infections can cause abnormalities in the valves between the chambers of the heart. Heart valve problems generally fall into two categories—the valve fails to open fully, or it fails to close completely. In either case, blood flow through the heart is impaired.

Treatment for heart valve disorders depends on their location and severity; serious problems may be treated with surgery to repair or replace a valve. People with certain types of heart valve defects are advised to take antibiotics before some types of dental and surgical procedures to prevent bacteria, which may be dislodged into the bloodstream during the procedure, from infecting the defective valve.

The most common heart valve disorder is **mitral valve prolapse (MVP)**, which occurs in about 2.7 percent of the Canadian population. MVP is characterized by a billowing of the mitral valve, which separates the left ventricle and left atrium during ventricular contraction; in some cases, blood leaks from the ventricle into the atrium. Most people with MVP have no symptoms; they have the same ability to exercise and live as long as people without MVP. The condition is often diagnosed during a routine medical exam when an extra heart sound (a click) or murmur is heard; the diagnosis can be confirmed with echocardiography. Treatment for MVP is usually unnecessary, although surgery may be needed in the rare cases where leakage through the faulty valve is severe.

> **mitral valve prolapse (MVP)**
> A condition in which the mitral valve billows out during ventricular contraction, possibly allowing leakage of blood from the left ventricle into the left atrium.

Protecting Yourself Against Cardiovascular Disease

You can take steps now to lower your risk of developing CVD (see "Strategies for Reducing Your Risk of Cardiovascular Disease" on connect). CVD can begin very early in life. For example, fatty streaks (very early atherosclerosis) can be seen on the aorta in children younger than age 10. Also, young adults with relatively low cholesterol levels go on to live substantially longer than those with higher levels. Reducing CVD risk factors when you are young can pay off with many extra years of life and health (see the Assess Yourself box).

 QUESTIONS FOR CRITICAL THINKING AND REFLECTION

Has anyone you know ever had a heart attack? If so, was the onset gradual or sudden? Were appropriate steps taken to help the person (for example, did anyone call 9-1-1, give CPR, or use an AED)? Do you feel comfortable dealing with a cardiac emergency? If not, what can you do to improve your readiness? What would be important about you taking/updating your CPR training?

Eat Heart Healthy

For most Canadians, eating a heart-healthy diet involves many of the changes suggested in *Eating Well with Canada's Food Guide*. See Chapter 5 for a detailed discussion of nutrition and dietary guidelines. Suggestions include the following:

- Decrease fat and cholesterol intake. (See the Take Charge box at the end of the chapter for ways to decrease your saturated fat and trans fat intake.)
- Eat a high-fibre diet.

Assess YOURSELF

Are You at Risk for CVD?

Your chances of suffering an early heart attack or stroke depend on a variety of factors, many of which are under your control. The best time to identify your risk factors and change your behaviour to lower your risk is when you are young. You can significantly affect your future health and quality of life if you adopt healthy behaviours. To help identify your risk factors, circle the response for each risk category that best describes you.

1. Gender and age
   - 0 Female age 55 or younger or male age 45 or younger
   - 2 Female age 55 or older or male age 45 or older

2. Heredity
   - 0 Neither parent suffered a heart attack or stroke before age 60
   - 3 One parent suffered a heart attack or stroke before age 60
   - 7 Both parents suffered a heart attack or stroke before age 60

3. Smoking
   - 0 Never smoked
   - 3 Quit more than two years ago and lifetime smoking is less than five pack-years*
   - 6 Quit less than two years ago or lifetime smoking is greater than five pack-years*
   - 8 Smoke less than half a pack per day
   - 13 Smoke more than half a pack per day
   - 15 Smoke more than one pack per day

4. Environmental tobacco smoke
   - 0 Do not live or work with smokers
   - 2 Exposed to ETS at work
   - 3 Live with a smoker
   - 4 Both live and work with smokers

5. Blood pressure
   If available, average your last three readings:
   - 0 120/80 or below
   - 1 121/81–130/85
   - 3 Don't know
   - 5 131/86–150/90
   - 9 151/91–170/100
   - 13 Above 170/100

6. Total cholesterol (mmol/L)
   Your physician has told you that you have
   - 0 Low total cholesterol
   - 3 Minimally high cholesterol
   - 5 High cholesterol
   - 6 Very high cholesterol

7. HDL Cholesterol (mmol/L)
   Your physician has told you that you have
   - 0 Very high HDL
   - 1 High HDL
   - 3 Moderate HDL
   - 5 Low HDL
   - 10 Very low HDL

8. Exercise
   - 0 Exercise three times a week
   - 1 Exercise once or twice a week
   - 2 Occasional exercise less than once a week
   - 7 Rarely exercise

9. Diabetes
   - 0 No personal or family history
   - 2 One parent with diabetes
   - 6 Two parents with diabetes
   - 9 Non-insulin-dependent diabetes
   - 13 Insulin-dependent diabetes

10. Body mass index (using the formula provided in Chapter 4)
    - 0 < 23.0
    - 1 23.0–24.9
    - 2 25.0–28.9
    - 3 29.0–34.9
    - 5 35.0–39.9
    - 7 ≥ 40

11. Stress
    - 0 Relaxed most of the time
    - 1 Occasionally stressed and angry
    - 2 Frequently stressed and angry
    - 3 Usually stressed and angry

Scoring

Total your risk factor points. Refer to the list below to get an approximate rating of your risk of suffering an early heart attack or stroke.

Score	Estimated Risk
Less than 20	Low risk
20–29	Moderate risk
30–45	High risk
Over 45	Extremely high risk

*Pack-years can be calculated by multiplying the number of packs you smoked per day by the number of years you smoked. For example, if you smoked a pack and a half a day for 5 years, you would have smoked the equivalent of 1.5 x 5 = 7.5 pack-years.

- Reduce sodium intake and increase potassium intake.
- Avoid excessive alcohol consumption.
- Eat foods rich in omega-3 fatty acids.

In addition to these familiar guidelines, a few specifics pertain to heart health:

- *Plant stanols and sterols:* These substances, found in some types of trans-fat–free margarines and other products, reduce the absorption of cholesterol in the body and help lower LDL levels. For people with high LDL levels that do not respond to changes in fat intake, experts suggest an intake of 2 grams per day of plant stanols or sterols.
- *Folic acid, vitamin B-6, and vitamin B-12:* These vitamins lower homocysteine levels, and folic acid has also been found to reduce the risk of hypertension.
- *Calcium:* Diets rich in calcium may help prevent hypertension and possibly stroke by reducing insulin resistance and platelet aggregation. Good sources of calcium are low-fat and fat-free dairy products.
- *Soy protein:* Although soy itself doesn't seem to have much effect on cholesterol, replacing some animal proteins with soy protein (such as tofu) may help lower LDL cholesterol.
- *Healthy carbohydrates:* Healthy carbohydrate choices include whole grains, fruits, and non-starchy vegetables. Healthy carbohydrates are important for people with insulin resistance, pre-diabetes, or diabetes.
- *Total calories:* Some studies have found that reducing energy intake can improve cholesterol and triglyceride levels as much as reducing fat intake does. Reduced calorie intake also helps control body weight—an extremely important risk factor for CVD.

Increased Fibre Intake

Fibre traps the bile acids the liver needs to manufacture cholesterol and carries them to the large intestine, where they are excreted. It slows the production of proteins that promote blood clotting. Fibre may also interfere with the absorption of dietary fat and may help you cut total food intake because foods rich in fibre tend to be filling. Studies have shown that a high-fibre diet is associated with a 40–50 percent reduction in the risk of heart attack and stroke; in 2013, researchers found that every 7 gram increase in total dietary fibre is associated with a 7 percent lower risk for first-time stroke.

To get the recommended 21–38 grams of dietary fibre per day, eat whole grains, fruits, and vegetables. Good sources of fibre include oatmeal, some breakfast cereals, barley, legumes, and most fruits and vegetables.

Decreased Sodium Intake and Increased Potassium Intake

Reducing sodium intake to recommended levels, while also increasing potassium intake, can help reduce blood pressure for many people. The recommended limit for sodium intake is 2300 milligrams per day; for population groups at special risk, the recommended limit is 1500 milligrams per day.

Potassium is also important in controlling blood pressure, and many North Americans consume less than recommended amounts of the mineral. Good food sources include leafy green vegetables (e.g., spinach and beet greens), root vegetables (e.g., white and sweet potatoes), vine fruits (e.g., cantaloupe and honeydew melon), winter squash, bananas, many dried fruits, and tomato sauce.

Moderate Alcohol Consumption (For Some)

Guidelines for Canadians state that moderate alcohol consumption may lower the risk of CVD among middle-aged and older adults. Moderate means no more than one drink per day for women and two drinks per day for men. Moderate alcohol use may increase HDL cholesterol; it may also reduce stroke risk, possibly by dampening the inflammatory response or by affecting blood clotting.

For most people under age 45, however, the risks of alcohol use probably outweigh any health benefit. Excessive alcohol consumption increases the risk of a variety of serious health problems, including hypertension, stroke, some cancers, liver disease, alcohol dependence, and injuries. See Chapter 15 for a detailed discussion of alcohol use, the effects of alcohol, and the importance of moderation in drinking.

Other Dietary Factors

Researchers have identified other dietary factors that may affect CVD risk. For example, *Omega-3 fatty acids,* found in fish, shellfish, and some plant foods (e.g., nuts and canola, soybean, and flaxseed oils), may reduce clotting, abnormal heart rhythms, and inflammation, and may have other heart-healthy effects, such as lowering triglycerides. Eating fish two or more times a week is often recommended; fish oil capsules may be appropriate for some people who won't eat fish or who have certain CVD risk factors. Note that omega-3 fatty acids may raise LDL levels and some fish sources may be high in mercury. Plant sources of omega-3 fatty acids are also a good choice.

Most experts recommend against taking nutritional supplements as a way to prevent heart disease. In fact, a 10-year-long study ending in 2008 revealed that vitamin C and E supplements provided no protection against heart disease in men. In some of the study's subjects, vitamin E supplementation was associated with an increased risk of stroke. An estimated 15 percent of Canadians take vitamin C and E supplements, and many people do so because of a long-standing yet unproven theory that these antioxidants protect against heart disease. Some evidence suggests that vitamin D deficiency may increase the risk of heart disease, especially in men, but experts do not currently advise taking vitamin D supplements to prevent CVD. If you are concerned about your heart health and may not be getting the nutrition you need, ask your physician or a registered dietitian for advice.

Exercise Regularly

You can significantly reduce your risk of CVD with a moderate amount of physical activity. Follow the guidelines for physical activity and exercise described in Chapter 6. Strength training in addition to aerobic exercise is recommended for building and maintaining cardiovascular health. Strength training helps lower blood pressure, reduce body fat, and improve lipid levels and glucose metabolism.

Avoid Tobacco

The number-one risk factor for CVD that you can control is smoking. If you smoke, quit. If you don't smoke, don't start. If you live or work with people who smoke, encourage them to quit—for their sake and yours. Exposure to ETS raises your risk of CVD, and no level of exposure is safe. If you find yourself breathing in smoke, take steps to prevent or stop the exposure. See Chapter 16 for detailed information on the effects of smoking and strategies for quitting.

Know and Manage your Blood Pressure

If you have no CVD risk factors, have your blood pressure measured by a trained professional at least once every two years; yearly tests are recommended if you have other risk factors. If your blood pressure is high, follow your physician's advice on how to lower it. For those with hypertension that is not readily controlled with lifestyle changes, many antihypertension medications are available.

QUICK STATS

A stroke survivor has a 20% chance of having another stroke within 2 years.

—Heart and Stroke Foundation of Canada, 2009

QUESTIONS FOR CRITICAL THINKING AND REFLECTION

Do you know what your blood pressure and cholesterol levels are? If not, is there a reason you don't know? Is there something preventing you from getting this information about yourself? How can you motivate yourself to have these easy but important health checks?

Know and Manage your Cholesterol Levels

All people ages 20 and older should talk with their physician about having their cholesterol checked. It is a good idea to get a fasting lipoprotein profile that measures total cholesterol, HDL, LDL, and triglyceride levels. Once you know your baseline numbers, you and your physician can develop an LDL goal and lifestyle plan.

Develop Effective Ways to Handle Stress and Anger

To reduce the psychological and social risk factors for CVD, develop effective strategies for handling the stress in your life. Shore up your social support network, and try some of the techniques described in Chapter 3 for managing stress.

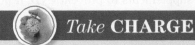 *Take* CHARGE

Reducing the Saturated and Trans Fats in Your Diet

No more than 7 percent of the calories in your diet should come from saturated fats, and no more than 1 percent should come from trans fats. Foods high in saturated fat include meat, poultry skin, full-fat dairy products, coconut and palm oils, and hydrogenated vegetable oils. Hydrogenated fats and products, such as snack foods that are made with them and deep-fried fast food, are high in trans fats.

Monitor your Current Diet

To see how your diet measures up, keep track in your health journal of everything you eat for three days. Information about the calorie and saturated fat content of foods is available on many food labels, in books, and on the Internet. The list below gives a few average values for foods that are rich sources of trans fats in the Canadian diet. However, food companies are trying to reduce or eliminate trans fats from their products, so it's important to read the labels.

At the end of the monitoring period, record the calories and grams of saturated and trans fat for as many of the foods you have eaten as possible. Determine the percentage of daily calories as fat that you consumed for each day: Multiply grams of saturated and trans fats by 9 (fat has 9 calories per gram) and then divide by total calories. For example, if you consumed 30 grams of saturated and trans fats and 2100 calories on a particular day, then your saturated and trans fat consumption as a percentage of total calories would be 30 x 9 = 270 calories of fat ÷ 2100 total calories = 0.13, or 13 percent. If you have trouble obtaining all the data you need to do the calculations, you can still estimate whether your diet is high in saturated and trans fats by seeing how many servings of foods high in unhealthy fats you typically consume on a daily basis (see the list).

	Grams of Trans Fat Per Serving
Pot pie	6
French fries (large)	5
Pound cake	5
Fish sticks	5
Doughnut	4
Biscuit	4
Fried, breaded chicken	3
Danish pastry	3
Vegetable shortening	3
Margarine (stick)	2
Microwave popcorn	2
Sandwich cookies	2
Snack crackers	2
Margarine (tub)	1

Making Heart-healthy Changes

To reduce your intake of unhealthy fats, you may want to set a limit on the number of servings of foods high in saturated and trans fats that you consume each day. Or you may want to set a more precise goal and then continue to monitor your daily consumption. The 7 percent limit corresponds to 12 grams of saturated and trans fats in a 1600-calorie diet, 17 grams in a 2200-calorie diet, and 22 grams in a 2800-calorie diet.

To plan healthy changes, take a close look at your food record. Do you choose many foods high in saturated and trans fats? Do you limit your portion sizes to those recommended by *Eating Well with Canada's Food Guide*? Try making healthy substitutions. Do you have a salami and cheese sandwich for lunch? Try turkey for a change. Do you always order French fries when you eat out? Try half a plain baked potato or a different vegetable next time. Do you snack on pastries, cookies, doughnuts, chips, or fatty crackers? Try fresh fruits and vegetables instead. If you frequently eat in fast-food restaurants or other places where the majority of the menu is heavy in saturated and trans fats, trying finding an appealing alternative—and recruit some friends to join you.

When you choose foods that are rich in saturated and trans fats, *watch your portion sizes carefully*. Choose cuts of meat that have the least amount of visible fat, and trim off what you see. And try to balance your choices throughout the day. For example, if your lunch includes a hamburger and fries, choose broiled fish or poultry or a vegetarian pasta dish for dinner. Plenty of delicious choices are low in saturated and trans fats. Plan your diet around a variety of whole grains, vegetables, legumes, and fruits, which are nearly always low in fats and high in nutrients.

Instead of	Try
Butter, stick margarine, vegetable shortening, coconut and palm oils	Vegetable oils, trans-fat-free tub or squeeze margarines
Whole or 2 percent milk; regular cheese, mayonnaise, and sour cream	Fat-free or 1 percent milk; low-fat cheese, fat-free or low-fat sour cream, yogourt, or mayonnaise
Chips, cheese puffs, crackers, buttered popcorn	Fruits, vegetables, rice cakes, plain popcorn, pretzels, fat-free chips, baked crackers
Cakes, cookies, pastries, doughnuts, cinnamon rolls, pie, regular ice cream	Fruit or a *small* serving of a low-fat sweet (angel food cake; fat-free ice cream, frozen yogourt, sherbet, or sorbet)
Biscuits, croissants, fried tortillas, regular granola, muffins, coffee cake	Whole-grain breads and rolls, baked tortillas, low-fat granola or cold cereal, English muffin, bagel
Creamy or cheesy sauces and soups	Tomato- and other vegetable-based sauces, clam sauce, clear soups
Ground beef, hamburger patty, meatloaf, ribs, T-bone or flank steak, prime grades of beef	Ground turkey, veggie burger, extra-lean ground beef, round steak, sirloin, choice or select grades of beef
Pork chops, roast, or ribs; bone-in ham; lamb chops or ribs	Pork sirloin or tenderloin; boneless ham; veal chops and cutlets; leg of lamb
Bacon, sausage, lunch meats, hot dogs	Canadian bacon; turkey, ham, or pastrami; other low-fat lunch meats
Poultry with skin; fried chicken or fish	Skinless poultry, especially breast or drumstick; baked, broiled, grilled, or roasted poultry or fish; ground turkey
French fries, onion rings	Baked potato or other non-fried vegetable, rice
Pizza, pot pie, macaroni and cheese, and other high-fat convenience foods	Vegetarian or turkey chili, pasta with vegetables, grilled poultry and fish dishes

Sources: New heart dos and don'ts. 2006. *Consumer Reports Health*, March, 49; American Heart Association. 2000. *An Eating Plan for Healthy Americans: The New 2000 Food Guidelines.* Dallas, Tex.: American Heart Association; U.S. Department of Agriculture and U.S. Department of Health and Human Services. 2000. *Nutrition and Your Health: Dietary Guidelines for Americans*, 5th ed. Home and Garden Bulletin No. 232.

SUMMARY

- The cardiovascular system pumps and circulates blood throughout the body. The heart pumps blood to the lungs via the pulmonary artery and to the body via the aorta.
- The exchange of nutrients and waste products takes place between the capillaries and the tissues.
- The six major risk factors for CVD that can be changed are smoking, high blood pressure, unhealthy cholesterol levels, inactivity, overweight and obesity, and diabetes.
- Effects of smoking include lower HDL levels, increased blood pressure and heart rate, accelerated plaque formation, and increased risk of blood clots.
- Hypertension occurs when blood pressure exceeds normal limits most of the time. It weakens the heart, scars and hardens arteries, and can damage the eyes and kidneys.
- High LDL and low HDL cholesterol levels contribute to clogged arteries and increase the risk of CVD.
- Physical inactivity, obesity, and diabetes are interrelated and are associated with high blood pressure and unhealthy cholesterol levels.
- Contributing risk factors that can be changed include high triglyceride levels and psychological and social factors.
- Risk factors for CVD that can't be changed include being over age 65, being male, being a woman experiencing menopause, being Aboriginal or of South Asian or African descent, and having a family history of CVD.
- Atherosclerosis is a progressive hardening and narrowing of arteries that can lead to restricted blood flow and even complete blockage.
- Heart attacks are usually the result of a long-term disease process. Warning signs of a heart attack include chest discomfort, shortness of breath, nausea, and sweating.
- A stroke occurs when the blood supply to the brain is cut off by a blood clot or hemorrhage. A transient ischemic attack (TIA) is a warning sign of stroke.
- Congestive heart failure occurs when the heart's pumping action becomes less efficient and fluid collects in the lungs or in other parts of the body.
- Dietary changes that can protect against CVD include decreasing your intake of fat, especially saturated and trans fats, and cholesterol, and increasing your intake of fibre by eating more fruits, vegetables, and whole grains.
- CVD risk can also be reduced by engaging in regular exercise, avoiding tobacco and environmental tobacco smoke, knowing and managing your blood pressure and cholesterol levels, and developing effective ways of handling stress and anger.

FOR MORE INFORMATION

BOOKS

Freeman, M. W., and C. E. Junge. 2005. Harvard *Medical School Guide to Lowering Your Cholesterol*. New York: McGraw-Hill. Information about cholesterol, including lifestyle changes and medication for improving cholesterol levels.

Heller, M. 2005. *The DASH Diet Action Plan, Based on the National Institutes of Health Research: Dietary Approaches to Stop Hypertension*. Northbrook, Ill.: Amidon Press. Background information and guidelines for adopting the DASH diet, along with meal plans to suit differing caloric needs and recipes.

Lipsky, M. S., et al. 2008. *American Medical Association Guide to Preventing and Treating Heart Disease*. New York: Wiley. A team of doctors provides advice for heart health to consumers.

Mostyn, B. 2007. *Pocket Guide to Low Sodium Foods*, 2nd ed. Olympia, Wash.: InData Publishing. Lists thousands of low-sodium products that can be purchased in supermarkets, as well as low-sodium choices available in many restaurants.

Phibbs, B. 2007. *The Human Heart: A Basic Guide to Heart Disease.* Philadelphia: Lippincott Williams & Wilkins. Information about heart disease, treatments, and recovery for patients and their families.

Romaine, D. S., and O. S. Randall. 2005. *The Encyclopedia of Heart and Heart Disease.* New York: Facts on File. Includes entries on the functioning of the cardiovascular system, types and causes of heart disease, and prevention and treatment.

ORGANIZATIONS, HOTLINES, AND WEBSITES

The Internet addresses listed here were accurate at the time of publication.

Canadian Hypertension Society. Provides information on the research and management of hypertension in Canada.
   http://www.hypertension.ca

Canadian Red Cross. Provides information about CPR and First Aid courses, as well as information pertaining to their mission of improving the lives of vulnerable people by mobilizing the power of humanity in Canada and around the world.
   http://www.redcross.ca/

Dietitians of Canada. Provides resources for consumers and health professionals, including articles, news events, and nutrition facts.
   http://www.dietitians.ca

Health Canada. Provides information and resources for healthy living among Canadians, including *Eating Well with Canada's Food Guide.*
   http://www.hc-sc.gc.ca

Heart and Stroke Foundation of Canada. Provides information about heart, stroke, and healthy living in Canada.
   http://www.heartandstroke.ca

The Human Heart: An On-Line Exploration. An online museum exhibit containing information on the structure and function of the heart, how to monitor your heart's health, and how to maintain a healthy heart.
   http://learn.fi.edu/learn/heart/index.html

MyHeartCentral.com. Provides information for heart patients and others interested in learning how to identify and reduce their risk factors for heart disease; includes links to many related sites.
   http://www.healthcentral.com/heart-disease

MedlinePlus: Blood, Heart, and Circulation Topics. Provides links to reliable sources of information on many topics relating to cardiovascular health.
   http://www.nlm.nih.gov/medlineplus/heartandcirculation.html

Public Health Agency of Canada. Provides information on a variety of diseases in Canada, including population statistics for heart disease and stroke.
   http://www.phac-aspc.gc.ca

U.S. National Heart, Lung, and Blood Institute. Provides information on and interactive applications for a variety of topics relating to cardiovascular health and disease, including cholesterol, smoking, obesity, hypertension, and the DASH diet.
   http://www.nhlbi.nih.gov

U.S. National Stroke Association. Provides information and referrals for people who have had a stroke and their families; includes a stroke risk assessment.
   http://www.stroke.org

See also the listings for Chapters 2–6.

SELECTED BIBLIOGRAPHY

Abramson, J.D., et al. 2013. Should people at low risk of cardiovascular disease take a statin? *BMJ* 347: f6123.

Albert, C. M., et al. 2008. Effect of folic acid and B vitamins on risk of cardio-vascular events and total mortality among women at high risk for cardio-vascular disease: A randomized trial. *Journal of the American Medical Association* 299(17): 2027–2036.

American Heart Association. 2012. *Heart Disease and Stroke Statistics—2012 Update.* Dallas: American Heart Association.

Berger, J. S., et al. 2006. Aspirin for the primary prevention of cardiovascular events in women and men: A sex-specific meta-analysis of randomized controlled trials. *Journal of the American Medical Association* 295(3): 306–313.

Bonaa, K. H., et al. 2006. Homocysteine lowering and cardiovascular events after acute myocardial infarction. *New England Journal of Medicine* 354(15): 1578–1588.

Brien, S. E., and P. T. Katzmarzyk. 2006. Physical activity and the metabolic syndrome in Canada. *Applied Physiology, Nutrition, and Metabolism* 31: 40–47.

Campbell, N. R. C. 2010. *The 2010 Canadian Hypertension Education Program Recommendations,* http://hypertension.ca/chep/wp-content/uploads/2010/08/FullRec2010_BMSbooklet_EN.pdf (retrieved April 6, 2015).

Colihan, D. 2008. *Silent Strokes Take a Toll,* http://www.webmd.com/stroke/news/20080626/silent-strokes-take-a-toll (retrieved November 10, 2015).

Conference Board of Canada. (2010, February). The Canadian Heart Health Strategy: Risk Factors and Future Cost Implications Report.

Cooper, R. S., et al. 2005. An international comparative study of blood pressure in populations of European vs. African descent. *BMC Medicine* 3(1): 2.

de Torbal, A., et al. 2006. Incidence of recognized and unrecognized myocardial infarction in men and women aged 55 and older: The Rotterdam Study. *European Heart Journal* 27(6): 729–736.

Elliott, P., et al. 2006. Association between protein intake and blood pressure: The INTERMAP study. *Archives of Internal Medicine* 166(1): 79–87.

Forman, J. P., et al. 2005. Folate intake and risk of incident hypertension among U.S. women. *Journal of the American Medical Association* 293(3): 320–329.

Giovannucci, E., et al. 2008. 25-hydroxyvitamin D and risk of myocardial infarction in men; a prospective study. *Archives of Internal Medicine* 168(11): 1174–1180.

Grundy, S. M., et al. 2004. Definition of metabolic syndrome: Report of the National Heart, Lung, and Blood Institute/American Heart Association conference on scientific issues related to definition. *Circulation* 109: 433–438.

Harvard Medical School. 2008. The status of statins. *Harvard Women's Health Watch* 15(6): 1–3.

Heart and Stroke Foundation of Canada. 2014. Getting your blood pressure in check, http://www.heartandstroke.com/site/c.ikIQLcMWJtE/b.3484023/ (retrieved March 13, 2015).

Hypertension Canada. 2014. Fact Sheet: The case for sodium reduction in Canada, https://www.hypertension.ca/images/whatsnew/Final%20Sodium%20Fact%20Sheet_2014.pdf (retrieved March 13, 2015).

Jenkins, D. J., et al. 2006. Assessment of the longer-term effects of a dietary portfolio of cholesterol-lowering foods in hypercholesterolemia. *American Journal of Clinical Nutrition* 83(3): 582–591.

Nissen, S. E., et al. 2005. Statin therapy, LDL cholesterol, C-reactive protein, and coronary artery disease. *New England Journal of Medicine* 352(1): 29–38.

OECD (2011), "Cardiac procedures (coronary angioplasty)," in Health at a Glance 2011: OECD Indicators, OECD Publishing, http://dx.doi.org/10.1787/health_glance-2011-34-en.

Ostrom, M. P., et al. 2008. Mortality incidence and the severity of coronary atherosclerosis assessed by computed tomography angiography. *Journal of the American College of Cardiology* 52(16): 1335–1343.

Pickering, T. G., et al. 2008. Call to action on use and reimbursement for home blood pressure monitoring: A joint scientific statement from the American Heart Association, American Society of Hypertension, and Preventive Cardiovascular Nurses Association. *Hypertension* 52(1): 10–29.

Public Health Agency of Canada. 2009. Tracking Heart Disease and Stroke in Canada, 2009, http://www.phac-aspc.gc.ca/publicat/2009/cvd-avc/pdf/cvd-avs-2009-eng.pdf (retrieved March 13, 2015).

Public Health Agency of Canada, 2009. Report from the National Diabetes Surveillance System: Diabetes in Canada, 2009, http://www.phac-aspc.gc.ca/publicat/2009/ndssdic-snsddac-09/2-5-eng.php (retrieved March 13, 2015).

Raggi, P., et al. 2008. Coronary artery calcium to predict all-cause mortality in elderly men and women. *Journal of the American College of Cardiology* 52(1): 17–23.

Refsum, H., et al. 2006. The Hordaland Homocysteine Study: A community-based study of homocysteine, its determinants, and associations with disease. *Journal of Nutrition* 136(6 Suppl.): 1731S–1740S.

Ridker, P. M., et al. 2005. C-reactive protein levels and outcomes after statin therapy. *New England Journal of Medicine* 352(1): 20–28.

Ridker, P. M., et al. 2005. A randomized trial of low-dose aspirin in the primary prevention of cardiovascular disease in women. *New England Journal of Medicine,* 7 March [epub].

Ridker, P. M., et al. 2008. Rosuvastatin to prevent vascular events in men and women with elevated C-reactive protein. *New England Journal of Medicine* 359(21): 2195–2207.

Riediger, N.D. & Clara, I. 2011. Prevalence of metabolic syndrome in the Canadian adult population. *CMAJ* 2011. DOI:10.1503/cmaj.110070.

Rothwell, P. M., and C. P. Warlow. 2005. Timing of TIAs preceding stroke: Time window for prevention is very short. *Neurology* 64(5): 817–820.

Rozanski, A. S., et al. 2005. The epidemiology, pathophysiology, and management of psychosocial risk factors in cardiac practice: The emerging field of behavioral cardiology. *Journal of the American College of Cardiology* 45(5): 637–651.

Sesso, H. D., et al. 2008. Vitamins E and C in the prevention of cardiovascular disease in men: Physician's Health Study II randomized controlled trial. *Journal of the American Medical Association* 300(18): 2123–2133.

Statistics Canada, Canadian Vital Statistics, Death Database (CANSIM table 102-0561). 2012, http://www.statcan.gc.ca/pub/84-215-x/2012001/tbl/t001-eng.htm (retrieved March 13, 2015).

Statistics Canada. (2012, December). Canada Health Measures Survey – Cholesterol levels of Canadians, 2009-2011, hhttp://www.statcan.gc.ca/pub/82-625-x/2012001/article/11732-eng.htm (retrieved March 13, 2015).

Tufts University. 2006. Pendulum swings on estrogen and women's heart health risk. *Health & Nutrition Newsletter* 24(3): 1–2.

Turhan, H., et al. 2005. High prevalence of metabolic syndrome among young women with premature coronary artery disease. *Coronary Artery Disease* 16(1): 37–40.

University of California, Berkeley. 2008. Heart tests: low- to high-tech. University of California, Berkeley, *Wellness Letter* August, 5.

Watkins, L.L., et al. 2013. Association of anxiety and depression with all-cause mortality in individuals with coronary heart disease. *Journal of the American heart Association 2:e000068* doi: 10.1161/JAHA.112.000068.

Webb, D. 2005. Supplements for a healthy heart: What works, what doesn't. *Environmental Nutrition* 28(12): 1, 4.3

Wilkins, K., et al. 2010. Blood pressure in Canadian adults. *Health Reports* 21(1), http://www.statcan.gc.ca/pub/82-003-x/2010001/article/11118-eng.pdf (retrieved March 13, 2015).

Willingham, S. A., and E. S. Kilpatrick. 2005. Evidence of gender bias when applying the new diagnostic criteria for myocardial infarction. *Heart* 91(2): 237–238.

Wittstein, I. S., et al. 2005. Neurohumoral features of myocardial stunning due to sudden emotional stress. *New England Journal of Medicine* 352(6): 539–548.

World Heart Federation. 2014. Diabetes, http://www.world-heart-federation.org/cardiovascular-health/cardiovascular-disease-risk-factors/diabetes/ (retrieved March 13, 2015).

Yusuf, S., et al. 2005. Obesity and the risk of myocardial infarction in 27,000 participants from 52 countries: A case-control study. *Lancet* 366(9497): 1640–1649.

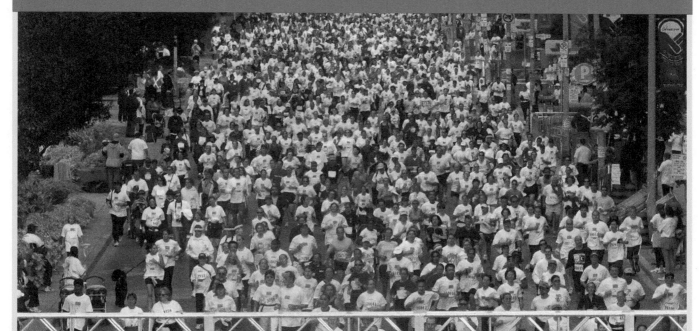

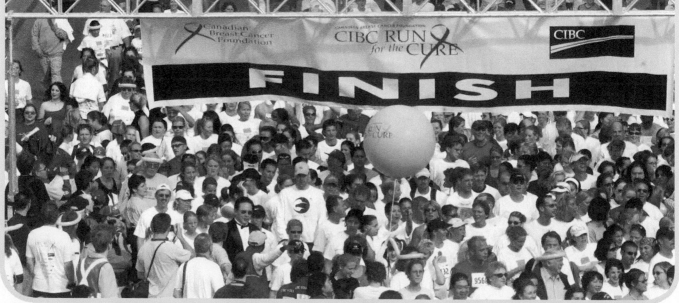

CHAPTER 8

Cancer

LOOKING AHEAD

After you have read and studied this chapter, you should be able to:

LO1 Explain what cancer is and how it spreads

LO2 List and describe common cancers: their risk factors, signs and symptoms, treatments, and approaches to prevention

LO3 Discuss some of the causes of cancer and how they can be avoided or minimized

LO4 Describe how cancer can be detected, diagnosed, and treated

LO5 List specific actions you can take to lower your risk of cancer

TEST YOUR KNOWLEDGE

1. Which type of cancer kills the most women each year?
a. breast cancer b. lung cancer c. ovarian cancer

2. Which type of cancer kills the most men each year?
a. prostate cancer b. lung cancer c. colon cancer

3. Testicular cancer is the most common cancer in men under age 30.
True or false?

4. The use of condoms during sexual intercourse can prevent cervical cancer in women.
True or false?

5. Eating which of these foods may help prevent cancer?
a. chili peppers b. broccoli c. oranges

ANSWERS

1. b.   There are more cases of breast cancer each year, but lung cancer kills more women. Smoking is the primary risk factor for lung cancer.

2. b.   There are more cases of prostate cancer, but lung cancer kills about three times as many men as prostate cancer does each year.

3. TRUE.   Although rare, testicular cancer is tied with non-Hodgkin lymphoma as the most common cancer in men ages 15–29. Regular self-exams may aid in its detection.

4. TRUE.   The primary cause of cervical cancer is infection with human papillomavirus (HPV), a sexually transmitted pathogen. The use of condoms helps prevent HPV infection.

5. ALL THREE.   These and many other fruit and vegetables are rich in phytochemicals, naturally occurring substances that may have anti-cancer effects.

Cancer is the leading cause of death in our country. In Canada, cancer is responsible for one in four deaths, claiming approximately 75 000 lives annually—more than 1450 each week. Iit was estimated that 191 300 new cases of cancer would be diagnosed in 2014; that means about 520 Canadians were being diagnosed with some form of cancer each day.

Even as medical science struggles to find a cure for cancer, mounting evidence indicates that most cancers can be prevented through simple changes in lifestyle. Tobacco use, for example, is responsible for about 25 percent of all cancer deaths worldwide, making it the single greatest avoidable risk factor for cancer (see Figure 8.1). Through behaviour and lifestyle changes, such as healthy dietary and physical activity habits, about 33 percent of 12 major cancers can be prevented. Such evidence proves that individual behaviour is a significant determinant of cancer risk.

This chapter introduces you to cancer, explains how the disease progresses, and identifies the factors that put people at risk for developing cancer. The following sections also discuss the lifestyle factors that can help you reduce your risk for cancer.

What is Cancer?

Cancer is the abnormal, uncontrolled multiplication of cells that, if left untreated, can ultimately cause death.

cancer
Abnormal, uncontrolled cellular multiplication.

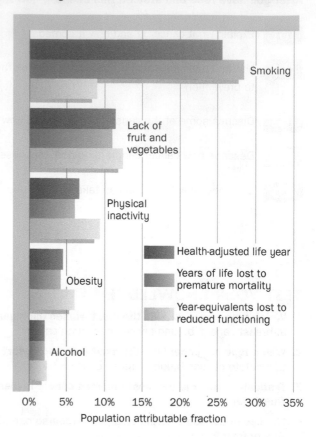

FIGURE 8.1

The Impact of Five Risk Factors on Cancer

Legend:
- Health-adjusted life year
- Years of life lost to premature mortality
- Year-equivalents lost to reduced functioning

X-axis: 0% 5% 10% 15% 20% 25% 30% 35%
Population attributable fraction

Categories: Smoking, Lack of fruit and vegetables, Physical inactivity, Obesity, Alcohol

Source: McIntosh, C. N. 2006. Population Health Impact of Cancer in Canada, 2001. Figure I. (http://www.statcan.gc.ca/pub/82-005-x/82-005-x2006001-eng.htm; retrieved April 8, 2015). Used with permission of Statistics Canada.

Tumours

Most cancers take the form of tumours, although not all tumours are cancerous. A **tumour** (or *neoplasm*) is simply a mass of tissue that serves no physiological purpose. It can be benign, like a wart, or malignant, like most lung cancers.

tumour
A mass of tissue that serves no physiological purpose; also called a *neoplasm*.

Benign (non-cancerous) **tumours** are made up of cells similar to the surrounding normal cells and are enclosed in a membrane that prevents them from penetrating neighbouring tissues. They are dangerous only if their physical presence interferes with body functions. A benign brain tumour, for example, can cause death if it blocks the blood supply to the brain.

benign tumour
A mass of tissue that is not cancerous.

QUICK STATS

The economic burden of cancer in Canada is about $22.5 billion annually.
—Thomson & Greve Young, 2009

The term **malignant tumour** is synonymous with cancer. A malignant tumour can invade surrounding structures, including blood vessels, the **lymphatic system**, and nerves. It can also spread to distant sites via the blood and lymphatic circulation, producing invasive tumours in almost any part of the body. A few cancers, such as leukemia (cancer of the blood), do not produce a mass but still have the fundamental property of rapid, uncontrolled cell multiplication; for this reason, such diseases are malignant and are considered to be a form of cancer.

malignant tumour
A mass of tissue that is cancerous and capable of spreading.

lymphatic system
A network of vessels that returns proteins, lipids, and other substances from fluid in the tissues to the circulatory system.

Every case of cancer begins as a change in a cell that allows it to grow and divide when it should not. Normally (in adults), cells divide and grow at a rate just sufficient to replace dying cells. In contrast, a malignant cell divides without regard for normal control mechanisms and gradually produces a mass of abnormal cells or a tumour. It takes about a billion cells to make a mass the size of a pea, so a single tumour cell must go through many divisions, often taking years, before the tumour grows to a noticeable size (see Figure 8.2).

FIGURE 8.2

Tumour Development Occurs in Stages

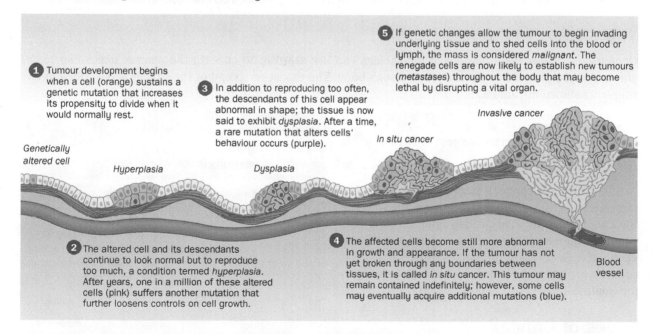

1 Tumour development begins when a cell (orange) sustains a genetic mutation that increases its propensity to divide when it would normally rest.

2 The altered cell and its descendants continue to look normal but to reproduce too much, a condition termed *hyperplasia*. After years, one in a million of these altered cells (pink) suffers another mutation that further loosens controls on cell growth.

3 In addition to reproducing too often, the descendants of this cell appear abnormal in shape; the tissue is now said to exhibit *dysplasia*. After a time, a rare mutation that alters cells' behaviour occurs (purple).

4 The affected cells become still more abnormal in growth and appearance. If the tumour has not yet broken through any boundaries between tissues, it is called *in situ* cancer. This tumour may remain contained indefinitely; however, some cells may eventually acquire additional mutations (blue).

5 If genetic changes allow the tumour to begin invading underlying tissue and to shed cells into the blood or lymph, the mass is considered *malignant*. The renegade cells are now likely to establish new tumours (*metastases*) throughout the body that may become lethal by disrupting a vital organ.

Genetically altered cell — Hyperplasia — Dysplasia — *In situ* cancer — *Invasive cancer* — Blood vessel

Source: Weinberg, R. A. 1996. How cancer arises. *Scientific American,* September. Copyright © 1996 by Dana Burns-Pizer. Reprinted with permission.

Eventually a tumour produces a sign or symptom that is determined by its location in the body. In the breast, for example, a tumour may be felt as a lump and diagnosed as cancer by an X-ray or a **biopsy**. In less accessible locations, such as the lung, ovary, or intestine, a tumour may be noticed only after considerable growth has taken place and may then be detected only by an indirect symptom—for instance, a persistent cough or unexplained bleeding or pain. In the case of leukemia, there is no lump, but the changes in the blood will eventually be noticed as increasing fatigue, infection, or abnormal bleeding.

> **biopsy**
> The removal and examination of a small piece of body tissue; a needle biopsy uses a needle to remove a small sample, but some biopsies require surgery.

Metastasis

Metastasis, the spreading of cancer cells from one part of the body to another, occurs because cancer cells do not stick to each other as strongly as normal cells do and therefore may not remain at the site of the *primary tumour* (the cancer's original location). They break away and can pass through the lining of lymph or blood vessels to invade nearby tissue. Once it is established, the tumour can recruit normal cells—such as bone marrow cells—modify them, and use them as envoys to travel to different parts of the body and prepare other sites to receive travelling cancer cells. The envoy cells work by creating proteins that attract the free-floating cancer cells, allowing them to gather at a new site and resume replicating. This travelling and seeding process is called *metastasizing*, and the new tumours are called *secondary tumours*, or *metastases*.

> **metastasis**
> The spread of cancer cells from one part of the body to another.

The ability of cancer cells to metastasize makes early cancer detection critical. To control the cancer, every cancerous cell must be removed. Once cancer cells enter either the lymphatic system or the bloodstream, it is extremely difficult to stop their spread to other organs of the body. In fact, counting the number of lymph nodes that contain cancer cells is one of the principal methods of predicting the outcome of the disease; the probability of a cure is much greater when the lymph nodes do not contain cancer cells.

The Stages of Cancer

Once a cancer has been diagnosed, physicians can use **staging** to classify the disease according to the amount of progress it has made in the person's body. The extent or spread of the cancer is described in five stages, as shown in Table 8.1.

> **staging**
> A method of classifying the progress or extent of a cancer in a person.

To identify a cancer's stage, physicians assess the size or extent of the primary tumour, whether the cancer has invaded nearby lymph nodes, and whether any metastases are present. By judging the extent of each criterion, physicians can determine the cancer's current stage and choose the most appropriate treatment based on the disease's progress.

Types of Cancer

The behaviour of tumours arising in different body organs is characteristic of the tissue of origin.

TABLE 8.1

Cancer Stages

Stage	Description
0	Early cancer, present only in the layer of cells where it originated
I, II, III	More extensive cancer, with higher numbers indicating greater tumour size and/or the degree to which the cancer has spread to nearby lymph nodes or organs adjacent to the primary tumour
IV	Advanced cancer that has spread to another organ

Source: U.S. National Institutes of Health, National Cancer Institute. 2004. Staging: Questions and Answers, http://www.cancer.gov/cancertopics/factsheet/detection/staging (retrieved May 29, 2015).

(Figure 8.3 shows the major cancer sites and the incidence of each type.) Because each cancer begins as a single altered cell with a specific function in the body, the cancer retains some of the properties of the normal cell for a time. For instance, cancer of the thyroid gland may produce too much thyroid hormone and cause hyperthyroidism as well as cancer. Usually, however, cancer cells lose their resemblance to normal tissue as they continue to multiply, becoming groups of rogue cells with increasingly unpredictable behaviour.

Malignant tumours are classified according to the types of cells that give rise to them:

- **Carcinomas** arise from **epithelia**, tissues that cover external body surfaces, line internal tubes and cavities, and form the secreting portion of glands. They are the most common type of cancers; major sites include the skin, breast, uterus, prostate, lungs, and gastrointestinal tract.
- **Sarcomas** arise from connective and fibrous tissues, such as muscle, bone, cartilage, and the membranes covering muscles and fat.
- **Lymphomas** are cancers of the lymph nodes, part of the body's infection-fighting system.
- **Leukemias** are cancers of the blood-forming cells, which reside chiefly in the **bone marrow**.

FIGURE 8.3

Cancer Cases and Deaths by Site and Sex

The "New cases" column indicates the number of cancers that occur annually in each site; the "Percent distribution of cancer deaths" column indicates the number of cancer deaths that are annually attributed to each type.

New cases	Percent distribution of cancer deaths	Male		Female	New cases	Percent distribution of cancer deaths
1 700	2.9	Brain/CNS		Brain/CNS	1 250	2.2
2 900	2.0	Oral		Oral	1 400	1.0
3 500	1.6	Skin (melanoma)		Skin (melanoma)	3 000	1.1
13 400	27.0	Lung		Lung	12 700	26.5
210	0.2	Breast		Breast	24 400	13.8
2 100	3.2	Stomach		Stomach	1 200	2.2
1 600	2.0	Liver		Liver	530	0.7
2 400	5.5	Pancreas		Pancreas	2 300	6.0
3 800	2.8	Kidney		Kidney	2 300	1.8
13 500	12.8	Colorectal		Colorectal	10 800	11.5
6 000	3.8	Bladder*		Bladder*	2 000	1.8
23 600	10.0	Prostate		Ovary	2 700	4.7
1 000	n/a	Testes		Body of Uterus	6 000	2.5
1 450	1.9	Multiple Myeloma		Cervix	1 450	1.0
3 400	3.8	Leukemia		Multiple Myeloma	1 100	1.7
540	n/a	Hodgkin lymphoma		Leukemia	2 600	3.1
4 400	3.6	Non-Hodgkin lymphoma		Hodgkin lymphoma	450	n/a
8 600	12.2	Other		Non-Hodgkin lymphoma	3 600	3.3
97 700		Total*		Other	8 500	13.7
				Total*	93 600	

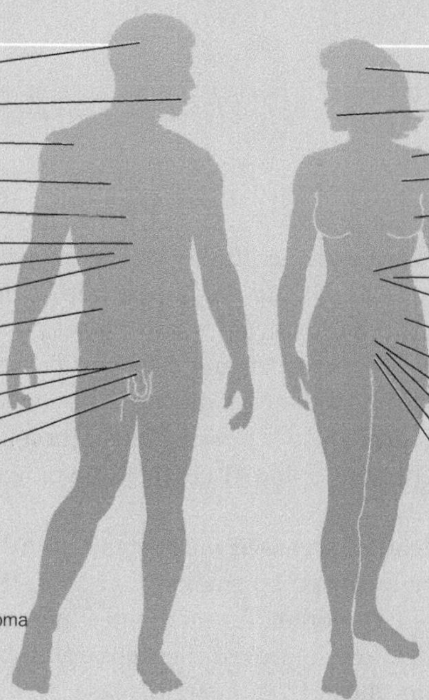

CNS = Central Nervous system
*Ontario does not currently report in situ bladder cancer.
**Column totals may not sum to row totals because of rounding; n/a = not available

CNS = Central Nervous system

*Ontario does not currently report *in situ* bladder cancer.

**Column totals may not sum to row totals because of rounding; n/a = not available

Source: Canadian Cancer Statistics 2014. Produced by Canadian Cancer Society, Statistics Canada, Public Health Agency of Canada, Provincial/Territorial Cancer Registries, http://www.cancer.ca/~/media/cancer.ca/CW/cancer%20information/cancer%20101/Canadian%20cancer%20statistics/Canadian-Cancer-Statistics-2014-EN.pdf. Figure 3.2 (p. 24) and Table 1.2 (p. 38).

carcinomas
Cancers that originate in epithelial tissue (skin, glands, and lining of internal organs).

epithelia
Tissue that covers a surface or lines a tube or cavity of the body, enclosing and protecting other parts of the body.

sarcomas
Cancers arising from bone, cartilage, or striated muscle.

lymphomas
Tumours originating from lymphatic tissue.

leukemias
Cancers of the blood or the blood-forming cells.

bone marrow
Soft vascular tissue in the interior cavities of bones that produces blood cells.

Cancers vary greatly in how easily they can be detected and how well they respond to treatment. For example, certain types of skin cancer are easily detected, grow slowly, and are very easy to remove; virtually all of these cancers are cured. Cancer of the pancreas, conversely, is very difficult to detect or treat, and very few patients survive the disease. In general, it is very difficult for an **oncologist** or a **hematologist** to predict how a specific cancer will behave because each one arises from a unique set of changes in a single cell.

oncologist
A medical specialist in the study of tumours.

hematologist
A medical specialist in the study of blood disorders, including cancers, such as leukemia and lymphoma.

The Incidence of Cancer

About 93 600 women and 97 000 men were expected to be diagnosed with cancer in Canada in 2014—this translates into approximately 3700 Canadians being diagnosed with cancer each week. Most were cured or were able to live years longer. In fact, the Canadian Cancer Society estimates that the five-year survival rate for all cancers that were diagnosed between 2006 and 2008 was 63 percent. This is a 7 percent increase over the five-year relative survival rate for all cancers diagnosed between 1992 and 1994. These statistics exclude almost 82 000 cases of the most curable types of skin cancer (non-melanoma skin cancers). At current Canadian incident rates, nearly 46 percent of men and 41 percent of women will develop cancer at some point in their lives (see the Gender Matters box).

Until 1991, the number of cancer deaths increased fairly steadily in North America, largely because of a wave of lethal lung cancers among men caused by smoking. In 1991, the death rate began to fall slowly; between 1998 and 2007 it dropped about 21 percent in men and 9 percent in women. This trend suggests that efforts at prevention, early detection, and improved therapy are all bearing fruit. However, death rates from cancer are not declining as fast as those from heart disease, in large part because of the differing effects that quitting smoking has on disease risk. Heart damage from smoking reverses more quickly and more significantly than the cancer-related damage from smoking. Smoking-related gene mutations cannot be reversed, although other mechanisms can sometimes control cellular changes. Heart disease also has other risk factors, such as high cholesterol and blood pressure, that can be tested for and controlled. As noted in Chapter 1, because heart disease death rates have continued to decline faster than cancer death rates, cancer has now overtaken heart disease as the leading cause of death among Canadians of all ages.

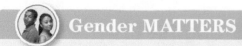

Gender MATTERS

Gender and Cancer

Men and women share most major risk factors for cancer, but they have a different experience because nearly a third of all cancers occur in sex organs (prostate, testes, breast, ovary, uterus, and cervix). In 2013, more 58 000 new cases of cancers in these organs were expected among Canadians.

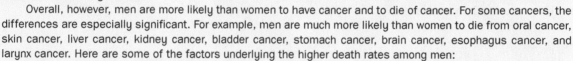

For women, this means that in addition to lifestyle factors such as smoking, diet, and exercise, hormonal factors relating to their menstrual and childbearing history are also important risk considerations. Women may also have a greater biological vulnerability to certain carcinogens, such as those in cigarettes.

Overall, however, men are more likely than women to have cancer and to die of cancer. For some cancers, the differences are especially significant. For example, men are much more likely than women to die from oral cancer, skin cancer, liver cancer, kidney cancer, bladder cancer, stomach cancer, brain cancer, esophagus cancer, and larynx cancer. Here are some of the factors underlying the higher death rates among men:

- *Higher rates of tobacco use:* Particularly in the past, men had significantly higher rates of smoking than women, leading to much higher rates of the many cancers linked to smoking, including oral and bladder cancers. Men also have much higher rates of spit tobacco and cigar use. Lung cancer rates among men increased dramatically following significantly increased smoking rates beginning in the early 1900s (inexpensive machine-produced cigarettes were developed in the late 1800s). The lung cancer rate levelled off and (for men) started to decline after smoking rates began dropping. The smoking-related increase in lung cancer among women occurred about 20–30 years after that seen in men, as smoking among women became more socially acceptable and widespread beginning in the 1930s and 1940s. Rates of lung cancer are now about the same in men and women.

- *Higher rates of alcohol use and abuse:* With 25 percent of Canadian males (compared to 10 percent of females) reporting heavy drinking, alcohol abuse is more common in men and is a risk factor for several cancers, including oral and liver cancers.

- *Greater occupational exposure to carcinogens:* Men are more likely to work in jobs where they are exposed to chemicals—including asbestos, arsenic, coal tar, pitch, and dyes—or radiation, and such exposure is a risk factor for cancers of the bladder, lung, and skin. Men are also more likely to have outdoor jobs involving frequent sun exposure.

- *Less use of preventive measures and less contact with health care providers:* Traditional gender roles may make men more likely to minimize symptoms and less likely to seek help or to discuss cancer-related worries with a health care provider. Men may place a low status on preventive care or screenings, such as using sunscreen and wearing hats to protect the skin from the sun or performing self-exams.

Many of the factors underlying men's greater risk for cancer are controllable. It is important for both men and women to remember that there are many concrete steps they can take to significantly reduce their risk of cancer.

Still, many more people could be saved from cancer. Researchers estimate that 78 percent of skin cancer could be prevented by protecting the skin from the rays of the sun during the first 18 years of life, and 85 percent of lung cancer could be prevented by avoiding exposure to tobacco smoke. Thousands of cases of colon, breast, and uterine cancer could be prevented by improving diet and controlling body weight. Regular screenings and self-examinations have the potential to save an additional 100 000 lives per year. Although cancer may seem like a mysterious disease, many concrete strategies can reduce the risk.

Common Cancers

A discussion of all types of cancer is beyond the scope of this book. In this section we look at some of the most common cancers and their causes, prevention, and treatment.

QUESTIONS FOR CRITICAL THINKING AND REFLECTION

Have you or anyone you know had an experience with cancer? If so, what was the experience like for you/that person, and what was outcome? Have you ever considered whether you might be at risk for some type of cancer? What steps are important for you to take in order to reduce your risk?

Lung Cancer

Lung cancer accounts for approximately 14 percent of all new cancer diagnoses and is the most common cause of cancer death in Canada. It is responsible for more than 20 000 deaths each year, which breaks down to about 388 deaths each week. Since the early 1990s, lung cancer has surpassed breast cancer as the leading cause of cancer death in women.

QUICK STATS

Worldwide, in 2008, 12 million new cases of cancer were diagnosed, 7 million deaths from cancer occurred, and 25 million people were living with a diagnosis of cancer.

—World Health Organization, 2008

Risk Factors

The chief risk factor for lung cancer is tobacco smoke, which currently accounts for 30 percent of all cancer deaths and more than 85 percent of lung cancer deaths. When smoking is combined with exposure to other carcinogens, such as asbestos particles or certain pollutants, the risk of cancer can be multiplied by a factor of 10 or more.

The smoker is not the only one at risk. Environmental tobacco smoke (ETS) is a human carcinogen; even brief exposure can cause serious harm. Long-term exposure to ETS increases the risk of lung cancer. It is estimated that exposure to ETS increases a non-smoker's risk of developing lung cancer by 20–30 percent as compared with people who are not exposed.

Detection and Treatment

Lung cancer is difficult to detect at an early stage and hard to cure even when detected early. Symptoms of lung cancer do not usually appear until the disease has advanced to the invasive stage. Signals such as a persistent cough, chest pain, or recurring bronchitis may be the first indication of a tumour's presence.

Studies suggest that spiral CT (computed tomography) scans, a computer-assisted body imaging technique, can detect lung cancer significantly earlier than chest X-rays. In cases where CT scanning is not available, a diagnosis can usually be made by chest X-ray or by studying the cells in sputum. Because almost all lung cancers arise from the cells that line the bronchi, tumours can

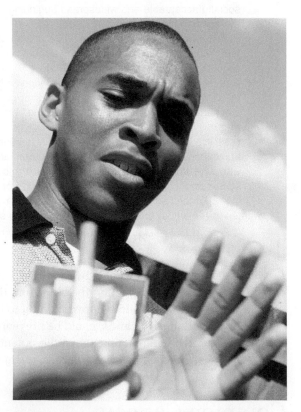

Smoking is responsible for about 30 percent of all cancer deaths. The benefits of quitting are substantial: Lung cancer risk decreases significantly after one smoke-free year and drops to half that of continuing smokers after 10 smoke-free years.

sometimes be visualized by fibre-optic bronchoscopy, a test in which a flexible lighted tube is inserted into the windpipe and the surfaces of the lung passages are directly inspected.

Treatment for lung cancer depends on the type and stage of the cancer. If caught early, localized cancers can be treated with surgery. But because only about 16 percent of lung cancers are detected before they spread, radiation and **chemotherapy** are often used in addition to surgery. For cases detected early, more than half (53 percent) of patients are alive five years after diagnosis; but overall, the five-year survival rate is only 17 percent. Phototherapy, gene therapy, and immunotherapy (a vaccine) are being studied in the hope of improving these statistics. In addition, one form of lung cancer, known as small-cell lung cancer and accounting for about 15 percent of cases, can be treated fairly successfully with chemotherapy, alone or in combination with radiation. A large percentage of cases go into **remission**, which in some cases lasts for years.

chemotherapy
The treatment of cancer with chemicals that selectively destroy cancerous cells.

remission
A period during the course of cancer in which there are no symptoms or other evidence of disease.

Colon and Rectal Cancer

Another common cancer in Canada is colon and rectal cancer (also called *colorectal cancer*). Although we have effective screening methods for colorectal cancer, it is the third most common type of cancer in Canada.

Risk Factors

Age is a key risk factor for colon and rectal cancer, with more than half of cases diagnosed in people age 70 and older. Heredity also plays a role. Many cancers arise from preexisting **polyps**, small growths on the wall of the colon that may gradually develop into malignancies. The tendency to form colon polyps appears to be determined by specific genes, so many colon cancers may be due to inherited gene mutations. Chronic bowel inflammation and type 2 diabetes increase the risk of colon cancer.

polyps
Small, usually harmless, masses of tissue that project from the inner surface of a mucous membrane, such as the colon or rectum.

Lifestyle is also a risk factor for colon and rectal cancer. Excessive alcohol use and smoking may increase the risk of colorectal cancer. Regular physical activity appears to reduce a person's risk, whereas obesity increases it. A diet rich in red and processed meats increases risk, whereas eating fruit, vegetables, and whole grains is associated with lower risk. However, research findings on whether dietary fibre prevents colon cancer have been mixed. Studies have suggested a protective role for folic acid, magnesium, vitamin D, and calcium; in contrast, high intake of refined carbohydrates, simple sugars, and smoked meats and fish may increase risk. The problematic role of simple (refined) sugars in a variety of cancers is a current focus of research; everyone can benefit from reducing refined sugar intake regardless of cancer risk/status.

Use of oral contraceptives or hormone replacement therapy may reduce risk in women. Regular use of non-steroidal anti-inflammatory drugs, such as Aspirin and ibuprofen, may decrease the risk of colon cancer and other cancers of the digestive tract.

Detection and Treatment

If identified early, precancerous polyps and early-stage cancers can be removed before they become malignant or spread. Because polyps may bleed as they progress, the standard warning signs of colon cancer are bleeding from the rectum and a change in bowel habits.

Regular screening tests are recommended beginning at age 50 (earlier for people with a family history of the disease). A yearly stool blood test can detect small amounts of blood in the stool long before obvious bleeding would be noticed. More involved screening tests are recommended at 5-year or 10-year intervals. In sigmoidoscopy or colonoscopy (see Figure 8.4), a flexible fibre-optic device is inserted through the rectum; the colon can be examined and polyps can be biopsied or removed without major surgery. Screening is effective; studies show it could prevent up to 76–90 percent of colon cancers. Still, only about one-half of Canadian adults ages 50–74 are up-to-date with their screenings, with women more likely (53 percent) than men (48 percent) to obtain screening.

Surgery is the primary treatment for colon and rectal cancer. Radiation and chemotherapy may be used before surgery to shrink a tumour or after surgery to destroy any remaining cancerous cells. For advanced cancer, treatment with chemotherapy or monoclonal antibodies in combination is an option. This treatment inhibits the growth of new blood vessels (angiogenesis) in tumours. The five-year survival rate for colorectal cancer is 64 percent for men and 65 percent for women.

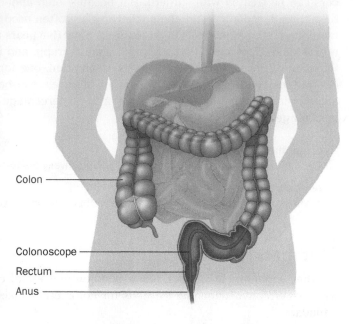

FIGURE 8.4

Colonoscopy

Colon

Colonoscope

Rectum

Anus

Breast Cancer

In Canada, breast cancer is the most common cancer in women and causes about half as many deaths in women as lung cancer. In men, breast cancer occurs only rarely (about 210 estimated cases in 2014). In this country, about 1 woman in 9 will develop breast cancer during her lifetime, and 1 woman in 29 will die from the disease. About 24 600 Canadian women will be diagnosed with breast cancer in the next year, and about 5000 women are expected to die from it in the same time period.

In Canada, fewer than 1 percent of breast cancer cases occur in women under age 30, but a woman's risk increases quickly with age. While fewer than 4 percent of new breast cancer diagnoses are made in women under age 40, the incidence more than triples to 15 percent among those ages 40–49. It nearly doubles again to about 25 percent of new diagnoses made in women ages 50–59, and the highest incidence is found in women ages 60 an older, where 57 percent of new cases are found. This translates into more than 80 percent of breast cancers being diagnosed among women over 50.

Risk Factors

Breast cancer has a strong genetic component. A woman with one first-degree relative (such as a mother or sister) with breast cancer has about twice the risk of developing the disease than those who with no close relatives with it. Those with two close relatives with breast cancer have about a three-fold increased risk. However, even though genetic factors are important, only about 15 percent of cancers occur in women with a family history of breast cancer.

Other risk factors include early onset of menstruation, late onset of menopause, having no children or having a first child after age 30, current use of hormone replacement therapy (HT), obesity, and alcohol use. Estrogen may be a unifying element for many of these risk factors. Estrogen circulates in a woman's body in high concentrations between puberty and menopause. Fat cells also produce estrogen, and estrogen levels are higher in obese women. Alcohol can interfere with estrogen metabolism in the liver and increase estrogen levels in the blood. Estrogen promotes the growth of cells in responsive sites, including the breast and the uterus, so any factor that increases estrogen exposure may raise breast cancer risk. A dramatic drop in rates of breast cancer between 2001 and 2004 was attributed in part to reduced use of HT by women over 50 beginning in July 2002. Millions of women stopped taking the hormones after research linked HT with an increased risk of breast cancer and heart disease.

Although some of the risk factors for breast cancer cannot be changed, important lifestyle risk factors can be controlled. Eating a low-fat, vegetable-rich diet, exercising regularly, limiting alcohol intake, and maintaining a healthy body weight can minimize the chance of developing breast cancer, even for women at risk from family history or other factors. Some research has also found that long-term use of Aspirin and other non-steroidal anti-inflammatory drugs reduces risk, possibly by affecting estrogen synthesis.

Early Detection

A cure is most likely if breast cancer is detected early, so regular screening is a good idea, even for younger women. The Canadian Cancer Society advises the use of the following guidelines for the early detection of breast cancer:

- A ***mammogram*** *(low-dose breast X-ray) at least every two years for women over 50* (see Figure 8.5): Mammography is especially valuable as an early detection tool because it can identify about 85–90 percent of breast cancers at an early stage, before physical symptoms develop. Studies show that magnetic resonance imaging (MRI) may be better than mammography at detecting breast abnormalities in some women, specifically those at high risk or those with dense breast tissue. A number of factors determine a woman's risk for developing breast cancer, and every woman should discuss her risk factors with a physician to determine what kinds of screening tests are warranted.

mammogram
Low-dose X-ray of the breasts used to check for early signs of breast cancer.

Unlike traditional mammography, digital mammograms are recorded on a computer disk rather than film. Digital mammograms can be enhanced and analyzed in more ways than traditional mammograms. Although digital mammography has not yet proved to be more effective at catching breast cancer in all women, there is evidence that it is more effective at spotting tumours in dense breast tissue. A National Cancer Institute study showed that digital mammography might be a better screening tool for women under age 50 who have dense breasts. Although the benefits of early detection and treatment of breast cancer are apparent, mammography is not without risk: It exposes women to X-rays, and X-ray radiation is linked to cancer. A woman's exposure to radiation from screening mammograms depends on the

FIGURE 8.5

Mammogram Image Depicting a Breast Cancer Tumour

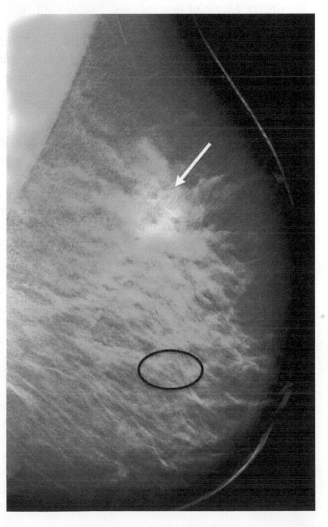

number of tests she has; however, X-ray technicians are well positioned to reduce women's radiation exposure. Research suggests the incidence of a new cancer forming because of radiation from breast screening mammography is very low. Therefore, the benefits of mammograms (i.e., early diagnosis and management of breast cancer) dramatically outweigh the potential threat associated with the small exposure to radiation resulting from a mammogram.

Ultrasound technology uses sound waves to create images of soft tissue. Although ultrasound is not often used as a standard screening tool for breast cancer, it is sometimes used as a follow-up investigational tool if a mammogram reveals an abnormality in breast tissue.

- *Clinical breast exam:* Women between the ages of 40 and 49 should have a clinical breast exam completed by a health professional every two years. Women age 40 and older should have one every year before their scheduled mammogram.
- *Breast awareness:* Breast self-exam (BSE) allows a woman to become familiar with her breasts, so she can alert her health care provider to any changes. For decades, BSE was heavily promoted as a way to detect breast cancer early. However, in 2007 the Canadian Cancer Society stopped recommending routine BSEs as a means of finding cancer. Research indicates that in the absence of mammography, BSE is not likely to reduce breast cancer mortality and can increase the number of benign breast biopsies conducted. In addition to the possible physical risks of biopsies, women face the emotional distress of undergoing a medically invasive procedure only to receive a benign result. Women who choose to continue practising BSE should be informed of its limitations. Beginning at age 20, women are now encouraged to become familiar with their breasts and to recognize what looks and feels normal for them. Women should become "breast aware," know the early symptoms of breast cancer, and notify their doctor of any changes. Unlike with BSE, women do not need to follow a particular technique or schedule.

Breast pain or tenderness is usually associated with benign conditions, such as menstruation, rather than with breast cancer. The first physical signs of breast cancer are more likely to be a lump, swelling, or thickening; skin irritation or dimpling; or nipple pain, scaliness, or retraction. Although most breast lumps are benign, any breast lump should be brought to the attention of a health care provider.

Treatment

If a lump is detected, it may be scanned by **ultrasonography** and biopsied to see if it is cancerous. In 90 percent of cases, the lump is found to be a cyst or other harmless growth, and no further treatment is needed. If the lump contains cancer cells, a variety of surgeries may be called for, ranging from a lumpectomy (removal of the lump and surrounding tissue) to a mastectomy (removal of the breast). For small tumours, lumpectomy is as effective as mastectomy. To determine whether the cancer has spread, lymph nodes from the armpit may be removed and examined. If cancer cells are found, tumour cells remaining in the body can often be slowed or killed by additional therapy, such as radiation, chemotherapy, or both.

> **ultrasonography**
> An imaging method in which sound waves are bounced off body structures to create an image on a TV monitor; also called *ultrasound.*

Survival rates from breast cancer vary depending on the nature of the tumour and whether it has metastasized. If the tumour is discovered before it has spread to the adjacent lymph nodes, the patient has about a 98 percent chance of surviving more than five years. The survival rate for all stages is 88 percent at five years and 82 percent at ten years.

New Strategies for Treatment and Prevention

A number of new drugs have been developed for the treatment or prevention of breast cancer. A family of drugs called selective estrogen-receptor modulators, or SERMs, act like estrogen in some tissues of the body but block estrogen's effects in others. One SERM, tamoxifen, has long been used in breast cancer treatment because it blocks the action of estrogen in breast tissue. In 1998, tamoxifen was approved to reduce the risk of breast cancer in healthy women who are at high risk for the disease. However, the drug has serious potential side effects, including increased risk of blood clots and uterine cancer, and its long-term effects are unknown. Another SERM currently being tested as a potential preventive agent is raloxifene, an osteoporosis drug that has fewer side effects than tamoxifen. Although still controversial, the use of SERMs in the prevention of breast cancer is a major breakthrough.

Women may take tamoxifen, anastrozole, or other drugs or undergo chemotherapy to help reduce the risk of recurrence. A genetic test can help predict the risk of breast cancer recurrence and help identify women who will benefit most from chemotherapy; women can then make more informed treatment decisions. For advanced cancer, treatment with trastuzumab, a monoclonal antibody, is an option for some women. Antibodies, discussed in Chapter 9, are proteins produced by the immune system that recognize and bind to foreign substances, such as bacteria; monoclonal antibodies are a special type of antibody that is produced in the laboratory and designed to bind to a specific cancer-related target.

QUICK STATS

88% of new cancer cases in Canada are diagnosed in people ages 50 and older.
—Canadian Cancer Society, 2013

Prostate Cancer

The prostate gland is situated at the base of the bladder in men and completely surrounds the male's urethra. It produces seminal fluid; if enlarged, it can block the flow of urine. Prostate cancer is the most common cancer in men and the third leading cause of cancer death in men. Approximately 23 600 new cases are diagnosed, and more than 3900 Canadian men die from the disease each year.

Risk Factors

Age is the strongest predictor of the risk, with about 89 percent of cases of prostate cancer diagnosed in men over age 60. Inherited genetic predisposition may be responsible for 5–20 percent of cases, and men with a family history of the disease should be particularly vigilant about screening.

Diets high in calories, dairy products, and animal fats and low in plant foods have also been implicated as possible culprits, as have obesity, inactivity, and a history of sexually transmitted diseases. Type 2 diabetes and insulin resistance are also associated with prostate cancer. Soy foods, tomatoes, and cruciferous vegetables are being investigated for their possible protective effects.

Detection

Early prostate cancer usually has no symptoms. Warning signs of prostate cancer can include changes in urinary frequency, weak or interrupted urine flow, painful urination, and blood in the urine.

Techniques for early detection include a digital rectal examination and the **prostate-specific antigen (PSA) blood test**. The Canadian Cancer Society recommends that men be provided information about the benefits and limitations of the tests and that men over 50 years of age talk with their doctor about screening for prostate cancer. Men at high risk, including North Americans of African descent and those with a family history of the disease, should speak with their doctor about the appropriateness of being tested earlier.

prostate-specific antigen (PSA) blood test
A diagnostic test for prostate cancer that measures blood levels of prostate-specific antigen (PSA).

During a digital rectal exam, a physician feels the prostate gland through the rectum to determine if the gland is enlarged or if lumps are present. The PSA blood test may detect an elevated level or a rapid increase in PSA. The PSA test can help catch early prostate cancer, but it also can register benign conditions (more than half of men over age 50 have benign prostate disease) and very slow-growing cancers that are unlikely to kill affected individuals. Further, it is not rare for men with normal PSA levels to have prostate cancer.

Because PSA tests can yield false-positive results, they may lead men to receive further testing or treatment that is not needed. Researchers are looking for ways to make the PSA test more sensitive. A new approach involves measuring the percentage of PSA that is free floating in the blood. PSA made by cancer cells is more likely to circulate bound to other proteins, whereas PSA from healthy prostate cells is more likely to be unbound. Thus, a low proportion of unbound or free PSA indicates greater risk, while a high proportion of free PSA is associated with lower risk.

PSA testing has been a subject of controversy among experts for several years because of its tendency to yield misleading results, leading to further testing that can lead to harm. This is especially a concern for men over age 75, who are more likely to die of other causes even if they have slow-growing prostate cancer. In older men, most prostate cancers are not deadly, making treatments pointless and potentially harmful. The Canadian Task Force on Preventive Health Care recommends against PSA screening; however, the Canadian Cancer Society recommends that men over age 50 should talk to their doctor about getting tested for prostate cancer.

Ultrasound is being used increasingly as a follow-up to detect lumps too small to be felt and to determine their size, shape, and properties. A needle biopsy of suspicious lumps can be performed relatively painlessly, and whether the biopsied cells are malignant or benign can be determined by examining them under a microscope.

Treatment

Treatments vary based on the stage of the cancer and the age of the patient. A small, slow-growing tumour in an older man may be treated with watchful waiting because he is more likely to die from another cause before his cancer becomes life threatening; however, a recent study shows that older men who undergo treatment live longer than those who don't. More aggressive treatment would be indicated for younger men or those with more advanced cancers. Treatment usually involves radical prostatectomy, in which the prostate is removed surgically. Although radical surgery has an excellent cure rate, it is major surgery and often results in **incontinence** or erectile dysfunction.

incontinence
The inability to control the flow of urine.

A less-invasive alternative involves surgical implantation of radioactive seeds. Radiation from the seeds destroys the tumour and much of the normal prostate tissue but leaves surrounding tissue relatively untouched. Alternative or additional treatments include external radiation, hormones that shrink tumours, cryotherapy, and chemotherapy. Survival rates for all stages of this cancer have improved steadily over the last two decades; the five-year survival rate is now 96 percent.

Cancers of the Female Reproductive Tract

Because the uterus, cervix, and ovaries are subject to similar hormonal influences, the cancers of these organs can be discussed as a group.

QUICK STATS

9650 cases of female genital system cancers were expected to be diagnosed in 2013.
—Statistics Canada, 2013

Cervical Cancer

Cancer of the cervix occurs frequently in women in their thirties or even twenties. In Canada, more than 1400 women are diagnosed with cervical cancer each year; the disease kills 380 annually.

Cervical cancer is at least in part a sexually transmitted infection. Almost all cases of cervical cancer stem from infection by the human papillomavirus (HPV), a group of about 100 related viruses that cause both common warts and genital warts. When certain types of HPV are introduced into the cervix, usually by an infected sex partner, the virus infects cervical cells, causing the cells to divide and grow. If unchecked, this growth can develop into cervical cancer. Cervical cancer is associated with multiple sex partners and is extremely rare in women who have not had heterosexual intercourse. Of those Canadian men and women who are sexually active, it is estimated that more than 70 percent will develop at least one HPV infection during their lifetime. The regular use of condoms can reduce the risk of transmitting HPV. Studies also suggest that women whose sexual partners are circumcised may be at reduced risk because circumcised men are less likely to be infected with HPV and to pass it to their partners.

Because only a very small percentage of HPV-infected women ever get cervical cancer, other factors must be involved. Two of the most important seem to be smoking and infection with genital herpes (discussed in Chapter 13 with other STIs). Both smoking and herpes infection can cause cancerous changes in cells in the laboratory and can speed and intensify the cancerous changes begun by HPV. Research suggests that women with high levels of HPV 16, a specific form of HPV, are at particularly high risk for the infection to develop into cancer. Some studies show that past exposure to the bacterium that causes the STI chlamydia may be a risk factor for cervical cancer that operates independently of HPV.

Screening for the changes in cervical cells that precede cancer is done chiefly by means of the **Pap test**. During a pelvic exam, cells are scraped from the cervix and examined under a microscope to see whether they are normal. If cells are abnormal but not yet cancerous, a condition commonly referred to as *cervical dysplasia*, the Pap test is repeated at intervals. Sometimes cervical cells spontaneously return to normal, but in about one-third of cases, the cellular changes progress toward malignancy. If this happens, the abnormal cells must be removed, either surgically or by destroying them with a cryoscopic (ultra-cold) probe or localized laser treatment. When the abnormal cells are in a precancerous state, the small patch of dangerous cells can be completely removed.

Pap test
A scraping of cells from the cervix for examination under a microscope to detect cancer.

Without timely surgery, the malignant patch of cells goes on to invade the wall of the cervix and spreads to adjacent lymph nodes and to the uterus. At this stage, chemotherapy may be used with radiation to kill the fast-growing cancer cells, but chances for a complete cure are lower. Even when a cure can be achieved, it often means surgical removal of the uterus.

Because the Pap test is highly effective, all sexually active women and women between ages 18 and 65 should be tested. The recommended schedule for testing depends on risk factors, the type of Pap test performed, and whether the Pap test is combined with HPV testing.

A vaccine called Gardasil that protects against four types of HPV viruses, including two that cause about 70 percent of cervical cancer cases, has been approved for use in Canada. Studies show that the vaccine, given in three doses over six months, also protects against cancers of the vagina and vulva. Vaccination works best when given to girls before they become sexually active, but the recommendation also allows for vaccination of girls and women ages 9–26. In 2010, Health Canada also approved the Gardasil vaccine for boys and men ages 9–26 to prevent genital warts. Cervarix, which prevents certain types of HPV, has also been approved for use in Canada among females ages 10–25.

Preliminary studies are providing good support for Gardasil's ability to prevent HPV among vaccinated females. However, vaccinated females are still encouraged to have a Pap test at regular intervals since the vaccine does not protect against all types of HPV. In March 2007, the Government of Canada announced $300 million for provinces and territories to establish an HPV immunization program. In Ontario, the government has created an immunization program that entitles all Grade 8 students to receive the vaccine free (Gardasil is an expensive vaccine at $135/dose).

QUICK STATS

4 million Pap tests are performed each year in Canada; about 8% are abnormal and require medical follow-up.
—Canadian Women's Health Network, 2012

Uterine, or Endometrial, Cancer

Cancer of the lining of the uterus, or endometrium, most often occurs after the age of 55. Uterine cancer affects about 5600 Canadian women annually and kills about 890 women each year. The risk factors are similar to those for breast cancer, including prolonged exposure to estrogen, early onset of menstruation, late menopause, never having been pregnant, and obesity. Type 2 diabetes is also associated with increased risk. The use of oral contraceptives, which combine estrogen and progestin, appears to provide protection.

Endometrial cancer is usually detectable by pelvic examination. It is treated surgically, commonly by hysterectomy (removal of the uterus). Radiation treatment, hormones, and chemotherapy may be used in addition to surgery. Of those diagnosed with uterine cancer, about 85 percent of patients are alive and disease-free five years later.

Ovarian Cancer

Although ovarian cancer is rare compared with cervical or uterine cancer, it causes more deaths than the other two combined. Ovarian cancer often has no warning signs. Early clues may include increased abdominal size and bloating, urinary urgency, and pelvic pain. It cannot be detected by Pap tests or any other simple screening method, and is often diagnosed only late in its development, when surgery and other therapies are unlikely to be successful.

The risk factors are similar to those for breast and endometrial cancer: increasing age (most ovarian cancer occurs after age 60), never having been pregnant, a family history of breast or ovarian cancer, obesity, and specific genetic mutations. A high number of ovulations appears to increase the chance that a cancer-causing genetic mutation will occur, so anything that lowers the number of lifetime ovulation cycles—pregnancy, breastfeeding, or use of oral contraceptives—reduces a woman's risk of ovarian cancer. A diet rich in fruit and vegetables may be associated with reduced risk.

Women with symptoms or who are at high risk because of family history or because they harbour a mutant gene should have thorough pelvic exams at regular intervals, as recommended by their physician. Pelvic exams may include the use of ultrasound to view the ovaries.

Ovarian cancer is treated by surgical removal of both ovaries, the fallopian tubes, and the uterus. Radiation and chemotherapy are sometimes used in addition to surgery. The five-year survival rate is only 45 percent, reflecting the difficulty of early detection.

Skin Cancer

Skin cancer is the most common cancer when cases of the highly curable forms are included in the count. (Usually these forms are not included, precisely because they are easily treated. Treatments are usually simple and successful when the cancers are caught early.) But of the 81 700 cases of skin cancer diagnosed each year, 6000 are of the most serious type, **melanoma**.

> **melanoma**
> A malignant tumour of the skin that arises from pigmented cells, usually a mole.

QUICK STATS

People with more than 50 moles are at increased risk for skin cancer.
—Canadian Dermatology Association, 2014

Risk Factors

Almost all cases of skin cancer can be traced to excessive exposure to **ultraviolet (UV) radiation** from the sun, including longer-wavelength ultraviolet A (UVA) and shorter-wavelength ultraviolet B (UVB) radiation. UVB radiation causes sunburns and can damage the eyes and the immune system. UVA is less likely to cause an immediate sunburn, but by damaging connective tissue it leads to premature aging of the skin, giving it a wrinkled, leathery appearance. (Tanning lamps and tanning-salon beds emit mostly UVA radiation.) Both UVA and UVB radiation have been linked to the development of skin cancer, and both solar and artificial sources of UV radiation, including sunlamps and tanning beds, are known human carcinogens.

> **ultraviolet (UV) radiation**
> Light rays of a specific wavelength emitted by the sun; most UV rays are blocked by the ozone layer in the upper atmosphere.

Both severe, acute sun reactions (sunburns) and chronic low-level sun reactions (suntans) can lead to skin cancer. People with fair skin have less natural protection against skin damage from the sun and a higher risk of developing skin cancer; people with naturally dark skin have a considerable degree of protection (see the Assess Yourself box). Melanoma is more common among Caucasians, particularly those with light-coloured skin. For example, in the United States, the annual average incidence rates for melanoma in 1999–2010 were 0.9 per 100 000 for black people, 3.8 per 100 000 for Hispanics, and 19.1 per 100 000 for white people. Although the statistics are likely similar in Canada, the Canadian Cancer Registry does not record ethnicity of the 6000 Canadians affected, and so race-specific rates cannot be estimated for the Canadian population. In general, men are more likely to develop and die from melanoma.

Severe sunburns in childhood have been linked to a greatly increased risk of skin cancer in later life, so children in particular should be protected. The risk of skin cancer increases in people who have had sunburns during childhood. In fact, the earlier in life a child is burned, the greater their risk for developing skin cancer later in life. Because of damage to the ozone layer of the atmosphere (discussed in Chapter 21), we may all be exposed to increasing amounts of UV radiation in the future.

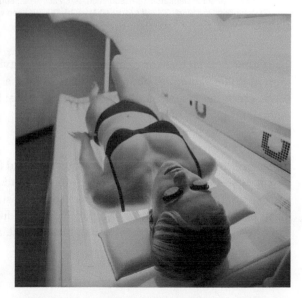

Tanning, either under direct sunlight or in a tanning bed, is a known cause of skin cancer.

Assess YOURSELF

Sun Sensitivity Test

Your risk for developing skin cancer depends on:
- How much sun you get at work and during recreation
- How much your skin reacts to the sun

Try the **Sun Sensitivity Test** to determine your risk of developing skin cancer.

	Yes	No
I have red or blonde hair.	☐	☐
I have light-coloured eyes—blue, green, or grey.	☐	☐
I freckle easily.	☐	☐
I always burn before I tan.	☐	☐
I have many moles.	☐	☐
I had two or more blistering sunburns before the age of 18.	☐	☐
I lived or had long vacations in a tropical climate as a child.	☐	☐
There is a family history of skin cancer.	☐	☐
I work outdoors in spring and summer.	☐	☐
I spend a lot of time in outdoor recreation.	☐	☐
Score 10 points for each "Yes."		

Scores

70–100 You are in the high-risk zone for skin cancer and other skin damage. Be careful and protect your skin from the sun.

40–60 You are increased risk for skin cancer. Pick up tips on sun protection.

10–30 You are still at risk. Carry on being careful.

Source: Canadian Dermatology Association. n.d. *Fact Sheet: Sun Sensitivity Test*, http://www.dermatology.ca/wp-content/uploads/2012/01/SunSensitivityTest_EN.pdf (retrieved May 28, 2015). Used with permission of The Canadian Dermatology Association.

Other risk factors for skin cancer include having many moles, particularly large ones; spending time at high altitudes; and a family history of the disease. Skin cancer may also be caused by exposure to coal tar, pitch, creosote, arsenic, and radioactive materials; but compared with sunlight, these agents account for only a small proportion of cases.

Types of Skin Cancer

There are three main types of skin cancer, named for the types of skin cells from which they develop. **Basal cell** and **squamous cell carcinomas** together account for about 93 percent of the skin cancers diagnosed each year. They are usually found in chronically sun-exposed areas, such as the face, neck, hands, and arms. They usually appear as pale, waxlike, pearly nodules or red, scaly, sharply outlined patches. These cancers are often painless, although they may bleed, crust, and form an open sore on the skin.

basal cell carcinoma
Cancer of the deepest layers of the skin.

squamous cell carcinoma
Cancer of the surface layers of the skin.

Melanoma is by far the most dangerous skin cancer because it spreads so rapidly. It can occur anywhere on the body, but the most common sites are the back, chest, abdomen, and lower legs. A melanoma usually appears at the site of a preexisting mole. The mole may begin to enlarge, become mottled or varied in colour (colours can include grey or blue, pink or red, and white), or develop an irregular surface or irregular borders. Tissue invaded by melanoma may also itch, burn, or bleed easily.

Prevention

One of the major steps you can take to protect yourself against all forms of skin cancer is to avoid overexposure to sunlight. Blistering, peeling sunburns from unprotected sun exposure are particularly dangerous, but suntans—whether from sunlight or tanning lamps—also increase your risk of developing skin cancer later in life. People of every age, especially babies and children, need to be protected from the sun with sunscreen and protective clothing. For a closer look at sunlight and skin cancer, see the Critical Consumer box.

Detection and Treatment

The only sure way to avoid a serious outcome from skin cancer is to make sure it is recognized and diagnosed early. Make it a habit to examine your skin regularly. Most of the spots, freckles, moles, and blemishes on your body are normal; you were born with some of them, and others appear and disappear throughout your life. But if you notice an unusual growth, discoloration, a sore that does not heal, or a mole that undergoes a sudden or progressive change, see your physician or a dermatologist immediately.

The characteristics that may signal a skin lesion as a melanoma—asymmetry, border irregularity, colour change, and a diameter greater than 0.5 centimetres—are shown in Figure 8.6. A mole that changes in size, shape, or colour is also of concern. In addition, if someone in your family has had numerous skin cancers or melanoma, consult a dermatologist for a complete skin examination and discussion of your particular risk.

If you have an unusual skin lesion, your physician will examine it and possibly perform a biopsy. If the lesion is cancerous, it is usually removed surgically, a procedure that can almost always be performed in the physician's office using a local anaesthetic. Occasionally, other forms of treatment may be used. Even for melanoma, the outlook after removal in the early stages is good, with a five-year survival rate of almost 90 percent.

FIGURE 8.6

The ABCDE Test for Melanoma

To see a variety of photos of melanoma and benign moles, visit SkinCancerGuide.ca (http://www.skincancerguide.ca/sitemap.html).

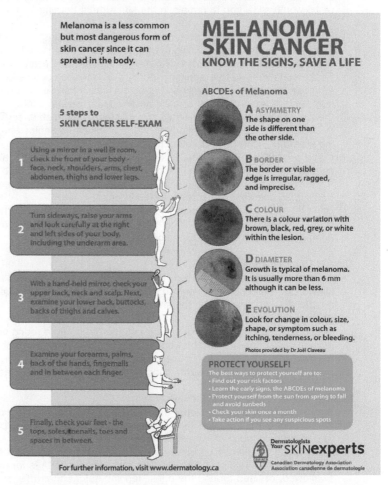

Source: Canadian Dermatology Association. 2009. *Melanoma Skin Cancer: Know the Signs, Save a Life,* http://www.dermatology.ca/wp-content/uploads/2012/01/MMPoster2009-EN.pdf (retrieved May 29, 2015).

Critical CONSUMER

Choosing and Using Sunscreen and Sun-Protective Clothing

With consistent use of the proper clothing, sunscreen, and common sense, you can lead an active outdoor life *and* protect your skin against most sun-induced damage.

Clothing

- *Wear long-sleeved shirts and long pants.* Dark-coloured, tightly woven fabrics provide reasonable protection from the sun. Another good choice is clothing made from special sun-protective fabrics; these garments have an ultraviolet protection factor (UPF) rating, similar to the sun protection factor (SPF) for sunscreen. For example, a fabric with a UPF rating of 20 allows only one-twentieth of the sun's UV radiation to pass through. There are three categories of UPF protection: A UPF of 15–24 provides good UV protection; a UPF of 25–39 provides very good protection; and a UPF of 40–50 provides excellent protection. By comparison, typical shirts provide a UPF of only 5–9, a value that drops when clothing is wet.
- *Wear a hat.* Your face, ears, neck, and scalp are especially vulnerable to the sun's harmful effects, making hats essential. A good choice is a broad-brimmed hat or a legionnaire-style cap that covers the ears and neck. Wear sunscreen on your face even if you are wearing a hat.
- *Wear sunglasses.* Exposure to UV rays can damage the eyes and cause cataracts.

Sunscreen

- Use a sunscreen and lip balm with a SPF of 15 or higher. (An SPF rating refers to the amount of time you can stay out in the sun before you burn, compared with not using sunscreen. For example, a product with an SPF of 15 would allow you to remain in the sun without burning 15 times as long, on average, as you could if you didn't apply sunscreen.)
- Choose a broad-spectrum sunscreen that protects against both UVA and UVB radiation. The SPF rating of a sunscreen currently applies only to UVB, but a number of ingredients, especially titanium dioxide and zinc oxide, are effective at blocking most UVA radiation. Use a water-resistant sunscreen if you swim or sweat a great deal.
- Shake sunscreen before applying. Apply it 30 minutes before exposure to allow it time to bond to the skin. Reapply sunscreen frequently and generously to all sun-exposed areas (many people overlook their temples, ears, and sides and backs of their necks). Most people use less than half as much as they need to attain the full SPF rating. Thirty millilitres of sunscreen is enough to cover an average-size adult wearing a swimsuit. Reapply sunscreen 15–30 minutes after sun exposure begins and then every two hours after that and following activities, such as swimming, that could remove sunscreen.
- If you are taking medications, ask your physician or pharmacist about possible reactions to sunlight or interactions with sunscreens. Medications for acne, allergies, and diabetes are just a few of the products that can trigger reactions. If you are using sunscreen and an insect repellent containing DEET, use extra sunscreen (DEET may decrease sunscreen's effectiveness).
- Don't let sunscreens give you a false sense of security. Most of the sunscreens currently on the market allow considerable UVA radiation to penetrate the skin, with the potential for causing skin cancers (especially melanoma), wrinkles, and other forms of skin damage.

Time of Day and Location

- Avoid sun exposure between 10 a.m. and 4 p.m., when the sun's rays are most intense. While a clear sky allows 100 percent of UV rays to reach the skin, scattered clouds still allow as much as 89 percent of UV rays to get through. Stay in the shade when you can.
- Consult the day's UV Index, which predicts UV levels on a 0–10+ scale, to get a sense of the amount of sun protection you will need; take special care on days with a rating of 5 or above. UV Index ratings are available in local newspapers, from the weather bureau, or from certain websites.
- Be aware that UV rays can penetrate at least 9 metres in water, so swimmers should wear water-resistant sunscreens. Snow, sand, water, concrete, and white-painted surfaces are also highly reflective.

Tanning Salons and Sunless Tanning Products

- Stay away from tanning salons! Despite advertising claims to the contrary, the lights used in tanning parlours are damaging to your skin. Tanning beds and lamps emit mostly UVA radiation, increasing your risk of premature skin aging (such as wrinkles) and skin cancer.
- If you really want a tan, consider using a sunless tanning product. Lotions, creams, and sprays containing the colour additive dihydroxyacetone (DHA) are available. DHA is for external use only and should not be inhaled, swallowed, or used around the eyes. Tanning salons that offer spraying or misting with DHA need to ensure that customers are protected from exposure to the eyes, lips, and mucous membranes, as well as internal exposure. Most sunless tanning products do not contain sunscreen, so if you use them in the sun, be sure to wear sunscreen.

Oral Cancer

Oral cancer—cancers of the lip, tongue, mouth, and throat—can be traced principally to cigarette, cigar, or pipe smoking, the use of spit tobacco, and the excessive consumption of alcohol. These risk factors work together to multiply a person's risk of oral cancer. The incidence of oral cancer is twice as great in men as in women and most frequent in men over 40. Some prominent sufferers of oral cancer have included Sigmund Freud and Fidel Castro, both notorious cigar smokers. Sports figures who have cultivated a taste for spit tobacco are now also increasingly being diagnosed with oral cancer. Among long-term snuff users, the excess risk of cancers of the cheek, tongue, and gum is nearly 50-fold (see Chapter 16 for more on cigars and spit tobacco).

Oral cancers are fairly easy to detect but are often hard to cure. And among those who survive, a significant number will develop another primary cancer of the head and neck. The main methods of treatment are surgery and radiation. The five-year survival rate is about 63 percent.

Testicular Cancer

Testicular cancer is relatively rare, accounting for only 1.1 percent of cancer in men (about 960 cases per year), but it is particularly prevalent among men ages 15–49. In general, testicular cancer has the lowest rates among Asian and black populations, while rates are increased among men whose father or brother had testicular cancer. Men with undescended testicles are at increased risk for testicular cancer, and for this reason the condition should be corrected in early childhood. Men whose mothers took DES (diethylstilbestrol, a synthetic form of estrogen) during pregnancy have an increased risk of undescended testicles and other genital anomalies. Thus, they may have a higher risk of testicular cancer.

Self-examination may help in the early detection of testicular cancer (see the Take Charge box). Tumours are treated by surgical removal of the testicle and, if the tumour has spread, by chemotherapy. The five-year survival rate for testicular cancer is 97 percent.

 Take **CHARGE**

Testicle Self-Examination

The best time to perform a testicular self-exam is after a warm shower or bath, when the scrotum is relaxed. First, stand in front of a mirror and look for any swelling of the scrotum. Then examine each testicle with both hands. Place the index and middle fingers under the testicle and the thumbs on top; roll the testicle gently between the fingers and thumbs. Don't worry if one testicle seems slightly larger than the other—that's common. Also, expect to feel the epididymis, the soft, sperm-carrying tube at the rear of the testicle.

Perform the self-exam each month. If you find a lump, swelling, or nodule, consult a physician right away. The abnormality may not be cancer, but only a physician can make a diagnosis. Other possible signs of testicular cancer include a change in the way a testicle feels, a sudden collection of fluid in the scrotum, a dull ache in the lower abdomen or groin, a feeling of heaviness in the scrotum, or pain in a testicle or the scrotum.

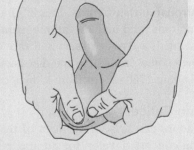

Source: Testicular Cancer Resource Center. 2009. *How to Do a Testicular Self Examination*, http://tcrc.acor.org/tcexam.html (retrieved May 28, 2015).

Other Cancers

Several other cancers affect a significant number of people each year. Some have identifiable risk factors, particularly smoking and obesity, that are controllable; the causes of others are still under investigation.

Pancreatic Cancer

The pancreas, a gland found deep within the abdomen behind the stomach, produces both digestive enzymes and insulin. Because of the gland's hidden location, pancreatic cancer is usually well advanced before symptoms become noticeable. Each year there are about 4700 new cases and about 4300 deaths from pancreatic cancer in Canada. About 20–30 percent of cases are linked to smoking. Other risk factors include being male, obese, sedentary, or over age 65; inheriting a disorder, such as hereditary pancreatitis; having diabetes; and eating a diet high in fat and meat and low in vegetables. Pancreatic cancer can be treated in many ways, but the disease is seldom cured.

Stomach Cancer

In many parts of the world, stomach cancer is the most common form of cancer. It is relatively unusual in Canada, with about 3300 new cases and 2000 deaths each year. It tends to occur after age 50 and is more than twice as common in men as in women. Risk factors include infection with the bacterium *Helicobacter pylori*, which has also been linked to the development of ulcers, and a diet high in smoked, salted, or pickled fish or meat. Bacteria, including *H. pylori*, can convert the nitrites in preserved foods into carcinogenic amines, and salt can break down the normal protective stomach coating, allowing these carcinogenic compounds access to the cells of the stomach wall. However, the great majority of people with *H. pylori* infection do not develop stomach cancer, particularly if they maintain a low-salt diet with plenty of fruit, vegetables, and whole grains.

There is no screening test for stomach cancer; it is usually recognized only after it has spread, and the five-year survival rate is only 25 percent for all stages.

Bladder Cancer

Bladder cancer is more than three times as common in men as in women, and smoking is the key risk factor. Smokers are 2.2 times as likely to develop bladder cancer as are non-smokers. People living in urban areas and workers exposed to chemicals used in the dye, rubber, and leather industries are also at increased risk.

There is no screening test for bladder cancer. The first symptoms are likely to be blood in the urine or increased frequency of urination. These symptoms can also signal a urinary tract infection but should trigger a visit to a physician, who can evaluate the possibility of cancer. With early detection, more than 90 percent of cases are curable. There are about 7900 new cases and about 2100 deaths from bladder cancer each year in Canada.

Kidney Cancer

Although kidney cancer usually occurs in people over age 50, anyone can develop it, and there are few controllable risk factors. Smoking and obesity are mild risk factors, as is a family history of the disease. Symptoms may include fatigue, pain in the side, and blood in the urine. Kidney cancer has been difficult to treat, with a five-year survival rate of only 68 percent for all stages. Recently, immune cell therapies have shown some promise in the disease's advanced stage. In Canada, there are about 5900 new cases each year and about 1750 deaths from kidney cancer.

Brain Cancer

Tumours can arise from most of the many types of cells that are found in the brain. The vast majority of brain cancers develop for no apparent reason; one of the few established risk factors is ionizing radiation, such as X-rays. Before the risks were recognized, children with ringworm of the scalp (a fungal infection) often received low-dose radiation therapy, which substantially increased their risk of brain tumours later in life. Symptoms are often non-specific and include headaches, fatigue, behavioural changes, and sometimes seizures. The incidence of these tumours has increased slightly over the past 20 years, but this increase may be due to improved methods of diagnosis. Some brain tumours are curable by surgery or by radiation and chemotherapy, but most are not. Survival time varies, depending on the type of the tumour, from one to eight years. In Canada each year, there are about 2900 new cases and 1950 deaths.

Leukemia

Leukemia, cancer of the white blood cells, can affect both children and adults. It starts in the bone marrow but can then spread to the lymph nodes, spleen, liver, other organs, and central nervous system. Like brain cancer, it is a complex disease with many different types and subtypes. Most people with leukemia have no known risk factors. About 20 percent of cases of adult leukemia are related to smoking; other possible risk factors include radiation and certain chemicals and infections. Most symptoms occur because leukemia cells crowd out the production of normal blood cells; the result can be fatigue, anemia, weight loss, and increased risk of infection. Treatment and survival rates vary, depending on the exact type and other factors. There are about 5800 new cases and 2600 deaths from leukemia each year in Canada.

Lymphoma

Arising from the lymph cells, lymphoma begins in the lymph nodes and then may spread to almost any part of the body. There are two types: Hodgkin's disease and non-Hodgkin's lymphoma (NHL). NHL is the more common and more deadly form of the disease. It is the sixth most common cancer in Canada, with about 7800 people diagnosed annually; just fewer than half of all patients will eventually die from the disease. Risk factors for NHL are not well understood, but people with compromised immune systems are at much greater risk, especially when exposed to radiation or certain infections and chemicals. A new therapy based on the use of antibodies has shown promise in treating patients. Rates of Hodgkin's disease in Canada have fallen by more than 50 percent since the early 1970s, and there are now about 1000 cases in Canada each year.

Multiple Myeloma

Normal plasma cells play an important role in the immune system, producing antibodies. Malignant plasma cells may produce tumours in several sites, particularly in the bone marrow; when they grow in multiple sites, they are referred to as multiple myeloma (MM). By crowding out normal bone marrow cells, MM can lead to anemia, excessive bleeding, and decreased resistance to infection. There is no single cause of multiple myeloma, however age appears to be a significant factor: those 60 years or older are at increased risk. Other risk factors are not well understood, although MM is more common among black people. Obesity has been associated with MM. There are about 2500 new cases in Canada each year and 1350 deaths.

QUESTIONS FOR CRITICAL THINKING AND REFLECTION

How many people do you know who have been diagnosed with cancer? Based on the information presented so far in this chapter, which known risk factors did the person/people have for the disease? What have you learned so far about reducing your personal risk factors for cancer?

The Causes of Cancer

Although scientists do not know everything about what causes cancer, they have identified genetic, environmental, and lifestyle factors.

The Role of DNA

Heredity and genetics are important factors in a person's risk of cancer. Certain genes may predispose some people to cancer, and specific genetic mutations have been associated with cancer.

DNA Basics

The nucleus of each cell in your body contains 23 pairs of **chromosomes**, which are made up of tightly packed coils of **DNA** (deoxyribonucleic acid). DNA consists of two long strands wound around each other in a spiral structure, like a twisted ladder; scientists refer to this spiral as a double helix. The rungs of the ladder are made from four different nucleotide bases: adenine, thymine, cytosine, and guanine, or A, T, C, and G. The arrangement of nucleotide bases along the double helix constitutes the genetic code. You can think of this code as a set of instructions for building, operating, and repairing your body.

chromosomes
The threadlike bodies in a cell nucleus that contain molecules of DNA; most human cells contain 23 pairs of chromosomes.

DNA
Deoxyribonucleic acid, a chemical substance that carries genetic information.

A *gene*, as described in Chapter 1, is a smaller unit of DNA made up of a specific sequence of nucleotide bases. Each chromosome contains hundreds, and in some cases thousands, of genes; you have about 25 000 genes in all. Each of your genes controls the production of a particular protein. The makeup of each protein—which amino acids it contains and in what sequence—is determined by its precise sequence of A, T, C, and G. Proteins build cells and make them work: They serve both as the structural material for your body and as the regulators of all chemical reactions and metabolic processes. By making different proteins at different times, genes can act as switches to alter the ways a cell works.

Cells reproduce by dividing in two, and your body makes billions of new cells every day. When a cell divides, the DNA replicates itself so that each new cell has a complete set of chromosomes. Through the proteins for which they code, some genes are responsible for controlling the rate of cell division, and some types of cells divide much more rapidly than others. Genes that control the rate of cell division often play a critical role in the development of cancer.

QUICK STATS

About 5–10% of all cancers have a strong hereditary component.
—Canadian Cancer Society, 2014

DNA Mutations and Cancer

A *mutation* is any change in the normal makeup of a gene. Some mutations are inherited. If the egg or sperm cell that produces a child contains a mutation, so will every one of the child's 30 trillion cells. Environmental agents can also produce mutational damage; these **mutagens** include radiation, certain viruses, and chemical substances in the air we breathe. (When a mutagen also causes cancer, it is called a *carcinogen*.) Some mutations are the result of copying errors that occur when DNA replicates itself as part of cell division.

mutagens
Environmental factors that can cause mutation, such as radiation and atmospheric chemicals.

A mutated gene no longer contains the proper code for producing its protein. Because a cell has two copies of each gene, it can sometimes get by with only one functioning version. In this case, the mutation may have no effect on health. However, if both copies of a gene are damaged or if the cell needs two normal copies to function properly, then the cell will cease to behave normally.

It usually takes several mutational changes over several years before a normal cell takes on the properties of a cancer cell. Genes in which mutations are associated with the conversion of a normal cell into a cancer cell are known as **oncogenes**. In their undamaged form, many oncogenes play a role in controlling or restricting cell growth; these are **tumour suppressor genes**. Mutational damage to these genes releases the brake on growth and leads to rapid and uncontrolled cell division—a precondition for the development of cancer.

oncogenes
Genes involved in the transformation of a normal cell into a cancer cell.

tumour suppressor genes
A type of oncogene that normally functions to restrain cellular growth.

A good example of how a series of mutational changes can produce cancer is provided by the *p53* gene, located on chromosome 17. In its normal form, the protein that is coded for by this gene actually helps prevent cancer: If a cell's DNA is damaged, the *p53* protein can either kill the cell outright or stop it from replicating until the damaged DNA is repaired. For example, if a skin cell's DNA is mutated by exposure to sunlight, the *p53* protein activates the cell's "suicide" machinery. By thus preventing the replication of damaged DNA, the *p53* protein keeps cells from progressing toward cancer. However, if the *p53* gene itself undergoes a mutation, these controls are lost, and the cell can become cancerous. In fact, the damaged version of *p53* can actually promote cell division and the spread of cancer. Researchers believe that damage to the *p53* gene and protein may be involved, directly and indirectly, in as many as 50–60 percent of cancers of all types.

Hereditary Cancer Risks

One way to obtain a mutated oncogene is to inherit it. One example is *BRCA1* (breast cancer gene 1): Women who inherit a damaged copy of this suppressor gene face a significantly increased risk of breast and ovarian cancer. In most cases, however, mutational damage occurs after birth. Although some specific genes do increase the risk for some cancers, many researchers say it is unlikely that science will identify genes that increase the risk of cancer in general. For example, only about 5–10 percent of breast cancer cases can be traced to inherited copies of a damaged *BRCA1* gene. Lifestyle decisions are still important even for those who have inherited a damaged suppressor gene.

Testing and identification of hereditary cancer risks can be helpful for some people, especially if it leads to increased attention to controllable risk factors and better medical screening. For more on hereditary cancer risks and the issues involved in genetic testing, see the In Focus box.

Cancer Promoters

Substances known as *cancer promoters* make up another important piece of the cancer puzzle. Carcinogenic agents, such as UV radiation, that cause mutational changes in the DNA of oncogenes are known as *cancer initiators*. Cancer promoters, conversely, don't directly produce DNA mutations. Instead, they accelerate the growth of cells without damaging or permanently altering their DNA. However, a faster growth rate means less time for a cell to repair DNA damage caused by initiators, so errors are more likely to be passed on. Estrogen, which stimulates cellular growth in the female reproductive organs, is an example of a cancer promoter. Cigarette smoke is a complete carcinogen because it acts as both an initiator and a promoter.

Although much still needs to be learned about the role of genetics in cancer, it's clear that minimizing mutation damage to our DNA will lower our risk of many cancers. Unfortunately, a great many substances produce cancer-causing mutations, and we can't escape them all. However, by identifying the important carcinogens and understanding how they produce their effects, we can help keep our DNA intact and avoid activating sleeping oncogenes. The careful study of oncogenes should also lead to more precise methods of assessing cancer risk and to new methods of diagnosis and treatment.

Tobacco Use

Smoking is responsible for 85 percent of lung cancers and for about 30 percent of all cancer deaths. Research has identified several types of cancer. In addition to lung and bronchial cancer (discussed earlier in this chapter and in Chapter 16), tobacco use is known to cause cancer of the larynx, mouth, pharynx, esophagus, stomach, pancreas, kidneys, bladder, and cervix. A direct causal relationship has also been established between tobacco use and acute myelogenous leukemia (AML).

The Canadian Cancer Society states that about 21 000 cases of tobacco-related cancer are diagnosed annually in Canada, killing about 37 000 citizens—about one of every five deaths each year. The Ontario Ministry of Health and Long-Term Care estimates the direct economic burden of tobacco use at $1.6 billion annually. With an additional $4.4 billion resulting from lost productivity, the total cost for tobacco-related diseases is actually $6.0 billion per year.

For more information on tobacco, tobacco products, and the toxic chemicals contained in these products, see Chapter 16.

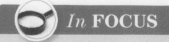

In FOCUS

Genetic Testing for Breast Cancer

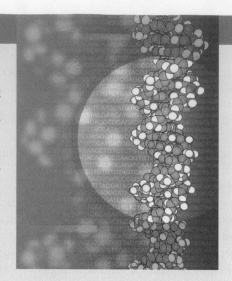

Recent discoveries of disease-related genes are opening up a host of issues related to genetic testing and associated legal, financial, and ethical concerns. Tests for hereditary mutations in breast cancer genes are now available, but who should be tested?

Researchers identified *BRCA1* in 1994 and *BRCA2* in 1995. About 1 or 2 in 1000 women in the general population carry a mutant copy of *BRCA1* or *BRCA2*, but in certain groups, most notably women of Ashkenazi (Eastern European) Jewish descent, as many as 3 in 100 may carry an altered gene. Defects in these genes cause breast cancer in as many as 50–70 percent of affected women; they also increase the risk of ovarian and other gynecological cancers. Women with an altered *BRCA* gene tend to develop breast cancer at younger ages than other women, and the cancers that develop are more malignant. The situation is complex, however, because hundreds of different mutations of *BRCA1* and *BRCA2* have been identified, and not all of them carry the same risks. Additional genes influencing risk have been identified—*TSG101* in 1997, *BRAF35* in 2001, *BASE* in 2003, *CHEK2* in 2005—and others will no doubt be found in the future.

Genetic analysis of DNA from a blood sample can identify mutant copies of *BRCA1* and *BRCA2*. Good news from a genetic test is reassuring, but it doesn't guarantee freedom from disease. Only 5–10 percent of all cases of breast cancer occur among women who inherit an altered version of *BRCA1* or *BRCA2*. And a woman with a family history of breast cancer must still be monitored closely, even if she carries normal versions of *BRCA1* and *BRCA2*; the cancer-causing genetic defect in her family could be located on another gene.

What about women who test positive for an altered copy of the gene? Options include close monitoring, drug treatment with a SERM, such as tamoxifen, and surgical removal of currently healthy breasts or ovaries. A 2008 study showed that when women with a *BRCA1* or *BRCA2* gene mutation had their ovaries removed as a preventive measure, their risk of breast cancer fell by 47 percent and their risk of other gynecologic cancers fell by 88 percent. The benefits of such pre-emptive surgery appear to be much greater among women with a mutation in the *BRCA2* gene than among those with a defective *BRCA1* gene. None of these strategies completely eliminates risk, and they may expose a woman to a dangerous or drastic treatment that is actually unnecessary.

The results and implications of genetic testing are multifaceted. Because a positive test may result in a challenging decision about appropriate prevention measures, genetic testing typically occurs in conjunction with professional counselling services in the provinces that offer testing. Counselling can provide women with an understanding of the impact of a positive test, both for themselves and for their families, which can help them to make an informed decision about whether to have testing done.

Dietary Factors

Diet is one of the most important factors in cancer prevention, but it is also one of the most complex and controversial. The foods you eat contain many biologically active compounds, and your food choices affect your cancer risk by both exposing you to potentially dangerous compounds and depriving you of potentially protective ones. In general, what we choose to put into our bodies will either support or detract from their abilities to help protect us from cancer and other ailments. Eating poorly and expecting our bodies to maintain optimal functioning is not dissimilar from putting poor quality gasoline in a car and expecting it to win a race (or even just keep going).

The following sections examine some of the dietary factors that may affect cancer risk. For a complete discussion of nutrition, see Chapter 5.

Dietary Fat and Meat

The Canadian Cancer Society encourages everyone to follow the guidelines in *Eating Well with Canada's Food Guide.* Specific recommendations include limiting consumption of processed and red meats, choosing high-fibre foods, and eating five to ten servings of fruit and vegetables each day. Diets high in fat and meat appear to contribute to certain cancers, including colon, stomach, and prostate. As is true with heart disease, certain types of fats may be riskier than others. Diets favouring omega-6 polyunsaturated fats are associated with a higher risk of certain cancers than are diets favouring the omega-3 forms of fat commonly found in fish and canola oil.

Refined Sugar

The role of refined sugars in cancer is a growing focus of research studies. Currently, the evidence is pointing toward a positive relationship between the consumption of sugary foods and drinks and the risk for a variety of cancers including, but not limited to, endometrial, colorectal, and pancreatic cancer. Furthermore, because high intakes of refined sugars are known contributors to obesity, and obesity itself is a risk for a variety of cancers, reducing refined sugar intake is a good idea all around.

Alcohol

Alcohol is associated with an increased incidence of several cancers. An average alcohol intake of two to five drinks per day is associated with one and a half times the risk of breast cancer, compared to women who do not drink alcohol. Alcohol and tobacco interact as risk factors for oral cancer, and heavy users of both alcohol and tobacco have a risk of oral cancer that ranges from 15 to 100 times as great as that of people who don't drink or smoke. Alcohol also increases the risk of colon cancer. For more information on alcohol, see Chapter 15.

Fried Foods

Scientists have found high levels of the chemical acrylamide (a probable human carcinogen) in starch-based foods that had been fried or baked at high temperatures, especially French fries and certain types of snack chips and crackers. Studies are ongoing, but the World Health Organization has urged food companies to lower the acrylamide content of foods to reduce any risk to public health. Acrylamide levels vary widely in foods, and there are currently no warnings against eating specific foods. The wisest course may be to eat a variety of foods and avoid overindulging in any single class of foods, particularly such foods as French fries and potato chips, which may contain other unhealthy substances, such as saturated and trans fats. You can also limit your exposure to acrylamide by not smoking—you would likely get much more of the chemical from smoking than from food.

Fibre

Various potential cancer-fighting actions have been proposed for fibre, but none of these actions has been firmly established. Further study is needed to clarify the relationship between fibre intake and cancer risk, and experts still recommend a high-fibre diet for its overall positive effect on health.

Fruit and Vegetables

Exactly which constituents of fruit and vegetables are responsible for reducing cancer risk is not clear, but researchers have identified many mechanisms by which food components may act against cancer. Some may prevent carcinogens from forming in the first place or block them from reaching or acting on target cells. Others boost enzymes that detoxify carcinogens and render them harmless. Still other anti-cancer agents act on cells that have already been exposed to carcinogens, slowing the development of cancer or starving cancer cells of oxygen and nutrients by cutting off their blood supply.

Some essential nutrients act as **anticarcinogens**. For example, vitamin C, vitamin E, selenium, and the **carotenoids** (vitamin A precursors) may help block cancer by acting as antioxidants. As described in Chapter 5, antioxidants prevent free radicals from damaging DNA and other cell components. Vitamin C may also block the conversion of nitrites (food preservatives) into cancer-causing agents. Folic acid may inhibit the transformation of normal cells into malignant cells and strengthen immune function. Calcium inhibits cell growth in the colon and may slow the spread of potentially cancerous cells.

anticarcinogens
Agents that destroy or otherwise block the action of carcinogens.

carotenoids
Any of a group of yellow-to-red plant pigments that can be converted to vitamin A by the liver, including beta-carotene, lutein, lycopene, and zeaxanthin; many act as antioxidants or have other anti-cancer effects.

Many other anti-cancer agents in the diet fall under the broader heading of *phytochemicals*, substances in plants that help protect against chronic diseases. One of the first to be identified was sulphoraphane, a potent anticarcinogen found in broccoli. Sulphoraphane induces the cells of the liver and kidney to produce higher levels of protective enzymes, which then neutralize dietary carcinogens. Most fruit and vegetables contain beneficial phytochemicals, and researchers are just beginning to identify them. Some of the most promising are listed in Table 8.2.

To increase your intake of these potential cancer fighters, eat a wide variety of fruit, vegetables, legumes, and grains. Don't rely on supplements. Some practical suggestions for increasing your intake of anti-cancer agents are included in the Take Charge box at the end of the chapter.

TABLE 8.2

Foods with Phytochemicals

Food	Phytochemical	Potential Anti-cancer Effects
Chili peppers (the hotter the pepper, the more capsaicin it contains)	Capsaicin	Neutralizes effect of nitrosamines; may block carcinogens in cigarette smoke from acting on cells
Oranges, lemons, limes, onions, apples, berries, eggplant	Flavonoids	Act as antioxidants; block access of carcinogens to cells; suppress malignant changes in cells; prevent cancer cells from multiplying
Citrus fruit, cherries	Monoterpenes	Help detoxify carcinogens; inhibit spread of cancer cells
Cruciferous vegetables (broccoli, cabbage, bok choy, cauliflower, kale, Brussels sprouts, collards)	Isothiocyanates	Boost production of cancer-fighting enzymes; suppress tumour growth; block effects of estrogen on cell growth
Garlic, onions, leeks, shallots, chives	Allyl sulphides	Increase levels of enzymes that break down potential carcinogens; boost activity of cancer-fighting immune cells
Grapes, red wine, peanuts	Resveratrol	Acts as an antioxidant; suppresses tumour growth
Green, oolong, and black teas (note that drinking very hot tea may *increase* the risk of some cancers), grapes, wine, turmeric	Polyphenols	Increase antioxidant activity; prevent cancer cells from multiplying; help speed excretion of carcinogens from body
Orange, deep yellow, red, pink, and dark green vegetables; some fruit	Carotenoids	Act as antioxidants; reduce levels of cancer-promoting enzymes; inhibit spread of cancer cells
Soy foods, whole grains, flax seeds, nuts	Phytoestrogens	Block effects of estrogen on cell growth; lower blood levels of estrogen
Whole grains, legumes	Phytic acid	Binds iron, which may prevent it from creating cell-damaging free radicals

Inactivity and Obesity

The Canadian Cancer Society recommends maintaining a healthy weight throughout life by balancing caloric intake with physical activity and by achieving and maintaining a healthy weight if you are currently overweight or obese. Being overweight or obese is linked with increased risk of several kinds of cancer, including breast and colon cancer (see Figure 8.7). See Chapters 4 and 6 for detailed information on weight management, physical activity, and exercise.

About one-third of 12 major cancers could be prevented through behaviour changes, such as engaging in regular physical activity, eating healthy, and maintaining a healthy bodyweight. Many people are unaware of the link between obesity and cancer; see the In the News box for more facts on cancer.

FIGURE 8.7

Body Weight and Cancer Mortality

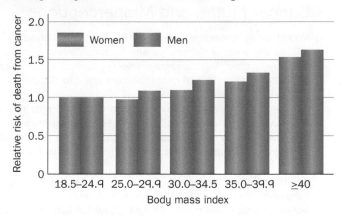

Source: McMillan, D. C., et al. 2006. ABC of obesity: obesity and cancer. *British Medical Journal* 333(7578). 1109–1111.

Carcinogens in the Environment

Some carcinogens occur naturally in the environment, such as viruses and the sun's UV rays. Others are manufactured or synthetic substances that show up occasionally in the general environment but more often in the work environments of specific industries.

Microbes

It is estimated that about 15–20 percent of the world's cancers are caused by microbes, including viruses, bacteria, and parasites, although the percentage is much lower in developed countries, such as Canada. As discussed earlier, certain types of human papillomavirus cause many cases of cervical cancer, and the *Helicobacter pylori* bacterium has been definitely linked to stomach cancer.

Viruses seem to be the main cancer causers. The Epstein-Barr virus, best known for causing mononucleosis, is also suspected of contributing to Hodgkin's disease, cancer of the pharynx, and some stomach cancers. Human herpes-virus 8 has been linked to Kaposi's sarcoma and certain types of lymphoma. Hepatitis viruses B and C together cause as many as 80 percent of the world's liver cancers.

Ingested Chemicals

The food industry uses preservatives and other additives to prevent food from becoming spoiled or stale (see Chapter 5). Some of these compounds are antioxidants and may actually decrease any cancer-causing properties the food might have.

Other compounds, such as the nitrates and nitrites found in processed meat, are potentially more dangerous. The nitrites inhibit the growth of bacteria, which could otherwise cause food poisoning. They also preserve the pink colour of the meat, which has no bearing on taste but looks more appetizing to many people. While nitrates and nitrites are not themselves carcinogenic, they can combine with dietary substances in the stomach and be converted to nitrosamines, which are highly potent carcinogens. Foods cured with nitrites, as well as those cured by salt or smoke, have been linked to esophageal and stomach cancer, and they should be eaten only in modest amounts.

Environmental and Industrial Pollution

Pollutants in urban air have long been suspected of contributing to the incidence of lung cancer. Fossil fuels and their combustion products, such as complex hydrocarbons, have been of special concern.

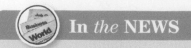

In *the* NEWS

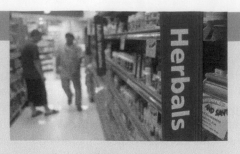

Cancer Myths and Misperceptions

Almost daily, cancer receives wide-ranging media coverage as it affects the lives of its victims and as breakthroughs create new hope for a cure. During regular checkups, doctors and dentists routinely look for signs of cancer and are quick to discuss the risks of developing cancer.

Remarkably, even as we are being inundated with information about cancer, studies show that many North Americans do not understand basic facts about the disease. Indeed, many still believe myths about cancer that were disproved long ago. Such misperceptions are leading North Americans to ignore good advice on cancer prevention and to continue lifestyle habits that increase the risk of cancer.

Healthier Cigarettes?

Scientists have concluded that so-called low-tar, low-nicotine, and light cigarettes are no safer than regular cigarettes. In fact, some brands of light cigarettes contain just as much nicotine and additives as regular cigarettes. Further, users of light cigarettes tend to smoke more frequently and inhale more deeply than smokers of regular cigarettes—often in the misguided belief that their chosen brand won't hurt them. In a 2006 survey, 72 percent of women and 63 percent of men said they believed light cigarettes were not as harmful as regular cigarettes. Meanwhile, smoking remains the leading preventable cause of cancer. Similarly, many smokers have switched to smokeless tobacco products (such as chewing tobacco), thinking they pose no health risks. Smokeless tobacco products contribute to head, throat, and oral cancers.

Obesity and Cancer

A survey published in 2011 showed that only 31 percent of Canadians were aware of the link between obesity and cancer. In another recent survey of North Americans, only about 15 percent of respondents knew their own BMI; most overweight and obese people surveyed did not view themselves as being too heavy.

As is the case with heart disease, maintaining a healthy weight and body composition can help reduce the risk of cancer. Although scientists are not sure how body fat works to increase cancer risk, evidence shows that overweight and obese people are in greater danger of breast, prostate, colorectal, and other cancers. In fact, obesity is considered in close competition with tobacco as the most preventable cause of death.

Prevailing Myths

In light of such findings, it may not be surprising to learn that many Canadians accept some myths about cancer, such as the following:

- *Antiperspirants and breast cancer:* The Canadian Cancer Society holds that no direct causal relationship has been found between antiperspirant use and breast cancer incidence.
- *Bras and breast cancer:* Currently, no reliable, scientific evidence shows a link between wearing a bra and developing breast cancer.
- *Microwaves and plastic containers:* Canadians believe that heating food in a microwave by using plastic dishes or plastic wrap will increase the risk of developing cancer. Some scientific evidence suggests that substances used to manufacture plastic products may transfer from the container into the food and that some of these products may be carcinogenic. Health Canada recommends not using plastic bowls or wrap in the microwave unless they are labelled as microwave safe.
- *Oyster sauce and soy sauce:* The production process for these products can lead to the formation of 3-MCPD, a chemical that has been identified as a possible carcinogen in humans. After completing its research, Health Canada has concluded that there is no immediate health risk to Canadians from consumption of soy and oyster sauces. However, Health Canada has identified that lifetime exposure to high levels of 3-MCPD could pose a health risk. Consequently, Health Canada has established 1.0 part per million (ppm) guideline for manufacturers of these sauces to reduce Canadians' long-term exposure to this chemical (this is considered to be a very safe level).
- *Reusing disposable water bottles:* Although many people are using non-plastic water bottles for environmental reasons, some people believe that disposable plastic water bottles can cause cancer if they are frozen or left in the car and exposed to heat. According to the Canadian Cancer Society, no evidence shows that reusing disposable plastic water bottles causes cancer.

Belief in these myths may be cause for concern. The first step in preventing and treating cancer is finding good sources of reliable information and following a qualified physician's advice.

The best available data indicate that less than 2 percent of cancer deaths are caused by general environmental pollution, such as substances in our air and water. Exposure to carcinogenic materials in the workplace is a more serious problem. Occupational exposure to specific carcinogens accounts for about 10 percent of cancer deaths among men and 1.3 percent among women. With increasing industry and government regulation, we can anticipate that the industrial sources of cancer risk will continue to diminish, at least in North America. In contrast, in the former Soviet Union and Eastern European countries, where environmental concerns were sacrificed to industrial productivity for decades, cancer rates from industrial pollution continue to climb.

Radiation

All sources of radiation are potentially carcinogenic, including medical X-rays, radioactive substances (radioisotopes), and UV rays from the sun. Most physicians and dentists are quite aware of the risk of radiation, and successful efforts have been made to reduce the amount of radiation needed for mammograms, dental X-rays, and other necessary medical X-rays. Full-body CT scans are sometimes advertised for routine screening in otherwise well individuals to look for tumours. Such screening is not recommended; it is typically expensive and may have false-positive findings that lead to unnecessary and invasive additional tests. Also, the radiation in these full-body X-rays may itself raise the risk of cancer; the radiation dose of one full-body CT scan is nearly 100 times that of a typical mammogram.

Sunlight is a very important source of radiation, but because its rays penetrate only a millimetre or so into the skin, it could be considered a surface carcinogen. Most cases of skin cancer are the relatively benign and highly curable basal cell carcinomas, but a substantial minority are the potentially deadly malignant melanomas. As discussed earlier, all types of skin cancer are increased by early and excessive exposure to the sun, and severe sunburn early in childhood appears to carry with it an added risk of melanoma later in life.

QUESTIONS FOR CRITICAL THINKING AND REFLECTION

What's important to you about knowing and managing (to the extent possible) your risks for cancer? How do your diet and exercise habits contribute to cancer prevention? What can you do to further reduce your risks?

QUICK STATS

Worldwide, 7.6 million people died of cancer in 2008.
—World Health Organization, 2013

Detecting, Diagnosing, and Treating Cancer

Early cancer detection often depends on our willingness to be aware of changes in our own body and to make sure we keep up with recommended diagnostic tests. Although treatment success varies with individual cancers, cure rates have increased—sometimes dramatically—in this century.

Detecting Cancer

Unlike those of some other diseases, early signs of cancer are usually not apparent to anyone but the person who has them. Even pain is not a reliable guide to early detection, because the initial stages of cancer may be painless. Self-monitoring is the first line of defence, and you can watch for the seven major warning signs shown in Figure 8.8. Remember them by the acronym CAUTION.

Although none of the warning signs is a sure indication of cancer, the appearance of any one should send you to see your physician. By being aware of the risk factors in your own life, your immediate family's cancer history, and your own history, you may bring a problem to the attention of a physician long before it would have been detected at a routine physical.

In addition to self-monitoring, the Canadian Cancer Society recommends routine cancer check-ups, as well as specific screening tests for certain cancers (see Table 8.3).

Diagnosing Cancer

Detection of a cancer by physical examination is only the beginning. Methods for determining the location, type, and degree of malignancy of a cancer continue to improve. Knowledge of the precise location and size of a tumour is necessary for effective surgery or radiation therapy. This is especially true in cases where the tumour may be hard to reach, as in the brain.

Imaging studies or exploratory surgery may be performed to identify a cancer's stage. A biopsy may be performed to confirm the type of tumour. Several

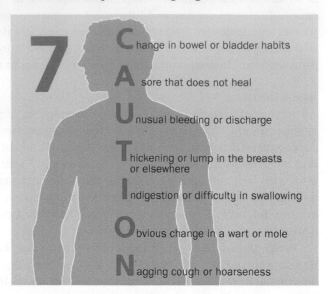

FIGURE 8.8

The Seven Major Warning Signs of Cancer

7

C hange in bowel or bladder habits

A sore that does not heal

U nusual bleeding or discharge

T hickening or lump in the breasts or elsewhere

I ndigestion or difficulty in swallowing

O bvious change in a wart or mole

N agging cough or hoarseness

diagnostic imaging techniques have replaced exploratory surgery for some patients. In magnetic resonance imaging (MRI), a huge electromagnet is used to detect hidden tumours by mapping, on a computer screen, the vibrations of different atoms in the body. Computed tomography (CT) scanning uses X-rays to examine the brain and other parts of the body. The process allows the construction of cross-sections, which show a

TABLE 8.3

Early Detection Screening Guidelines

Site	Recommendation
Breast	• Mammograms every second year are recommended starting at age 50. The age at which screening should be stopped should be individualized by considering the potential risks and benefits of screening in the context of overall health status and longevity. • A clinical breast exam should be part of a health exam about every 2 years for women age 40 and older. • Women should know how their breasts normally feel and report any breast change promptly to their health care providers. Breast self-exam is an option for women starting in their twenties.
Cervix	• Annual screening is recommended for women who are sexually active or at age 18. • After 2 normal smears, Pap tests should be completed every 3 years to age 69. • The HPV vaccine prevents HPV infection but should occur in addition to, not instead of, cervical cancer screening.
Colon and rectum	Beginning at age 50, men and women should begin screening: • A fecal occult blood test (FOBT) or fecal immunochemical test (FIT) every 2 years. • If a test is positive for blood, a colonoscopy should be performed to determine the cause of bleeding.
Prostate	• Men over 50 should talk to their doctor about being tested for prostate cancer. The PSA test and the digital rectal examination are methods to screen for prostate cancer. • Men at high risk (black men and men with a strong family history of one or more first-degree relatives diagnosed with prostate cancer at an early age) should talk to their doctor to see if they should be examined at an earlier age. • For men at both average risk and high risk, information should be provided about what is known and what is uncertain about the benefits and limitations of early detection and treatment of prostate cancer so that they can make an informed decision about testing.

Sources: Canadian Cancer Society. 2014. Various pages on site, http://www.cancer.ca (retrieved June 4, 2015).

tumour's shape and location more accurately than is possible with conventional X-rays. For patients undergoing radiation therapy, CT scanning enables the therapist to pinpoint the tumour more precisely, thereby providing more accurate radiation dosage while sparing normal tissue.

Ultrasonography has also been used increasingly in the past few years to view tumours. It has several advantages: It can be used in the physician's office, it is less expensive than other imaging methods, and it is completely safe. Prostate ultrasound (a rectal probe that uses ultrasonic waves to produce an image of the prostate gland) is being investigated for its ability to detect small, hidden tumours that would be missed by a digital rectal exam.

THINKING ABOUT THE ENVIRONMENT

Research suggests that about 7 percent of cancer deaths in North America stem from exposure to carcinogens in the environment. According to this estimate, almost 6 percent of deaths result from occupational exposure to carcinogens (10 percent among men and 1.3 percent among women); the remaining 2 percent result from human-made or naturally occurring pollutants in the larger environment.

These cancer-inducing or cancer-promoting agents come from a wide variety of sources. Radon, for example, is an invisible radioactive element that rises into the atmosphere from the ground in some areas. Exposure to radon is known to cause lung cancer, and radon is present in many buildings and homes. Asbestos, which is tightly controlled but still present in many older buildings, is another known carcinogen that affects people who are regularly exposed to it.

Other environmental carcinogens include some agricultural chemicals, industrial pollutants, and waste products that are not properly disposed of (such as certain materials used in electronic devices). Although it's impossible to avoid all these things completely, it is a good idea to be aware of them and minimize contact.

See Chapter 21 for more information on the environment and environmental health.

Treating Cancer

The ideal cancer therapy would kill or remove all cancerous cells while leaving normal tissue untouched. Sometimes this is almost possible, as when a surgeon removes a small superficial tumour of the skin. Usually the tumour is less accessible, and some combination of surgery, radiation therapy, and chemotherapy must be applied instead. Some patients choose to combine conventional therapies with alternative treatments (see the Critical Consumer box for more information).

Surgery

For most cancers, surgery is the most useful treatment. In many cases, the organ containing the tumour is not essential for life and can be partially or completely removed. This is true especially for localized breast, prostate, or testicular cancer, where the surgical removal of one breast, the prostate gland, or one testicle may give a long-lasting cure. Surgery is less effective when the tumour involves cells of the immune system, which are widely distributed throughout the body, or when the cancer has already metastasized. In such cases, surgery must be combined with other techniques.

Chemotherapy

Chemotherapy, or the use of cell-killing drugs to destroy rapidly growing cancer cells, has been in use since the 1940s. Many of these drugs work by interfering with DNA synthesis and replication in rapidly dividing cells. Normal cells, which usually grow slowly, are not destroyed by these drugs. However, some normal tissues, such as intestinal, hair, and blood-forming cells, are always growing, and damage to these tissues produces the unpleasant side effects of chemotherapy, including nausea, vomiting, diarrhea, and hair loss.

Chemotherapy drugs are often used in combinations or with surgery. Recently, in a procedure called **induction chemotherapy**, physicians have begun to use chemotherapy before surgery, both to shrink the tumour and to kill any existing small metastases as soon as possible.

Critical CONSUMER

Including Complementary Cancer Care

Sometimes conventional treatments for cancer are simply not enough, or are not in line with a person's beliefs or values. A patient may be told that there is little conventional therapy can do, other than providing medication to ease pain. When therapy is available, it may be painful and even intolerable to some people. Not surprisingly, many people with cancer look for complementary and alternative therapies. As many as 80 percent of cancer patients report combining conventional treatments with some type of mind–body technique. A much smaller number of patients look for alternatives to the more conventional therapies. These may be therapies within the bounds of legitimate medical practice that have not yet proven themselves in clinical trials. Or, at the extreme, alternative therapies may be scientifically unsound and dangerous, as well as expensive.

Complementary therapies, such as yoga, massage, acupuncture, meditation, music therapy, tai chi, and prayer, can have positive physical and psychological benefits for patients and improve quality of life as people deal with illness and the often difficult treatments for cancer. Mind–body practices can reduce pain and anxiety, improve sleep, and give people a sense of control and participation in their treatment; such practices may also enhance the immune system. (See Chapter 3 for more on stress and relaxation techniques.) Mind–body practices typically can be used in combination with conventional cancer therapies. There is some proof that these techniques may be helpful as complementary therapies to conventional cancer treatment.

For other types of therapies, the Canadian Cancer Society suggests several ways people with cancer can make safe and informed decisions:

- Understand the differences among conventional, complementary, integrative, and alternative therapies.
- Find out as much as you can about complementary or alternative therapies you are thinking about, including the possible benefits and risks.
- Talk to your health care team about complementary therapy or alternative therapies and how they may interact with the care you are receiving.
- Be especially cautious when evaluating cancer remedies promoted online; one recent study found that as many as one-third of cancer-related alternative medicine sites offered advice that was harmful or potentially dangerous.

One danger of alternative medicine is the very real possibility that proven therapies will be neglected while unproven, faddish alternative approaches are pursued; if alternate therapies delay proven therapies, lives may be lost. Another danger is that complementary therapies may counteract or affect conventional therapies; for example, some herbal supplements have been found to affect how cancer drugs are absorbed and used by the body. Further, some of these alternative therapies are expensive, and many patients are concerned about the cost of unproven therapies. A recent study revealed that 70 percent of patients using complementary therapies did not inform their physicians. However, it is essential for physicians to have this information so any side effects or harmful interactions can be prevented.

Sources: Canadian Cancer Society. 2014. *Complementary and Alternative Therapies*, http://www.cancer.ca/en/cancer-information/diagnosis-and-treatment/complementary-therapies/?region=on (retrieved May 28, 2015); National Cancer Institute. 2013. *Complementary and Alternative Medicine in Cancer Treatment: Questions and Answers*, http://www.cancer.gov/cancertopics/factsheet/therapy/CAM (retrieved May 28, 2015).

induction chemotherapy
The use of chemotherapy before surgery to shrink a cancerous tumour and prevent metastasis; sometimes eliminates the need for radical surgery.

Radiation

In cancer radiation therapy, a beam of X-rays or gamma rays is directed at the tumour, and the tumour cells are killed. Occasionally, when an organ is small enough, radioactive seeds are surgically placed inside the cancerous organ to destroy the tumour and then removed later if necessary. Radiation destroys both normal and cancerous cells, but because it can be precisely directed at the tumour it is usually less toxic for the patient than either surgery or chemotherapy, and it can often be performed on an outpatient basis. Radiation may be used as an exclusive treatment or in combination with surgery and chemotherapy.

New and Experimental Techniques

Many new and exciting possibilities for cancer therapy promise alternatives to the options of surgery, radiation, and chemotherapy. The research into alternatives is ongoing. One Canadian devoted to finding a cure for cancer was Terry Fox. Terry Fox's cancer journey raised awareness and money and left a lasting legacy (see the In Focus box). Although it is impossible to predict which of these new approaches will be most successful, researchers hope that cancer therapy overall will become increasingly safer and more effective:

- *Gene therapy:* Completion of the sequencing of the human genome in 2000 offered many new insights into cancer. Scientists have already discovered important new subtypes of tumours for breast cancer, melanoma, leukemia, and lymphomas based on patterns of gene expression. **Gene therapy** is the manipulation of gene expression in human cells. Gene therapy offers a potential treatment or cure for cancer, as well as for various genetic diseases. For gene therapy to succeed, new genes must be delivered to defective cells without disturbing the overall functioning of the cells. In the treatment of cancer, gene therapy would turn off the genes responsible for causing cells to divide rapidly and become malignant. By using this approach, researchers hope to develop targeted therapies for specific cancers.

gene therapy
The manipulation of gene expression in human cells; offers a potential treatment or cure for cancer by turning off the genes responsible for causing cells to divide rapidly and become malignant.

QUICK STATS

28 100 Ontarians were expected to die from cancer in 2014, making Ontario the leading province for cancer deaths.

—Canadian Cancer Society, 2014

 In FOCUS

Cancer Research in Canada: The Efforts of Terry Fox

In 1977, at the age of 18, a young sports enthusiast named Terry Fox was diagnosed with osteogenic sarcoma (bone cancer). As a result of his cancer, Terry had his right leg amputated 15 centimetres above the knee. But rather than dwelling on his own circumstances, he found himself moved by the stories of other people with cancer and the terrible treatments they endured. His compassion motivated Terry to run across Canada and raise money for cancer research. His goal was a lofty one: to raise $1 million.

Terry started his journey on April 12, 1980, in St. John's, Newfoundland, running with one strong leg and one artificial leg. In the beginning, not many people were aware of the run, but it soon began to attract attention and donations. His journey was quickly named the Marathon of Hope.

However, after running 5373 kilometres in 143 days, and crossing six provinces, Terry's journey came to an end in Thunder Bay, Ontario. His cancer had metastasized to his lungs. Although he couldn't finish his run across Canada, his spirit had touched Canadians and the donations continued.

On his return to British Columbia, Terry was honoured with numerous awards, including those from the American Cancer Society and the Province of British Columbia. Terry is also the youngest Champion of the Order of Canada. On June 28, 1981, at the age of 22, Terry lost his battle with cancer. His Marathon of Hope had raised $24.17 million.

More than 30 years later, Terry's legacy lives on. To date, more than $500 million has been raised for cancer research in Terry's name.

Sources: The Terry Fox Foundation. 2011. *Terry Fox and the Foundation*, http://www.terryfox.org/TerryFox; and Mayo Clinic. 2013. *Bone Cancer*, http://www.mayoclinic.org/diseases-conditions/bone-cancer/home/ovc-20126418 (retrieved May 29, 2015).

- *Bone marrow and stem cell transplants:* In cancers of the blood-forming cells or lymph cells, a patient's own bone marrow may have to be eliminated by radiation or chemotherapy to rid the body of cancer cells. Bone marrow can then be restored by transplanting healthy bone marrow cells from a compatible donor. Transplant incompatibility can be a problem, but progress on this front has been made through the use of **stem cells**. These unique, unspecialized cells can divide and produce more specialized cell types, including bone marrow cells (see Chapter 17). These stem cells can be identified, purified, and grown outside the body and then transplanted back into the person with cancer. This technique would allow for safe repopulation of bone marrow after radiation.

stem cells
Unspecialized cells that can divide and produce cells that differentiate into the many different types of specialized cells in the body (brain cells, muscle cells, skin cells, blood cells, and so on).

- *Biological therapies:* Biological therapies are based on enhancing the immune system's reaction to a tumour. Techniques include cancer vaccines, genetic modification of the body's immune cells, and the use of genetically engineered cytokines, which enhance immune cell function. Melanomas seem particularly susceptible to these biological approaches. Cancer vaccines are also under study for kidney cancer, lymphoma, lung cancer, and other cancers.
- *Proteasome inhibitors:* Proteasomes help control the cell cycle—the process through which cells divide. If proteasomes malfunction, as is often the case in cancer cells, then cells may begin multiplying out of control. Proteasome inhibitors block the action of proteasomes, halting cell division and killing the cells. One proteasome inhibitor is now being used against certain cancers, and other such drugs are in development.
- *Anti-angiogenesis drugs:* To obtain nutrients, cancer cells signal the body to produce new blood vessels, a process called angiogenesis. Drugs that block angiogenesis could keep tumours from growing and spreading.
- *Enzyme activators/blockers:* Normal cells die after dividing a given number of times. Scientists believe that the enzyme caspase triggers the death of normally functioning cells. In cancer cells, caspase activity may be blocked. Conversely, if the enzyme telomerase becomes active in cancer cells, the life-death cycle stops and the cells duplicate indefinitely. In effect, inactive caspase or active telomerase may keep cancer cells alive. Researchers are studying compounds that can either activate caspase or deactivate telomerase; either type of drug might lead cancer cells to self-destruct. No such drugs are now in clinical use.

QUESTIONS FOR CRITICAL THINKING AND REFLECTION

Do you know how to perform self-examinations? Has your doctor ever suggested that you do so, or given you instructions on proper technique? Given what you know about yourself and your family's medical history, which self-exams would be important for you?

Living with Cancer

Nearly 838 725 people in Canada survived cancer in the previous 10 years. However, the fear of cancer never disappears; recurrence is always a possibility.

Psychological support is an important factor during treatment for cancer (see the Mind Body Spirit box). For some patients, family, friends, and a caring physician or nurse provide all the support that is necessary. For many people, an organized support group can help provide needed social and psychological support.

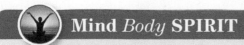

Mind *Body* SPIRIT

Coping with Cancer

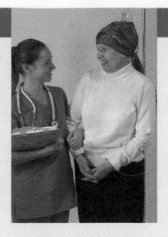

A cancer diagnosis was once viewed as a death sentence, and patients and families were often left to face their fears alone. People were sometimes reluctant to admit to the diagnosis of cancer or share it with others because of feelings of hopelessness or irrational guilt.

Since about the 1970s, a cultural shift has taken place. Improved diagnostic methods and therapies have increased survival times and cures. Media attention on positive developments has created a better understanding of the scientific basis of cancer. Some of the mystery about and dread of cancer have begun to abate, leading to a more positive atmosphere for people with cancer and their families.

If You Have Cancer

Each person's experience with cancer is unique, based on his or her own personality and values. Some people turn to their friends and family members for support, whereas others prefer help from other people with cancer, professional counsellors, or faith-based groups. If you have cancer, it is important to do what is right for you. Here are some strategies for dealing with the difficult emotions that may accompany a cancer diagnosis:

- Remember that cancer doesn't always mean death. Many cancers are curable or controllable for long periods, and people return to a normal, healthy life. Hope and optimism are important elements in cancer survival.
- Focus on controlling what you can. Be informed and involved with your medical care, keep your appointments, and make healthy changes in your lifestyle.
- Work toward having a positive attitude, but don't feel guilty if you can't maintain it all the time. Having cancer is difficult, and low moods will occur no matter how good you are at coping. If they become frequent or severe, seek help.
- Use strategies that have helped you solve problems and manage your emotions in the past. Some people respond to information gathering, talking with others, and prayer or meditation. Physical activity, music, art, and sharing personal stories may help lessen stress.
- Confide feelings and worries to someone close to you. Don't bottle up your feelings to spare your loved ones. If you don't feel comfortable sharing with others, consider expressing your emotions in a journal.

Finding a Support Group

Support groups may be led by cancer survivors, group members, or trained professionals. These groups typically present information, teach coping skills, and give people with cancer a place to share common concerns and obtain emotional support. Support groups may focus on education, behavioural training, or group interaction. Behavioural training can involve meditation and other techniques to reduce stress or the effects of chemotherapy or radiation therapy.

Research has shown that support groups can enhance quality of life in very practical ways. For instance, patients in breast cancer support groups were found to have improved psychological symptoms, less pain, and improved family relationships compared with patients in a control group.

Support groups vary in quality, and people with cancer may find that a support group fails to discuss topics relevant to their personal situation. Some people may find a support group upsetting because it stirs up too many uncomfortable feelings or because the leader is not skilled. Find a group that is right for you.

Online support groups can be very helpful for people living in rural areas or confined to their homes. Medical information on the Internet is highly variable in quality, however; you should check with your physician before making any decisions based on online information.

Supporting a Person with Cancer

There is no one right way to act with a person facing cancer. Reassure the person of your love, and let him or her know that you are available for both practical and emotional support. A person with cancer may want you to be very involved in treatment or coping, or he or she may want your help in maintaining a more normal routine. Guidelines for visiting a person with cancer include the following:

- Before you visit, call to ask if it's a good time. Surprise visits are often not welcome. Don't overstay.

- Be a good listener. Allow the person to express all his or her feelings, and don't discount fears or minimize the seriousness of the situation. Let the person with cancer decide whether the two of you talk about the illness. It's human to want to laugh and talk about other things sometimes.
- Ask "What can I get you?" or "How can I help?" instead of saying "Let me know if I can help." Make specific offers: to clean the bathroom, go grocery shopping, do laundry, or give caregivers a break.
- Refrain from offering advice. You may have heard about the latest treatment or hottest physician, but unless you are asked for suggestions, keep them to yourself.
- If you want to take food, ask about dietary restrictions ahead of time. Use a disposable container so the person won't have to return it.
- Don't be put off if your first visit gets a lukewarm reception. Many people with cancer are on an emotional roller coaster, and their feelings and needs will change over time.

   Support groups also exist for friends and family members of people with cancer. These groups give people a place to express their fears about many issues, such as relationship changes, financial problems, and ways to provide emotional support for the person with cancer.

Palliative Care

Palliative care, while not postponing death, enhances the quality of life for people who have been diagnosed with terminal cancer and their families. An essential component of cancer management, it provides pain and symptom relief, along with psychosocial support. This holistic approach to end-of-life care begins at diagnosis and continues through to death, where dying is considered a normal part of life. Drawing on music, relaxation, and art therapy, palliative care strives to enhance emotional well-being. As a result, studies show that palliative care can positively influence a patient's disease progression. A comprehensive, multidisciplinary approach, involving both family and community resources, is required for effective palliative care.

Sources: Kissane, D. W., et al. 2004. Effect of cognitive-existential group therapy on survival in early-stage breast cancer. *Journal of Clinical Oncology* 22(21): 4255–4260; National Cancer Institute. 2002. *Facing Forward: Life After Cancer Treatment,* http://www.cancer.gov/cancertopics/coping/life-after-treatment/page6 (retrieved May 29, 2015); Goodwin, P. J., et al. 2001. The effect of group psychosocial support on survival in metastatic breast cancer. *New England Journal of Medicine* 345(24): 1719–1726; Life with cancer: How to provide support. 1996. *Women's Health Advocate,* September; Holland, J. C. 1996. Cancer's psychological challenges. *Scientific American,* September; Nainis, N., et al. 2006. Relieving symptoms in cancer: Innovative use of art therapy. *Journal of Pain and Symptom Management* 31(2): 162–169; and World Health Organization. 2010. *Cancer: Palliative Care,* http://www.who.int/cancer/palliative/en/ (retrieved May 29, 2015).

Preventing Cancer

As mentioned throughout this chapter, your lifestyle choices can radically lower your cancer risks (see Figure 8.9). Here are some guidelines:

- *Avoid tobacco.* The bloodstream carries carcinogens from tobacco smoke throughout the body, making smoking a risk for many forms of cancer other than lung cancer. The use of spit tobacco increases the risk of cancers of the mouth, larynx, throat, and esophagus. It is also important to avoid exposure to environmental tobacco smoke.
- *Control diet and weight.* About one-third of all cancers are in some way linked to what we eat. Choose a low-(refined) sugar, plant-based diet containing a wide variety of fruit, vegetables, and whole grains rich in phytochemicals. Drink alcohol only in moderation, if at all. Maintain a healthy weight.
- *Exercise.* Regular exercise is linked to lower rates of some cancers. It also helps control weight and reduce risk factors for other diseases.
- *Protect your skin.* Almost all cases of skin cancer are sun related. Wear protective clothing when you are out in the sun, and use a sunscreen with an SPF rating of 15 or higher. Don't go to tanning salons or use tanning booths.
- *Avoid environmental and occupational carcinogens.* Try to avoid exposure to cancer-causing agents in the environment, especially in the workplace. These agents can range from second-hand smoke to pesticides and other chemicals.

   Also, follow the Canadian Cancer Society's recommendations for cancer screenings. Your doctor can help you determine the most appropriate timing and methods for screenings.

FIGURE 8.9

Strategies for Reducing your Risk of Cancer

Do More
- Eat a varied, plant-based diet that is high in fibre-rich foods, such as legumes and whole grains.
- Eat five to ten servings of fruits and vegetables every day, favouring foods from the following categories:
    Cruciferous vegetables
    Citrus fruits
    Berries
    Dark green leafy vegetables
    Dark yellow, orange, or red fruits and vegetables
- Be physically active.
- Maintain a healthy weight.
- Practise safer sex (to avoid HPV infection).
- Protect your skin from the sun with appropriate clothing and sunscreen.
- Perform regular self-exams (testicular self-exam, skin self-exam).
- Obtain recommended screening tests and discuss with your physician any family history of cancer.

Do Less
- Don't use tobacco in any form:
    Cigarettes
    Spit tobacco
    Cigars and pipes
    Bidis and clove cigarettes
- Avoid exposure to environmental tobacco smoke.
- Limit consumption of fatty meats and other sources of saturated fat.
- Avoid excessive alcohol consumption.
- Limit consumption of salt.
- Don't eat charred foods, and limit consumption of cured and smoked meats and meat and fish grilled in a direct flame.
- Limit exposure to UV radiation from sunlight or tanning lamps or beds.
- Avoid occupational exposure to carcinogens.

QUESTIONS FOR CRITICAL THINKING AND REFLECTION

Review the guidelines just listed for preventing cancer. How many of these things do you do regularly? How often do you think about them? For example, do you often forget to use sunscreen before going outdoors or do you ever hang out in places where people smoke? What do you want to do differently?

 Take **CHARGE**

Incorporating More Fruit and Vegetables into Your Diet

When we think about the health benefits of fruit and vegetables, we usually focus on the fact that they are rich in carbohydrates, dietary fibre, and vitamins and low in fat. A benefit that we may overlook is that they contain specific cancer-fighting compounds, phytochemicals that help slow, stop, or even reverse the process of cancer. In line with *Eating Well with Canada's Food Guide*, the Canadian Cancer Society recommends eating five to ten servings of fruit and vegetables each day, in an effort to reduce a person's risk of cancer. However, most Canadians are not meeting these guidelines. In 2012, nearly 60 percent of Canadians did not consume the suggested number of fruit and vegetables each day, varying from 52.2 percent in Quebec to 74.2 percent in Nunavut. Fruit and vegetable consumption also varies with age and sex. Consistently, men tend to eat fewer servings than their female counterparts in all age groups; those 55 years of age and older consume the largest amount of fruit and vegetables.

Most Canadians need to increase the amount of fruit and vegetables they eat every day. Begin by monitoring your diet for one to two weeks to assess your current intake; then look for ways to incorporate these foods into your diet in easy and tasty ways. Here are some tips to get you started.

Breakfast
- Drink 100 percent juice every morning (a mix of vegetable and fruit together is great combination).
- Add berries or sliced fruit to cereal or no/low-sugar yogurt. Top bagels with tomato slices.
- Try a fruit smoothie made from fresh or frozen fruit, a splash of orange juice, and no/low-sugar yogurt. Adding green vegetables to smoothies is a great way to increase vegetable intake.

Lunch
- Choose vegetable soup or salad with your meal.

- Replace potato chips or French fries with cut-up vegetables.
- Add extra chunks of fruit and vegetables to salads.
- Try adding vegetables, such as roasted peppers, cucumber slices, shredded carrots, avocado, or salsa, to sandwiches.
- Drink tomato or vegetable juice instead of soft drinks (watch for excess sodium).

Dinner
- Choose a vegetarian main course, such as stir-fry or vegetable stew. Have at least two servings of vegetables with every dinner.
- Microwave vegetables and sprinkle them with a little bit of Parmesan cheese.
- Substitute vegetables for meat in casseroles and pasta and chili recipes.
- At the salad bar, pile your plate with healthy vegetables and use olive oil, vinegar, and herbs as dressing.

Snacks and On the Go
- Keep ready-to-eat-fruit and vegetables on hand (apples, plums, pears, and carrots).
- Keep small packages of dried fruit in the car (try dried apricots, peaches, pears, and raisins).
- Make ice cubes from 100 percent fruit juice and drop them into regular or sparkling water.
- Freeze grapes for a cool summer treat.

In the Grocery Store
- Stock up on canned, frozen, and dried fruit and vegetables when they go on sale.
- Buy fresh fruit and vegetables in season; they will taste best and be less expensive.
- To save on preparation time, buy pre-cut vegetables and fruit and packaged salads.
- Try a new fresh fruit or vegetable every week.

The All-Stars
Different fruit and vegetables contribute different vitamins, phytochemicals, and other nutrients, so be sure to get a variety. The following types of produce are particularly rich in nutrients and phytochemicals:
- Cruciferous vegetables (broccoli, cauliflower, cabbage, kale, etc.)
- Citrus fruit (oranges, lemons, limes, grapefruit, tangerines, etc.)
- Berries (strawberries, raspberries, blueberries, etc.)
- Dark green leafy vegetables (spinach, chard, collards, beet greens, kale, mustard greens, romaine and other dark lettuces, etc.)
- Deep yellow, orange, and red fruit and vegetables (carrots, pumpkin, sweet potatoes, winter squash, red and yellow bell peppers, apricots, cantaloupe, mangoes, papayas, etc.)

SUMMARY

- A malignant tumour can invade surrounding structures and spread to distant sites via the blood and lymphatic system, producing additional tumours.
- A malignant cell divides without regard for normal growth. As tumours grow, they produce signs or symptoms that are determined by their location in the body.
- One in two men and one in three women will develop cancer.
- Lung cancer kills more people than any other type of cancer. Tobacco smoke is the primary cause.
- Colon and rectal cancer are linked to age, heredity, obesity, and a diet rich in red meat and low in fruit and vegetables. Most colon cancers arise from preexisting polyps.
- Breast cancer affects about one in nine women in Canada. Although breast cancer has a genetic component, diet and hormones are also risk factors.
- Prostate cancer is chiefly a disease of aging; diet and lifestyle probably are factors in its occurrence. Early detection is possible through rectal examinations, PSA blood tests, and sometimes ultrasound.

- Cancers of the female reproductive tract include cervical, uterine, and ovarian cancer. The Pap test is an effective screening test for cervical cancer.
- Abnormal cellular changes in the epidermis, often a result of exposure to the sun, cause skin cancer, as does chronic exposure to certain chemicals. Skin cancers occur as basal cell carcinoma, squamous cell carcinoma, and melanoma.
- Oral cancer is caused primarily by smoking, excess alcohol consumption, and use of spit tobacco. Oral cancers are easy to detect but often hard to treat.
- Testicular cancer can be detected early through self-examination.
- Mutational damage to a cell's DNA can lead to rapid and uncontrolled growth of cells; mutagens include radiation, viral infection, and chemical substances in food and air.
- Cancer-promoting dietary factors include meat, certain types of fats, and alcohol.
- Diets high in fruit and vegetables are linked to a lower risk of cancer.
- Other possible causes of cancer include inactivity and obesity, certain types of infections and chemicals, and radiation.
- Self-monitoring and regular screening tests are essential to early cancer detection.
- Methods of cancer diagnosis include magnetic resonance imaging, computed tomography, and ultrasound.
- Treatment methods usually consist of some combination of surgery, chemotherapy, and radiation. Gene therapy, bone marrow and stem cell transplants, proteasome inhibitors, biological therapies, and drugs that inhibit angiogenesis or telomerase also hold promise as effective treatments.
- Strategies for preventing cancer include avoiding tobacco; eating a varied, moderate diet and controlling weight; exercising regularly; protecting skin from the sun; avoiding exposure to environmental and occupational carcinogens; and getting recommended cancer screening tests.

FOR MORE INFORMATION

BOOKS

American Cancer Society. 2009. *The American Cancer Society Complete Guide to Complementary & Alternative Cancer Therapies.* Atlanta: American Cancer Society. In-depth information about cancer therapies being used alongside traditional Western medicine in treating cancer.

Beliveau, R., and D. Gingras, 2006. *Foods That Fight Cancer: Preventing Cancer through Diet.* New York: DK Publishing. Information about appropriate foods to fight cancer.

Cotter, A. 1999. *From This Moment On: A Guide for Those Recently Diagnosed with Cancer.* MacMillan Canada. Information on the experience of having cancer.

Hartmann, L. C., C. L. Loprinzi, and B. S. Gostout. 2005. *Mayo Clinic: Guide to Women's Cancers.* New York: Kensington. Information about a variety of women's cancers.

McKinnell, R. G., et al. 2006. *The Biological Basis of Cancer,* 2nd ed. Boston: Cambridge University Press. The underlying causes of cancer and actual cases of the disease and its impact on patients and families.

Oh, W. 2006. *Prostate Cancer: An Issue of Hematology/Oncology Clinics.* Toronto: Elsevier Canada. Information on prostate cancer.

Rosenbaum, E., et al. 2008. *Everyone's Guide to Cancer Therapy,* rev. 5th ed. Riverside, N.J.: Andrews McMeel. Articles on the known causes, diagnoses, and treatments for many types of cancer reviewed by a panel of more than 100 oncologists.

Servan-Schreiber, D. 2008. *The Anti-Cancer Life: A New Way of Life.* Toronto: HarperCollins Publishers. Information on both the personal experience and the research of a physician diagnosed with cancer, discussing both conventional treatments and alternative therapies.

Turkington, C., and W. LiPera. 2005. *The Encyclopedia of Cancer.* New York: Facts on File. Entries on a variety of topics relating to cancer causes, prevention, diagnosis, and treatment.

Williams, P. 2006. *Breast Cancer.* Toronto: Penguin Group Canada. Information about breast cancer.

ORGANIZATIONS, HOTLINES, AND WEBSITES

The Internet addresses listed here were accurate at the time of publication.

Breast Cancer Society of Canada. Provides information on breast cancer.
http://www.bcsc.ca

Canadian Breast Cancer Foundation. Provides information about breast cancer.
http://www.cbcf.org

Cancer Care Ontario. Provides information on the prevention and care of cancer in Ontario.
http://www.cancercare.on.ca

Canadian Cancer Research Alliance. Provides information about organizations devoted to cancer work.
http://www.ccra-acrc.ca

Canadian Cancer Society. Provides information on cancer, treatments, prevention, and research.
http://www.cancer.ca

Canadian Dermatology Association. Provides information on skin cancer.
http://www.dermatology.ca

Cancer Guide: Steve Dunn's Cancer Information Page. Links to many online cancer resources and advice about how to make the best use of information.
http://www.cancerguide.org

Cancer News. Provides links to news and information on many types of cancer.
http://www.cancernews.com

Clinical Trials. Information about clinical trials for new cancer treatments can be accessed at the following sites:
http://www.cancer.gov/clinicaltrials
http://www.centerwatch.com

Colorectcal Cancer Association of Canada. Provides information on treatment, screening, and statistics.
http://www.colorectal-cancer.ca

Harvard School of Public Health: Disease Risk Index. Includes interactive risk assessments and tips for preventing common cancers.
http://www.diseaseriskindex.harvard.edu/update/

Lung Cancer Canada. Provides detailed information about lung cancer.
http://www.lungcancercanada.ca

MedlinePlus Cancer Information. Provides news and links to reliable information on a variety of cancers and cancer treatment.
http://www.nlm.nih.gov/medlineplus/cancers.html

National Comprehensive Cancer Network. Presents treatment guidelines for physicians and patients related to the treatment of various cancers; these guidelines were developed by a group of leading cancer centres.
http://www.nccn.org

Ovarian Cancer Canada. Presents information on ovarian cancer and treatment options.
http://www.ovariancanada.org

Prostate Cancer Canada. Contains facts, statistics, and treatment on prostate cancer.
http://www.prostatecancer.ca

Public Health Agency of Canada. Provides information about the various forms of cancer.
http://www.phac-aspc.gc.ca/cd-mc/cancer/index-eng.php

U.S. National Cancer Institute. Provides information on treatment options, screening, and clinical trials.
http://www.cancer.gov

U.S. National Toxicology Program. Provides regular reports listing those substances that are known or reasonably assumed to cause cancer in humans.
http://ntp-server.niehs.nih.gov

See also the listings in Chapters 4–6, 15, and 16.

SELECTED BIBLIOGRAPHY

Abbasi, N. R., et al. 2004. Early diagnosis of cutaneous melanoma. *Journal of the American Medical Association* 292(22): 2771–2776.

Alberta Health Services. 2008. *Melanoma,* http://www.albertahealthservices.ca/2273.asp (retrieved April 9, 2015).

Baker, S., and J. Kaprio. 2006. Common susceptibility genes for cancer: Search for the end of the rainbow. *British Medical Journal* 332(7550): 1150–1152.

Bjorge, T., S. Tretli, and A. Engeland. 2004. Relation of height and body mass index to renal cell carcinoma in two million Norwegian men and women. *American Journal of Epidemiology* 60(12): 1168–1176.

Brand, T. C., et al. 2006. Prostate cancer detection strategies. *Current Urology Reports* 7(3): 181–185.

Brenner, D. J., et al. 2004. Estimated radiation risks potentially associated with full-body CT screening. *Radiology* 232(3): 735–738.

Canadian Cancer Society. 2014. *Inherited Cancer Risk,* http://www.cancer.ca/en/cancer-information/cancer-101/what-is-a-risk-factor/genetic-risk/inherited-cancer-risk/?region=on (retrieved May 29, 2015).

Canadian Cancer Society's Advisory Committee on Cancer Statistics. Canadian Cancer Statistics 2013. Toronto ON: Canadian Cancer Society; ISSN 0835-2976.

Canadian Cancer Society's Advisory Committee on Cancer Statistics. Canadian Cancer Statistics 2014. Toronto, ON: Canadian Cancer Society; 2014. ISSN 0835-2976.

Centers for Disease Control and Prevention. 2013. *Skin cancer rates by race and ethnicity,* http://www.cdc.gov/cancer/skin/statistics/race.htm (retrieved May 29, 2015).

Chao, A., et al. 2005. Meat consumption and risk of colorectal cancer. *Journal of the American Medical Association* 293(2): 172–182.

Chia, K. S., et al. 2005. Profound changes in breast cancer incidence may reflect changes into a Westernized lifestyle: A comparative population-based study in Singapore and Sweden. *International Journal of Cancer* 113(2): 302–306.

de Vries, S. H., et al. 2004. Prostate cancer characteristics and prostate specific antigen changes in screening detected patients initially treated with a watchful waiting policy. *Journal of Urology* 172 (6 Pt 1): 2193–2196.

Ellison, L.F., et al. 2010. *An update on cancer survival.* Statistics Canada, Catalogue no. 82-003-XPE. Health Reports 21(3): 1–6.

Elmore, J. G., et al. 2005. Screening for breast cancer. *Journal of the American Medical Association* 293(10): 1245–1256.

Flood, A., et al. 2005. Calcium from diet and supplements is associated with reduced risk of colorectal cancer in a prospective cohort of women. *Cancer Epidemiology, Biomarkers and Prevention* 14(1): 126–132.

Garland, S. 2006. Efficacy of a quadrivalent HPV (types 6, 11, 16, 18) L1 VLP vaccine against external genital disease: Future 1 analysis. *European Journal of Obstetrics, Gynecology, and Reproductive Biology* 107(1): 18–27.

Goff, B. A., et al. 2004. Frequency of symptoms of ovarian cancer in women presenting to primary care clinics. *Journal of the American Medical Association* 291(22): 2705–2712.

Harper, D. M., et al. 2004. Efficacy of a bivalent L1 virus-like particle vaccine in prevention of infection with human papillomavirus types 16 and 18 in young women: A randomised controlled trial. *Lancet* 364(9447): 1757–1765.

Hou, L., et al. 2004. Computing physical activity and risk of colon cancer in Shanghai, China. *American Journal of Epidemiology* 160(9): 860–867.

Jee, S. H., et al. 2005. Fasting serum glucose level and cancer risk in Korean men and women. *Journal of the American Medical Association* 293(2): 194–202.

Jemal, A., et al. 2005. Cancer Statistics, 2005. *CA: A Cancer Journal for Clinicians* 55(1): 10–30.

Kaplan, R. N., et al. 2005. VEGFR1-positive haematopoietic bone marrow progenitors initiate the pre-metastatic niche. *Nature* 438(7069): 820–827.

Kauff, N. D., et al. 2008. Risk-reducing salpingo-oophorectomy for the prevention of *BRCA1*- and *BRCA2*-associated breast and gynecologic cancer: A multicenter, prospective study. *Journal of Clinical Oncology* 26(8): 1331–1337.

King, M.G., et al. 2013. Consumption of sugary foods and drinks and risk of endometrial cancer. *Cancer Causes and Control* 24(7): 1427–1436.

Kroenke, C. H., et al. 2005. Weight, weight gain, and survival after breast cancer diagnosis. *Journal of Clinical Oncology* 23(7): 1370–1378.

Laaksonen, D. E., et al. 2004. Serum linoleic and total polyunsaturated fatty acids in relation to prostate and other cancers: A population-based cohort study. *International Journal of Cancer* 111(3): 444–450.

Larsson, S.C., et al. 2006. Consumption of sugar and sugar-sweetened foods and the risk of pancreatic cancer in a prospective study. *American Journal of Clinical Nutrition* 84: 1171–1176.

Mandelblatt, J. S., K. A. Cronin, S. Bailey S, et al. 2009. Effects of mammography screening under different screening schedules: model estimates of potential benefits and harms. *Annals of Internal Medicine*, 151(10): 738–747.

Martinez, M. E. 2005. Primary prevention of colorectal cancer: Lifestyle, nutrition, exercise. *Recent Results in Cancer Research* 166: 177–211.

Mayo Clinic. 2006. Skin cancer epidemic. Take steps to avoid sun damage. *Mayo Clinic Health Letter* 24(4): 1–3.

Mayo Clinic. 2008. Bladder cancer: Early discovery, vigilance are key. *Mayo Clinic Health Letter* 26(10): 1–3.

Mayo Clinic. 2008. Breast imaging: Advances in earlier cancer detection. *Mayo Clinic Health Letter* 26(2): 1–3.

Mayo Clinic. 2014. *Cancer survival rate: What it means for your prognosis*, http://www.mayoclinic.org/diseases-conditions/cancer/in-depth/cancer/art-20044517 (retrieved May 29, 2015).

Meadows, M. 2004. Cancer vaccines: Training the immune system to fight cancer. *FDA Consumer*, September/October.

Melanoma. 2004. *Journal of the American Medical Association* 292(22): 2800.

Mor, G., et al. 2005. Serum protein markers for early detection of ovarian cancer. *Proceedings of the National Academy of Sciences USA*, May 12 [epub].

Nainis, N., et al. 2006. Relieving symptoms in cancer: Innovative use of art therapy. *Journal of Pain and Symptom Management* 31(2): 162–169.

National Toxicology Program. 2005. *Report on Carcinogens,* 11th ed. Research Triangle Park, N.C.: National Toxicology Program.

Occupational Cancer Research Centre. 2011. Research Day 2011: The Burden of Occupational Cancer, http://occupationalcancer.ca/wp-content/uploads/2011/03/Burden-Backgrounder-Final.pdf (retrieved May 29, 2015).

Ontario Ministry of Health and Long-Term Care. 2013. *Tobacco Legislation Facts and Myths,* http://www.mhp.gov.on.ca/en/smoke-free/legislation/clearning-air.asp (retrieved May 29, 2015).

Ontario Ministry of Health Promotion. 2010. *Comprehensive Tobacco Control Guidance Document.* Queen's Printer for Ontario: ISBN: 978-1-4435-2910-5, http://www.health.gov.on.ca/en/pro/programs/publichealth/oph_standards/docs/guidance/ComprehensiveTobaccoControl.pdf (retrieved May 29, 2015).

Osborn, N. K., and D. A. Ahlquist. 2005. Stool screening for colorectal cancer: Molecular approaches. *Gastroenterology* 128(1): 192–206.

Paik, S., et al. 2004. A multigene assay to predict recurrence of tamoxifen-treated, node-negative breast cancer. *New England Journal of Medicine* 351(27): 2817–2826.

Parmet, S. 2004. Genetics and breast cancer. *Journal of the American Medical Association* 292(4): 522.

Pelucchi, C., et al. 2004. Fibre intake and prostate cancer risk. *International Journal of Cancer* 109(2): 278–280.

Putt, K. S., et al. 2006. Small-molecule activation of procaspase-3 to caspase-3 as a personalized anticancer strategy. *Nature Chemical Biology* 2: 543–550, http://www.nature.com/nchembio/journal/v2/n10/full/nchembio814.html (retrieved May 29, 2015).

Roden, R. B., et al. 2004. Vaccination to prevent and treat cervical cancer. *Human Pathology* 35(8): 971–982.

Seeff, L. C., et al. 2004. How many endoscopies are performed for colorectal cancer screening? Results from CDC's survey of endoscopic capacity. *Gastroenterology* 127(6): 1670–1677.

Terry, M. B., et al. 2004. Association of frequency and duration of aspirin use and hormone receptor status with breast cancer risk. *Journal of the American Medical Association* 291(20): 2433–2440.

Trimble, C. L., et al. 2005. Active and passive cigarette smoking and the risk of cervical neoplasia. *Obstetrics and Gynecology* 105(1): 174–181.

U.S. Preventive Services Task Force. 2008. Screening for prostate cancer: U.S. Preventive Services Task Force recommendation statement. *Annals of Internal Medicine* 149(3): 185–191.

Van Gils, C. H., et al. 2005. Consumption of vegetables and fruits and risk of breast cancer. *Journal of the American Medical Association* 293(3): 183–193.

Vecchia, C. L., et al. 1993. Refined-sugar intake and the risk of colorectal cancer in humans. *International Journal of Cancer* 55(3): 386–389.

Velicer, C. M., et al. 2004. Antibiotic use in relation to the risk of breast cancer. *Journal of the American Medical Association* 291(7): 827–835.

Weinstein, S. J., et al. 2005. Serum alpha-tocopherol and gamma-tocopherol in relation to prostate cancer risk in a prospective study. *Journal of the National Cancer Institute* 97(5): 396–399.

Wellness facts. 2006. *Wellness Letter* 22(5): 1.

World Health Organization. 2009. *Preventing cancer: promoting a healthy diet and physical activity in childhood* http://www.who.int/cancer/prevention/children/en/ (retrieved May 29, 2015).

World Health Organization. 2014. *Cancer: Palliative Care,* http://www.who.int/cancer/palliative/en/ (retrieved May 29, 2015).

World Health Organization. 2014. *Cancer,* http://www.who.int/cancer/en/ (retrieved May 29, 2015).

World Health Organization: International Agency for Research on Cancer. 2014. *World Cancer Report 2014,* http://www.iarc.fr/en/publications/pdfs-online/wcr/ (retrieved May 29, 2015).

CHAPTER 9

Immunity and Infection

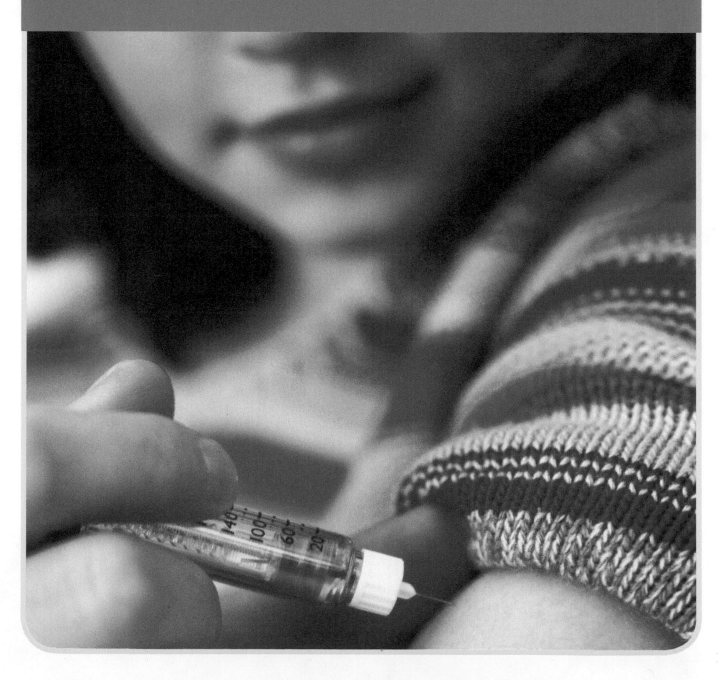

LOOKING AHEAD

After you have read and studied this chapter, you should be able to:

LO1   Describe the step-by-step process by which infectious diseases are transmitted

LO2   Identify the body's physical and chemical barriers to infection

LO3   Explain how the immune system responds to an invading microorganism

LO4   Identify the major types of pathogens and describe the common diseases they cause

LO5   Discuss steps you can take to prevent infections and strengthen your immune system

TEST YOUR KNOWLEDGE

1. **Which of the following can transmit disease-causing pathogens (such as bacteria or viruses) from one person to another?**
   a. mosquitoes b. doorknobs c. soil

2. **When taking a prescription antibiotic, you should always finish the entire course of medication, even if you start feeling better before running out of medicine.**
   True or false?

3. **Which of the following can recognize and eliminate specific microbes (such as bacteria) that invade the body?**
   a. antigens b. antibodies c. antidotes

4. **Because medical facilities are sanitary, patients rarely catch bacterial infections in hospitals.**
   True or false?

5. **You can reduce your chances of getting sick by doing which of the following?**
   a. washing your hands frequently
   b. keeping your immunizations up to date
   c. getting enough sleep

ANSWERS

1. ALL THREE.   Pathogens can be transmitted directly (by contact with a sick person) or indirectly (by contact with an infected animal or insect or a contaminated object like a doorknob).

2. TRUE.   Failing to take all your medication can lead to a relapse of the illness; taking antibiotics incorrectly also contributes to the development of antibiotic-resistant bacteria.

3. b.   Antibodies are specialized proteins produced by the immune system, which can recognize and target specific invading organisms.

4. FALSE.   Thousands of people die each year from infections contracted in health care settings.

5. ALL THREE.   Frequent handwashing prevents the spread of many disease-causing agents. Immunizations prime the body to tackle an invading organism. Sleep helps support a healthy immune system.

Countless microscopic organisms live around, on, and in us. Although most microbes are beneficial, many of them can cause disease. But the constant vigilance of our immune system keeps them at bay and our bodies intact and healthy. The immune system works to keep the body from being overwhelmed not just by external invaders that cause **infections,** but also by internal changes, such as cancer.

infections
Invasion of the body by microorganisms.

Most people don't notice these internal skirmishes unless they become sick. But people today are more knowledgeable about the complexities of immunity because they have heard about or had experience with *human immunodeficiency virus* (*HIV*) infection, which directly attacks the immune system. The rise in other infections has caught the public's attention, too. Old scourges, such as tuberculosis, are making comebacks—in stronger, drug-resistant forms.

This chapter introduces you to the mechanisms of immunity and infection and shows how to keep yourself well in a world of disease-causing microorganisms.

The Chain of Infection

Infectious diseases are transmitted from one person to another through a series of steps—a chain of infection (see Figure 9.1). New infections can be prevented by interfering with any step in this process.

Links in the Chain

The chain of infection has six major links: the pathogen, its reservoir, a portal of exit, a means of transmission, a portal of entry, and a new host.

Pathogen

The infectious disease cycle begins with a pathogen, a microorganism that causes disease. HIV (the virus that causes acquired immune deficiency syndrome, commonly known as *AIDS*) and the tuberculosis bacterium are examples of pathogens. Many pathogens cause illness because they produce **toxins** that harm human tissue; others do so by directly invading body cells.

FIGURE 9.1

The Chain of Infection

Any break in the chain of infection can prevent disease.

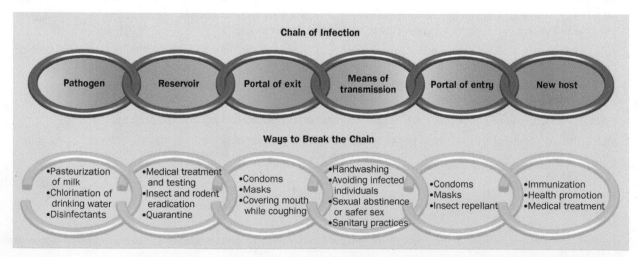

> **toxins**
> Poisonous substances.

Reservoir

The pathogen has a natural environment—called a **reservoir**—in which it typically lives. This reservoir can be a person, an animal, or an environmental component, such as soil or water. A person who is the reservoir for a pathogen may be ill or may be an asymptomatic carrier who, although having no symptoms, can spread infection.

> **reservoir**
> A natural environment in which a pathogen typically lives.

Portal of Exit

To transmit infection, the pathogen must leave the reservoir through some portal of exit. In the case of a human reservoir, portals of exit include saliva (for mumps, for example), the mucous membranes (for many sexually transmitted infections), blood (for HIV and hepatitis), feces (for intestinal infections), and nose and throat discharges (for colds and influenza).

Means of Transmission

Transmission can occur directly or indirectly. In direct transmission, the pathogen is passed from one person to another without an intermediary. Direct transmission usually requires fairly close association with an infected host, but not necessarily physical contact. For example, sneezing and coughing can discharge infectious particles into the air, where they can be inhaled by someone nearby. Most common respiratory infections and many intestinal infections are passed directly—for example, when a person with an infectious agent on his or her hands touches someone else. In addition to coughing and sneezing into the crook of the arm, proper handwashing is also key. See Figure 9.2 for proper handwashing techniques to help reduce transmission opportunities. Other means of direct transmission include sexual contact and contact with blood.

Transmission can also occur indirectly. Animals and insects, such as rats, ticks, and mosquitoes, can serve as **vectors**, carrying the pathogen from one host to another. Pathogens can also be transmitted via contaminated soil, food, or water or from inanimate objects, such as eating utensils, doorknobs, and handkerchiefs. Some pathogens float in the air for long periods, suspended on tiny particles of dust or droplets that can travel long distances before they are inhaled and cause infection.

> **vectors**
> Insects, rodents, or other organisms that carry and transmit a pathogen from one host to another.

Portal of Entry

To infect a new host, a pathogen must have a portal of entry into the body. Pathogens can enter in one of three general ways:
1. Direct contact with or penetration of the skin
2. Inhalation through the mouth or nose
3. Ingestion of contaminated food or water

Pathogens that enter the skin or mucous membranes can cause a local infection of the tissue, or they may penetrate into the bloodstream or lymphatic system, thereby causing a more extensive **systemic infection**. Agents that cause sexually transmitted infections (STIs) usually enter the body through the mucous membranes lining the urethra (in males) or the cervix (in females). Organisms that are transmitted via respiratory secretions may cause upper respiratory infections or pneumonia, or they may enter the bloodstream and cause systemic infection. Food-borne and water-borne organisms enter the mouth and travel to the location that will best support their reproduction. They may attack the cells of the small intestine or the colon, causing diarrhea, or they may enter the bloodstream via the digestive system and travel to other parts of the body.

FIGURE 9.2

Proper Handwashing Techniques

Handwashing with soap and water

1. Remove jewellery and wet hands and wrists with warm water.

2. Use 1 or 2 squirts of liquid or foam soap.

3. Lather soap and scrub hands well, palm to palm.

4. Scrub in between and around fingers.

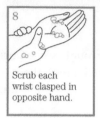

5. Scrub back of each hand with palm of other hand.

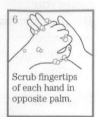

6. Scrub fingertips of each hand in opposite palm.

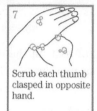

7. Scrub each thumb clasped in opposite hand.

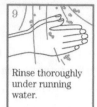

8. Scrub each wrist clasped in opposite hand.

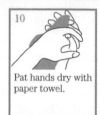

9. Rinse thoroughly under running water.

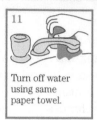

10. Pat hands dry with paper towel.

11. Turn off water using same paper towel.

Cleaning with alcohol-based hand rub

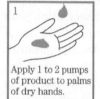

1. Apply 1 to 2 pumps of product to palms of dry hands.

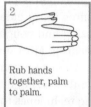

2. Rub hands together, palm to palm.

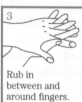

3. Rub in between and around fingers.

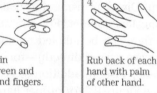

4. Rub back of each hand with palm of other hand.

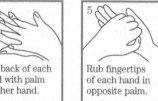

5. Rub fingertips of each hand in opposite palm.

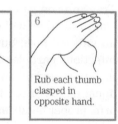

6. Rub each thumb clasped in opposite hand.

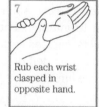

7. Rub each wrist clasped in opposite hand.

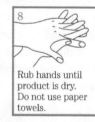

8. Rub hands until product is dry. Do not use paper towels.

Source: Ontario Ministry of Health and Long-Term Care. 2007. *Handwashing*, http://www.southwesthealthline.ca/healthlibrary_docs/C.5.Handwashing.pdf (retrieved June 10, 2015). Catalogue No. CIB-4446797 March 2007. © Queen's Printer for Ontario, 2007. Reproduced with permission.

---

systemic infection
An invasion by a microorganism that spreads though the blood or lymphatic system to large portions of the body.

The New Host

Once in the new host, a variety of factors determine whether the pathogen will be able to establish itself and cause infection. People with a strong immune system or resistance to a particular pathogen are less likely to become ill than people with poor immunity (the concept of immunity will be discussed later in the chapter). The number of pathogens that enter the new host is also important; the body's defences may be able to overcome a few bacteria, for example, but may be overwhelmed by thousands. If conditions are right, the pathogen will multiply and produce disease in the new host. In such a case, the new host may become a reservoir from which a new chain of infection can be started.

Breaking the Chain

Interrupting the chain of infection at any point can prevent disease. Strategies for breaking the chain include a mix of public health measures and individual action. For example, a pathogen's reservoir can be isolated or destroyed, as when a sick individual is placed under quarantine or when insects or animals carrying pathogens are killed. Public sanitation practices, such as sewage treatment and the chlorination of drinking water, can also kill pathogens. Transmission can be disrupted through various strategies, such as handwashing and the use of facemasks. Immunization and the treatment of infected hosts can stop the pathogen from multiplying, producing a serious disease, and being passed on to a new host. Some methods of breaking the chain of infection are listed in Figure 9.1.

QUESTIONS FOR CRITICAL THINKING AND REFLECTION

Think about the last time you were sick with a cold, the flu, or an intestinal infection. Can you identify the reservoir from which the infection came? What vector, if any, transmitted the illness to you? Did you pass the infection to anyone else? If so, how? What could you do differently to avoid infecting others?

The Body's Defence System

Our bodies have very effective ways of protecting themselves against invasion by foreign organisms, especially pathogens. The body's first line of defence is a formidable array of physical and chemical barriers. When these barriers are breached, the body's **immune system** comes into play. Together, these defences provide an effective response to nearly all the challenges and invasions our bodies will ever experience.

immune system
The body's collective physical and chemical defences against foreign organisms and pathogens.

Physical and Chemical Barriers

The skin, the body's largest organ, prevents many microorganisms from entering the body. Although many bacterial and fungal organisms live on the surface of the skin, very few can penetrate it except through a cut or break.

Wherever there is an opening in the body, or an area without skin, other barriers exist. The mouth is lined with mucous membranes, which contain cells designed to prevent the passage of unwanted organisms and particles. Body openings and the fluids that cover them (for example, tears, saliva, and vaginal secretions) are rich in antibodies (discussed in detail later in the chapter) and in enzymes that break down and destroy many microorganisms.

The respiratory tract is lined not only with mucous membranes, but also with cells that have hair-like protrusions called *cilia*. The cilia sweep foreign matter up and out of the respiratory tract. Particles that are not caught by this mechanism may be expelled from the system by a cough. If the ciliated cells are damaged or destroyed, a cough is the body's only way of ridding the airways of foreign particles. This is one reason smokers generally have a chronic cough—to compensate for damaged airways.

The Immune System

The immune system operates through a remarkable information network involving billions of cellular defenders that rush to protect the body when a threat arises. Once the body has been invaded by a foreign organism, an elaborate system of responses is activated. Two of these responses are the inflammatory response and the immune response.

Immunological Defenders

The immune response is carried out by different types of white blood cells, which are continuously being produced in the bone marrow.

- **Neutrophils**, one type of white blood cell, travel in the bloodstream to areas of invasion, attacking and ingesting pathogens.
- **Macrophages**, or "big eaters," take up stations in tissues and act as scavengers, devouring pathogens and worn-out cells.
- **Natural killer cells** directly destroy virus-infected cells and cells that have turned cancerous.
- **Dendritic cells**, which reside in tissues, eat pathogens and activate lymphocytes.
- **Lymphocytes**, of which there are several types, are white blood cells that travel in both the bloodstream and the lymphatic system.

neutrophils
A type of white blood cell that engulfs foreign organisms and infected, damaged, or aged cells; particularly prevalent during the inflammatory response.

macrophages
Large phagocytic (cell-eating) cells that devour foreign particles.

natural killer cells
A type of white blood cell that directly destroys virus-infected cells and cancer cells.

dendritic cells
A type of white blood cell specialized to activate T and B cells.

lymphocytes
A type of white blood cell that works in both the bloodstream and the lymphatic system.

At various places in the lymphatic system are lymph nodes (or glands), where macrophages and dendritic cells congregate and filter bacteria and other substances from the lymph (see Figure 9.3). When these nodes are actively involved in fighting an invasion of microorganisms, they fill with cells; physicians use the location of swollen lymph nodes as a clue to the location and cause of an infection.

The two main types of lymphocytes are **T cells** and **B cells**. T cells are further differentiated into **helper T cells**, **killer T cells**, and **suppressor T cells** (also called *regulatory T cells*). B cells are lymphocytes that produce **antibodies**. The first time T cells and B cells encounter a specific invader, some of them are reserved as **memory T and B cells**, enabling the body to mount a rapid response should the same invader appear again in the future. These cells and cell products—macrophages, natural killer cells, dendritic cells, T cells, B cells and antibodies, and memory cells—are the primary players in the body's immune response.

T cells
A type of lymphocyte that arises in bone marrow and matures in the thymus (thus its name).

B cells
A type of lymphocyte that matures in the bone marrow and produces antibodies.

helper T cells
Lymphocytes that help activate other T cells and may help B cells produce antibodies.

killer T cells
Lymphocytes that kill body cells that have been invaded by foreign organisms; also can kill cells that have turned cancerous.

suppressor T cells
Lymphocytes that inhibit the growth of other lymphocytes; also called *regulatory T cells*.

antibodies
Specialized proteins produced by white blood cells that can recognize and neutralize specific microbes.

memory T and B cells
Lymphocytes generated during an initial infection that circulate in the body for years, remembering the specific antigens that caused the infection and quickly destroying them if they appear again.

The immune system is built on a remarkable feature of these defenders: the ability to distinguish foreign cells from the body's own cells. Because lymphocytes are capable of great destruction, it is essential that they not attack the body itself. When they do, they cause **autoimmune diseases**, such as lupus and rheumatoid arthritis.

autoimmune diseases
Diseases in which the immune system attacks the person's own body.

All the cells in your body display markers on their surfaces—tiny molecular shapes—that identify them as "self" to lymphocytes that encounter them. Invading microorganisms also display markers on their surface; lymphocytes identify these as foreign, or "non-self." Non-self markers that trigger the immune response are known as **antigens**.

antigens
Markers on the surface of a foreign substance that immune system cells recognize as non-self and that trigger the immune response.

Antibodies have complementary surface markers that work with antigens like a lock and key. When an antigen appears in the body, it eventually encounters an antibody with a complementary pattern. The antibody locks onto the antigen, triggering a series of events designed to destroy the invading pathogen. The truly astonishing thing is that the body does not synthesize the appropriate antibody lock after it comes into contact with the antigen key. Rather, antibodies already exist for millions, if not billions, of possible antigens.

FIGURE 9.3

The Lymphatic System

The lymphatic system consists of a network of vessels and organs, including the spleen, lymph nodes, thymus, and tonsils. The vessels pick up excess fluid and proteins, lipids, and other particles from body tissues. These pass through the lymph nodes, where macrophages and dendritic cells help clear the lymph (fluid) of debris and bacteria and other pathogens. The cleansed lymph is then returned to the bloodstream. The lymphatic organs are production centres for infection-fighting cells and sites for some immune responses.

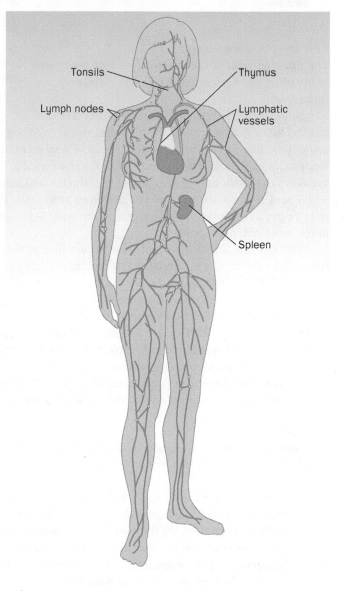

The Inflammatory Response

When the body has been injured or infected, one of the body's responses is the inflammatory response. Special cells in the area of invasion or injury release **histamine** and other substances that cause blood vessels to dilate and fluid to flow out of capillaries into the injured tissue. This produces increased heat, swelling, and redness in the affected area. White blood cells, including neutrophils, dendritic cells, and macrophages, are drawn to the area and attack the invaders—in many cases, destroying them. At the site of infection there may be *pus*, a collection of dead white blood cells and debris resulting from the encounter.

histamine
A chemical responsible for the dilation and increased permeability of blood vessels in allergic reactions.

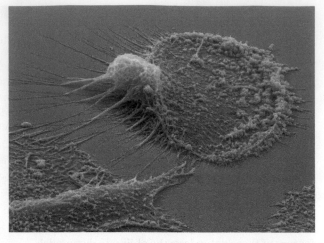

Dendritic cells are white blood cells that engulf foreign cells and display their antigens, thereby activating T and B cells. The dendritic cell shown in this scanning electron micrograph is magnified 2700 times.

The Immune Response

The immune system makes two types of responses to invading pathogens: natural (innate) and acquired (adaptive).

Neutrophils, macrophages, dendritic cells, and natural killer cells are part of the natural response. They recognize pathogens as "foreign" but have no memory of past infections; they respond the same way no matter how many times a pathogen invades. These cells essentially eat the invaders, destroying them internally. Natural killer cells also destroy infected body cells, breaking the chain of reproduction of a pathogen and helping to stop an infection.

T and B cells are part of the acquired response. They change after one contact with the pathogen, developing a memory for the antigen. If the body is invaded again, they recognize the pathogen and mount a much more potent response.

Think of the immune response as having four phases, as shown in Figure 9.4. In each phase, the system takes steps to destroy the invader and restore the body to health.

- *Phase 1:* Dendritic cells are drawn to the site of the injury and consume the foreign cells; they then provide information about the pathogen by displaying its antigen on their surfaces. Helper T cells read this information and rush to respond.
- *Phase 2:* Helper T cells multiply rapidly and trigger the production of killer T cells and B cells in the spleen and lymph nodes. **Cytokines**, chemical messengers secreted by lymphocytes, help regulate and coordinate the immune response; *interleukins* and *interferons* are two examples of cytokines. They stimulate increased production of T cells, B cells, and antibodies; promote the activities of natural killer cells; produce fever; and have special antipathogenic properties themselves.

cytokines
Chemical messengers produced by a variety of cell types that help regulate many cell functions; immune system cells release cytokines that help amplify and coordinate the immune response.

- *Phase 3:* Killer T cells strike at foreign cells and body cells that have been invaded and infected, identifying them by the antigens displayed on the cell surfaces. Puncturing the cell membrane, they sacrifice body cells to destroy the foreign organism within. This type of action is known as a *cell-mediated immune response* because the attack is carried out by cells. Killer T cells also trigger an amplified inflammatory response and recruit more macrophages to help clean up the site.

    B cells work in a different way. Stimulated to multiply by helper T cells, they produce large quantities of antibody molecules, which are released in the bloodstream and tissues. Antibodies are Y-shaped protein molecules that bind to antigen-bearing targets and mark them for destruction by macrophages. This type of response is known as an *antibody-mediated immune response*. Antibodies work against bacteria, viruses, and other substances when they are in the body but outside cells. They do not work against infected body cells or viruses that are replicating inside cells.

FIGURE 9.4

The Immune Response

Once invaded by a pathogen, the body mounts a complex series of reactions to eliminate the invader. Pictured here are the principal elements of the immune response to a virus; not shown are the many types of cytokines that help coordinate the actions of different types of defenders.

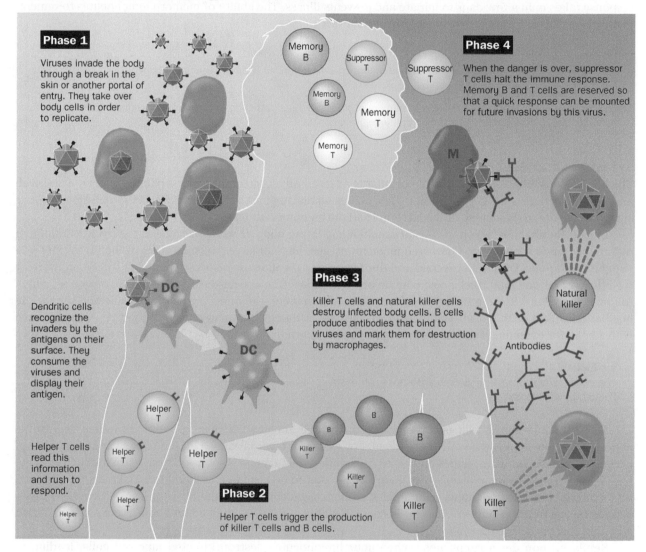

- *Phase 4:* The last phase of the immune response is a slowdown of activity. During the course of the immune response, regulatory molecules and cells inhibit lymphocyte proliferation and induce lymphocyte death; this process restores resting levels of B and T cells. The dead cells, killed pathogens, and other debris that result from the immune response are scavenged by certain types of white blood cells; filtered out of circulation by the liver, spleen, and kidneys; and excreted from the body.

QUICK STATS

Worldwide, 1100 epidemics of different diseases were identified between 2002 and 2007.

—World Health Organization, 2007

Immunity

After an infection, survival often confers **immunity**; that is, an infected person will never get the same illness again. This is because some of the lymphocytes created during the second phase of the immune response are reserved as memory T and B cells. As part of the acquired immune response, they continue to circulate in the blood and lymphatic system for years or even for the rest of the person's life. If the same antigen enters the body again, the memory T and B cells recognize and destroy it before it can cause illness. This subsequent response takes only a few days to initiate and prevents illness. The ability of memory lymphocytes to remember previous infections is known as **acquired immunity.**

> **immunity**
> Mechanisms that defend the body against infection; specific defences against specific pathogens.
>
> **acquired immunity**
> The body's ability to mobilize the cellular memory of an attack by a pathogen to throw off subsequent attacks; acquired through vaccination and the normal immune response.

Symptoms and Contagion

The immune system is operating at the cellular level at all times, maintaining its vigilance when you are well and fighting invaders when you are sick. How does it all feel to you, the host for these activities? How do your symptoms relate to the course of the infection and the immune response?

During **incubation**, when viruses are multiplying in the body or when bacteria are actively multiplying before the immune system has gathered momentum, you may not have any symptoms of the illness, but you may be contagious. During the second and third phases of the immune response, you may still be unaware of the infection, or you may "feel a cold coming on." Symptoms first appear during the *prodromal period*, which follows incubation. If the infected host has acquired immunity, the infection may be eradicated during the incubation period or the prodromal period. In this case, although you may have felt you were coming down with a cold, for example, it does not develop into a full-blown illness.

> **incubation**
> The period when bacteria or viruses are actively multiplying inside the body's cells; usually a period without symptoms of illness.

Many symptoms of an illness are actually due to the immune response of the body rather than to the actions or products of the invading organism. For example, fever is caused by the release and activation of certain cytokines in macrophages and other cells during the immune response. These cytokines travel in the bloodstream to the brain and cause the body's thermostat to be reset to a higher level. The resulting elevated temperature helps the body in its fight against pathogens by enhancing immune responses. During an illness, it is necessary to lower a fever only if it is uncomfortably high (more than 38.6°C) or if it occurs in an infant who is at risk for seizures from fever.

Similarly, you get a runny nose when your lymphocytes destroy infected mucosal cells, leading to increased mucus production. The malaise and fatigue of the flu are caused by pro-inflammatory cytokines.

You are contagious when you have infectious microbes in your body and they can gain access to another person. This may be before a vigorous immune response has occurred, so at times you may be contagious before experiencing any symptoms. This means that you can transmit an illness without knowing you are infected or catch an illness from someone who doesn't appear to be sick. Conversely, your symptoms may continue after the pathogens have been mostly destroyed, when you are no longer infectious.

Immunization

The ability of the immune system to remember previously encountered organisms and retain its strength against them is the basis for **immunization**. When a person is immunized, the immune system is primed with an antigen similar to the pathogenic organism but not as dangerous. The body responds by producing antibodies, which prevent serious infection when and if the person is exposed to the disease organism itself. The preparation used to manipulate the immune system is known as a **vaccine** (see Table 9.1).

immunization
The process of conferring immunity to a pathogen by administering a vaccine.

vaccine
A preparation of killed or weakened microorganisms, inactivated toxins, or components of microorganisms that is administered to stimulate an immune response; a vaccine protects against future infection by the pathogen.

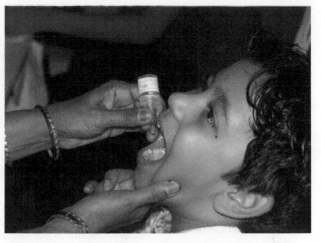

Oral vaccines have made it easier to immunize children in remote and impoverished areas of the world.

Types of Vaccines

Vaccines can be made in several ways. In some cases, microbes are cultured in the laboratory in a way that attenuates (weakens) them. These live, attenuated organisms are used in vaccines against several diseases, such as measles, mumps, and rubella (German measles). In other cases, when it is not possible to breed attenuated organisms, vaccines are made from pathogens that have been killed in the laboratory but that still retain their ability to stimulate the production of antibodies. Vaccines composed of killed viruses are used against influenza viruses, among others.

Vaccines confer what is known as *active immunity*—that is, the vaccinated person produces his or her own antibodies to the microorganism. Another type of injection confers *passive immunity*. In this case, a person exposed to a disease is injected with the antibodies themselves, produced by other human beings or animals who have recovered from the disease. Injections of gamma globulin—a product made from the blood plasma of many individuals containing all the antibodies they have ever made—are sometimes given to people to create a rapid but temporary immunity to a particular disease. Gamma globulin is also sometimes used to treat antibody deficiency syndromes.

QUICK STATS

27 common diseases can be prevented by vaccines, including 16 harmful diseases that target children and youth.

—CDC, 2007; 2013

VACCINE SAFETY   Side effects from immunization, such as soreness at the injection site, are usually mild. It is estimated that an allergic reaction may occur in less than 1 in 1 million doses. Any risk from vaccines must be balanced against the risk posed by the diseases they prevent; for example, the death rate from diphtheria is about 5–10 percent.

The Public Health Agency of Canada monitors reports of adverse reactions to vaccines, and new formulations or types of vaccines are being developed to increase safety. For example, oral polio vaccine, which contains live but weakened poliovirus, has been replaced by inactivated poliovirus, which contains killed virus. The oral vaccine is somewhat more effective, but in about 1 in 2.7 million cases, it causes polio; because of the low risk for polio in Canada, the oral vaccine is no longer used.

TABLE 9.1

Immunizations for Canadian Children and Adults

Vaccine	People for Whom Immunization Is Recommended
Diphtheria, tetanus, acellular pertussis, and inactivated polio virus vaccine (DTAP-IPV)	All children up to 6 years. Infants receive it starting at 2 months. Booster shots are recommended at age 4, 6, and 12 months, at age 4–6 years, and every 10 years thereafter.
Haemophilus influenzae type b conjugate (Hib)	All children up to 5 years of age. All infants starting at 2 months up to 18 months. Older children and adults who have had a splenectomy or bone marrow transplant, have sickle-cell disease or HIV/AIDS, or are undergoing immunosuppressant drug therapy.
HPV vaccine	Females and males between 9 and 13 years of age, before the onset of sexual intercourse. Females and males between the ages of 14 and 26 years of age, even if they are already sexually active. Females who have had previous pap abnormalities. Males who have sex with other males. Either sex who have had a previous HPV infection.
Measles, mumps, and rubella (MMR)	All children. First dose is given when the child is 12–15 months old. Second dose at 18 months of age or any time thereafter; for convenience it should be given at school entry (4–6 years). All children at age 11–18 years or at high-school entry. Unvaccinated first-year post-secondary students living in dormitories, military recruits, and others at increased risk.
Varicella (Var)	Children ages 12–15 months should receive first dose. Second dose at 18 months of age or after, ideally prior to school entry. Susceptible individuals 13 years of age should receive two doses at least 28 days apart. All adults if no record or unclear, doses 1 and 2, at least 4 weeks apart for susceptible adults (no history of natural disease or seronegativity).
Hepatitis A	Occupational risk, lifestyle, travel, and living in areas lacking adequate sanitation. Outbreak control, post-exposure immunoprophylaxis. Patients with chronic liver disease.
Hepatitis B	All children 9–17 years of age. For infants born to chronic carriers, the first dose should be given at birth. Those with occupational risk, lifestyle risk, post-exposure immunoprophylaxis, patients with chronic liver disease, and health care workers.
Pneumococcal conjugate-13-valent (Pneu-C-7)	All children under 2 years of age. First dose is given at 2 months.
Pneumococcyl polysaccharide (Pneu-P-23)	Adults 65 years. Adults < 65 years who have conditions putting them at increased risk of pneumococcal disease.
Meningococcal C conjugate (Men-C)	Children under 5 years of age, adolescents, and young adults. The recommended schedule depends on the age of the individual.
Influenza (Inf)	Annually for all individuals age 6 months and older.
Diphtheria, tetanus (Td)	All adults. Booster is recommended every 10 years. If no record or unclear, then doses 1 and 2, 4–8 weeks apart, and dose 3 at 6–12 months later; one of the doses should be given as Tdap for pertussis protection.

NOTE: This guide is for information purposes only. All parents and adults should discuss their personal immunization schedule recommendations with their physician.

Source: Public Healthy Agency of Canada. *Canadian Immunization Guide, 2014*. Reproduced with permission from the Minister of Health, 2015. All rights reserved. HYPERLINK "http://www.phac-aspc.gc.ca/publicat/cig-gci/index-eng.php" \l "toc"http://www.phac-aspc.gc.ca/publicat/cig-gci/index-eng.php#toc

QUICK STATS

Worldwide, 1.5 million children die each year of vaccine-preventable diseases.
—WHO, 2012

A possible link was proposed in the past between immunization and autism, a severe developmental disorder characterized by behavioural problems and impaired social and communication skills. However, a 2004 Institute of Medicine report concluded that evidence does not support such a link; a large 2006 study confirmed this conclusion. Thimerosal, a mercury-containing preservative, was withdrawn from most pediatric vaccines in Canada, although no clear link has been found between vaccines containing thimerosal and autism.

QUESTIONS FOR CRITICAL THINKING AND REFLECTION

What are your views on government-required child vaccinations? What has shaped your views on this issue?

Allergy: The Body's Defence System Gone Haywire

Many Canadians are affected by **allergies**. Allergies result from a hypersensitive and overactive immune system. The immune system typically defends the body against only genuinely harmful pathogens, such as viruses and bacteria. However, in someone with an allergy, the immune system also mounts a response to a harmless substance, such as pollen or animal dander. Allergy symptoms—stuffy nose, sneezing, wheezing, skin rashes, and so on—result primarily from the immune response rather than from the substances that provoke the response.

> **allergies**
> A disorder caused by the body's exaggerated response to foreign chemicals and proteins; also called *hypersensitivity*.

Allergens

Substances that provoke allergies are known as **allergens**; they may cause a response if they are inhaled or swallowed or if they come in contact with the skin. Different people have allergic reactions to different substances, but many Canadians react to at least one common allergen, such as one of the following:

- *Pollen:* Referred to as hay fever or allergic rhinitis, pollen allergies are widespread; weeds, grasses, and trees are common producers of allergenic pollen.
- *Animal dander:* People with animal allergies are usually allergic not to fur but to dander (dead skin flakes), urine, or a protein found in saliva; allergies to mice, dogs, and cats are common.
- *Dust mites and cockroaches:* The droppings of cockroaches and microscopic dust mites can trigger allergies; mites live in carpets, upholstered furniture, and bedding.
- *Moulds and mildew:* The small spores produced by these fungi can trigger allergy symptoms; moulds and mildew thrive in damp areas of buildings.
- *Foods:* The most common food allergens in adults include peanuts, tree nuts, fish, and shellfish.
- *Insect stings:* The venom of insects, such as yellow jackets, honeybees, hornets, paper wasps, and fire ants, causes allergic reactions in some people.

> **allergens**
> Substances that trigger an allergic reaction.

People may also be allergic to certain medications; plants, such as poison oak; latex; metals, such as nickel; and compounds found in cosmetics.

The Allergic Response

Most allergic reactions are due to the production of a special type of antibody known as immunoglobulin E (IgE). Initial exposure to a particular allergen may cause little response, but it sensitizes the immune system by causing the production of allergen-specific IgE, which binds to mast cells (see Figure 9.5). Mast cells are part of the immune system and play a role in healing, the immune response, and allergic reactions. When the

FIGURE 9.5

The Allergic Response

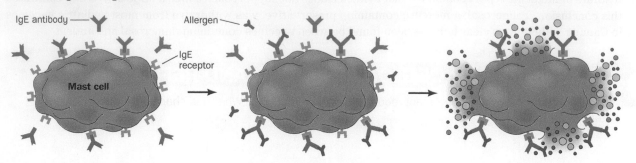

During sensitization, allergens, such as pollen, trigger the production of IgE antibodies, which bind to mast cells.

During an allergic reaction, the allergens enter the bloodstream and are recognized and bound by the IgE antibodies.

The IgE-allergen combination causes mast cells to release histamine and other compounds into surrounding tissue, producing allergy symptoms.

body is subsequently exposed to the allergen, the allergen binds to IgE, causing the mast cells to release large amounts of histamine and other compounds into surrounding tissues.

Histamine has many effects, including increasing the inflammatory response and stimulating mucus production. The precise symptoms depend on what part of the body is affected. In the nose, histamine may cause congestion and sneezing; in the eyes, itchiness and tearing; in the skin, redness, swelling, and itching; in the intestines, bloating and cramping; and in the lungs, coughing, wheezing, and shortness of breath. In some people, an allergen can trigger an asthma attack (see the Dimensions of Diversity box). Symptoms often occur immediately, within minutes of exposure, but inflammatory reactions may take hours or days to develop and then may persist for several days.

The most serious, but rare, kind of allergic reaction is **anaphylaxis**, which results from a release of histamine throughout the body. Anaphylactic reactions can be life threatening because symptoms may include swelling of the throat, extremely low blood pressure, fainting, heart arrhythmia, and seizures. Anaphylaxis is a medical emergency, and treatment requires immediate injection of epinephrine. People at risk for anaphylaxis should wear MedicAlert identification and keep self-administrable epinephrine readily available.

anaphylaxis
A severe systemic hypersensitive reaction to an allergen characterized by difficulty breathing, low blood pressure, heart arrhythmia, seizure, and sometimes death.

 Dimensions *of* DIVERSITY

Environment, Ethnicity, and Asthma

Asthma is caused by both inflammation of the airways and spasm of the muscles surrounding the airways. The spasm causes constriction, and the inflammation causes the airway linings to swell and secrete extra mucus, which further obstructs the passages. The inflammation can become chronic, making airways even more sensitive to triggers. The symptoms of asthma—wheezing, tightness in the chest, and shortness of breath—may be mild and occur only occasionally, or they may be severe and occur daily.

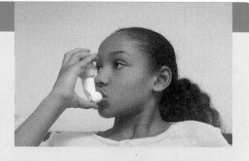

An asthma attack begins when something sets off inflammation of the bronchial tubes. Usually it's an allergic reaction to an inhaled allergen, most commonly dust mites, mould, animal dander, or pollen. Anything that irritates or overtaxes the bronchial airways can also trigger spasms, such as exercise, cold air, pollutants, tobacco smoke, infection, or stress. In females with asthma, hormonal changes that occur as menstruation starts may increase vulnerability to attacks.

Patterns and Prevalence

The prevalence of asthma is increasing. In Canada, more than 2.3 million adults and nearly a half million children (ages 4 to 11 years) have asthma; each year asthma is responsible for almost 150 000 emergency department visits and somewhere between 250 and 500 deaths. Between 1994 and 2001, the number of Canadian children with asthma increased by 2 percent, representing 70 000 children, and despite better treatment options, the death rate remains worrisome.

The tendency to develop asthma may be hereditary, but some patterns appear to link it to the increased Westernization of environmental factors, such as changes in maternal diet and increased exposures to household allergens, pets, environmental tobacco smoke, and environmental pollution. Although research is ongoing, it is clear that the environment is an important determinant of asthma.

With regard to ethnicity, Canadian researchers recently found that children of Asian and African descent are at greater risk of being misdiagnosed with asthma and, therefore, being overmedicated for the condition. The reason for this misdiagnosis has to do with an increasingly popular diagnostic test—assessing the amount of nitric oxide in exhaled breath—to detect and manage the disease. Children of Asian and African descent have higher levels of nitric oxide than other children, leading to a diagnosis of asthma in some children who do not actually have it. More research is needed to better identify the typical levels of nitric oxide among various groups, thus avoiding potential misdiagnosis and treatment.

Treatment and Prevention of Attacks

Inhaling a muscle-relaxing medication from a bronchodilator can relieve an asthma attack immediately by opening the bronchial tubes. Inhaling an anti-inflammatory drug can treat the underlying inflammation. Both types of treatments may be needed to get asthma under control. Other medications for asthma block the actions of molecules involved in the body's inflammatory response. Asthmatics can monitor their condition by testing their peak airflow several times a day; a drop in peak airflow can signal an upcoming attack.

It's also a good idea to avoid allergens when possible. A recent study of urban children found that relatively small changes can reduce asthma symptoms and health care visits. In this study, allergen exposures were reduced by covering the mattresses and pillows with special covers; using HEPA filters in vacuum cleaners and room air purifiers; and employing professional pest control. Other researchers have found that many children with asthma live in households in which simple allergen control methods haven't been taken, including closing windows to keep pollen out, avoiding environmental tobacco smoke, and reducing or eliminating exposure to pets.

Sources: Asthma Society of Canada. *Asthma Facts and Statistics,* http://www.asthma.ca/corp/newsroom/pdf/asthmastats.pdf (retrieved June 10, 2015); Kovesi, T., Y. Kulka, and R. Dales. 2008. Exhaled nitric oxide concentrationis affected by age, height, and race in healthy 9–12-year-old children. *CHEST* 133: 169–175; Garner, R., and D. Kohen. 2008. Changes in the prevalence of asthma among Canadian children. *Health Reports* 19(2), http://www.statcan.gc.ca/pub/82-003-x/2008002/article/10551-eng.htm (retrieved June 10, 2015); and Wang, H.-Y., et al. 2008. Prevalence of asthma among Chinese adolescents living in Canada and in China. *Canadian Medical Association Journal* 179(11): 1133–1142 http://www.cmaj.ca/cgi/content/full/179/11/1133 (retrieved June 10, 2015).

Dealing with Allergies

If you suspect you might have an allergy, visit your physician or an allergy specialist. You have three general strategies for dealing with allergies:

- *Avoidance:* You may be able to avoid or minimize exposure to allergens by making changes in your environment or behaviour. For example, removing carpets from the bedroom and using special bedding can reduce dust mite contact. Pollen exposure can be limited by avoiding outdoor activities during peak pollination times, keeping windows shut, and showering and changing clothes following outdoor activities. If you can't part with a pet, keep pets out of bedrooms and frequently vacuum or damp-mop floors.
- *Medication:* A variety of medications are available for allergy sufferers. Many over-the-counter antihistamines are effective at controlling symptoms, such as blocked nasal, sinus, or middle ear passages. Prescription corticosteroids delivered by aerosol markedly reduce allergy symptoms, increase effectiveness, and help limit systemic absorption and side effects.
- *Immunotherapy:* Referred to as allergy shots, immunotherapy desensitizes a person to a particular allergen through the administration of gradually increasing doses of the allergen over months or years.

Pathogens and Disease

When pathogens enter body tissue, they can cause illness and sometimes death to the host. Worldwide, infectious diseases are responsible for more than 25 percent or about 15 million deaths each year (see Table 9.2).

Pathogens include bacteria, viruses, fungi, protozoa, parasitic worms, and prions (see Figure 9.6). Infections can occur almost anywhere in or on the body. Common types of infection include bronchitis, infection of the airways (bronchi); meningitis, infection of the tissue surrounding the brain and spinal cord; conjunctivitis, infection of the layer of cells surrounding the eyes; pharyngitis, or sore throat; pneumonia, infection of the lung; gastroenteritis, infection of the gastrointestinal tract; cellulitis, infection of the soft tissues; osteomyelitis, infection of the bones; and so on, for every tissue and organ.

TABLE 9.2

Most Prevalent Infectious Diseases Worldwide

Disease	Approximate Number of Deaths per Year
Pneumonia	3 884 000
HIV/AIDS	2 777 000
Diarrheal diseases	1 798 000
Tuberculosis	1 300 000–2 000 000
Malaria	1 272 000
Measles	611 000
Pertussis (whooping cough)	294 000
Tetanus	214 000
Meningitis	173 000
Syphilis	157 000

Sources: World Health Organization. 2004. *The World Health Report 2004*; Geneva: World Health Organization; and Fauci et al. 2005. Emerging infectious diseases: a 10-year perspective from the National Institute of Allergy and Infectious Diseases. *Emerging Infectious Diseases*, http://wwwnc.cdc.gov/eid/article/11/4/04-1167.htm (retrieved June 9, 2015).

Bacteria

The most abundant living things on Earth are **bacteria**, single-celled organisms that usually reproduce by splitting in two to create a pair of identical cells. Many species of bacteria feed on dead matter and play an important role in the recycling of nutrients for other organisms; other species feed on living things and may cause disease. Bacteria are often classified according to their shape: They may be bacilli (rod shaped), cocci (spherical), spirochete (spiral), or vibrios (comma shaped).

bacteria (bacterium, singular)
Microscopic single-celled organisms; about 100 bacterial species can cause disease in humans.

We harbour both helpful and harmful bacteria on our skin and in our gastrointestinal and reproductive tracts. The human colon contains friendly bacteria that produce certain vitamins and help digest nutrients. (A large portion of feces consists of bacteria.) Friendly bacteria also keep harmful bacteria in check by competing for food and resources and secreting substances toxic to pathogenic bacteria. For example, *Lactobacillus acidophilus* resides in the vagina and produces chemicals that kill yeast and bacteria that cause vaginal infections.

Not all bacteria found in the body are beneficial, however. Pathogenic bacteria in food or drink can disrupt the normal harmony in the intestines by invading cells or producing damaging toxins. Sexual activity can introduce pathogenic bacteria into the reproductive tract. Within the bloodstream, tissues, and organs, the human body is usually aseptic—devoid of bacteria. If bacteria find their way into these areas, infection may result.

Pneumonia

Inflammation of the lungs, called **pneumonia**, may be caused by infection with bacteria, viruses, or fungi or by contact with chemical toxins or irritants. Pneumonia can be serious if the alveoli (air sacs) become clogged with fluid, thus preventing oxygen from reaching the bloodstream. Pneumonia often follows another illness, such as a cold or the flu, but the symptoms are typically more severe: fever, chills, shortness of breath, increased mucus production, and cough. Pneumonia grouped with influenza ranks eighth among the leading causes of death for Canadians; people most at risk for severe infection include those under age 2 and over age 75 and those with chronic health problems, such as heart disease, asthma, or HIV. Bacterial pneumonia can be treated with antibiotics.

FIGURE 9.6

Pathogens and Associated Infectious Diseases

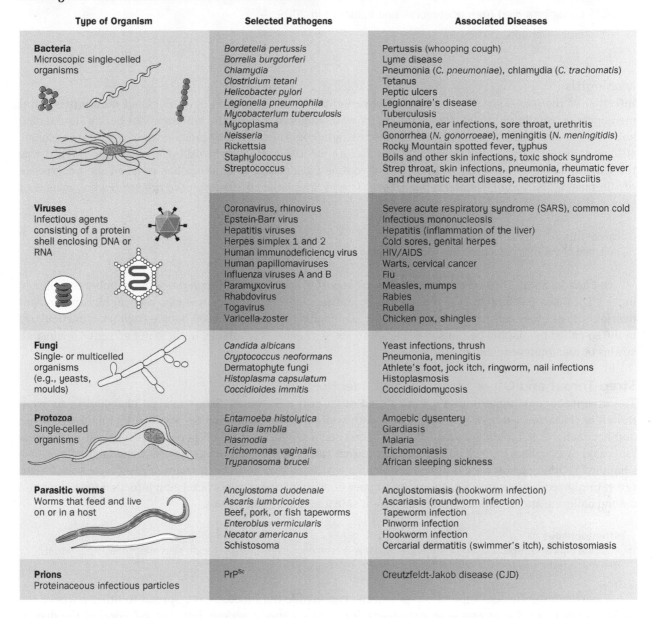

Type of Organism	Selected Pathogens	Associated Diseases
Bacteria Microscopic single-celled organisms	*Bordetella pertussis* *Borrelia burgdorferi* *Chlamydia* *Clostridium tetani* *Helicobacter pylori* *Legionella pneumophila* *Mycobacterium tuberculosis* *Mycoplasma* *Neisseria* Rickettsia Staphylococcus Streptococcus	Pertussis (whooping cough) Lyme disease Pneumonia (*C. pneumoniae*), chlamydia (*C. trachomatis*) Tetanus Peptic ulcers Legionnaire's disease Tuberculosis Pneumonia, ear infections, sore throat, urethritis Gonorrhea (*N. gonorroeae*), meningitis (*N. meningitidis*) Rocky Mountain spotted fever, typhus Boils and other skin infections, toxic shock syndrome Strep throat, skin infections, pneumonia, rheumatic fever and rheumatic heart disease, necrotizing fasciitis
Viruses Infectious agents consisting of a protein shell enclosing DNA or RNA	Coronavirus, rhinovirus Epstein-Barr virus Hepatitis viruses Herpes simplex 1 and 2 Human immunodeficiency virus Human papillomaviruses Influenza viruses A and B Paramyxovirus Rhabdovirus Togavirus Varicella-zoster	Severe acute respiratory syndrome (SARS), common cold Infectious mononucleosis Hepatitis (inflammation of the liver) Cold sores, genital herpes HIV/AIDS Warts, cervical cancer Flu Measles, mumps Rabies Rubella Chicken pox, shingles
Fungi Single- or multicelled organisms (e.g., yeasts, moulds)	*Candida albicans* *Cryptococcus neoformans* Dermatophyte fungi *Histoplasma capsulatum* *Coccidioides immitis*	Yeast infections, thrush Pneumonia, meningitis Athlete's foot, jock itch, ringworm, nail infections Histoplasmosis Coccidioidomycosis
Protozoa Single-celled organisms	*Entamoeba histolytica* *Giardia lamblia* *Plasmodia* *Trichomonas vaginalis* *Trypanosoma brucei*	Amoebic dysentery Giardiasis Malaria Trichomoniasis African sleeping sickness
Parasitic worms Worms that feed and live on or in a host	*Ancylostoma duodenale* *Ascaris lumbricoides* Beef, pork, or fish tapeworms *Enterobius vermicularis* *Necator americanus* Schistosoma	Ancylostomiasis (hookworm infection) Ascariasis (roundworm infection) Tapeworm infection Pinworm infection Hookworm infection Cercarial dermatitis (swimmer's itch), schistosomiasis
Prions Proteinaceous infectious particles	PrP^{Sc}	Creutzfeldt-Jakob disease (CJD)

pneumonia
Inflammation of the lungs, typically caused by infection or exposure to chemical toxins or irritants.

Pneumococcus bacteria are the most common cause of bacterial pneumonia; a vaccine is available and recommended for all adults age 65 and older and others at risk. Other bacteria that may cause pneumonia include *Streptococcus pneumoniae*, *Chlamydia pneumoniae*, and **mycoplasmas**. Outbreaks of infection with mycoplasmas are relatively common among young adults, especially in crowded settings, such as dormitories.

mycoplasmas
Small bacteria with an incomplete cell wall that may cause sore throats, ear infections, and pneumonia.

5826 Canadians died from pneumonia and influenza in 2009.
—Statistics Canada, 2012

Meningitis

Infection of the *meninges*, the membranes covering the brain and spinal cord, is called **meningitis**. Viral meningitis is usually mild and goes away on its own; bacterial meningitis, however, can be life threatening and requires immediate treatment with antibiotics. Symptoms of meningitis include fever, a severe headache, stiff neck, sensitivity to light, and confusion. Before the 1990s, *Haemophilus Influenzae* type b (Hib) was the leading cause of bacterial meningitis, but routine vaccination of children has reduced the occurrence of Hib meningitis. Today, *Neisseria meningitidis* and *Streptococcus pneumoniae* are the leading causes of bacterial meningitis.

meningitis
Infection of the meninges (membranes covering the brain and spinal cord).

In Canada, about 1000 cases of meningitis are reported each year, although the actual number is probably higher. The disease is fatal in 11 percent of cases, and about 20 percent of people who recover have permanent hearing loss or other serious effects. Worldwide, meningitis kills about 135 000 people each year, particularly in the so-called meningitis belt in sub-Saharan Africa. A vaccine is available, but it is not effective against all strains of meningitis-causing bacteria.

Strep Throat and Other Streptococcal Infections

The **streptococcus** bacterium is spherical and often grows in chains. Streptococcal pharyngitis, or strep throat, is characterized by a red, sore throat with white patches on the tonsils, swollen lymph nodes, fever, and headache. It is typically spread through close contact with an infected person via respiratory droplets (sneezing or coughing). If left untreated, strep throat can develop into the more serious rheumatic fever (see Chapter 7). Other streptococcal infections include scarletina (scarlet fever), characterized by a sore throat, fever, bright red tongue, and a rash over the upper body; impetigo, a superficial skin infection most common among children; and erysipelas, inflammation of skin and underlying tissues.

streptococcus
Any of a genus (Streptococcus) of spherical bacteria; streptococcal species can cause skin infections, strep throat, rheumatic fever, pneumonia, scarlet fever, and other diseases.

A particularly virulent type of streptococcus can invade the bloodstream, spread to other parts of the body, and produce dangerous systemic illness. It can also cause a serious but rare infection of the deeper layers of the skin, a condition called necrotizing fasciitis, or "flesh-eating strep." This dangerous infection is characterized by tissue death and is treated with antibiotics and removal of the infected tissue or limb. Other species of streptococci are implicated in pneumonia, endocarditis (infection of the heart lining and valves), and serious infections in pregnant women and newborns.

Toxic Shock Syndrome and Other Staphylococcal Infections

The spherical **staphylococcus** bacterium often grows in small clusters. It is commonly found on the skin and in the nasal passages of healthy people. Occasionally, staphylococci enter the body and cause an infection, ranging from minor skin infections, such as boils, to very serious conditions, such as blood infections and pneumonia. The strain known as methicillin-resistant *Staphylococcus aureus* (MRSA) has become the most common cause of skin infections treated in emergency rooms (see the In the News box for more information). This antibiotic-resistant strain causes painful skin lesions that resemble infected spider bites.

staphylococcus

Any of a genus (Staphylococcus) of spherical, clustered bacteria commonly found on the skin or in the nasal passages; staphylococcal species may enter the body and cause several conditions, such as boils, pneumonia, and toxic shock syndrome.

Staphylococcus aureus is also responsible for many cases of toxic shock syndrome (TSS). The bacteria produce a deadly toxin that causes shock (potentially life-threatening low blood pressure), high fever, a peeling skin rash, and inflammation of several organ systems. TSS was first diagnosed in women using highly absorbent tampons, which appear to allow the growth of staphylococci; however, less than half of all cases occur in men and in women not using tampons. (See Chapter 11 for information on TSS, as it relates to contraception.)

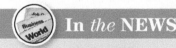 **In *the* NEWS**

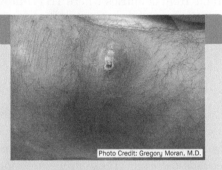

Photo Credit: Gregory Moran, M.D.

MRSA: The Superbug?

Staphylococcus (often shortened to staph) infections are certainly nothing new; people have been dealing with minor staph infections for generations. In fact, it is estimated that as many as 30 percent of people carry the staph bacteria in their bodies. Most of us come into contact with the germ many times during our lives, usually with little or no consequences.

In recent years, however, an antibiotic-resistant strain of staph—called methicillin-resistant *Staphylococcus aureus* (MRSA)—has changed the public's perception of staph as a relatively harmless germ. Medical experts have dubbed MRSA a *superbug* because it is highly resistant to several first-line medicines normally used to treat staph infections. These drugs include methicillin, penicillin, oxacillin, and amoxicillin, among others. MRSA is virulent, and it can be deadly.

In Canada, just fewer than 6000 cases of MRSA are reported annually. About 85 percent of these infections affect patients in health care facilities or those who have recently left a health care setting. People who contract health-care-associated MRSA typically have undergone an invasive surgical procedure or have an immune system weakened by illness or treatment for another disease. Experts say invasive MRSA is now the leading cause of surgical site infections, bloodstream infections, and pneumonia in hospitals and nursing homes.

Although less common, MRSA also affects people who have not been exposed to a health care facility; such infections are called *community-associated MRSA (CA-MRSA)* infections. CA-MRSA is usually not invasive, meaning it doesn't enter the soft tissues under the skin. Instead, most community-associated infections take the form of surface abscesses and pus-filled lesions. Even though their numbers are low, community-based infections are a growing concern because they may indicate that MRSA is gaining strength "in the wild," making it more difficult to manage.

In the age of antibiotics, it's hard to imagine being infected by a germ that can't be killed. But epidemiologists say the overuse of antibiotics is one of the main reasons that bugs, such as MRSA, have become so strong. When people take antibiotics inappropriately or incorrectly, as North Americans have been doing for decades, bacteria have an opportunity to adapt. As a result, they can become resistant to antibiotics and the drugs lose their effectiveness.

Doctors also say that MRSA is a powerful reminder of a valuable lesson: Wash your hands. Frequent handwashing may be the most effective way to avoid infections—not just from MRSA, but also from a host of other germs. Other simple but important methods for preventing infections also apply to MRSA:

- When washing your hands, use lots of soap and scrub briskly for at least 20 seconds.
- If soap and water aren't available, carry an alcohol-based hand sanitizer with you and use it often.
- Keep your hands away from your face.
- If you have an open wound, keep it clean, dry, and covered with a bandage.
- Don't share personal items, such as towels, razors, and tweezers; they can harbour germs and spread infection.
- If you have a skin lesion that resembles a spider bite, have it checked by a physician right away.

Sources: Centers for Disease Control and Prevention. 2013. *General Information About MRSA in the Community,* http://www.cdc.gov/mrsa/ (retrieved June 10, 2015); Klevens, R. M., et al. 2007. Invasive methicillin-resistant *Staphylococcus aureus* infections in the United States. *Journal of the American Medical Association* 298(15): 1763–1771; and Public Health Agency of Canada. 2012. *Canadian Nosocomial Infection Surveillance Program (CNISP),* http://www.phac-aspc.gc.ca/nois-sinp/survprog-eng.php (retrieved June 10, 2015).

Tuberculosis

Caused by the bacterium *Mycobacterium tuberculosis*, **tuberculosis (TB)** is a chronic bacterial infection that usually affects the lungs. TB is spread via the respiratory route. Symptoms include coughing, fatigue, night sweats, weight loss, and fever.

> **tuberculosis (TB)**
> A chronic bacterial infection that usually affects the lungs.

About 1600 Canadians are infected with TB annually. Only about 5–10 percent of people with latent TB infections actually develop an active case of the disease; their immune system prevents the disease from becoming active. In Canada, active TB is most common among Aboriginal peoples and foreign-born immigrants from countries where TB is **endemic**. TB accounted for 37 Canadian deaths in 2008. Worldwide, about 2 billion people—one-third of the population—are infected with TB, and in 2012 about 8.6 million developed active TB and more than 1.3 million died.

> **endemic**
> Persistent and relatively widespread in a given population.

Many strains of tuberculosis respond to antibiotics, but only over a course of treatment lasting 6–12 months. Failure to complete treatment can lead to relapse and the development of strains of antibiotic-resistant bacteria. Of particular concern is the emergence of *M. tuberculosis* with extensive resistance to second-line drugs. These drugs are more toxic than first-line drugs—the drugs primarily used against bacterial infections. In 2008 in Canada, 7 percent of TB bacteria isolated in labs were mono-resistant, and 1 percent were multidrug resistant (MDR). None of the resistant cases were extensively drug resistant (XDR), which is a promising finding given that XDR TB is geographically widespread and is a serious threat to public health.

Tick-Borne Infections

Some diseases are transmitted via insect vectors. Lyme disease is one such infection, and it accounts for more than 95 percent of all reported vector-borne illness in North America. It is spread by the bite of a tick of the genus *Ixodes* that is infected with the spiral bacterium *Borrelia burgdorferi*. Ticks acquire the spirochete by ingesting the blood of an infected animal; they can then transmit the microbe to their next host. The deer tick is responsible for transmitting Lyme disease bacteria to humans in the northeastern and north-central areas of North America; on the Pacific Coast, the culprit is the western black-legged tick, as shown in Figure 9.7. Lyme disease is not a nationally reported disease in Canada, which makes incidence rates difficult to determine. It is thought to be uncommon here, with, for example, only 95 cases being reported in Ontario between in 2010.

Symptoms of Lyme disease vary but typically occur in three stages. In the first stage, about 70–80 percent of victims develop a bull's-eye-shaped red rash expanding from the area of the bite, usually about two weeks after the bite occurs. The second stage occurs weeks to months later in 10–20 percent of untreated patients; symptoms may involve the nervous and cardiovascular systems and can include impaired coordination, partial facial paralysis, and heart rhythm abnormalities. These symptoms usually disappear on their own within a few weeks. The third stage, which occurs in about half of untreated people, can develop months or years after the tick bite and usually consists of chronic or recurring arthritis. Lyme disease can also cause fetal damage or death at any stage of pregnancy. Lyme disease is treatable at all stages, although arthritis symptoms may not completely resolve. Lyme disease is preventable by avoiding contact with ticks or by removing a tick before it has had the chance to transmit the infection.

Rocky Mountain spotted fever and typhus are caused by the *rickettsias* bacterium and are also transmitted via tick bites. Rocky Mountain spotted fever is characterized by sudden onset of fever, headache, and muscle pain, followed by development of a spotted rash. Ehrlichiosis, another tick-borne disease, typically causes less severe symptoms.

FIGURE 9.7

Deer Tick (actual size)

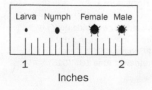

Larva Nymph Female Male

1   2
Inches

Ulcers

At some point in their lifetime, about 10 percent of Canadians will have an ulcer, a sore in the lining of the stomach or the first part of the small intestine (duodenum). Some ulcers are caused by long-term use of non-steroidal anti-inflammatory drugs (NSAIDs). In addition, up to 90 percent of ulcers are caused by infection with *Helicobacter pylori*. Ulcer symptoms include gnawing or burning pain in the abdomen, nausea, and loss of appetite. If tests show the presence of *H. pylori*, antibiotics often cure the infection and the ulcers.

Other Bacterial Infections

The following are a few of the many other infections caused by bacteria:

- *Tetanus:* Also known as *lockjaw*, tetanus is caused by the bacterium *Clostridium tetani*, which thrives in deep puncture wounds and produces a deadly toxin. The toxin causes muscular stiffness and spasms, and infection is fatal in about 10–20 percent of cases. Because of widespread vaccination, tetanus is rare in the Canada. Worldwide, however, about 180 000 people die from tetanus each year, primarily newborns infected through the unsterile cutting of the umbilical cord.

- *C. diff:* Another type of *Clostridium bacteria*, called *Clostridium difficile (C. diff)*, has joined MRSA as a major emerging threat in North American health care settings. Several varieties of *C. diff* have been known for decades to exist, and they generally cause illnesses ranging from diarrhea to life-threatening colitis. Most *C. diff* bugs do their harm by damaging the mucous lining of the intestine. Since 2000, however, one specific strain of *C. diff*—named NAP1—has emerged as a growing problem in hospitals. The NAP1 variant of *C. diff* is especially dangerous because it produces multiple toxins and generates them many times faster than other types of *C. diff*. Further, NAP1 is resistant to a wide range of antibiotics. Some experts previously described the trend in *C. diff* NAP1 infections as an **epidemic** because infections were increasing at a rate of about 10 percent annually. However, between 2005 and 2010, there was a 26.7 percent reduction in the number of cases reported in Canada. Most *C. diff* infections occur in hospitals and commonly affect people who are already being treated with antibiotics for other infections. However, community-based infections are also on the rise, indicating that *C. diff* is spread via person-to-person contact. More than 2 percent of infected people die from the disease. The infection can be treated with a few powerful antibiotics, and treatment is most successful when the infection is caught early. The best ways to avoid *C. diff* infection are to wash your hands frequently and take antibiotics only when absolutely necessary.

epidemic
The occurrence in a particular community or region of more than the expected number of cases of a particular disease.

- *Pertussis:* Also known as *whooping cough*, pertussis is a highly contagious respiratory illness caused by a toxin produced by the bacterium *Bordetella pertussis*. Pertussis is characterized by bursts of rapid coughing, followed by a long attempt at inhalation that is often accompanied by a high-pitched whoop; symptoms may persist for two to eight weeks. Over the past decade, the frequency of cases of pertussis in Canada have ranged from 600 to 5000. Those at high risk include infants and children who are too young to be fully vaccinated and those who have not completed the primary vaccination series. One to three Canadian infants die each year from whooping cough. Adolescents and adults become susceptible when immunity from vaccination wanes, so a booster shot is recommended every 10 years. Adults and adolescents account for about 28 percent of whooping cough cases.

- *Urinary tract infections (UTIs):* Infection of the bladder and urethra is most common among sexually active women, but can occur in anyone. The bacterium *Escherichi coli* is the most common infectious agent, responsible for about 80 percent of all UTIs. Infection most often occurs when bacteria from the digestive tract that live on the skin around the anus get pushed toward the opening of the urethra during sexual intercourse; then, the bacteria travel up the urethra and into the bladder. Women who are particularly susceptible may be given a supply of antibiotics to use after intercourse or at the first sign of infection; urinating before and after intercourse may also help prevent UTIs.

Bacteria responsible for food-borne illness are described in Chapter 5; Chapter 13 discusses sexually-transmitted bacterial infections, such as chlamydia.

Antibiotic Treatments

The body's immune system can fight off many, if not most, bacterial infections. However, while the body musters its defences, some bacteria can cause a great deal of damage: Inflammation, caused by the gathering of white blood cells, may lead to scarring and permanently damaged tissues. To help the body deal with these infections, science and medicine have made a considerable contribution: antibiotics.

ACTIONS OF ANTIBIOTICS **Antibiotics** are both naturally occurring and synthetic substances that can kill bacteria. Most antibiotics work in a similar fashion: They interrupt the production of new bacteria by damaging some part of their reproductive cycle or by causing faulty parts of new bacteria to be made. Penicillin inhibits the formation of the cell wall when bacteria divide to form new cells. Other antibiotics inhibit the production of certain proteins by the bacteria, and still others interfere directly with the reading of genetic material (DNA) during the process of bacterial reproduction. Antibiotics are among the most widely prescribed and effective drugs.

> **antibiotics**
> Synthetic or naturally occurring substances used as drugs to kill bacteria.

ANTIBIOTIC RESISTANCE When antibiotics are misused or overused, the pathogens they are designed to treat can become resistant to their effects. A bacterium can become resistant from a chance genetic mutation or through the transfer of genetic material from one bacterium to another. When exposed to antibiotics, resistant bacteria can grow and flourish, while the antibiotic-sensitive bacteria die off. Eventually, an entire colony of bacteria can become resistant to one or more antibiotics and can become very difficult to treat. Antibiotic-resistant strains of many common bacteria have developed, including strains of gonorrhea (an STI) and salmonellosis (a food-borne illness). One strain of tuberculosis is resistant to seven different antibiotics. Antibiotic resistance is a major factor contributing to the recent rise in problematic infectious diseases.

The more often bacteria encounter antibiotics, the more likely they are to develop resistance. Resistance is promoted when people fail to take the full course of an antibiotic or when they inappropriately take antibiotics for viral infections. Another possible source of resistance is the substantial use of antibiotics in agriculture. At least four species of antibiotic-resistant bacteria are documented to have been transmitted from food animals to humans. Limits may be placed on using drugs used in human medicine in animals as last resorts for serious or life-threatening disease.

You can help prevent the development of antibiotic-resistant strains of bacteria by using antibiotics properly:

- Don't take an antibiotic every time you get sick. They are mainly helpful for bacterial infections; they are ineffective against viruses.
- Use antibiotics as directed, and finish the full course of medication even if you begin to feel better. This helps ensure that all targeted bacteria are killed off.
- Never take an antibiotic without a prescription. If you take an antibiotic for a viral infection, take the wrong one, or take an insufficient dose, your illness will not improve, and you will give bacteria the opportunity to develop resistance.

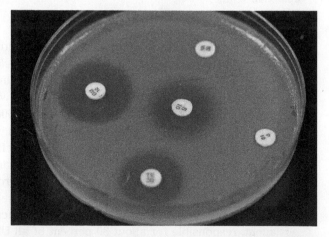

One of the dangers of antibiotic overuse is the development of bacteria resistant to drugs. Cultures of *E. coli* (a bacterium normally present in the human intestine) in this laboratory dish are sensitive to four different types of antibiotics, as indicated by the wide circles where no bacteria are growing, but they are resistant to two other types, which have no effect on their growth.

Viruses

Visible only with an electron (high-magnification) microscope, **viruses** lack all the enzymes essential to energy production and protein synthesis in normal animal cells, and they cannot grow or reproduce by themselves. Viruses are **parasites**; they take what they need for growth and reproduction from the cells they invade. Once a virus is inside the host cell, it sheds its protein covering, and its genetic material takes control of the cell and manufactures more viruses like itself (see Figure 9.8). To fight viruses, the cellular immunity system produces several substances, such as interferon; these same substances are also responsible for most of the symptoms of a viral illness.

viruses
Very small infectious agents composed of nucleic acid (DNA or RNA) surrounded by a protein coat; lack an independent metabolism and reproduce only within a host cell.

parasites
Organisms that live on or in a living host; the relationship benefits the parasite and harms the host.

Illnesses caused by viruses are the most common forms of **contagious disease**. Different viruses affect different kinds of cells, and the seriousness of the disease they cause depends greatly on which kind of cell is affected. The viruses that cause colds, for example, attack upper respiratory tract cells, which are constantly cast off and replaced; the disease is therefore mild. Poliovirus, in contrast, attacks nerve cells that cannot be replaced, and the consequences, such as paralysis, are severe. HIV infection, a viral illness that destroys immune system cells, can destroy the body's ability to fight infectious diseases (see Chapter 13).

contagious disease
A disease that can be transmitted from one person to another; most are viral diseases, such as the common cold and flu.

FIGURE 9.8

Life Cycle of a Virus

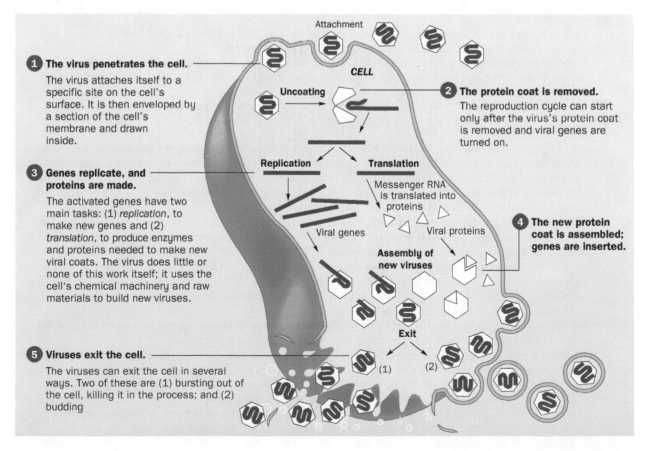

1 The virus penetrates the cell.
The virus attaches itself to a specific site on the cell's surface. It is then enveloped by a section of the cell's membrane and drawn inside.

2 The protein coat is removed.
The reproduction cycle can start only after the virus's protein coat is removed and viral genes are turned on.

3 Genes replicate, and proteins are made.
The activated genes have two main tasks: (1) *replication*, to make new genes and (2) *translation*, to produce enzymes and proteins needed to make new viral coats. The virus does little or none of this work itself; it uses the cell's chemical machinery and raw materials to build new viruses.

4 The new protein coat is assembled; genes are inserted.

5 Viruses exit the cell.
The viruses can exit the cell in several ways. Two of these are (1) bursting out of the cell, killing it in the process; and (2) budding

Attachment

CELL

Uncoating

Replication   Translation

Messenger RNA is translated into proteins

Viral genes   Viral proteins

Assembly of new viruses

Exit
(1)   (2)

The Common Cold

Although generally brief, lasting only one to two weeks, colds are nonetheless irritating and often interfere with our normal activities. A cold may be caused by any of more than 200 different viruses that attack the lining of the nasal passages; rhinoviruses and coronaviruses cause a large percentage of all colds among adults.

Cold viruses are almost always transmitted by hand-to-hand contact. To lessen your risk of contracting a cold, wash your hands frequently; if you touch someone else, avoid touching your face until after you have washed your hands. Colds are not caused by exposure to cold weather or by being chilled or overheated; more colds occur in the fall and winter months, probably because of the opening of school season (children contract more colds than adults) and because people spend more time indoors in the fall and winter months, making person-to-person transmission of viruses more likely.

If you catch a cold, over-the-counter cold remedies may help treat your symptoms but do not directly attack the viral cause (see the Critical Consumer box). Sometimes it is difficult to determine whether your symptoms are due to a virus (as for colds, flu, and some sinus infections), a bacterium (as for other sinus infections), or an allergy, but this information is important for appropriate treatment, as shown in Table 9.3. For example, antibiotics will not help treat a cold, but will help treat a bacterial sinus infection.

 Critical CONSUMER

Preventing and Treating the Common Cold

Prevention

Colds are usually spread by hand-to-hand contact with another person or with objects, such as doorknobs and telephones, which an infected person may have handled. The best way to avoid transmission is to wash your hands frequently with warm water and soap. Keeping your immune system strong is another good prevention strategy (see the guidelines provided later in the chapter).

Home Treatments

- Get some extra rest. It isn't usually necessary to stay home in bed, but you will need to slow down a little from your usual routine to give your body a chance to fight the infection.
- Drink plenty of liquids to prevent dehydration. Hot liquids, such as herbal tea and clear chicken soup, will soothe a sore throat and loosen secretions; gargling with a glass of slightly salty water may also help. Avoid alcoholic beverages when you have a cold.
- Hot showers or the use of a humidifier can help eliminate nasal stuffiness and soothe inflamed membranes.

Over-the-Counter Treatments

Avoid multisymptom cold remedies. Because these products include drugs to treat symptoms you may not even have, you risk suffering from side effects from medications you don't need. It's better to treat each symptom separately:

- *Analgesics*—Aspirin, acetaminophen (Tylenol), ibuprofen (Advil or Motrin), and naproxen sodium (Aleve)—all help lower fever and relieve muscle aches. Use of Aspirin is associated with an increased risk of a serious condition called Reye's syndrome in children and teenagers; for this reason, Aspirin should be given only to adults.
- *Decongestants* shrink nasal blood vessels, relieving swelling and congestion. However, they may dry out mucous membranes in the throat and make a sore throat worse. Nasal sprays shouldn't be used for more than two or three days to avoid rebound congestion.
- *Cough medicines* may be helpful when your cough is non-productive (not bringing up mucus) or if it disrupts your sleep or work. Expectorants make coughs more productive by increasing the volume of mucus and decreasing its thickness, thereby helping remove irritants from the respiratory airways. Suppressants (antitussives) reduce the frequency of coughing.
- *Antihistamines* decrease nasal secretions caused by the effects of histamine, so they are much more useful in treating allergies than colds. *Caution:* Many antihistamines can make you drowsy.

  Antibiotics will not help a cold unless a bacterial infection, such as strep throat, is also present, and overuse of antibiotics leads to the development of drug resistance. The jury is still out on whether other remedies, including zinc gluconate lozenges, echinacea, and vitamin C, will relieve symptoms or shorten the duration of a cold. Researchers are also studying antiviral drugs that target the most common types of cold viruses.

  Sometimes a cold leads to a more serious complication, such as bronchitis, pneumonia, or strep throat. If a fever of 38.8°C or higher persists, or if cold symptoms don't get better after two weeks, see your health care provider.

TABLE 9.3

What's Causing My Symptoms?

Symptoms	Influenza	Common Cold	Allergy	Sinusitis
Headache	Usually	Occasionally	Occasionally	Usually
Muscle aches	Usually (severe)	Usually (mild)	Rarely	Rarely
Fatigue, weakness	Usually (severe; sudden onset; may last several weeks)	Usually (mild)	Rarely	Rarely
Fever	Usually (high, typically 38.8–40°C; sudden onset; lasts 3–4 days)	Occasionally (mild)	Never	Occasionally
Cough	Usually (often severe)	Occasionally	Occasionally	Usually
Runny, stuffy nose	Occasionally	Usually	Usually	Usually (stuffy)
Nasal discharge	Occasionally	Usually (thick, clear to yellowish green)	Usually (watery, clear)	Usually (thick, yellowish green)
Sneezing	Occasionally	Occasionally	Usually	Rarely
Sore throat	Occasionally	Usually	Occasionally	Rarely
Itchy eyes, nose, throat	Rarely	Rarely	Usually	Never

Source: Copyright © 2000. Excerpted from "Is it the flu?" by Consumers Union of U.S., Inc. Yonkers, NY 10703-1057, a non-profit organization. Reprinted with permission from the November 2000 issue of *Consumer Reports*® for educational purposes only. No commercial use or reproduction permitted (http://www.ConsumerReportsHealth.org).

Influenza

Commonly called *the flu*, **influenza** is an infection of the respiratory tract caused by the influenza virus. (Many people use the term "stomach flu" to describe gastrointestinal illnesses, but these infections are actually caused by organisms other than influenza viruses). Compared with the common cold, influenza is a more serious illness, usually including a fever and extreme fatigue. Most people who get the flu recover within one to two weeks, but some develop potentially life-threatening complications, such as pneumonia. The highest rates of infection occur in children. Influenza is highly contagious and is spread via respiratory droplets (see the In Focus box).

influenza
Infection of the respiratory tract by the influenza virus, which is highly infectious and adaptable; the form changes so easily that every year new strains arise, making treatment difficult; commonly known as *the flu*.

The most effective way of preventing the flu is through annual vaccination. The influenza vaccine consists of killed virus and provides protection against the strains of the virus currently circulating; it is updated each year in response to changes in the virus. Vaccination can be appropriate for anyone age 6 months or older who wants to reduce risk of the flu. A number of medications are used to treat influenza, but in most cases they can shorten the duration of illness by little more than a day and then only if treatment begins within one to two days after onset of symptoms. Several medications are also effective in reducing the risk of illness from influenza; however, they are less effective than the vaccine.

QUICK STATS

The flu results in an average of 20 000 hospitalizations and 4000 deaths in Canada each year.
—Public Health Agency of Canada, 2012

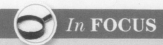 *In* FOCUS

The H1N1 Flu Pandemic

In April 2009, the H1N1 flu virus emerged as a new strain of *pandemic* influenza, which differed from the seasonal flu. (A pandemic is a disease epidemic that is unusually severe or widespread.) People had no natural immunity to protect against virus. Surveillance of its spread showed that it affected more young and healthy people than the regular seasonal flu, which normally affects seniors and young children. People with underlying medical conditions and pregnant women were at a greater risk for severe illness.

H1N1 flu virus has been reported around the world and was a strain of the influenza virus that had previously primarily affected pigs. In the spring of 2009, it emerged in people in North America and spread to humans in regions around the world. This was a new strain of influenza and humans had little to no natural immunity to this virus. The WHO declared H1N1 a pandemic in June 2009. The H1N1 flu virus is still circulating in Canada and other countries, including the United States.

Like seasonal influenza strains, the H1N1 flu virus is contagious and can be spread when an infected person coughs or sneezes and the germs enter the nose, eyes, or throat of another person. These germs can also rest on hard surfaces, like counters and doorknobs, and can be picked up on hands and transmitted to the respiratory system when people touch their mouth and/or nose. It is not possible to catch it through blood transfusions.

Symptoms

More investigation is needed on how long a person can be infectious (able to spread the virus to others); however, it is believed that this period is for one day before the onset of symptoms and continues for approximately seven days after symptoms have started. The table shows the frequency of H1N1 symptoms.

Almost Always	Common	Sometimes
Cough and fever	Fatigue	Nausea
	Muscle aches	Vomiting
	Sore throat	Diarrhea
	Headache	
	Decreased appetite	
	Runny nose	

Prevention

To help minimize the spread of influenza, the Public Health Agency advises Canadians to:
- Wash hands often with soap and warm water for at least 20 seconds, or use hand sanitizer.
- Keep your hands away from your face.
- Cough and sneeze into your arm, not your hand. If you use a tissue, dispose of it as soon as possible and wash your hands.
- Get immunized.
- Keep common surface areas—for example, doorknobs, light switches, telephones, and keyboards—clean and disinfected.
- Eat healthy foods and stay physically active to keep your immune system strong.
- Keep doing what you normally do, but if you get sick, stay home.

Treatment

If you get flu-like symptoms and are otherwise healthy, you should stay home to recover. If your symptoms worsen or you experience difficulty breathing or serious shortness of breath, it is important to seek medical attention.

Antivirals

Antivirals are prescription medications used to treat viral illnesses, including the flu. If taken shortly after getting sick (within the first 24 to 48 hours), they can reduce flu symptoms, shorten the length of illness, and may reduce serious complications. They are available in two forms: a pill (called oseltamivir or Tamiflu) or an inhaler (called zanamivir or Relenza). Antivirals are recommended for the treatment of moderate to severe illness, and for people at risk of severe disease. Your doctor will decide if treatment is right for you.

Vaccination

The Public Health Agency of Canada encourages all Canadians to get vaccinated against the flu to protect themselves and their families. For instance, the 2013/14 seasonal flu vaccine provided protection against a number of flu viruses, including the H1N1 flu virus strain. Even if you received the H1N1 flu shot or had H1N1 influenza during the pandemic in 2009, you cannot assume you are still protected.

Source: *Key Facts on H1N1 Flu Virus.* Public Health Agency of Canada. Reproduced with the permission of the Minister of Health, 2011. Public Health Agency of Canada. 2014. *Influenza: Seasonal Influenza,* http://www.phac-aspc.gc.ca/influenza/index-eng.php (retrieved June 10, 2015).

Measles, Mumps, and Rubella

Three childhood viral illnesses that have waned in Canada because of effective vaccines are measles, mumps, and rubella (German measles). Measles and rubella are generally characterized by rash and fever. Measles can occasionally cause more severe illness, including liver or brain infection or pneumonia; worldwide in 2012, 122 000 people died from measles, making it the leading killer of children whose deaths could have been prevented by vaccines. Measles is a highly contagious disease, and before the introduction of vaccines, 300 000–400 000 Canadians contracted the measles annually. In 2011, 750 cases were reported, which is a substantial increase over the ten previous years.

Rubella, if it infects a pregnant woman, can be transmitted to a fetus, causing miscarriage, stillbirth, and severe birth defects, including deafness, eye and heart defects, and mental impairment.

Mumps generally causes swelling of the parotid (salivary) glands, located just below and in front of the ears. This virus can also cause meningitis and, in males, inflammation of the testes.

Chicken Pox, Cold Sores, and Other Herpesvirus Infections

The **herpesviruses** are a large group of viruses. Once infected, the host is never free of the virus. The virus lies latent within certain cells and becomes active periodically, producing symptoms. Herpesviruses are particularly dangerous for people with a depressed immune system, as in the case of HIV infection. The family of herpesviruses includes the following:

- *Varicella-zoster virus*, which causes chicken pox and shingles. Chicken pox is a highly contagious childhood disease characterized by an itchy rash made up of small blisters. The infection is usually mild, although complications are more likely to occur in young infants and adults. After the rash resolves, the virus becomes latent, living in sensory nerves. Many years later, the virus may reactivate and cause shingles; symptoms of shingles include pain in the affected nerves and a rash on the skin that follows the pattern of the nerve pathways (often a band over the ribs on one side of the body). A vaccine is available that prevents chicken pox in the majority of cases and results in milder illness if the disease does occur.
- *Herpes simplex virus (HSV) types 1 and 2*, which cause cold sores and the STI herpes (Chapter 13). Herpes infections are characterized by small, painful ulcers in the area around the mouth or genitals, at the site where a person first contracts the virus. Following the initial infection, HSV becomes latent and may reactivate again and again over time. Many infected people do not know they are infected, and the virus can be transmitted even when sores are not apparent. Antiviral medications are available to prevent recurrences of genital herpes.
- *Epstein-Barr virus (EBV)*, which causes infectious mononucleosis. Mono, as it is commonly called, is characterized by fever, sore throat, swollen lymph nodes, and fatigue. It is usually spread by intimate contact with the saliva of an infected person—hence the name "kissing disease." Mono most often affects adolescents and young adults. Although EBV does reactivate throughout life, it generally does not cause any further symptoms. In a few people, especially those with HIV infection, EBV is associated with the development of cancers of the lymph system (see "Are All Diseases Infectious?" on ☐ connect).

---

herpesvirus
A family of viruses responsible for cold sores, mononucleosis, chicken pox, and the STI known as herpes; frequently causes latent infections.

Two herpes viruses that can cause severe infections in people with a suppressed immune system are cytomegalovirus (CMV), which infects the lungs, brain, colon, and eyes, and human herpesvirus 8 (HHV-8), which has been linked to Kaposi's sarcoma.

Viral Encephalitis

HSV type 1 is a possible cause of viral **encephalitis**, inflammation of brain tissue caused by a viral infection. Other possible causes include HIV and several mosquito-borne viruses, including Japanese encephalitis virus, equine encephalomyelitis virus, and West Nile virus. Mild cases of encephalitis may cause fever, headache, nausea, and lethargy; severe cases are characterized by memory loss, delirium, diminished speech function, and seizures, and they may result in permanent brain damage or death. Although rare, it is difficult to determine the exact prevalence of encephalitis because it is often underreported.

> **encephalitis**
> Inflammation of the brain; fever, headache, nausea, and lethargy are common initial symptoms, followed in some cases by memory loss, seizures, brain damage, and death.

QUICK STATS

More than 242 000 Canadians have hepatitis C; 21% don't know they have it.
—Public Health Agency of Canada, 2011; Canadian Liver Foundation, 2012

Viral Hepatitis

Viral **hepatitis** is a term used to describe several different infections that cause inflammation of the liver. Hepatitis is usually caused by one of the three most common hepatitis viruses.

- *Hepatitis A virus (HAV)* causes the mildest form of the disease and is usually transmitted by food or water contaminated by sewage or an infected person.
- *Hepatitis B virus (HBV)* is usually transmitted sexually; it is discussed in detail in Chapter 13.
- *Hepatitis C virus (HCV)* can also be transmitted sexually, but it is much more commonly passed through direct contact with infected blood via injection drug use or, before the development of screening tests, blood transfusions. HBV and, to a lesser extent, HCV, can also be passed from a pregnant woman to her child.

> **hepatitis**
> Inflammation of the liver, which can be caused by infection, drugs, or toxins.

There are effective vaccines for hepatitis A and B, but new cases of hepatitis occur in Canada each year. Symptoms of acute hepatitis infection can include fatigue, **jaundice**, abdominal pain, loss of appetite, nausea, and diarrhea. Most people recover from hepatitis A within a month or so. However, 5–10 percent of people infected with HBV and 85–90 percent of people infected with HCV become chronic carriers of the virus, capable of infecting others for the rest of their lives. Some chronic carriers remain asymptomatic, while others slowly develop chronic liver disease, cirrhosis, or liver cancer. An estimated 500 million people worldwide may be chronic carriers of hepatitis. In addition, many of the 618 000 deaths from liver cancer each year can be traced to viral hepatitis.

> **jaundice**
> Increased bile pigment levels in the blood, characterized by yellowing of the skin and the whites of the eyes.

The extent of HCV infection has only recently been recognized, and many infected people are unaware of their condition. To ensure proper treatment and prevention, testing for HCV may be recommended for people at risk, including people who have ever injected drugs (even once), who received a blood transfusion or a donated organ before July 1992, who have engaged in high-risk sexual behaviour, or who have had body piercing, tattoos, or acupuncture involving unsterile equipment (see the Critical Consumer box). Antiviral drugs are available to treat chronic hepatitis, but they are not completely effective and may have significant side effects.

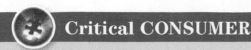

Critical CONSUMER

Tattoos and Body Piercing

Because tattooing and body piercing involve the use of needles, they carry health risks. If you are considering either procedure, you can reduce the risks by carefully choosing a body artist and following aftercare directions.

Tattoos are permanent marks applied with an electrically powered instrument that injects dye into the second layer of the skin. Pain and a little bleeding are common; a tattoo typically takes a week or two to heal and should be protected from sun exposure until then.

In piercing, the artist pushes a needle through the skin; a piece of jewellery holds the piercing open. Earlobe piercing is the most common, but people also pierce the upper ear, eyebrow, tongue, lip, nose, navel, nipples, and genitals. Healing time varies depending on the site of the piercing and other factors. Some pain and swelling are common; prolonged bleeding may follow oral piercing because the tongue contains so many blood vessels.

Potential Health Issues

- *Infection:* People are at risk from the transmission of blood-borne infectious agents, such as hepatitis and HIV, if instruments are not sterilized properly. No cases of HIV infection have been traced to tattooing or piercing. In 2006, an outbreak of MRSA occurred among customers of tattoo parlours in several U.S. states. In most cases, investigators found that the tattooists had not followed proper hygiene procedures, such as changing gloves between customers. Because of the potential risks of infection, people currently cannot donate blood for 12 months following application of body art, including tattoos and some body piercings. People with heart valve problems should check with a physician before body piercing to determine if they should take antibiotics before the procedure.
- *Allergic reactions:* Some people may be allergic to pigments used in tattooing or to metals used in body-piercing jewellery. All jewellery should be of non-corrosive materials, such as stainless steel or titanium; avoid jewellery that contains nickel.
- *Nodules and scars:* Some people may develop granulomas (nodules) or keloids (a type of scar) following tattooing or body piercing.
- *Problems relating to placement:* Tattoos may become swollen or burn if the wearer undergoes magnetic resonance imaging (MRI), and tattoos may also interfere with the quality of MRI images. Oral ornaments may obscure dental problems in dental X-rays; they may also damage teeth and fillings and interfere with speech and chewing. Navel piercings may become infected more easily because tight-fitting clothes allow moisture to collect in the area.

Tattoos are meant to be permanent and so are expensive and very difficult (or impossible) to remove completely. Tattoo removal may involve scraping or cutting off the layers of tattooed skin or using a laser to break up the pigment in the tattoo; some scarring can occur. Body piercings may close and heal once the jewellery is removed, but they may leave a permanent scar.

Choosing a Body Artist and Studio

A body art studio should be clean and have an autoclave for sterilizing instruments. Needles should be sterilized and disposable; piercing guns should not be used, as they cannot be adequately sterilized. The body artist should wear disposable latex gloves throughout the procedure. Leftover tattoo ink should be thrown away and not reused. Ask to see references and aftercare instructions beforehand.

Poliomyelitis

An infectious viral disease that affects the nervous system, **poliomyelitis** (polio) can cause irreversible paralysis and death in some affected individuals. As with other vaccine-preventable diseases, the incidence of polio declined dramatically in Canada following the introduction of the vaccine, and North and South America are now considered free of the disease.

poliomyelitis
A disease of the nervous system, sometimes crippling; vaccines now prevent most cases of polio.

QUICK STATS

Polio remains endemic in only 3 countries: Afghanistan, Nigeria, and Pakistan (down from more than 125 countries in 1988).

—World Health Organization, 2014

Rabies

Caused by a rhabdovirus, rabies is a potentially fatal infection of the central nervous system that is most often transmitted through an animal bite. Canadian rabies-related deaths among humans declined dramatically during the twentieth century because of the widespread vaccination of domestic animals and the development of a highly effective vaccine regimen that provides immunity following exposure (post-exposure prophylaxis, or PEP).

Although rabies is rare in Canada (only 23 people have died of rabies since 1924), most recent cases have been traced to bats. It is recommended that PEP be considered for anyone who has had direct contact with a bat, including someone who has been in the same room with a bat and who might be unaware that contact has occurred (a sleeping child, for example). PEP consists of one dose of immunoglobulin and five doses of rabies vaccine over a 28-day period.

Human Papillomavirus (HPV)

The more than 100 different types of HPV cause a variety of warts (non-cancerous skin tumours), including common warts on the hands, plantar warts on the soles of the feet, and genital warts around the genitalia. Depending on their location, warts may be removed by using over-the-counter preparations or professional methods, such as laser surgery or cryosurgery. Because HPV infection is chronic, warts can reappear despite treatment. As described in Chapter 8, HPV causes the majority of cases of cervical cancer. A vaccine was approved for use by Health Canada in 2006 for females ages 9–26 and in 2010 for males in the same age range. A second vaccine option is now available for females only, ages 10–25.

Treating Viral Illnesses

Antiviral drugs typically work by interfering with some part of the viral life cycle; for example, they may prevent a virus from entering body cells or from successfully reproducing within cells. Antivirals are currently available to fight infections caused by HIV, influenza, herpes simplex, varicella-zoster, HBV, and HCV. Most other viral diseases must simply run their course.

Fungi

A **fungus** is an organism that absorbs food from organic matter. Fungi may be multicellular (like moulds) or unicellular (like yeasts). Mushrooms and the moulds that form on bread and cheese are all fungi. Only about 50 fungi out of many thousands of species cause disease in humans, and these diseases are usually restricted to the skin, mucous membranes, and lungs. Some fungal diseases are extremely difficult to treat because some fungi form spores, an especially resistant dormant stage of the organism.

---

fungus

A single-celled or multicelled organism that absorbs food from living or dead organic matter; examples include moulds, mushrooms, and yeasts; fungal diseases include yeast infections, athlete's foot, and ringworm.

Candida albicans is a common fungus found naturally in the vagina of most women. When excessive growth occurs, the result is itching and discomfort, commonly known as a *yeast infection*. Factors that increase the growth of *C. albicans* include the use of antibiotics, clothing that keeps the vaginal area excessively warm and moist, pregnancy, oral contraceptive use, and certain diseases, including diabetes and HIV infection. The most common symptom is usually a thick white or yellowish discharge. Prescription and OTC treatments are available. Women should not self-treat unless they are certain from a past medical diagnosis that they have a yeast infection. (Misdiagnosis could mean that a different and more severe infection goes untreated.) *C. albicans* overgrowth can occur in other areas of the body, especially in the mouth in infants (a condition known as thrush).

Other common fungal conditions, including athlete's foot, jock itch, and ringworm, affect the skin. These three conditions are usually mild and easy to cure.

Fungi can also cause systemic diseases that are severe, life threatening, and extremely difficult to treat. Histoplasmosis, or valley fever, causes pulmonary and sometimes systemic disease and is most common in the St. Lawrence River Valley where 20–30 percent of people test positive. In North America, more than 50 million people have tested positive. Fungal infections can be especially deadly in people with an impaired immune system.

Protozoa

Another group of pathogens is single-celled organisms known as **protozoa**. Millions of people in developing countries have protozoal infections.

> **protozoa** (protozoan, singular)
> Microscopic single-celled organisms that often produce recurrent, cyclical attacks of disease.

Malaria, caused by a protozoan of the genus *Plasmodium*, is characterized by recurrent attacks of severe flu-like symptoms (chills, fever, headache, nausea, and vomiting) and may cause anemia. The protozoan is injected into the bloodstream via a mosquito bite. Although relatively rare in Canada, malaria is a major killer worldwide; in 2012, about 207 million cases of malaria occurred along with 627 000 deaths, mostly among infants and children in Africa. Drugs are available to prevent and treat malaria, but in the poorest, most remote areas, conditions make it difficult to distribute drugs. Drug-resistant strains of malaria have emerged, requiring new medicines.

> **malaria**
> A severe, recurrent, mosquito-borne infection caused by the protozoan *Plasmodium*.

QUICK STATS

In developing countries, more than 10% of children's deaths are due to malaria. In 2012, that translated into 482 000 children under age 5 (1300/day or one child a minute).

—CDC, 2007; World Health Organization, 2013

Giardiasis is caused by *Giardia lamblia*, a single-celled parasite that lives in the intestines of humans and animals. Giardiasis is characterized by nausea, diarrhea, bloating, and abdominal cramps, and it is among the most common water-borne diseases in North America. People may become infected with *Giardia* if they consume contaminated food or water or pick up the parasite from the contaminated surface of an object, such as a bathroom fixture, diaper pail, or toy. People at risk include child care workers, children who attend daycare, international travellers, and hikers and campers who drink untreated water. Giardiasis is rarely serious and can be treated with prescription medications.

> **giardiasis**
> An intestinal disease caused by the protozoan *Giardia lamblia*.

Other protozoal infections include the following:
- *Trichomoniasis (trich)* is a common vaginal infection. Although usually mild and treatable, trich may increase the risk of HIV transmission (see Chapter 13).

- *Trypanosomiasis* (African sleeping sickness) is transmitted through the bite of an infected tsetse fly and causes extreme fatigue, fever, rash, severe headache, central nervous system damage, and death.
- *Amoebic dysentery* is a severe form of amebiasis, infection of the intestines with the parasite *Entamoeba histolytica*. It is characterized by bloody diarrhea, stomach pain, and fever.

Parasitic Worms

Parasitic worms are the largest organisms that can enter the body to cause infection. The tapeworm, for example, can grow several metres long. Worms, including intestinal parasites, such as the tapeworm and hookworm, cause a variety of relatively mild infections. Pinworm, the most common worm infection in Canada, primarily affects young children. Pinworms are white and about the size of a staple and live in the rectum of humans; they can cause itching and difficulty sleeping. Smaller worms known as flukes infect organs, such as the liver and lungs, and in large numbers can be deadly. Worm infections generally originate from contaminated food or drink and can be controlled by careful attention to hygiene.

> **parasitic worms**
> Pathogens that cause intestinal and other infections; include tapeworms, hookworms, pinworms, and flukes.

Prions

In recent years, several fatal degenerative disorders of the central nervous system have been linked to **prions**, or proteinaceous infectious particles. Unlike all other infectious agents, prions appear to lack DNA or RNA and to consist only of protein; their presence in the body does not trigger an immune response. Prions have an abnormal shape and form deposits in the brain. They may spread by triggering normal proteins to change their structure to the abnormal and damaging form.

> **prions**
> Proteinaceous infectious particles thought to be responsible for a class of neurodegenerative diseases known as transmissible spongiform encephalopathies; Creutzfeldt-Jakob disease (CJD) in humans and bovine spongiform encephalopathy (BSE, or mad cow disease) are prion diseases.

Prions are associated with a class of diseases known as *transmissible spongiform encephalopathies (TSEs)*, which are characterized by sponge-like holes in the brain. Symptoms of TSEs include loss of coordination, weakness, dementia, and death. Known prion diseases include Creutzfeldt-Jakob disease (CJD) in humans; bovine spongiform encephalopathy (BSE), or mad cow disease, in cattle; and scrapie in sheep. Some prion diseases are inherited or the result of spontaneous genetic mutations, whereas others are the result of eating infected tissue or being exposed to prions during medical procedures, such as organ transplants. A variant form of CJD referred to as vCJD occurs in humans who are infected by eating beef from cows with BSE.

Between 1996 and 2011, 224 cases of vCJD were reported worldwide, with 175 of those cases occurring in the United Kingdom. The first indigenous Canadian BSE case was identified in 2003 (the first case in Canada was found in 1993 in a cow originally imported from Britain, as discussed in Chapter 5). Steps have been taken or proposed to reduce the number of BSE-infected cows and the likelihood of meat from an infected animal entering the human food supply. These include increasing surveillance, limiting or banning the use of cattle products in feed for other cattle, prohibiting meat imports from countries with BSE-infected cattle, restricting certain people from giving blood, and banning the use of downer (non-ambulatory) cattle for food for human consumption. Prions present special challenges because they are resistant to heat, radiation, and chemicals that kill other pathogens and because the diseases they cause have a long incubation period. In fact, experts say BSE can take 50 years to incubate. Authorities are now concerned that many more people may harbour BSE than estimated, leading to an epidemic of vCJD in coming decades. Scientists are working to develop new tests that would detect low levels of dangerous prions in asymptomatic cattle.

Emerging Infectious Diseases

Emerging infectious diseases are those infections whose incidence in humans has increased or threatens to increase in the near future. They include both known diseases that have experienced a resurgence, such as tuberculosis and cholera, and diseases that were previously unknown or confined to specific areas, such as the Ebola and West Nile viruses.

Selected Infections of Concern

Although the chances of the average Canadian contracting an exotic infection are very low, emerging infections are a concern to public health officials and represent a challenge to all nations in the future.

WEST NILE VIRUS A mini-outbreak of encephalitis in North America in 1999 led to the identification of West Nile virus, which had previously been restricted to Africa, the Middle East, and parts of Europe. In Canada, more than 2000 cases were confirmed in 2007, and only 447 cases in 2012. West Nile virus is carried by birds and then passed to humans when mosquitoes bite first an infected bird and then a person. Most people who are bitten have few or no symptoms, but the virus can cause permanent brain damage or death in some. Vaccines are being developed for West Nile virus, but it is important to protect yourself from mosquito bites.

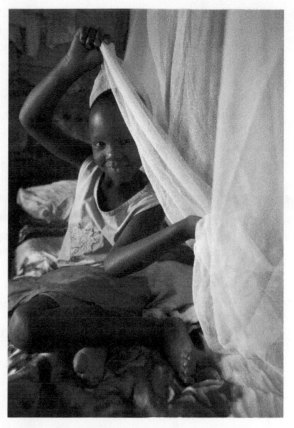

Insecticides, repellents, protective clothing, and screens are helpful in reducing mosquito bites. In developing countries, nets are a first line of defence against mosquitoes.

SEVERE ACUTE RESPIRATORY SYNDROME (SARS) In February 2003, SARS appeared in southern China and quickly spread to more than 15 countries; it is a form of pneumonia that is fatal in about 4 percent of cases. SARS is caused by a new type of coronavirus found in wildlife that may have crossed the species barrier when certain wildlife species were consumed as delicacies. By 2004, SARS had been responsible for more than 8000 illnesses and 800 deaths. No new cases have been reported since 2004.

ROTAVIRUS The leading viral cause of gastroenteritis, an intestinal inflammation that results in vomiting and diarrhea, rotavirus infects almost every child at one time or another. Worldwide, the virus kills about 500 000 children each year, mostly in developing countries. Left untreated, rotavirus-induced diarrhea can become severe and lead to dehydration, which can be fatal. Rotavirus spreads through poor hygiene and sanitation practices.

***ESCHERICHIA COLI* O157:H7** This potentially deadly strain of *E. coli*, transmitted in contaminated food, can cause bloody diarrhea and kidney damage. In 2000, more than 2000 people in Walkerton, Ontario, became ill, 68 were hospitalized, and 7 died from drinking well water contaminated by cattle fecal matter following heavy rains. Other outbreaks have been linked to spinach, lettuce, alfalfa sprouts, unpasteurized juice, petting zoos, and contaminated public swimming pools.

HANTAVIRUS   Since first being recognized in 1993, 61 cases of hantavirus pulmonary syndrome (HPS) have been reported in Canada with at least 20 deaths. HPS is caused by the rodent-borne Sin Nombre virus (SNV) and is spread primarily through airborne viral particles from rodent urine, droppings, or saliva. It is characterized by a dangerous fluid buildup in the lungs and is fatal in about 38 percent of cases.

EBOLA   Human outbreaks of the often fatal Ebola hemorrhagic fever (EHF) have occurred only in Africa. The Ebola virus is transmitted by contact with infected blood or other body secretions, and many cases of EHF have been linked to unsanitary conditions in medical facilities. Because symptoms appear quickly and depending on the strain, 25–90 percent of victims die, usually within a few days, the virus tends not to spread widely.

THINKING ABOUT THE ENVIRONMENT

Many environmental factors contribute to the spread of infectious diseases. Here are a few examples:
- In poverty-stricken regions, many people become ill as a result of unsanitary conditions and a lack of clean drinking water.
- Unsustainable development practices, such as clearing forests and draining wetlands, disturb the ecosystem and force many disease-carrying vectors (such as vermin and insects) out of their natural habitats and into contact with people.
- A shift in rainfall patterns (perhaps caused by global warming) may allow mosquito-borne diseases, such as malaria, to spread from the tropics into the temperate zones. Since many species of mosquito in North America can carry malaria, such changes could someday make malaria a widespread health threat to Canada.

For more information on the environment and environmental health, see Chapter 21.

Factors Contributing to Emerging Infections

What's behind this rising tide of infectious diseases? Contributing factors are complex and interrelated.

DRUG RESISTANCE   New or increasing drug resistance has been found in organisms that cause malaria, tuberculosis, gonorrhea, influenza, AIDS, and pneumococcal and staphylococcal infections. Infections caused by drug-resistant organisms prolong illness, and—if not treated in time with more effective, expensive drugs—they can cause death. Some bacterial strains now appear to be resistant to all available antibiotics.

POVERTY   More than 1 billion people live in extreme poverty, and one-third of the world's population have no reliable access to essential drugs. In parts of Africa and Asia, this terrible fact is true for half of the population. Population growth, urbanization, overcrowding, and migration (including the movement of refugees) also spread infectious diseases.

BREAKDOWN OF PUBLIC HEALTH MEASURES   A poor public health infrastructure is often associated with poverty and social upheaval, but other problems, such as contaminated water supplies, can occur even in industrial countries. Inadequate vaccination has led to the re-emergence of some diseases, such as diphtheria and pertussis. Natural disasters, such as floods and hurricanes, also disrupt the public health infrastructure, leaving survivors with contaminated water and food supplies and no shelter from disease-carrying insects.

TRAVEL AND COMMERCE   In 2012, experts estimated that more than one billion travellers crossed national borders, and by 2030 that rate is expected to rise to 1.8 billion annually. As a result, international tourism and trade have opened the world to infectious agents. SARS was quickly spread throughout the world by infected air travellers. The reintroduction of cholera into the western hemisphere is thought to have occurred through the discharge of bilge water from a Chinese freighter into the waters off Peru.

MASS FOOD PRODUCTION AND DISTRIBUTION Food now travels long distances to our table, and microbes are transmitted along with it. Mass production of food increases the likelihood that a chance contamination can lead to mass illness.

HUMAN BEHAVIOURS Changes in patterns of human behaviour also influence the spread of infectious diseases. The widespread use of injectable drugs rapidly transmits HIV infection and hepatitis. Changes in sexual behaviour over the past 30 years have led to a proliferation of old and new STIs. The use of daycare facilities for children has led to increases in the incidence of several infections that cause diarrhea.

BIOTERRORISM The deliberate release of deadly infectious agents is an ongoing concern, although Canadians' experience has, to date, been one of witness to what has happened to our southern neighbours. In 2001, infectious anthrax spores sent through the mail sickened 11 and killed 5 people in the United States. Potential bioterrorism agents that have been categorized as a highest concern are those that can be easily disseminated or transmitted from person to person and that have a high mortality rate and the potential for a major public health impact; these include anthrax, smallpox, plague, botulism, and viral hemorrhagic fevers, such as Ebola.

QUICK STATS

Nearly all major bacterial infections are becoming resistant to common antibiotics.
—FDA, 2013

Other Immune Disorders: Cancer and Autoimmune Diseases

The immune system has evolved to protect the body from invasion by foreign microorganisms. Sometimes, as in the case of cancer, the body comes under attack by its own cells. As explained in Chapter 8, cancer cells cease to cooperate normally with the rest of the body and multiply uncontrollably. The immune system can often detect cells that have recently become cancerous and then destroy them just as it would a foreign microorganism. But if the immune system breaks down, as it may when people get older, when they have certain immune disorders (including HIV infection), or when they are receiving chemotherapy for other diseases, the cancer cells may multiply out of control before the immune system recognizes the danger. By the time the immune system gears up to destroy the cancerous cells, it may be too late.

Another immune disorder occurs when the body confuses its own cells with foreign organisms. As described earlier, the immune system must recognize many thousands of antigens as foreign and then be able to recognize the same antigens again and again. Our own tissue cells also are antigenic; that is, they would be recognized by another person's immune system as foreign. A delicate balance must be maintained to ensure that our immune system recognizes only truly foreign antigens as enemies; erroneous recognition of our own cells as foreign produces havoc.

This is what happens in autoimmune diseases, such as rheumatoid arthritis and systemic lupus erythematosus. In this type of malady, the immune system seems to be a bit too sensitive and begins to misapprehend itself as non-self. For reasons not well understood, these conditions are much more common in women than in men (see the Gender Matters box).

QUESTIONS FOR CRITICAL THINKING AND REFLECTION

Have you ever had any of the illnesses described in the preceding section? How were you exposed to the disease? Could you have taken any precautions to avoid it? What will you do differently now?

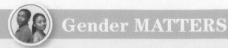

Gender MATTERS

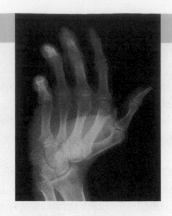

Women and Autoimmune Diseases

Although the immune systems of men and women are essentially the same, women have much higher rates of many autoimmune diseases. The reason gender is a determinant of autoimmune diseases is somewhat of a mystery. One clue may come from pregnancy: To conceive and carry a baby to term, a woman's body must temporarily suppress its immune response so it doesn't attack the sperm or the fetus. Another factor seems to be related to estrogen. Estrogen receptors have been found on suppressor T cells, pointing to a possible link between the glands controlling immunity and those controlling sex hormones. Women also appear to have somewhat enhanced immunity compared with men, a factor that could be linked to both longer lifespans and higher rates of autoimmune disorders.

Systemic lupus erythematosus is an autoimmune disease in which the immune system attacks the body's normal tissue, causing inflammation of the joints, blood vessels, heart, lungs, brain, and kidneys. Its symptoms include painful swollen joints, a rash on the nose and cheeks, sensitivity to sunlight, chest pain, fatigue, and dizziness. About 50 000 Canadians are known to have lupus, and 80 percent of them are women; the disorder is especially common among Aboriginal peoples and black women. Lupus usually begins before menopause and may flare up during pregnancy. For some women, symptoms also increase in severity during menstruation or with the use of oral contraceptives. A link between these exacerbating factors is increased levels of estrogen, but this connection is not well understood. Researchers have also identified genetic mutations that may be associated with lupus.

In rheumatoid arthritis, the body's immune system attacks the membranes lining the joints, causing pain and swelling. Among the estimated 300 000 Canadians with rheumatoid arthritis, women outnumber men three to one. The causes of the disease are not well understood. Researchers have hypothesized that an as-yet-unidentified virus may stimulate the immune system and trigger the disease. When the disease is present in younger women, symptoms often improve during pregnancy, when estrogen levels are higher—the opposite of what is seen in the case of lupus. Therefore, although estrogen levels may play a role in these disorders, its effects appear to be influenced by many other factors.

Other autoimmune disorders more common among women than men include multiple sclerosis, a neurological disease caused by the destruction of the protective coating around nerves; scleroderma, a connective tissue disease characterized by thickening, hardening, and tightening of the skin; and Graves' disease, characterized by an increase in the production of thyroid hormone, which affects metabolism and many body systems.

Supporting Your Immune System

Pathogens threaten everyone's wellness, but you can take steps to prevent them from compromising your health. Here are some general guidelines for keeping pathogens at bay:

- Eat a balanced diet and maintain a healthy weight, as discussed in Chapters 4 and 5.
- Get enough sleep. Most people need six to eight hours every night. Sleep helps your body replenish itself and encourages the production of immune-system cells. Lack of sleep can actually increase your chances of getting sick.
- Exercise, but not when you are sick. Exercise helps you stay healthy, as discussed in Chapter 6. It also staves off stress, which can weaken your immune system. For more information, see the Mind Body Spirit box.
- Don't smoke. Smoking decreases the levels of some immune cells (see Chapter 16).
- If you drink alcohol, do so only in moderation (see Chapter 14). Excessive drinking can interfere with normal immune system functioning.
- Make sure that you have sufficient vitamin D in your diet. Vitamin D deficiency has been implicated in several allergic and autoimmune disorders. The RDI for vitamin D is 600 IU per day, but some experts recommend up to 2000 (but no more than 4000) IU per day.

Mind *Body* **SPIRIT**

Immunity and Stress

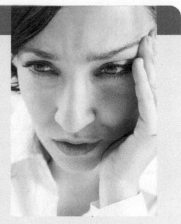

Studies have shown that rates of illness are higher for weeks or even months in people who have experienced the severe emotional trauma of divorce or the death of a loved one. But can commonplace anxieties and stresses also cause measurable changes in the immune system? And can common stress-management techniques boost the immune system? The answer to these questions appears to be yes. Consider the following research findings:

- Medical students taking final exams showed a much weaker immune response to a hepatitis vaccination than unstressed students. In other studies, stress was associated with lower T-cell responses and antibody levels following influenza vaccinations.
- People with higher levels of stress and who had a negative or pessimistic outlook developed more colds during a yearlong study than did individuals with lower levels of stress and a more positive outlook.
- In a study of caregivers, relaxation sessions were associated with increased secretion of cytokines in minor wounds, thus speeding healing. Relaxation and imagery have been shown to increase T-cell levels in some people.
- A study comparing parents of children with cancer (who presumably had high stress levels) with parents of healthy children found that stress appears to interfere with the body's ability to shut down the inflammatory response after it gets started. Continuing high levels of cytokines and inflammation could harm health. The same study found that social support is a determinant of improved immune response.

In seeking to explain these effects, researchers are looking at the connections among stress, hormones, and immunity. Some hormones, such as cortisol, appear to impair the ability of immune cells to multiply and function. Others, such as prolactin, seem to give immune cells a boost. By matching stress levels and hormonal changes to the ups and downs of immune function, researchers hope to gain a better grasp of the shifting chemistry of mind and immunity.

- Wash your hands frequently, as advised throughout this chapter. Antibacterial soap has not been proven to reduce the risk of infection any better than regular soap, especially if you wash properly. Use hand sanitizer when soap and water aren't available; make sure the product is at least 60 percent alcohol.
- Avoid contact with people who are contagious with an infectious disease.
- Make sure you drink water only from clean sources. Unpurified water from lakes and streams can carry pathogens, even if it seems pristine.
- Avoid contact with disease carriers, such as rodents, mosquitoes, and ticks. Never touch or feed wild animals or rodents.
- Practise safer sex (as described in Chapter 13).
- Do not use injectable drugs of any kind (see Chapter 14).
- Make sure you have received all your recommended vaccinations, and keep them up to date. Your physician can tell you exactly what immunizations you need and when you should have them.

SUMMARY

- The step-by-step process by which infections are transmitted from one person to another involves the pathogen, its reservoir, a portal of exit, a means of transmission, a portal of entry, and a new host.
- Infection can be prevented by breaking the chain at any point. Strategies include public health measures, such as treatment of drinking water, and individual actions, such as handwashing.
- Physical and chemical barriers to microorganisms include skin, mucous membranes, and the cilia lining the respiratory tract.
- The immune response is carried out by white blood cells that are continuously produced in the bone marrow. These include neutrophils, macrophages, dendritic cells, natural killer cells, and lymphocytes.
- The immune response has four stages: recognition of the invading pathogen; rapid replication of killer T cells and B cells; attack by killer T cells and macrophages; and suppression of the immune response.
- Immunization is based on the body's ability to remember previously encountered organisms and retain its strength against them.
- Allergic reactions occur when the immune system responds to harmless substances as if they were dangerous antigens.
- Bacteria are single-celled organisms; some cause disease in humans. Bacterial infections include pneumonia, meningitis, strep throat, toxic shock syndrome, tuberculosis, Lyme disease, and ulcers.
- Most antibiotics work by interrupting the production of new bacteria; they do *not* work against viruses. Bacteria can become resistant to antibiotics.
- Viruses cannot grow or reproduce themselves; different viruses cause the common cold, influenza, measles, mumps, rubella, chicken pox, cold sores, mononucleosis, encephalitis, hepatitis, polio, and warts.
- Other diseases are caused by certain types of fungi, protozoa, parasitic worms, and prions.
- Autoimmune diseases occur when the body identifies its own cells as foreign.
- The immune system needs little help other than adequate nutrition and rest, a moderate lifestyle, and protection from excessive stress. Vaccinations also help protect against disease.

FOR MORE INFORMATION

BOOKS

Barry, J. 2005. *The Great Influenza: The Epic Story of the Deadliest Plague in History*. New York: Penguin. A compelling account of the medical, social, and political aspects of the Influenza epidemic of 1918–1919.

Nakazawa, D. J. 2009. *The Autoimmune Epidemic*. New York: Touchstone. The potential links between autoimmune disorders and environmental toxins.

Roitt, I. M., et al. 2006. *Roitt's Essential Immunology*, 11th ed. London: Blackwell. A highly readable introduction to the science of immunology.

Siegel, M. 2006. *Bird Flu: Everything You Need to Know About the Next Pandemic*. New York: Wiley. An examination of the potential threat of an avian flu outbreak and the measures we can take to protect ourselves.

Sompayrac, L. M. 2012. *How the Immune System Works*. 4th ed. Malden, MA: Blackwell Science. A highly readable overview of basic concepts of immunity.

ORGANIZATIONS, HOTLINES, AND WEBSITES

The Internet addresses listed here were accurate at the time of publication.

Alliance for the Prudent Use of Antibiotics. Provides information on the proper use of antibiotics and tips for avoiding infections.
http://www.tufts.edu/med/apua

Arthritis Society of Canada. Provides leadership and funding for research, advocacy, and solutions to improve the quality of life for Canadians affected by arthritis.
https://www.arthritis.ca

Canadian Cancer Society: The Human Papillomavirus and Cervical Cancer. Provides information about HPV.
http://www.cancer.ca/en/cancer-information/cancer-101/what-is-a-risk-factor/viruses-bacteria-and-other-infectious-agents/hpv/?region=on *Canadian Digestive Health Foundation.* Provides advice and support to the millions of Canadians who suffer from digestive disorders.
http://www.cdhf.ca/en/

Cells Alive! Includes micrographs of immune cells and pathogens at work.
http://www.cellsalive.com

Health Canada: Hepatitis. Provides information about hepatitis in Canada.
http://www.hc-sc.gc.ca/hc-ps/dc-ma/hep-eng.php

Health Canada: STI—Sexually Transmitted Infections. Provides information and resources about sexual health and STIs in Canada.
http://www.phac-aspc.gc.ca/publicat/std-mts/index-eng.php

Immunize Canada. Provides information about vaccinations, vaccine safety, and resources for increasing awareness of the benefits and risks of immunization for all ages.
http://immunize.ca/en/default.aspx

Lupus Canada. Provides information and resources about lupus in Canada.
http://www.lupuscanada.org

Public Health Agency of Canada: Infectious Diseases. Provides information about infectious diseases.
http://www.phac-aspc.gc.ca/id-mi/index-eng.php

Public Health Agency of Canada: Immunization Schedules. Provides information about recommended immunizations for Canadian children and adults.
http://www.phac-aspc.gc.ca/im/is-vc-eng.php

Public Health Agency of Canada: Travel Health. Provides travel health information, including advisories, notices, and travel-related diseases.
http://www.phac-aspc.gc.ca/tmp-pmv/index-eng.php

U.S. National Foundation for Infectious Diseases. Provides information about a variety of diseases and disease issues.
http://www.nfid.org

U.S. National Institute of Allergy and Infectious Diseases. Includes fact sheets about many topics relating to allergies and infectious diseases, including tuberculosis and STIs.
http://www.niaid.nih.gov

World Health Organization: Infectious Diseases. Provides fact sheets about many emerging and tropical diseases as well as information about current outbreaks.
http://www.who.int/topics/infectious_diseases/en/

See also the listings in Chapters 5 and 13.

SELECTED BIBLIOGRAPHY

Blaser, M. 2011. Antibiotic overuse: Stop the killing of beneficial bacteria. Nature 476: 393–394.Cashman, N. R., and B. Caughey. 2004. Prion diseases—Close to an effective therapy? *Nature Reviews: Drug Discovery* 3(12): 874–884.

Canadian Institutes of Health Research. 2014. *About CIHR's Antibiotic Resistance Initiatives*, http://www.cihr-irsc.gc.ca/e/40485.html (retrieved June 10, 2015).

Chhabra, N., et al. 2012. Pharmacotherapy for mulitdrug resistant tuberculosis. *Journal of Pharmacology and Pharmacotherapy* 3(2): 98–104.

Cieslak, P. R., K. Hedberg, and L. E. Lee. 2004. Chickenpox outbreak in a highly vaccinated school population: In reply. *Pediatrics* 114(4): 1131.

Daneman, N., T. A. Stukel, X. Ma,, M. Vermeulen, and A. Guttmann. 2012. Reduction in Clostridium difficile Infection Rates after Mandatory Hospital Public Reporting: Findings from a Longitudinal Cohort Study in Canada. *PLoS Med 9(7):* e1001268. doi:10.1371/journal.pmed.1001268

Do Prado, M. F., et al. 2012. Antimicrobial efficacy of alcohol-based gels with a 30-s application. *Letters in Applied Microbiology* 54(6): 564–567.

Fairweather, D., and N. R. Rose. 2004. Women and autoimmune diseases. *Emerging Infectious Diseases* 10(11): 2005–2011.

Fauci, A. S. 2004. Emerging infectious diseases: A clear and present danger to humanity. *Journal of the American Medical Association* 292(15): 1887–1888.

Fauci A. S., N. A. Touchette, and G. K. Folkers. 2005. Emerging infectious diseases: a 10-year perspective from the National Institute of Allergy and Infectious Diseases. *Emerging Infectious Diseases*, http://wwwnc.cdc.gov/eid/article/11/4/04-1167.htm (retrieved June 9, 2015).

Frieri, M., and A. Valluri. 2011. Vitamin D deficiency as a risk factor for allergic disorders and immune mechanisms. *Allergy Asthma Proceedings* 32(6): 438–444.

Government of Canada. 2014. *Tuberculosis*, http://healthycanadians.gc.ca/health-sante/disease-maladie/tuberculosis-tuberculose-eng.php (retrieved June 10, 2015).

International Federation of Pharmaceutical Manufacturers & Associations. 2012. *The Changing Landscape on Access to Medicines*, http://www.ifpma.org/fileadmin/content/Publication/2012/ChangingLandscapes-Web.pdf (retrieved June 10, 2015).

Lamb, A. K., et al. 2011. Reducing asthma disparities by addressing environmental inequities: a case study of regional asthma management and prevention's advocacy efforts. *Family & Community Health* 34: S54–S62.

Lehtinen, M., et al. 2012. Overall efficacy of HPV-16/18 AS04-adjuvanted vaccine against grade 3 or greater cervical intraepithelial neoplasia: 4-year end-of-study analysis of the randomised, double-blind PATRICIA trial. *Lancet Oncology* 13(1): 89–99.

Levy, S. B., and B. Marshall. 2004. Antibacterial resistance worldwide: Causes, challenges, and responses. *Nature Medicine* 10(12 Suppl.): S122–S129.

Parker, S. K., et al. 2004. Thimerosal-containing vaccines and autistic spectrum disorder: A critical review of published original data. *Pediatrics* 114(3): 793–804.

Public Health Agency of Canada. 2011. *Human Papillomavirus (HPV) Prevention and HPV Vaccines: Questions and Answers*, http://www.phac-aspc.gc.ca/std-mts/hpv-vph/hpv-vph-vaccine-eng.php (retrieved June 10, 2015).

Public Health Agency of Canada. 2011. *Rabies Virus: pathogen safety data sheet – infectious substances*, http://www.phac-aspc.gc.ca/lab-bio/res/psds-ftss/rab-eng.php (retrieved June 10, 2015).

Public Health Agency of Canada. 2011. *Hepatitis C in Canada: 2005-2010 Surveillance Report*. Centre for Communicable Diseases and Infection Control, Infectious Disease Prevention and Control Branch, Public Health Agency of Canada.

Public Health Agency of Canada. 2012. *Tuberculosis in Canada 2008*. Ottawa (Canada): Minister of Public Works and Government Services Canada, http://publications.gc.ca/collections/collection_2012/aspc-phac/HP37-5-2008-eng.pdf (retrieved June 9, 2015).

Public Health Agency of Canada. 2013. Statement on Seasonal Influenza Vaccine for 2013-2014. *Canada Communicable Disease Report CCDR 39* (ASC-4), http://www.phac-aspc.gc.ca/publicat/ccdr-rmtc/13vol39/acs-dcc-4/index-eng.php (retrieved June 14, 2015).

Public Health Agency of Canada. 2014. *Canadian Immunization Guide,* http://www.phac-aspc.gc.ca/publicat/cig-gci/index-eng.php (retrieved June 10, 2015).

Public Health Agency of Canada. 2014. *Measles,* http://www.phac-aspc.gc.ca/im/vpd-mev/measles-rougeole/surveillance-eng.php (retrieved June 10, 2015).

Sider, D., et al. 2012. *Technical Report: Update on Lyme Disease Prevention and Control.* Public Health Ontario, http://www.publichealthontario.ca/en/eRepository/PHO%20Technical%20Report%20-%20Update%20on%20Lyme%20Disease%20Prevention%20and%20Control%20Final%20030212.pdf (retrieved June 10, 2015).

Smeeth, L., et al. 2004. MMR vaccination and pervasive developmental disorders: A case-control study. *Lancet* 364(9438): 963–969.

Tohme, R., and S. D. Holmberg. 2012. Transmission of hepatitis C virus infection through tattooing and piercing: a critical review. *Clinical Infectious Diseases* 54(8): 1167–1178.

Vazquez, M., et al. 2004. Effectiveness over time of varicella vaccine. *Journal of the American Medical Association* 291(7): 851–855.

World Health Organization. 2004. *WHO Guidelines for the Global Surveillance of Severe Acute Respiratory Syndrome (SARS), Updated Recommendations.* Geneva: World Health Organization, http://www.who.int/csr/resources/publications/WHO_CDS_CSR_ARO_2004_1/en/ (retrieved June 10, 2015).

World Health Organization. 2012. *Variant Creutzfeldt-Jakob Disease: Fact Sheet No° 180,* http://www.who.int/mediacentre/factsheets/fs180/en/ (retrieved June 10, 2015).

World Health Organization. 2013. *Malaria Report 2013.* Geneva: World Health Organization, http://www.who.int/malaria/publications/world_malaria_report_2013/report/en/ (retrieved June 10, 2015).

World Health Organization. 2013. *The World Health Report 2013: Research for Universal Health Coverage.* Geneva: World Health Organization, http://www.who.int/whr/en/ (retrieved June 10, 2015).

World Health Organization. 2014. *Poliomyelitis: Fact Sheet N°114,* http://www.who.int/mediacentre/factsheets/fs114/en/index.html (retrieved June 10, 2015).

World Health Organization. 2014. *Measles: Fact Sheet N°286,* http://www.who.int/mediacentre/factsheets/fs286/en/ (retrieved June 10, 2015).

CHAPTER 10

Healthy Relationships and Communication

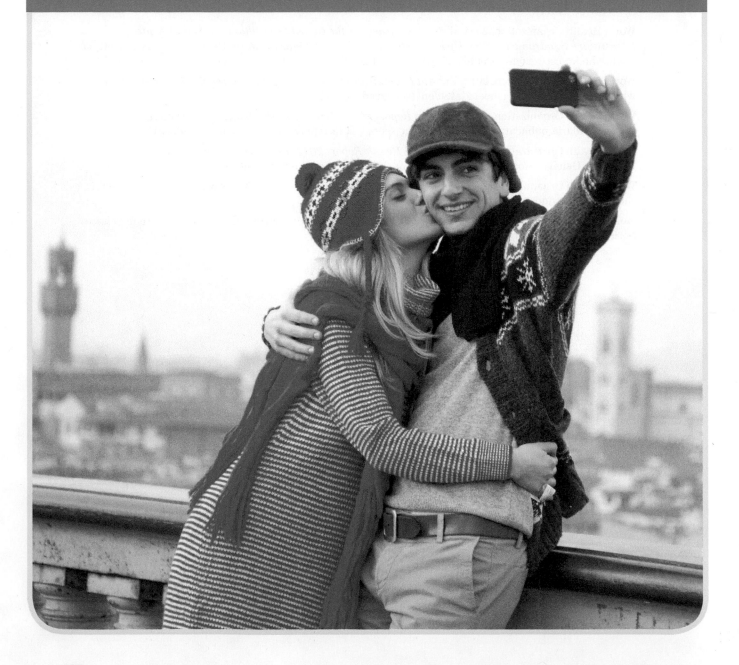

LOOKING AHEAD

After you have read and studied this chapter, you should be able to:

LO1 Explain the qualities that help people develop intimate relationships

LO2 Describe different types of love relationships and the stages they often go through

LO3 Identify common challenges of forming and maintaining intimate relationships

LO4 Explain some elements of healthy and productive communication

LO5 List some characteristics of successful families and some problems families may face

TEST YOUR KNOWLEDGE

1. **What percentage of Canadians report having no one to confide in?**
   a. 10 percent b. 15 percent c. 20 percent

2. **In a typical long-term intimate relationship, commitment tends to increase over time.**
   True or false?

3. **Jealousy is a good indicator of what?**
   a. love b. insecurity c. passion

4. **What percentage of Canadian children live in a single-parent home?**
   a. 2.5 percent b. 5 percent c. 16.3 percent

ANSWERS

1. c.   One in five Canadians (20 percent) say they don't have anyone with whom they can share intimate thoughts. The average person's circle of close friends has steadily shrunk over the last two decades.

2. TRUE.   Although passion and physical attraction tend to decline over time, most couples become increasingly committed to their relationship as time goes by.

3. b.   Some people think that the existence of jealousy proves the existence of love, but jealousy is actually a more accurate yardstick for measuring insecurity or possessiveness. Jealousy can destroy a relationship.

4. c.   About one-sixth of Canadian families with children are single-parent families. About 80 percent of those children live with their mother, while about 3.5 percent live with their father.

Human beings need social relationships; we cannot thrive as solitary creatures. Nor could the human species survive if adults didn't cherish and support each other, if we didn't form strong mutual attachments with our infants, and if we didn't create families in which to raise children. Simply put, people need people.

Although people are held together in relationships by a variety of factors, the foundation of many relationships is the ability to both give and receive love. Love in its many forms—romantic, passionate, platonic, parental—is the wellspring from which much of life's meaning and delight flows. In our culture, it binds us together as partners, parents, children, and friends.

Just as important is developing a healthy relationship with ourselves, which includes the ability to self-soothe, to regulate our emotions, and to be alone with ourselves at times.

Developing Close Relationships

People who develop successful close, often called intimate, relationships believe in themselves and in the people around them. They are willing to give of themselves—to share their ideas, feelings, time, needs—and to accept what others want to give them.

Self-Concept and Self-Esteem

The principal element that we all bring to our relationships is our *selves*. To have successful relationships, we must first accept and feel good about ourselves. A positive self-concept and a healthy level of self-esteem help us love and respect others.

As discussed in Chapter 2, the roots of our identity and sense of self can be found in childhood, in the relationships we had with our parents and other family members. As adults, we probably have a sense that we are basically lovable, worthwhile people and that we can trust others if, as babies and children, we experienced the following:

- We felt loved, valued, and respected.
- Adults responded to our needs in a reasonably appropriate way.
- Adults gave us the freedom to explore and develop a sense of being separate individuals.

Gender Role

Another thing we learn in early childhood is our *gender role*—the activities, abilities, and characteristics that our culture deems appropriate for us based on whether we are male or female. In our society, men have traditionally been expected to work and provide for their families; to be aggressive, competitive, and power oriented; and to use thinking and logic to solve problems. Women have been expected to take care of the home and children; to be cooperative, supportive, and nurturing; and to approach life emotionally and intuitively. Although much more egalitarian gender roles are emerging in our society, the stereotypes we absorb in childhood tend to be deeply ingrained.

Attachment

Our ways of relating to others may also be rooted in childhood. Although our ways of being with people can be affected by a variety of factors, some researchers, known as attachment theorists, have suggested that our adult styles of loving may be based on the style of **attachment** we established in infancy with our mother, father, siblings, or other primary caregiver. Much work has been done on attachment theory, and as a general overview, people who are *secure* in their intimate relationships probably had a secure, trusting, mutually satisfying attachment to their mother, father, or other parenting figure. As adults, they may find it relatively easy to get close to others. They don't worry about being abandoned or having someone get too close to them. They feel that other people like them and are generally well intentioned.

attachment
The emotional tie between an infant and his or her caregiver or between two people in a close relationship.

People who are clinging and dependent in their relationships may have had an *anxious/ambivalent* attachment, in which a parent's inconsistent responses made them unsure that their needs would be met. As adults, they may worry about whether their partners really love them and will stay with them. They tend to feel that others don't want to get as close as they do. They may want to merge completely with another person, which sometimes scares others away.

People who seem to run from relationships may have had an *anxious/avoidant* attachment, in which a parent's inappropriate responses made them want to escape from his or her sphere of influence. As adults, they feel uncomfortable being close to others. They may be distrustful and fearful of becoming dependent. Their partners usually want more intimacy than they do.

Even if people's earliest experiences and relationships were less than ideal, however, they can still establish satisfying relationships in adulthood. In fact, relationships in adolescence and adulthood give us an excellent opportunity to work on and through unresolved issues and conflicts from the past. After all, very few people have perfect parents and perfect siblings, and no one grows up without experiencing some sort of personal pain and conflict.

People can be resilient and flexible. They have the capacity to change their ideas, beliefs, and behaviour patterns. They can learn ways to raise their self-esteem; they can become more trusting, accepting, and appreciative of others; and they can acquire the communication and conflict-resolution skills required for maintaining successful relationships. Although it helps to have a good start in life, it may be even more important to begin again, right from where you are. Most important is to be accepting of and kind to ourselves as we are in the present and to do our best to grow and develop emotionally.

Friendship

The first relationships we form outside the family are friendships. The friendships we form in childhood are important in our development; through them we learn about tolerance, sharing, and trust. Friendships usually include most or all of the following characteristics:

- *Companionship:* Friends are usually relaxed and happy in each other's company. They typically have common values and interests and make plans to spend time together. But real friends are also able to be tense and unhappy with each other. Unlike fair-weather friends, we need to be able to support others as we would want support from them, even on bad days.
- *Respect:* Friends have a basic respect for each other's humanity and individuality. Good friends respect each other's feelings and opinions and work to resolve their differences without demeaning or insulting each other. They also show their respect by being honest with each other (see "Being a Good Friend" on ⊒**connect**).
- *Acceptance:* Friends accept each other, flaws and all. They feel free to be themselves and express their feelings without fear of ridicule or criticism.
- *Help:* Sharing time, energy, and even material goods is important to friendship. Friends know they can rely on each other in times of need.
- *Trust:* Friends are secure in the knowledge that they will not intentionally hurt each other. They feel safe confiding in each other.
- *Loyalty:* Friends can count on each other. They stand up for each other in both word and deed.
- *Mutuality:* Friends retain their individual identities, but close friendships are characterized by a sense of mutuality: "What affects you affects me." Friends share the ups and downs in each other's lives.
- *Reciprocity:* Friendships are reciprocal. There is give-and-take between friends and the feeling that both share joys and burdens more or less equally over time.

Intimate romantic partnerships are like friendships in many ways, but they have additional characteristics. These relationships usually include sexual desire and expression, a greater demand for exclusiveness, and deeper levels of caring. Friendships are usually considered both more stable and longer lasting than intimate partnerships. Friends are often more accepting and less critical than lovers, probably because their expectations are different. Like love relationships, friendships bind society together, providing people with emotional support and buffering them from stress.

As important as friendships are, however, the average Canadian's social circle is shrinking—to the point that 20 percent say they have no one they want to confide in. In 2006, sociological researchers released details of a study confirming the issue. According to the study, people have fewer close friends than ever before. Most have only two friends they consider close enough to discuss problems with. (In 1985, the average was three confidants per person.) That being said, in a recent Canadian study of more than 1700 university students, researchers found students to be more satisfied with their social health, including their connections with friends, family members, and romantic partners, than with any other aspect of their health. The value of having close friends and confidants is important for both emotional and physical health. In fact, a Canadian study published in the journal *Canadian Family Physician* found that the lack of a confidant was associated with not having a regular doctor.

Love, Sex, and Intimacy

Love is one of the most basic and profound human emotions. It is a powerful force in all our intimate relationships. Love encompasses opposites: affection and anger, excitement and boredom, stability and change, bonds and freedom. Love does not give us perfect happiness, but it does give our lives meaning.

In many kinds of adult relationships, love is closely intertwined with sexuality. In the past, marriage was considered the only acceptable context for sexual activities. However, for many people today, sex is legitimized by love. Many couples, heterosexual and gay or lesbian, live together in committed relationships. We now use personal standards rather than social norms to make decisions about sex. Many people, however, worry about this trend toward personal responsibility and the bypassing of traditional norms and values. They fear that the prevailing attitude about sexuality has resulted in a greater emphasis on sex over love and a permissiveness that has undermined the commitment needed to make a true loving relationship work. This casual attitude toward sex may also make it easier for people to sexualize their dependency needs.

For most people, love, sex, and commitment are closely linked ideals in intimate relationships. Love reflects the positive factors that draw people together and sustain them in a relationship. It includes trust, caring, respect, loyalty, interest in the other, and concern for the other's well-being. Sex brings excitement and passion to the relationship. It intensifies the relationship and adds fascination and pleasure.

Commitment, the determination to continue, reflects the stable factors that help maintain the relationship. Responsibility, reliability, and faithfulness are characteristics of commitment. Although love, sex, and commitment are related, they are not necessarily connected. One can exist without the others. Despite the various faces of love, sex, and commitment, most of us long for a special relationship that contains them all.

Other elements can be identified as features of love, such as euphoria, preoccupation with the loved one, idealization or devaluation of the loved one, and so on, but these tend to be temporary. These characteristics may include **infatuation**, which will fade or deepen into something more substantial. As relationships progress, the central aspects of love and commitment take on more importance.

infatuation
An idealizing, obsessive attraction, characterized by a high degree of physical arousal.

Men and women tend to have different views of the relationship between love (or intimacy) and sex (or passion). Numerous studies have found that men can separate love from sex rather easily, although many men find that their most erotic sexual experiences occur in the context of a love relationship. Women generally view sex from the point of view of a relationship. Some people believe you can have satisfying sex without love—with friends, acquaintances, or strangers. Although sex with love is an important norm in our culture, it is frequently disregarded in practice, as the high incidence of extra-relational affairs attests.

QUICK STATS

15–18% of married people will have an affair during their marriage.

—National Opinion Research Center, 2006

The Pleasure and Pain of Love

The experience of intense love has confused and tormented lovers throughout history. They live in a tumultuous state of excitement, subject to wildly fluctuating feelings of joy and despair. They lose their appetite, can't sleep, and can think of nothing but the loved one. Is this happiness? Misery? Or both?

The contradictory nature of passionate love can be understood by recognizing that human emotions have two components: physiological arousal and an emotional explanation for the arousal. Love is just one of many emotions accompanied by physiological arousal; numerous unpleasant ones can also generate arousal, such as fear, rejection, frustration, and challenge. Although some experiences, such as attraction and sexual desire, are pleasant, extreme excitement is similar to fear and is unpleasant. For this reason, passionate love may be too intense to enjoy. Over time, the physical intensity and excitement tend to diminish. When this happens, pleasure may actually increase.

The Transformation of Love

All human relationships change over time, and love relationships are no exception. At first, love is likely to be characterized by high levels of passion and rapidly increasing intimacy. After a while, passion decreases as we become habituated to it and to the person. The diminishing of romance or passionate love is often experienced as a crisis in a relationship. If a more lasting love fails to emerge, the relationship will likely break up.

Unlike passion, however, commitment does not necessarily diminish over time. When intensity diminishes, partners often discover a more enduring love. They can now move from absorption in each other to a relationship that includes external goals and projects, friends, and family. In this kind of intimate, more secure love, satisfaction comes not just from the relationship itself, but also from achieving other creative goals, such as work or child rearing. The key to successful relationships is in transforming passion into an intimate love, based on closeness, caring, and the promise of a shared future.

Challenges in Relationships

Many people believe that love naturally makes an intimate relationship easy to begin and maintain, but in fact, obstacles arise and challenges occur. Even in the best of circumstances, a loving relationship will be tested. Individuals bring to a relationship diverse needs and wants, some of which emerge only at times of change or stress. Common relationship challenges relate to self-disclosure, commitment, expectations, competitiveness, and jealousy.

Is There Hidden Treasure in Our Relationships?

Obviously, we have relationships for fun, companionship, children, and support. But is that all there is to it? Is there hidden meaning to be found in our intimate relationships? Do they repeat issues and conflicts from our past *as well as* offer a way to heal and grow beyond these early-life difficulties? Some experts contend that, as adults, we unconsciously recreate relationships with others that play out the dramas of childhood. In doing so, they say, we attempt to work through and master problems from the past.

At various points in our lives, we may unconsciously play the part of our younger selves—or the part of another person (such as a parent or a sibling)—with the new emotional figure in our lives. We play these roles in the hope of getting emotionally what we didn't get as children or of giving back what we did get.

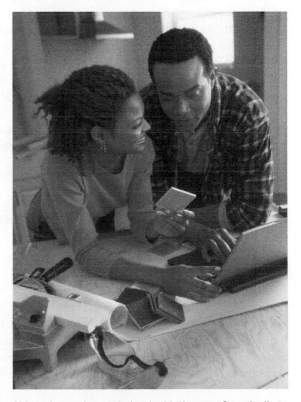

Although passion and physical intimacy often decline with time, other aspects of a relationship—such as commitment—tend to grow as the relationship matures.

Quite often, conflicts in our later-life relationships have to do with our feelings and needs. We tend to expect too much, offer too little, or simply feel confused when it comes to our and the other's emotions. Problems in relationships are not always reflective of incompatibility and may sometimes indicate issues that are just very emotionally difficult because of past frustrations or hurt.

The good news is that our problems in relationships are the potential path to our growth as individuals as well as a couple. A man who feels he doesn't receive enough love from his partner (and didn't from his parents) may benefit from cultivating additional platonic relationships rather than hoping for complete satisfaction from one person. A woman who feels the need for more independence in a relationship (which she didn't have growing up) may grow from learning to stay with her discomfort around intimacy and see if she is gradually able to tolerate more closeness without becoming frightened or pulling back.

Ultimately, it seems that the best relationships are those in which we can be both securely connected and then separate and be on our own at times. Developmental psychology suggests that the healthiest infants are able to feel comforted by their mother without being engulfed and can be apart from her without feeling abandoned. Most important seems to be the mother's ability to be empathically attuned to the child to know when to comfort and when to let go.

Relationships in which we can be open, expressive, and understood offer us the greatest chance to grow, develop our potential, and awaken to as much life as possible. Perhaps the larger, hidden meaning of relationships is to help us cultivate the intimacy and freedom that may have been in short supply while we were growing up. We can help ourselves and others to heal and grow by offering and asking for love and compassion. We can free ourselves from the limits imposed on us from the past by challenging ourselves to see where we are afraid to go in our relationships and then going there with our partners.

Honesty and Openness

Everyone looks for honesty and openness in an intimate relationship. However, especially at the beginning of a relationship, partners may engage in a certain amount of pretense in an effort to present themselves in the best possible manner. Although obvious when considering what is important in a relationship, for people in the excitement of a new relationship, it may be easy to forget that it is usually best to be yourself from the start to give both you and your potential partner a chance to find out if you are comfortable with each other's beliefs, interests, and lifestyles.

Getting close to another person by sharing thoughts and feelings may feel emotionally risky, but it is necessary for a relationship to deepen. In general, it is a good idea to take your time, and self-disclose at a slow but steady rate—one that doesn't make you feel too vulnerable or your partner too uncomfortable. Over time, you and your partner will learn more about each other and feel more comfortable sharing. In fact, intimate familiarity with your partner's life is a key characteristic of successful long-term relationships.

QUICK STATS

About 13% of university students say that relationship problems affect their academic performance.

—*National College Health Assessment II*, 2013

Unequal or Premature Commitment

Sometimes one person in an intimate partnership becomes more serious about the relationship than the other partner. In this situation, it can be very difficult to maintain a friendship without hurting the other person. Sometimes a couple makes a premature commitment, and then one of the partners has second thoughts and wants to break off the relationship. Sometimes both partners begin to realize that something is wrong, but each is afraid to tell the other. Most such problems can be dealt with only by honest and sensitive communication.

Unrealistic Expectations

Each partner brings hopes and expectations to a relationship, some of which may be unrealistic, unfair, and, ultimately, very damaging to the relationship (see the Assess Yourself box). For example, if you believe that

Assess YOURSELF

Are You Emotionally Intelligent?

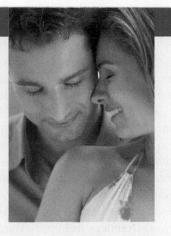

Emotional intelligence (also known as EQ or EIQ) can be defined as the degree to which we can skillfully and adaptively deal with our emotions and those of others.

More specifically, EQ involves the following:

1. Recognizing feelings as they occur
2. Responding to feelings with neither impulsive, aggressive reactivity, nor suppression, denial, distraction, or avoidance
3. Being able to tolerate and contain strong emotions and soothe yourself in the presence of powerful feelings
4. Being able to use the energy of strong emotions to motivate yourself and respond skillfully to the situation at hand
5. Being able to perceive the content of feelings to connect the emotion to its source and understand why you are feeling a particular emotion
6. Being able to recognize and bear the feelings of others without needing to distance yourself or dissuade the other person from having their feelings
7. Being able to persist in the face of fear or frustration and cultivate resilience
8. Being able to delay gratification
9. Being able to be curious and stay open to feelings rather than close down, tighten up, or turn away from emotions
10. Being able to express a wide range of emotions in a way that is natural and to a degree that is appropriate to the particular situation

How do you cultivate emotional intelligence? The key lies in the ability to develop the overarching skill of *mindfulness*—the ability to dispassionately observe thoughts and feelings as they occur and while they are occurring. This skill is aided by cultivating a *witness* or a *watcher* in your mind and noting the arising of strong reactions with a certain detachment. By holding our reactions in a larger mental space, we can make more measured, wise, and skillful responses to the situation at hand.

Mindfulness can be cultivated by simply paying more attention to the operation of our minds, slowing down our lives enough to make more detailed observations, and staying in the moment to maximize awareness of ourselves and others. Although we often have a limited ability to control external events, it turns out that we have a great deal of ability to discipline, focus, and train our minds. With practice, we not only can become more emotionally intelligent, but also may be able to cultivate an ongoing peace of mind that many people find so elusive.

love will eliminate all your problems, you may start to blame your partner for anything that goes wrong in your life. Other unrealistic expectations include the following:

- *Expecting your partner to change:* There are probably some things about your partner that you like more than other things. It's OK to discuss them with your partner; however, it's unfair to demand that your partner change to meet all of your expectations. Accept the differences between your ideal and reality.
- *Assuming that your partner has all the same opinions, priorities, interests, and goals as you:* Don't assume that you think the same about everything—or that you must if the relationship is to succeed. Agreement on key issues is important, but differences can enhance a relationship as long as partners understand and respect each other's points of view.
- *Believing that a relationship will fulfill all of your personal, financial, intellectual, and social needs:* Expecting a relationship to fulfill all your needs places too much pressure on your partner and on your relationship, and it will inevitably lead to disappointment. For your own well-being, it's important to maintain some degree of autonomy and self-sufficiency.

Competitiveness

Games and competitive sports add flavour to the bonding process—as long as the focus is on fun. If one partner always feels the strong need to compete and win, it can detract from the sense of connectedness, interdependence, equality, and mutuality between partners. The same can be said for a perfectionistic need to be right in every instance—to win every argument.

If competitiveness is a problem for you, ask yourself if your need to win is more important than your partner's feelings or the future of your relationship. Try non-competitive activities or an activity where you are a beginner and your partner excels. Accept that your partner's views may be just as valid and important to your partner as your own views are to you.

Balancing Time Spent Together and Apart

You may enjoy time together with your partner, but you may also want to spend time alone or with other friends. If you or your partner interprets time apart as rejection or lack of commitment, it can damage a relationship. Talk with your partner about what time apart means and share your feelings about what you expect from the relationship in terms of time together. Consider your partner's feelings carefully, and try to reach a compromise that satisfies both of you.

Differences in expectations about time spent together can mirror differences in ideas about emotional closeness. Any romantic relationship involves giving up some degree of autonomy in order to develop an identity as a couple. But remember that every person is unique and has different needs for distance and closeness in a relationship.

Jealousy

Jealousy is the angry, painful response to a partner's real, imagined, or likely involvement with a third person. Some people think that the existence of jealousy proves the existence of love, but jealousy is actually a sign of insecurity or possessiveness.

In its irrational and extreme forms, jealousy can destroy a relationship by its insistent demands and attempts at control. Jealousy is a factor in precipitating violence in dating relationships among both high school and college/university students, and abusive spouses often use jealousy to justify their violence. (Problems with control and violence in relationships are discussed in Chapter 20.)

People with a healthy level of self-esteem are less likely to feel jealous. When jealousy occurs in a relationship, it's important for the partners to communicate clearly with each other about their feelings.

Supportiveness

Another key to successful relationships is the ability to ask for and give support. Partners need to know that they can count on each other during difficult times. If you are having trouble getting or giving the support that you or your partner needs, try some of the suggestions in the Take Charge box.

Unhealthy Relationships

Everyone should be able to recognize when a relationship is unhealthy. Relatively extreme examples of unhealthy relationships are those that involve codependency or that are physically or emotionally abusive; strategies for addressing these problems are presented in Chapters 14 and 20, respectively.

Even relationships that are not abusive or codependent can still be unhealthy. If your relationship lacks love and respect and places little value on the time you and your partner or friend have spent together, it may be time to get professional help or to end the partnership.

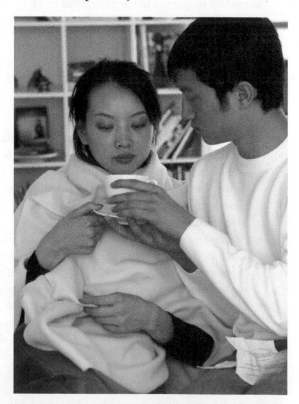

Supportiveness is a sign of commitment and compassion and is an important part of any healthy relationship.

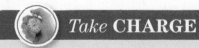

Take CHARGE

Strategies for Enhancing Support in Relationships

- *Be aware of the importance of support.* Time and energy spent on support will help both you and your partner deal with stress and create a positive atmosphere that will help when differences or conflicts do occur.
- *Learn to ask for help from your partner.* Try different ways of asking for help and support from your partner and make note of which approaches work best for your relationship.
- *Help your partner the way she or he would like to be helped.* Some people prefer empathy and emotional support, whereas others like more practical help with problems.
- *Avoid negativity, especially when being asked for help.* Asking for help puts a person in a vulnerable position. If your partner asks for your aid, be gracious and supportive; don't use phrases like "I told you so" or "You should have just . . ." Otherwise, your partner may learn not to ask for your help or support at all.
- *Make positive attributions.* If you're unsure about the reasons for your partner's behaviour, give her or him the benefit of the doubt. For example, if your partner arrives for a date 30 minutes late and in a bad mood, assume it's because she or he had a bad day rather than attributing it to a character flaw or relationship problem. Offer appropriate support.
- *Help yourself.* Develop coping strategies for times your partner won't be available. These might include things you can do for yourself, such as going for a walk, or other people you can turn to for support.
- *Keep relationship problems separate.* Avoid bringing up relationship problems when you are offering or asking for help.
- *Avoid giving advice.* Immediately offering advice when asked for help implies that you are smarter or more capable than your partner at solving your partner's difficulty. Begin by providing emotional support and validating your partner's feelings. Then, if asked, help brainstorm solutions.

Source: Plante, T., and K. Sullivan. 2000. *Getting Together and Staying Together: The Stanford Course on Intimate Relationships.* Bloomington, Ind.: 1st Books Library. Reprinted with permission of the author.

(Partnerships can refer to both romantic relationships and platonic friendships.) Further, if your relationship is characterized by communication styles that include criticism, contempt, defensiveness, and withdrawal—despite real efforts to repair these destructive patterns—the relationship may not be salvageable. Consider these questions:

- Do you and your partner have more negative than positive experiences and interactions?
- Are there old hurts that you or your partner cannot forgive?
- Do you feel disrespected or unloved?
- Do you find it hard to feel positive feelings of affection for your partner?
- Does it feel as if your relationship has been a waste of time?

Spiritual leaders suggest that relationships are unhealthy when you feel that your sense of spontaneity, your potential for inner growth and joy, and your connection to your spiritual life is deadened. Being in an unhappy relationship has negative physical and mental consequences of; although breaking up is painful and difficult, it is ultimately better than living in a toxic relationship.

Ending a Relationship

Even when a couple starts out with the best of intentions, an intimate relationship may not last. Some break-ups occur quickly following direct action by one or both partners, but many others occur over an extended period as the couple goes through a cycle of separating and reconciling.

Ending an intimate relationship is usually difficult and painful. Both partners may feel attacked and abandoned, but feelings of distress are likely to be more acute for the rejected partner. If you are involved in a breakup, the following suggestions may help make the ending easier:

- *Give the relationship a fair chance before breaking up.* If it's still not working, you will know you did everything you could.
- *Be fair and honest.* If you are initiating the breakup, don't try to make your partner feel responsible.

- *Be tactful and compassionate.* You can leave the relationship without deliberately damaging your partner's self-esteem. Emphasize your mutual incompatibility, and admit your own contributions to the problem.
- *If you are the rejected person, give yourself time to resolve your anger and pain.* Mobilize your coping resources, including social support and other stress-management techniques. You may go through a process of mourning the relationship, experiencing disbelief, anger, sadness, and finally acceptance. Remember that there are actually many people with whom you can potentially have an intimate relationship.
- *Recognize the value in the experience.* You honour the feelings that you shared with your partner by validating the relationship as a worthwhile experience. Ending a close relationship can teach you valuable lessons about your needs, preferences, strengths, and weaknesses. Use your insights to increase your chance of success in your next relationship.

Use the recovery period following a breakup for self-renewal. Redirect more of your attention to yourself, and reconnect with people and areas of your life that may have been neglected as a result of the relationship. Time will help heal the pain of the loss of the relationship.

 QUESTIONS FOR CRITICAL THINKING AND REFLECTION

Have you ever ended an intimate relationship? If so, how did you handle it? How did you feel after the breakup? How did the breakup affect your former partner? What did you learn about yourself? In what ways has the experience helped you in other relationships?

Communication

The key to developing and maintaining any type of intimate relationship is good communication. Most of the time, we don't actually think about communicating; we simply talk and behave naturally. But when problems arise—when we feel others don't understand us or when someone accuses us of not listening—we become aware of our limitations or, more commonly, what we think are other people's limitations. Miscommunication creates frustration and distances us from our friends and partners.

Non-Verbal Communication

Even when we are silent, we are communicating. We send messages when we look at someone or look away, lean forward or sit back, smile or frown. Especially important forms of non-verbal communication are touch, eye contact, and proximity. If someone we are talking to touches our hand or arm, looks into our eyes, and leans toward us when we talk, we get the message that the person is interested in us and cares about what we are saying. If a person keeps looking around the room while we are talking or takes a step backward, we get the impression the person is uninterested or wants to end the conversation.

The ability to interpret non-verbal messages correctly is important to the success of relationships. It's also important, when sending messages, to make sure our body language agrees with our words. When our verbal and non-verbal messages don't correspond, we send a mixed message.

QUICK STATS

As much as 65% of communication is non-verbal.

—Ray Birdwhistell, Anthropologist, 1970

Communication Skills

Three keys to good communication in relationships are self-disclosure, listening, and feedback.

- *Self-disclosure* involves revealing personal information that we ordinarily wouldn't reveal because of the risk involved. It usually increases feelings of closeness and moves the relationship to a deeper level of intimacy. Friends often disclose the most to each other, sharing feelings, experiences, hopes, and disappointments; married couples sometimes share less because they think they already know everything there is to know about each other.

- *Listening*, the second key to good communication, is a rare skill. Good listening skills require that we spend more time and energy trying to fully understand another person's story and less time judging, evaluating, blaming, advising, analyzing, or trying to control. Empathy, warmth, respect, and genuineness are qualities of skillful listeners. Attentive listening encourages friends or partners to share more and, in turn, to be attentive listeners. To connect with other people and develop real emotional intimacy, listening is essential.

- *Feedback*, a constructive response to another's self-disclosure, is the third key to good communication. Giving positive feedback means acknowledging that the friend's or partner's feelings are valid—no matter how upsetting or troubling—and offering self-disclosure in response. If, for example, your partner discloses unhappiness about your relationship, it is more constructive to say that you are concerned or saddened by that and want to hear more about it than to get angry, to blame, to try to inflict pain, or to withdraw. Self-disclosure and feedback can open the door to change, whereas other responses block communication and change. (For tips on improving your skills, see the Take Charge box.)

Take CHARGE

Guidelines for Effective Communication

Getting Started

- When you want to have a serious discussion with your partner, find an appropriate time and place. Choose a block of time when you will not be interrupted or rushed and a place that is private.
- Face your partner and maintain eye contact. Use non-verbal feedback to show that you are interested and involved in the communication process.

Being an Effective Speaker

- State your concern or issue as clearly as you can.
- Use "I" statements—statements about how *you* feel—rather than statements beginning with "You," which tell the other person how you think he or she feels. When you use "I" statements, you are taking responsibility for your feelings. "You" statements are often blaming or accusatory and will probably get a defensive or resentful response. The statement "I feel unloved," for example, sends a clearer, less blaming message than the statement "You don't love me."
- Focus on a specific behaviour rather than on the whole person. Be specific about the behaviour you like or don't like. Avoid generalizations beginning with "You always" or "You never." Such statements make people feel defensive.
- Make constructive requests. Opening your request with "I would like" keeps the focus on your needs rather than your partner's supposed deficiencies.
- Avoid blaming, accusing, and belittling. Even if you are right, you have little to gain by putting your partner down. Studies have shown that when people feel criticized or attacked, they are less able to think rationally or solve problems constructively.
- Ask for action ahead of time, not after the fact. Tell your partner what you would like to have happen in the future; don't wait for him or her to blow it and then express anger or disappointment.

Being an Effective Listener

- Provide appropriate non-verbal feedback (nodding, smiling, making eye contact, and so on).
- Don't interrupt.

- Develop the skill of reflective listening. Don't judge, evaluate, analyze, or offer solutions (unless asked to do so). Your partner may just need to have you there to sort out some feelings. By jumping in right away to fix the problem, you may actually be cutting off communication.
- Don't give unsolicited advice. Giving advice implies that you know more about what a person needs to do than he or she does; therefore, it often evokes anger or resentment.
- Clarify your understanding of what your partner is saying by restating it in your own words and asking if your understanding is correct. "I think you're saying that you would feel uncomfortable having dinner with my parents and that you would prefer to meet them in a more casual setting. Is that right?" This type of specific feedback prevents misunderstandings and helps validate the speaker's feelings and message.
- Be sure you are really listening, not off somewhere in your mind rehearsing your reply. Try to tune in to your partner's feelings as well as the words.
- Let your partner know that you value what he or she is saying and want to understand. Respect for the other person is the cornerstone of effective communication.

Gender and Communication

Some of the difficulties people encounter in relationships can be traced to common gender differences in communication. Many experts believe that, because of the way they have been raised, men and women generally approach conversation and communication differently. According to this view, men may be more inclined to use conversation in a *competitive* way, perhaps hoping to establish dominance in relationships. When male conversations are over, men may find themselves in a one-up or a one-down position. Women may be more inclined to use conversation in a more *affiliative* way, perhaps hoping to establish friendships. They negotiate various degrees of closeness, seeking to give and receive support. Men may talk more—though without disclosing more—and listen less. Women may be more inclined to use good listening skills, such as eye contact, frequent nodding, focused attention, and asking relevant questions.

Although these are generalized patterns, they can translate into problems in specific conversations. Even when a man and a woman are talking about the same subject, their unconscious goals may be very different. The woman may be looking for understanding and closeness, while the man may be trying to demonstrate his competence by giving advice and solving problems. Both styles are valid; the problem comes when differences in style result in poor communication and misunderstanding. See the Gender Matters box for more information.

Sometimes communication is not the problem in a relationship—the partners understand each other all too well. The problem is that they are unable or unwilling to change or compromise. Although good communication can't salvage a bad relationship, it does enable couples to see their differences and make more informed decisions.

Conflict and Conflict Resolution

Conflict is natural in intimate relationships. No matter how close two people become, they still remain separate individuals with their own needs, desires, past experiences, and ways of seeing the world. In fact, the closer the relationship, the more differences and the more opportunities for conflict there will be.

Conflict itself isn't dangerous to a relationship; in fact, it may indicate that the relationship is growing. But if it

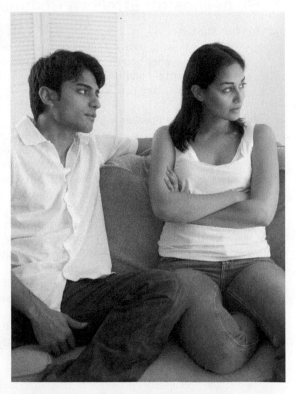

Conflict is an inevitable part of any intimate relationship. Couples need to develop constructive ways of resolving conflicts in order to maintain a healthy relationship.

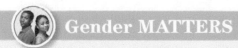

Gender MATTERS

Gender and Communication

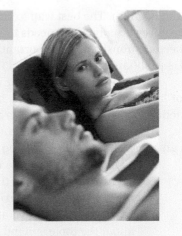

From an early age, parents, teachers, and society send different messages to girls and boys regarding emotion; that is, researchers have found that males and females are socialized to communicate in different ways. Boys tend to learn to suppress and bury their feelings, especially fear and other emotions that make them feel vulnerable. Girls are generally encouraged to express and talk about their feelings.

These differences are further reinforced by peer groups. Gender segregation is already apparent in preschool and increases throughout middle childhood for most children. Boys and girls spend most of their time with peers of the same gender, and their communication styles are very different. For example, when conflict arises, girls tend to care more about preserving their relationships, and boys care more about maintaining the game they were playing.

Research also shows that men have a more intense physiological response to certain emotions. In discussions around conflict, a man's blood pressure and heart rate rise higher and remain elevated longer. Part of the reason may be that a man's internal dialogue repeats upsetting thoughts (for example, "How could she say that? I can't take this!"). When anyone is physiologically or emotionally overwhelmed ("flooded"), productive communication is impossible.

A common pattern that can arise between men and women is called "confront–withdraw." A woman often approaches her male partner because she is upset and wants to talk about it. The man tries to calm her down, provides solutions he sees as rational, and withdraws. This response may make his partner even more upset and demanding, which causes the man to further shut down. Given what we know about gender differences, we might understand the man's response as one of self-protection, because he is entering territory that is both unknown and physically unpleasant.

To enjoy intimacy, men and women must work to better understand each other and develop a more compatible communication style. Insufficient research exists currently to identify typical patterns in same-sex relationships. It may be advisable for sex-same partners to see which (if either) common pattern is more relevant for themselves and their partner.

Advice for Men

- When your partner raises an emotional topic, be aware of uncomfortable feelings and the desire to retreat.
- Do not run away (physically or emotionally)! Telling her to "calm down" will likely create the opposite response.
- Find a way to stay connected. This is the only way to deescalate the conflict.
- Empathize: Listen to what she is saying, and even if you disagree, communicate to her that you understand how she is feeling and where she is coming from. Often when a person feels genuinely heard, that is enough.
- Try not to think of her comments as personal attacks; instead, continue to empathize.
- You may need to calm yourself. Try taking long deep breaths, telling yourself that your partner needs to air her feelings, and remembering that she, too, wants the conflict to end.
- In some cases, a 20-minute break—during which you soothe yourself rather than think upsetting thoughts—can be helpful.

Advice for Women

- Try to be calm when approaching conflict; practise similar relaxation techniques to those described in "Advice for Men."
- Try to speak in ways that will not provoke defensiveness; complain rather than criticize, be specific, and use "I" statements.
- Try not to be critical of your partner's responses or his attempts to communicate.
- Be aware if he is withdrawing, and, if appropriate, help him to relax by using methods you have discussed previously.

Source: Gottman, J. 1994. *Why Marriages Succeed or Fail ... and How You Can Make Yours Last.* New York: Simon & Schuster.

isn't handled in a constructive way, conflict can damage—and ultimately destroy—the relationship. Consider the following guidelines, but remember that different couples communicate in different ways around conflict.

Conflict is often accompanied by anger—a natural emotion, but one that can be difficult to handle. If we express anger aggressively, we run the risk of creating distrust, fear, and distance; if we act it out without thinking things through, we can cause the conflict to escalate; if we suppress anger, it turns into resentment and hostility. The best way to handle anger in a relationship is to recognize it as a symptom of something that requires attention and needs to be changed. When angry, partners should exercise restraint in order to not to become abusive. It is important to express anger skillfully and not in a way that is out of proportion to the issue at hand.

The sources of conflict for couples change over time, but they primarily revolve around the basic tasks of living together: dividing the housework, handling money, spending time together, and so on. Sexual interaction is also a source of disagreement for many couples.

Although there are numerous theories on and approaches to conflict resolution, the following strategies can be helpful when negotiating with a partner:

1. *Clarify the issue.* Take responsibility for thinking through your feelings and discovering what's really bothering you. Agree that one partner will speak first and have the chance to speak fully while the other listens. Then reverse the roles. Try to understand your partner's position fully by repeating what you have heard and asking questions to clarify or elicit more information. Agree to talk only about the topic at hand and not get distracted by other issues. Sum up what your partner has said.

2. *Find out what each person wants.* Ask your partner to express his or her desires. Don't assume you know what your partner wants and don't speak for him or her.

3. *Determine how you both can get what you want.* Brainstorm to generate a variety of options.

4. *Decide how to negotiate.* Work out a plan for change; for example, one partner will do one task and the other will do another task, or one partner will do a task in exchange for something he or she wants. Be willing to compromise, and avoid trying to win.

5. *Solidify the agreements.* Go over the plan verbally and write it down, if necessary, to ensure that you both understand and agree to it.

6. *Review and renegotiate.* Decide on a time frame for trying out your plan, and set a time to discuss how it's working. Make adjustments as needed.

To resolve conflicts, partners have to feel safe in voicing disagreements. They have to trust that the discussion won't get out of control, that they won't be abandoned by the other, and that the partner won't take advantage of their vulnerability. Partners should follow some basic ground rules when they argue, such as avoiding ultimatums, resisting the urge to give the silent treatment, refusing to "hit below the belt," and not using sex to smooth over disagreements.

When you argue, maintain a spirit of goodwill and avoid being harshly critical or contemptuous. Remember—you care about your partner and want things to work out. See the disagreement as a difficulty that the two of you have together rather than as something your partner does to you. Finish serious discussions on a positive note by expressing your respect and affection for your partner and your appreciation for having been listened to. If you and your partner find that you argue repeatedly over the same issue, it may be better to stop trying to resolve that problem and instead come to accept the differences between you.

QUESTIONS FOR CRITICAL THINKING AND REFLECTION

How do you handle conflict in your relationships? Do you fight intensely and then make up? Discuss, negotiate, and compromise? Avoid conflict altogether? Whatever your pattern of conflict resolution (or avoidance), where do you think you learned it? How effective is it for you? How do you want it to be? If it isn't working well, what ideas do you have for improvement?

Pairing and Singlehood

Although most people eventually marry or commit to a partner, everyone spends some time as a single person, and nearly all make some attempt, consciously or unconsciously, to find a partner. Intimate relationships are as important for singles as for couples.

Choosing a Partner

Most men and women select partners for long-term relationships through a fairly predictable process, although they may not be consciously aware of it. First attraction is based on easily observable characteristics: looks, dress, social status, and reciprocated interest. Most people pair with someone who lives in the same geographic area, is from a similar ethnic and socioeconomic background, has similar educational attainment, lives a similar lifestyle, and is like them in terms of physical attraction.

Once the euphoria of romantic love winds down, personality traits and behaviours become more significant factors in how the partners view each other. The emphasis shifts to basic values and future aspirations regarding career, family, and children. At some point, they decide whether the relationship feels viable and is worthy of their continued commitment.

Perhaps the most important question for potential mates to ask is, "How much do we have in common?" Although differences add interest to a relationship, similarities increase the chances of a relationship's success. Areas in which differences can affect a relationship include values, religion, ethnicity, attitudes toward sexuality and gender roles, socioeconomic status, familiarity with each other's culture, and interactions with the extended family (see the Dimensions of Diversity box). Acceptance and communication skills go a long way toward making a relationship work, no matter how different the partners.

 Dimensions *of* DIVERSITY

Interfaith and Intrafaith Partnerships

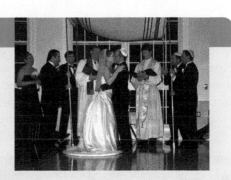

Culture can be a determinant of partnership choices, but this is not always the case. Interfaith marriage is becoming more common among Canadians; in 2001, 19 percent of couples were in an interfaith marriage, up from 15 percent in 1981. With this increasing trend, we can expect that when the government releases more recent statistics, even more couples will be in interfaith unions. There are many types of interfaith partnerships, including partners from (1) two completely different religions, (2) two religions with similar roots, (3) two divisions of the same religion, or (4) two denominations from the same religious division. The latter two are often called intrafaith partnerships.

Marrying someone of a different faith can broaden the partners' worldview and enrich their lives; however, it can also be a potential stressor and a challenge to a relationship.

The impact of being an interfaith couple depends on how religious the partners are. There is no specifically correct way to address religious diversity in a partnership, but the following are some potential approaches:

- *Withdrawal:* In some couples, both partners withdraw from their respective religions. Religious differences may be minimized, but the withdrawal may not last. If a partner was observant before the relationship, it is likely that she or he will want to become actively involved again. This often occurs with a significant life event, such as the birth of a child or death of a parent.
- *Conversion:* In some interfaith couples, one partner converts to the religion of the other. Religious differences are decreased, but problems can occur if the partner who converts develops resentment, has difficulties with her or his family of origin, misses the old religion, or experiences feelings of guilt or betrayal.
- *Compromise:* Some couples convert together to a new religion, possibly to a religion or denomination at a midpoint between their two religions. The couple may find a happy medium that is satisfying to both. However, both may experience the problems associated with conversion.
- *Multifaith:* Some couples join both religions—formally or informally. They may alternate places of worship weekly or make other creative arrangements. The advantage of this pattern is that both partners maintain their religions and learn more about each other. Problems may arise if the religions have conflicting values or practices.
- *Ecumenical:* In some relationships, partners merge their religions. They may combine the best of each or observe only the areas in which the religions intersect. They may get the best of both worlds or discover that their religions have more in common than they thought. In some cases, however, the original religious institutions may condemn compromise.

- *Diversity:* In some couples, each partner chooses to follow his or her own religion. If both partners are very religious, they do not then have to give up an important part of their lives. However, some partners consider this approach undesirable because it means more time spent apart.
- *Do nothing:* Some couples find no need to address religious differences because neither partner is observant or committed to a religion to an extent that it is a relationship challenge. They address specific issues if and when they arise.

Couples often handle their religious differences without a problem until they marry or have children. Planning an interfaith wedding can be fraught with unique stressors, such as differing rituals and the expectations of guests from different faiths. When children arrive, decisions may need to be made about many issues, such as baptism, circumcision, and religious upbringing.

To maintain a successful partnership, couples should communicate about religious issues before getting married and having children. Discuss the importance of your religions and religious needs. Consider ways that you can honour each other's religious traditions. Learn to discuss issues relating to religion and spirituality in ways that bring you closer together.

Sources: Statistics Canada. 2006. Study: Interreligious unions. *The Daily*, October 3, http://www.statcan.gc.ca/daily-quotidien/061003/dq061003b-eng.htm (retrieved June 30, 2015); Robinson, B. A. 2007. *Inter-Faith Marriages*, http://www.religioustolerance.org/ifm_menu.htm (retrieved June 30, 2015); and Robinson, B. A. 1999. *How Inter-Faith and Intra-Faith Couples Handle Religious Differences*, http://www.religioustolerance.org/ifm_diff.htm (retrieved June 30, 2015).

Dating

Every culture has certain rituals for pairing and finding mates. Parent-arranged marriages, still the norm in many cultures, are often very stable and permanent. Although the Canadian cultural norm is personal choice in courtship and mate selection, the popularity of dating services and online matchmaking suggests that many people want help finding a suitable partner (see the In Focus box).

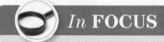 *In* **FOCUS**

Online Relationships

Worldwide, tens of millions of people use the World Wide Web to network and to find friends and partners. Social networking websites, such as Facebook, MySpace, and Friendster, offer places for profiles, photos, blogs, music, videos, and email to vast numbers of people, mostly teens and young adults, seeking to connect online.

Online dating sites and forums, such as Match.com or Lavalife, are also popular, especially among those recently out of college or university who are seeking an intimate partner or an expanded circle of friends. In fact, nearly 1.2 million Canadians have visited an online dating service.

Connecting with people online has its advantages and its drawbacks. It allows people to communicate in a relaxed way, to try out different personas, and to share things they might not share with family or friends face to face. Many find that it offers a sense of privacy, safety, and comfort. It is easy to put yourself out there without too much investment—you can get to know someone from the comfort of your own home, set your own pace, and start and end the relationships at any time. With millions of singles using dating forums that allow them to outline exactly what they are seeking, the Internet can increase a person's chance of finding a good match.

Meeting people online has drawbacks, however. People often misrepresent themselves, pretending to be very different—older or younger or even of a different sex—than they really are. Investing time and emotional resources in such relationships can be painful. In some instances, online romances have become dangerous or even deadly (see Chapter 20 for information on cyberstalking).

Because people have greater freedom to reveal only what they want to, users should also be aware of a greater tendency to idealize online partners—setting themselves up for later disappointment. If you find that your online friend seems perfect, consider that a warning sign. Looking for partners online can become like shopping: The choices available may increase your tendency to search for perfection or find fault quickly, thereby keeping you from giving people a chance. Remember what is most important to you and keep your expectations realistic.

When looking for friends and partners online, you are also missing important and powerful sources of information: chemistry and in-person intuition. Much of our communication is transmitted through body language and tone, which are not available online and cannot be fully captured even by Web cams. Trust your feelings regarding the process of the relationship. Are you revealing more than the other person? Is there a balance in the amount of time spent talking by each of you? Is the other person respecting your boundaries? Just as in real-life dating, online relationships require you to use common sense and to trust your instincts.

If you decide to pursue an online relationship, here are some strategies that can help you have a positive experience and stay safe:

- To improve your chances of meeting people interested in you as a person, avoid sexually oriented websites.
- Know what you are looking for as well as what you have to offer someone else. If you are looking for a relationship, make that fact clear. About 80 percent of Canadian users of online dating services are single. Find out the other person's situation and intentions.
- Many websites let users upload photos. Know, however, that your photo can be downloaded by anyone, distributed to other individuals or sites, and even altered. Don't post photos unless you are completely comfortable with the potential consequences.
- Don't give out personal information, including your real full name, school, or place of employment, until you feel sure that you are giving the information to someone who is trustworthy. Do not give anyone your address or phone number over the Internet.
- Consider setting up a second email account for sending and receiving dating-related emails.
- If someone does not respond to a message, try not to take it personally. There are many reasons why a person may not pursue the connection. Do not send multiple messages to an unresponsive person; doing so could lead to an accusation of stalking. If someone stops responding to your messages, drop the interaction completely.
- Before deciding whether to meet an online friend in person, arrange to talk over the phone a few times.
- Don't agree to meet someone face to face unless you feel completely comfortable about it. Always meet initially in a very public place—a museum, a coffee shop, or a restaurant—not in private, and especially not at your home. Bring along a friend to further increase your safety, let a friend know where you will be, or plan to have a friend call you during the date.

If you pursue online relationships, don't let them interfere with your other interpersonal relationships and social activities. Online dating can have an addictive element that can become unhealthy. To maximize your emotional and interpersonal wellness, use the Internet to widen your circle of friends, not shrink it.

Most Canadians find romantic partners through some form of dating. They narrow the field through a process of getting to know each other. Dating often revolves around a mutually enjoyable activity, such as seeing a movie or having dinner. Traditionally, in the male–female dating pattern, the man took the lead, initiating the date, while the woman waited to be called. In this pattern, casual dating might evolve into steady or exclusive dating, then engagement, and finally marriage.

For many young people today, traditional dating has given way to a more casual form of getting together in groups. Greater equality between the sexes is at the root of this change. People go out in groups, rather than strictly as couples, and each person pays his or her way. A man and woman may begin to spend more time together, but often in the group context. If sexual involvement develops, it is more likely to be based on friendship, respect, and common interests than on expectations related to gender roles. In this model, mate selection may progress from getting together to living together to marriage.

Instead of traditional dating, some young people today are having casual sexual encounters with no commitment or emotional intimacy, referred to as *hooking up*. See the In Focus box for more information.

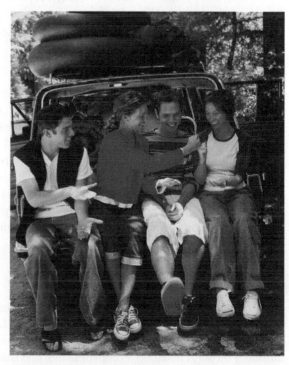

For many college and university students today, group activities have replaced dating as a way to meet and get to know potential partners.

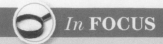

In FOCUS

Hooking Up

A current trend among teenagers, young adults, and college and university students is *hooking up*—having casual sexual encounters with acquaintances or strangers with no commitment or investment in a relationship. The sexual activity can be anything from kissing to intercourse, but the key element is the lack of emotional intimacy. Although casual sex is not new, the difference today is that hooking up seems to be the main form of sexual activity for many people, as opposed to sexual activity within a relationship. Some data indicate that more than 80 percent of college/university students have had at least one hookup experience. If dating occurs at all, it happens after people have had sex and become a couple.

Hooking up most likely has its roots in the changing social and sexual patterns of the 1960s. Since then, changes in college and university policies have contributed to the shift, such as the move away from post-secondary institutions acting *in loco parentis* (in the place of parents), the trend toward coed dorms, and the increase in the percentage of women in student populations and the decreased availability of men. This behaviour addresses the desire for "instant intimacy," but also protects the participants from the risk or responsibility of emotional involvement.

Because hooking up is often fueled by alcohol, it is associated with sexual risk taking and negative health effects, including the risk of acquiring a sexually transmitted disease. In 2007, for example, young adults aged 15 to 24 had rates of chlamydia that were 4 to 5.5 times the overall incidence rate for the general population, according to the Centers for Disease Control. Hooking up can also have emotional and mental health consequences, including sexual regret, negative emotional reactions, psychological distress, depression, and anxiety. Women are more likely to suffer these reactions after hooking up, but men experience them too. Biological anthropologists suggest that having sex—even casual sex—sets off hormones that cause feelings of bonding and attachment, which are inevitably thwarted in a hookup.

On some campuses, a backlash against hooking up has taken place. In some cases, individuals are deciding they don't want to be part of the hook-up culture. In other cases, groups and organizations have formed to call for a return to traditional dating, or at least some middle ground between dating and hooking up that doesn't have the potential to cause physical and emotional harm. The existence of alternative social and sexual norms can help students think twice about their sexual activities.

Sources: Downing-Matibag, T. M., and B. Geisenger. 2009. Hooking up and sexual risk taking among college students: a health belief model perspective. *Qualitative Health Research* 19(9): 1196–1209; Bachtel, M. Is dating really dead? Emerging evidence on the college hookup culture and health issues. *Action Newsletter, American College Health Association* 49(2): 16–18; and Chen, S. 2010. *No hooking up, no sex for some coeds*, http://www.cnn.com/2010/LIVING/04/19/college.anti.hookup.culture/index.html?hpt=Sbin (retrieved July 3, 2015).

Living Together

About 80 percent of Canadian adult couples are in opposite-sex marriages and 19.4 percent are in common-law relationships. Nearly 43 560 Canadians are in same-sex common-law partnerships, and approximately 21 015 are in same-sex marriages (representing 0.3 percent of all married couples in Canada). The decision to live together in a **common-law** or **cohabitating relationship** is one of the most rapid and dramatic social changes that has ever occurred in our society (see Figure 10.1). It seems to be gaining acceptance as part of the normal mate-selection process. Today, about 60 percent of couples live together prior to marrying. Several factors are involved in this change, including greater acceptance of premarital sex, increased availability of contraceptives, the tendency for people to wait longer before getting married, and a larger pool of single and divorced individuals.

common-law or cohabitating relationship
Living together in a sexual relationship without being married.

Cohabitation is more popular among younger people than older, although a significant number of older couples live together without marrying as well. Living together provides many of the benefits of marriage: companionship; a setting for an enjoyable and meaningful relationship; the opportunity to develop greater intimacy through learning, compromising, and sharing; a satisfying sex life; and a way to save on living costs.

Living together has certain advantages over marriage. For one thing, it can give the partners a greater sense of autonomy. Not bound by the social rules and expectations that are part of the institution of marriage, partners may find it easier to keep their identity and more of their independence. Cohabitation doesn't incur

FIGURE 10.1

Distribution (in Percentage) of Census Families by Family Structure, Canada, 1961 to 2011

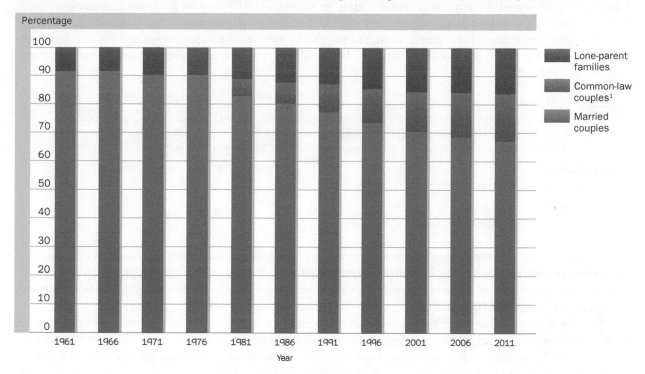

Note: Historical comparisons for census families, particularly lone-parent families, must be interpreted with caution due to conceptual changes in 2001. For more information, see "Concepts and Definitions" in *Family Portrait: Continuity and Change in Canadian Families and Households in 2006, 2006 Census,* http://wwwl2.statcan. gc.ca/census-recensement/2006/as-sa/97-553/index-eng.cfm, Catalogue no. 97-553-X2006001.

[1]Data on common-law couples are not available prior to the 1981 Census.

Source: Statistics Canada, Censuses of population, 1961 to 2011, http://wwwl2.statcan.gc.ca/census-recensement/2011/as-sa/98-312-x/2011003/fig/fig3_1-1-eng.cfm.

the same obligations as marriage. If things don't work out, the partners may find it easier to leave a relationship that hasn't been legally sanctioned.

But living together has some liabilities, too. In some cases, the legal protections of marriage are absent, such as health benefits and property and inheritance rights. These considerations can be particularly serious if the couple has children, from either former relationships or the current one. Couples may feel social or family pressure to marry or otherwise change their living arrangements, especially if they have young children. The general trend, however, is toward legitimizing non-marital partnerships; for example, employers, communities, and provinces and territories now typically extend benefits to unmarried domestic partners.

Although many people choose cohabitation as a kind of trial marriage, unmarried partnerships tend to be less stable than marriages. In a survey of women ages 15–44 who had cohabited, fewer than half were still living—married (37 percent) or unmarried (10 percent)—with their first live-in partner, 34 percent had dissolved the relationship before marriage, and 21 percent had married and then divorced their partner. There is little evidence that cohabitation before marriage leads to happier or longer-lasting marriages; in fact, some studies have found slightly less marital satisfaction and slightly higher divorce rates among couples who had previously cohabited.

QUICK STATS

About 40% of cohabiting couples get married.

—Centers for Disease Control and Prevention, 2013

Same-Sex Partnerships

Regardless of **sexual orientation**, most people look for love in a close, satisfying, committed relationship. A person whose sexual orientation is **lesbian**, **gay**, or bisexual (LGB) may be involved in a same-sex relationship. Same-sex couples have many similarities with **heterosexual** couples (those who seek members of the other sex). According to one study, most gay men and lesbians have experienced at least one long-term relationship with a single partner. Like any intimate relationship, same-sex partnerships provide intimacy, passion, and security.

> **sexual orientation**
> A consistent pattern of emotional and sexual attraction based on biological sex; it exists along a continuum that ranges from being exclusively heterosexual (attracted to people of the other sex), to being bisexual (attracted to people of both sexes), to being exclusively gay or lesbian (attracted to people of your own sex).
>
> **gay** or **lesbian**
> Emotional and sexual attraction to people of your own sex.
>
> **heterosexual**
> Emotional and sexual attraction to people of the other sex.

One difference between heterosexual and same-sex couples is that same-sex partnerships may be more egalitarian (equal) and less organized around traditional gender roles. Same-sex couples may put greater emphasis on partnership than on role assignment. Domestic tasks may be shared or split, and both partners often support themselves financially.

Another difference between heterosexual and same-sex relationships is that same-sex partners often have to deal with societal hostility or ambivalence toward their relationship, in contrast to the societal approval and rights given to heterosexual couples (see the In the News box). *Homophobia*, fear or hatred of gay people, can be obvious, as in the case of violence or discrimination, or more subtle, as in the way same-sex couples are portrayed in the media. Additional stress on a same-sex partnership may occur if an LGB individual is a member of a family or ethnic group that is not entirely accepting of her or his sexual orientation.

Bisexual individuals involved in heterosexual relationships may feel shame or guilt around the acceptance and privileges afforded to them by their heterosexual relationship. Because of the impact of societal disapproval, community resources and support may be more important for same-sex couples as a source of identity and social support than they are for heterosexuals. Many communities offer support groups for same-sex partners and families to help them build social networks and a sense of pride and acceptance.

Although many challenges for same-sex partnerships are common to all relationships, some issues are unique to LGB partnerships. Because men may not be socialized to communicate about interpersonal and emotional issues, communication problems may be particularly common or acute in gay relationships. Some researchers suggest that the process of female socialization, with its emphasis on creating and maintaining intimacy, makes lesbian relationships more likely to be characterized by fusion, enmeshment, and a blurring of boundaries. Problems may

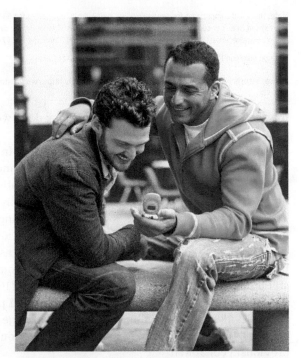

Greater openness has made gay men and lesbians more visible than they used to be, although they still constitute a minority of the population. Most gay people have experienced at least one long-term relationship with one partner.

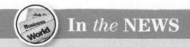 **In *the* NEWS**

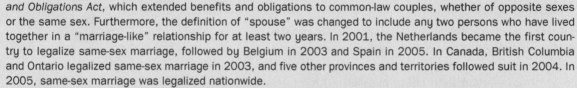

Same-Sex Marriage and Civil Unions

Marriage is often viewed primarily as a social or religious institution, but it is in fact an institution defined by governmental statutes that confer legal and economic rights and responsibilities. Many laws include a distinction based on marriage. Marital status affects tax status, inheritance, medical decision making, and many other aspects of life.

The push for legal recognition of same-sex partnerships began decades ago, but it was brought to the forefront of public debate beginning in the 1990s. Supporters of same-sex marriage rights, however, met with stiff opposition at provincial, territorial, and federal levels.

In 2000, the Canadian Parliament enacted the *Modernization of Benefits and Obligations Act*, which extended benefits and obligations to common-law couples, whether of opposite sexes or the same sex. Furthermore, the definition of "spouse" was changed to include any two persons who have lived together in a "marriage-like" relationship for at least two years. In 2001, the Netherlands became the first country to legalize same-sex marriage, followed by Belgium in 2003 and Spain in 2005. In Canada, British Columbia and Ontario legalized same-sex marriage in 2003, and five other provinces and territories followed suit in 2004. In 2005, same-sex marriage was legalized nationwide.

Across Canada, same-sex couples are permitted to legally marry. This was safeguarded in legislation when the *Civil Marriage Act*, which was passed by Parliament, came into force on July 20, 2005. Before passage of the Act, courts in nine jurisdictions, representing 89 percent of Canada's population, had already extended equal civil marriage to same-sex couples. Following the *Civil Marriage Act* ruling of 2005, members of Parliament were asked to reopen the equal marriage debate. The motion was rejected on December 7, 2006, and same-sex marriage in Canada seems to no longer be an issue for legal debate. The court ruling to recognize same-sex marriages in Canada was based on the finding that excluding same-sex couples from civil marriage is unjustifiable discrimination, which violates section 15 of the Canadian Charter of Rights and Freedoms.

What cases are made for and against civil union and same-sex marriage? Opponents put forth numerous arguments, including that the purpose of marriage is to procreate, that the Bible forbids same-sex unions, that gay people are seeking special rights, that it's bad for children and families, and that the majority of the population opposes such unions. The primary argument, however, is that same-sex marriage undermines the sanctity and validity of marriage as it is traditionally understood and thus undermines society. Rules and restrictions on who can marry preserve the value of the institution of marriage, according to this view. The underlying assumption of this position is that gay men and lesbians make a choice and that people can change their orientation, though the process may be difficult.

Proponents of civil unions and same-sex marriage believe that sexual orientation is outside the control of the individual and results from genetic and environmental factors that create an unchangeable orientation. The issue of same-sex union is then seen as one of basic civil rights, in which a group is being denied rights—to publicly express their commitment to one another, to provide security for their children, and to receive the legal and economic benefits afforded to married heterosexual couples—on the basis of something as unalterable as skin colour. Both opponents and proponents of same-sex marriage point out that marriage is healthy for both men and women and is the main social institution promoting family values; both sides see this assertion as supportive of their position. Today in Canada, 9.4 percent of same-sex couples are raising children (80.3 percent of whom are female couples and 19.7 percent are male couples).

Sources: Ambert, A. 2005. Same-sex couples and same-sex-parent families: Relationships, parenting, and issues of marriage. The Vanier Institute of the Family. *Contemporary Family Trends,* http://www.ibrarian.net/navon/paper/Contemporary_Family_Trends. pdf?paperid=3288548 (retrieved April 17, 2015); CBC News. 2006. *MPs Defeat Bid the Reopen Same-Sex Marriage Debate,* http:// www.cbc.ca/news/canada/mps-defeat-bid-to-reopen-same-sex-marriage-debate-1.599856 (retrieved November 16, 2015); and Same-Sex Families Raising Children. 2013. *Fascinating Families,* http://www.vanierinstitute.ca/include/get.php?nodeid=2817 (retrieved July 3, 2015).

also arise when one member of a same-sex relationship has come out, or publicly identified as LGB, earlier than the other; consequently, the more experienced individual may wonder and worry whether the partner's sexual orientation is transient. The less experienced member of the relationship may feel threatened by the partner's level of "outness" or involvement in the LGB community. If same-sex couples decide to seek counselling, it is important to find a therapist who is an ally of the LGB community and who has training and experience working with LGB couples.

See Chapter 11 for more information on sexual orientation, gender identity, and sexual behaviour.

Singlehood

Despite the prevalence and popularity of marriage, a significant and growing number of adults in our society are unmarried—for the first time in Canada, being single is more common than being married, with 53 percent of Canadians (age 15+) being unmarried. Out of all unmarried adults, most have never been married (see Figure 10.2).

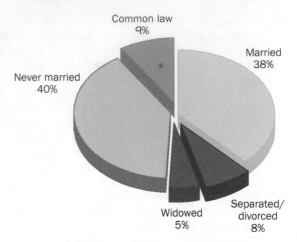

FIGURE 10.2

Marital Status of the Canadian Population

Common law 9%
Married 38%
Never married 40%
Widowed 5%
Separated/ divorced 8%

Note: Estimates are final post-censal for 2008 and 2009, updated post-censal for 2010 and 2011, and preliminary post-censal for 2012.

Source: Statistics Canada, CANSIM, table 051-0042, http://www5.statcan.gc.ca/cansim/a26?lang=eng&retrLang=eng&id=0510042&tabMode=dataTable&srchLan=-1&p1=-1&p2=9.

Several factors contribute to the growing number of single people. One is the changing view of singlehood, which is increasingly being viewed as a legitimate alternative to marriage. Education and careers are delaying the age at which young people are marrying. The average age for a first marriage in Canada is now 31.1 years for men and 29.1 years for women. More young people are living with their parents as they complete their education, seek jobs, or strive for financial independence. Many other single people live together without being married. High divorce rates mean more singles, and people who have experienced divorce in their families may have more negative attitudes about marriage and more positive attitudes about singlehood.

Being single doesn't mean not having close relationships, however. Single people date, enjoy active and fulfilling social lives, and have a variety of sexual experiences and relationships. Other advantages of being single include more opportunities for personal and career development without concern for family obligations and more freedom and control in making life choices. Disadvantages include loneliness and a lack of companionship, as well as economic hardships (mainly for single women). Single men and women alike experience some discrimination and often are pressured to get married.

Nearly everyone has at least one episode of being single in adult life, whether before marriage, between marriages, following divorce or the death of a spouse, or for the person's entire life. How enjoyable and valuable this single time is depends on several factors, including how deliberately the person has chosen it; how satisfied the person is with his or her social relationships, standard of living, and job; how comfortable the person feels when alone; and how resourceful and energetic the person is about creating an interesting and fulfilling life.

QUESTIONS FOR CRITICAL THINKING AND REFLECTION

How have your life's experiences influenced your views on marriage and singlehood? If you are single now, do you plan to get married, or do you have doubts about it? If you are married, do you enjoy it? Do you have regrets? How do you explain these feelings? What could you do to make your relationships more fulfilling?

Marriage

The majority of Canadians marry at some time in their life. Marriage continues to remain popular because it satisfies several basic needs. Marriage has many important social, moral, economic, and political aspects, all of which have changed over the years. In the past, people married mainly for practical reasons, such as raising children or forming an economic unit. Today, people marry more for personal and emotional reasons.

Benefits of Marriage

The primary functions and benefits of marriage are those of any intimate relationship: affection, personal affirmation, companionship, sexual fulfillment, and emotional growth. Marriage also provides a setting in which to raise children, although an increasing number of couples choose to remain without children, and people can also choose to raise children without being married. Marriage is also important for providing for the future. By committing themselves to the relationship, people establish themselves with lifelong companions as well as some insurance for their later years.

Good marriages have been shown to have myriad positive effects on individuals' health (see the Mind Body Spirit box).

 Mind *Body* SPIRIT

Are Intimate Relationships Good for Your Health?

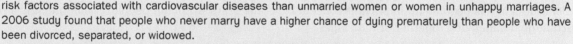

Findings suggest that marriage has intrinsic benefits. Married people, on average, live longer than unmarried people—whether single, divorced, or widowed— and they score higher on measures of mental health. They have a lower prevalence of headaches, low-back pain, inactivity, and psychological distress. Married people consistently report being happier than unmarried people.

The benefits of intimate relationships have been demonstrated for a range of conditions. For example, people with strong social support are less likely to catch colds. They recover better from heart attacks, live longer with heart disease, and have higher survival rates for certain cancers. Among men with prostate cancer, those who are married live significantly longer than those who are single, divorced, or widowed. Women in satisfying marriages are less likely to develop risk factors associated with cardiovascular diseases than unmarried women or women in unhappy marriages. A 2006 study found that people who never marry have a higher chance of dying prematurely than people who have been divorced, separated, or widowed.

What is it about social relationships that supports wellness? Some studies suggest that friends and partners may encourage and reinforce healthy habits, such as exercising, eating right, and seeing a physician when needed. In times of illness, a loving partner can provide both practical help (sometimes financial) and emotional support. Feeling loved, esteemed, and valued brings comfort at a time of vulnerability, reduces anxiety, and mitigates the damaging effects of stress and risks of social isolation.

Although good relationships may help the sick get better, bad relationships may have the opposite effect. The impact of relationship quality on the course of illness may be partly explained by effects of the immune system: A study of married couples whose fighting went beyond normal conflict and into criticism and name-calling found them to have weaker immune responses than couples whose arguments were more civil. Hostile couples need more time for injuries to heal; their systems tend to contain higher levels of inflammatory agents, which have been linked to long-term illness. New research shows that high marital stress is linked with risky lifestyle choices and behaviours and non-adherence to medical regimens. Similarly, unhappy marriages are associated with risk factors for heart disease, such as depression, hostility, and anger.

Marriage, of course, isn't the only support system available. Whether married, in a committed partnership, or single, if you have supportive people in your life, you are likely to enjoy better physical and emotional health than if you feel isolated and alone. So when you start planning lifestyle changes to improve your health and well-being, don't forget to nurture your relationships with family and friends. Relationships are powerful medicine.

Issues in Marriage

Although we might like to believe otherwise, love is not enough to make a successful marriage. Couples have to be strong and successful in their relationship before getting married, because relationship problems will be magnified rather than solved by marriage. The following relationship characteristics appear to be the best predictors of a happy marriage:

- The partners have realistic expectations about their relationship.
- Each feels good about the personality of the other. ·
- They communicate well.
- They have effective ways of resolving conflicts.
- They agree on religious and ethical values.
- They have an egalitarian role relationship.
- They have a good balance of individual versus joint interests and leisure activities.

Once married, couples must provide each other with emotional support, negotiate and establish marital roles, establish domestic and career priorities, handle their finances, make sexual adjustments, manage boundaries and relationships with their extended family, and participate in the larger community.

Marital roles and responsibilities have undergone profound changes in recent years. Many couples no longer accept traditional role assumptions, such as that the husband is solely responsible for supporting the family and the wife is solely responsible for domestic work. Today, many husbands share domestic tasks, and many wives work outside the home. In fact, more than 75 percent of women (ages 20–64 years) who are either married or living in a common-law relationship are in the labour force, including women with babies less than one year of age. Although women still take most of the responsibility for home and children even when they work, and although men still suffer more job-related stress and health problems than women do, the trend is toward an equalization of responsibilities.

The Role of Commitment

Coping with all these challenges requires that couples be committed to remaining in the relationship through its inevitable ups and downs. They need to be tolerant of each other's imperfections and keep their perspective and sense of humour. Commitment is based on conscious choice rather than on feelings, which, by their very nature, are transitory. Commitment is a promise of a shared future, a promise to be together, come what may. Committed partners put effort and energy into the relationship, no matter how they feel. They take time to attend to their partner, give compliments, and deal with conflict when necessary.

Commitment has become an important concept in recent years. To many people, commitment is a more important goal than living together or marriage.

QUESTIONS FOR CRITICAL THINKING AND REFLECTION

How do you define "commitment" in a relationship? Is it simply a matter of staying faithful to a partner, or is there more? In your own relationships, what signs of commitment do you look for from your partner? What signs of commitment does your partner see in you? What's important about commitment in your relationships?

Separation and Divorce

According to Statistics Canada, by the year 2035, about 38 percent of couples who married in 2004 will be divorced. The high rate of divorce in Canada reflects our extremely high expectations for emotional fulfillment and satisfaction in marriage (see Figure 10.3). It also indicates that we no longer believe in the permanence of marriage.

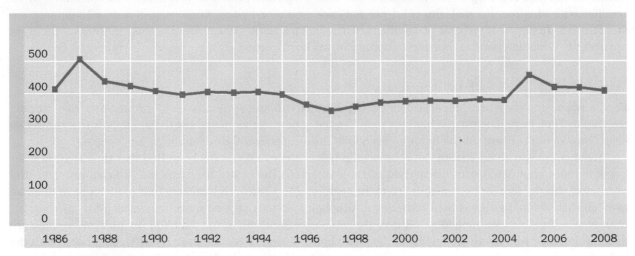

FIGURE 10.3

30 Year Total Divorce Rate, Canada 1986–2008 (per 1000 marriages)

Note: Statistics Canada did not calculate divorce rates by marriage duration and total divorces rates for 2005.

Source: For 1986 to 1996, Statistics Canada: *Vital statistics compendium, 1996.* Ottawa: Statistics Canada, Health Statistics Division, 1999 (Cat. No. 84-214-XPE); for 1997 to 2003: Statistics Canada. *Divorces. Shelf tables.* Ottawa: Statistics Canada, 1999-2005; for 2004: *30 and 50 year total divorce rates per 1,000 marriages, Canada, provinces and territories, annual (rate per 1,000 marriages)* (CANSIM Table 101-6511). Ottawa: Statistics Canada, 2008; and for 2006 to 2008: Statistics Canada, Health Statistics Division, Canadian Vital Statistics, *Divorce Database and Marriage Database.* Ottawa: Statistics Canada, 2011.

The process of divorce usually begins with an emotional separation. Often one partner is unhappy and looks beyond the relationship for other forms of validation. Dissatisfaction increases until the unhappy partner decides he or she can no longer stay. Physical separation follows, although it may take some time for the relationship to be over emotionally.

Except for the death of a spouse or family member, divorce is the greatest stress-producing event in life. Research shows that divorced women are more likely to develop heart disease than married, remarried, or widowed women. Both men and women experience turmoil, depression, and lowered self-esteem during and after divorce. People experience separation distress and loneliness for about a year, and then begin a recovery period of one to three years. During this time they gradually construct a post-divorce identity, along with a new pattern of life. Most people are surprised by how long it takes to recover from divorce.

Children are especially vulnerable to the trauma of divorce, and sometimes counselling is appropriate to help them adjust to the changes in their lives. However, recent research has found that children who spend substantial time with both parents are usually better adjusted than those in sole custody arrangements and as well adjusted as their peers from intact families.

Despite the distress of separation and divorce, the negative effects are usually balanced sooner or later by the possibility of finding a more suitable partner, constructing a new life, and developing new aspects of the self. About 75 percent of all people who divorce remarry, often within five years. More Canadian men than women want to remarry following divorce. One result of the high divorce and remarriage rate is a growing number of stepfamilies (discussed in the next section).

QUICK STATS

74% of Canadians consider extramarital affairs to be immoral.

—Leger Marketing, 2006

Family Life

Canadian families are very different today from what they were even a few decades ago. Currently, of all families with children, the majority (87.4 percent) are considered intact families, and nearly 13 percent are stepfamilies. Just over 16 percent of families are headed by a single parent. Despite the tremendous variation apparent in Canadian families, certain patterns can still be discerned.

Becoming a Parent

Few new parents have any preparation for the job of parenting, yet they have to assume that role literally overnight. They have to learn quickly how to hold a baby, how to change it, how to feed it, how to interpret its cries. No wonder the birth of the first child is one of the most stressful transitions for any couple.

Even couples with an egalitarian relationship before their first child is born find that their marital roles become more traditional with the arrival of the new baby. The father becomes the primary provider and protector, and the mother becomes the primary nurturer. Most research indicates that mothers have to make greater changes in their lives than fathers do. Although men today spend more time caring for their infants than ever before, women typically still take the ultimate responsibility for the baby. In addition, women are usually the ones who make job changes; they may quit working or reduce their hours to stay home with the baby for several months or more, or they may try to juggle the multiple roles of mother, homemaker, and employer/employee, and feel guilty that they never have enough time to do justice to any of these roles.

Not surprisingly, marital satisfaction often declines after the birth of the first child. The wife who has stopped working may feel she is cut off from the world, and may feel overburdened and resentful from trying to fulfill duties both at home and on the job. The husband may have a hard time adjusting to having to share his wife's love and attention with the baby.

But marital dissatisfaction after the baby is born is not inevitable. Couples who successfully weather the stresses of a new baby seem to have these three characteristics in common:

1. They had developed a strong relationship before the baby was born.
2. They had planned to have the child and want it very much.
3. They communicate well about their feelings and expectations.

Parenting

Sometimes being a parent is a source of unparalleled pleasure and pride: the first smile (at you), the first word, the first home run. But at other times parenting can seem like an overwhelming responsibility.

Parenting Styles

Most parents worry about their ability to raise a healthy, responsible, and well-adjusted child. Parents may wonder about the long-term impact of each decision they make on their child's well-being and personality. According to parenting experts, no one action or decision (within limits) will determine a child's personality or development; instead, what is most important is the *parenting style*, or overall approach to parenting.

Research has revealed four general styles of parenting. The four styles vary primarily according to the levels of two characteristics of the parents:

- *Demandingness* encompasses the use of discipline and supervision, the expectation that children act responsibly and maturely, and the direct response to disobedience.

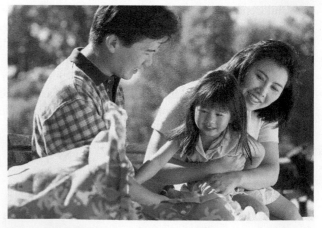

Setting clear boundaries, holding children to high expectations, and responding with warmth to children's needs are all positive parenting strategies.

- *Responsiveness* refers to a parent's warmth and his or her intent to facilitate independence and self-confidence in a child by being supportive, connected, and understanding of the child's needs. Most parents use a blend of the four general styles but tend toward one style.

AUTHORITARIAN *Authoritarian* parents are high in demandingness and low in responsiveness. They give orders and expect them to be obeyed, giving very little warmth or consideration to their children's special needs. They maintain a structured environment where the rules are explicit and set without input or discussion with the child. Children of authoritarian parents rate low on social competence, self-esteem, intellectual curiosity, spontaneity, and initiative. They perform fairly well in school and do not exhibit a lot of problem behaviour; however, they have higher levels of depression.

AUTHORITATIVE *Authoritative* parents are high in both demandingness and responsiveness. They set clear boundaries and expectations, but they are also loving, supportive, and attuned to their children's needs. They are firm in their decisions but allow for a give-and-take in discussions with the intent of fostering independent thinking.

Both authoritarian and authoritative parents hold their children to high expectations. The difference is that authoritarian parents expect their children to follow their commands without question or comment, and authoritative parents are more likely to explain their reasoning and allow children to express themselves. Research consistently shows that children of authoritative parents are the best adjusted and rate particularly high in social competence.

PERMISSIVE (OR INDULGENT) *Permissive* parents are high in responsiveness and low in demandingness. They do not expect their children to act maturely, but instead allow them to follow their own impulses. They are very warm, patient, and accepting, and they are focused on not stifling their child's innate creativity. They use little discipline and are often non-traditional. Children of permissive parents have difficulty with impulse control, are immature, perform more poorly in school, have more problem behaviours, and take less responsibility for their actions. They also have higher self-esteem, better social skills, and lower levels of depression.

UNINVOLVED *Uninvolved* parents are low in both demandingness and responsiveness. They require little from their children and respond with little attention, frequency, or effort. In extreme cases, this style might reach the level of child neglect. Research has found that children of uninvolved parents perform worse in all areas measured compared with children of parents who use the other styles.

Children's Temperaments

Every child has a tendency toward certain moods and a style of reacting—a temperament—that is apparent from infancy and often lasts into adulthood. Research has identified three basic temperament types; most children show aspects of different temperaments but tend toward one.

- *Easy children* are happy, content, and have regular sleeping and eating habits. They are adaptable and not easily upset.
- *Difficult children* are fussy, fearful in new situations or with strangers, and have irregular sleeping and feeding habits. They are easily upset and often hard to soothe.
- *Slow-to-warm-up children* are somewhat fussy and tend to react negatively or fearfully to new people or situations; however, they slowly warm up and adapt positively.

A match between parental style and child temperament is ideal. Difficulties tend to arise when a mismatch occurs in temperaments and styles and the parent is not versed in parenting skills. For example, a parent who expects quick action in response to a command may not be a good match for a slow-to-respond child. Parents should be attuned to their child's distinct style and do their best to support the child.

According to psychologists, "optimal attunement" of the parent to the child involves allowing the child to feel close and connected without feeling engulfed or impinged on, while also allowing for separation and aloneness without the child feeling abandoned or rejected. *Attachment parenting* advocates believe that if children are consistently held, attended to, and not allowed to be unhappy for any length of time, they will internalize the parents' consistent care and support and grow up more able to provide this for themselves and others.

QUICK STATS

The size of the Canadian family has declined from an average of 4.3 persons in 1921, to 3.9 in 1961, to 2.9 in 2011.

—Human Resources and Skills Development Canada, 2011; Statistics Canada, 2012

Parenting and the Family Life Cycle

Parenting that is responsive and demanding is the most beneficial for children. Providing a balance of firm limits and clear structure along with high levels of warmth, nurturance, and respect for the child's own special needs and temperament, as well as her or his growing independence, is the best predictor for raising a healthy child. The important thing is to keep seeking ways to promote satisfaction for all family members—including the parents! It is also important for parents to develop and maintain confidence in their parenting skills, their common sense—and, above all, their love for their children.

At each stage of the family life cycle, the relationship between parents and children changes. And with those changes come new challenges. The parents' primary responsibility to a small, helpless baby is to ensure its physical well-being around the clock. As babies grow into toddlers and begin to crawl and walk and talk, they begin to be able to take care of some of their own physical needs. For parents, the challenge at this stage is to strike a balance between giving children the freedom to explore and setting limits that will keep the children safe and secure. As children grow toward adolescence, parents need to give them increasing independence and gradually be willing to let them risk success or failure on their own.

Marital satisfaction for most couples tends to decline somewhat while the children are in school. Reasons include the financial and emotional pressures of a growing family and the increased job and community responsibilities of parents in their thirties, forties, and fifties. Once the last child has left home, marital satisfaction usually increases because couples have time to enjoy each other once more.

Single Parents

Today the family life cycle for many women is marriage, motherhood, divorce, single parenthood, remarriage, and widowhood.

In some single-parent families, the traditional family life cycle is reversed and the baby comes before the marriage. In some of these families, the single parent is a teenage mother; she may be of a lower socioeconomic status, and she may never get married or may not marry for several years. The number of Canadian women with children who are single and have never been married is also increasing. These lone parents of today tend to be older, on average, than their counterparts were in the past. In 2001, 30 percent of these lone parents were ages 35–44, up from 15 percent in 1981.

Economic difficulties are the primary problem for single mothers, especially for unmarried mothers who have not finished high school and have difficulty finding work. Divorced mothers usually experience a sharp drop in income the first few years on their own, but if they have job skills or education they usually can eventually support themselves and their children adequately. Other problems for single mothers are the often-conflicting demands of playing both father and mother and the difficulty of satisfying their own needs for adult companionship and affection.

Financial pressures are also a complaint of single fathers, but they do not experience them to the extent that single mothers do. Because they are likely to have less practice than mothers in juggling parental and professional roles, they may worry that they do not spend enough time with their children. Because single fatherhood is not as common as single motherhood, however, the men who choose it are likely to be stable, established, and strongly motivated to be with their children.

Research about the effect on children of growing up in a single-parent family is inconclusive. Evidence seems to indicate that these children tend to have less success in school and in their careers than children from two-parent families, but these effects may be associated more strongly with low educational attainment of the single parent than with the absence of the second parent. Two-parent families are not necessarily better if one of the parents spends little time relating to the children or is physically or emotionally abusive.

Stepfamilies

Single parenthood is usually a transitional stage: About three out of four divorced women and about four out of five divorced men will ultimately remarry. Rates are lower for widowed men and women, but overall, many of the marriages in North America are remarriages for the husband, the wife, or both. If either partner brings children from a previous marriage into the new family unit, a stepfamily (or blended family) is formed.

Stepfamilies are significantly different from primary families and should not be expected to duplicate the emotions and relationships of a primary family. Research has shown that healthy stepfamilies are less cohesive and more adaptable than healthy primary families; they have a greater capacity to allow for individual differences and accept that biologically related family members will have emotionally closer relationships. Stepfamilies gradually gain more of a sense of being a family as they build a history of shared daily experiences and major life events.

Successful Families

Family life can be extremely challenging. A strong family is not a family without problems; it's a family that copes successfully with stress and crisis (see "Strategies of Strong Families" on ⊟ connect). Successful families are intentionally connected—members share experiences and meanings.

An excellent way to build strong family ties is to develop family rituals and routines: organized, repeated activities that have meaning for family members. Families with regular routines and rituals have healthier children, more satisfying marriages, and stronger family relationships. Some of the most common routines identified in research studies are dinnertime, a regular bedtime, and household chores; common rituals include birthdays, religious and other holidays, and Sunday activities. Family routines may even serve as protective factors, balancing out potential risk factors associated with single-parent families and families with divorce and remarriage. You may want to consider incorporating a regular family mealtime into your family routine, as it allows parents and children to develop closer relationships and leads to better parenting, healthier children, and better school performance.

Although Canadian families have tremendous variation, researchers have proposed that six major qualities or themes appear in strong families:

1. *Commitment:* The family is very important to its members; sexual fidelity between partners is included in commitment.
2. *Appreciation:* Family members care about one another and express their appreciation. The home is a positive place for family members.
3. *Communication:* Family members spend time listening to one another and enjoying one another's company. They talk about disagreements and attempt to solve problems.
4. *Time together:* Family members do things together, often simple activities that don't cost money.
5. *Spiritual wellness:* The family promotes sharing, love, and compassion for other human beings.
6. *Coping with stress and crisis:* When faced with illness, death, marital conflict, or other crises, family members pull together, seek help, and use other coping strategies to meet the challenge.

It may surprise some people that members of strong families are often seen at counselling centres. They know that the smartest thing to do in some situations is to get help. Many resources are available for individuals and families seeking counselling; people can turn to physicians, clergy, marriage and family counsellors, psychologists, or other trained professionals.

THINKING ABOUT THE ENVIRONMENT

Parents can instil a lifelong sense of environmental stewardship in their children by teaching them these simple habits:

- Recycle waste as much as possible.
- Purchase environmentally friendly products that are manufactured from recyclable materials.
- Turn off lights and appliances when they are not needed.
- Shop for locally grown foods that are raised through environmentally sustainable practices.

For more information on the environment, see Chapter 21.

QUESTIONS FOR CRITICAL THINKING AND REFLECTION

In what ways is your own family successful? In what ways is your own family challenged in terms of members' relationships? What could you do to make your relationships in your family more successful? What could be different if you focused on improving both the easy and the challenging relationships within your family?

SUMMARY

- Healthy intimate relationships are an important component of the well-being of both individuals and society. Many intimate relationships are held together by love.
- Successful relationships begin with a positive sense of self and reasonably high self-esteem. Personal identity, gender roles, and styles of attachment are all rooted in childhood experiences.
- The characteristics of friendship include companionship, respect, acceptance, help, trust, loyalty, and reciprocity.
- Love, sex, and commitment are closely linked ideals in intimate relationships. Love includes trust, caring, respect, and loyalty. Sex brings excitement, fascination, and passion to the relationship.
- Common challenges in relationships relate to issues of self-disclosure, commitment, expectations, competitiveness, balancing time spent together and apart, and jealousy. Partners in successful relationships have strong communication skills and support each other in difficult times.
- The keys to good communication in relationships are self-disclosure, listening, and feedback.
- Conflict is inevitable in intimate relationships; partners need to have constructive ways to negotiate their differences.
- People usually choose partners like themselves. If partners are very different, acceptance and good communication skills are necessary to maintain the relationship.
- Most Canadians find partners through dating or getting together in groups. Cohabitation is a growing social pattern that allows partners to get to know each other intimately without being married.
- Gay and lesbian partnerships are similar to heterosexual partnerships, with some differences. Partners often don't conform to traditional gender roles, and they may experience hostility or ambivalence rather than approval toward their partnership from society.
- Singlehood is a growing option in our society. Advantages include greater variety in sex partners and more freedom in making life decisions; disadvantages include loneliness and possible economic hardship, especially for single women.

- Marriage fulfills many functions for individuals and society. It can provide people with affection, affirmation, and sexual fulfillment; a context for child rearing; and the promise of lifelong companionship.
- Love isn't enough to ensure a successful marriage. Partners have to be realistic, feel good about each other, have communication and conflict-resolution skills, share values, and have a balance of individual and joint interests.
- When problems can't be worked out, people often separate and divorce. Divorce is traumatic for all involved, especially children, but the negative effects are usually balanced in time by positive ones.
- Four general parenting styles are authoritarian, authoritative, permissive, and uninvolved; the authoritative style is usually associated with the best outcomes.
- At each stage of the family life cycle, relationships change. Marital satisfaction may be lower during the child-rearing years and higher later.
- Many families today are single-parent families. Problems for single parents include economic difficulties, conflicting demands, and time pressures.
- Stepfamilies are formed when single, divorced, or widowed people remarry and create new family units. Stepfamilies gradually gain more of a sense of being a family as they build a history of shared experiences.
- Important qualities of successful families include commitment to the family, appreciation of family members, communication, time spent together, spiritual wellness, and effective methods of dealing with stress.

FOR MORE INFORMATION

For resources in your area, check your campus directory for a counselling centre or peer counselling program, or search for community mental health agencies online.

BOOKS

Brooks, J. B. 2010. *The Process of Parenting*, 8th ed. New York: McGraw-Hill. A description of how parents and caregivers can translate their love and concern for children into effective parenting behaviour.

DeGenova, M. K., F. P. Rice. N. Stinnett, and N. Stinnett. 2010. *Intimate Relationships, Marriages, and Families*, 8th ed. New York: McGraw-Hill. A comprehensive introduction to relationships.

McKay, M., P. Fanning, and K. Paleg. 2007. *Couple Skills: Making Your Relationship Work*, 2nd rev. ed. New York: New Harbinger. A comprehensive guide to improving communication, resolving conflict, and developing greater intimacy and commitment in relationships.

Miller, R., 2011. *Intimate Relationships*, 6th ed. New York: McGraw-Hill. A balanced presentation of both the positive and the problematic aspects of intimate relationships.

Olson, D., J. DeFrain and L. Skogrand. 2010. *Marriages and Families: Intimacy, Diversity, and Strengths*, 7th ed. New York: McGraw-Hill. A comprehensive introduction to relationships and families.

ORGANIZATIONS AND WEBSITES

The Internet addresses listed here were accurate at the time of publication.

Association for Couples in Marriage Enrichment. Promotes activities to strengthen marriage; a resource for books, tapes, and other materials.
http://www.bettermarriages.org

Canadians for Equal Marriage. Includes information about a nationwide, bilingual campaign made up of individuals and organizations from all walks of Canadian life committed to upholding equal marriage rights for couples of any sexual orientation.
http://www.equal-marriage.ca

Charity Village Nonprofit Neighbourhood. Includes links to information and support for lesbian, gay, bisexual, and transgendered (LGBT) people.
　　http://www.charityvillage.com/cv/nonpr/nonpr27.html

Conflict Resolution Information Source. Provides links to a broad range of Internet resources on conflict resolution. Information covers interpersonal, marriage, family, and other types of conflicts.
　　http://www.crinfo.org

Family Education Network. Provides information about education, safety, health, and other family-related issues.
　　http://www.familyeducation.com

Gottman Institute. Includes tips and suggestions for relationships and parenting, including an online relationships quiz.
　　http://www.gottman.com

Life Innovations. Provides materials for premarital counselling and marital enrichment.
　　http://www.prepare-enrich.com

Parents Without Partners. Provides educational programs, literature, and support groups for single parents and their children. Search the online directory for a referral to a local chapter.
　　http://www.parentswithoutpartners.org

Registry of Marriage and Family Therapists in Canada. Provides information about the profession, resources, and links to therapists in different area of Canada.
　　http://www.marriageandfamily.ca

Vanier Institute of the Family. Provides research, resources, consultation, and policy development regarding the importance of families to Canadian society.
　　http://www.vifamily.ca

See also the listings for Chapters 2 and 12.

SELECTED BIBLIOGRAPHY

Beaupré, P. 2008. I do… Take two? Changes in intentions to remarry among divorced Canadians during the past 20 years. *Matter of Fact* 5, http://dsp-psd.tpsgc.gc.ca/collection_2008/statcan/89-630-X/89-630-XIE2008005.pdf (retrieved July 3, 2105).

Christakis, N. A., et al. 2006. Mortality after hospitalization of a spouse. *New England Journal of Medicine* 354(7): 719–730.

Copen et al. 2013. First premarital cohabitation in the United States: 2006-2010 National survey of Family Growth. *National Health Statistics Reports* (64), http://www.cdc.gov/nchs/data/nhsr/nhsr064.pdf (retrieved July 3, 2015).

Employment and Social Development Canada. 2014. *Well-being in Canada; Family Life – Marriage,* http://www4.hrsdc.gc.ca/.3ndic.1t.4r@-eng.jsp?iid=78 (retrieved July 3, 2015).

Employment and Social Development Canada. 2014. *Well-being in Canada; Family Life – Divorce,* http://www4.hrsdc.gc.ca/.3ndic.1t.4r@-eng.jsp?iid=76 (retrieved July 3, 2015).

Holt-Lunstad, J., W. Birmingham, and B. Q. Jones. 2008. Is there something unique about marriage? *Annals of Behavioral Medicine* 35(2): 239–244.

Lichter, D. T., R. N. Turner, and S. Sassler. 2010. National estimates of the rise in serial cohabitation. *Social Science Research* 39(5): 754–765.

Lu, Y. & Morissette, R. 2010. Women's participation and economic downturns. *Perspectives*. Catalogue no. 75-001-X, http://www.statcan.gc.ca/pub/75-001-x/2010105/pdf/11160-eng.pdf (retrieved July 3, 2015).

McPherson, M., L. Smith-Lovin, and M. Brashears. 2006. Social isolation in America: Changes in core discussion networks over two decades. *American Sociological Review* 71: 353–375.

Medical memo: Marital stress and the heart. 2004. *Harvard Men's Health Watch*, May.

Mookadam, F., and H. M. Arthur. 2004. Social support and its relationship to morbidity and mortality after acute myocardial infarction: Systematic overview. *Archives of Internal Medicine* 164(14): 1514–1518.

Najib, A., et al. 2004. Regional brain activity in women grieving a romantic relationship breakup. *American Journal of Psychiatry* 161(12): 2245–2256.

Pleis, J. R., and M. Lethbridge-Cejku. 2007. Summary health statistics for U.S. adults: National Health Interview Survey, 2006. *Vital and Health Statistics* 10(235): 1–153.

Public Health Agency of Canada. 2013. What makes Canadians healthy or unhealthy? http://www.phac-aspc.gc.ca/ph-sp/determinants/determinants-eng.php (retrieved July 3, 2015).

Roisman, G. I., et al. 2008. Adult romantic relationships as contexts of human development: A multimethod comparison of same-sex couples with opposite-sex dating, engaged, and married dyads. *Developmental Psychology* 44(1): 91–101.

Schoen, R., et al. 2007. Family transitions in young adulthood. *Demography* 44(4): 807–820.

Statistics Canada. 2005. *Women in Canada: A Gender-Based Statistical Report*, 5th ed., http://www.statcan.gc.ca/pub/89-503-x/89-503-x2005001-eng.pdf (retrieved July 3, 2015).

Statistics Canada. 2011. Divorces and crude divorce rates, Canada, provinces and territories, annual. (CANSIM table 101-6501) (in Excel format). Ottawa: Statistics Canada.

Statistics Canada. 2012. *Portrait of Families and Living Arrangements in Canada; Families, households and marital status, 2011 Census of Population.* Catalogue no. 98-312-X2011001, http://www12.statcan.gc.ca/census-recensement/2011/as-sa/98-312-x/98-312-x2011001-eng.pdf (retrieved July 3, 2015).

Statistics Canada. 2014. Population by marital status and sex. CANSIM, table 051-0042, http://www.statcan.gc.ca/tables-tableaux/sum-som/l01/cst01/famil01-eng.htm (retrieved July 3, 2015).

Strong, B., et al. 2005. *Human Sexuality: Diversity in Contemporary America*, 5th ed. New York: McGraw-Hill.

Talbot, Y., et al. 2001. Canadians without regular medical doctors. Who are they? *Canadian Family Physician* 47(1), 58–64.

Tucker, P. and J. Irwin. 2011. University students' satisfaction with, interest in improving, and receptivity to attending programs aimed at health and well-being. *Health Promotion Practice 12(3), 388–395. doi: 10.1177/1524839908330814.*

Vanier Institute. 2013. Same-sex families raising children. *Fascinating Families* (51), http://www.vanier-institute.ca/include/get.php?nodeid=2817 (retrieved July 3, 2015).

Wainright, J. L., S. T. Russell, and C. J. Patterson. 2004. Psychosocial adjustment, school outcomes, and romantic relationships of adolescents with same-sex parents. *Child Development* 75(6): 1886–1898.

Whisman, M. A., L. A. Uebelacker, and L. M. Weinstock. 2004. Psychopathology and marital satisfaction: The importance of evaluating both partners. *Journal of Consulting and Clinical Psychology* 72(5): 830–838.

Yarber, W., B. Sayad, and B. Strong. 2010. *Human Sexuality: Diversity in Contemporary America*, 7th ed. New York: McGraw-Hill.

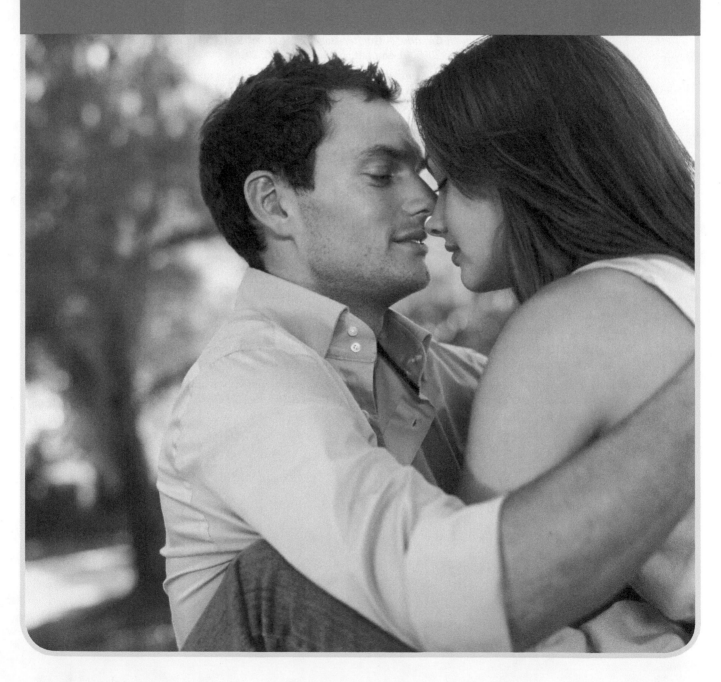

CHAPTER 11

Healthy Sexuality

LOOKING AHEAD

After you have read and studied this chapter, you should be able to:

LO1 Describe the structure and function of the female and male sex organs

LO2 Explain the changes in sexual functioning that occur during a person's life

LO3 Describe how the sex organs function during sexual activity

LO4 Identify common causes of sexual problems

LO5 Outline the factors that influence sexual behaviour and the various ways human sexuality can be expressed

LO6 Describe guidelines for safe, responsible sexual behaviour

LO7 Identify the advantages, disadvantages, and level of effectiveness of commonly used reversible contraceptive methods

LO8 Understand the different types of abortion procedures

TEST YOUR KNOWLEDGE

1. **Although testosterone is the primary male hormone, it is also produced in women.**
   True or false?

2. **Which of the following is a risk factor for erectile dysfunction (impotence)?**
   a. smoking b. overweight c. physical inactivity

3. **Calcium supplements may reduce symptoms of premenstrual syndrome (PMS) in some women.**
   True or false?

4. **Alcohol consumption by young people is associated with unplanned, unprotected sexual activity and higher rates of sexually transmitted infections (STIs).**
   True or false?

5. **Sperm can survive only about 24 hours inside a woman's body.**
   True or false?

6. **Abortion is illegal in some parts of Canada.**
   True of false?

ANSWERS

1. TRUE.   Testosterone is produced in small amounts by a woman's ovaries.

2. ALL THREE.   70–80 percent of cases of erectile dysfunction are thought to involve physical factors.

3. TRUE.   Other self-help strategies for PMS include exercise, stress reduction, and a diet low in fat and rich in complex carbohydrates.

4. TRUE.   Studies have shown that raising the drinking age and increasing the price of beer (through taxes) leads to a decrease in STI rates among young adults.

5. FALSE.   Sperm usually live about 72 hours inside the woman's body but can live up to six or seven days.

6. FALSE.   Abortion is legal throughout every province and territory in Canada.

Humans are sexual beings. Sexual activity is the source of our most intense physical pleasures, a central ingredient in many of our intimate emotional relationships, and the key to reproduction.

Sexuality is more than just sexual behaviour. It is a complex, interacting group of inborn, biological characteristics and acquired behaviours people learn in the course of growing up in a particular family, community, and society. Sexuality includes biological sex (being biologically male or female), gender (masculine and feminine behaviours), sexual anatomy and physiology, sexual functioning and practices, and social and sexual interactions with others. Our individual sense of identity is powerfully influenced by our sexuality. We think of ourselves in fundamental ways as male or female; as heterosexual, gay, or lesbian; as single, attached, married, or divorced.

> **sexuality**
> A dimension of personality shaped by biological, psychosocial, and cultural forces and concerning all aspects of sexual behaviour.

Because it can arouse intense feelings, sexuality can be an emotionally charged topic. In many communities, sexual expression is regulated with restrictions and taboos, specifying which functions and behaviours are acceptable and "normal" and which are unacceptable and "abnormal." Young people in Canada are bombarded with conflicting messages about sex. The mass media suggest that the average person is a sexual athlete who continually jumps in and out of bed without using contraception, producing offspring, or contracting disease. Although parents, educators, and other responsible adults may try to present a more balanced picture, they often convey their own hidden messages as well. Ignorance, confusion, and fear are frequently the result.

Basic information about the body, sexual functioning, and sexual behaviour is vital to healthy adult life. Once we understand the facts, we have a better basis for evaluating the messages we get and for making informed, responsible choices about our sexual activities. If you have questions about some aspects of your physical sexuality, this chapter will provide you with answers.

Sexual Anatomy

In spite of their different appearances, the sex organs of men and women arise from the same structures and fulfill similar functions. Each person has a pair of **gonads**; ovaries are the female gonads, and testes are the male gonads. The gonads produce **germ cells** and sex hormones. The germ cells are **ova** (eggs) in females and **sperm** in males. Ova and sperm are the basic units of reproduction; their union results in the creation of a new life.

> **gonads**
> The primary reproductive organs that produce germ cells and sex hormones; the ovaries and testes.
>
> **germ cells**
> Sperm and ova.
>
> **ovum** (ova, plural)
> A germ cell produced by a female, which combines with a male germ cell (sperm) to create a fetus; also called an *egg*.
>
> **sperm**
> A germ cell produced by a male, which combines with a female germ cell (ovum) to create a fetus.

Female Sex Organs

The external sex organs, or genitals, of the female are called the **vulva** (see Figure 11.1). The mons pubis, a rounded mass of fatty tissue over the pubic bone, becomes covered with hair during puberty (biological maturation). Below it are two paired folds of skin called the labia majora (major lips) and the labia minora (minor lips). Enclosed within these folds are the clitoris, the opening of the urethra, and the opening of the vagina.

> **vulva**
> The external female genitals or sex organs.

FIGURE 11.1

FIGURE 11.1

The Female Sex Organs

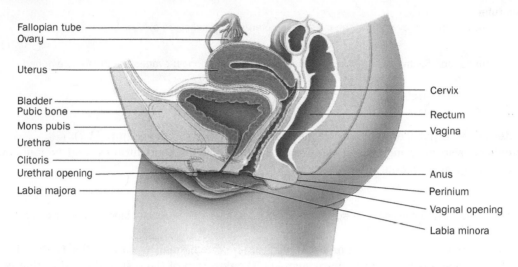

The **clitoris** is highly sensitive to touch and plays an important role in female sexual arousal and orgasm. The clitoris consists of a shaft, glans, and spongy tissue that fill with blood during sexual excitement. The glans is the most sensitive part of the clitoris and is covered by the clitoral hood, or **prepuce**, which is formed from the upper portion of the labia minora.

clitoris
The highly sensitive female genital structure.

prepuce
The foreskin of the clitoris or penis.

The female **urethra** is a duct that leads directly from the urinary bladder to its opening between the clitoris and the opening of the vagina; it conducts urine from the bladder to the outside of the body. The female urethra is independent of the genitals.

urethra
The duct that carries urine from the bladder to the outside of the body.

The vaginal opening is partially covered by a membrane called the **hymen**. This membrane can be stretched or torn during athletic activity or when a woman has sexual intercourse for the first time. (The idea that an intact hymen is the sign of virginity is a myth.) The **vagina** is the passage that leads to the internal reproductive organs. It is the female structure for heterosexual sexual intercourse and also serves as the birth canal.

hymen
A membrane that partially covers the vaginal opening.

vagina
The passage leading from the female genitals to the internal reproductive organs; the birth canal.

Projecting into the upper part of the vagina is the **cervix**, which is the opening of the **uterus**—or *womb*—where a fertilized egg is implanted and grows into a *fetus*.

cervix
The end of the uterus opening toward the vagina.

uterus
The hollow, thick-walled, muscular organ in which the fertilized egg develops; the womb.

A pair of **fallopian tubes** (or *oviducts*) extends from the top of the uterus. The end of each oviduct surrounds an **ovary** and guides the mature ovum down into the uterus after the egg exits the ovary.

> **fallopian tube**
> A duct that guides a mature ovum from the ovary to the uterus; also called an *oviduct*.
>
> **ovary**
> One of two female reproductive glands that produce ova and sex hormones; ovaries are the female gonads.

Male Sex Organs

A man's external sex organs, or genitals, are the penis and the scrotum (see Figure 11.2).

The **penis** consists of spongy tissue that becomes engorged with blood during sexual excitement, causing the organ to enlarge and become erect.

> **penis**
> The male genital structure consisting of spongy tissue that becomes engorged with blood during sexual excitement.

The **scrotum** is a pouch that contains a pair of sperm-producing male gonads, called **testes**. The scrotum maintains the testes at a temperature approximately 3°C below that of the rest of the body—that is, at about 34°C. The process of sperm production is extremely heat sensitive. In hot temperatures the muscles in the scrotum relax, and the testes move away from the heat of the body. This ability to regulate the temperature of the testes is important because elevated testicular temperature can interfere with normal sperm production.

> **scrotum**
> The loose sac of skin and muscle fibres that contains the testes.
>
> **testis** (testes, plural)
> One of two male gonads, the site of sperm production; also called a *testicle*.

Through the entire length of the penis runs the urethra, which can carry both urine and *semen*, the sperm-carrying fluid, to the opening at the tip of the penis. Although urine and semen share a common passage, they are prevented from mixing together by muscles that control their entry into the urethra.

FIGURE 11.2

The Male Sex Organs

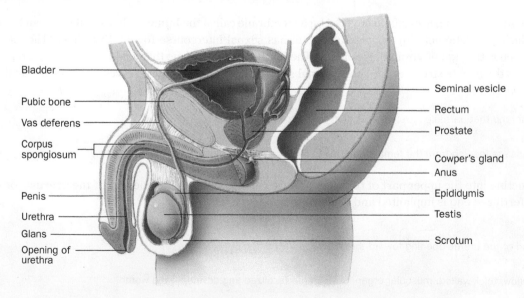

During its brief lifetime, a sperm takes the following route:

1. Sperm are produced inside a maze of tiny, tightly packed tubules within the testes. As they begin to mature, sperm flow into a single storage tube called the **epididymis**, which lies on the surface of each testis.
2. Sperm move from each epididymis into another tube called the **vas deferens**, which carries them upward into the abdominal cavity and through an organ called the **prostate gland**. This gland produces some of the fluid in semen, which helps transport and nourish the sperm.
3. The two *vasa deferentia* eventually merge into a pair of **seminal vesicles**, whose secretions provide nutrients for the semen.
4. On the final stage of their journey, sperm flow into the **ejaculatory ducts**, which join the urethra.

epididymis
A storage duct for maturing sperm, located on the surface of each testis.

vas deferens (vasa deferentia, plural)
A tube that carries sperm from the epididymis through the prostate gland to the seminal vesicles.

prostate gland
An organ in the male reproductive system; produces some of the fluid in semen, which helps transport and nourish sperm.

seminal vesicle
A tube leading from the vas deferens to the ejaculatory duct; secretes nutrients for the semen.

ejaculatory duct
A tube that carries mature sperm to the urethra so they can exit the body on ejaculation.

The **Cowper's glands** are two small structures flanking the urethra. During sexual arousal, these glands secrete a clear, mucus-like fluid that appears at the tip of the penis. The exact purpose of pre-ejaculatory fluid is not known, but it is thought to help lubricate the urethra to facilitate the passage of sperm. In some men, pre-ejaculatory fluid may contain sperm, so withdrawal of the penis before ejaculation is not a reliable form of contraception.

Cowper's gland
In the male reproductive system, a small organ that produces pre-ejaculatory fluid.

QUICK STATS

A normal sperm count ranges from 15 million to more than 200 million sperm per millilitre of semen.
—Mayo Clinic, 2014

Circumcision

The smooth, rounded tip of the penis is the highly sensitive **glans**, an important component in sexual arousal (see Figure 11.3). The glans is partially covered by the foreskin, or prepuce, a retractable fold of skin that is removed by **circumcision** in about 9 percent of newborn males in Canada. Circumcision is performed for cultural, religious, and hygienic reasons, and rates of circumcision vary widely among different groups. Worldwide, the rate is about 30 percent. Most Europeans, Asians, South and Central Americans, and Africans do not perform circumcision; Jews and Muslims are the major groups who circumcise for religious reasons.

glans
The rounded head of the penis or the clitoris.

circumcision
Surgical removal of the foreskin of the penis.

FIGURE 11.3

Circumcised and Uncircumcised Penis

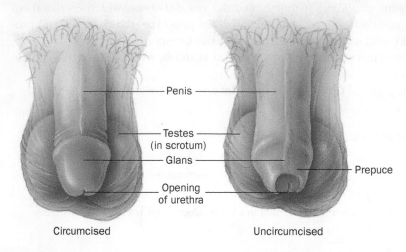

Penis

Testes (in scrotum)

Glans

Opening of urethra

Prepuce

Circumcised   Uncircumcised

The pros and cons of this simple procedure have been widely debated. Citing research findings, proponents argue that it promotes cleanliness and reduces the risk of urinary tract infections in newborns and the risk of sexually transmitted infections (STIs), including HIV, later in life. STI education and the practice of abstinence or low-risk sexual behaviours have a far greater impact on the transmission of STIs than does circumcision. However, where safer sex practices are not adhered to, circumcision can have a protective effect. Recent studies in countries with high rates of HIV infection and AIDS have shown that circumcision can reduce the risk of acquiring HIV through heterosexual contact in men by as much as 60 percent.

In 2007, an expert panel from the World Health Organization (WHO) recognized that male circumcision is an effective intervention for decreasing the spread of HIV, but stressed that circumcision provides only partial protection and must be combined with other preventive strategies, such as condom use and limiting the number of sexual partners.

Opponents of circumcision state that it is an unnecessary surgical procedure that causes pain and puts a baby at risk for complications. They also argue that, by removing the foreskin, circumcision exposes the glans of the penis to constant irritation by clothing, thereby reducing its sensitivity; research into this issue has been inconclusive.

The Canadian Paediatric Association (CPS) takes the position (opposed by some physicians) that although circumcision has potential medical benefits, the research is not sufficient to recommend the procedure routinely. The CPS issued a statement that "circumcision of newborns should *not* be routinely performed." All provincial health insurance plans have now removed non-therapeutic circumcision from the list of procedures covered, because of the lack of health benefits.

QUESTIONS FOR CRITICAL THINKING AND REFLECTION

What are your personal views on circumcision? Who or what has influenced those opinions? Are the bases of your views primarily cultural, moral, or medical?

THINKING ABOUT THE ENVIRONMENT

Research points to several possible environmental causes for sexual problems, but because studies have been scattered and have produced conflicting results, scientists are now beginning exhaustive studies into these issues. Still, some researchers contend that environmental contaminants may cause a variety of sexual problems in humans. For example,

- Prenatal exposure to chemicals called phthalates may interfere with the development of sex organs in the male fetus.
- Adult exposure to pesticides may reduce sperm quality and quantity in men.
- Exposure to a number of common cleaning solvents (such as acetone) may increase a woman's chance of miscarriage.

For more information on the environment and environmental health, see Chapter 21.

Hormones and the Reproductive Life Cycle

Many cultural and personal factors help shape the expression of your sexuality, but biology also plays an important role. The sex hormones produced by the ovaries or testes have a major influence on the development and function of the reproductive system throughout life.

The sex hormones made by the testes are called **androgens**, the most important of which is *testosterone*. The female sex hormones, produced by the ovaries, belong to two groups: **estrogens** and **progestins**, the most important of which is *progesterone*. The ovaries also produce a small amount of testosterone. The cortex of the **adrenal glands** also produces androgens in both males and females.

androgens
Male sex hormones produced by the testes in males and by the adrenal glands in both sexes.

estrogens
A class of female sex hormones, produced by the ovaries, that bring about sexual maturation at puberty and maintain reproductive functions.

progestins
A class of female sex hormones, produced by the ovaries, that sustain reproductive functions.

adrenal glands
Endocrine glands, located over the kidneys, that produce androgens (among other hormones).

The hormones produced by the testes, the ovaries, and the adrenal glands are regulated by the hormones of the **pituitary gland**, located at the base of the brain. This gland in turn is controlled by hormones produced by the **hypothalamus** in the brain.

pituitary gland
An endocrine gland at the base of the brain that produces follicle-stimulating hormone (FSH) and luteinizing hormone (LH), among others.

hypothalamus
A region of the brain above the pituitary gland whose hormones control the secretions of the pituitary; also involved in the nervous control of sexual functions.

Differentiation of the Embryo

The biological sex of an individual is determined by the fertilizing sperm at the time of conception. All human cells normally contain 23 pairs of chromosomes. In 22 of the pairs, the two partner chromosomes match. But in the twenty-third pair, the **sex chromosomes**, two configurations are possible. Individuals with two matching X chromosomes are female, and individuals with one X and one Y chromosome are male. Thus, at the time of conception, the genetic sex is established: Females are XX and males are XY (see the Gender Matters box).

sex chromosomes
The X and Y chromosomes, which determine an individual's biological sex.

Genetic sex dictates whether the undifferentiated gonads become ovaries or testes. If a Y chromosome is present, the gonads become testes; the testes will produce the male hormone **testosterone**. Testosterone circulates throughout the body and causes the undifferentiated reproductive structures to develop into male sex organs (penis, scrotum, and so on). If a Y chromosome is not present, there is no testosterone and the gonads become ovaries and the reproductive structures develop into female sex organs (clitoris, labia, and so on).

testosterone
The most important androgen (male sex hormone); stimulates an embryo to develop into a male and induces the development of male secondary sex characteristics during puberty.

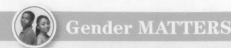 Gender **MATTERS**

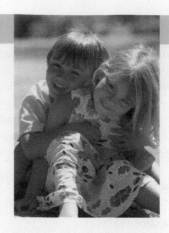

Sexual Differentiation, Hormones, and the Brain

Males and females are different from each other in many ways, but we are also very similar. We develop from the same embryonic tissue. The presence or absence of androgens determines how the sex organs develop. The entire process is known as *sexual differentiation*.

As described in the chapter, each male and female reproductive structure develops from the same undifferentiated tissue, so every structure in one sex has its counterpart in the other. For example, the tissue that gives rise to the clitoris in females becomes the penis in males, and the tissue that gives rise to the labia majora in females becomes the scrotum in males. The appearance of the genitals is sometimes called *gonadal* sex.

Exposure to hormones affects more than just the reproductive organs; it also influences development of the brain. It has been demonstrated many times that males tend to perform better than females at tasks requiring spatial skills and females perform better than males on tests of verbal skills. If androgens are involved in this gender difference, we would expect genetic females exposed to androgens to do better at spatial skills and genetic males deprived of androgens to do worse—and this is exactly what we find.

In a condition known as androgen insensitivity syndrome, genetic males do not have cell receptors for male hormones and they develop physically as females—and their spatial skills are more like those of females than males. The converse occurs when genetic females are exposed before birth to excess male hormones. In a fascinating study of twins, it was found that in opposite-sex pairs, female twins had a more masculine pattern of skills and behaviour compared with same-sex female twins. In opposite-sex twins, the female twin is exposed in utero to some of the androgens produced by her male twin, and these androgens influence her brain organization and thus her spatial skills.

Each person is the product of biological events that act on the cells in the body, including the brain. However, the physical and social environment then shapes this biological foundation to produce unique individuals. Some researchers point to the human past as a way to explain sex differences in language and visual-spatial skills. For example, the early division of labour with men as hunters and women as food gatherers, camp organizers, and child raisers may have selected for different skills based on gender, including visual-spatial skills in men and communication skills in women.

Sources: Cohen-Bendahan, C., et al. 2004. Prenatal exposure to testosterone and functional lateralization: A study in same-sex and opposite-sex twin girls. *Psychoneuroendocrinology* 29(7): 911–916; Sinisi, A., et al. 2003. Sexual differentiation. *Journal of Endocrinological Investigation* 26(3 Suppl.): 23–28; and Joseph, R. 2000. The evolution of sex differences in language, sexuality, and visual-spatial skills. *Archives of Sexual Behavior* 29(1): 35–66.

Female Sexual Maturation

Although humans are fully sexually differentiated at birth, the differences between males and females are accentuated at **puberty**, the period during which the reproductive system matures, secondary sex characteristics develop, and the bodies of males and females begin to appear more distinctive. The changes of puberty are induced by testosterone in the male and estrogen and **progesterone** in the female.

puberty
The period of biological maturation during adolescence.

progesterone
The most important progestin (female sex hormone); induces the development of female secondary sex characteristics during puberty, regulates the menstrual cycle, and sustains pregnancy.

Physical Changes

The first sign of puberty in girls is breast development, followed by a rounding of the hips and buttocks. As the breasts develop, hair appears in the pubic region and later in the underarms. Shortly after the onset of breast development, girls show an increase in growth rate. Breast development usually begins between ages 8 and 13, and the time of rapid body growth occurs between ages 9 and 15.

The Menstrual Cycle

A major landmark of puberty for young women is the onset of the **menstrual cycle**, the monthly ovarian cycle that leads to menstruation (loss of blood and tissue lining the uterus) in the absence of pregnancy. The timing of **menarche** (the first *menstrual period*) varies with several factors, including ethnicity, genetics, and nutritional status. The "normal" range for the onset of menstruation is wide; some girls experience menarche when they are as young as 9 or 10 years of age, and others when they are 16 or 17 years old. The current average age of menarche in Canada is around 12.7 years of age. Two hundred years ago, the average age of menarche was closer to 17 years. The earlier onset of menarche is probably due in large part to nutritional factors. When age at menarche is examined worldwide, menarche tends to come later to girls who live in relative poverty with diets lacking in protein and calories. Obesity is strongly correlated with earlier menarche, which may explain the current trend for earlier menarche in Canada and many other countries. Some experts worry that exposure to estrogen-like chemicals in the environment may also be contributing to earlier menarche.

menstrual cycle
The monthly ovarian cycle, regulated by hormones; in the absence of pregnancy, menstruation occurs.

menarche
The first menstrual period, experienced by most young women at some point during adolescence.

The day of the onset of bleeding is day 1 of the menstrual cycle. For the purposes of our discussion, a cycle of 28 days will be used; however, normal cycles vary in length from 21 to 35 days. The menstrual cycle consists of the following four phases (see Figure 11.4):

FIGURE 11.4

The Menstrual Cycle

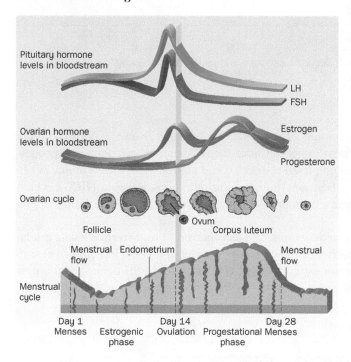

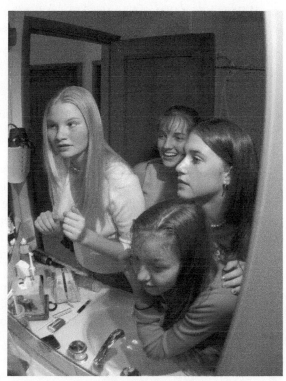

Once they reach puberty, these adolescents are biologically adults, but it will take several more years for them to become adults in social and psychological terms.

1. Menses

During **menses**, characterized by the menstrual flow, blood levels of hormones from the ovaries and the pituitary gland are relatively low. This phase of the cycle usually lasts from day one to about day five.

> **menses**
> The portion of the menstrual cycle characterized by menstrual flow.

2. Estrogenic Phase

The estrogenic phase begins when the menstrual flow ceases and the pituitary gland begins to produce increasing amounts of follicle-stimulating hormone (FSH) and luteinizing hormone (LH). Under the influence of FSH, an egg-containing ovarian **follicle** begins to mature, producing increasingly higher amounts of estrogens. Stimulated by estrogen, the **endometrium**, the uterine lining, thickens with large numbers of blood vessels and uterine glands.

> **follicle**
> A saclike structure within the ovary, in which eggs (ova) mature.
>
> **endometrium**
> The lining of the uterus.

3. Ovulation

A surge of a potent estrogen called *estradiol* from the follicle causes the pituitary to release a large burst of LH and a smaller amount of FSH. The high concentration of LH stimulates the developing follicle to release its ovum. This event is known as **ovulation**. After ovulation, the follicle is transformed into the **corpus luteum**, which produces progesterone and estrogen. Ovulation usually occurs about 14 days before the onset of menstrual flow, a fact that can be used to predict the most fertile time during the menstrual cycle, useful in both fertility treatment and natural family planning methods.

> **ovulation**
> The release of a mature egg (ovum) from an ovary.
>
> **corpus luteum**
> The part of the ovarian follicle left after ovulation, which secretes estrogen and progesterone during the second half of the menstrual cycle.

4. Progestational Phase

During the progestational phase of the cycle, the amount of progesterone secreted from the corpus luteum increases and remains high until the onset of the next menses. Under the influence of estrogen and progesterone, the endometrium continues to develop, readying itself to receive and nourish a fertilized ovum. When pregnancy occurs, the fertilized egg produces the hormone human chorionic gonadotropin (HCG), which maintains the corpus luteum. Thus, levels of ovarian hormones remain high and the uterine lining is preserved, preventing menses.

If pregnancy does not occur, the corpus luteum degenerates, and estrogen and progesterone levels gradually fall. Below certain hormonal levels, the endometrium can no longer be maintained, and it begins to slough off, initiating menses. As the levels of ovarian hormones fall, a slight rise in LH and FSH occurs, and a new menstrual cycle begins.

QUICK STATS

75% of women experience premenstrual symptoms during their childbearing years.

—National Institutes of Health, 2012

MENSTRUAL PROBLEMS   Menstruation is a normal biological process, but it may cause physical or psychological problems. **Dysmenorrhea** is characterized by cramps in the lower abdomen, backache, vomiting, nausea, a bloated feeling, diarrhea, and loss of appetite. Some of these symptoms can be attributed to uterine muscular contractions caused by chemicals called *prostaglandins*. Any drug that blocks the effects of prostaglandins, such as Aspirin or ibuprofen, will usually alleviate some of the symptoms of dysmenorrhea.

dysmenorrhea
Painful or problematic menstruation.

Many women experience transient physical and emotional symptoms before the onset of their menstrual flow. Depending on their severity, these symptoms may be categorized along a continuum from **premenstrual tension** through **premenstrual syndrome (PMS)** to **premenstrual dysphoric disorder (PMDD)**. Premenstrual tension symptoms are mild and may include negative mood changes and physical symptoms, such as abdominal cramping and backache. More severe symptoms are classified as PMS; very severe symptoms that cause impairment in social functioning and work-related activities are classified as PMDD. All three conditions share a definite pattern: Symptoms appear before the onset of menses and disappear within a few days after the start of menstruation.

premenstrual tension
Mild physical and emotional changes associated with the time before the onset of menses; symptoms can include abdominal cramping and backache.

premenstrual syndrome (PMS)
A disorder characterized by physical discomfort, psychological distress, and behavioural changes that begin after ovulation and cease when menstruation begins.

premenstrual dysphoric disorder (PMDD)
Severe form of PMS, characterized by symptoms serious enough to interfere with work or school or with social activities and relationships.

Symptoms associated with PMS and PMDD include physical changes, such as breast tenderness, water retention (bloating), headache, and fatigue; insomnia or excessive sleep; appetite changes and food cravings; irritability, anger, and increased interpersonal conflict; mood swings; depression and sadness; anxiety and tearfulness; inability to concentrate; social withdrawal; and the sense that one is out of control or overwhelmed. The key to diagnosing PMS and PMDD is to keep a daily diary of symptoms over several menstrual cycles. PMDD is distinguished from PMS by the severity of symptoms, which in PMDD interfere significantly with work or school and with usual social activities and relationships.

Despite many research studies, the causes of PMS and PMDD are still unknown, and it is unclear why some women are more vulnerable than others. Research has focused on a variety of substances in the body that may fluctuate with the menstrual cycle. Most researchers feel that PMS is probably caused by a combination of hormonal, nutritional, and psychological factors.

Selective serotonin reuptake inhibitors (SSRIs), including Zoloft, Paxil, and Celexa, are the first-line treatment for PMDD. Until recently, women using SSRIs took the medication throughout the entire menstrual cycle, but it has now been shown that taking the medication during just the progestational phase of the cycle is similarly effective. Progestational phase use reduces the exposure to the drug and its associated side effects. Antianxiety medications and progesterone have also been tested for progestational phase administration but show little positive effect in easing symptoms.

Other drug treatments include estrogen, certain oral contraceptives, diuretics to minimize water retention, and drugs, such as Aspirin, ibuprofen, and more potent prescription prostaglandin inhibitors that block the effects of prostaglandins. In 2009, the Yaz birth control pill was approved by Health Canada. In addition to birth control, Yaz helped to reduce PMDD. Yaz, and a similar oral contraceptive, Yasmin, contain drospirenone, a synthetic progestin that is similar to natural progesterone and has a diuretic effect that seems to counteract some premenstrual symptoms. Yaz also reduced moderate acne in women who wanted an oral contraceptive for birth control. However, in 2011, Health Canada completed a safety review of these drospirenone-containing drugs with respect to the risk of blood clots, and determined that they may be associated with a risk of clots 1.5 to 3 times higher than other birth control pills. Recently, these pills have been the subject of a number of Canadian-based news reports pertaining to suspected associated deaths and a class action lawsuit against the maker of the pills. If you are considering taking these or any medication, it is critical to have a thorough conversation with your physician about the pros and the cons. It is also important to recognize that a number of vitamins, minerals, and other dietary supplements have also been studied for PMS relief. Only one supplement, calcium, has been shown in rigorous clinical studies to provide relief; several others show promise, but more research is needed.

The following strategies provide relief for many women, and all of them can contribute to a healthy lifestyle at any time:

- *Limit salt intake.* Salt promotes water retention and bloating.
- *Exercise.* Women who exercise experience fewer symptoms before and after menstrual periods.
- *Don't use alcohol or tobacco.* Alcohol and tobacco may aggravate certain symptoms of PMS and PMDD.
- *Eat a nutritious diet.* Choose a low-fat diet rich in complex carbohydrates from vegetables, fruits, and whole grain breads, cereals, and pasta. Get enough calcium from calcium-rich foods and, if needed, supplements. Minimize your intake of sugar and caffeine, and avoid chocolate, which is rich in both.
- *Relax.* Stress reduction is always beneficial, and stressful events can trigger PMS symptoms. Try relaxation techniques during the premenstrual time.

If symptoms persist, keep a daily diary to track both the types of symptoms you experience and their severity. See your physician for an evaluation and to learn more about treatments that are available only with a prescription.

Male Sexual Maturation

Reproductive maturation of boys occurs about two years later than that of girls, usually at about age 10 or 11. Testicular growth is usually the first obvious sign of sexual maturity in boys. The penis also grows at this time, reaching adult size by about age 18. Pubic hair begins to develop after the genitals begin to increase in size, with underarm and facial hair gradually appearing. Hair on the chest, back, and abdomen increases later in development. The voice deepens as a result of the lengthening and thickening of the vocal chords. A small amount of breast development occurs in many boys during puberty. This is called *gynecomastia*, and it usually decreases after puberty. Excessive breast growth can occur in some boys, especially if they are overweight. Boys grow taller for about six years after the first signs of puberty, with a very rapid period of growth about two years after puberty starts.

Acne

A not-so-welcome aspect of puberty for many boys and girls is the development of acne, technically called *acne vulgaris*. During adolescence, acne is typically worse in males; in adulthood, women tend to have more acne than men. The production of male hormones in puberty is the initial trigger for acne in most boys and girls. Acne is caused by multiple factors, including hormones, excess oil production, plugging of hair follicles (pores), infection with the bacterium *Propionibacterium acnes*, and inflammation. Fortunately, many treatments for acne exist, making control of this skin disease possible in nearly all cases.

QUICK STATS

85–100% of all people are affected by acne at some point during their lives.
—eMedicine.com, 2008

Aging and Human Sexuality

Changes in hormone production and sexual functioning occur as we age. As a woman approaches age 50, her ovaries gradually cease to function and she enters **menopause**, the cessation of menstruation. For some women, the associated drop in hormone production causes symptoms that are troublesome. The most common physical symptom of menopause is hot flashes, sensations of warmth rising to the face from the upper chest, with or without perspiration and chills. Other symptoms include headaches, dizziness, palpitations, and joint pains. Osteoporosis—decreasing bone density—can develop, making older women more vulnerable to fractures. Some menopausal women become moody, even markedly depressed, and they may also experience fatigue, irritability, and forgetfulness.

menopause
The cessation of menstruation, occurring gradually around age 50.

To alleviate the symptoms of menopause and reduce the risk of heart disease and osteoporosis, millions of women have been prescribed hormone therapy (HT), a regimen of hormones that includes estrogen and progesterone. In 2002, an ongoing study of HT involving more than 16 000 women was halted because the women in the study who had been taking HT for long periods had more strokes, heart attacks, and blood clots and had a higher incidence of breast cancer than women in the study taking a placebo. The risks for such health problems were small but significant enough to halt the study. The positive findings from this study were a reduction in hip fractures and a reduced risk of colon cancer among the women taking HT. Many women who were taking HT stopped and many more never started as a result of the publicity surrounding the 2002 study.

In 2007, analysis of data on breast cancer in Canada showed a decline in 2003 and 2004, possibly because fewer women took HT (although other factors may also be responsible for the decline in breast cancer). At around the same time, scientists reanalyzed the original 2002 data on HT and found that women who started HT close to the time of menopause tended to have a reduced risk of cardiovascular disease, while women who took HT several years after going through menopause had a higher risk of heart disease. As a result of these findings, women taking HT were advised to consult their health care providers about their personal risks and benefits. (See Chapters 5, 7, 8, and 17 for more information on osteoporosis, heart disease, breast cancer, and HT.)

As a result of decreased estrogen production during menopause, the vaginal walls become thin, and lubrication in response to sexual arousal diminishes; sexual intercourse may become painful. Hormonal treatment or the use of lubricants during intercourse can minimize these problems.

Between the ages of 35 and 65, men experience a gradual decline in testosterone production resulting in the aging male syndrome, sometimes referred to as *male menopause* or *andropause*. Experts generally prefer the term *aging male syndrome* because the process is much more gradual than female menopause.

Symptoms vary widely among men, but most men experience at least some of the following symptoms as they age: loss of muscle mass, increased fat mass, decreased sex drive, erectile problems, depressed mood, irritability, difficulties with concentration, increased urination, loss of bone mineral density, and sleep difficulties. In some cases, treatment with testosterone can help. Although taking testosterone can be very harmful in young healthy men, older men with low testosterone levels may benefit from carefully prescribed testosterone treatment.

As men get older, they depend more on direct physical stimulation for sexual arousal. They take longer to achieve an erection and find it more difficult to maintain one; orgasmic contractions are less intense. Older men with erectile dysfunction are often prescribed medications, such as Viagra, or even more successful therapies that combine medication with a testosterone gel applied to the skin; see the section on sexual dysfunction later in the chapter for more information.

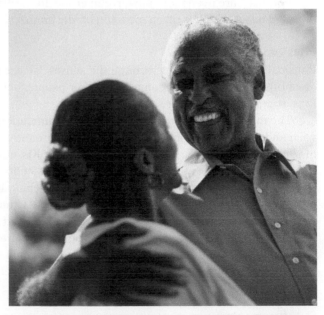

Although sexual physiology changes as people get older, many men and women readily adjust to these alterations.

Unlike women, who are born with all the eggs they will ever have and stop being fertile at menopause, men continue to produce sperm throughout their lives and can sometimes father children when they are well into their eighties and even nineties. Starting at about age 30, however, men become gradually less fertile. Regardless of the age of their female partners, couples in which the male is over age 35 have a 50 percent lower pregnancy rate than couples in which the man is 30 years old or younger. Men who are over age 40 are more likely to produce children with health problems, such as autism, schizophrenia, and Down syndrome.

As women and men age, sexual activity can continue to be a source of pleasure and satisfaction for them. A recent study of sexuality in older adults found that three-fourths of those 57–64 years old were sexually active (defined as having at least one sexual partner in the last year). Half of those 65–74 years old, and about one-fourth of those 75–85, remained sexually active.

QUESTIONS FOR CRITICAL THINKING AND REFLECTION

Think about your own experience as you matured sexually during puberty and adolescence. In what ways did these changes affect your life? How did they contribute to the person you are today? What do you wish you had known then that you know now?

Sexual Functioning

In this section, we discuss sexual physiology—how the sex organs function during sexual activity—and problems that can occur with sexual functioning. Sexual activity is based on stimulus and response. Erotic stimulation leads to sexual arousal (excitement), which may culminate in the intensely pleasurable experience of orgasm. But sexual activity should not be thought of only in terms of the sex organs. Responses to sexual stimulation involve not just the genitals, but also the entire body—and the mind as well.

Sexual Stimulation

Sexual excitement can come from many sources, both physical and psychological. Although physical stimuli have an obvious and direct effect, some people believe psychological stimuli—thoughts, fantasies, desires, perceptions—are even more powerfully erotic. Regardless of the source of erotic stimuli, all stimulation has a physical basis, which is given meaning by the brain.

Physical Stimulation

Physical stimulation comes through the senses: We are aroused by things we see, hear, taste, smell, and feel. Most often, sexual stimuli come from other people, but they may also come from books, photographs, paintings, songs, films, or other sources.

The most obvious and effective physical stimulation is touching. Even though culturally defined practices vary and individual people have different preferences, most sexual encounters eventually involve some form of touching with hands, lips, and body surfaces. Kissing, caressing, fondling, and hugging are as much a part of sexual encounters as they are of expressing affection.

The most intense form of stimulation by touching involves the genitals. The clitoris and the glans of the penis are particularly sensitive to such stimulation. Other highly responsive areas include the vaginal opening, the nipples, the breasts, the insides of the thighs, the buttocks, the anal region, the scrotum, the lips, and the earlobes. Such sexually sensitive areas, or **erogenous zones**, are especially susceptible to sexual arousal for most people, most of the time. Often, though, what determines the response is not *what* is touched but how, for how long, and by whom. Under the right circumstances, touching any part of the body can cause sexual arousal.

erogenous zone
Any region of the body highly responsive to sexual stimulation.

Psychological Stimulation

Sexual arousal also has an important psychological component, regardless of the nature of the physical stimulation. Fantasies, ideas, memories of past experiences, and mood can all generate sexual excitement. Erotic thoughts may be linked to an imagined person or situation or to a sexual experience from the past. Fantasies may involve activities a person doesn't actually want to experience in reality, usually because they are dangerous, frightening, or forbidden.

Arousal is also powerfully influenced by emotions. How you feel about a person and how the person feels about you matter tremendously in how sexually responsive you are likely to be. Even the most direct forms of physical stimulation carry emotional overtones. Kissing, caressing, and fondling express affection and caring. The emotional charge they give to a sexual interaction is at least as significant to sexual arousal as the purely physical stimulation achieved by touching.

The Sexual Response Cycle

Men and women respond physiologically with a predictable set of reactions, regardless of the nature of the stimulation.

Two physiological mechanisms explain most genital and bodily reactions during sexual arousal and orgasm. These mechanisms are vasocongestion and muscular tension. **Vasocongestion** is the engorgement of tissues that results when more blood flows into an organ than is flowing out. Thus, the penis becomes erect on the same principle that makes a garden hose become stiff when the water is turned on. Increased muscular tension culminates in rhythmical muscular contractions during orgasm.

vasocongestion
The accumulation of blood in tissues and organs.

In the late 1960s, Masters and Johnson first identified the four phases that characterize the sexual response cycle, and these four phases are still known to be accurate today:

1. In the *excitement phase*, the penis becomes erect as its tissues become engorged with blood. The testes expand and are pulled upward within the scrotum. In women, the clitoris, labia, and vaginal walls are similarly engorged with blood. Tension increases in the vaginal muscles, and the vaginal walls become moist with lubricating fluid.
2. The *plateau phase* is an extension of the excitement phase. Reactions become more marked. In men, the penis becomes harder, and the testes become larger. In women, the lower part of the vagina swells, as its upper end expands and vaginal lubrication increases.
3. In the *orgasmic phase*, or **orgasm**, rhythmic contractions occur along the man's penis, urethra, prostate gland, seminal vesicles, and muscles in the pelvic and anal regions. These involuntary muscular contractions lead to the ejaculation of **semen**, which consists of sperm cells from the testes and secretions from the prostate gland and seminal vesicles. In women, contractions occur in the lower part of the vagina and in the uterus, as well as in the pelvic region and the anus.
4. In the *resolution phase*, all the changes initiated during the excitement phase are reversed. Excess blood drains from tissues, the muscles in the region relax, and the genital structures return to their unstimulated state.

orgasm
The discharge of accumulated sexual tension with characteristic genital and bodily manifestations and a subjective sensation of intense pleasure.

semen
Seminal fluid, consisting of sperm cells and secretions from the prostate gland and seminal vesicles.

More general physical reactions accompany the genital changes in both men and women. Beginning with the excitement phase, nipples become erect, the woman's breasts begin to swell, and in both sexes the skin of the chest becomes flushed; these changes are more marked in women. The heart rate doubles by the plateau phase, and respiration becomes faster. During orgasm, breathing becomes irregular and the person may moan or cry out. A feeling of warmth leads to increased sweating during the resolution phase. Deep relaxation and a sense of well-being pervade the body and the mind.

Male and female reactions during the sexual response cycle differ somewhat. Generally, the male pattern is more uniform, whereas the female pattern is more varied. For instance, the female excitement phase may lead directly to orgasm, or orgasmic and plateau phases may be fused.

Male orgasm is marked by the ejaculation of semen. After ejaculation, men enter a *refractory period*, during which they cannot be restimulated to orgasm. Women do not have a refractory period, and immediate restimulation to orgasm is possible for some women.

Sexual Problems

Both physical and psychological factors can interfere with sexual functioning. Disturbances in sexual desire, performance, or satisfaction are referred to as **sexual dysfunctions**.

> **sexual dysfunction**
> A disturbance in sexual desire, performance, or satisfaction.

Common Sexual Health Problems

Some problems with sexual functioning are due to treatable or preventable infections or other sexual health problems. Conditions that affect women include the following:

- *Vaginitis*, inflammation of the vagina, is caused by a variety of organisms: *Candida* (yeast infection), *Trichomonas* (trichomoniasis), and the overgrowth of a variety of bacteria (bacterial vaginosis). Symptoms include vaginal discharge, vaginal irritation, and pain during intercourse. (See Chapters 9 and 13 for more information.)
- *Endometriosis* is the growth of endometrial tissue (tissue normally found lining the uterus) outside the uterus. It occurs most often in women of childbearing age, and pain in the lower abdomen and pelvis is the most common symptom. Pain with premenstrual intercourse may occur. Endometriosis can cause serious problems if left untreated because the endometrial tissue can scar and partially or completely block the oviducts, causing infertility (difficulty conceiving) or sterility (the inability to conceive). Endometriosis is treated with hormone therapy or surgery.
- *Pelvic inflammatory disease (PID)* is an infection of the uterus, oviducts, or ovaries caused when microorganisms spread to these areas from the vagina. Approximately 50–75 percent of PID cases are caused by sexually transmitted organisms associated with diseases, such as gonorrhea and chlamydia. PID can cause scarring of the oviducts, resulting in infertility or sterility. Symptoms include pain in the abdomen and pelvis, fever, and possibly pain during intercourse. Sexually transmitted infections are discussed in detail in Chapter 13.

Sexual health problems that affect men include the following:

- *Prostatitis* is inflammation or infection of the prostate gland. Prostatitis can be acute (sudden) or chronic (gradual and long-lasting). The symptoms of *acute bacterial prostatitis* usually appear suddenly and may include fever, chills, flulike symptoms, pain in the lower back or groin, problems with urination, and painful ejaculation. Acute prostatitis is treated with antibiotics. It is potentially serious, so any man with these symptoms needs to seek immediate medical attention.
- *Chronic prostatitis* is more common in men over age 40. It can be caused by infection or inflammation of the prostate and is sometimes difficult to diagnose and treat.
- *Testicular cancer* occurs most commonly in men in their twenties and thirties. A rare cancer, it has a very high cure rate if detected early. Every man should perform testicular self-exams regularly (see Chapter 8).

Sexual Dysfunctions

The term *sexual dysfunction* encompasses disturbances in sexual desire, performance, or satisfaction. A wide variety of physical conditions and drugs may interfere with sexual functioning; psychological causes and problems in intimate relationships can be important factors in many cases.

COMMON SEXUAL DYSFUNCTIONS   Common sexual dysfunctions in men include **erectile dysfunction** (previously called *impotence*), the inability to have or maintain an erection sufficient for sexual intercourse; **premature ejaculation**, ejaculation before or just on penetration of the vagina or anus; and **retarded ejaculation**, the inability to ejaculate once an erection is achieved. Many men experience occasional difficulty achieving an erection or ejaculating because of excessive alcohol consumption, fatigue, or stress.

> **erectile dysfunction**
> The inability to have or maintain an erection.
>
> **premature ejaculation**
> Involuntary orgasm before or shortly after the penis enters the vagina or anus; ejaculation that takes place sooner than desired.
>
> **retarded ejaculation**
> The inability to ejaculate when desired during intercourse.

Female sexual problems generally involve either a lack of desire to have sex, the failure to become physically aroused even when sex is desired, the failure to have an orgasm (**orgasmic dysfunction**), or pain during sexual contact. All of these problems can have physical and psychological components. Many medical problems can influence a woman's desire and ability to respond sexually. Hormonal factors, especially menopause, also have a major influence. Psychological and social issues, such as relationship difficulties, family stresses, depression, and past sexual trauma, are all frequent causes of sexual dysfunction.

> **orgasmic dysfunction**
> The inability to experience orgasm.

Orgasmic dysfunction has been the subject of a great deal of discussion over the years, as people debated the nature of the female orgasm and what constitutes dysfunction in women. Many women experience orgasm but not during intercourse, or they experience orgasm during intercourse only if the clitoris is directly stimulated at the same time. In general, the inability to experience orgasm under certain circumstances is a problem only if the woman considers it so.

TREATING SEXUAL DYSFUNCTION   Most forms of sexual dysfunction are treatable. The first step is to have a physical examination to find a possible medical cause. Heart disease and diabetes, for example, may cause erectile dysfunction; in fact, erectile dysfunction is often the first sign of a serious medical condition. This is one reason men who buy drugs online to treat their erectile dysfunction without first getting a good medical evaluation may be missing out on the opportunity to diagnose and treat a potentially life-threatening disease. Up to 80 percent of all erectile problems are thought to be due to physical factors, particularly vascular problems involving restriction of blood flow. Smoking affects blood flow in the penis and is an independent risk factor for erectile dysfunction.

Alcohol and many prescription and non-prescription drugs can inhibit sexual response. In particular, antidepressant drugs (especially the widely used SSRIs, such as Prozac) are believed to cause sexual dysfunction in up to half the people who take them. Switching to a different antidepressant often helps, and sometimes other drugs, such as Viagra, are used to counteract the side effects of antidepressants.

Other common medications that can inhibit sexual response include certain drugs that treat high blood pressure. Patients are sometimes reluctant to tell their physician that they are having sexual problems and may even stop taking their blood pressure medication for this reason. Letting the doctor know about sexual and other side effects is crucial because most of the time the problem can be solved by switching to a different medication. Newer antihypertensive drugs are highly effective and do not usually have sexual side effects.

Many treatments are available, particularly for erectile dysfunction. In 1999, Viagra (sildenafil citrate), the first-ever prescription pill for erectile dysfunction, was approved for use by Health Canada. Since then, two other oral medications with actions similar to Viagra, Cialis (tadalafil) and Levitra (vardenafil), have been approved. All three work by enhancing the effects of nitric oxide, a chemical that relaxes smooth muscles in the penis. This increases the amount of blood flow and allows a natural erection to occur in response to sexual stimulation. The medications are generally safe for healthy men, but they should not be used by men who have a high risk of heart attack or stroke. They are effective in about 70 percent of users, but they have potential side effects, including headaches, indigestion, facial flushing, back pain, visual and hearing disturbances, and changes in blood pressure. Viagra, Cialis, and Levitra should never be taken by anyone who takes nitrate medication (usually prescribed for heart problems). Also, the recreational drugs amyl nitrate or nitrite (sometimes called "poppers") should never be combined with drugs for erectile dysfunction. The combination of nitrates and Viagra-like drugs can cause a sudden potentially lethal drop in blood pressure.

Viagra use by men between the ages of 18 and 45 has risen dramatically—possibly due to use of the drug for recreational purposes (see Figure 11.5). The drug may cut the refractory period in men who do not have erectile dysfunction; younger men may also be using it to cope with performance anxiety or the effects of other drugs, such as antidepressants.

FIGURE 11.5

Total Erectile Dysfunction Dispensed Units in Canada by Province

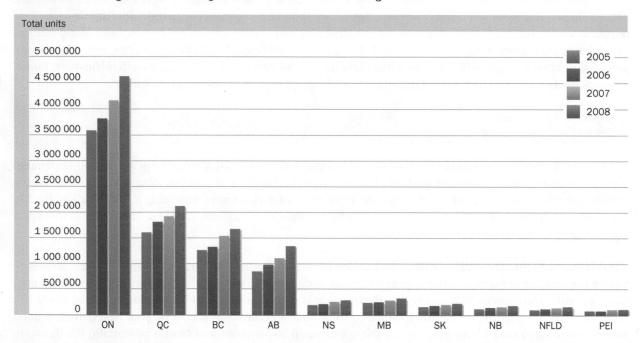

Source: *Therapeutic Trends, Erectile Dysfunction and Its Treatments.* Figure 3,http://www.stacommunications.com/journals/cpm/2009/09-September%2009/043 Therapeutic%20Trends.pdf.

QUICK STATS

About 3 million Canadian men over age 40 are affected by erectile dysfunction.
—*Elliot, S.L., 2011*

Although Viagra is not approved for use by women, a growing number of women are trying the drug. Research findings are mixed as to whether Viagra can increase sex drive and satisfaction levels in women. Recent studies have shown, however, that the drug can help women with sexual dysfunction caused by the use of antidepressant drugs.

Other treatments for erectile dysfunction in men are available. Medications, with the active ingredient alprostadil, can be administered with a fine needle into the penis or placed into the tip of the penis as a tiny suppository about the size of a grain of rice; it works by relaxing the smooth muscles lining the blood vessels in the penis. A topical cream can also be applied to the penis to improve erectile function. For a small number of men with testosterone deficiency, hormone replacement therapy is an option. There are also vacuum devices that pull blood into the penis, and in cases where other treatments are unsuccessful, penile implants can be used. Exercise may also help improve erectile function, especially exercises that target the muscles of the pelvic floor.

Even when sexual dysfunction has a physical cause, emotional and social factors frequently compound the problem. Many people with no obvious physical disorder have sexual problems because of psychological and social issues. Too often, sexual difficulties are treated with drugs when non-drug strategies may be more appropriate. Psychosocial causes of dysfunction include troubled relationships, a lack of sexual skills, irrational attitudes and beliefs, anxiety, and psychosexual trauma, such as sexual abuse or rape. Many of these problems can be addressed by sex therapy. A therapist may recommend books or films to help counter sexual myths and teach sexual skills. A therapist can also promote open discussion between partners and suggest specific techniques. .

Women who seek treatment for orgasmic dysfunction often have not learned what types of stimulation will excite them and bring them to orgasm. Most sex therapists treat this problem with **masturbation** (genital self-stimulation). Women are taught about their own anatomy and sexual responses and then are encouraged to experiment with masturbation until they experience orgasm. Once they can masturbate to orgasm, they can transfer this learning to sexual intercourse with a partner.

> **masturbation**
> Self-stimulation for the purpose of sexual arousal and orgasm.

Substances being tested for the treatment of female sexual dysfunction include prostaglandin creams and testosterone patches. A prostaglandin cream that improves blood flow to the clitoris is currently being developed under the name Femprox, and may soon be available to treat female sexual arousal disorder. Another option is a device that creates suction over the clitoris to increase blood flow and sensitivity.

QUESTIONS FOR CRITICAL THINKING AND REFLECTION

If you are sexually active, would you consider using a product such as Viagra even if you didn't need it? Are you fully aware of the potential side effects of such products? In your opinion, would the potential benefits outweigh the risks? How do you think your views might change (if at all) as you get older?

Sexual Behaviour

Many behaviours stem from sexual impulses, and sexual expression takes a variety of forms. Probably the most basic aspect of sexuality is reproduction. But sexual excitement and satisfaction are aspects of sexual behaviour separate from reproduction. The intensely pleasurable sensations of arousal and orgasm are probably the strongest motivators for human sexual behaviour. People are infinitely varied in the ways they seek to experience erotic pleasure.

The Development of Sexual Behaviour

Sexual behaviour is a product of many factors, including genetics, physiology, psychology, and social and cultural influences. Our behaviour is shaped by the interplay of our biological predispositions and our life experiences.

Gender Roles and Gender Identity

As mentioned in Chapters 3 and 10, your *gender role* is everything you do in your daily life that expresses your maleness or femaleness to others, including dress, speech patterns, and mannerisms. Your **gender identity** is your personal, inner sense of being male or female.

gender identity
A person's personal, internal sense of maleness or femaleness.

Biological sex, gender role, and gender identity are usually in agreement, but some people experience conflict among them. For example, a male who feels trapped in the body of a male and who wants to be a female appears to others as a male, but his gender identity is that of a female. The umbrella term *transgender* is often used to describe any individual whose appearance, personal characteristics, or behaviour differs from the social and cultural norms for males and females. Transgender individuals include the following:

- *Transsexual* men and women, who feel their biological sex does not match their gender identity. Transsexuals may seek sex reassignment, which involves surgery to change the appearance of the genitals and hormonal treatments to induce secondary sex characteristics, such as breasts or facial hair.
- *Transvestites*, who enjoy wearing clothing identified with the other gender. Cross-dressing covers a broad range of behaviours, from wearing one article of clothing of the other sex in a private location to wearing an entire outfit in public.
- *Intersexed individuals*, who were born with ambiguous genitals—neither fully female nor fully male—because of genetic or hormonal abnormalities. Intersexed individuals may or may not have undergone surgery as infants to assign them to a particular sex.
- Men or women, regardless of sexual orientation, whose appearance, characteristics, or behaviour is perceived as gender atypical in their society or culture.

BIOLOGICAL AND CULTURAL INFLUENCES Some gender characteristics are determined biologically, such as the genitals a person is born with and the secondary sex characteristics that develop at puberty. Others are defined by society and learned in the course of growing up. From birth, children are encouraged to behave in ways their culture deems appropriate for one sex or the other. In Canadian society, parents usually give children gender-specific names, clothes, and toys, and children may model their own behaviour after their same-sex parent. Family and friends create an environment that teaches the child how to act appropriately as a girl or a boy. Teachers, television, books, and even strangers model these gender roles.

Gender roles vary from one society to another and from one time to another. In Canada today, for example, many women shave their legs and wear makeup; in some Muslim countries, women wear robes and veils that conceal their face and body. Each set of behaviours expresses some learned aspect of the female gender role in that society, and each set may be inappropriate in the other society. Standards of sexual attractiveness also vary from one culture to another.

An extreme example of how cultural traditions can affect gender roles and sexual activity is female genital mutilation, or "female circumcision." Each year in 28 African countries, parts of Asia and the Middle East, and immigrant communities elsewhere, 3 million female children undergo this procedure. In some cases, only the hood of the clitoris is removed. In others, the entire clitoris, the labia minora, and parts of the labia majora are removed. The sides of the labia majora may be sewn together, leaving only a small opening for the passage of urine and menstrual blood. The effects of these painful procedures

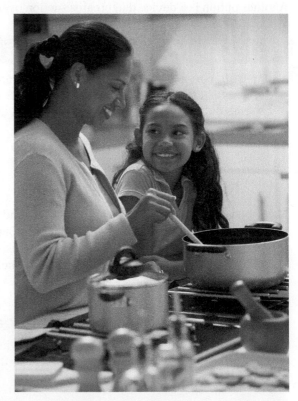

Our sense of gender identity and many of our gender-role behaviours are overwhelmingly influenced by cultural factors. This young girl is learning gender-specific behaviours by imitating her mother.

can include bleeding, infection, the inability to enjoy sex, and infertility. Women who have endured genital mutilation commonly have difficulty during labour and childbirth. Children of such women are at far greater risk of dying during or after childbirth.

The practice probably developed as a way of controlling women's sexuality and ensuring that a woman would be a virgin when she married. After marriage, her husband reopens the labia to allow intercourse and childbirth.

Many countries now have laws against female genital mutilation. The WHO and other groups are trying to educate people about the negative medical consequences of this practice.

QUICK STATS

More than 125 million girls and women have endured ritualized female genital mutilation (FGM) in the 29 countries in Africa and the Middle East where FGM is most concentrated.

—Unicef Statistics, 2014

GENDER-ROLE FLEXIBILITY Historically, gender roles have tended to emphasize the differences between males and females, but new gender roles are emerging in our society that reflect more of a mix of male and female characteristics and behaviours. This tendency toward **androgyny** greatly broadens the range of experiences available to both males and females. Androgynous adults are less stereotyped in their thinking; in how they look, dress, and act; in how they divide work in the home; in how they think about jobs and careers; and in how they express themselves sexually. Women in our society today are able, and even expected, to be much more assertive, competitive, ambitious, and powerful than they were allowed to be in the past; likewise, men can be more sensitive, articulate, nurturing, and emotionally expressive.

androgyny
The state of being neither overtly male nor female.

Gender, Sexuality, and the Mass Media

Many of our ideas about sexuality and gender roles are shaped by the mass media. Media images of sexuality are often more influential than the family in shaping the sexual attitudes and behaviours of adolescents and university students. Yet these images are usually unrealistic and help perpetuate stereotypes of women and men in our society. The mass media rarely portray people negotiating safer sex or communicating seriously about other sexual issues.

Childhood Sexual Behaviour

The capacity to respond sexually is present at birth. Ultrasound studies suggest that boys experience erections in the uterus. After birth, both sexes have the capacity for orgasm, though many babies may not experience it. As people grow, many discover this capacity through self-exploration. Sexual behaviours gradually emerge in childhood; self-exploration and touching the genitals are common forms of play, observed among infants as young as six months. They gradually lead to more deliberate forms of masturbation, with or without orgasm.

Children often engage in sexual play with playmates by exploring each other's genitals. These activities are often part of games like "playing house" or "playing doctor." By age 12, 40 percent of boys have engaged in sex play; the peak exploration age for girls is age 9, by which time 14 percent have had such experiences.

Adolescent Sexuality

A person who has experienced puberty is biologically an adult. But in psychological and social terms, people take five to ten more years to attain full adult status. This discrepancy between biological and social maturity creates considerable confusion over what constitutes appropriate sexual behaviour during adolescence.

Sexual fantasies and dreams become more common and explicit in adolescence than at earlier ages, often as an accompaniment to masturbation. Research has shown that about 80 percent of teenage boys and 55 percent of teenage girls masturbate more or less regularly. Once puberty is reached, orgasm in boys is accompanied by ejaculation. Teenage boys also experience **nocturnal emissions** ("wet dreams"). Some girls also have orgasmic dreams.

> **nocturnal emissions**
> Orgasm and ejaculation (wet dream) during sleep.

Sexual interaction during adolescence usually takes place between peers in the context of dating. Sexual intimacy is usually expressed in such relationships through petting and necking, which may involve kissing, caressing, and stimulating the breasts and genitals. These activities lead to arousal but may not culminate in orgasm.

Many Canadian teenagers also engage in premarital sexual relations. Recent surveys indicate that the average age of first sexual intercourse in Canada is about 16.5 years old. Twenty-eight percent of 15–19-year-olds in Canada have had sex at least once. Rates for premarital sex vary considerably from one group to another, however, based on ethnic, educational, socioeconomic, religious, geographic, and other factors. First-time intercourse is affected by these same factors, plus psychological readiness, fear of consequences, being in love, going steady, peer pressure, and the need to act like an adult, gain popularity, or rebel. A mother's relationship with her daughter influences the timing of first intercourse. Girls who perceive that their mother disapproves of their having sex are more likely to delay first intercourse.

Adolescent sexual behaviours are not confined to heterosexual relationships. Beginning in childhood, sex play involves members of one's own sex as well as of the other sex. Same-sex attractions, with or without sexual encounters, are common in adolescence. For many these are youthful experiments and don't mean that participants will ultimately be gay or lesbian. For some, they may be a factor in adult sexual orientation. Most adult gay men and women trace their orientation to childhood.

Adult Sexuality

Early adulthood is a time when people make important life choices—a time of increasing responsibility in terms of interpersonal relationships and family life (see the Mind Body Spirit box). In recent years, there has

 Mind *Body* SPIRIT

Sexual Decision Making

Choosing to have sex can change a relationship and a person's life. In making decisions about sexual activity, you owe it to yourself and your partner to think and talk honestly about your choices. Consider the following issues:

- *Your background, beliefs, and goals:* What are your religious, moral, or personal values regarding relationships and sex? What are your priorities at this time, and how will a sexual relationship fit into your goals and plans for the future? Are you physically, emotionally, and financially ready to accept the potential consequences of the choices you make?
- *Your relationship with your partner:* How do you feel about your partner and your relationship? Do you respect and trust each other? Do you feel comfortable talking about sexual issues, and have you discussed contraception, pregnancy, and safer sex? How do you think having sex will affect your relationship and how you feel about yourself and your partner? What does having sex mean to each of you?
- *Your reasons for having sex:* What reasons do you have for moving into a sexual relationship? Are you being honest with yourself and your partner about this?

  Personal decisions about sex should always be respected. You have the right to make your own choices and to do only what you feel comfortable with. When you make choices about sex based on self-respect, along with physical, emotional, and spiritual considerations, you will be more likely to feel good about your decisions—now and in the future.

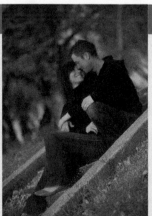

been a trend toward marriage at a later age than in past decades. And before marriage, more young adults are driven by a need to become sexually knowledgeable (see the In Focus box). Today, more people in their twenties believe that becoming sexually experienced rather than preserving virginity is an important prelude to selecting a mate.

Individual motivations for engaging in sexual activities change with age. Younger men state that they engage in sex for physical reasons, whereas women of the same age state that they engage in sex for emotional reasons. As men and women get older, their motives change; men more often engage in sex for emotional reasons, and women more often for physical reasons. In the oldest age groups, women's and men's motives for sex are actually the reverse of those of the earliest age groups. In addition to age, other factors, such as ethnicity, educational attainment, and living arrangements, also influence adult choices about sexuality. Take the quiz in the Assess Yourself box to explore your own beliefs and opinions about sex.

Sexuality in Illness and Disability

Any disease or disability that affects mobility, well-being, self-esteem, or body image has the potential to affect sexual expression. People with chronic diseases or disabilities often have special needs regarding their sexual behaviour. They may also confront the perception that they are asexual. Sexuality is integral to all of us, regardless of our physical status.

The diagnosis of a chronic illness or the onset of a disability usually requires major adjustments in many areas of life, including sexuality. At first, sexual activity may take a low priority because of fear and the loss

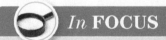

Sexual Activity Among Post-Secondary Students

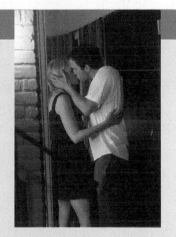

The popular perception of university and college students is that they are young, attractive, and highly sexually active. But how close are these stereotypes to reality? In a recent survey of nearly 95 000 students, about one-third of the respondents said they had never had a sexual partner or were currently not sexually active. Of those students who reported having sex with a partner, the vast majority said they had only one partner. Only a small group—about 1 in 10 students—reported having had three or more sexual partners in the last year.

Students tend to grossly overestimate the sexual activity level of their peers, mirroring the popular perception of university and college students. In the survey, students guessed that their peers had more than twice as many sex partners as they actually did.

Slightly more than half of all students said they had not had sexual intercourse in the past 30 days. When asked what types of intercourse they engaged in, most sexually active students reported participating in either vaginal or oral intercourse. Anal intercourse was relatively rare, with only about 1 in 20 students reporting having had anal sex one or more times in the last month. Once again, students wildly overestimated the frequency of all types of intercourse among their fellow students; more than half of the students who were polled guessed that the typical student at their institution was participating in anal sex, while in reality only a small minority of students reported having had anal sex.

Judging from the results of this large survey, condom use among students is far from consistent. Only about 18 percent of students reported using a condom every time they had vaginal intercourse in the last month. Birth control pills were the most popular contraceptive, with condoms a close second. The vast majority of students do not use condoms when they engage in oral sex. When asked about condom use during anal sex—which is among the riskiest of all sexual behaviours in terms of acquiring a sexually transmitted infection—the majority of students who reported this activity did not use a condom the last time they had anal sex.

Among the men polled in this study, 93 percent described themselves as heterosexual, as did 95 percent of women. About 4 percent of men identified themselves as gay and 1 percent of women identified themselves as lesbian. Another 2 percent of university men and 3 percent of women classified themselves as bisexual. Less than 1 percent of students described themselves as transgender.

Assess YOURSELF

Your Sexual Attitudes

For each statement, circle the response that most closely reflects your position:

	Agree	Not sure	Disagree
1. Sex education encourages young people to make good decisions about sex.	3	2	1
2. Same-sex attraction is a healthy, normal expression of sexuality.	3	2	1
3. Members of the other sex will think more highly of you if you remain mysterious.	3	2	1
4. It's better to wait until marriage to have sex.	3	2	1
5. Abortion should be a personal, private choice for a woman.	3	2	1
6. It's natural for men to have more sexual freedom than women.	3	2	1
7. Condoms should be made available to teenagers.	3	2	1
8. Access to pornography should not be restricted for adults.	3	2	1
9. A woman who is raped usually does something to provoke it.	3	2	1
10. Contraception is the woman's responsibility.	3	2	1
11. Feminism has had a positive influence on society.	3	2	1
12. Masturbation is a healthy expression of sexuality.	3	2	1
13. I have many friends of the other sex.	3	2	1
14. Prostitution should be legalized.	3	2	1
15. Women use sex for love; men use love for sex.	3	2	1
16. Our society is too sexually uptight.	3	2	1
17. The man should be the undisputed head of the household.	3	2	1
18. Having sex just for pleasure is OK.	3	2	1

Scoring
1–18:   Traditional attitude about sexuality
19–36:   Ambivalent attitude about sexuality
37–54:   Open, progressive attitude about sexuality

of self-esteem. Individuals and couples can learn to become creative about sexual expression and develop new approaches based on the limitations of the disability. Developing a positive body image is often a particularly important, and difficult, adjustment for people with physical illness or limitations.

Sexual Orientation

Sexual orientation is a consistent pattern of emotional and sexual attraction based on biological sex. It exists along a continuum that ranges from being exclusively heterosexual (attracted to people of the other sex), to being bisexual (attracted to people of both sexes), to being exclusively gay or lesbian (attracted to people of your own sex). The term *straight* is often used to refer to heterosexuals, and the preferred terms in the gay community are *gay men* (for men), *gay people* (for both men and women), and *lesbians* (for women). The terms *homosexual* and *homosexuality* are outdated and offensive to many gay people.

Sexual orientation involves feelings and self-concept, and individuals may or may not express their sexual orientation in their behaviour. In national surveys, about 2–6 percent of men identify themselves as gay and about 1.5 percent of women identify themselves as lesbians. It is difficult to gauge the accuracy of these estimates because people may not tell the truth in surveys that probe very sensitive and private aspects of their lives.

Heterosexuality

The great majority of people are heterosexual. The heterosexual lifestyle usually includes all the behaviour and relationship patterns described in Chapter 10: dating, engagement or living together, and marriage.

Same-Sex Attraction

Same-sex attraction exists in almost all cultures. The major difference between heterosexuals and gay people is in their sex partners. Gay people are as varied and different from one another as are heterosexuals. Just like heterosexuals, lesbians and gay men may be in long-term, committed relationships or they may date different people.

Bisexuality

Some bisexual individuals are involved with partners of both sexes at the same time, whereas others may alternate between same-sex partners and partners of the other sex ("serial bisexuality"). The largest group of bisexuals consists of married men who have secret sexual involvements with men but who rarely have female sexual contacts outside marriage.

The Origins of Sexual Orientation

Many theories try to account for the development of sexual orientation. At this time, most experts agree that sexual orientation results from multiple genetic, biological, cultural, social, and psychological factors.

Scientists are now looking for genetic markers associated with sexual orientation in males. This study, funded by the National Institutes of Health, will examine the DNA of 1000 pairs of gay brothers and their families. Twin studies are another way of looking at the genetic contribution to sexual identity. Identical twins share the same DNA, so if sexual orientation were entirely genetically determined, we would expect that if one identical twin was gay or lesbian, the other would be as well. But studies of many identical twins (both gay men and lesbians) show that the odds are between 30 percent and 50 percent that both twins will have the same sexual orientation. These studies provide evidence that our genes make an important but limited contribution to our sexual orientation.

Exposure to hormones before birth also has a major impact on sexual orientation. Experiments with mice show that exposure to sex hormones early in development determines whether they will ultimately be sexually attracted to male or female mice. The situation is much more complicated in humans, but most researchers believe that the hormonal environment in the womb probably has an important influence on sexual orientation.

Researchers have also compared the brain structure of gay and heterosexual men. Although some differences have been found, they are not consistent across all studies. Also, even if brain structure differences exist, it is unclear whether they are the cause or an effect of differences in sexual orientation.

Several studies have shown that the more older brothers a boy has, the more likely he will grow up to be gay. The odds of being gay go up 33 percent with each older brother. There are numerous theories to explain this phenomenon. One intriguing, but unproven, theory suggests that mothers with multiple biological sons may develop antibodies against proteins produced by male fetuses. The immune response by the mother may affect the fetal development of later sons, resulting in an increased chance of being gay.

Many psychological theories have also been proposed. Researchers have looked at how much contact children have with members of the two sexes, at the types of relationships children have with their parents, and at family dynamics. Early negative experiences with heterosexuality or positive experiences with same-sex attraction have also been proposed as possible influences. The significant growth of single-parent families over the past 40 years has not been accompanied by large shifts in sexual orientation among Canadians, so it is unlikely that family dynamics or early learning experiences are strong factors in determining sexual orientation. In addition, parents' sexual orientation seems to have little impact on children's sexual orientation. Studies of children raised by gay or lesbian parents show that these children's ultimate sexual orientation is similar to that of children raised by heterosexual parents.

So far, most studies on the origin of sexual orientation have focused on males. The factors that determine sexual orientation in women may be even more complex. Perhaps the most important message is that sexual orientation is most likely the result of the complex interaction of biological, psychological, and social factors, possibly different ones in each individual.

Varieties of Human Sexual Behaviour

Some sexual behaviours are aimed at self-stimulation only, whereas other practices involve interaction with a partner. Some people choose not to express their sexuality at all.

Celibacy

Continuous abstention from sexual activities, termed **celibacy**, can be a conscious and deliberate choice, or it can be necessitated by circumstances. Health considerations and religious and moral beliefs may lead some people to celibacy, particularly until marriage or until an acceptable partner appears.

> **celibacy**
> Continuous abstention from sexual activity.

Many people use the related term *abstinence* to refer to avoidance of just one sexual activity—intercourse. Abstinence can also be chosen as a method to prevent pregnancy and sexually transmitted infections.

Autoeroticism and Masturbation

The most common form of **autoeroticism** is **erotic fantasy**, creating imaginary experiences that range from fleeting thoughts to elaborate scenarios.

> **autoeroticism**
> Behaviour aimed at sexual self-stimulation.
>
> **erotic fantasy**
> Sexually arousing thoughts and daydreams.

Masturbation involves manually stimulating the genitals, rubbing them against objects, or using stimulating devices, such as vibrators. Although commonly associated with adolescence, masturbation is practised by many throughout adult life. It may be used as a substitute for sexual intercourse or as part of sexual activity with a partner. Masturbation gives a person control over the pace, time, and method of sexual release and pleasure.

Touching and Foreplay

Touching is integral to sexual experiences, whether in the form of massage, kissing, fondling, or holding. Our entire body surface is a sensory organ, and touching almost anywhere can enhance intimacy and sexual arousal. Touching can convey a variety of messages, including affection, comfort, and a desire for further sexual contact.

During arousal, many men and women manually and orally stimulate each other by touching, stroking, and caressing their partner's genitals. Men and women vary greatly in their preferences for the type, pacing, and vigour of such **foreplay**. Working out the details to

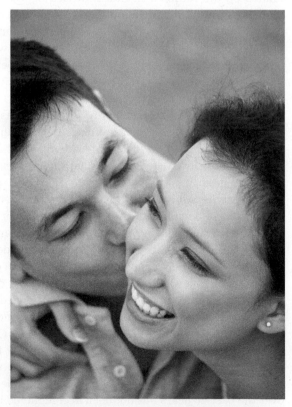

This couple's physical experiences together will be powerfully affected by their emotions, ideas, and values and by the quality of their relationship.

accommodate each other's pleasure is a key to enjoying these activities. Direct communication about preferences can enhance sexual pleasure and protect both partners from physical and psychological discomfort.

> **foreplay**
> Kissing, touching, and any form of oral or genital contact that stimulates people toward intercourse.

Oral-Genital Stimulation

Cunnilingus (the stimulation of the female genitals with the lips and tongue) and **fellatio** (the stimulation of the penis with the mouth) are common practices. Oral sex may be practised either as part of foreplay or as a sex act culminating in orgasm. Although prevalence varies in different populations, 90 percent of men, 88 percent of women, and more than 50 percent of teens report that they have engaged in oral sex. A recent study showed that more teens ages 15–19 had engaged in oral sex than in vaginal intercourse. The most common reasons given for postponing vaginal sex were avoidance of pregnancy and the desire to remain technically a virgin.

> **cunnilingus**
> Oral stimulation of the female genitals.
>
> **fellatio**
> Oral stimulation of the penis.

Like all acts of sexual expression between two people, oral sex requires the cooperation and consent of both partners. If they disagree about its acceptability, they need to discuss their feelings and try to reach a mutually pleasing solution.

Anal Intercourse

About 10 percent of heterosexuals and 50 percent of gay males regularly practise anal stimulation and penetration by the penis or a finger. The receiver does not usually reach orgasm from anal intercourse, though men usually experience orgasm while penetrating.

Because the anus is composed of delicate tissues that tear easily under such pressure, anal intercourse is one of the riskiest of sexual behaviours associated with the transmission of HIV and all other sexually-transmitted infections. Anal intercourse is also associated with increased risk of anal cancer, hemorrhoids, anal fissures, prolapsed rectum, and fecal incontinence. The use of condoms is highly recommended for anyone engaging in anal sex. Special care and precaution should be exercised if anal sex is practised—cleanliness, lubrication, and gentle entry at the very least. Anything that is inserted into the anus should not subsequently be put into the vagina unless it has been thoroughly washed. Bacteria normally present in the anus can cause vaginal infections.

Sexual Intercourse

For most adults, most of the time, **sexual intercourse** (*coitus*) is the ultimate sexual experience. Men and women engage in vaginal intercourse to fulfill both sexual and psychological needs. In a 2006 study, 87 of men ages 15–44 and 98 percent of women in the same age group reported having had vaginal intercourse. The most common heterosexual practice is the man inserting his erect penis into the woman's dilated and lubricated vagina after sufficient arousal.

> **sexual intercourse**
> Sexual relations involving genital union; also called *coitus* and also known as *making love*.

Much has been written on how to enhance pleasure through various coital techniques, positions, and practices. For a woman, the key factor in physical readiness for coitus is adequate vaginal lubrication, and in psychological readiness, being aroused and receptive. For a man, the setting and the partner must arouse him to attain and maintain an erection. Psychological factors and the quality of the relationship are more important to overall sexual satisfaction than sophisticated or exotic sexual techniques.

Atypical and Problematic Sexual Behaviours

In Canadian culture, many kinds of sexual behaviour are accepted. However, some types of sexual expression are considered harmful; they may be illegal, classified as mental disorders, or both. Because sexual behaviour occurs on a continuum, it is sometimes difficult to differentiate a behaviour that is simply atypical from one that is harmful. When attempting to evaluate an unusual sexual behaviour, experts consider the issues of consent between partners and whether physical or psychological harm is done to the individual or to others.

The term *paraphilia* is used to describe certain sexual behaviours that are atypical and cause harm to the self or others. Clinically, the term may be used for a sexual behaviour that causes significant distress to the individual involved or to other people. Paraphilias of clinical concern are characterized by recurring, intense sexual fantasies and urges that involve non-human objects, the suffering or humiliation of oneself or a partner, or children or non-consenting individuals. Examples are peeping into strangers' homes, making obscene phone calls, and having sexual contact with children. The effects of paraphilic behaviour on others range from minor upset to serious physical and long-term psychological harm. Paraphilias are considered mental disorders according to the *Diagnostic and Statistical Manual of Mental Disorders*, the guidebook used by mental health care professionals in Canada and many other countries.

The use of force and coercion in sexual relationships is one of the most serious problems in human interactions. The most extreme manifestation of **sexual coercion**—forcing a person to submit to another's sexual desires—is rape, but sexual coercion occurs in many subtler forms, such as sexual harassment. Sexual coercion—including rape, the sexual abuse of children, and sexual harassment—is discussed in detail in Chapter 20.

sexual coercion
The use of physical or psychological force or intimidation to make a person submit to sexual demands.

Responsible Sexual Behaviour

Healthy sexuality is an important part of adult life. It can be a source of pleasurable experiences and emotions and an important part of intimate partnerships. But sexual behaviour also carries many responsibilities, as well as potential consequences, such as pregnancy, STIs, and emotional changes in the relationship. Every sexually active person should be aware of these consequences and accept responsibility for them.

Open, Honest Communication
Each partner needs to clearly indicate what sexual involvement means to him or her. Does it mean love, fun, a permanent commitment, or something else? The intentions of both partners should be clear. For strategies on talking about sexual issues with your partner, see the Take Charge box.

Agreed-On Sexual Activities
No one should pressure or coerce a partner. Sexual behaviours should be consistent with the sexual values, preferences, and comfort level of both partners. Everyone has the right to refuse sexual activity at any time.

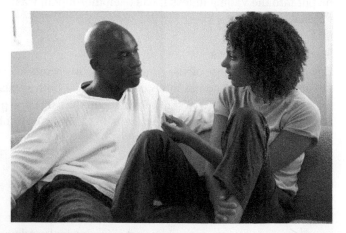
Responsible sexual behaviour includes discussing potential consequences openly and honestly.

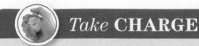

Take CHARGE

Communicating About Sexuality

To talk with your partner about sexuality, follow the general suggestions for effective communication given in Chapter 10. Getting started may be the most difficult part. Some people feel more comfortable if they begin by talking about talking—that is, initiating a discussion about why people are so uncomfortable talking about sexuality. Talking about sexual histories—how partners first learned about sex or how family and cultural background influenced sexual values and attitudes—is another way to get started. Reading about sex can also be a good beginning: Partners can read an article or a book and then discuss their reactions.

Be honest about what you feel and what you want from your partner. Cultural and personal obstacles to discussing sexual subjects can be difficult to overcome, but self-disclosure is important for successful relationships. Research indicates that when one partner openly discusses attitudes and feelings, the other partner is more likely to do the same. If your partner seems hesitant to open up, try asking open-ended or either/or questions: "Where do you like to be touched?" or "Would you like to talk about this now or wait until later?"

If something is bothering you about your sexual relationship, choose a good time to initiate a discussion with your partner. Be specific and direct, but also tactful. Focus on what you actually observe, rather than on what you think the behaviour means. "You didn't touch or hug me when your friends were around" is an observation. "You're ashamed of me around your friends" is an inference about your partner's feelings. Try focusing on a specific behaviour that concerns you rather than on the person as a whole—your partner can change behaviours but not his or her entire personality. For example, you could say "I'd like you to take a few minutes away from studying to kiss me" instead of "You're so caught up in your work, you never have time for me."

If you are going to make a statement that your partner may interpret as criticism, try mixing it with something positive: "I love spending time with you, but I feel annoyed when you . . ." Similarly, if your partner says something that upsets you, don't lash out. An aggressive response may make you feel better in the short run, but it will not help the communication process or the quality of the relationship.

If you want to say no to some sexual activity, say no unequivocally. Don't send mixed messages. If you are afraid of hurting your partner's feelings, offer an alternative if it's appropriate: "I am uncomfortable with that. How about . . .?"

If you are in love, you may think that the sexual aspects of a relationship will work out magically without discussion. However, partners who never talk about sex deny themselves the opportunity to increase their closeness and improve their relationship.

Sexual Privacy

Intimate relationships involving sexual activity are based on trust, and that trust can be violated if partners reveal private information about the relationship to others. Sexual privacy also involves respecting other people—not engaging in activities in the presence of others that would make them uncomfortable. The question of how to handle bringing a partner back to a shared residence room is something that many university students must address. Roommates should be respectful of one another and discuss the situation in advance to avoid embarrassing encounters.

Using Contraception

If pregnancy is not desired, contraception should be used during sexual intercourse. Both partners need to take responsibility for protecting against unwanted pregnancy. Partners should discuss contraception before sexual involvement begins. (Contraception is discussed in the next section of this chapter.)

Safer Sex

Both partners should be aware of and practise safer sex to guard against sexually transmitted infections (STIs). Canada faces a significant challenge to the sexual health of its people because of the high numbers of STIs. Many sexual behaviours carry the risk of STIs, including HIV infection. Partners should be honest about their health and any medical conditions and work out a plan for protection. (For more information on STIs and safer sex practices, see Chapter 13.)

Sober Sex

The use of alcohol or drugs in sexual situations increases the risk of unplanned, unprotected sexual activity. This is particularly true of young adults, many of whom engage in episodes of binge drinking during social events. The link between intoxication and unsafe sex is illustrated by a recent study that found that areas with higher drinking ages and higher beer taxes have lower rates of STIs. Alcohol and drugs impair judgment and should not be used in association with sexual activity.

Aside from the dangers of mixing alcohol and sex, alcohol has a negative impact on sexual performance in both men and women. Although alcohol may lower sexual inhibition and make people more likely to attempt a sexual encounter, too much alcohol makes it difficult for a man to achieve or keep an erection, decreases vaginal lubrication in women, and makes orgasm more difficult to achieve in both sexes. Chronic overuse of alcohol reduces testosterone in men, ultimately causing erectile dysfunction, infertility, and body changes, such as enlarged breasts. Women who overuse alcohol often experience menstrual abnormalities and decreased sexual function. Similarly, cigarette smoking has a powerful negative effect on sexual function, primarily because it decreases blood flow to the genitals.

QUESTIONS FOR CRITICAL THINKING AND REFLECTION

If you are sexually active or plan to become active soon, how open have you been about communicating with your partner? Are you aware of your partner's feelings about sex and his or her comfort level with certain activities? Do you and your partner share the same views on contraception, STI prevention, and ethical issues about sex? What's important to you about having open dialogue with your partner about sex?

Contraception

People have always had a compelling interest in managing fertility and preventing unwanted pregnancies, a practice commonly known as **birth control**. Records dating to the fourth century BCE describe the use of foods, herbs, drugs, douches, and sponges to prevent **conception**, which is the fusion of an ovum and a sperm that creates a fertilized egg. Early attempts at **contraception** (blocking conception through the use of a device, substance, or method) were based on the same principle as many modern birth control methods.

birth control
The practice of managing fertility and preventing unwanted pregnancies.

conception
The fusion of ovum and sperm, resulting in a fertilized egg, or zygote.

contraception
The prevention of conception through the use of a device, substance, or method.

Today, women and men can choose from many different types of **contraceptives** to avoid unwanted pregnancies. Modern contraceptives take a wide variety of forms and work in different ways. Modern contraceptive methods are much more predictable and effective than in the past, and people in developed countries now have many options when it comes to making decisions about their sexual and contraceptive behaviour.

contraceptives
Any agent or method that can prevent conception.

Worldwide, however, the situation is quite different. People in many countries have little access to contraceptive information and supplies. The World Health Organization estimates that 80 million women worldwide have unintended or unwanted pregnancies every year and 500 000 women die from complications of pregnancy and childbirth.

Principles of Contraception

There are a variety of effective approaches to contraception, including the following:

- **Barrier methods** work by physically blocking the sperm from reaching the egg. Diaphragms, condoms, and several other methods are based on this principle.
- **Hormonal methods**, such as oral contraceptives (birth control pills), alter the biochemistry of the woman's body, preventing ovulation (the release of the egg) and producing changes that make it more difficult for the sperm to reach the egg if ovulation does occur.
- **Natural methods** of contraception are based on the fact that egg and sperm have to be present at the same time if fertilization is to occur.
- **Surgical methods**—female (**tubal sterilization** or **tubal ligation**, or **hysterectomy**) and male (**vasectomy**) **sterilization**—more or less permanently prevent transport of the sperm or eggs to the site of conception.

barrier methods
A contraceptive that acts as a physical barrier, blocking the sperm from reaching the egg.

hormonal methods
A contraceptive that alters the biochemistry of the woman's body, preventing ovulation and making it more difficult for the sperm to reach the egg if ovulation does occur.

natural methods
An approach to contraception that does not use drugs or devices; requires avoiding intercourse during the time in a woman's menstrual cycle when an egg is likely to be present at the site of conception and the risk of pregnancy is greatest.

surgical methods
Sterilization of a male or female to permanently prevent the transport of sperm or eggs to the site of conception.

tubal sterilization
Severing or blocking the oviducts to prevent eggs from reaching the uterus; also called *tubal ligation*.

hysterectomy
Surgical removal of the uterus.

vasectomy
The surgical severing of the ducts that carry sperm to the ejaculatory duct.

sterilization
Surgically altering the reproductive system to prevent pregnancy.

All contraceptive methods have advantages and disadvantages that make them appropriate for some people but not for others or the best choice at one period of life but not at another. Factors that affect the choice of method include effectiveness, convenience, cost, reversibility, side effects and risks, and protection against STIs. (See the In Focus box to make sure you are not basing your current choices on common misinformation.)

QUESTIONS FOR CRITICAL THINKING AND REFLECTION

Before reading this section, how familiar were you with the principles of contraception? Did you know as much as you thought? Does this kind of information make you feel as though you should be more or less directly responsible for the contraceptive choices in your life?

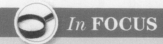 *In* FOCUS

Myths about Contraception

Myth Taking birth control pills for a few days before having sex gives reliable protection against pregnancy.

Fact Instructions for taking birth control pills must be followed carefully to provide effective contraception. With most pills, this means starting them with a menstrual period and then taking one every day.

Myth Pregnancy never occurs when unprotected intercourse takes place just before or just after a menstrual period.

Fact Menstrual cycles may be irregular, and ovulation may be unpredictable.

Myth During sexual relations, sperm enter the vagina only during ejaculation and never before.

Fact The small amount of fluid secreted before ejaculation may contain sperm. This is why withdrawing the penis from the vagina just before ejaculation is not an effective method of contraception.

Myth If semen is deposited just outside the vaginal entrance, pregnancy cannot occur.

Fact Although sperm usually live about 72 hours within the woman's body, they can live up to six or seven days and are capable of travelling through the vagina and up into the uterus and oviducts.

Myth Douching immediately after sexual relations can prevent sperm from reaching and fertilizing an egg.

Fact During ejaculation (within the vagina), some sperm begin to enter the cervix and uterus. Because these sperm are no longer in the vagina, it is impossible to remove them by douching after sexual relations. Douching may actually push the sperm up farther.

Myth A woman who is breastfeeding does not have to use any contraceptive method to prevent pregnancy.

Fact Frequent and regular breastfeeding may at times prevent ovulation, but not consistently and reliably. Ovulation and pregnancy may occur before the first period after delivering a baby.

Myth Women can't become pregnant the first time they have intercourse.

Fact Any time intercourse without protection takes place, pregnancy may result. There is nothing unique about first intercourse that prevents this.

Myth Taking a break from the pill periodically is necessary for safety.

Fact Taking a prolonged break from oral contraceptive use has no known medical benefits; the risks and benefits of ongoing pill use should be evaluated for each individual. Pregnancy commonly occurs when one method of contraception is stopped and not immediately replaced by another method.

Myth Pregnancy is impossible if partners have sex while standing up.

Fact Sperm can travel and reach the egg regardless of body position.

Reversible Contraception

Reversibility is an extremely important consideration for young adults when they choose a contraceptive method, because most people either plan to have children or at least want to keep their options open until they are older.

Oral Contraceptives: The Pill

About a century ago, a researcher noted that ovulation does not occur during pregnancy. Further research revealed the hormonal mechanism: During pregnancy, the corpus luteum secretes progesterone and estrogen in amounts high enough to suppress ovulation. **Oral contraceptives (OCs)**, or *birth control pills*, prevent ovulation by mimicking the hormonal activity of the corpus luteum. The active ingredients in OCs are estrogen and progestins, laboratory-made compounds that are closely related to progesterone. Today, OCs are the most widely used form of contraception among unmarried women and are second only to sterilization among married women.

> **oral contraceptives (OCs)**
> Any of various hormone compounds (estrogen and progestins) in pill form that prevent conception by preventing ovulation.

In addition to preventing ovulation, the birth control pill has other backup contraceptive effects. It inhibits the movement of sperm by thickening the cervical mucus, alters the rate of ovum transport by means of its hormonal effects on the oviducts, and may prevent implantation by changing the lining of the uterus, in the unlikely event that a fertilized ovum reaches that area.

The most common type of OC is the *combination pill*. Each one-month packet contains a three-week supply of pills that combine varying types and amounts of estrogen and progestin. Some packets also include a one-week supply of inactive pills to be taken following the hormone pills; others simply instruct the woman to take no pills at all for one week before starting the next cycle. During the week in which no hormones are taken, a light menstrual period occurs. Many different types of combination pills are available.

Advantages

OCs are very effective in preventing pregnancy. Nearly all unplanned pregnancies result because the pills were not taken as directed. The pill is relatively simple to use and does not hinder sexual spontaneity. Most women also enjoy the predictable regularity of periods, as well as the decrease in cramps and blood loss. For young women, the reversibility of the pill is especially important; **fertility**—the ability to reproduce—returns after the pill is discontinued (although not always immediately).

> **fertility**
> The ability to reproduce.

Medical advantages include a decreased incidence of benign breast disease, iron-deficiency anemia, pelvic inflammatory disease (PID), ectopic pregnancy, colon and rectal cancer, endometrial cancer (in the lining of the uterus), and ovarian cancer. Women who have never used the pill are twice as likely to develop endometrial or ovarian cancer as those who have taken it for at least five years.

Disadvantages

Although OCs lower the risk of PID, they do not protect against HIV infection or other STIs in the lower reproductive tract. OCs have been associated with increased cervical chlamydia. Regular condom use is recommended for an OC user, unless she is in a long-term, mutually monogamous relationship with an uninfected partner.

The hormones in birth control pills influence all tissues of the body and can lead to a variety of disturbances. Symptoms of early pregnancy—morning nausea and swollen breasts, for example—may appear during the first few months of OC use. They usually disappear by the fourth cycle. Other side effects include depression, nervousness, changes in sex drive, dizziness, generalized headaches, migraine, bleeding between periods, and changes in the lining of the walls of the vagina, with an increase in clear or white vaginal discharge. Melasma, or "mask of pregnancy," sometimes occurs, causing brown pigmentation to appear on the face. Acne may develop or worsen but, in most women, using the pill causes acne to clear up, and it is sometimes prescribed for that purpose.

Serious side effects have been reported in a small number of women. These include blood clots, stroke, and heart attack, concentrated mostly in older women who smoke or have a history of circulatory disease. Recent studies have shown no increased risk of stroke or heart attack for healthy, young, non-smoking women on lower-dosage pills. OC users may be slightly more prone to high blood pressure, blood clots in the legs and arms, and benign liver tumours that may rupture and bleed.

OC use is associated with little, if any, increase in breast cancer and a slight increase in cervical cancer; however, earlier detection and other variables, such as number of sexual partners, may account for much of this increase. The link between OC use and cervical cancer appears to pertain primarily to women infected with human papillomavirus, an STI.

Birth control pills are not recommended for women with a history of blood clots (or a close family member with unexplained blood clots at an early age), heart disease or stroke, migraines with changes in vision, any form of cancer or liver tumour, or impaired liver function. Women with certain other health conditions or behaviours, including migraines without changes in vision, high blood pressure, cigarette smoking, and sickle-cell disease, require close monitoring.

Reversible hormonal contraceptives are available in several forms. Shown here are a variety of birth control pill options.

Effectiveness

OC effectiveness varies substantially because it depends so much on individual factors. If taken exactly as directed, the failure rate is extremely low (0.3 percent). However, among average users, lapses, such as forgetting to take a pill, do occur, and a typical first-year failure rate is 8.7 percent. The continuation rate for OCs also varies; the average rate is 68 percent after one year.

Contraceptive Skin Patch

The contraceptive skin patch, Ortho Evra, is a thin, 4.5 centimetre by 4.5 centimetre patch that slowly releases an estrogen and a progestin into the bloodstream. The contraceptive patch prevents pregnancy in the same way as combination OCs, following a similar schedule. Each patch is worn continuously for one week and is replaced on the same day of the week for three consecutive weeks. The fourth week is patch free, allowing a woman to have her menstrual period.

The patch can be worn on the upper outer arm, abdomen, buttocks, or upper torso (excluding the breasts); it is designed to stick to skin even during bathing or swimming. If a patch should fall off for more than a day, it is advisable to start a new four-week cycle of patches and use a backup method of contraception for the first week. Patches should be discarded according to the manufacturer's directions to avoid leakage of hormones into the environment.

Advantages

With both perfect and typical use, the patch is as effective as OCs in preventing pregnancy. Compliance seems to be higher with the patch than with OCs, probably because the patch requires weekly instead of daily action. Medical benefits are likely to be comparable to those of OCs.

Disadvantages

With patch use, additional measures must be taken to protect against STIs. Minor side effects are similar to those of OCs, although breast discomfort may be more common in patch users. Some women also experience skin irritation around the patch. More serious complications are thought to be similar to those of OCs, including an increased risk of side effects among women who smoke. However, because Ortho Evra exposes users to higher doses of estrogen than most OCs, patch use may further increase the risk of blood clots and other adverse effects.

Effectiveness

With perfect use, the patch's failure rate is very low (0.3 percent) in the first year of use. The typical failure rate is assumed to be lower than the pill's 8.7 percent, because consistent use is better among patch users. The product appears to be less effective when used by women weighing more than 90 kilograms.

Vaginal Contraceptive Ring

The NuvaRing is a vaginal ring that is moulded with a mixture of progestin and estrogen. The five-centimetre ring slowly releases hormones and maintains blood hormone levels comparable to those found with OC use; it prevents pregnancy in the same way as OCs. A woman inserts the ring anytime during the first five days of her menstrual period and leaves it in place for three weeks. During the fourth week, which is ring-free, her next menstrual period occurs. A new ring is then inserted. Rings should be discarded according to the manufacturer's directions to avoid leakage of hormones into the environment.

Backup contraception must be used for the first seven days of the first ring use or if the ring has been removed for more than three hours during use. A diaphragm is not recommended as a backup contraceptive with the NuvaRing because the ring may interfere with the placement of a diaphragm. Diaphragm use is discussed later in this chapter.

Advantages

The NuvaRing offers one month of protection with no daily or weekly action required. It does not require a fitting by a clinician, and exact placement in the vagina is not critical as it is with a diaphragm. Medical benefits are probably similar to those of OCs.

Disadvantages

The NuvaRing gives no protection against STIs. Side effects are roughly comparable to those seen with OC use, except for a lower incidence of nausea and vomiting. Other side effects may include vaginal discharge, vaginitis, and vaginal irritation. Medical risks also are similar to those found with OC use.

Effectiveness

As with the pill and patch, the perfect use failure rate is around 0.3 percent and the typical use failure rate is likely to be lower than the pill's 8.7 percent.

Contraceptive Implant

Contraceptive implants are placed under the skin of the upper arm and deliver a small but steady dose of progestin (a synthetic progesterone) over a period of years.

The progestins in implants have several contraceptive effects. They cause hormonal shifts that may inhibit ovulation and affect development of the uterine lining. The hormones also thicken the cervical mucus, inhibiting the movement of sperm. Finally, they may slow the transport of the egg through the fallopian tubes. Contraceptive implants are best suited for women who want continuous and long-term protection against pregnancy.

Advantages

Contraceptive implants are highly effective. After insertion of the implants, no further action is required; contraceptive effects are quickly reversed on removal. Because implants, unlike the combination pill, contain no estrogen, they carry a lower risk of certain side effects, such as blood clots and other cardiovascular complications. In addition, the progestin is released at a steady rate, in smaller quantities than are found in oral contraceptives. The thickened cervical mucus resulting from implant use has a protective effect against PID.

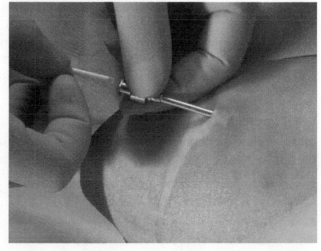

Only trained health professionals can insert a contraceptive implant.

Disadvantages

Like the pill, an implant provides no protection against HIV infection and STIs in the lower reproductive tract. Although the implants are barely visible, their appearance may bother some women. Only specially trained practitioners can insert or remove the implants, and removal is sometimes difficult.

The most common side effects of contraceptive implants are menstrual irregularities, including longer menstrual periods, spotting between periods, or no bleeding at all. The menstrual cycle usually becomes more regular after one year of use. Less common side effects include headaches, weight gain, breast tenderness, nausea, acne, and mood swings. Cautions and more serious health concerns are similar to those associated with oral contraceptives but are less common.

Effectiveness

The overall failure rate is estimated at about 0.1 percent.

Injectable Contraceptives

Hormonal contraceptive injections were developed in the 1960s and are currently being used in at least 80 countries throughout the world. The first injectable contraceptive approved for use in Canada was Depo-Provera, which uses long-acting progestins. Injected into the arm or buttocks, Depo-Provera is usually given every 12 weeks, although it actually provides effective contraception for a few weeks beyond that. As another progestin-only contraceptive, it prevents pregnancy in the same ways as implants.

Advantages

Injectable contraceptives are highly effective and require little action on the part of the user. Because the injections leave no trace and involve no ongoing supplies, injectables allow women almost total privacy in their decision to use contraception. Depo-Provera has no estrogen-related side effects; it requires only periodic injections rather than the minor surgical procedures of implant insertion and removal.

Disadvantages

Injectable contraceptives provide no protection against HIV infection and STIs in the lower reproductive tract. A woman must visit a health care facility every three months to receive the injections. The side effects of Depo-Provera are similar to those of implants; menstrual irregularities are the most common, and after one year of using Depo-Provera many women have no menstrual bleeding at all. Weight gain is a common side effect. After discontinuing the use of Depo-Provera, women may experience temporary infertility for up to 12 months.

Reasons for not using Depo-Provera are similar to those for not using implants. Extended use of Depo-Provera is associated with decreased bone density, a risk factor for osteoporosis (see Chapter 5); women who use Depo-Provera are advised to do weight-bearing exercise and take 1000 milligrams of calcium daily. Women are advised to use Depo-Provera as a long-term contraceptive (longer than two years, for example) only if other methods are inadequate. Studies have found that bone density rebounds when use of Depo-Provera stops.

Effectiveness

The perfect use failure rate is 0.3 percent for Depo-Provera. With typical use, the failure rate increases to 6.7 percent in the first year of use. The one-year continuation rate for Depo-Provera is about 56 percent.

Emergency Contraception

Emergency contraception refers to postcoital methods—those used after unprotected sexual intercourse. An emergency contraceptive may be appropriate if a regularly used method has failed (for example, if a condom breaks) or if unprotected sex has occurred. Sometimes called the "morning-after pill," emergency contraceptives are designed only for emergency use and should not be relied on as a regular birth control method.

emergency contraception
A birth control method used after unprotected sexual intercourse has occurred.

Until recently the most frequently used emergency contraceptive was a two-dose regimen of certain oral contraceptives. Researchers are still uncertain precisely how OCs work as emergency contraceptives. Opponents of their use argue that if they act by preventing implantation of a fertilized egg, they may actually be **abortifacients**; however, recent evidence indicates that prevention of implantation is not their primary mode of action. Postcoital pills appear to work primarily by inhibiting or delaying ovulation and by altering the transport of sperm or eggs; they do not affect a fertilized egg already implanted in the uterus.

abortifacient
An agent or a substance that induces abortion.

Plan B is a newer product specifically designed for emergency contraception. It is available over the counter in Canada and contains two progestin-only pills. The first pill should be taken as soon as possible (no more than 120 hours) after inadequately protected sex. The second pill should be taken 12 hours after the first. Both pills may be taken together in a single dose with little change in effectiveness or side effects. If taken within 24 hours after intercourse, Plan B may prevent as many as 95 percent of expected pregnancies. Overall, Plan B reduces pregnancy risk by about 89 percent. It is most effective if initiated in the first 12 hours. Possible side effects are similar to those associated with the OC regimen and can include nausea, stomach pain, headache, dizziness, and breast tenderness.

Easy access to emergency contraception is important because the sooner the drug is taken, the more effective it is. Some clinicians advise women to keep a package of emergency contraception on hand in case their regular contraception method fails. Research has found that ready access to emergency contraception does not lead to an increase in unprotected intercourse, unintended pregnancies, or STIs.

Intrauterine devices, discussed in the next section, can also be used for emergency contraception: If inserted within five days of unprotected intercourse, they are even more effective than OCs. However, because their use is more complicated, they are not used nearly as frequently.

The Intrauterine Device (IUD)

The **intrauterine device (IUD)** is a small device placed in the uterus as a contraceptive. There are two types of IUDs in Canada, and they are effective for about five years.

intrauterine device (IUD)
A plastic device inserted into the uterus as a contraceptive.

Researchers do not know exactly how IUDs prevent pregnancy. Current evidence suggests that they work primarily by preventing fertilization. IUDs may cause biochemical changes in the uterus and affect the movement of sperm and eggs; although less likely, they may also interfere with implantation of fertilized eggs. Some IUDs slowly release very small amounts of hormones, which impede fertilization or implantation.

An IUD must be inserted and removed by a trained professional. It can be inserted at any time during the menstrual cycle, as long as the woman is not pregnant. The device is threaded into a sterile inserter, which is introduced through the cervix; a plunger pushes the IUD into the uterus. The threads protruding from the cervix are trimmed so that only 2.5–4 centimetres remain in the upper vagina.

Advantages

Intrauterine devices are highly reliable and are simple and convenient to use, requiring no attention except for a periodic check of the string position. They do not require the woman to anticipate or interrupt sexual activity. According to researchers, IUD use reduces the risk of developing endometrial cancer by as much as 40 percent. Usually IUDs have only localized side effects, and in the absence of complications they are considered a fully reversible contraceptive. In most cases, fertility is restored as soon as the IUD is removed. The risks of ectopic pregnancy and uterine cancer are both decreased with IUD use.

Disadvantages

Most side effects of IUD use are limited to the genital tract. Heavy menstrual flow and bleeding and spotting between periods may occur, although with some IUDs menstrual periods tend to become shorter and lighter over time. Another side effect is pain, particularly uterine cramps and backache, which seem to occur most often in women who have never been pregnant. Spontaneous expulsion of the IUD happens to 5–6 percent of women within the first year, most commonly during the first months after insertion. The older the woman is and the more children she has had, the less likely she is to expel the device. In about 1 of 1000 insertions, the IUD punctures the wall of the uterus and may migrate into the abdominal cavity.

A serious but rare complication of IUD use is pelvic inflammatory disease (PID). Most pelvic infections among IUD users occur shortly after insertion, are relatively mild, and can be treated successfully with antibiotics. However, early and adequate treatment is critical—a lingering infection can lead to tubal scarring and subsequent infertility.

Some physicians advise against the use of IUDs by young women who have never been pregnant because of the increased incidence of side effects in this group and the risk of infection with the possibility of subsequent infertility.

IUDs are not recommended for women of any age who are at high risk for STIs. They are also unsuitable for women with suspected pregnancy, large tumours of the uterus or other anatomical abnormalities, irregular or unexplained bleeding, or rheumatic heart disease. No evidence has been found linking IUD use to an increased risk of cancer. IUDs offer no protection against STIs.

Early IUD danger signals are abdominal pain, fever, chills, foul-smelling vaginal discharge, irregular menstrual periods, and other unusual vaginal bleeding. A change in string length should also be noted. An annual checkup is important and should include a Pap test and a blood check for anemia if menstrual flow has increased.

Effectiveness

The typical failure rate of IUDs during the first year of use is 0.1–0.6 percent. Effectiveness can be increased by periodically checking to see that the device is in place and by using a backup method for the first few months after IUD insertion. If pregnancy occurs, the IUD should be removed to safeguard the health of the woman and to maintain the pregnancy. The continuation rate of IUDs is about 80 percent after one year of use.

Male Condoms

The male condom is a thin sheath designed to cover the penis during sexual intercourse. Most brands available in Canada are made of latex, although condoms made of polyurethane are also now available. Condoms prevent sperm from entering the vagina and provide protection against disease. Condoms are the most widely used barrier method and the third most popular of all contraceptive methods used in North America, after the pill and female sterilization.

Condom sales have increased dramatically in recent years, primarily because they are the only method that provides substantial protection against HIV infection as well as some protection against other STIs. At least one-third of all male condoms are bought by women.

Advantages

Condoms are easy to purchase and are available without prescription or medical supervision. In addition to being free of medical side effects (other than occasional allergic reactions), latex condoms help protect against STIs. A recent study determined that condoms may also protect women from human papilloma virus (HPV), which causes cervical cancer. Condoms made of polyurethane are appropriate for people who are allergic to latex. However, they are more likely to slip or break than latex condoms and therefore may give less protection against STIs and pregnancy. (Lambskin condoms permit the passage of HIV and other disease-causing organisms, so they can be used only for pregnancy prevention, not the prevention of STIs.)

Except for abstinence, correct and consistent use of latex male condoms offers the most reliable available protection against the transmission of HIV. (See Figure 11.6 for the proper way to use a condom.)

Disadvantages

The two most common complaints about condoms are that they diminish sensation and interfere with spontaneity. Although some people find these drawbacks serious, others consider them only minor disadvantages. Many couples learn to creatively integrate condom use into their sexual practices. Indeed, it can be a way to improve communication and share responsibility in a relationship.

Effectiveness

In actual use, the failure rate of condoms varies considerably. First-year rates among typical users average about 17.4 percent. With perfect use, the first-year failure rate is about 2 percent. At least some pregnancies happen because the condom is carelessly removed after ejaculation. Some may also occur because of breakage or slippage, which may happen 1–2 times in every 100 instances of use for latex condoms and up to 10 times in every 100 instances for polyurethane condoms. Breakage is more common among inexperienced users. Other contributing factors include poorly fitting condoms, insufficient lubrication, excessively vigorous sex, and improper storage (because heat destroys rubber, latex condoms should not be stored for long periods in a wallet or a car's glove compartment). To help ensure quality, condoms should not be used past their expiration date or more than five years past their date of manufacture (two years for those with spermicide).

If a condom breaks or is carelessly removed, the risk of pregnancy can be reduced somewhat by the immediate use of a vaginal spermicide. Some clinicians recommend keeping emergency contraceptive pills on hand. If the emergency contraceptive Plan B is taken within one hour of inadequately protected sex, the failure rate is only about 0.14 percent. The most common cause of pregnancy with condom users is "taking a chance"—that is, occasionally not using a condom at all—or waiting to use it until after preejaculate fluid (which may contain some sperm) has already entered the vagina.

FIGURE 11.6

Use of the Male Condom

(a) Check the expiration date and check to see that the package is intact. Put the condom on before any genital contact. If uncircumcised, pull back the foreskin. Cover the head of the penis with the condom. Leave some space at the tip for ejaculate, but gently press out any air. This will reduce the risk of breakage. **(b)** Unroll the condom so that the entire erect penis is covered all the way to the base. If needed, you may generously apply a water-based or silicone lubricant to the outside of the condom before penetration. Do not use oil-based lubricants. To prevent slippage, hold the condom at the base of the penis when withdrawing. **(c)** After ejaculation occurs, withdraw the penis before it gets soft. Hold onto the condom to prevent slippage. Throw the condom away.

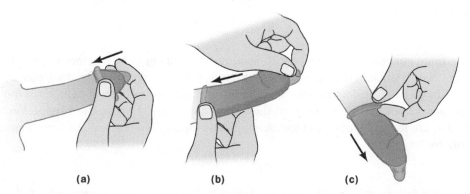

(a) (b) (c)

Source: McKinley Health Center, University of Illinois at Urbana-Champaign. 2004. *How to Use a Condom and Spermicidal Jelly for Intercourse*, http://www.mckinley.illinois.edu/handouts/condom_spermicidal_jelly/condom_spermicidal_jelly.html (retrieved July 22, 2015).

Female Condoms

A female condom is a latex or polyurethane pouch that can be inserted into a woman's vagina. Although the female condom is preferred in certain situations because it requires less participation on the part of the male partner, its overall popularity remains far below that of the male condom.

The female condom currently available is a disposable device that comes in one size and consists of a soft, loose-fitting polyurethane sheath with two flexible rings (see Figure 11.7). The ring at the closed end is inserted into the vagina and placed at the cervix, much like a diaphragm. The ring at the open end remains outside the vagina. The walls of the condom protect the inside of the vagina.

The directions that accompany the condom should be followed closely. It can be inserted up to eight hours before intercourse and should be used with the supplied lubricant or a spermicide to prevent penile irritation. As with male condoms, users need to take care not to tear the condom during insertion or removal. Following intercourse, the woman should remove the condom immediately, before standing up. By twisting and squeezing the outer ring, she can prevent the spilling of semen. A new condom should be used for each act of sexual intercourse. A female condom should not be used with a male condom because when the two are used together slippage is more likely to occur.

FIGURE 11.7

The Female Condom Properly Positioned

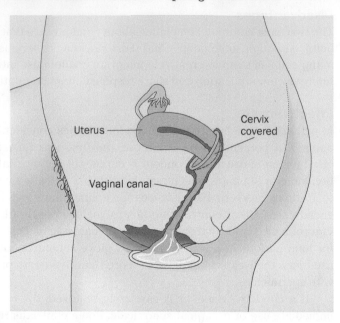

Uterus

Cervix covered

Vaginal canal

Advantages

For many women, the greatest advantage of the female condom is the control it gives them over contraception and STI prevention. (Partner cooperation is still important, however.) Female condoms can be inserted before sexual activity and are thus less disruptive than male condoms. Because the outer part of the condom covers the area around the vaginal opening as well as the base of the penis during intercourse, it offers potentially better protection against genital warts or herpes. The polyurethane pouch can be used by people who are allergic to latex. And because polyurethane is thin and pliable, little loss of sensation occurs.

When used correctly, the female condom should theoretically provide protection against HIV transmission and STIs comparable to that of the latex male condom. However, in research involving typical users, the female condom was less effective in preventing both pregnancy and STIs. With careful instruction and practice, effectiveness can be improved.

Disadvantages

As with the traditional condom, interference with spontaneity is likely to be a common complaint. The outer ring, which hangs visibly outside the vagina, may be bothersome during foreplay; if so, couples may choose to put the device in just before intercourse. During coitus, both partners must take care that the penis is inserted into the pouch, not outside it, and that the device does not slip inside the vagina. Female condoms, like male condoms, are made for one-time use. A single female condom costs about four times as much as a single male condom.

Effectiveness

The typical first-year failure rate of the female condom is 27 percent. For women who follow instructions carefully and consistently, the failure rate is considerably lower—about 5 percent. Although the female condom rarely breaks during use, slippage occurs in nearly one in ten users. The risk of being exposed to semen is higher if the relationship is new or short-term, if intercourse is very active, and if there is a large disparity between vagina and penis sizes. Having Plan B available as a backup contraceptive is recommended.

The Diaphragm with Spermicide

Before oral contraceptives were introduced, about 25 percent of all North American couples who used any form of contraception relied on the **diaphragm**. Many diaphragm users switched to the pill or IUDs, but the diaphragm offers advantages that are important to some couples.

> **diaphragm**
> A contraceptive device consisting of a flexible, dome-shaped cup that covers the cervix and prevents sperm from entering the uterus.

The diaphragm is a dome-shaped cup of thin rubber stretched over a collapsible metal ring. When correctly used with spermicidal cream or jelly, the diaphragm covers the cervix, blocking sperm from entering the uterus.

Diaphragms are available only by prescription. Because of individual anatomical differences among women, a diaphragm must be carefully fitted by a trained clinician to ensure both comfort and effectiveness. The fitting should be checked with each routine annual medical examination, as well as after childbirth, abortion, or a weight change of more than 4.5 kilograms.

The woman spreads spermicidal jelly or cream on the diaphragm before inserting it and checking its placement (see Figure 11.8). If more than six hours elapse between the time of insertion and the time of intercourse, additional spermicide must be applied. The diaphragm must be left in place for at least six hours after the last act of coitus to give the spermicide enough time to kill all the sperm. With repeated intercourse, a condom should be used for additional protection.

To remove the diaphragm, the woman simply hooks the front rim down from the pubic bone with one finger and pulls it out. She should wash it with mild soap and water, rinse it, pat it dry, and then examine it for holes or cracks. Defects would most likely develop near the rim and can be spotted by looking at the diaphragm in front of a bright light. After inspecting the diaphragm, she should store it in its case.

FIGURE 11.8

Use of the Diaphragm

Wash your hands with soap and water before inserting the diaphragm. It can be inserted while squatting, lying down, or standing with one foot raised. **(a)** Place about 15 millilitres (a tablespoon) of spermicidal jelly or cream in the concave side of the diaphragm, and spread it around the inside of the diaphragm and around the rim. **(b)** Squeeze the diaphragm into a long, narrow shape between the thumb and forefinger. Insert it into the vagina, and push it up along the back wall of the vagina as far as it will go. **(c)** Check its position to make sure the cervix is completely covered and that the front rim of the diaphragm is tucked behind the pubic bone.

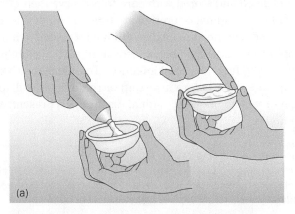
(a)

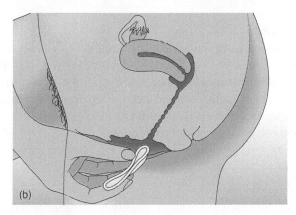
(b)

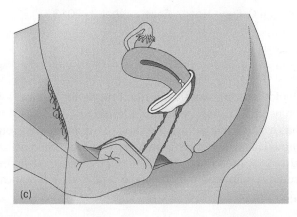
(c)

Advantages

Diaphragm use is less intrusive than male condom use because a diaphragm can be inserted up to six hours before intercourse. Its use can be limited to times of sexual activity only, and it allows for immediate and total reversibility. The diaphragm is free of medical side effects (other than rare allergic reactions).

When used along with spermicidal jelly or cream, it offers significant protection against gonorrhea and possibly chlamydia, STIs that are transmitted only by semen and for which the cervix is the sole site of entry. Diaphragm use can also protect the cervix from semen infected with the human papillomavirus, which causes cervical cancer. However, the diaphragm is unlikely to protect against STIs that can be transmitted through vaginal or vulvar surfaces (in addition to the cervix), including HIV infection, genital herpes, and syphilis.

Disadvantages

Diaphragms must always be used with a spermicide, so a woman must keep both of these somewhat bulky supplies with her whenever she anticipates sexual activity. Diaphragms require extra attention, since they must be cleaned and stored with care to preserve their effectiveness. Some women cannot wear a diaphragm because of their vaginal or uterine anatomy. In other women, diaphragm use can cause an increase in bladder infections and may need to be discontinued if repeated infections occur.

Diaphragms have also been associated with a slightly increased risk of **toxic shock syndrome (TSS)**, an occasionally fatal bacterial infection. To reduce the risk of TSS, a woman should wash her hands carefully with soap and water before inserting or removing the diaphragm, should not use the diaphragm during menstruation or when abnormal vaginal discharge is present, and should never leave the device in place for more than 24 hours.

toxic shock syndrome (TSS)
A bacterial disease usually associated with tampon use; can also occur in men; symptoms include weakness, cold and clammy hands, fever, nausea, and headache. TSS can progress to life-threatening complications, including very low blood pressure (shock) and kidney and liver failure.

Effectiveness

The diaphragm's effectiveness depends mainly on whether it is used properly. In actual practice, women rarely use it correctly every time they have intercourse. With perfect use, the failure rate is about 6 percent. Typical failure rates are 16 percent during the first year of use. The main causes of failure are incorrect insertion, inconsistent use, and inaccurate fitting. Sometimes, too, the vaginal walls expand during sexual stimulation, causing the diaphragm to be dislodged. If a diaphragm slips during intercourse, a woman may choose to use emergency contraception.

QUICK STATS

17% of Canadian university students have experienced unprotected sex when drinking alcohol.
—National College Health Assessment II, 2013

Lea's Shield

Lea's Shield is a one-size-fits-all diaphragm-like device, available by prescription. Made of silicone rubber, it can be used by women who are allergic to latex, and it is not damaged by petroleum-based products. The shield has a valve that allows the flow of air and fluids from the cervix as well as a loop that aids in insertion and removal. The device may be inserted at any time before intercourse, but should be left in place for eight hours after last intercourse; it can be worn for up to 48 hours. Like the diaphragm, it must be used with spermicide. Studies completed thus far have reported advantages, disadvantages, and failure rates similar to those of the diaphragm.

FemCap

FemCap, another barrier device, is a small flexible cup that fits snugly over the cervix and is held in place by suction. This cervical cap is a clear silicone cup with a brim around the dome to hold spermicide and trap sperm and a removal strap over the dome. It comes in three sizes and must be fitted by a trained clinician. It is used like a diaphragm, with a small amount of spermicide placed in the cup and on the brim before insertion.

> **FemCap**
> A small flexible cup that fits over the cervix, to be used with spermicide.

Advantages

Advantages of the cervical cap are similar to those associated with diaphragm use and include partial STI protection. It is an alternative for women who cannot use a diaphragm because of anatomical reasons or recurrent urinary tract infections. Because the cap fits tightly, it does not require backup condom use with repeated intercourse. It may be left in place for up to 48 hours.

Disadvantages

Along with most of the disadvantages associated with the diaphragm, difficulty with insertion and removal is more common for cervical cap users. Because there may be a slightly increased risk of TSS with prolonged use, the cap should not be left in place for more than 48 hours.

Effectiveness

Studies indicate that the average failure rate for the cervical cap is 16 percent for women who have never had a child and 32 percent for women who have had a child. Failure rates drop significantly with perfect use.

The Contraceptive Sponge

The **sponge** is a round, absorbent device about five centimetres in diameter with a polyester loop on one side (for removal) and a concave dimple on the other side, which helps it fit snugly over the cervix. The sponge is made of polyurethane and is presaturated with the same spermicide that is used in contraceptive creams and foams. The spermicide is activated when moistened with a small amount of water just before insertion. The sponge, which can be used only once, acts as a barrier, as a spermicide, and as a seminal fluid absorbent.

> **sponge**
> A contraceptive device about five centimetres in diameter that fits over the cervix and acts as a barrier, spermicide, and seminal fluid absorbent.

Advantages

The sponge offers advantages similar to those of the diaphragm and cervical cap, including partial protection against some STIs. In addition, sponges can be obtained without a prescription or professional fitting, and they may be safely left in place for 24 hours without the addition of spermicide for repeated intercourse.

Disadvantages

Reported disadvantages include difficulty with removal and an unpleasant odour if the sponge is left in place for more than 18 hours. Allergic reactions, such as irritation of the vagina, are more common with the sponge than with other spermicide products, probably because the overall dose contained in each sponge is significantly higher than that used with other methods. (A sponge contains 1 gram of spermicide compared with the 60–100 milligrams present in one application of other spermicidal products.) If irritation of the vaginal lining occurs, the risk of yeast infections and STIs (including HIV) may increase.

Because the sponge has also been associated with toxic shock syndrome, the same precautions must be taken as described for diaphragm use. A sponge user should be especially alert for symptoms of TSS when the sponge has been difficult to remove or was not removed intact.

Effectiveness

The typical effectiveness of the sponge is the same as the diaphragm (16 percent failure rate during the first year of use) for women who have never experienced childbirth. For women who have had a child, however, sponges are significantly less effective than diaphragms. One possible explanation is that the sponge's size may be insufficient to adequately cover the cervix after childbirth. To ensure effectiveness, the user should carefully check the expiration date on each sponge, as shelf life is limited.

Vaginal Spermicides

Spermicidal compounds developed for use with a diaphragm have been adapted for use without a diaphragm by combining them with a bulky base. Foams, creams, jellies, suppositories, and films are all available. Foam is sold in an aerosol bottle or a metal container with an applicator that fits on the nozzle. Creams and jellies are sold in tubes with an applicator that can be screwed onto the opening of the tube.

Foams, creams, and jellies must be placed deep in the vagina near the cervical entrance and must be inserted no more than 60 minutes before intercourse. After an hour, their effectiveness is drastically reduced, and a new dose must be inserted. Another application is also required before each repeated act of coitus. If the woman wants to **douche**, she should wait for at least six hours after the last intercourse to make sure that there has been time for the spermicide to kill all the sperm; douching is not recommended, however, because it can irritate vaginal tissue and increase the risk of various infections.

> **douche**
> To apply a stream of water or other solutions to a body part or cavity, such as the vagina; not a contraceptive technique.

The spermicidal suppository is small and easily inserted like a tampon. Because body heat is needed to dissolve and activate the suppository, it is important to wait at least 15 minutes after insertion before having intercourse. The suppository's spermicidal effects are limited in time, and coitus should take place within one hour of insertion. A new suppository is required for every act of intercourse.

Vaginal contraceptive film (VCF) is a paper-thin five centimetre by five centimetre film that contains spermicide. It is folded over one or two fingers and placed high in the vagina, as close to the cervix as possible. In about 15 minutes the film dissolves into a spermicidal gel that is effective for up to one hour. A new film must be inserted for each act of intercourse.

Advantages

The use of vaginal spermicides is relatively simple and can be limited to times of sexual activity. They are readily available in most drugstores and do not require a prescription or a pelvic examination. Spermicides allow for complete and immediate reversibility, and the only medical side effects are occasional allergic reactions. Vaginal spermicides may provide limited protection against some STIs but should never be used instead of condoms for reliable protection.

Disadvantages

When used alone, vaginal spermicides must be inserted shortly before intercourse, so their use may be seen as an annoying disruption. Some women find the slight increase in vaginal fluids after spermicide use unpleasant. Spermicides can alter the balance of bacteria in the vagina. Because this may increase the occurrence of yeast infections and urinary tract infections, women who are especially prone to these infections may want to avoid spermicides. Also, this method does not protect against gonorrhea, chlamydia, or HIV. Overuse of spermicides can irritate vaginal tissues; if this occurs, the risk of HIV transmission may increase.

Effectiveness

The effectiveness rates of vaginal spermicides vary widely, depending partly on how consistently and carefully instructions are followed. The typical failure rate is about 29 percent during the first year of use. Foam is probably the most effective form of spermicide, because its effervescent mass forms a denser and more

QUESTIONS FOR CRITICAL THINKING AND REFLECTION

What are the most important factors influencing your personal decisions about contraception? List these factors in order of their priority to you, and determine whether you have given each factor full consideration in choosing a contraceptive method.

evenly distributed barrier to the cervical opening. Creams and jellies provide only minimal protection unless used with a diaphragm or cervical cap.

Spermicide is generally recommended only in combination with other barrier methods or as a backup to other contraceptives. Plan B provides a better backup than spermicides, however.

Whatever your needs, circumstances, or beliefs, *do* make a choice about contraception. Not choosing anything is the one method known *not* to work. This is an area in which taking charge of your health has immediate and profound implications for your future. The method you choose today won't necessarily be the one you will want to use your whole life, or even next year. But it should be one that works for you right now.

Even with the vast array of contraceptive options available to Canadians, unwanted pregnancies do occur for various reasons. When this happens, abortion may need to be considered.

Abortion

Few issues are as complex and emotionally charged as abortion. In Canada, public attention has focused on the legal definition of abortion and the issue of restricting its practice. These far-reaching questions are important, but the most difficult aspects of abortion are personal—especially for women who must decide whether to have an abortion.

Because most women who undergo abortions are young, many university and college students have personal experience with unintended pregnancy and abortion. Therefore, students are in a good position not just to debate the larger issues surrounding abortion, but also to address the complex human factors involved in preventing pregnancy and dealing with unintended pregnancy.

Abortion is legal in throughout Canada; the number of abortions by province and territory in 2010 are shown in Table 11.1.

TABLE 11.1

Number of Induced Abortions* Reported in Canada[†] in 2010

Province	Number of Abortions
Newfoundland and Labrador	1 068
Prince Edward Island[†]	0
Nova Scotia	2 125[§]
New Brunswick	1 098
Quebec	26 106**
Ontario	28 765**
Manitoba	4 150
Saskatchewan	1 915[§]
Alberta	13 084
British Columbia	12 149[††]
Yukon Territory	147[§]
Northwest Territories	40[§]
Nunavut	100[§]
Total induced abortions	90 747[††]

Notes

*Induced abortion is defined as the medical termination of pregnancy. Equivalent terms include artificial abortion, therapeutic abortion, voluntary termination of pregnancy, elective termination of pregnancy, and active termination of pregnancy.

[†]Figures include induced abortions performed in a hospital or clinic setting in Canada (numbers are presented by the province/territory in which the abortion was performed).

[‡]Induced abortions are not performed in Prince Edward Island. Prince Edward Island residents who received an induced abortion in a hospital travelled to another province/territory.

[§]Induced abortions are not performed in clinics in Nova Scotia, Saskatchewan, Yukon, the Northwest Territories, or Nunavut.

**Ontario (clinic data only) and Quebec (clinic and hospital data) include only induced abortions covered by their respective provincial health insurance plans. Data from all other provinces/territories (including Ontario hospital data) include all induced abortions, whether paid for by the patient or by a different health insurance plan. For example, patients with coverage under Quebec's health insurance plan receiving care in Manitoba are reported by Manitoba. However, patients with coverage under Manitoba's health insurance plan receiving care in Quebec are not reported (by either Quebec or Manitoba).

[††]Hospitals are mandated by their provincial/territorial ministry of health to report all hospital activity (not limited to abortions); therefore, coverage of abortions performed in Canadian hospitals can be considered complete. However, there is no such legislative requirement for clinics to report their activity (reporting is voluntary). For 2010, clinic data for British Columbia is incomplete.

Source: Canadian Institute for Health Information. 2014. *Number of Induced Abortions* Reported in Canada† in 2010, http://www.cihi.ca/CIHI-ext-portal/pdf/internet/TA_IO_ALLDATATABLES20120417_EN (retrieved July 22, 2015).

The word **abortion**, by strict definition, means the expulsion of an embryo or a fetus from the uterus before it is sufficiently developed to survive outside the uterus. As commonly used, however, the term *abortion* refers only to those expulsions that are artificially induced by mechanical means or drugs.

> **abortion**
> The artificially induced expulsion of an embryo or a fetus from the uterus.

Methods of Abortion

Abortion methods can be divided into two categories: surgical and medical. Surgical abortion is by far the most common.

Suction Curettage

First developed in China in 1958, **suction curettage** (commonly known as *dilation and curettage*, or D&C) is the most common method for abortions performed from the sixth to the twelfth week of pregnancy. The procedure can be done quickly, usually on an outpatient basis, and the risk of complications is small.

> **suction curettage**
> Removal of the embryo or fetus by means of suction; also called *dilation and curettage (D&C)*.

A sedative may be given, along with a local anaesthetic. A speculum is inserted into the vagina, and the cervix is cleansed with a surgical solution. The cervix is dilated and a suction curette, a specially designed tube, is then inserted into the uterus (see Figure 11.9). The curette is attached to the rubber tubing of an electric pump, and suction is applied. In 20–30 seconds, the uterus is emptied. Moderate cramping is common during evacuation. To ensure that no fragments of tissue are left in the uterus, the doctor usually scrapes the uterine lining with a metal curette, an instrument with a spoonlike tip. The entire suction curettage procedure takes five to ten minutes.

After a few hours in a recovery area, the woman can return home. She is usually instructed not to have intercourse or use tampons for several weeks after the abortion and to return for a post-abortion examination. This follow-up exam is important to verify that the abortion was complete and that no signs of infection are present.

Manual Vacuum Aspiration

For more than 30 years, gynecologists have used **manual vacuum aspiration (MVA)** to manage incomplete abortions, for endometrial sampling in non-pregnant women, and for elective abortion. During this procedure, as in suction curettage, the woman receives a local anaesthesia and her cervix is dilated. A plastic tube

FIGURE 11.9

Suction Curettage

This procedure takes five to ten minutes and can be performed up to the twelfth week of pregnancy.

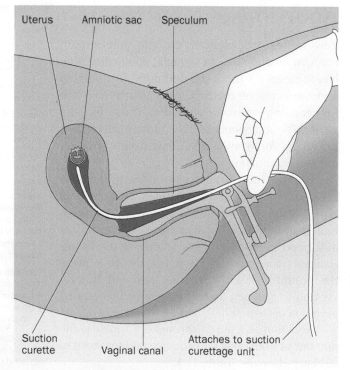

attached to a handheld syringe is inserted through the cervix and into the uterus. The syringe provides gentle suction, which empties the uterus.

> **manual vacuum aspiration (MVA)**
> The vacuum aspiration of uterine contents shortly after a missed period by using a handheld syringe.

MVA has several advantages over the traditional D&C. Manual vacuum aspiration may be used earlier in pregnancy, can be performed in the office, and does not require an electric pump or additional equipment. It is also significantly cheaper than suction curettage, does not require electricity, and can be performed by mid-level providers, such as midwives and nurses. For these reasons, MVA is ideal for low-resource settings. A number of recent studies have shown that the two techniques have equivalent safety profiles and low rates of complications when done up to 10 weeks of gestation.

Medical Abortion

Medical abortion is generally used in very early pregnancy, within 49 days of the last menstrual period. The combination of drugs that is given causes the embryo and products of conception to be passed out through the vagina, as in a natural miscarriage. An ultrasound may be performed before giving the medication to make sure that the pregnancy dates are accurate, because complication rates for medical abortion are higher if the pregnancy is more advanced.

Advantages and Disadvantages of Medical Abortion

Medical abortion is generally safer than surgical abortion because it involves no anaesthesia or surgical risks. Some women feel that medical abortion allows them to take more control of the procedure and gives them more privacy than a surgical abortion would. Medical abortion can also be done very early in pregnancy.

The major disadvantages of medical abortion are that the process takes days or even weeks to complete (early surgical abortion generally takes less than an hour and can be done under sedation), and that bleeding after the procedure is often heavier and lasts longer than with surgical abortion. Medical abortion also generally requires more clinic visits than surgical abortion.

Possible Psychological Effects

After an exhaustive review completed in 1988, it was concluded that the available evidence failed to demonstrate either a negative or a positive long-term impact of abortion on mental health. More recent research has resulted in the same general conclusion. The frequency of any psychiatric diagnosis in women who have undergone an abortion procedure is no higher than in women with no such history.

The psychological side effects of abortion, however, are less clearly defined than the physical ones. Responses vary and depend on the individual woman's psychological makeup, family background, current personal and social relationships, cultural attitudes, and many other factors. A woman who has specific goals with a somewhat structured life may be able to incorporate her decision to have an abortion as the unequivocally best and most acceptable course more easily than a woman who feels uncertain about her future.

Although many women experience great relief after an abortion and virtually no negative feelings, some go through a period of ambivalence. Along with relief, they often feel a mixture of other responses, such as guilt, regret, loss, sadness, and anger. When a woman feels she was pressured into sexual intercourse or into the abortion, she may feel bitter. If she strongly believes abortion to be immoral, she may wonder if she is still a good person. Many of these feelings are strongest immediately after the abortion, when hormonal shifts are occurring; such feelings often pass quite rapidly. Others take time to resolve and fade only slowly. It is important for a woman to realize that a mixture of feelings is natural. The decision-making process and feelings about abortion can be very complex for some women.

For a woman who experiences psychological or emotional effects after an abortion, talking with a close friend or family member can be very helpful. Supportive people can help her feel positive about herself and her decision. Although a legal and relatively common procedure in Canada, abortion is still treated very secretively in most of our society, so it is easy for a woman to feel isolated and alone. Many clinical centres that offer abortions make peer counselling available. Other women find they can identify with case histories in books written on abortion, which can help them deal with their own reactions. Unresolved emotions may persist, and a woman should seek professional counselling.

QUESTIONS FOR CRITICAL THINKING AND REFLECTION

What is your stand on the issue of late-term abortion? Do you feel it is never acceptable, or is it acceptable under certain circumstances? If so, what are those circumstances?

SUMMARY

- The female external sex organs are called the vulva; the clitoris plays an important role in sexual arousal and orgasm.
- The vagina leads to the internal sex organs, including the uterus, oviducts, and ovaries.
- The male external sex organs are the penis and the scrotum; the glans of the penis is an important site of sexual arousal.
- Internal sexual structures include the testes, vasa deferentia, seminal vesicles, and prostate gland.
- The fertilizing sperm determines the sex of the individual. Specialized genes on the Y chromosome initiate the process of male sexual differentiation in the embryo.
- Hormones initiate the changes that occur during puberty: The reproductive system matures, secondary sex characteristics develop, and the bodies of males and females become more distinctive.
- The menstrual cycle consists of four phases: menses, the estrogenic phase, ovulation, and the progestational phase.
- The ovaries gradually cease to function as women approach age 50 and enter menopause. The pattern of male sexual responses changes with age, and testosterone production gradually decreases.
- Sexual activity is based on stimulus and response. Stimulation may be physical or psychological.
- Vasocongestion and muscle tension are the primary physiological mechanisms of sexual arousal.
- The sexual response cycle has four stages: excitement, plateau, orgasm, and resolution.
- Physical and psychological problems can both interfere with sexual functioning.
- A treatment for sexual dysfunction first addresses any underlying medical conditions and then looks at psychosocial problems.
- Some gender characteristics are determined biologically, and others are defined by society. Children learn traits and behaviours traditionally deemed appropriate for one sex or the other.
- The ability to respond sexually is present at birth. Sexual behaviours emerging in childhood include self-exploration, perhaps leading to masturbation.
- Although puberty defines biological adulthood, people take five to ten more years to reach social maturity.
- Sexual fantasies and dreams and nocturnal emissions characterize adolescent sexuality.
- A person's sexual orientation can be heterosexual, gay or lesbian, or bisexual. Possible influences include genetics, hormonal factors, and early childhood experiences.
- Human sexual behaviours include celibacy, erotic fantasy, masturbation, touching, cunnilingus, fellatio, anal intercourse, and coitus.
- To evaluate whether an atypical sexual behaviour is problematic, experts consider the issues of consent between partners and whether the behaviour results in physical or psychological harm.

- Responsible sexuality includes open, honest communication; agreed-on sexual activities; sexual privacy; the use of contraception; safer sex practices; sober sex; and the taking of responsibility for consequences.
- Barrier methods of contraception physically prevent sperm from reaching the egg; hormonal methods are designed to prevent ovulation, fertilization, or implantation; and surgical methods permanently block the movement of sperm or eggs to the site of conception.
- The choice of contraceptive method depends on effectiveness, convenience, cost, reversibility, side effects and risk factors, and protection against STIs. Measures of effectiveness include failure rate and continuation rate.
- Hormonal methods of contraception include a combination of estrogen and progestins or progesterone alone. Hormones may be delivered via pills, patch, vaginal ring, implants, or injections.
- Hormonal methods of contraception prevent ovulation, inhibit the movement of sperm, and affect the uterine lining so that implantation is prevented.
- The most commonly used emergency contraceptives are two-dose regimens of oral contraceptives and Plan B, which is now available without a prescription to women 18 and older.
- How IUDs work is not clearly understood; they may cause biochemical changes in the uterus, affect movement of sperm and eggs, or interfere with the implantation of the egg in the uterus.
- Male condoms are simple to use, immediately reversible, and provide STI protection; female condoms are available but are more difficult to use.
- The diaphragm, Lea's Shield, cervical cap, and contraceptive sponge cover the cervix and block sperm from entering; all are used with or contain spermicide.
- Vaginal spermicides come in the form of foams, creams, jellies, suppositories, and film.
- Abortion is legal in Canada, and the procedure can be either surgical or medical.
- Psychological effects may be experienced by some women who undergo abortion; having a supportive friend, partner, or family is important to help with these challenges. Professional counselling may also be advised.

FOR MORE INFORMATION

BOOKS

Bogle, K. 2008. *Hooking Up: Sex, Dating and Relationships on Campus.* New York: New York University Press. An examination of the "hookup" culture on university and college campuses today.

Halbreich, U. 2003. New advances in premenstrual syndromes (PMS/PMDD). *Psychoneuroendocrinology* [Special Issue] 28(3 Suppl.). An entire issue devoted to all aspects of PMS and PMDD, including symptoms, treatments, and possible causes.

Kelly, G. F. 2011. *Sexuality Today,* 10th ed. New York: McGraw-Hill. An accessible approach that highlights cross-cultural examples, popular topics and issues, and case studies featuring university- and college-age individuals.

Marcus, E. 2005. *Is It a Choice? Answers to 300 of the Most Frequently Asked Questions About Gay and Lesbian People,* 3rd ed. San Francisco: Harper. Candid and informative information on coming out, family roles, and politics.

Meston, C., and D. Buss. 2009. *Why Women Have Sex.* New York: Times Books. A fascinating, readable, yet scholarly book about all aspects of female sexuality, especially sexual desire.

Omoto, A. M., and H. S. Kurtzman, eds. 2006. *Sexual Orientation and Mental Health: Examining Identity and Development in Lesbian, Gay, and Bisexual People.* Washington, D.C.: American Psychological Association. Topics in mental health as well as sexual behaviour, work satisfaction, and the well-being of children of same-sex couples.

Strong, B., et al. 2008. *Human Sexuality: Diversity in Contemporary America,* 6th ed. New York: McGraw-Hill. A comprehensive introduction to human sexuality.

Taverner, W. J. 2009. *Taking Sides: Clashing Views on Controversial Issues in Human Sexuality*, 11th ed. New York: McGraw-Hill. Pro and con position statements on sexuality issues relating to biology, behaviour, and legal and social issues.

ORGANIZATIONS, HOTLINES, AND WEBSITES

The Internet addresses listed here were accurate at the time of publication.

Center for Young Women's Health. Includes information about many topics, such as menstruation, gynecological exams, eating disorders, body piercing, and sexual health.
http://www.youngwomenshealth.org

Children Now. Provides advice for parents about talking with children about difficult issues, including sex, relationships, and STIs.
http://www.childrennow.org/parenting-resources/

International Planned Parenthood Federation. Provides information from a global service provider and a leading advocate of sexual and reproductive health and rights for all.
http://www.ippf.org

The Kinsey Institute for Research in Sex, Gender, and Reproduction. Provides information from one of the oldest and most respected institutions doing research on sexuality.
http://www.kinseyinstitute.org

Public Health Agency of Canada. Includes information about different methods of birth control.
http://www.sexualityandu.ca/birth-control/birth_control_methods_contraception

Sexuality and U. Provides credible and up-to-date information and education on sexual health.
http://www.sexualityandu.ca

Sex Information and Education Council of Canada. Fosters professional education and public knowledge about sexuality and sexual health.
http://www.sieccan.org

Sexuality Information and Education Council of the United States. Provides information on many aspects of sexuality including an extensive library and numerous publications.
http://www.siecus.org

World Association for Sexual Health. Works to promote sexual health for all.
http://www.worldsexualhealth.org

See also the listings for Chapters 10, 12, and 13.

SELECTED BIBLIOGRAPHY

Advance provision of emergency contraception for pregnancy prevention (full review). 2007. *Cochrane Database of Systematic Reviews* (2): CD005497.

Agot, K. E., et al. 2004. Risk of HIV-1 in rural Kenya: A comparison of circumcised and uncircumcised men. *Epidemiology* 15(2): 157–163.

Al-Sahab, B. et al. 2010. Age at menarche in Canada: results from the National Longitudinal Survey of Children & Youth. *BMC Public Health* 10: 736, http://www.biomedcentral.com/1471-2458/10/736.

Anawalt, B. D. 2007. Update on the development of male hormonal contraceptives. *Current Opinion in Investigational Drugs* 8(4): 318–323.

Ashok, P. W., et al. 2005. Patient preference in a randomized study comparing medical and surgical abortion at 10–13 weeks gestation. *Contraception* 71(2): 143–148.

Beckman, L. J., et al. 2006. Women's acceptance of the diaphragm: The role of relationship factors. *Journal of Sex Research* 43(4): 297–306.

Beksinska, M. E., et al. 2007. Bone mineral density in adolescents using norethisterone enanthate, depot-medroxyprogesterone acetate or combined oral contraceptives for contraception. *Contraception* 75(6): 438–443.

Bogaert, A. F. 2006. Biological versus nonbiological older brothers and men's sexual orientation. *Proceedings of the National Academy of Sciences* 103(28): 10771–10774.

Brohet, R. M., et al. 2007. Oral contraceptives and breast cancer risk in the international BRCA 1/2 carrier cohort study: A report from EMBRACE, GENEPSO, GEO-HEBON, and the IBCCS Collaborating Group. *Journal of Clinical Oncology* 25(25): 3831–3836.

Burkman, R. T. 2007. Transdermal hormonal contraception: Benefits and risks. *American Journal of Obstetrics and Gynecology* 197(2): 134.e1–134.e6.

Canadian Institutes for Health Information. 2014. Number of Induced Abortions Reported in Canada in 2010, by Province/Territory of Hospital or Clinic, http://www.cihi.ca/CIHI-ext-portal/pdf/internet/TA_10_ALLDATATABLES20120417_EN (retrieved July 22, 2015).

Chamley, L. W., and G. N. Clarke. 2007. Antisperm antibodies and conception. *Seminars in Immunopathology* 29(2): 169–184.

Coffee, A. L., et al. 2007. Long-term assessment of symptomatology and satisfaction of an extended oral contraceptive regimen. *Contraception* 75(6): 444–449.

Consumer Reports On Health. 2009. *Healthy Sex: His and Hers*, http://www.consumerreports.org/health/conditions-and-treatments/sex-health/overview/sexual-health-ov.htm (retrieved July 22, 2015).

Curtis, K. M., et al. 2007. Neoplasia with use of intrauterine devices. *Contraception* 75(6 Suppl.): S60–S69.

Dailar, Cynthia. 2006. *Guttmacher Policy Review*, http://www.guttmacher.org/pubs/gpr/09/3/gpr090312.html (retrieved July 22, 2015).

Elliot, S.L. 2011. Hot topics in erectile dysfunction. *BC Medical Journal* 53(9): 480–486.

Fazio, L., and G. Brock. 2004. Erectile dysfunction: management update. *Canadian Medical Association Journal* 170(9): 1429–1437.

Frye, C. A. 2006. An overview of oral contraceptives: Mechanism of action and clinical use. *Neurology* 66(6 Suppl.): S29–S36.

Gades, N. M., et al. 2005. Association between smoking and erectile dysfunction: A population-based study. *American Journal of Epidemiology* 161(4): 346–351.

Gilliam, M., et al. 2007. Factors associated with willingness to use the contraceptive vaginal ring. *Contraception* 76(1): 30–34.

Gordon, L., et al. 2007. Clinical inquiries. What hormonal contraception is most effective for obese women? *Journal of Family Practice* 56(6): 471–473.

Harris, M. A., J. C. Prior, and M. Koehoorn. 2008. Age at menarche in the Canadian population: Secular trends and relationship to adulthood BMI. *Journal of Adolescent Health* 43(6): 548–554.

Health Canada. 2006. *It's Your Health: Seniors and Aging—Sexual Activity*, http://www.serc.mb.ca/sites/default/files/resources/SeniorsAging_Sexual_Activity.pdf (retrieved April 21, 2015).

Hershberger, S. L., and N. L. Segal. 2004. The cognitive, behavioral, and personality profiles of male monozygotic triplet set discordant for sexual orientation. *Archives of Sexual Behavior* 33(5): 497–514.

Hijazi, R. A., and G. R. Cunningham. 2004. Andropause: Is androgen replacement therapy indicated for the aging male? *Annual Review of Medicine* 56: 117–137.

Hutcheson, J. C. 2004. Male neonatal circumcision: Indications, controversies and complications. *Urologic Clinics of North America* 31(3): 461–471.

Isley, M. M., and A. Edelman. 2007. Contraceptive implants: An overview and update. *Obstetrics and Gynecology Clinics of North America* 34(1): 73–90.

Jick, S., et al. 2007. Further results on the risk of nonfatal venous thromboembolism in users of the contraceptive transdermal patch compared to users of oral contraceptives containing norgestimate and 35 micrograms of ethinyl estradiol. *Contraception* 76(1): 4–7.

Kalmuss, D., and C. Tatum. 2007. Patterns of men's use of sexual and reproductive health services. *Perspectives on Sexual and Reproductive Health* 39(2): 74–81.

Laumann, E. O., et al. 2005. Sexual problems among women and men aged 40–80 y: Prevalence and correlates identified in the Global Study of Sexual Attitudes and Behaviors. *International Journal of Impotence Research* 17(1): 39–57.

Lee, J. M., et al. 2007. Weight status in young girls and the onset of puberty. *Pediatrics* 119(3): 624–630.

Lewis, B. H., et al. 2006. Medical implications of the male biological clock. *Journal of the American Medical Association* 296(19): 2369–2371.

Lurie, G., et al. 2007. Association of estrogen and progestin potency of oral contraceptives with ovarian carcinoma risk. *Obstetrics and Gynecology* 109(3): 597–607.

Macaluso, M., et al. 2007. Efficacy of the male latex condom and of the female polyurethane condom as barriers to semen during intercourse: A randomized clinical trial. *American Journal of Epidemiology* 166(1): 88–96.

MacIsaac, L., and E. Espey. 2007. Intrauterine contraception: The pendulum swings back. *Obstetrics and Gynecology Clinics of North America* 34(1): 91–111.

Margolis, K. L., et al. 2007. A prospective study of oral contraceptive use and risk of myocardial infarction among Swedish women. *Fertility and Sterility* 88(2): 310–316.

Meirik, O., and T. M. Farley. 2007. Risk of cancer and the oral contraceptive pill. *British Medical Journal* 335(7621): 621–622.

Moreau, C., et al. 2007. Oral contraceptive tolerance: Does the type of pill matter? *Obstetrics and Gynecology* 109(6): 1277–1285.

National Institutes of Health. 2007. *Decrease in Breast Cancer Rates Related to Reduction in Use of Hormone Replacement Therapy,* http://www.nih.gov/news/pr/apr2007/nci-18a.htm (retrieved July 21, 2015).

Nettleman, M. D., et al. 2007. Reasons for unprotected intercourse: Analysis of the PRAMS survey. *Contraception* 75(5): 361–366.

Padian, N. S., et al. 2007. Diaphragm and lubricant gel for prevention of HIV acquisition in southern African women: A randomized controlled trial. *Lancet* 370(9583): 251–261.

Prine, L. 2007. Emergency contraception, myths and facts. *Obstetrics and Gynecology Clinics of North American* 34(1): 127–136.

Rates of circumcision slashed in past 30 years. 2006. *The Gazette.* March 23: A13, http://www.cirp.org/news/2006-03-23montrealgazette/ (retrieved July 21, 2015).

Rossouw, J. E., et al. 2007. Postmenopausal hormone therapy and risk of cardiovascular disease by age and years since menopause. *Journal of the American Medical Association* 297(13): 1465–1477.

Roumen, F. J. 2007. The contraceptive vaginal ring compared with the combined oral contraceptive pill: A comprehensive review of randomized controlled trials. *Contraception* 75(6): 420–429.

Sanderson, C. A., and D. J. Yopyk. 2007. Improving condom use intentions and behavior by changing perceived partner norms: An evaluation of condom promotion videos for college students. *Health Psychology* 26(4): 481–487.

Shtarkshall, R. A., et al. 2007. Sex education and sexual socialization: Roles for educators and parents. *Perspectives on Sexual and Reproductive Health* 39(2): 116–119.Swica, Y. 2007. The transdermal patch and the vaginal ring: Two novel methods of combined hormonal contraception. *Obstetrics and Gynecology Clinics of North America* 34(1): 31–42.

Sulak, P. J., et al. 2006. Impact of an adolescent sex education program that was implemented by an academic medical center. *American Journal of Obstetrics and Gynecology* 195(1): 78–84.

Unicef Statistics and Monitoring Section. 2014. Female genital mutilation/cutting: a statistical overview and exploration of the dynamics of change, http://data.unicef.org/corecode/uploads/document6/uploaded_pdfs/corecode/FGMC_Lo_res_Final_26.pdf (retrieved July 21, 2015).

Wang, L., et al. 2004. Stress and dysmenorrhoea: A population based prospective study. *Occupational and Environmental Medicine* 61(12): 1021–1026.

WebMD. 2007. *Acne vulgaris,* http://www.emedicine.com/derm/topic2.htm (retrieved July 21, 2015).

Westhoff, C., et al. 2007. Initiation of oral contraceptives using a quick start compared with a conventional start: A randomized controlled trial. *Obstetrics and Gynecology* 109(6): 1270–1276.

Witte, S. S., et al. 2006. Promoting female condom use to heterosexual couples: Findings from a randomized clinical trial. *Perspectives on Sexual and Reproductive Health* 38(3): 148–154.

World Health Organization. 2007. *WHO and UNAIDS Announce Recommendations from Expert Consultation on Male Circumcision for HIV Prevention,* http://www.who.int/hiv/mediacentre/news68/en/print.html (retrieved July 22, 2015).

Zurawin, R. K., and L. Ayensu-Coker. 2007. Innovations in contraception: A review. *Clinical Obstetrics and Gynecology* 50(2): 425–439.

CHAPTER 12

Pregnancy and Childbirth

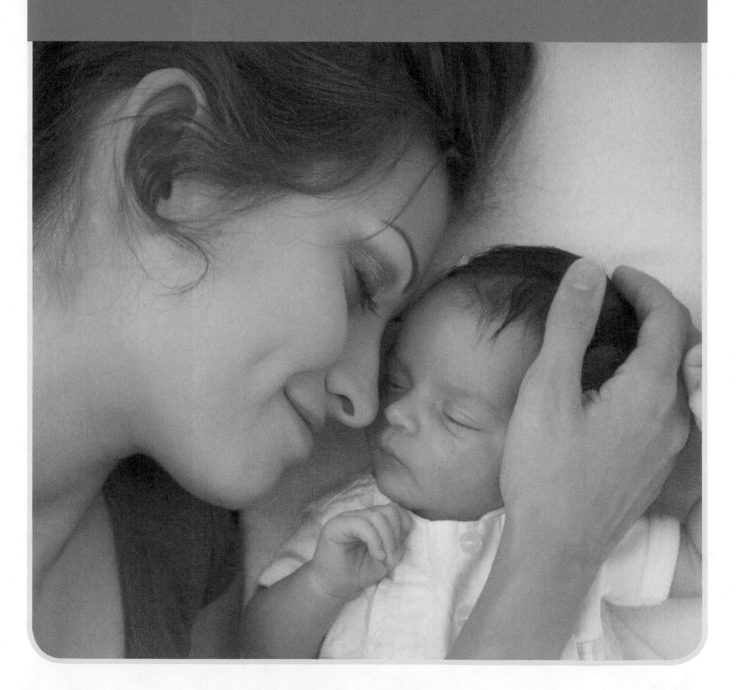

LOOKING AHEAD

After you have read and studied this chapter, you should be able to:

LO1 List key issues to consider when deciding about parenthood

LO2 Explain the process of conception, and describe the most common causes of and treatments for infertility

LO3 Describe the physical and emotional changes a pregnant woman typically experiences

LO4 Discuss the stages of fetal development

LO5 List the important components of good prenatal care

LO6 Describe the process of labour and delivery

TEST YOUR KNOWLEDGE

1. What is the average age of first-time mothers in Canada?
a. 23.6 b. 25.9 c. 28.5

2. What is the leading cause of female infertility?
a. growths in the uterus
b. exposure to radiation
c. tubal factors, such as blockages and previous infection

3. Before conception and in the early weeks of pregnancy, adequate intake of which of the following nutrients can reduce the risk of spina bifida and other neural tube defects?
a. iron b. folic acid c. calcium

4. Cigarette smoking before or during pregnancy is linked to which of the following?
a. congenital anomalies b. low birth weight c. miscarriage d. central nervous system defects e. all of the above

ANSWERS

1. c.   According to Statistics Canada, the average age of first-time mothers in 2011 was 28.5 years. The average age of first-time mothers in 1961 and 1991 was 23.6 and 25.9 years, respectively.

2. c.   If left untreated, the sexually transmitted infections (STIs) gonorrhea and chlamydia can lead to tubal scarring and blockage.

3. b.   It is recommended that all reproductive-age women consume 400 micrograms of folic acid from fortified foods and supplements each day to reduce the risk of spina bifida and other neural tube defects.

4. e.   Maternal smoking during pregnancy is associated with many types of birth defects and low birth weight. Lower measured intelligence levels and increased frequencies of behavioural and psychological abnormalities have been reported in children and adults whose mothers smoked cigarettes during pregnancy. Also, the risk of having a miscarriage is 20–80 percent higher among women who smoke cigarettes during pregnancy than it is in non-smokers.

Deciding whether to become a parent is one of the most important choices a person can ever make. Yet many people approach this decision with only a vague notion of what is involved in pregnancy and childbirth. This may help explain why about half of the pregnancies in Canada are unintentional.

Previous generations of Canadians assumed that virtually every married couple would have children. Today, however, with changing cultural expectations and more sophisticated contraceptive technology, you can choose whether and when to have a child. As a result of these changes, the average age of first-time mothers in Canada has steadily increased over the past 50 years. From 1961 to 2011, the average age of first-time mothers increased from 23.6 to 28.5 years. Figure 12.1 illustrates these trends. The more you know about conception and pregnancy, fetal development and prenatal care, and childbirth and parenting, the more capable you will be of making intelligent, informed decisions about them. This chapter presents information you can use both now and later in life to make the choices about pregnancy and childbirth that are right for you.

FIGURE 12.1

Average Age of Mother by Birth Order, Canada, 1945–2011

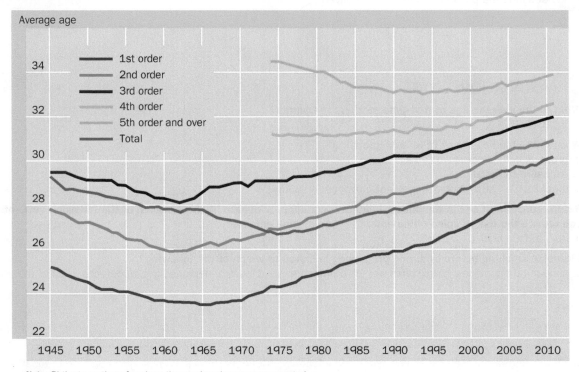

Note: Births to mothers for whom the age is unknown were prorated.

Sources: Statistics Canada, Canadian Vital Statistics, Births Database, 1945 to 2011, Survey 3231 and Demography Division, demographic estimates, http://www.statcan. gc.ca/pub/91-209-x/2013001/article/11784/c-g/fig03-eng.htm (retrieved September 26, 2015).

Preparation for Parenthood

Before you decide whether or when to become a parent, you should consider your suitability and readiness. If you elect to have a child, you can take some actions before the pregnancy begins to help ensure a healthy outcome.

Deciding to Become a Parent

Many factors must be taken into account when you are considering parenthood. Some issues are relevant to both men and women; others apply only to women.

Health and Age

Generally speaking, healthier women tend to have more trouble-free pregnancies and healthier babies. Women who are considering motherhood should see their doctor for a complete medical checkup to catch problems that might interfere with pregnancy or childbirth. For example, high blood pressure and diabetes may require ongoing attention; if uncontrolled, these health problems can pose life-threatening dangers to mother or child.

A mother's age can also be a factor in pregnancy and childbirth. Teenagers and women over age 35 have a higher incidence of certain problems that can affect the health of both mother and baby. In fact, most experts automatically classify a pregnancy as high-risk if the mother is over age 35, especially if it is her first pregnancy.

QUICK STATS

Across Canada, in 2011, the youngest average age of first-time mother was in Nunavut (22.1 years) and the oldest was in British Columbia (29.5 years).

—Statistics Canada, 2013

Emotional Preparedness

Just as they need to be physically prepared, parents also need to be emotionally ready to have a child. A new baby is helpless and relies on adults for everything. For parents, this means being strong and stable enough to handle the responsibility and being mature enough to give up certain freedoms to care for a child.

Financial Circumstances

Parenthood is financially draining, even for families with steady incomes. If you are planning to have a child, try to make sure you are prepared financially—especially during the first few years, when the costs of diapers, furniture, and other necessities quickly add up. It makes good sense for all expecting parents to consult with a financial planner, regardless of income level. A qualified financial planner can help new parents see their larger financial picture and focus on important issues, such as taxes, insurance needs, and saving for long-term goals and emergencies. A good rule of thumb is to prepare to spend approximately $10 000 per year per child.

Relationships

The stress and expense of child rearing can strain any relationship, even a healthy one, which is why it is important for couples to plan for parenting. Through open, honest discussion, partners should make sure they are both ready to take the step of having a child. Both should be equally committed to parenthood and agree on matters of child care, housework, and other day-to-day responsibilities. Couples with relationship problems should work together to resolve their issues—with professional help, if necessary—before adding a child to the mix.

New parents also need a strong support network of friends and family members who can lend a hand when things get tough. Many first-time parents count on their own parents and siblings for aid with child care or household chores. It can be easy, however, to alienate family and friends with too many requests for assistance. To avoid this problem, parents-to-be should include members of their support network in the planning process to figure out who will be able to help, in what ways, and at what times.

Future Plans

Having a child can put other life plans on hold, especially if the pregnancy is unintended. Anyone considering parenthood should make sure that it will fit with other goals. Otherwise, it may be necessary to postpone or cancel educational or career plans.

An important aspect of this planning is child care. New parents should figure out whether they will need child care services (such as a daycare centre or a private caregiver) in order to work or attend school.

The cost and availability of such services can be a deciding factor in determining whether parents can pursue their future plans. Canadian child care costs range from approximately $25 to $100 per day depending on the type of child care service; however, lower rates are often available for those in need of financial assistance.

Attitude and Aptitude

Before having a child, it's important for parents to recognize whether they have the right attitude about child rearing. If one parent is devoted to a child but the other views parenting as a burden, the partnership and the child will suffer. Before deciding to become a parent, it's a good idea to spend time with young children and see how you respond to them. It is also wise to talk to people who have raised children, and see if their experiences strike a positive chord in you.

Parents-to-be should also ask themselves how much they know about caring for a child and seek help according to their needs. Certain skills—such as diaper changing, bathing, and feeding—are essential but easy to learn and quickly become routine with a little practice. Other important parenting attributes, such as patience and the ability to stay calm in a crisis, aren't easily acquired if you don't already have them.

Luckily, many good sources of information are available for first-time parents. The best place to start is a family physician or pediatrician. Many hospitals and health units offer free or low-cost classes on labour, delivery, breastfeeding, and basic child care for expecting parents.

Pre-conception Care

The birth of a healthy baby depends in part on the mother's overall wellness before conception. The Society of Obstetricians and Gynaecologists of Canada (SOGC) recommends that all women receive health care to help them prepare for pregnancy. **Pre-conception care** should include an assessment of health risks, the promotion of healthy lifestyle behaviours, and any treatments necessary to reduce risk. The following are some of the issues, tests, and treatments involved during pre-conception care:

- *Pre-existing conditions:* Medical conditions, such as diabetes, epilepsy, asthma, high blood pressure, and anemia, can cause problems during pregnancy. These conditions should be treated and monitored closely throughout pregnancy.
- *Medications:* Some medications and dietary supplements harm the **fetus** (the unborn baby from the ninth week after conception to the moment of birth), so a pregnant woman may need to change or stop taking certain drugs.
- *Prior pregnancies:* Problems with previous pregnancies or deliveries—such as miscarriage, premature birth, or delivery complications—may be due to a treatable physical condition.

pre-conception care
Health care in preparation for pregnancy.

fetus
The developmental stage of a human from the ninth week after conception to the moment of birth.

- *Age:* As mentioned earlier, a woman's age may place her at risk for certain problems during pregnancy. A pregnant teenager, for example, may require special nutrition to meet her own growing body's needs and those of her baby. A woman over age 35 may need genetic testing because of the increased risk of her baby developing Down syndrome.

QUICK STATS

In 2011, the average age of fathers at the time of the birth of their first biological child was 28.3 years.

—Social and Aboriginal Statistics Division, Statistics Canada

- *Tobacco, alcohol, and caffeine use:* These substances can harm a developing fetus. Women who smoke, drink, or consume caffeine should stop before becoming pregnant. (See Chapters 14–16 for more information on these and other substances.)
- *Infections:* A woman who has any type of infection should be treated for the infection before getting pregnant, if possible. This is good advice for men, too, to avoid transmitting an infection to their partner. A woman may need to be vaccinated against hepatitis B, rubella (German measles), varicella (chicken pox), and other communicable diseases if she is at risk for them. Testing for tuberculosis and some STIs can ensure treatment before pregnancy. (See Chapters 9 and 13 for more on infectious diseases and STIs.)
- *HIV:* Any woman who is at risk of HIV infection should be tested before getting pregnant; her partner should be tested as well. (See Chapter 13 for more on HIV and AIDS.)
- *Diet:* Good nutrition is essential to a healthy pregnancy. Nutritional counselling can help a woman create a plan for healthy eating before and during pregnancy. Diet is especially important for any woman with special nutritional needs or an eating disorder, or who is overweight or obese. Physicians commonly prescribe prenatal vitamin supplements to pregnant women. The SOGC recommends that all women of childbearing age take extra folic acid to reduce the risk of neural tube defects that can arise in the fetus. (See Chapter 5 for more information on nutrition.)
- *Multiple births:* If twins or multiple births run in a woman's family, she is more likely to have multiple births, too. Multiple births are also more prevalent in mothers who are obese, over 40, or using certain reproductive technologies to get pregnant.
- *Genetic diseases:* If either partner has a family history of any genetic disease, then genetic counselling may be in order before pregnancy. Genetic testing can determine whether the mother or father is a carrier for a specific disease. With counselling, a couple can decide how best to deal with the possibility of transferring a disease to a child. Members of some ethnic groups are at higher risk for genetic disorders; for more information on these disorders, see the Dimensions of Diversity box.

Additional tests or changes in behaviour may be recommended for prospective parents who have recently travelled outside Canada; who work with chemicals, radiation, or toxic substances; who participate in physically demanding or hazardous activities or occupations; or who face significant psychosocial risks, including homelessness, an unsafe home environment, or mental illness.

 Dimensions *of* DIVERSITY

Ethnicity and Genetic Diseases

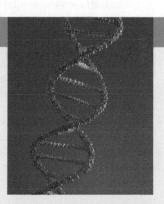

Genes carry the chemical instructions that determine the development of hundreds of individual traits, including disease risks, in every human being. Many traits and conditions involve multiple genes and environmental influences. Some diseases, however, can be traced to a mutation in a single gene.

Children inherit one set of genes from each parent. If only one copy of an abnormal gene is necessary to produce a disease, then it is called a *dominant* gene. Diseases caused by dominant genes seldom skip a generation; anyone who carries the gene will probably get the disease.

If two copies of an abnormal gene (one from each parent) are necessary for a disease to occur, then the gene is called *recessive*. Many diseases caused by recessive genes occur disproportionately in certain ethnic groups. Prospective parents who come from the same ethnic group can be tested for any recessive diseases that are known to occur in that group. If both parents are carriers, each of their children will have about a 25 percent chance of developing the disease.

The following list describes a few common conditions with proven genetic links in certain ethnic populations. If there is a history of any of these conditions in your family and you plan to have children, genetic tests and counselling can help assess the risk to your prospective offspring.

- *Sickle-cell disease* is common in the African-descended population of North America. It affects millions of people worldwide, primarily those whose ancestors come from sub-Saharan Africa, South America, Cuba,

Central America, Saudi Arabia, India, and Mediterranean countries (Turkey, Greece, and Italy). In this disease, red blood cells, which carry oxygen to the body's tissues, change shape; the normally disc-shaped cells become sickle-shaped. The altered cells carry less oxygen and can block small blood vessels. People who inherit one gene for sickle-cell disease experience only mild symptoms; those with two genes become severely, often fatally, ill. If you are at risk for sickle-cell disease, you should take care to reduce stress and respond to minor infections because red blood cells become sickle-shaped when the body is under stress. You should also have regular checkups and appropriate treatment, if required.

- *Hemochromatosis* (iron overload) affects about 1 in 200 people. At highest risk are people of Northern European (especially Irish), Mediterranean, and Hispanic descent. In hemochromatosis, the body absorbs and stores up to ten times the normal amount of iron. Iron deposits form in the joints, liver, heart, and pancreas. If untreated, the disease can cause organ failure and death. Early symptoms are often vague and include weakness, lethargy, darkening of the skin, and joint pain. Early detection and treatment are necessary to prevent damage. Treatment involves reducing iron stores by removing blood from the body (a process known as phlebotomy or "bloodletting"). Sometimes, if the person is eligible, donating blood on a regular basis can serve as the treatment.

- *Tay-Sachs disease*, another recessive disorder, occurs in about 1 in 3000 Jewish people of Eastern European ancestry. People with Tay-Sachs disease cannot properly metabolize fat. As a result, the brain and other nerve tissues deteriorate. Affected children show weakness in their movements and eventually develop blindness (by age 12–18 months) and seizures. This disease is fatal, and death usually occurs by age 6. No effective treatment is currently available.

- *Cystic fibrosis* occurs in 1 in 2500–3000 Caucasians; about 1 in 29 carries one copy of the cystic fibrosis gene. Because essential enzymes of the pancreas are deficient, the body cannot properly absorb nutrients. Thick mucus impairs functioning in the lungs and intestinal tracts of people with this disease. Cystic fibrosis is often fatal in early childhood, but treatments are increasingly effective in reducing symptoms and prolonging life. In some cases, symptoms do not appear until early adulthood.

- *Thalassemia* is a blood disease found most often among Italians, Greeks, and to a lesser extent people of African and Asian descent. When inherited from one parent, this form of anemia is mild; when two genes are present, the disease is severe and can cause fetal death. Children with this condition require repeated blood transfusions, eventually resulting in a damaging iron build-up. New interventions, such as genetic engineering, bone marrow transplants, and chemicals that bind with excess iron and remove it from the body, offer promise. Transplantation of stem cells from the umbilical cord blood of an unaffected sibling or donor is already being used in some cases. If you are at risk of carrying thalassemia, you should get regular checkups and monitor your health for symptoms, and learn ways to manage symptoms if they start to occur.

- *Lactose intolerance*, or intolerance to lactose-containing foods (primarily dairy products), is a common problem that often has a genetic component. Clinical symptoms of lactose intolerance include diarrhea, abdominal pain, and flatulence after ingestion of milk or milk-containing products. These symptoms result from low intestinal lactase levels, which are commonly caused by the reduced genetic expression of the enzyme lactase-phlorizin hydrolase. Genetically regulated reduction of lactase activity determined by racial or ethnic factors is the underlying mechanism of lactose malabsorption in healthy individuals. If you suspect lactose intolerance, see your doctor for a lactose absorption test. In the absence of a correctable underlying disease, lactose malabsorption is treated by reducing lactose intake, finding alternatives to foods containing lactose, taking an enzyme substitute, and maintaining calcium and vitamin D intake.

Other health problems that have a hereditary component and that disproportionately affect certain ethnic groups include diabetes, osteoporosis, high blood pressure, alcoholism, and certain cancers. Other chapters in this text discuss many of these links.

Understanding Fertility

Conceiving a child is a highly complex process. Although many couples conceive readily, others can testify to the difficulties that can be encountered.

Conception

The process of conception involves the **fertilization** of an ovum (egg) from a woman by a sperm from a man (see Figure 12.2). Every month during a woman's fertile years, her body prepares itself for conception and pregnancy. In one of her ovaries an egg matures and is released from its follicle. The egg, about the size of a pinpoint, travels through an oviduct, or fallopian tube, to the uterus in three to four days. The endometrium, or lining of the uterus, has already thickened for the implantation of a **fertilized egg**, or *zygote*. If the egg is not fertilized, it lasts about 24 hours and then disintegrates. It is expelled along with the uterine lining during menstruation.

fertilization
The initiation of biological reproduction: the union of the nucleus of an egg cell with the nucleus of a sperm cell.

fertilized egg
The egg after penetration by a sperm; a zygote.

FIGURE 12.2

Fertilization and Early Development of the Embryo

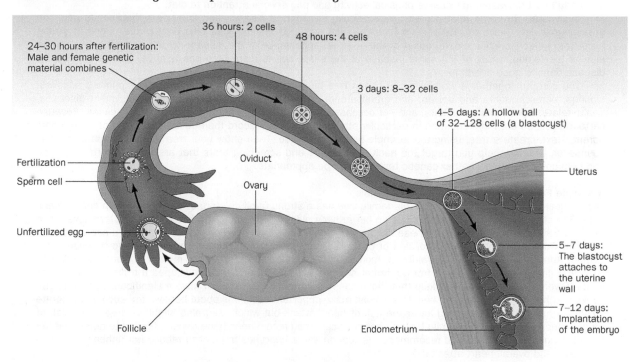

Sperm cells are produced in the man's testes and ejaculated from his penis into the woman's vagina during sexual intercourse (except in cases of artificial insemination or assisted reproduction). Sperm cells are much smaller than eggs. The typical ejaculate contains millions of sperm, but only a few complete the journey through the uterus and up the fallopian tube to the egg. Many sperm cells do not survive the acidic environment of the vagina.

Once through the cervix and into the uterus, many sperm cells are diverted to the wrong oviduct or get stuck along the way. Of those that reach the egg, only one will penetrate its hard outer layer. As sperm approach the egg, they release enzymes that soften this outer layer. Enzymes from hundreds of sperm must be released for the egg's outer layer to soften enough to allow one sperm cell to penetrate. The first sperm cell that bumps into a spot that is soft enough can swim into the egg cell. It then merges with the nucleus of the egg, and fertilization occurs. The sperm's tail, its means of locomotion, gets stuck in the outer membrane and drops off, leaving the sperm head inside the egg. The egg then releases a chemical that makes it impenetrable by other sperm.

The ovum carries the hereditary characteristics of the mother and her ancestors; sperm cells carry the hereditary characteristics of the father and his ancestors. Each parent cell—egg or sperm—contains 23 chromosomes, each of which contains genes, packages of chemical instructions for the developing baby. Genes provide the blueprint for a unique individual (see the Assess Yourself box for more information about genetics).

Assess YOURSELF

Creating a Family Health Tree

The genetic inheritance that each of us receives from our parents—and that our children receive from us—contains more than just physical characteristics, such as eye and hair colour. Heredity also contributes to our risk of developing certain diseases and disorders. For certain uncommon illnesses, such as hemophilia and sickle-cell disease, heredity is the primary cause; if your parents pass on the necessary genes, you will get the disease. But heredity plays a subtler role in many other diseases, which are caused at least in part by environmental influences, such as infection, cancer-causing chemicals, and physical inactivity. Although your genes alone will not produce those diseases, they can determine how susceptible you are. Researchers have found a genetic influence in many common disorders, including heart disease, diabetes, depression, asthma, alcoholism, and certain forms of cancer.

Knowing that a specific disease runs in your family can save your life. It allows you to watch for early warning signs and get screening tests more often than you otherwise would. Changing health habits, too, can be valuable for people with a family history of certain diseases. An individual with a family history of high cholesterol and early heart disease can increase physical activity and pay special attention to diet.

In general, the more relatives with a genetically transmitted disease and the closer they are to you, the greater your risk. However, non-genetic factors—such as health habits—can also play a role. Signs of strong hereditary influence include early onset of the disease, appearance of the disease largely or exclusively on one side of the family, onset of the same disease at the same age in more than one relative, and developing the disease despite good health habits.

You can put together a simple family health tree by compiling a few key facts on your primary relatives: siblings, parents, aunts and uncles, and grandparents. Those facts include the date of birth, major diseases, health-related conditions and habits, and, for deceased relatives, the age at death as well as the cause. Because certain diseases are more common in particular ethnic groups, also record the ethnic background of each grandparent. Next, create a tree, using the example below as a guide. Then show your tree to a physician or genetic counsellor, who can help you target the health behaviours and screening tests that are most important for you and help you determine whether genetic testing might be appropriate.

A Sample Family Health Tree and What It Means

The 55-year-old woman who prepared this family tree has a strong family history of osteoporosis on her mother's side. She also has several close relatives on her father's side of the family who had high cholesterol levels and had heart attacks at an early age. These risk factors significantly increase her chance of having a heart attack.

The woman has two aunts who died of breast cancer, but there are several reasons not to be overly concerned. Aunts are second-degree relatives, more distantly related to her than her mother or sister (first-degree relatives). In addition, they came from different sides of the family, and they developed the disease quite late in life. Given these factors, it is likely that these cases of breast cancer did not have a significant genetic origin. Looking at her family history can help this woman make important decisions about behaviours, such as moderate alcohol consumption, which may lower the risk of heart attack but which may also slightly increase the risk of breast cancer. Based on her family history, her physician may recommend bone density testing to determine her risk of dangerous fractures and recommend medication and a heart-healthy diet to reduce her unhealthy cholesterol level and overall heart attack risk.

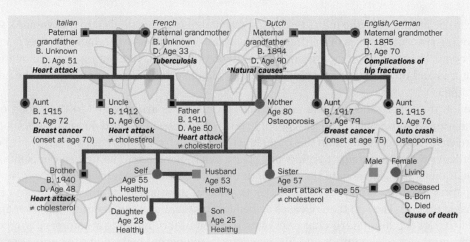

Sources: From "Prepare for the Future: Know Your Ancestors" and "Creating a Family Health Tree" © 1999 by Consumers Union of U.S., Inc. Yonkers, NY 10703-1057, a nonprofit organization. Reprinted with permission from the September 1999 issue of *Consumer Reports on Health*® for educational purposes only. No commercial use or reproduction permitted. (http://www.ConsumerReports.org)

As soon as fertilization occurs, the zygote starts to undergo the cell division that begins the growth process. It continues to divide as it travels through the oviduct to the uterus. On reaching the uterus, the cluster of cells, now called a *blastocyst*, becomes implanted in the endometrium.

The usual course of events is that one egg and one sperm unite to produce one fertilized egg and one baby. But if the ovaries release two (or more) eggs during ovulation and if both eggs are fertilized, twins will develop. These twins will be no more alike than siblings from different pregnancies, because each will have come from a different fertilized egg. Twins who develop this way are referred to as **fraternal twins**; they may be the same sex or different sexes. About 70 percent of twins are fraternal. Twins can also develop from the division of a single fertilized egg into two cells that develop separately. Because these babies share all genetic material, they are **identical twins**. The most serious complication of multiple births is preterm delivery (delivery before the fetuses are adequately mature). Studies show that the more fetuses a woman carries simultaneously, the shorter the gestational period will be. In 1934, the Dionne quintuplets were born in a northern Ontario farmhouse. This was Canada's most famous multiple birth because these quintuplets were the first in the world to be conceived and born naturally (before the advent of fertility medications) and to survive through infancy.

fraternal twins
Twins who develop from separate fertilized eggs; not genetically identical.

identical twins
Twins who develop from the division of a single zygote; genetically identical.

QUESTIONS FOR CRITICAL THINKING AND REFLECTION

If you don't have children now, do you plan to have them someday? Have you given any thought to the skills and qualities that make a good parent? Given what you know about yourself today, do you think you will make a good parent? What skills or qualities do you think you need to develop?

QUICK STATS

In 2011, about 3% of births in Canada were multiples.
—Statistics Canada, 2013

Infertility

Millions of couples have difficulty conceiving. **Infertility** is defined as the inability to conceive after trying for a year or more. It affects about 15 percent of the reproductive-age population of Canada. Many couples seek treatment for infertility each year. Although the focus is often on women (where the cause of infertility is found in 40 percent of cases), 20 percent of the factors contributing to infertility are male, and in 30 percent of infertile couples, both partners have problems. No cause can be found in 10 percent of cases. It is important that each individual be evaluated.

infertility
The inability to conceive after trying for a year or more.

Female Infertility

Female infertility usually results from one of two key causes—tubal blockage (40 percent) or failure to ovulate (40 percent). An additional 10 percent of cases of infertility are due to anatomical abnormalities, benign growths in the uterus, thyroid disease, and other uncommon conditions; the remaining 10 percent of cases are unexplained. Unexplained infertility implies that a cause for the infertility has not been found after completing all relevant investigations. This is often very frustrating for the couple involved.

Blocked fallopian tubes are most commonly the result of *pelvic inflammatory disease (PID)*, a serious complication of several sexually transmitted infections. Most cases of PID are associated with untreated cases of chlamydia or gonorrhea. The Public Health Agency of Canada reports that there are approximately 100 000 cases of symptomatic PID per year in Canada; however, since PID is often asymptomatic and is not reportable, up to two-thirds of cases go unrecognized. It is estimated that 10–15 percent of reproductive-age females have had PID. One episode of PID can result in infertility in 13 percent of patients. With a second infection, the risk increases to 36 percent and to 75 percent with a third infection. Tubal blockages can also be caused by prior surgery or by *endometriosis*, a condition in which endometrial (uterine) tissue grows outside of the uterus. This tissue responds to hormones and can cause pelvic pain, bleeding, scarring, and adhesions. Endometriosis is typically treated with hormonal therapy and surgery.

Age affects fertility; beginning at around age 30, a woman's fertility naturally begins to decline. Age is probably the main factor in ovulation failure. Exposure to toxic chemicals or radiation also appears to reduce fertility, as does cigarette smoking.

Male Infertility

Male factor infertility accounts for about 20 percent of infertile couples. The leading causes of male infertility can be divided into four main categories: hypothalamic pituitary disease or congenital disorders, testicular disease, disorders of sperm transport, and unexplained. Some acquired disorders of the testes can lead to infertility, such as damage from the following causes:

- Drug use (large doses of marijuana, for example, cause lower sperm counts and suppress certain reproductive hormones)
- Radiation
- Infection (such as having had mumps as a child)
- Environmental toxins
- Hyperthermia
- Smoking

Studies have identified a link between infertility and overweight and obesity in men, although the mechanism responsible for the relationship is not clear.

Treating Infertility

The cause of infertility can be determined for about 90 percent of infertile couples. Most cases of infertility are treated with conventional medical therapies. Surgery can repair oviducts, clear up endometriosis, and correct anatomical problems in both men and women. Fertility drugs can help women ovulate, although they may cause multiple births. If these conventional treatments don't work, couples can turn to **assisted reproductive technology (ART)** techniques, as described in the following sections.

assisted reproductive technology (ART)
Advanced medical techniques used to treat infertility.

Most infertility treatments are expensive and emotionally draining, however, and their success is hard to predict. Some infertile couples choose not to try to have children, while others turn to adoption. One measure you can take now to avoid infertility is to protect yourself against STIs and to treat promptly and completely any disease you do contract. Also, couples who are ready should consider trying to conceive before the woman's late 30s to decrease the probability of age-related infertility.

INTRAUTERINE INSEMINATION Male infertility can sometimes be overcome by collecting and concentrating the man's sperm and introducing it by syringe into a woman's vagina or uterus, a procedure known as **artificial (intrauterine) insemination**. To increase the probability of success, the woman is often given fertility drugs to induce ovulation before the insemination procedure. The sperm can be provided by the woman's partner or, if there are severe problems with his sperm or he carries a serious genetic disorder, by a donor. Donor sperm are also used by single women and lesbian couples who want to conceive by using artificial insemination. The success rate is about 60–70 percent.

> **artificial (intrauterine) insemination**
> The introduction of semen into the vagina by artificial means, usually by syringe.

IVF, GIFT, AND ZIFT Three related techniques for overcoming infertility involve removing mature eggs from a woman's ovary.
- In **in vitro fertilization (IVF)**, the harvested eggs are mixed with sperm in a laboratory dish. If eggs are successfully fertilized, one or more of the resulting embryos are inserted into the woman's uterus. IVF is often used by women with blocked oviducts.
- In **gamete intrafallopian transfer (GIFT)**, eggs and sperm are surgically placed into the fallopian tubes before fertilization.
- In **zygote intrafallopian transfer (ZIFT)**, eggs are fertilized outside the woman's body and surgically introduced into the oviducts after they begin to divide.

> **in vitro fertilization (IVF)**
> Combining egg and sperm outside the body and inserting the fertilized egg into the uterus.
>
> **gamete intrafallopian transfer (GIFT)**
> Surgically introducing eggs and sperm into the fallopian tube before fertilization.
>
> **zygote intrafallopian transfer (ZIFT)**
> Surgically introducing a fertilized egg into the fallopian tube.

GIFT and ZIFT can be used by women who have at least one open fallopian tube. Variations on these three techniques are also becoming available (see the In the News box).

IVF, GIFT, and ZIFT have drawbacks. Success rates vary from about 27 percent to 51 percent. They cost between $5000 and $13 000 per procedure and may require five or more cycles to produce one live birth. They also increase the chance of multiple births, which in turn increases the risk of premature birth and maternal complications, including pregnancy-related hypertension and diabetes.

SURROGATE MOTHERHOOD Surrogate motherhood involves a contract between an infertile couple and a fertile woman who agrees to carry a fetus. The surrogate mother agrees to be artificially inseminated by the father's sperm or to undergo IVF with the couple's embryo to carry the baby to term, and to give it to the couple at birth. In many areas of the world, the couple pays the surrogate mother for her services. However, in 2004, the Assisted Human Reproduction Act was passed in Canada, which prohibits payment to a surrogate mother, unless it is to reimburse her for expenses, such as medications, travel, and clothing.

QUESTIONS FOR CRITICAL THINKING AND REFLECTION

What are your personal views on infertility treatments? Do you feel they are appropriate, or do you think infertile couples should opt to adopt a child? If you were faced with a diagnosis of infertility, which choices would you consider?

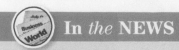

In *the* NEWS

Reproductive Technology

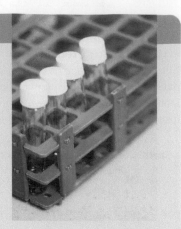

Research into the areas of genetics and cloning promise more breakthroughs for ART treatments. Below are a few of the most advanced techniques currently in use and under study.

Use of donor eggs, donor sperm, and donor embryos is fairly common in ART treatments. The use of donor eggs and embryos has allowed women in their fifties to complete pregnancy and deliver a baby. The resulting offspring is no more genetically related to the woman than an adopted child would be. Use of ART in women of this age is controversial.

Intracytoplasmic sperm injection (ICSI), in which a single sperm is injected into a mature egg, was originally developed to overcome cases of severe male infertility; it is now used for a broader range of conditions. Some studies have linked ICSI to an increase in genetic and birth defects in offspring. In addition, ICSI allows men who are infertile because of Y chromosome defects to have children, even though any sons they have will inherit the defect and also be infertile.

Cryopreservation of ovarian tissue and unfertilized eggs has been studied as a possible means of preserving fertility in women undergoing cancer therapy. In 2004, the first woman gave birth after having ovarian tissue removed and frozen before cancer chemotherapy and then reimplanted. This technique could potentially be used in women who choose to delay childbearing.

Freezing embryos is common in ART because multiple eggs are usually harvested and fertilized during IVF. If the initial IVF cycle is unsuccessful, the backup embryos can be used for additional attempts.

Preimplantation genetic diagnosis, in which embryos created through IVF undergo genetic analysis before implantation in the womb, was originally developed to help couples at risk for genetic diseases. According to the Assisted Human Reproduction Act, sex selection is prohibited in Canada, but outside Canada, some physicians now offer this technology for sex selection in couples who have no fertility problems.

Injection of cytoplasm (the material in a cell that surrounds the nucleus) from a younger woman's egg into an older woman's egg can be used as a possible means of reducing genetic errors in the older woman's egg. These errors occur in so-called mitochondrial DNA, genetic material in the cytoplasm of the cell that is passed along unchanged to offspring.

Nuclear transfer, a technique related to cytoplasm injection, uses cloning technology—the transfer of the nucleus from an older woman's egg into an egg from a younger woman from which the nucleus has been removed. In cytoplasm injection and nuclear transfer, the offspring carry DNA from two women—nuclear DNA from one woman and mitochondrial DNA from a second woman—and so have three genetic "parents."

Cloning is different from the techniques discussed here because it is a form of asexual reproduction in which offspring are genetically identical to one parent. In other words, a clone carries the genes of only one person, not two. However, as described above, the cloning technique of nuclear transfer could potentially be used in the treatment of infertility. Nuclear transfer could theoretically also be used to create a child that is the genetic offspring of two people of the same sex. However, under the Assisted Human Reproduction Act, any form of human cloning is illegal in Canada.

Emotional Responses to Infertility

Couples who seek treatment for infertility have often already confronted the possibility of not being able to become biological parents. Many infertile couples feel they have lost control over a major area of their lives. They may lose perspective on the rest of their lives as they focus more and more on the reasons for their infertility and on treatment. Infertile couples may need to set their own limits on how much treatment they are willing to undergo.

Support groups for infertile couples can provide help in this difficult situation, but there are few easy answers to infertility. If treatment is unsuccessful, couples must mourn the loss of the children they will never bear. They will need to make some kind of decision about their future—whether to pursue plans for adoption or another treatment or to adjust to childlessness and go on with their lives.

THINKING ABOUT THE ENVIRONMENT

Global studies indicate that sperm counts have dropped by as much as 50 percent in the past 30 years. Many researchers believe that exposure to toxic substances (such as lead, chemical pollutants, and radiation) may be the cause.

Of special interest is a class of chemicals called endocrine disrupters—substances found widely in the environment that mimic or interfere with the body's hormones. Endocrine disrupters may cause problems with reproduction, development, and fertility in humans; tests have linked these chemicals to reproductive problems in animals. Endocrine disrupters can be found in plastics, detergents, food, toys, cosmetics, pesticides, and other everyday products. The Government of Canada is taking national and international measures to investigate the effects of endocrine disruptors.

For more information on the environment and health, see Chapter 21.

Pregnancy

Pregnancy is usually discussed in terms of **trimesters**—three periods of about three months (or 13 weeks) each. During the first trimester, the mother experiences a few physical changes and some fairly common symptoms. During the second trimester, often the most peaceful time of pregnancy, the mother gains weight, looks noticeably pregnant, and may experience a general sense of well-being if she is happy about having a child. The third trimester is the hardest for the mother because she must breathe, digest, excrete, and circulate blood for herself and the growing fetus. The weight of the fetus, the pressure of its body on her organs, and its increased demands on her system can cause discomfort and fatigue and may make the mother increasingly impatient to give birth.

> **trimester**
> One of the three, three-month periods of pregnancy.

Pregnancy Tests

The earliest tests for pregnancy are chemical tests designed to detect the presence of **human chorionic gonadotropin (HCG)**, a hormone produced by the implanted fertilized egg. These tests may be performed as early as two weeks after fertilization.

> **human chorionic gonadotropin (HCG)**
> A hormone produced by the fertilized egg that can be detected in the urine or blood of the mother within a few weeks of conception.

Home pregnancy test kits, which are sold in drugstores without a prescription, include a small sample of red blood cells coated with HCG antibodies, to which the woman adds a small amount of her urine. If the concentration of HCG is great enough, it will clump together with the HCG antibodies, indicating that the woman is pregnant. Home pregnancy tests can be very reliable, but the instructions must be followed carefully. If a home test done at the time of a missed menstrual period is negative, retesting after another week is recommended. In the first day or two following a missed period, the concentration of HCG may be too low to be detected by the test.

Changes in the Woman's Body

Hormonal changes begin as soon as the egg is fertilized, and for the next nine months the woman's body nourishes the fetus and adjusts to its growth. Let's take a closer look at the changes of early, middle, and late pregnancy (see Figure 12.3).

Early Signs and Symptoms

Early recognition of pregnancy is important, especially for women with physical problems and nutritional deficiencies. The following symptoms are not absolute indications of pregnancy, but they are reasons to visit a health care provider:

- *A missed menstrual period:* If an egg has been fertilized and implanted in the uterine wall, the endometrium is retained to nourish the embryo. A woman who misses a period after having intercourse may be pregnant.
- *Slight bleeding:* Slight bleeding follows implantation of the fertilized egg in about 14 percent of pregnant women. Because this happens about the time a period is expected, the bleeding is sometimes mistaken for menstrual flow. It usually lasts only a few days.
- *Nausea:* About two-thirds of pregnant women feel nauseated, probably as a reaction to increased levels of progesterone and other hormones. Although this nausea is often called *morning sickness*, some women have it all day long. It frequently begins during the 6th week and disappears by the 12th week. In some cases, it lasts throughout the pregnancy.
- *Breast tenderness:* Some women experience breast tenderness, swelling, and tingling, usually described as different from the tenderness experienced before menstruation.
- *Increased urination:* Increased frequency of urination can occur soon after the missed period.
- *Sleepiness, fatigue, and emotional upset:* These symptoms result from hormonal changes. Fatigue can be surprisingly overwhelming in the first trimester, but usually improves significantly around the third month of pregnancy.

The first reliable physical signs of pregnancy can be distinguished about four weeks after a woman misses her menstrual period. A softening of the uterus just above the cervix, called *Hegar's sign*, and other changes in the cervix and pelvis are apparent during a pelvic examination. The labia minora and the cervix may take on a purple colour rather than their usual pink hue.

FIGURE 12.3

Physiological Changes during Pregnancy

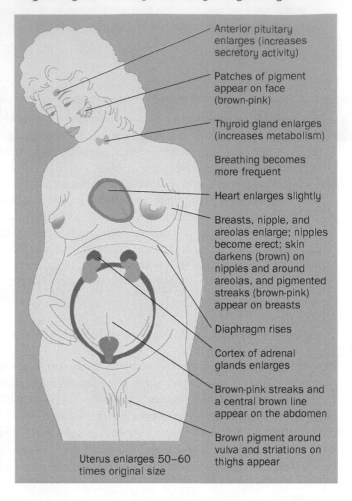

- Anterior pituitary enlarges (increases secretory activity)
- Patches of pigment appear on face (brown-pink)
- Thyroid gland enlarges (increases metabolism)
- Breathing becomes more frequent
- Heart enlarges slightly
- Breasts, nipple, and areolas enlarge; nipples become erect; skin darkens (brown) on nipples and around areolas, and pigmented streaks (brown-pink) appear on breasts
- Diaphragm rises
- Cortex of adrenal glands enlarges
- Brown-pink streaks and a central brown line appear on the abdomen
- Brown pigment around vulva and striations on thighs appear

Uterus enlarges 50–60 times original size

Four weeks after a woman misses her menstrual period, she would be considered to be about eight weeks pregnant because pregnancy is calculated from the time of a woman's last menstrual period rather than from the time of actual fertilization. (The timing of ovulation and fertilization is often difficult to determine.) Although a woman should see her physician to determine her due date, due dates can be approximated by subtracting three months from the date of the last menstrual period and then adding seven days. For example, a woman whose last menstrual period began on September 20 would have a due date of about June 27.

Continuing Changes in the Woman's Body

The most obvious changes during pregnancy occur in the reproductive organs. During the first three months, the uterus enlarges to about three times its non-pregnant size, but it still cannot be felt in the abdomen. By the fourth month, it is large enough to make the abdomen protrude. By the seventh or eighth month, the uterus pushes up into the rib cage, which makes breathing slightly more difficult. The breasts enlarge and are sensitive; by week eight, they may tingle or throb. The pigmented area around the nipple, the areola, darkens and broadens.

Other changes are going on as well. Early in pregnancy, the muscles and ligaments attached to bones begin to soften and stretch. The joints between the pelvic bones loosen and spread, making it easier to have a baby but harder to walk. The circulatory system becomes more efficient to accommodate the blood volume, which increases by 50 percent, and the heart pumps it more rapidly. Much of the increased blood flow goes to the uterus and placenta (the organ that exchanges nutrients and waste between mother and fetus). The mother's lungs also become more efficient, and her rib cage widens to permit her to inhale up to 40 percent more air. Much of the oxygen goes to the fetus. The kidneys become highly efficient, removing waste products from fetal circulation and producing large amounts of urine by mid-pregnancy.

The average weight gain during a healthy pregnancy is 12.5 kilograms (about 28 pounds), although actual weight change depends on the individual. According to Health Canada, the recommended weight gain in pregnancy is based on a woman's pre-pregnancy BMI (Body Mass Index). A pregnancy weight gain calculator can be found on Health Canada's website (search for it at www.hc-sc.gc.ca). About 60 percent of the weight gain is directly related to the baby (such as the fetus and placenta); the rest accumulates over the woman's body as fluid and fat.

As the woman's skin stretches, small breaks may occur in the elastic fibres of the lower layer of skin, producing *stretch marks* on her abdomen, hips, breasts, or thighs. Increased pigment production darkens the skin in 90 percent of pregnant women, especially in places that have stretched.

Changes During the Later Stages of Pregnancy

By the end of the sixth month, the increased needs of the fetus place a burden on the mother's lungs, heart, and kidneys. Her back may ache from the pressure of the baby's weight and from having to throw her shoulders back to keep her balance while standing, as shown in Figure 12.4. Her body retains more water, perhaps up to three extra litres of fluid. Her legs, hands, ankles, or feet may swell, and she may be bothered by leg cramps, heartburn, or constipation. Despite discomfort, both her digestion and her metabolism are working at top efficiency.

FIGURE 12.4

The Fetus during the Third Trimester of Pregnancy

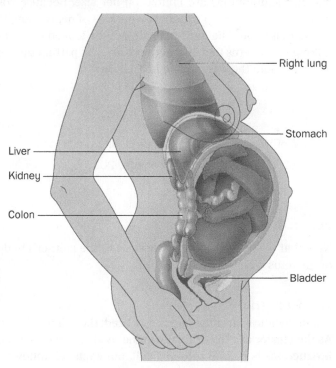

The uterus prepares for childbirth with preliminary contractions, called *Braxton Hicks contractions*. Unlike true labour contractions, these are usually short, irregular, and painless. The mother may only be aware that at times her abdomen is hard to the touch. These contractions become more frequent and intense as the delivery date approaches.

In the ninth month, the baby settles into the pelvic bones, usually head down, fitting snugly. This process, called **lightening**, allows the uterus to sink down about five centimetres, producing a visible change in the mother's profile. Pelvic pressure increases, and pressure on the diaphragm lightens. Breathing becomes easier; urination becomes more frequent. Sometimes, after a first pregnancy, the baby doesn't settle down into the pelvis until labour begins.

> **lightening**
> A process in which the uterus sinks down because the baby's head settles into the mother's pelvic area.

Emotional Responses to Pregnancy

Rapid changes in hormone levels can cause a pregnant woman to experience unpredictable emotions. A large part of pregnancy is beyond the woman's control—her changing appearance, her energy level, her variable moods—and some women need extra support and reassurance. Hormonal changes can also make women feel exhilarated and euphoric, although for some women such moods are temporary.

Like the physical changes that accompany pregnancy, emotional responses also change as the pregnancy develops. During the first trimester, the pregnant woman may fear that she may miscarry or that the child will not be normal. Education about pregnancy and childbirth and support from her partner, friends, relatives, and health care professionals are important antidotes to these fears (see the Gender Matters box).

During the second trimester, the pregnant woman can feel the fetus move within her, and worries about miscarriages usually begin to diminish. She may look and feel happy and be delighted as her pregnancy begins to show. However, she may also worry that her increasing size makes her unattractive. Reassurance from her partner can ease these fears.

The third trimester is the time of greatest physical stress during the pregnancy. A woman may find that her physical abilities are limited by her size. Because some women feel physically awkward and sexually unattractive, they may experience periods of depression. But many also feel a great deal of happy excitement and anticipation. The fetus may already be looked on as a member of the family, and both parents may begin talking to the fetus and interacting with it by patting the mother's belly. The upcoming birth will probably be a focus for both the woman and her partner.

QUICK STATS

10% of women have depression during pregnancy.

—Public Health Agency of Canada, 2012

Fetal Development

Now that we have seen what happens to the mother's body during pregnancy, let's consider the development of the fetus (see Figure 12.5).

The First Trimester

About 30 hours after the egg is fertilized, the cell divides, and this process of cell division repeats many times. As the cluster of cells drifts down the oviduct, several different kinds of cells emerge. The entire set of genetic instructions is passed to every cell, but each cell follows only certain instructions; if this were not the case,

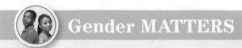

Gender MATTERS

Pregnancy Tasks for Fathers

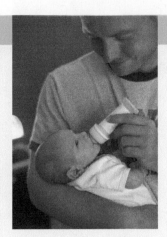

Before the Pregnancy

- *Consider your lifestyle and health habits.* A healthy lifestyle can help boost fertility and improve pregnancy outcome. Being too thin or too heavy may lower a man's sperm count, as may marijuana use. Men who smoke and drink have a lower concentration of sperm and a lower percentage of active sperm. Exposure to chemicals on the job may also affect pregnancy.
- *Check your budget and financial situation.* Make sure your finances are in order and that you have as much life, health, and disability insurance as you may need. See a financial planner for advice. Try putting away extra money every month now—both to practise living on a tighter budget and to save.
- *Get any necessary health checks and genetic counselling.* See the discussion of potential health concerns in the section "Pre-conception Care."

During the Pregnancy

- *Help your partner stay healthy during the pregnancy.* If you smoke, quit; second-hand smoke is dangerous for the developing fetus. Support your partner by making other lifestyle changes or joining her in any changes she is making; for example, drink non-alcoholic beverages, take walks with her, and get extra sleep.
- *Help around the home and with planning for the baby.* Help shop for necessities, and help get your home ready for a baby. Pregnancy is hard work, so providing extra help with household chores and errands can be an important element of support. For example, because of the risk of infection by toxoplasmosis, pregnant women should avoid handling cat litter; if you and your partner have a cat, emptying the litter box should be your job.
- *Be involved.* Go to all the prenatal visits, birth preparation or education classes, hospital tours, and so on. Learn more about pregnancy, childbirth, and parenting by reading books, visiting Internet sites, and talking with other parents.

After the Baby Arrives

- *Help meet your baby's needs.* If your job allows, take parental leave to help with the new baby. Support the new mother by helping with baby care (feeding, diaper changes), laundry, shopping, and other chores. Take turns or join the mother when the baby needs care or feeding during the night; one survey found that more than half of fathers continue to sleep or pretend to be asleep when their babies cry during the night.
- *Support your partner, and ask others for help.* It is normal for a new mother to be tired and to experience mood changes, and some men also experience anxiety about their new role. Good communication between partners and help from supportive relatives and friends can help new parents adjust.
- *Give your partner some time off.* A new mother needs time to recover from childbirth, even after she leaves the hospital or birthing centre. This is especially true if the delivery was difficult, if a Caesarean section was performed, or if an episiotomy was required. Aside from doing the daily chores, the father can help the mother's recuperation by taking the baby for a few hours at a time. If the baby is being bottle-fed, take charge for a morning, an afternoon, or even the entire day.

---

we would not have different organs or body parts. For example, all cells carry genes for hair colour and eye colour, but only the cells of the hair follicles and irises (of the eye) respond to that information.

Around the fourth day after fertilization, the cluster, now about 32–128 cells and hollow, arrives in the uterus; this is a **blastocyst**. On about the sixth or seventh day, the blastocyst attaches to the uterine wall, usually along the upper curve; over the next few days, it becomes firmly implanted and begins to draw nourishment from the endometrium, the uterine lining.

blastocyst
A stage of development, days 6–14, before the cell cluster becomes the embryo and placenta.

FIGURE 12.5

A Chronology of Milestones in Prenatal Development

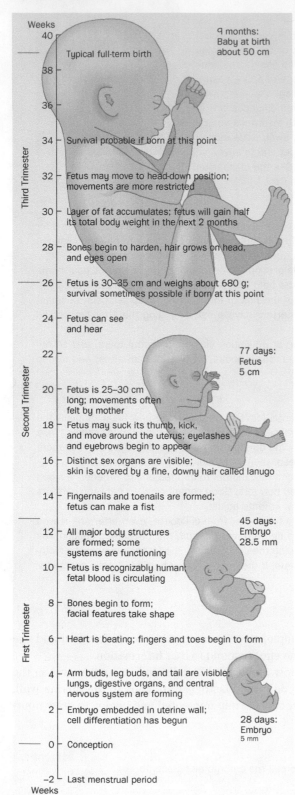

Weeks

40 — Typical full-term birth

9 months: Baby at birth about 50 cm

Third Trimester

38

36

34 — Survival probable if born at this point

32 — Fetus may move to head-down position; movements are more restricted

30 — Layer of fat accumulates; fetus will gain half its total body weight in the next 2 months

28 — Bones begin to harden, hair grows on head, and eyes open

26 — Fetus is 30–35 cm and weighs about 680 g; survival sometimes possible if born at this point

24 — Fetus can see and hear

Second Trimester

22

77 days: Fetus 5 cm

20 — Fetus is 25–30 cm long; movements often felt by mother

18 — Fetus may suck its thumb, kick, and move around the uterus; eyelashes and eyebrows begin to appear

16 — Distinct sex organs are visible; skin is covered by a fine, downy hair called lanugo

14 — Fingernails and toenails are formed; fetus can make a fist

First Trimester

12 — All major body structures are formed; some systems are functioning

45 days: Embryo 28.5 mm

10 — Fetus is recognizably human; fetal blood is circulating

8 — Bones begin to form; facial features take shape

6 — Heart is beating; fingers and toes begin to form

4 — Arm buds, leg buds, and tail are visible; lungs, digestive organs, and central nervous system are forming

2 — Embryo embedded in uterine wall; cell differentiation has begun

28 days: Embryo 5 mm

0 — Conception

–2 — Last menstrual period

Weeks

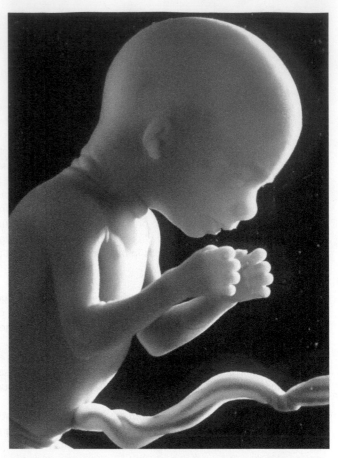

By the fourth month, the fetus is growing rapidly and is about 25 centimetres long. Weighing about 170 grams, it moves vigorously in the uterus and can suck its thumb, frown, and turn its head.

The blastocyst becomes an **embryo** by about the end of the second week after fertilization. The inner cells of the blastocyst separate into three layers. One layer becomes inner body parts, the digestive and respiratory systems; the middle layer becomes muscle, bone, blood, kidneys, and sex glands; and the third layer becomes the skin, hair, and nervous tissue.

embryo
The stage of development between blastocyst and fetus; about weeks two to eight.

The outermost shell of cells becomes the **placenta**, **umbilical cord**, and **amniotic sac**, as shown in Figure 12.6. A network of blood vessels called *chorionic villi* eventually forms the placenta. The human placenta allows a two-way exchange of nutrients and waste materials between the mother and the fetus. The placenta brings oxygen and nutrients to the fetus and transports waste products out. The placenta does not

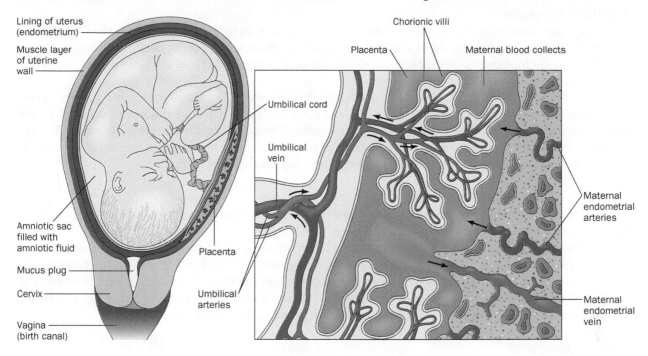

FIGURE 12.6

A Cross-sectional View of the Fetus in the Uterus and an Enlargement of the Placenta

provide a perfect barrier between the fetal circulation and the maternal circulation, however. Some blood cells are exchanged and certain substances, such as alcohol, pass freely from the maternal circulation through the placenta to the fetus.

placenta
The organ through which the fetus receives nourishment and empties waste via the mother's circulatory system; after birth, the placenta is expelled from the uterus.

umbilical cord
The cord connecting the placenta and fetus, through which nutrients pass.

amniotic sac
A membranous pouch enclosing and protecting the fetus; also holds amniotic fluid.

The period between weeks two and nine is a time of rapid differentiation and change. All the major body structures are formed during this time, including the heart, brain, liver, lungs, and sex organs; the eyes, nose, ears, arms, and legs also appear. Some organs begin to function—the heart begins to beat, and the liver starts producing blood cells. Because body structures are forming, the developing organism is vulnerable to damage from environmental influences, such as drugs and infections (discussed in detail in sections that follow).

By the end of the second month, the brain sends out impulses that coordinate the functioning of other organs. The embryo is now a fetus, and most further changes will be in the size and refinement of working body parts. In the third month, the fetus begins to be quite active. By the end of the first trimester, the fetus is about 2.5 centimetres long and weighs less than 30 grams.

The Second Trimester

To grow to about 35 centimetres and 680 grams during the second trimester, the fetus must have large amounts of food, oxygen, and water, which come from the mother through the placenta. All body systems are operating, and the fetal heartbeat can be heard with a stethoscope. The mother can detect fetal movements beginning in the fourth or fifth month. Against great odds, a fetus born prematurely at the end of the second trimester might survive.

The Third Trimester

The fetus gains most of its birth weight during the last three months. Some of the weight is fatty tissue under the skin that insulates the fetus and supplies food. The fetus needs a great deal of calcium, iron, and nitrogen from the food the mother eats. Some 85 percent of the calcium and iron she consumes goes into the fetal bloodstream.

Although the fetus may live if it is born during the seventh month, it needs the fat layer acquired in the eighth month and time for the organs, especially the respiratory and digestive organs, to develop. It also needs the immunity supplied by the antibodies in the mother's blood during the final three months. The antibodies protect the fetus against many of the diseases to which the mother has acquired immunity. Breast milk can help the baby further resist infections because it also contains maternal antibodies.

Diagnosing Fetal Abnormalities

About 3 percent of babies are born with a major birth defect. Information about the health and sex of a fetus can be obtained before birth through prenatal testing.

Ultrasonography (also called *ultrasound*) uses high-frequency sound waves to create a **sonogram**, or visual image, of the fetus in the uterus. Sonograms show the position of the fetus, its size and gestational age, and the presence of certain anatomical problems. Sonograms can sometimes be used to determine the sex of the fetus. Sonograms are considered safe for a pregnant woman and the fetus, but both the SOGC and Health Canada advise against "keepsake" sonograms performed for no medical purpose.

> **ultrasonography**
> The use of high-frequency sound waves to view the fetus in the uterus; also known as *ultrasound*.
>
> **sonogram**
> The visual image of the fetus produced by ultrasonography.

Amniocentesis involves the removal of fluid from the uterus with a long, thin needle inserted through the abdominal wall. It is usually performed between 15 and 18 weeks into the pregnancy, although earlier amniocentesis is available. A genetic analysis of the fetal cells in the fluid can reveal the presence of chromosomal disorders, such as Down syndrome, and some genetic diseases, including Tay-Sachs disease. The sex of the fetus can also be determined. Most amniocentesis tests are performed on pregnant women over age 35, who have a greater risk of chromosomal abnormalities, or in cases where the fetus is known to be at risk for a particular chromosomal or genetic defect. Amniocentesis carries a slight risk (a 0.3–0.7 percent chance) of miscarriage.

> **amniocentesis**
> A process in which amniotic fluid is removed and analyzed to detect possible birth defects.

Another prenatal test is **chorionic villus sampling (CVS)**, which can be performed earlier in pregnancy than amniocentesis, between weeks 10 and 12. This procedure involves removal through the cervix (by catheter) or abdomen (by needle) of a tiny section of chorionic villi,

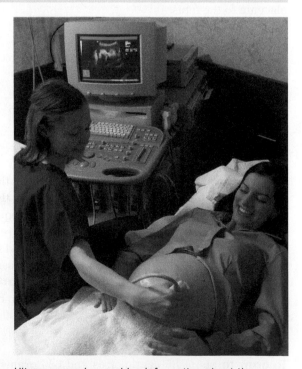

Ultrasonography provides information about the position, size, and physical condition of a fetus in the uterus.

which contain fetal cells that then can be analyzed. When CVS first became available, it was associated with a higher risk of miscarriage than amniocentesis, but by 2003 the two procedures were found to be equally safe.

chorionic villus sampling (CVS)
Surgical removal of a tiny section of chorionic villi to be analyzed for genetic defects.

Integrated prenatal screening (IPS) can be used to help identify fetuses with neural tube defects, Down syndrome, and other anomalies. IPS combines ultrasound evaluation of nuchal translucency (the thickness of the back of the fetus's neck) with two separate maternal blood tests done between the 11th and 14th week and the 15th and 18th week of pregnancy. The blood is analyzed for four hormone levels: human chorionic gonadotropin (HCG), unconjugated estriol, alpha-fetoprotein (AFP), and pregnancy associated plasma protein-A (PAPP-A). The hormone levels and ultrasound measurements are compared with appropriate standards, and the results are used to estimate the probability that the fetus has particular anomalies. IPS is a screening test rather than a diagnostic test and it has a false positive rate of about 2–4 percent. In the case of abnormal IPS results, parents may choose further testing, such as amniocentesis or CVS. The SOGC recommends that amniocentesis or CVS be performed only in women with an abnormal IPS result or in pregnant woman over 40 years of age.

integrated prenatal screen (IPS)
A combination of an ultrasound and two blood tests, used to assess the risk of fetal abnormalities.

Genetic counsellors explain the results of the different tests so that parents can understand their implications. If a fetus is found to have a defect, it may be carried to term, aborted, or, in rare instances, treated while still in the uterus. Results of most current screening tests are not available until after week 12 of pregnancy; consequently, if abortion is chosen, it is likely to involve one of the more medically complex and physically difficult methods (see Chapter 11). Researchers are searching for new fetal screening techniques that are less invasive and that can be done earlier in pregnancy.

QUICK STATS

In 2011, the infant mortality rate in Canada was about 5 in 1000.
—Statistics Canada, 2013

Fetal Programming

Amniocentesis, CVS, and IPS look for chromosomal, genetic, and other anomalies that typically cause immediate problems. A new area of study known as *fetal programming theory* focuses on how conditions in the womb may influence the risk of adult diseases. For example, researchers have linked low birth weight to an increased risk of heart disease, high blood pressure, obesity, diabetes, and schizophrenia; high birth weight in female infants, however, has been linked to an increased risk of breast cancer in later life.

How might conditions during gestation affect the risk of adult diseases? A number of studies have looked at groups of people born in areas of poverty or at times of famine, when pregnant women were unable to eat properly. The poor prenatal conditions that stunt the growth of a developing fetus and lead to low birth weight may also affect specific organs. For example, if energy is limited, resources may be directed toward the developing fetal brain and away from other organs, including the liver and kidneys. Later in life, a small liver may be unable to clear cholesterol from the bloodstream, thereby increasing cholesterol levels and raising the risk of heart disease; undersized kidneys may be less able to regulate blood pressure. The fetus may also respond to limited resources by developing a permanently thrifty metabolism that triggers increased appetite and fat storage—leading to a greater risk of adult obesity and diabetes. Stress, both physical and emotional, increases maternal levels of the hormone cortisol, which in turn may permanently affect an infant's system of blood pressure regulation (see the Mind Body Spirit box).

Mind *Body* SPIRIT

Stress and Pregnancy

High levels of stress can have the same adverse effects on a pregnant woman as they do on anyone else (see Chapter 3). However, recent research suggests that stress can also affect the course of pregnancy and the health of the fetus.

Researchers have linked high levels of stress to miscarriage, preterm labour, and low birth weight. In one study, women who reported high levels of job stress were found to have a risk of miscarriage two to three times as high as that of less-stressed women. Other studies have found that pregnant women who experience major life changes, traumatic experiences, or high levels of pregnancy-related anxiety are at greater risk for preterm labour and for having a low-birth-weight infant.

Stress hormones may constrict blood flow to the placenta, depriving the fetus of the oxygen and nutrients needed for growth and development. Stress hormones also play a role in triggering labour, so high hormone levels may also increase the risk of preterm labour.

Stress may also affect the behaviour of a pregnant woman. For example, negative coping techniques, such as use of tobacco, alcohol, and other drugs, can adversely affect a developing fetus. On the flip side, social support during pregnancy has been linked to improved fetal growth and healthy birth weight.

The time in pregnancy in which stress is experienced may be important in determining its effects. A study of earthquake survivors found that women who were in their first trimester when the earthquake occurred were at increased risk for preterm labour; women further along in their pregnancies experienced no such increase in risk. Researchers hypothesize that hormones produced in the later stages of pregnancy may protect both mother and fetus from the effects of stress.

High levels of stress have also been linked to birth defects. Although the overall risk of birth defects is very low, women who experience severe emotional trauma around the time of conception or during the first trimester are more likely to have an infant with defects of the skull, spine, palate, or limbs. The relationship between stress and birth defects has been found to be significantly greater in women with lower levels of education, suggesting that chronic stressors and behaviours that go along with low educational attainment and low income may increase the impact of stressful life events on fetal development.

Researchers have studied the long-term effects of stress by looking at children of pregnant Dutch women who experienced high levels of physical and emotional stress during the "Hunger Winter" of 1944–1945, when the Nazis blockaded the western Netherlands. Fetuses exposed to the famine early in development were found to be at increased risk of central nervous system defects and, as adults, obesity and schizophrenia.

Although most women in North America do not experience such extreme stressors during pregnancy, these studies reinforce the importance of adequate prenatal care, including stress management and social support.

Hormones may also be involved in the link between high birth weight and increased risk of breast cancer. Growth factors that contribute to high birth weight include leptin, insulin, and estrogen. Exposure to high levels of these in the womb may alter developing breast tissue in such a way that, when exposed to estrogen later in life, breast cells may be more likely to become malignant.

Although fetal programming theory is not yet embraced by all scientists, these studies emphasize that everything that occurs during pregnancy can have an impact on the developing fetus. In the future, people may be able to use information about their birth weight and other indicators of gestational conditions just as they can now use family history and genetic information—to alert them to special health risks and to help them improve their health.

The Importance of Prenatal Care

Adequate prenatal care—as described in the following sections—is essential to the health of both mother and baby. All physicians recommend that women start getting regular prenatal checkups as soon as they become pregnant. Typically, this means one checkup every four weeks during the first 30 weeks, checkups every second week until the 36th week, then weekly checkups until delivery.

Regular Checkups

In the woman's first visit to her health care provider, she will be asked for a detailed medical history of herself and her family. The physician or midwife will note any hereditary conditions that may assume increased significance during pregnancy. The tendency to develop gestational diabetes (diabetes during pregnancy only), for example, can be inherited; appropriate treatment during pregnancy reduces the risk of serious harm.

The woman is given a complete physical exam and is informed about appropriate diet. She returns for regular checkups throughout the pregnancy, during which her blood pressure and weight gain are measured, her urine is analyzed, and the size and position of the fetus are monitored. Regular prenatal visits also give the mother a chance to discuss her concerns and assure herself that everything is proceeding normally. Physicians, midwives, health educators, and teachers of prenatal and childbirth classes can provide the mother with invaluable information.

Blood Tests

A blood sample is taken during the initial prenatal visit to determine blood type and detect possible anemia or Rh incompatibilities. The **Rh factor** is a blood protein. If an Rh-positive father and an Rh-negative mother conceive an Rh-positive baby, the baby's blood will be incompatible with the mother's. If some of the baby's blood enters the mother's bloodstream during delivery, she will develop antibodies to it just as she would toward a virus. If she has subsequent Rh-positive babies, the antibodies in the mother's blood, passing through the placenta, will destroy the fetus's red blood cells, possibly leading to jaundice, anemia, intellectual disabilities, or death. This condition is completely treatable with a serum called Rh-immune globulin, which destroys Rh-positive cells as they enter the mother's body and prevents her from forming antibodies to them. Rh-immune globulin is given to Rh-negative mothers in the third trimester and again after the birth if the baby is found to be Rh-positive.

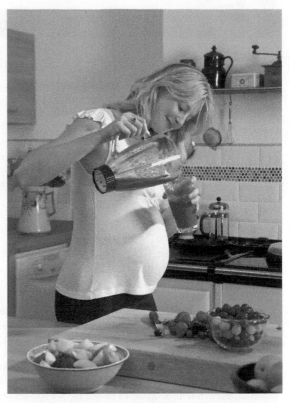

A woman's dietary needs change during pregnancy, so it's important to eat a nutritionally sound diet.

> **Rh factor**
> A protein found in blood; Rh incompatibility between a mother and fetus can jeopardize the fetus's health.

Blood may also be tested for evidence of hepatitis B, syphilis, rubella and varicella immunity, thyroid problems, and, with the mother's permission, HIV infection.

Prenatal Nutrition

A nutritious diet throughout pregnancy is essential for both the fetus and the mother. Not only does the baby get all its nutrients from the mother, but it also competes with her for nutrients not sufficiently available to meet both their needs. When a woman's diet is low in iron or calcium, the fetus receives most of it, and the mother may become deficient in the mineral. To meet the increased nutritional demands of her body, a pregnant woman shouldn't just eat more; she should make sure that her diet is nutritionally adequate (see the Take Charge box).

Avoiding Drugs and Other Environmental Hazards

In addition to the food the mother eats, the drugs she takes and the chemicals she is exposed to affect the fetus. Everything the mother ingests may eventually reach the fetus in some proportion. Some drugs harm the

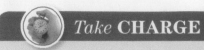

Take **CHARGE**

Healthy Eating During Pregnancy

To maintain her own health and help the fetus grow, a woman needs to consume about 250–500 extra calories per day during pregnancy. Breastfeeding an infant requires even more energy—about 500 or more extra calories per day.

Healthy Choices

To ensure a balanced intake of key nutrients, pregnant women should follow *Eating Well with Canada's Food Guide*, which is based on four basic food groups. Pregnant women should and include two to three extra servings per day from one of the food groups. For women of childbearing age, the daily recommended intake from each group is as follows:

- Vegetables and fruit: seven to eight servings; choose dark green and brightly coloured vegetables and fruit.
- Grain products: six to seven servings; choose whole grain breads, rice, and pasta.
- Meat and alternatives: two servings; choose lean meats and meat alternatives.
- Milk and alternatives: two servings; choose low-fat varieties of milk, yogourt, and cheese.

A copy of *Eating Well with Canada's Food Guide* and recommendations for pregnant women can be found on Health Canada's website (listed in the For More Information section at the end of the chapter). See Chapter 5 for a more detailed discussion of *Eating Well with Canada's Food Guide*.

Supplements

Some physicians may prescribe vitamin and mineral supplements for women who are pregnant or lactating or who are trying to get pregnant. Adequate vitamin and mineral intake is important for many reasons. For example, women with low levels of vitamin D are more likely to have low-birth-weight babies.

Adequate intake of the B vitamin folate before conception and during pregnancy has been shown to decrease the risk of neural tube defects, including spina bifida. Any woman capable of becoming pregnant should consume at least 400 micrograms (0.4 milligrams) of folic acid (the synthetic form of folate) daily from fortified foods or supplements, in addition to folate from a varied diet. Pregnant women should have 400–1000 micrograms every day. Women who have already had a pregnancy involving a fetus with a neural tube defect should consult with a physician about taking a much larger amount of folic acid (4 milligrams), starting one month before conception and continuing through the first trimester. Folate is found naturally in leafy green vegetables, legumes, citrus fruits, and most berries. In 1998, it became mandatory for enriched grain products to be fortified with folic acid. This adds approximately 100 micrograms of folic acid to an average woman's daily diet.

It is important that a pregnant woman not supplement beyond her physician's advice because some vitamins and minerals are harmful if taken in excess. It is also important not to take herbal dietary supplements without consulting a physician; few dietary supplements have been tested for safety during pregnancy, but some have been shown to be dangerous.

Food Safety

Pregnant women should pay special attention to food safety because food-borne pathogens can be particularly dangerous during pregnancy. Two such pathogens are *Listeria monocytogenes* and *Toxoplasma gondii*. *Listeria* is a bacterium most often found in undercooked or ready-to-eat meat, poultry, or seafood, soft cheeses, products made with unpasteurized milk, and unpasteurized juice. Listeriosis causes flu-like symptoms in pregnant women; if the fetus is infected, the result can be miscarriage, premature birth, or birth defects. According to the Government of Canada website (http://healthycanadians.gc.ca), if pregnant women are exposed to the bacteria they are twenty times more likely to develop Listeriosis compared to other healthy adults.

T. gondii, a parasite carried by cats, can also contaminate food or soil. Toxoplasmosis is typically caused by eating undercooked meat or poultry or unwashed fruits and vegetables, cleaning a litter box, or handling contaminated soil. Toxoplasmosis causes few symptoms in pregnant women, but if passed to the fetus it may cause miscarriage or mental impairment.

One further food safety recommendation for pregnant women relates to fish. Most types of fish are good choices for a healthy diet, but a few types can be contaminated with mercury or industrial pollutants. Health Canada recommends that pregnant women consume two food guide servings of fish per week (one serving is 75 grams). Fish contains important fats that are necessary for the development of a baby's brain, nerves, and eyes. Health Canada suggests consumption of the following fish as they have low levels of contaminants: salmon, trout, herring, haddock, canned light tuna, pollock (Boston bluefish), sole, flounder, anchovy, char, hake, mullet, smelt, Atlantic mackerel, and lake white fish. Certain types of fish should be limited or avoided during pregnancy including tuna (fresh, frozen, and canned albacore), shark, swordfish, marlin, orange roughy, and escolar. Health Canada recommends that pregnant women check with their provincial or territorial authority before consuming any fish caught in local waters.

For detailed information on food safety, see Chapter 5.

fetus but not the mother because the fetus is in the process of developing and because the proper dose for the mother is a massive dose for the fetus.

During the first trimester, when the major body structures are rapidly forming, the fetus is extremely vulnerable to environmental factors, such as viral infections, radiation, drugs, and other **teratogens**, any of which can cause **congenital malformations**, or birth defects. The most susceptible body parts are those growing most rapidly at the time of exposure. The rubella (German measles) virus, for example, can cause a congenital malformation of a delicate system, such as the eyes or ears, leading to blindness or deafness, if exposure occurs during the first trimester, but it does no damage later in the pregnancy. Similarly, the drug thalidomide taken early in pregnancy prevents the formation of arms and legs in fetuses, but taken later, when limbs are already formed, it causes no damage. Other drugs can cause damage throughout prenatal development.

teratogens
Agents or influences that cause physical defects in a developing fetus.

congenital malformations
Physical defects existing at the time of birth, either inherited or caused during gestation.

ALCOHOL   Alcohol is a potent teratogen. Getting drunk just one time during pregnancy may be enough to cause brain damage in a fetus. Alcohol consumption during pregnancy can be associated with miscarriages, stillbirths, and, in live babies, **fetal alcohol spectrum disorder (FASD)**. FASD includes several alcohol-related diagnoses, such as alcohol-related birth defects (ARBD), alcohol-related neurodevelopmental disorder (ARND), partial fetal alcohol syndrome (pFAS), and the most severe disease, fetal alcohol syndrome (FAS). Babies with FASD many have a wide range of disabilities, including physical, social, cognitive, and emotional problems. These children may have difficulties with learning, behaviour, and social situations. They may also have a small head and body size, unusual facial characteristics, congenital heart defects, defective joints, impaired vision, mental impairment, and abnormal behaviour patterns. According to the Public Health Agency of Canada, there is no safe amount of alcohol and no safe time to drink alcohol during pregnancy (see Chapter 15).

fetal alcohol spectrum disorder (FASD)
A combination of birth defects caused by alcohol consumption by the mother during pregnancy.

QUICK STATS

Approximately 1% of people living in Canada have FASD.
—Public Health Agency of Canada, 2014

TOBACCO   According to the Centre for Addiction and Mental Health (CAMH), 10.5 percent of women report smoking during their pregnancy. Pregnant women who smoke should quit, and non-smoking pregnant women should avoid places where people smoke. Smoking during pregnancy increases the risk of miscarriage, low birth weight, immune system impairment, and infant death; it may also cause genetic damage or physical deformations. If nicotine levels in a mother's bloodstream are high, fetal breathing rate and movement become more rapid. The fetus may also metabolize cancer-causing by-products of tobacco.

Infants of women who smoke during pregnancy have poorer lung function at birth, and exposure to second-hand smoke after birth increases a baby's susceptibility to pneumonia and bronchitis. If a mother who smokes also breastfeeds, her infant will be exposed to tobacco chemicals through breast milk. See Chapter 16 for more on the effects of smoking.

CAFFEINE   Caffeine, a powerful stimulant, puts both mother and fetus under stress by raising the level of the hormone epinephrine. Caffeine also reduces the blood supply to the uterus. One study found that consuming the amount of caffeine in five or more cups of coffee a day doubled the risk of miscarriage. Coffee, colas, strong black tea, and chocolate are high in caffeine, as are some over-the-counter medications. A pregnant woman should limit her caffeine intake to no more than 300 milligrams per day, which is the equivalent of about two cups of coffee.

DRUGS   Some prescription drugs, including some blood pressure medications, can harm the fetus, so they should be used only under medical supervision. Additionally, some babies born to women who use antidepressants during pregnancy suffer withdrawal symptoms after birth. Accutane, an anti-acne drug, may have caused more than 1000 cases of severe birth defects in the 1980s. Over-the-counter drugs should be used only under a physician's direction. Large doses of vitamin A, for example, can cause birth defects.

Recreational drugs, such as cocaine, are thought to increase the risk of major birth defects. Marijuana use may also interfere with fertility treatments, and methamphetamine use is associated with underweight babies.

STIs AND OTHER INFECTIONS   Infections, including those that are sexually transmitted, are another serious problem for the fetus. The most common cause of life-threatening infections in newborns is Group B streptococcus (GBS), a type of bacterium that can cause pneumonia, meningitis, and blood infections. About 25 percent of all pregnant women carry GBS but do not become ill, so routine screening close to the time of delivery is recommended. A woman who carries GBS or who develops a fever during labour will be given intravenous antibiotics at the time of labour to reduce the risk of passing GBS to her baby.

Syphilis can infect and kill a fetus; if the baby is born alive, it will have syphilis. Penicillin taken by the mother during pregnancy cures syphilis in both mother and fetus. Gonorrhea can infect the baby during delivery and cause blindness. Because gonorrhea is often asymptomatic, in Canada the eyes of newborns are routinely treated with erythromycin ointment to destroy gonorrheal bacteria. All pregnant women should be tested for hepatitis B, a virus that can pass from the mother to the infant at birth. Infants of infected mothers can be immunized shortly after birth.

Herpes simplex can damage the baby's eyes and brain and cause death, and no cure has yet been discovered for it. Genital herpes can be transmitted to the baby during delivery if the mother's infection is in the active phase. If this is the case, the baby may be delivered by Caesarean section. An initial outbreak of herpes can be dangerous if it occurs during pregnancy because the virus may pass through the placenta to the fetus. For this reason, it is important to know if the pregnant woman or her partner has a history of herpes.

The human immunodeficiency virus (HIV), which causes AIDS, can be passed to the fetus by an HIV-infected mother during pregnancy, labour and delivery, or breastfeeding. The babies most at risk are those whose mothers inject drugs or are the sex partners of men who inject drugs. HIV testing is critical for any woman at risk for HIV, and some physicians recommend routine testing for all pregnant women. Antiviral drugs, given to a mother infected with HIV during pregnancy and delivery and to her newborn immediately following birth, reduce the rate of HIV transmission from mother to infant from 25 percent to 5 percent or less. Of course, women should also take all the necessary precautions against HIV infection during pregnancy. (See Chapter 13 for more on HIV and other STIs.)

Environmental factors affecting fetal or infant development are summarized in Table 12.2.

Prenatal Activity and Exercise

Physical activity during pregnancy contributes to mental and physical wellness. Women can continue working at their jobs until late in their pregnancy, provided the work isn't so physically demanding that it jeopardizes their health. At the same time, pregnant women need more rest and sleep to maintain their own well-being and that of the fetus.

A moderate exercise program during pregnancy does not adversely affect pregnancy or birth; in fact, regular exercise appears to improve a woman's chance of an on-time delivery and may reduce the risk of pregnancy-related diabetes. The amniotic sac protects the fetus, and normal activities will not harm it. A woman who exercised before becoming pregnant can often continue her program, with appropriate modifications to maintain her comfort and safety. A pregnant woman who hasn't been exercising and wants to start should first consult a physician.

The SOGC recommends that all pregnant women engage in aerobic and strength conditioning exercises, unless they have a contraindication to exercise, and provided they are not embarking on a physical activity

TABLE 12.1

Selected Environmental Factors Associated with Problems in a Fetus or an Infant

Agent or Condition	Potential Effects
Isotretinoin (acne medication)	Small head, mental impairment, deformed or absent ears, heart defects, cleft lip and palate
Alcohol	Unusual facial characteristics, small head, heart defects, mental impairment, defective joints
Chlamydia	Eye infections, pneumonia
Cigarette smoking	Miscarriage, stillbirth, low birth weight, respiratory problems, sudden infant death
Cocaine	Miscarriage, stillbirth, low birth weight, small head, defects of genital and urinary tracts
Cytomegalovirus (CMV)	Small head, mental impairment, blindness
Diabetes (insulin-dependent)	Malformations of the brain, spine, and heart
Gonorrhea	Eye infection leading to blindness if untreated
Herpes	Brain damage, death
HIV infection	Impaired immunity, death
Lead	Reduced IQ, learning disorders
Marijuana	Impaired fetal growth, increase in alcohol-related fetal damage
Mercury	Brain damage
Propecia (hair loss medication)	Abnormalities of the male sex organs
Radiation (high dose)	Small head, growth and mental impairment, multiple birth defects
Rubella (German measles)	Malformation of eyes or ears causing deafness or blindness; small head; mental impairment
Syphilis	Fetal death and miscarriage, prematurity, physical deformities
Tetracycline	Pigmentation of teeth, underdevelopment of enamel
Vitamin A (excess)	Miscarriage, defects of the head, brain, spine, and urinary tract

regime for the first time. Walking, swimming, and stationary cycling are all good choices; more strenuous activities that could result in a fall are best delayed until after the birth.

Kegel exercises, to strengthen the pelvic floor muscles, are recommended for pregnant women. These exercises are performed by alternately contracting and releasing the muscles used to stop the flow of urine. Each contraction should be held for about five seconds. Kegel exercises should be done several times a day, for a total of about 50 repetitions daily.

Prenatal exercise classes are valuable because they teach exercises that tone the body muscles involved in birth, especially those of the abdomen, back, and legs. Toned-up muscles aid delivery and help the body regain its non-pregnant shape afterward.

Preparing for Birth

Childbirth (also called *prenatal*) classes are almost a routine part of the prenatal experience for both mothers and fathers these days. These classes typically teach the details of the birth process as well as relaxation techniques to help deal with the discomfort of labour and delivery. The mother learns and practises a variety of techniques so she will be able to choose what works best for her during labour when the time comes. The father typically acts as a coach, supporting his partner emotionally and helping her with her breathing and relaxing. He can remain with her throughout labour and delivery, even when a Caesarean section is performed.

Complications of Pregnancy and Pregnancy Loss

About 31 percent of mothers-to-be have complications during pregnancy. Some complications may prevent full-term development of the fetus or affect the health of the infant at birth. As discussed earlier in the chapter, exposure to harmful substances, such as alcohol or drugs, can harm the fetus. Other complications are caused by physiological problems or genetic abnormalities.

Ectopic Pregnancy

In an **ectopic pregnancy**, the fertilized egg implants and begins to develop outside of the uterus, usually in an oviduct (see Figure 12.7). The incidence of ectopic pregnancy is about 2 percent in the general population. Ectopic pregnancies account for about 4 percent of the annual pregnancy-related deaths in Canada.

> **ectopic pregnancy**
> A pregnancy in which the embryo develops outside of the uterus, usually in the fallopian tube.

FIGURE 12.7

Ectopic Pregnancy in a Fallopian Tube

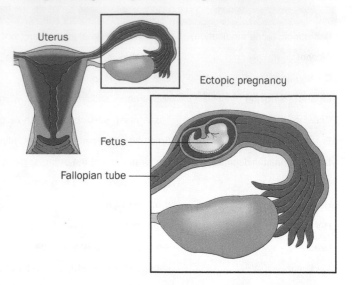

Ectopic pregnancies usually occur because the fallopian tube is blocked, most often as a result of pelvic inflammatory disease; smoking also increases a woman's risk for ectopic pregnancy. The embryo may spontaneously abort, or the embryo and placenta may continue to expand until they rupture the oviduct. Sharp pain on one side of the abdomen or in the lower back, usually in about the seventh or eighth week, may signal an ectopic pregnancy, and a woman may have irregular bleeding. If bleeding from a rupture is severe, the woman may go into shock, characterized by low blood pressure, a fast pulse, weakness, and fainting.

Surgical removal of the embryo and the oviduct may be necessary to save the mother's life, although microsurgery can sometimes be used to repair the damaged oviduct. If diagnosed early, before the oviduct ruptures, ectopic pregnancy can often be successfully treated without surgery. The incidence of ectopic pregnancy has more than quadrupled in the past 25 years.

Spontaneous Abortion

A spontaneous abortion, or miscarriage, is the termination of pregnancy before the 20th week. About 15–20 percent of all clinically diagnosed pregnancies end in miscarriage, and many women have miscarriages without knowing they were pregnant. About 30 percent of miscarriages occur before the 12th week of pregnancy. Most—about 60 percent—are due to chromosomal abnormalities in the fetus. Certain occupations that involve exposure to chemicals may increase the likelihood of a spontaneous abortion.

Vaginal bleeding (spotting) is usually the first sign that a pregnant woman may miscarry. She may also develop pelvic cramps, and her symptoms of pregnancy may disappear. (Note: Mild cramping is common in pregnancy and is usually not associated with miscarriage.)

One miscarriage doesn't mean that later pregnancies will be unsuccessful, and 70–90 percent of women who miscarry eventually become pregnant again. About 1 percent of women suffer three or more miscarriages, possibly because of anatomical, hormonal, genetic, or immunological factors.

Stillbirth

The terms *fetal death*, *fetal demise*, *stillbirth*, and *stillborn* all refer to the delivery of a fetus that shows no signs of life. Each year, more than 3 million stillbirths occur worldwide. In Canada, the stillbirth rate is a little more than 6 in 1000. Risk factors for stillbirth include smoking, advanced maternal age, obesity, multiple gestations, and chronic disease. Race is also a factor; black women have twice as many stillbirths as white women.

Preeclampsia

A disease unique to human pregnancy, **preeclampsia**, is characterized by elevated blood pressure and the appearance of protein in the urine. Symptoms include headache, right upper-quadrant abdominal pain, vision changes (referred to as *scotomata*), and notable increased swelling and weight gain. If preeclampsia is untreated, patients can develop seizures, a condition called **eclampsia**. Other potential complications of preeclampsia are liver and kidney damage, bleeding, fetal growth restriction, and even fetal death.

preeclampsia
A condition of pregnancy characterized by high blood pressure and protein in the urine.

eclampsia
A severe, potentially life-threatening form of preeclampsia, characterized by seizures.

The incidence of preeclampsia is commonly cited to be about 5 percent, but wide variations are reported. The incidence is related to race and ethnicity as well as to environmental factors and family history. It affects women at all reproductive ages. The incidence of preeclampsia in Canada is about 2.6 percent, and of these, 0.5 percent progress to eclampsia.

Women with mild preeclampsia may be monitored closely as outpatients and placed on home bed rest. More severe cases may require hospitalization for close medical management and early delivery.

Placenta Previa

In **placenta previa**, the placenta either completely or partially covers the cervical opening, preventing the mother from delivering the baby vaginally. As a result, the baby must be delivered by Caesarean section. This condition occurs in 1 in 250 live births. Risk factors include prior Caesarean delivery, multiple pregnancies, intrauterine surgery, smoking, multiple gestations, and advanced maternal age. Previas often present as painless bright red vaginal bleeding and may be associated with contractions. They account for 20 percent of bleeding in the third trimester.

placenta previa
A complication of pregnancy in which the placenta covers the cervical opening, preventing the mother from delivering the baby vaginally.

Placental Abruption

In **placental abruption**, a normally implanted placenta prematurely separates from the uterine wall. Women experience abdominal pain, vaginal bleeding, and uterine tenderness. It accounts for 30 percent of all bleeding in the third trimester. The condition also increases the risk of fetal death. The risk factors for developing a placental abruption are maternal age, tobacco smoking, cocaine use, multiple gestation, trauma, preeclampsia, hypertension, and preterm premature rupture of membranes.

placental abruption
A complication of pregnancy in which a normally implanted placenta prematurely separates from the uterine wall.

Gestational Diabetes

During gestation, about 4 percent of all pregnant women develop **gestational diabetes mellitus (GDM)**, in which the body loses its ability to use insulin properly. In these women, diabetes occurs only during pregnancy. The condition stems from placental secretion of certain hormones, including growth hormone, cortisol, placental lactogen, and progesterone. GDM arises when pancreatic function is not sufficient to overcome the insulin resistance created by these pregnancy-related hormones. Women diagnosed with GDM have an increased risk of developing type 2 diabetes later in life. It is important to accurately diagnose and treat GDM as it can lead to preeclampsia, polyhydramnios (increased levels of amniotic fluid), large fetuses, birth trauma, operative deliveries, perinatal mortality, and neonatal metabolic complications.

> **gestational diabetes mellitus (GDM)**
> A form of diabetes that occurs during pregnancy.

Preterm Labour

When a pregnant woman goes into labour before the 37th week of gestation, she is said to undergo *preterm labour*. Preterm labour is one of the most common reasons for hospitalizing pregnant women, but verifying true preterm labour can be difficult. About 30–50 percent of preterm labours resolve themselves, with the pregnancy continuing to full-term. In other cases, interventions may be required to delay labour and allow gestation to continue.

Labour Induction

If pregnancy continues well beyond the baby's due date, it may be necessary to induce labour artificially. This is one of the most common obstetrical procedures and is typically offered to pregnant women who have not delivered 7–14 days past their due date. Labour can be artificially induced in several ways.

Low Birth Weight and Premature Birth

A **low-birth-weight (LBW)** baby is one that weighs less than 2.5 kilograms at birth. LBW babies may be **premature** (born before the 37th week of pregnancy) or full-term. Babies who are born small even though they are full-term are referred to as *small-for-date* or *small-for-gestational-age* babies. Low birth weight affected about 6 percent of babies born in 2011 in Canada. About half of all cases are related to teenage pregnancy, cigarette smoking, poor nutrition, and poor maternal health. Other maternal factors include drug use, stress, depression, and anxiety. Adequate prenatal care is the best way to prevent LBW.

> **low birth weight (LBW)**
> Weighing less than 2.5 kilograms at birth, often the result of prematurity.
>
> **premature**
> Born before the 37th week of pregnancy.

Full-term LBW babies tend to have fewer problems than premature infants. In Canada in 2011–2012, about 8 percent of babies were born prematurely. Many premature infants' organs are not sufficiently developed. Even mild prematurity increases an infant's risk of dying in the first month or year of life. Premature infants are subject to respiratory problems and infections. They may have difficulty eating because they may be too small to suck a breast or bottle and their swallowing mechanism may be underdeveloped. As they get older, premature infants may have problems, such as learning difficulties, behaviour problems, poor hearing and vision, and physical awkwardness.

Infant Mortality

The Canadian rate of **infant mortality**, the death of a child of less than one year of age, is near its lowest point ever, however it remains far higher than that of most of the developed world. Canada ranks low among the world's developed countries for infant mortality, with about 5 deaths for every 1000 live births. Many experts agree that it is difficult to make international comparisons because birth registration and reporting procedures are not standardized across the globe. Table 12.3 shows the infant mortality rate across Canada from 2007–2011. Infant mortality rates are higher among Aboriginal peoples in Canada; poverty and inadequate health care are key causes.

> **infant mortality**
> The death of a child less than one year of age.

Other causes of infant death are congenital problems, infectious diseases, and injuries.

In **sudden infant death syndrome (SIDS)**, an apparently healthy infant dies suddenly while sleeping. The number of SIDS deaths has decreased since 1992, when the Back to Sleep campaign was instituted to make people aware that putting babies to bed on their backs rather than on their stomachs significantly reduces the risk of SIDS. Research suggests that abnormalities in the brainstem, the part of the brain that regulates breathing, heart rate, and other basic functions, underlie the risk for SIDS. Risk is greatly increased for infants with these innate differences if they are exposed to environmental risks, such as sleeping face down; being exposed to tobacco smoke, alcohol, or other drugs; or sleeping on a soft mattress or with fluffy bedding, pillows, or stuffed toys. Overbundling a baby or keeping a baby's room too warm also increases the risk of SIDS; because of this, SIDS deaths are more common in the colder months. Exposure to nitrous dioxide air pollution is also under investigation as a possible contributing factor. Several studies have found that the use of a pacifier significantly reduces the risk of SIDS.

TABLE 12.2

Infant Mortality Rates, 2007–2011

	2007	2008	2009	2010	2011
Both sexes					
Canada	**5.1**	**5.1**	**4.9**	**5.0**	**4.8**
Newfoundland and Labrador	7.5	5.1	6.3	5.3	6.3
Prince Edward Island	5.0	2.0	3.4	3.6	4.2
Nova Scotia	3.3	3.5	3.4	4.6	4.9
New Brunswick	4.3	3.2	5.8	3.4	3.5
Quebec	4.5	4.3	4.4	5.0	4.3
Ontario	5.2	5.3	5.0	5.0	4.6
Manitoba	7.3	6.5	6.3	6.7	7.7
Saskatchewan	5.8	6.2	6.7	5.9	6.7
Alberta	6.0	6.2	5.5	5.9	5.3
British Columbia	4.0	3.7	3.6	3.8	3.8
Yukon	8.5	5.4	7.8	5.2	0.0
Northwest Territories	4.1	9.7	15.5	1.4	7.2
Nunavut	15.1	16.1	14.8	14.5	26.3

Note: The infant mortality rate is calculated as the number of deaths of children less than one year of age per 1000 live births in the same year.

Source: Statistics Canada, CANSIM, table 102-0504.

sudden infant death syndrome (SIDS)
The sudden death of an apparently healthy infant during sleep.

Coping with Loss

Parents form a deep attachment to their children even before birth, and those who lose an infant before or during birth usually experience deep grief. Initial feelings of shocked disbelief and numbness may give way to sadness, anger, crying spells, and preoccupation with the loss. Physical sensations, such as tightness in the chest or stomach, loss of appetite, and sleeplessness, may also occur. For the mother, physical exhaustion and hormone imbalances can compound the emotional and physical stress.

Experiencing the pain of loss is part of the healing process. A support group or professional counselling is also often helpful. Planning the next pregnancy, with a physician's input, can be an important step toward recovery, as long as the mind and body are given time to heal.

QUESTIONS FOR CRITICAL THINKING AND REFLECTION

Do you know anyone who has lost a child to miscarriage, stillbirth, or a birth defect? If so, how did he or she cope with the loss? What would you do to help someone in this situation?

Childbirth

By the end of the ninth month of pregnancy, most women are tired of being pregnant; both parents are eager to start a new phase of their lives. Most couples find the actual process of birth to be an exciting and positive experience.

Choices in Childbirth

Many couples today can choose the type of practitioner and the environment they want for the birth of their child. A high-risk pregnancy is probably best handled by a specialist physician in a hospital with a nursery, but for low-risk births, many options are available.

Most babies in Canada are born in hospital. Parents can choose to have their baby delivered by a physician (an obstetrician or family practitioner) or by a registered midwife. In Canada, most babies are delivered by an obstetrician. The number of babies delivered by family physicians is decreasing, while the number delivered by midwives is increasing.

Midwives are health care providers who care for women and their babies during pregnancy, labour, delivery, and the postpartum period. Midwifery is regulated in Canada by provincial and territorial authorities. Midwives who are registered with these authorities use the title registered midwife (RM) or *sage-femme* (SF), and they are legally allowed to practise midwifery.

Some mothers-to-be are accompanied in the delivery room by a labour companion, called a *doula*. A doula is a woman who has either been through childbirth or has extensive experience with birth. She stays with the labouring woman continuously and provides emotional and tangible support, information, and advocacy. Supportive labour companions may improve labour progress by reducing maternal anxiety. Studies show that the presence of a knowledgeable doula can shorten the duration of labour, increase the rate of spontaneous vaginal birth, and reduce the use of narcotic painkillers, forceps delivery, and Caesarean birth.

It's important for prospective parents to discuss all aspects of labour and delivery with their physician or midwife beforehand so they can learn what to expect and can state their preferences. For more information, see the Critical Consumer box.

 Critical CONSUMER

Making a Birth Plan

A variety of birth situations can have positive physical and psychological outcomes. Parents should choose what is appropriate for their medical circumstances and what feels most comfortable to them. Prospective parents should discuss their preferences in the following areas with their physician or midwife:

1. Who will be present at the birth? The father? Friends? Children and other relatives? Will young siblings be allowed to visit the mother and new baby? What are the hospital/centre policies in terms of visitors and number of people present at the birth?
2. What type of room will the mother be in during labour, delivery, and recovery?
3. What types of tables, beds, or birthing chairs are available? What type of environment can be created for the birth? Can specific music be played?
4. Will the mother receive any routine preparation, such as an enema, intravenous feeding, or shaving of the pubic area?
5. What is the policy regarding food and drink during labour? Will the mother have the option of walking around or taking a shower or bath during labour?
6. Under what circumstances does the physician or midwife administer drugs to induce or augment labour? The use of these drugs tends to change the course of labour and carries a small risk.
7. How is the fetus monitored during labour? According to the SOGC, it is best to monitor the baby at regular intervals during labour; however, some circumstances require continuous monitoring.
8. Under what circumstances will an episiotomy, an incision at the base of the vaginal opening, be performed? Are any steps taken to avoid it? According to the SOGC, there is no reason to perform routine episiotomies.
9. Under what circumstances will forceps or vacuum extraction be used? In some cases of fetal distress, the use of forceps or vacuum extraction may be necessary to save the infant's life, but some authorities believe these techniques are overused.

10. What types of medications are typically used during labour and delivery? Some form of anaesthetic is usually administered during most hospital deliveries, as are hormones that intensify the contractions and shrink the uterus after delivery. Different types of anaesthetics, including short-acting narcotics, regional nerve blocks, and local anaesthetics, may be available; each has different effects on the mother and the fetus.
11. Under what conditions or circumstances does the physician perform a Caesarean section?
12. Who will "catch" the baby as she or he is born? Who will cut the umbilical cord?
13. What will be done to the baby immediately after birth? What kinds of tests and procedures will be done on the baby, and when?
14. How often will the baby be brought to the mother while they remain in the hospital or birthing centre? Can the baby stay in the mother's room rather than in a nursery? This practice is known as **rooming-in**. Research shows that rooming-in is best for babies and mothers. It gives the mother and baby an opportunity to bond, and the risk of infection is decreased for babies who room-in with their mother when compared with babies who stay in a nursery.
15. How will the baby be fed—by breast or bottle? Will feeding be on a schedule or on demand? Is there someone with breastfeeding expertise available to answer questions if necessary?

Labour and Delivery

The birth process occurs in three stages (see Figure 12.8). **Labour** begins when hormonal changes in both the mother and the baby cause strong, rhythmic uterine **contractions** to begin. These contractions exert pressure on the cervix and cause the lengthwise muscles of the uterus to pull on the circular muscles around the cervix, creating effacement (thinning) and dilation (opening) of the cervix. The contractions also pressure the baby to descend into the mother's pelvis, if it hasn't already. The entire process of labour and delivery usually takes between 2 and 36 hours, depending on the size of the baby, the baby's position in the uterus, the size of the mother's pelvis, the strength of the uterine contractions, the number of prior deliveries, and other factors. The length of labour is generally shorter for second and subsequent births.

labour
The act or process of giving birth to a child, expelling it with the placenta from the mother's body by means of uterine contractions.

contraction
Shortening of the muscles in the uterine wall, which causes effacement and dilation of the cervix and assists in expelling the fetus.

FIGURE 12.8

Birth: Labour and Delivery

(**a**) The first stage of labour; (**b**) the second stage of labour: delivery of the baby; (**c**) the third stage of labour: expulsion of the placenta.

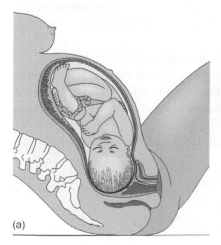
(a)

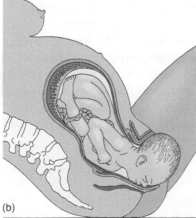
(b)

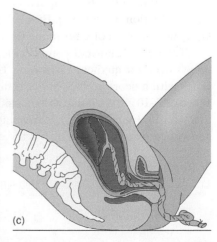
(c)

The First Stage of Labour

The first stage of labour averages 13 hours for a first birth, although wide variation exists among women. It begins with cervical effacement and dilation and continues until the cervix is completely dilated (10 centimetres). Contractions usually last about 30 seconds and occur every 15–20 minutes at first, more often later. The prepared mother relaxes as much as possible during these contractions to allow labour to proceed without being blocked by tension. Early in the first stage, a small amount of bleeding may occur as a plug of slightly bloody mucus that blocked the opening of the cervix during pregnancy is expelled. In some women, the amniotic sac ruptures and the fluid rushes out; this is sometimes referred to as the "water breaking."

The last part of the first stage of labour, called **transition**, is characterized by strong and frequent contractions, much more intense than in the early stages of labour. Contractions may last 60–90 seconds and occur every 1–3 minutes. During transition the cervix opens completely, to a diameter of about 10 centimetres. The head of the fetus usually measures 9–10 centimetres; thus once the cervix has dilated completely, the head can pass through. Many women report that transition, which normally lasts about 30–60 minutes, is the most difficult part of labour.

transition
The last part of the first stage of labour, during which the cervix becomes fully dilated; characterized by intense and frequent contractions.

The Second Stage of Labour

The second stage of labour begins with complete cervical dilation and ends with the delivery of the baby. The baby is slowly pushed down, through the bones of the pelvic ring, past the cervix, and into the vagina, which it stretches open. The mother bears down with the contractions to help push the baby down and out. Some women find this the most difficult part of labour; others find that the contractions and bearing down bring a sense of relief. The baby's back bends, the head turns to fit through the narrowest parts of the passageway, and the soft bones of the baby's skull move together and overlap as it is squeezed through the pelvis. When the top of the head appears at the vaginal opening, the baby is said to be crowning.

As the head of the baby emerges, the physician or midwife will remove any mucus from the mouth and nose, wipe the baby's face, and check to ensure that the umbilical cord is not around the neck. With a few more contractions, the baby's shoulders and body emerge. As the baby is squeezed through the pelvis, cervix, and vagina, the fluid in the lungs is forced out by the pressure on the baby's chest. Once this pressure is released as the baby emerges from the vagina, the chest expands and the lungs fill with air for the first time. The baby will still be connected to the mother via the umbilical cord, which is not cut until it stops pulsating. The baby will appear wet and often is covered with a cheese-like substance. The baby's head may be oddly shaped at first, because of the moulding of the soft plates of bone during birth, but it usually takes on a more rounded appearance within 24 hours.

The Third Stage of Labour

In the third stage of labour, the uterus continues to contract until the placenta is expelled. This stage usually takes 5–30 minutes. It is important that the entire placenta be expelled; if part remains in the uterus, it may cause infection or bleeding. Breastfeeding soon after delivery helps control uterine bleeding because it stimulates the secretion of a hormone that makes the uterus contract.

The baby's physical condition is assessed with the **Apgar score**, a formalized system for assessing the baby's need for medical assistance. Heart rate, respiration, colour, reflexes, and muscle tone are individually rated with a score of 0–2, and a total score between 0 and 10 is given at one and five minutes after birth. A score of 7–10 at five minutes is considered normal. Most newborns are also tested for at least 30 rare disorders that can be treated early, decreasing future health problems for the child. In Canada, many newborns are screened for such disorders, but the specific disorders screened for vary across provinces and territories.

Apgar score
A formalized system for assessing a newborn's need for medical assistance.

Pain Relief During Labour and Delivery

Women vary in how much pain they experience in childbirth. First babies are typically the most challenging to deliver, as the birth canal has never stretched to this extent before. It is recommended that women and their partners learn about labour and what kinds of choices are available for pain relief. Childbirth preparation courses are a good place to start, and communicating with the obstetrician or midwife is essential to assess the approaches that will be available. Breathing and relaxation techniques, such as Lamaze or Bradley, have been used effectively, and they are often modified by the labouring women to be even more effective. Forms of hypnosis can also be used.

The most commonly employed medical intervention for pain relief is the epidural. This procedure involves placing a thin plastic catheter between the vertebrae in the lower back. Medication that reduces the transmission of pain signals to the brain is given through this catheter. Local anaesthetic drugs are given in low concentration to minimize weakening of the leg muscles so that the mother can effectively push during the birth. The amount of medication given is quite low and does not accumulate in the baby or interfere with the baby's transition after birth. The mother is awake and is an active participant in the birth.

Women can also elect to have narcotics, such as morphine or demerol, given for pain relief during labour, but these medications usually provide less pain relief than the epidural and, if given shortly before the birth, can cause the baby to be less vigorous at birth. Local anaesthesia is available for repair of any tear or **episiotomy** if the mother has not used an epidural for the labour.

episiotomy
An incision made to widen the vaginal opening to facilitate birth and prevent uncontrolled tearing during delivery.

Caesarean Deliveries

In a **Caesarean section**, the baby is removed through a surgical incision in the abdominal wall and uterus. Caesarean sections are necessary when a baby cannot be delivered vaginally—for example, if the baby's head is bigger than the mother's pelvic girdle or if the baby is in an unusual position. If the mother has a serious health condition, such as high blood pressure, a Caesarean may be safer for her than labour and a vaginal delivery. Caesareans are more common among women who are overweight or have diabetes. Other reasons for Caesarean delivery include abnormal or difficult labour, fetal distress, and the presence of a dangerous infection, such as herpes, that can be passed to the baby during delivery. A growing number of Caesareans are performed on low-risk mothers; researchers hope further analysis will help determine if the trend is due to patient choice, physician choice, or a combination of the two.

Caesarean section
A surgical incision through the abdominal wall and uterus, performed to deliver a fetus.

According to Statistics Canada, the Caesarean delivery rate in Canada is the highest it has ever been, increasing from 5 percent of deliveries in the 1960s, to 20 percent in the 1980s, to more than 25 percent today. Like any major surgery, Caesarean sections carry some risk and should be performed only for valid medical reasons rather than for convenience. The SOGC encourages deliveries without interventions, such as Caesarean sections, unless medically necessary. Women who have Caesarean sections can remain conscious during the operation if they are given a regional anaesthetic, and the father or another person the mother chooses may be present.

Repeat Caesarean deliveries are also very common. In 2011–2012, about 82 percent of Canadian women who had had one child by Caesarean had subsequent children delivered the same way—an increase of 9 percent from 73 percent in 2001–2002. Although the risk of complications associated with a vaginal delivery after a previous Caesarean delivery is low, there is a small (1 percent) risk of serious complication to the mother and baby if the previous uterine scar opens during labour (uterine rupture). For this reason, women and their doctors may choose to deliver by elective repeat Caesarean.

The Postpartum Period

The **postpartum period**, a stage of about three months following childbirth, is a time of critical family adjustments. Parenthood begins literally overnight, and the transition can cause considerable stress.

> **postpartum period**
> The period of about three months after delivering a baby.

Following a vaginal delivery, mothers usually leave the hospital within one to three days (after a Caesarean section, they usually stay three to five days). Uterine contractions will occur from time to time for several days after delivery, especially during nursing, as the uterus begins to return to its pre-birth size. It usually takes six to eight weeks for a woman's reproductive organs to return to their pre-birth condition. She will have a bloody discharge called *lochia* for three to six weeks after the birth.

Within the first few days after birth, a baby will undergo newborn screening for certain rare disorders as noted above. The baby's head—if somewhat pointed following a vaginal delivery—will become more rounded within a few days. It takes about a week for the umbilical cord stump to shrivel and fall off. Regular infant checkups for health screenings and immunizations usually begin when the infant is only a few weeks old.

Breastfeeding

In 2011–2012, about 89 percent of Canadian mothers breastfed their infants after delivery. This is a slight increase from 85 percent in 2003. **Lactation**, the production of milk, begins about three days after childbirth. Before that time (sometimes as early as the second trimester), **colostrum** is secreted by the nipples. Colostrum contains antibodies that help protect the newborn from infectious diseases and is also high in protein.

> **lactation**
> The production of milk.
>
> **colostrum**
> A yellowish fluid secreted by the mammary glands around the time of childbirth until milk comes in, about the third day.

Health Canada and the Canadian Paediatric Society recommend breastfeeding exclusively for six months, then in combination with solid food up to two years of age, and then for as long after that as a mother and baby desire. Exclusive breastfeeding means that a baby is only fed breast milk and no other liquids or solids. In 2011–2012, 26 percent of Canadian mothers breastfed exclusively for at least 6 months, compared to 17 percent in 2003. Figure 12.9 illustrates the increase in breastfeeding rates from 2003 to 2011–2012 across Canada. Human milk is perfectly suited to the baby's nutritional needs and digestive capabilities, and it supplies the baby with antibodies. Breastfeeding decreases the incidence of infant ear infections, allergies, anemia, diarrhea, and bacterial meningitis. Preschoolers who were breastfed as babies are less likely to be overweight, and school-age children who were breastfed are less anxious and better able to cope with stress. Breastfeeding even has a beneficial effect on blood pressure and cholesterol levels later in life.

Breastfeeding is beneficial to the mother, as well. It stimulates contractions that help the uterus return to normal more rapidly, contributes to post-pregnancy weight loss, and may reduce the risk of ovarian cancer, breast cancer, and post-menopausal hip fracture. Nursing also provides a sense of closeness and emotional well-being for mother and child. For women who want to breastfeed but who have problems, help is available from support groups, books, or a lactation consultant.

For some women, physical problems, such as tenderness or infection of the nipples, can make breastfeeding difficult. If a woman has an illness or requires drug treatment, she may have to bottle-feed her baby because drugs and infectious agents may show up in breast milk. Breastfeeding can be restrictive, making it especially difficult for working mothers. Employers rarely provide nursing breaks, so bottle-feeding or the use of a breast pump (to express milk for use while the mother is away from her infant) may be the only practical alternatives. Bottle-feeding also allows the father or other caregiver to share in the nurturing process. Both breastfeeding and bottle-feeding can be part of loving, secure parent–child relationships.

When a mother doesn't nurse, menstruation usually begins within about 10 weeks. Breastfeeding can prevent the return of menstruation for six months or longer because the hormone prolactin, which aids milk production, suppresses hormones vital to the development of mature eggs. However, ovulation—and pregnancy—can occur before menstruation returns, so breastfeeding is not a reliable contraceptive method; if a woman wants to avoid pregnancy, she should use a more reliable method. If the mother becomes pregnant while still nursing, she needs to make sure that she is receiving adequate nutrition, because the energy requirement for both breastfeeding and gestating is immense. With proper counselling, breastfeeding can continue until near delivery.

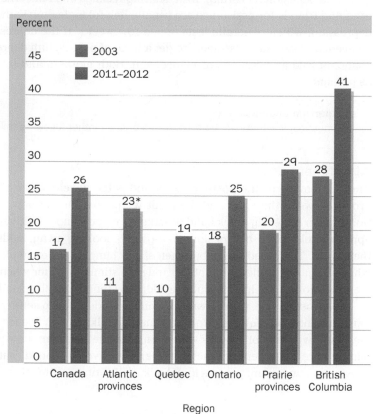

FIGURE 12.9

Rates of Exclusive Breastfeeding for Six Months or More, 2003 and 2011–2012

Percent

- 2003
- 2011–2012

Region	2003	2011–2012
Canada	17	26
Atlantic provinces	11	23*
Quebec	10	19
Ontario	18	25
Prairie provinces	20	29
British Columbia	28	41

Region

Source: Statistics Canada, *Canadian Community Health Survey,* 2003 and 2011-2012, http://www.statcan.gc.ca/pub/82-624-x/2013001/article/11879/c-g/c-g-03-eng.htm

QUICK STATS

51% of women in Canada exclusively breastfed their babies for at least 4 months in 2011–2012.

—Statistics Canada, 2013

Postpartum Depression

Many women experience fluctuating emotions during the postpartum period as hormone levels change. The physical stress of labour, as well as dehydration, blood loss, and other physical factors, lowers the woman's stamina. About 50–80 percent of new mothers experience "baby

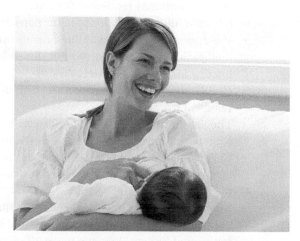

Breastfeeding can enhance the bond between mother and child. Health Canada and the Canadian Paediatric Society recommend breastfeeding exclusively for six months and then in combination with solid food up to 2 years of age and beyond.

blues," characterized by episodes of sadness, weeping, anxiety, headache, sleep disturbances, and irritability. A mother may feel lonely and anxious about caring for her infant. About 5–9 percent of new mothers experience **postpartum depression**, a more disabling syndrome characterized by despondency, mood swings, guilt, and occasional hostility. Rest, sharing feelings and concerns with others, and relying on supportive relatives and friends for assistance are usually helpful in dealing with mild cases of the baby blues or postpartum depression, which generally lasts only a few weeks. If the depression is serious, professional treatment may be needed. Some men also seem to get a form of postpartum depression, characterized by anxiety about their changing role and feelings of inadequacy. Both mothers and fathers need time to adjust to their new roles as parents.

> **postpartum depression**
> An emotional low that may be experienced by the mother following childbirth.

Attachment

Another feature of the postpartum period is the development of attachment—the strong emotional tie that grows between the baby and the adult who cares for the baby. Parents can foster secure attachment relationships in the early weeks and months by responding sensitively to the baby's needs. Parents who respond appropriately to the baby's signals of gazing, looking away, smiling, and crying establish feelings of trust in their child. They feed the baby when she is hungry, for example; respond when she cries; interact with her when she gazes, smiles, or babbles; and stop stimulating her when she frowns or looks away. A secure attachment relationship helps the child develop and function well socially, emotionally, and mentally.

For most people, the arrival of a child provides a deep sense of joy and accomplishment. However, adjusting to parenthood requires effort and energy. Talking with friends and relatives about their experiences during the first few weeks or months with a baby can help prepare new parents for the period when the baby's needs may require all the energy that both parents have to expend. But the pleasures of nurturing a new baby are substantial, and many parents look back on this time as one of the most significant and joyful of their lives.

SUMMARY

- Factors to consider when deciding if and when to have a child include physical health and age; financial circumstances; relationship with your partner; educational, career, and child care plans; emotional readiness for parenthood; social support system; personal qualities, attitudes toward children, and aptitude for parenting; and philosophical or religious beliefs.
- Pre-conception care examines many factors, such as preexisting medical conditions, current medications, age of the mother, lifestyle behaviours, infections, nutritional status, and family history of genetic disease.
- Fertilization is a complex process culminating when a sperm penetrates the membrane of the egg released from the woman's ovary.
- The leading causes of infertility in women are blocked oviducts and ovulation disorders. Exposure to toxins, injury to the testicles, and infection can cause infertility in men.
- Early signs and symptoms of pregnancy include a missed menstrual period; slight bleeding; nausea; breast tenderness; increased urination; fatigue and emotional upset; and a softening of the uterus just above the cervix.
- During pregnancy, the uterus enlarges until it pushes up into the rib cage; the breasts enlarge and may secrete colostrum; the muscles and ligaments soften and stretch; and the circulatory system, lungs, and kidneys become more efficient.
- The fetal anatomy is almost completely formed in the first trimester and is refined in the second; during the third trimester, the fetus grows and gains most of its weight, storing nutrients in fatty tissues.

- Prenatal tests include ultrasound, amniocentesis, chorionic villus sampling, and integrated prenatal screening.
- Health care during pregnancy includes a complete history and physical at the beginning, followed by regular checkups and monitoring of blood pressure, weight gain, and size and position of the fetus.
- Important elements of prenatal care include good nutrition; avoidance of drugs, alcohol, tobacco, infections, and other harmful environmental agents or conditions; regular physical activity; and childbirth or prenatal classes.
- Pregnancy usually proceeds without major complications. Problems that can occur include ectopic pregnancy, spontaneous abortion, preeclampsia, and low birth weight. The loss of a fetus or an infant is deeply felt by most parents, who need time to grieve and heal.
- Couples preparing for childbirth may have many options to choose from, including type of practitioner and facility.
- The first stage of labour begins with contractions that exert pressure on the cervix, causing effacement and dilation. The second stage begins with complete cervical dilation and ends when the baby emerges. The third stage of labour is expulsion of the placenta.
- During the postpartum period, the mother's body begins to return to its pre-pregnancy state, and she may begin to breastfeed. Both mother and father must adjust to their new roles as parents, as they develop a strong emotional tie to their baby.

FOR MORE INFORMATION

BOOKS

Beer, A. E., J. Kantecki, and L. Reed. 2006. *Is Your Body Baby-Friendly? Unexplained Infertility, Miscarriage, and IVF Failure Explained and Treated.* Chicago: AJR Publishing. Covers many issues facing women and couples who are trying to overcome infertility.

Lees, C., K. Reynolds, and G. McCarten. 2007. *Pregnancy and Birth: Your Questions Answered.* London: Dorling Kindersley. Answers hundreds of common questions about conception, pregnancy, and delivery.

Lichtman, R., L. Simpson, and A. Rosenfield. 2005. *Dr. Guttmacher's Pregnancy, Birth & Family Planning*, updated ed. New York: New American Library. A complete guide to contraception, conception, pregnancy, and childbirth.

Riley, L. 2006. *Healthy Eating During Pregnancy.* New York: Meredith Books. Up-to-date dietary information and meal-planning guides for pregnant women.

Schuurmans, N., V. Senikas, and A. B. Lalonde. 2009. *Healthy Beginnings: Giving Your Baby the Best Start from Preconception to Birth*, 4th ed. Toronto: John Wiley and Sons Canada. A step-by-step guide to pregnancy and childbirth.

Wynbrandt, J. 2007. *Encyclopedia of Genetic Disorders and Birth Defects.* New York: Facts on File. A detailed overview of many types of birth defects, both inherited and non-inherited.

ORGANIZATIONS AND WEBSITES

The Internet addresses listed here were accurate at the time of publication.

Canadian Agency for Drugs and Technologies in Health. Provides information relating to many health technologies, including those related to assisted reproduction.
http://www.cadth.ca

Canadian Association of Midwives. Provides information about midwifery in Canada.
http://www.canadianmidwives.org

Caring for Kids. Provides information from the Canadian Paediatric Society regarding health of babies and children, including safe sleep and reducing the risk of sudden infant death syndrome.
http://www.caringforkids.cps.ca

Childbirth.Org. Contains medical information and personal stories about all phases of pregnancy and birth.
> http://www.childbirth.org

Health Canada. Provides publications and other resources on many health issues including assisted human reproduction (AHR), healthy diet and pregnancy, and healthy babies.
> http://www.hc-sc.gc.ca

Health Canada. Provides a pregnancy weight gain calculator.
> http://www.hc-sc.gc.ca/fn-an/nutrition/prenatal/bmi/index-eng.php

International Council on Infertility Information Dissemination. Includes information on current research and treatments for infertility.
> http://www.inciid.org

La Leche League International. Provides advice and support for breastfeeding mothers.
> http://www.llli.org/

March of Dimes. Provides public education materials on many pregnancy-related topics, including pre-conception care, genetic screening, diet and exercise, and the effects of smoking and drinking during pregnancy.
> http://www.marchofdimes.com

Motherisk. Provides information about pregnancy and breastfeeding, with counsellors available by phone. Run by the Hospital for Sick Children in Toronto, Ontario.
> http://www.motherisk.org

Public Health Agency of Canada: The Sensible Guide to a Healthy Pregnancy. Reviews lifestyle choices to ensure a healthy pregnancy.
> http://www.phac-aspc.gc.ca/hp-gs/guide-eng.php

Society of Obstetricians and Gynaecologists of Canada. Provides up-to-date information on women's health topics including infertility, pregnancy, and childbirth.
> http://www.sogc.org

SELECTED BIBLIOGRAPHY

American Academy of Pediatrics Section on Breastfeeding. 2005. Breastfeeding and the use of human milk. *Pediatrics* 115(2): 496–506.

American Academy of Pediatrics Task Force on Sudden Infant Death Syndrome. 2005. The changing concept of sudden infant death syndrome. *Pediatrics* 116(5): 1245–1255.

Canadian Agency for Drugs and Technology in Health. 2009. *Health Technology Update 10: Assisted Reproductive Technologies in Canada,* http://www.cadth.ca/index.php/en/hta/reports-publications/health-technology-update/issue-10-september-2008/assisted-reproductive (retrieved September 28, 2015).

Canadian Council on Social Development. 2006. *Stats and Facts: Canadian Families—The Costs of Raising Children,* http://www.ccsd.ca/factsheets/family/index.htm (retrieved April 26, 2015).

Canadian Institute for Health Information. 2012. Highlights of 2010-2011 Selected indicators describing the birthing process in Canada, https://secure.cihi.ca/free_products/Childbirth_Highlights_2011-12_EN.pdf (retrieved September 28, 2015).

Case, A. M. 2003. Infertility evaluation and management. Strategies for family physicians. *Canadian Family Physician* 49(11): 1465–1472.

de la Chica, R. A., et al. 2005. Chromosomal instability in amniocytes from fetuses of mothers who smoke. *Journal of the American Medical Association* 293(10): 1212–1222.

Department of Justice of Canada. 2010. *Assisted Human Reproduction Act 2004,* http://laws.justice.gc.ca/en/A-13.4/FullText.html (retrieved September 28, 2015).

De Sutter, P. 2006. Rational diagnosis and treatment of infertility. *Best Practice & Research: Clinical Obstetrics and Gynaecology* 20: 647–664.

Does caffeine in pregnancy cause birth defects? 2006. *Child Health Alert* 24: 2.

Duncombe, D., et al. 2006. Vigorous exercise and birth outcomes in a sample of recreational exercisers: A prospective study across pregnancy. *The Australian & New Zealand Journal of Obstetrics & Gynaecology* 46(4): 288–292.

Gionet, L. 2013. "Breastfeeding trends in Canada," *Health at a Glance,* November. Statistics Canada Catalogue no. 82-624-X.

Gorman, C. 2006. What alcohol does to a child. *Time,* 5 June.

Harrison, E. C., and J. S. Taylor. 2006. IVF therapy for unexplained infertility. *American Family Physician* 73(1): 63–65.

Health Canada. 2007. *Pregnancy: Smoking and Your Body,* http://www.hc-sc.gc.ca/hc-ps/tobac-tabac/body-corps/preg-gros-eng.php (retrieved September 28, 2015).

Jimenez-Chillaron, J. C., et al. 2005. Beta-cell secretory dysfunction in the pathogenesis of low birth weight–associated diabetes. *Diabetes* 54(3): 702–711.

Leguizamon, G. F., and N. P. Zeff. 2006. Hypertension and the pregnancy complicated by diabetes. *Current Diabetes Reports* 6(4): 297–304.

Levine, R. J., et al. 2005. Urinary placental growth factor and risk of preeclampsia. *Journal of the American Medical Association* 293(1): 77–85.

Macfarlane, A., and D. Tuffnell. 2006. Diabetes and pregnancy. *British Medical Journal* 333(7560): 157–158.

Mannion, C. A., et al. 2006. Association of low intake of milk and vitamin D during pregnancy with decreased birth weight. *Canadian Medical Association Journal* 174(9): 1273–1277.

March of Dimes. 2009. *Pregnancy Complications: Depression,* http://www.marchofdimes.com/complications_depression.html (retrieved September 28, 2015).

McCormack, V. A., et al. 2005. Birth characteristics and adult cancer incidence: Swedish cohort of over 11,000 men and women. *International Journal of Cancer* 115: 611–617.

Murray, H., et al. 2005. Diagnosis and treatment of ectopic pregnancy. *Canadian Medical Association Journal* 173(8), http://www.cmaj.ca/cgi/content/full/173/8/905 (retrieved September 28, 2015).

Pattenden, S., et al. 2006. Parental smoking and children's respiratory health: Independent effects of prenatal and postnatal exposure. *Tobacco Control* 15(4): 294–301.

Public Health Agency of Canada. 2008. *The Sensible Guide to a Healthy Pregnancy,* http://www.phac-aspc.gc.ca/hp-gs/pdf/hpguide-eng.pdf (retrieved September 28, 2015).

Public Health Agency of Canada. 2012. Depression in Pregnancy, http://www.phac-aspc.gc.ca/mh-sm/preg_dep-eng.php (retrieved September 27, 2015).

Public Health Agency of Canada. 2014. Fetal Alcohol Spectrum Disorder, http://www.phac-aspc.gc.ca/hp-ps/dca-dea/prog-ini/fasd-etcaf/Index-eng.php (retrieved September 27, 2015).

Schuurmans, N., V. Senikas, and A. B. Lalonde. 2009. *Healthy Beginnings: Giving Your Baby the Best Start from Preconception to Birth,* 4th ed. Toronto: John Wiley and Sons Canada.

Scollan-Koliopoulos, M., et al. 2006. Gestational diabetes management: Guidelines to a healthy pregnancy. *Nurse Practitioner* 31(6): 14–23.

Statistics Canada. 2013. Infant Mortality Rates, by Province and territory, http://www.statcan.gc.ca/tables-tableaux/sum-som/l01/cst01/health21a-eng.htm (retrieved September 28, 2015).

Statistics Canada. 2013. Birth and total fertility rate, by province and territory, http://www.statcan.gc.ca/tables-tableaux/sum-som/l01/cst01/hlth85a-eng.htm (retrieved September 27, 2015).

Statistics Canada. 2013. Fertility Overview, 2009-2011, http://www.statcan.gc.ca/pub/91-209-x/2013001/article/11784-eng.htm (retrieved September 27, 2015).

Statistics Canada. 2014. Father's Day…by the numbers, http://www42.statcan.gc.ca/smr08/2014/smr08_187_2014-eng.htm (retrieved September 27, 2015).

UNICEF. 2009. *The State of the World's Children: Basic Indicators,* http://www.unicef.org/rightsite/sowc/statistics.php (retrieved April 26, 2015).

Voelker, R. 2005. The business of baby pictures: Controversy brews over "keepsake" fetal ultrasounds. *Journal of the American Medication Association* 293(1): 25–27.

World Health Organization. 2010. Genomic *Resource Centre: Genes and Human Disease,* http://www.who.int/genomics/public/geneticdiseases/en/index2.html (retrieved April 26, 2015).

CHAPTER 13

Sexually Transmitted Infections (STIs)

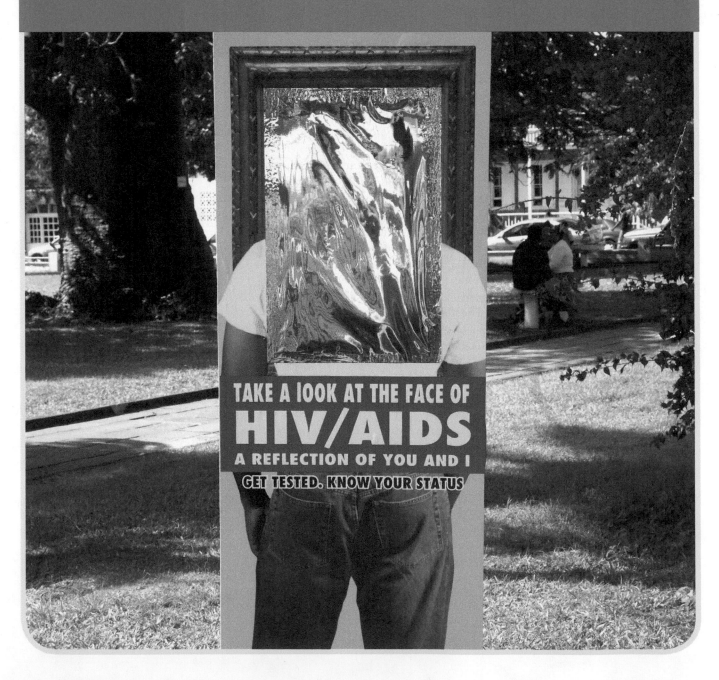

TAKE A lOOK AT THE FACE OF
HIV/AIDS
A REFLECTION OF YOU AND I
GET TESTED. KNOW YOUR STATUS

LOOKING AHEAD

After you have read and studied this chapter, you should be able to:

LO1 Discuss the symptoms of, risks for, and treatments for the major sexually transmitted infections (STIs)

LO2 Explain how different STIs affect the body and how they are transmitted and diagnosed

LO3 List strategies for protecting yourself from STIs

TEST YOUR KNOWLEDGE

1. **If you have a sexually transmitted infection (STI), you will know it.**
   True or false?

2. **About what percentage of Canadians living with HIV are unaware of their infection?**
   a. 5 percent b. 15 percent c. 25 percent d. 55 percent

3. **A man with an STI is more likely to transmit the infection to a female partner than vice versa.**
   True or false?

4. **After you have had an STI once, you become immune to that disease and cannot get it again.**
   True or false?

5. **Worldwide, HIV infection is spread primarily via which of the following?**
   a. injection drug use b. sex between men c. mother-to-child transmission d. heterosexual sex

ANSWERS

1. FALSE. Many people with STIs have no symptoms and do not know they are infected; however, they can still pass an infection to any partner.

2. c. It is estimated that 25 percent of Canadians living with HIV do not know they are carrying the virus that causes AIDS.

3. TRUE. For many STIs, infected men are at least twice as likely as infected women to transmit an STI to a partner.

4. FALSE. Reinfection with STIs is very common. For example, if you are treated for and cured of chlamydia and then you have sex with your untreated partner, the chances are very good that you will be infected again.

5. d. The vast majority of HIV infection cases worldwide result from heterosexual contact, and the majority of new cases occur in teenage girls and young women.

Considering the intimate nature of sexual activity, it is not surprising that many infections can be transmitted from one person to another through sexual contact. Of course, colds, influenza, and many other infections can spread from one sexual partner to another, but sexual contact is not the primary means of transmission for these illnesses. **Sexually transmitted infections (STIs)**—previously referred to as sexually transmitted diseases (STDs)—spread from person to person mainly through sexual activity.

> **sexually transmitted infection (STI)**
> An infection that can be transmitted by sexual contact; some can also be transmitted by other means.

STIs are a particularly insidious group of illnesses because a person can be infected and able to transmit the disease yet not look or feel sick; this is why the term *sexually transmitted infection (STI)* has replaced the term *sexually transmitted disease* in Canada. Everyone should have a clear understanding of what STIs are, how they are transmitted, and how they can be prevented. Many STIs can also be cured if treated early and properly. This chapter introduces the major forms of sexually transmitted infections; it also provides information about healthy, safer sexual behaviour to help you understand how to reduce the further spread of these infections.

The Major STIs

The following seven STIs pose a major health threat:
- Chlamydia
- Gonorrhea
- Syphilis
- Human papillomavirus (HPV)
- Genital herpes (HSV 1 and HSV 2)
- HIV/AIDS
- Hepatitis B (HBV)

These diseases are considered major threats because they are serious in themselves, cause serious complications if left untreated, and pose risks to a fetus or newborn. STIs can result in serious long-term consequences, including chronic pain, infertility, stillbirths, genital cancers, and death.

All these diseases have a relatively high incidence among Canadians, as shown in Table 13.1. In fact, a 2012 report from the Public Health Agency of Canada shows that many of the most common STIs are on the rise in Canada. To assess your current level of responsibility for STI prevention, complete the quiz in the Assess Yourself box.

Chlamydia

STIs are caused by more than 30 different organisms, including viruses, bacteria, fungi, and protozoa. *Chlamydia trachomatis* causes **chlamydia**, the most prevalent bacterial STI in Canada. According to the Public Health Agency of Canada, rates of chlamydia infection in Canada have been increasing steadily since 1997, with almost 95 000 cases reported in 2010. Many experts believe that the rise in the reported rates of chlamydia may also be due, in part, to improved detection. The highest rates of infection occur in single people ages 15–24; interestingly, however, an increase in the number of cases among middle-aged and older adults has also been reported. In 2010, similar to previous years, reported chlamydia rates were highest in Nunavut, the Northwest

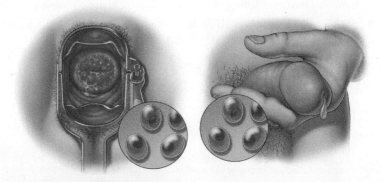

TABLE 13.1

Epidemiology of STIs in Canada

STI	How Common in Clinical Practice?	Trends in Incidence	Groups Most Affected
Chlamydia	• Most commonly diagnosed and reported bacterial STI • 94 690 cases reported in 2010	• Steadily increasing in Canada since 1997 • Between 2001 and 2010, the greatest relative rate increases were observed among women ages 40–59 and men ages 60+	• Young women and men ages 15–24
Gonorrhea	• Second most commonly diagnosed and reported bacterial STI • 11 397 cases reported in 2010	• Steadily increasing in Canada since 1997 • Rapid increase in quinolone (antibiotic) resistance from early 1990s to mid-2000s; as such, quinolones are no longer recommended for treatment of gonococcal infections in Canada • Between 2001 and 2010, the greatest relative rate increases were observed among males and females ages 10–14	• Young men ages 20–24 • Young women ages 15–24
Syphilis	• Previously rare in Canada • 1757 cases reported in 2010	• Dramatic national increases since 1997; between 2001 and 2010, overall increase in syphilis rates was 456.7 percent • Related to regional outbreaks across Canada • Between 2001 and 2010, the greatest relative rate increases were observed in males ages 15–19 and men ages 40–59	• Men ages 25–39 • Women ages 20–29 • In 2010, 90.5 percent of reported cases were males
Human papillomavirus (HPV)	• Very common • Estimated prevalence between 10–30 percent • 70 percent of the adult population will have had at least one genital HPV infection in their lifetime	• True incidence is not known as HPV is not a reportable STI	• Adolescent and young adult women and men (although it affects women and men of all ages)
Genital herpes (HSV 1 and HSV 2)	• Common	• True incidence is not known as HSV is not a reportable STI	• Very common in adolescent and adult men and women • Women are affected more often than men
HIV/AIDS	• Rare in general practice • 2623 new cases reported in Canada in 2008	• 7 percent rise in number of HIV-positive test reports from 2007–2008	• Men who have sex with men • Acquisition in endemic regions • People who inject drugs • Young women ages 15–19
Hepatitis B (HBV)	• Low to moderate in general practice and varies in different populations • Approximately 700 acute cases per year in Canada	• Acute HBV twice as high for men • Peak incidence rates are found in the 30–39 age group	• People who inject drugs and share equipment • People with multiple sexual partners • Acquisition in endemic regions • Sexual and household contacts of an acute or a chronic carrier • Infants born to hepatitis B surface antigen positive (HbsAg+) mothers

Sources: Public Health Agency of Canada. 2013. *Canadian Guidelines on Sexually Transmitted Infections,* http://www.phac-aspc.gc.ca/std-mts/sti-its/ (retrieved October 27, 2015); Public Health Agency of Canada. 2012. *Report on Sexually Transmitted Infections in Canada: 2010,* http://publications.gc.ca/collections/collection_2013/aspc-phac/HP37-10-2010-eng.pdf (retrieved October 27, 2015); and Public Health Agency of Canada. 2013. *Canadian Guidelines on Sexually Transmitted Infections: Gonococcal Infections Chapter,* http://www.phac-aspc.gc.ca/std-mts/sti-its/cgsti-ldcits/assets/pdf/section-5-6-eng.pdf (retrieved October 27, 2015).

Assess YOURSELF

Do Your Attitudes and Behaviours Put You at Risk for STIs?

To identify your STI risk factors, read the following statements and identify whether each one is true or false for you.

True or False
1. I have never been sexually active. (If false, continue. If true, you are not at risk; respond to the remaining statements based on how you realistically believe you would act.)
2. I am in a mutually monogamous relationship with an uninfected partner or am not currently sexually active. (If false, continue. If true, you are at minimal risk now; respond to the remaining statements according to your attitudes and past behaviours.)
3. I have only one sex partner.
4. I always use a condom for each act of intercourse, even if I am fairly certain my partner has no infections.
5. I do not use oil-based lubricants or other products with condoms.
6. I discuss STIs and prevention with new partners before having sex.
7. I do not use alcohol or other mood-altering drugs in sexual situations.
8. I would tell my partner if I thought I had been exposed to an STI.
9. I am familiar with the signs and symptoms of STIs.
10. I regularly perform genital self-examinations.
11. When I notice any sign or symptom of any STI or if I engage in risky sexual behaviour, I consult my physician immediately.
12. I obtain screening for HIV and STIs regularly. In addition (if female), I obtain yearly pelvic exams and Pap tests.
13. When diagnosed with an STI, I inform all recent partners.
14. When I have a sign or symptom of an STI that goes away on its own, I still consult my physician.
15. I do not use drugs prescribed for friends or partners or left over from other illnesses to treat STIs.
16. I do not share syringes or needles to inject drugs.

False answers indicate attitudes and behaviours that may put you at risk for contracting STIs or for suffering serious medical consequences from them. If you feel you are at risk of infection for any reason, contacting a health professional and getting tested will allow you to get the answers—and the treatments—you may need.

Territories, and Yukon. (Table 13.2 shows rates of common STIs in all provinces and territories). Both men and women are susceptible to chlamydia, but, as with most STIs, women bear the greater burden because of possible complications and consequences of the disease (see the Gender Matters box). *C. trachomatis* can be transmitted by oral sex as well as by other forms of sexual intercourse.

> **chlamydia**
> An STI transmitted by the pathogenic bacterium *Chlamydia trachomatis*.

In most women, chlamydia produces no early symptoms. If left untreated, it can lead to pelvic inflammatory disease (PID), which is discussed later in this chapter. Chlamydia also greatly increases a woman's risk for infertility and ectopic (tubal) pregnancy.

TABLE 13.2

Rates of Common STIs by Province and Territory, 2010

	Chlamydia	Gonorrhea	Syphilis
British Columbia	**261.9**	30.1	3.4
Alberta	**352.9**	**31.9**	4.5
Saskatchewan	**484.0**	**72.6**	3.4
Manitoba	**516.0**	**79.5**	1.4
Ontario	253.4	30.0	5.9
Quebec	219.1	26.1	6.8
New Brunswick	242.8	8.1	4.5
Nova Scotia	237.3	9.2 (NS/PEI)	1.9 (NS/PEI)
Prince Edward Island	149.7	see above	see above
Newfoundland and Labrador	126.3	2.4	0.8
Yukon	**666.2**	**89.8**	2.9
Northwest Territories	**2086.4**	**502.8**	18.3
Nunavut	**4193.3**	**1950.6**	0.0

Notes: Rates are per 100 000 population. Bolded numbers indicate rates above national average.

Source: Public Health Agency of Canada. 2012. *Report on Sexually Transmitted Infections in Canada: 2010.* Adapted and reproduced with permission from the Minister of Health, 2015. All rights reserved. (http://publications.gc.ca/collections/collection_2013/aspc-phac/HP37-10-2010-eng.pdf; retrieved October 27, 2015).

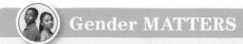

Gender MATTERS

Women Are Hit Hard by STIs

Sexually transmitted infections cause suffering for all who are infected, but in many ways, women and girls are the hardest hit, for both biological and social reasons.

Male-to-female transmission of many infections is more likely to occur than female-to-male transmission. This is particularly true of HIV: Studies show that it is three to eight times easier for a man infected with HIV to transmit the virus to a woman than it is for a woman with HIV to infect a man. Researchers have also found that after one episode of sexual intercourse, a female has a 60–90 percent chance of contracting gonorrhea from her infected male partner, whereas the risk of transmission from a woman to a man is 20–30 percent.

Young women have been hit especially hard by STIs. A 2010 report from the Public Health Agency of Canada shows that the highest rates of STIs are among Canadian women ages 15–24 (for chlamydia and gonorrhea) and 20–24 (for syphilis). Young women are more vulnerable to STIs than older women because the less mature cervix is more susceptible to injury and infection. As a woman ages, the type of cells at the opening of the cervix gradually changes so that the tissue becomes more resistant to infection. Young women are also more vulnerable for social and emotional reasons: Lack of control in relationships, fear of discussing condom use, and an older sex partner are all linked to increased STI risk.

Once infected, women tend to suffer more consequences of STIs than men. For example, gonorrhea and chlamydia can cause PID and permanent damage to the oviducts in women, but these infections tend to have less serious effects in men. HPV infection causes nearly all cases of cervical cancer. HPV infection is also associated with penile cancer in men, but penile cancer is much less common than cervical cancer. Women have the added concern of the potential effects of STIs during pregnancy.

Worldwide, as many women as men now die from AIDS each year, and in the hardest-hit regions of Africa, nearly 60 percent of adults infected with HIV are women. In Canada, the proportion of women with HIV has remained relatively stable for the past decade; in 2012, females accounted for 23.1 percent of all cases in the country. Women with HIV infection often face tremendous challenges when they are ill because they may be caring for family members who are also infected and ill. In addition, women may become sicker at lower viral loads than men do. Women and men with HIV do about equally well if they have similar access to treatment, but in many cases women are diagnosed later in the course of HIV infection, receive less treatment, and die sooner.

Social and economic factors play a large role in the transmission and consequences of STIs for women. Sexual violence against women is spreading STIs, as are such practices as very early marriage for women, often to much older men who have had many sexual partners. Cultural gender norms that promote premarital and extramarital relationships for men, combined with women's lack of power to negotiate safer sex, make STIs a risk even for women who are married and monogamous. In addition, lack of education and economic opportunities can force women into commercial sex work, placing them at high risk for STIs.

In some parts of the world, the stigma of having an STI hits women harder. For example, men with HIV are typically cared for by female family members, without being questioned about the source of their infection. Women, in contrast, may be accused of having had extramarital sex and receive less help and support. It is women who typically provide care to relatives with HIV as well as support the household financially when other earners are too ill to work. But if husbands die, women often do not inherit property and can be thrown deeper into poverty. Solutions to the STI crisis in women must include empowerment in the social sphere in addition to direct health care.

Sources: Dunkle, K. M., et al. 2004. Gender-based violence, relationship power, and risk of HIV infection in women attending antenatal clinics in South Africa. *Lancet* 363(9419): 1415–1421; Joint United Nations Programme on HIV/AIDS. 2004. *AIDS Epidemic Update, December 2004.* Geneva: UNAIDS; World Health Organization. 2003. *Gender and HIV/AIDS.* Geneva: World Health Organization; Wong, T., et al. 2004. Gender differences in bacterial STIs in Canada. *BMC Women's Health* 4(1 Suppl.): S26, http://www.biomedcentral.com/1472-6874/4/S1/S26 (retrieved October 27, 2015); Public Health Agency of Canada. 2013. *At a Glance – HIV and AIDS in Canada: Surveillance Report to December 31st, 2012,* http://www.phac-aspc.gc.ca/aids-sida/publication/survreport/2012/dec/index-eng.php (retrieved October 27, 2015); and Public Health Agency of Canada. 2012. *Report on Sexually Transmitted Infections in Canada: 2010,* http://publications.gc.ca/collections/collection_2013/aspc-phac/HP37-10-2010-eng.pdf (retrieved October 27, 2015).

Because rates of infection are high and most women with chlamydia have no symptoms, many physicians screen sexually active women at the time of their routine pelvic exam. Chlamydia can also lead to infertility in men, although not as often as in women. In men under age 35, chlamydia is the most common cause of **epididymitis**, inflammation of the sperm-carrying ducts. And up to half of all cases of **urethritis** (inflamation of the urethra) in men are caused by chlamydia. Despite these statistics, many infected men have no symptoms. The Public Health Agency of Canada currently recommends routine screening for all at-risk groups, including pregnant women and sexually active individuals 25 years old or younger.

> **epididymitis**
> An inflammation of the small body of sperm-carrying ducts that rests on the testes.
>
> **urethritis**
> An inflammation of the tube that carries urine from the bladder to the outside opening.

Infants of infected mothers can acquire the infection through contact with the pathogen in the birth canal during delivery. The Canadian Paediatric Society recommends routine prenatal screening for chlamydia; testing pregnant women and treating those infected is a highly effective way to prevent infection of newborns.

QUICK STATS

Chlamydia affects approximately twice as many women as men.
—Public Health Agency of Canada, 2012

Symptoms

In men, chlamydia symptoms include painful urination, a slight watery discharge from the penis, and sometimes pain around the testicles. Although most women with chlamydia are asymptomatic, some notice increased vaginal discharge, burning with urination, pain or bleeding with intercourse, and lower abdominal pain. Less common symptoms in both men and women include arthritis, conjunctivitis, sore throat, and rectal inflammation and pain (in people who become infected during receptive anal intercourse). Symptoms in both men and women can begin within five days of infection. However, most people experience few or no symptoms, increasing the likelihood that they will inadvertently spread the infection to their partners.

Diagnosis

Chlamydia is typically diagnosed through laboratory tests on a urine sample using NAAT or a small amount of fluid from the urethra or cervix.

Treatment

Once chlamydia has been diagnosed, the infected person and his or her partner(s) are given antibiotics—usually doxycycline, ofloxacin, or a newer drug, azithromycin, which can cure infection in one dose. Treatment of partners is important because people who have been treated for chlamydia are susceptible to getting the disease again if they have sexual contact with an infected person. Because the risk of repeat infection is so high, the Public Health Agency of Canada now recommends that all people who have been treated for chlamydia be retested six months after treatment is completed.

Gonorrhea

More than 11 000 cases of **gonorrhea** were reported to Health Canada in 2010. Like chlamydia, however, gonorrhea is underreported because it is often symptomless, so the number of actual cases is likely much higher. The highest incidence is among Canadians under the age of 30. Like chlamydia, untreated gonorrhea can cause PID in women and urethritis and epididymitis in men. It can also cause arthritis, rashes, and eye infections, and it occasionally involves internal organs. Being infected with gonorrhea increases the likelihood that HIV will be transmitted. A woman who is infected during pregnancy is at risk for preterm delivery and for having a baby with life threatening gonorrheal infection of the blood or joints. An infant passing through the birth canal of an infected mother may contract **gonococcal conjunctivitis**, an infection in the eyes that can cause blindness if not treated. In Canada, newborn babies are routinely treated with antimicrobial eyedrops to prevent eye infection.

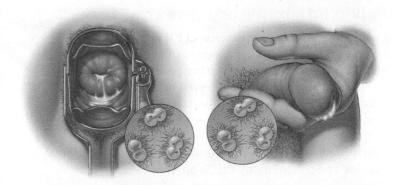

gonorrhea
A sexually transmitted bacterial infection that usually affects mucous membranes.

gonococcal conjunctivitis
An inflammation of the mucous membrane lining of the eyelids, caused by the gonococcus bacterium.

Gonorrhea is caused by the bacterium *Neisseria gonorrhoeae*, which flourishes in mucous membranes. The microbe cannot thrive outside the human body and dies within moments of exposure to light and air. Consequently, gonorrhea cannot be contracted from toilet seats, towels, or other objects.

Symptoms

In males, the incubation period for gonorrhea is brief, generally two to seven days. The first symptoms are due to urethritis, which causes urinary discomfort and a thick, yellowish-white or yellowish-green discharge from the penis. The lips of the urethral opening may become inflamed and swollen. In some cases, the lymph glands in the groin become enlarged and swollen. Up to half of males have minor symptoms or none at all.

Most females with gonorrhea are asymptomatic. Those who do have symptoms often experience pain with urination, increased vaginal discharge, and severe menstrual cramps. Up to 40 percent of women with untreated gonorrhea develop PID. Women may also develop painful abscesses in the Bartholin's glands, a pair of glands located on either side of the opening of the vagina.

Gonorrhea can also infect the throat or rectum of people who engage in oral or anal sex. Gonorrhea symptoms in the throat may be a sore throat or pus on the tonsils, and those in the rectum may be pus or blood in the feces or rectal pain and itching.

Diagnosis

Several tests—gram stain, detection of bacterial genes or DNA, or culture—may be performed; depending on the test, samples of urine or cervical, urethral, throat, or rectal fluids may be collected.

Treatment

Gonorrhea can be cured with antibiotics, but increasing drug resistance is a major concern. Today only one class of antibiotics, the cephalosporins, remains consistently effective against gonorrhea. People with gonorrhea often also have chlamydia, so additional antibiotics are typically given to treat chlamydia. Follow-up tests are sometimes performed to make sure the infection has been eradicated. If you have had gonorrhea and have been treated, you can still get the disease again if you have sexual contact with an infected partner.

QUICK STATS

After a tenfold drop in gonorrhea incidence between 1981 and 1995, rates of this STI are again rising in Canada.

—Public Health Agency of Canada, 2012

Pelvic Inflammatory Disease

Pelvic inflammatory disease (PID) is a major complication in 10–40 percent of women who have been infected with either gonorrhea or chlamydia and have not received adequate treatment. PID occurs when the initial infection with gonorrhea or chlamydia travels upward, often along with other bacteria, beyond the cervix into the uterus, oviducts, ovaries, and pelvic cavity. PID is often serious enough to require hospitalization and sometimes surgery. Even if the disease is treated successfully, about 25 percent of affected women will have long-term problems, such as a continuing susceptibility to infection, ectopic pregnancy, infertility, and chronic pelvic pain.

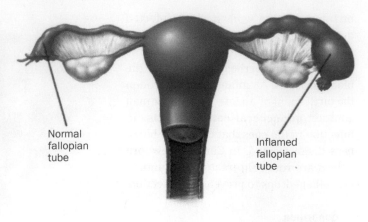

Normal fallopian tube

Inflamed fallopian tube

> **pelvic inflammatory disease (PID)**
> An infection that progresses from the vagina and cervix to the uterus, oviducts, and pelvic cavity.

PID is the leading cause of infertility in young women, often going undetected until the inability to become pregnant leads to further evaluation. Infertility occurs in 8 percent of women after one episode of PID, 20 percent after two episodes, and 40 percent after three episodes. The risk of ectopic pregnancy increases significantly in women who have had PID.

Women under age 25 are much more likely to develop PID than are older women. It is estimated that 100 000 women in Canada suffer from PID every year, although exact numbers are unknown as PID is not nationally reported (see the In Focus box). As with all STIs, the more sex partners a woman has had, the greater her risk of PID. Smokers have twice the risk of PID as non-smokers. Using intrauterine devices (IUDs) for contraception also increases the risk of PID. Research into whether the use of other contraceptives protects against PID has yielded mixed results, although oral contraceptive use may reduce the severity of PID symptoms.

Symptoms

Symptoms of PID vary greatly. Some women, especially those with chlamydia, may be asymptomatic; others may feel very ill with abdominal pain, fever, chills, nausea, and vomiting. Early symptoms are essentially the same as those described earlier for chlamydia and gonorrhea. Symptoms often begin or worsen during or soon after a woman's menstrual period. Many women have abnormal vaginal bleeding—either bleeding between periods or heavy and painful menstrual bleeding.

Diagnosis

Diagnosis of PID is made on the basis of symptoms, physical examination, ultrasound, and laboratory tests. Laparoscopy may be used to confirm the diagnosis and obtain material for cultures. Cultures from the rectum or cervix may also be taken to help identify the specific organism. The symptoms of PID, ectopic pregnancy, and appendicitis can be quite similar, so careful evaluation is required to make the correct diagnosis.

Treatment

Starting treatment of PID as quickly as possible is important to minimize damage to the reproductive organs. Antibiotics are usually started immediately; in severe cases, the woman may be hospitalized and antibiotics given intravenously. It is especially important that an infected woman's partners be treated. As many as 60 percent of the male contacts of women with PID are infected with the bacteria that caused the infection but are asymptomatic.

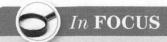

In FOCUS

Monitoring Infections in Canada

Surveillance is the ongoing and timely systematic collection, analysis, and interpretation of data essential to public health practice. The occurrences of infectious diseases that are deemed important (by the Advisory Committee on Epidemiology) need to be reported to public health officials. The reporting of notifiable diseases is mandated by provinces and territories and is voluntarily reported to the Canadian Notifiable Disease Surveillance System (CNDSS). The list of reported notifiable diseases is agreed upon by consensus among provincial, territorial, and federal health officials against specified criteria.

Canada monitors a range of STIs through the CNDSS. Some STIs have been tracked for many years, while others are more recent additions. For example, gonorrhea and infectious syphilis have been nationally notifiable infectious diseases since 1924, while chlamydia has only been a notifiable disease since 1990. All positive HIV test reports and AIDS cases have been legally reportable everywhere in Canada since 2003. Other STIs, such as genital herpes and human papillomavirus (HPV), are not nationally reported.

The number of STI cases reported to the CNDSS, and the population rates calculated as a result, do not account for all infections in the population. For example, an infected individual may not show symptoms and thus may not be tested and recorded. In addition, since women tend to interact more frequently with the health care system, they are more likely than men to be screened or to seek treatment for STIs. This may partly explain why more infections are diagnosed and reported among women than among men. Changes in rates over time must also be interpreted cautiously because they are subject to changes in both screening practices and laboratory technology and diagnostic capabilities. In addition, when the number of cases is very small, the rates are more prone to fluctuations over time.

Sources: Public Health Agency of Canada. 2010. *HIV/AIDS Epi Updates. July 2010,* http://www.phac-aspc.gc.ca/aids-sida/publication/epi/2010/4-eng.php (retrieved October 27, 2015); and Public Health Agency of Canada. 2013. *The Chief Public Health Officer's Report on the State of Public Health in Canada, 2013. Infectious Disease—The Never-ending Threat,* http://www.phac-aspc.gc.ca/cphorsphc-respcacsp/2013/sti-its-eng.php (retrieved October 27, 2015).

Syphilis

Syphilis, a disease that once caused death and disability for millions, can now be effectively treated with antibiotics. In 2010, close to 1800 cases of syphilis were reported in Canada. The number of new cases hit an all-time low from 1994 to 2000, but has been on the rise since then. Recent outbreaks of syphilis have been reported in a number of locations across Canada, including Calgary, Edmonton, Vancouver, Winnipeg, Toronto, Ottawa, Montreal, Halifax, Yukon, and

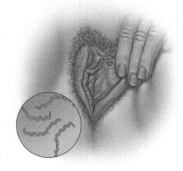
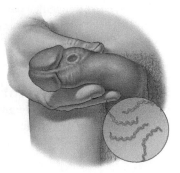

Northwest Territories. Aboriginal people are disproportionately affected by syphilis; although self-identified Aboriginal people make up 7 percent of the population in Canadian jurisdictions that report ethnicity data, they account for about 22 percent of syphilis cases in these locations. A number of factors have contributed to this trend, including a wide array of social and health inequities.

> **syphilis**
> A sexually transmitted bacterial infection caused by the spirochete *Treponema pallidum*.

The increase in syphilis has been greatest in men who are gay or bisexual, prompting health officials to call for increased education in safer sex practices among these groups. Some of the outbreaks have centred around sex workers and their clients, and others have been locally acquired infections in heterosexual individuals. Another recent trend is an increase in the proportion of cases of syphilis from oral sex. People with syphilis in the mouth may not have symptoms, or they may mistake the sores for another illness. The sores associated with syphilis, regardless of their location, dramatically increase the risk of acquiring HIV or transmitting it to someone else.

Syphilis is caused by a spirochete called *Treponema pallidum*, a thin, corkscrew-shaped bacterium. The disease is usually acquired through sexual contact, although infected pregnant women can transmit it to the fetus. The pathogen passes through any break or opening in the skin or mucous membranes and can be transmitted by kissing, vaginal or anal intercourse, or oral-genital contact. Although easy to treat, syphilis can be difficult to recognize, and if left untreated the disease can cause devastating damage to almost any system of the body.

Symptoms

Syphilis progresses through several stages. *Primary syphilis* is characterized by an ulcer called a **chancre** that appears within 3–90 days after exposure. The chancre is usually found at the site where the organism entered the body, such as the genital area, but it may also appear in other sites, such as the mouth, breasts, or fingers. Chancres contain large numbers of bacteria and make the disease highly contagious when present; they are often painless and typically heal on their own within a few weeks. If the disease is not treated during the primary stage, about a third of infected individuals progress to chronic stages of infections.

> **chancre**
> The sore produced by syphilis in its earliest stage.

Secondary syphilis is usually marked by mild, flu-like symptoms and a skin rash that appears three to six weeks after the chancre. The rash may cover the entire body or only a few areas, but the palms of the hands and soles of the feet are usually involved. Areas of skin affected by the rash are highly contagious but usually heal within several weeks or months.

If the disease remains untreated, the symptoms of secondary syphilis may recur over several years; affected individuals may then lapse into an asymptomatic *latent stage* in which they experience no further consequences of infection. However, in about a third of cases of untreated secondary syphilis, the individual develops *tertiary syphilis*. Tertiary syphilis can damage many organs of the body, possibly causing severe dementia, cardiovascular damage, blindness, and death.

In infected pregnant women, the syphilis bacterium can cross the placenta. If the mother is not treated, the probable result is stillbirth, prematurity, or congenital deformity. In many cases, the infant is also born infected (*congenital syphilis*) and requires treatment.

Diagnosis and Treatment

Syphilis is diagnosed by examination of infected tissues and with blood tests. All stages can be treated with antibiotics, but damage from tertiary syphilis can be permanent.

Human Papillomavirus

Human papillomavirus (HPV) infection is estimated to be one of the most common STIs in Canada and around the world (see the In the News box). HPV infection causes a variety of human diseases, including common warts, **genital warts**, and genital cancers. HPV is the cause of virtually all cervical cancer, but it also causes penile cancer and some forms of anal and oropharyngeal cancers. Genital HPV is usually spread from one person to another through sexual activity, including oral sex.

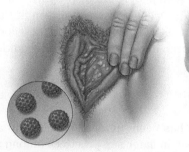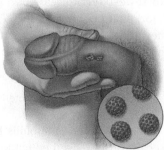

human papillomavirus (HPV)
The pathogen that causes human warts, including genital warts.

genital warts
A sexually transmitted viral infection characterized by growths on the genitals; also called *genital HPV infection* or *condyloma*.

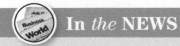
In *the* NEWS

STIs: A Growing Public Health Concern for All Canadians

The most recent statistics show that chlamydia, gonorrhea, and syphilis—three nationally reportable STIs—are all on the rise in Canada. Although chlamydia and gonorrhea rates continue to be higher among younger adults, rates of all three STIs have increased dramatically among middle-aged and older adults (ages 40+). For example, from 2001 to 2010, rates of chlamydia increased by 175.5 percent among middle-aged women (ages 40–59) and 180.8 percent among older men (ages 60+).

It is evident that STIs pose a major threat to the health and well-being of all Canadians. STIs are public health challenges for many reasons.

- *STIs are stealth diseases.* Many STIs, including chlamydia, genital herpes, trichomoniasis, HPV, and even early HIV infection, often have few, if any, recognizable symptoms. The large number of disease carriers who are unaware of their infection makes these diseases extremely difficult to control. Experts believe that in most cases, HIV is transmitted very early in the disease, before people are aware of the infection. The fact that most people are symptom-free for the first several years of HIV infection highlights the need to frequently test people who are at risk.
- *Viral STIs are persistent and incurable.* Even if detected, most viral STIs—genital herpes, HPV infection, and HIV infection—are not curable with current therapies. This means that the number of people capable of infecting others continues to grow. The best hope for controlling viral STIs is the development and widespread use of effective vaccines.
- *Screening tests may be underused.* Many individuals are unaware of or too embarrassed to request STI screening. Testing more people for STIs could potentially bring STI rates down; it would at least provide an opportunity to counsel people about risky sexual behaviours. Also potentially helpful would be media messages about the benefits and availability of confidential STI screening services.
- *Young people are particularly vulnerable to STIs.* Some of the highest rates and increases in STIs are in Canadians ages 15–24. Young adults are more likely to be uninformed about STIs and safer sex, embarrassed to ask for information, and unaware of how to access appropriate STI testing and treatment services. Many young adults are sexually active by age 25, but young people are more likely to be unmarried, have more than one partner over time, and have a partner who has an STI. Young people need medically accurate information about abstinence, condoms, and other contraceptive methods—and open communication and encouragement from family, friends, and the community to behave responsibly.

Until STIs are controllable with vaccines or effective screening and treatment, the only way to reduce your risk is to limit the number of sexual partners and to use condoms consistently. Those who choose abstinence or a mutually monogamous relationship with one uninfected partner have no risk of STIs.

The Society of Obstetricians and Gynaecologists of Canada (SOGC) estimates that 10–30 percent of Canadian adults are infected with HPV. It is also estimated that up to 70 percent of adults will have at least one HPV infection in their lifetime. Most people infected with HPV have no symptoms at all and are unaware that they are infected and contagious. The good news is that the immune system usually clears the virus, and the infection disappears without any treatment. But in some cases, the infection persists and causes genital warts or cancers.

QUICK STATS

In low- and middle-income countries, the vaccination of at least 70% of girls against HPV could prevent more than 4 million deaths from cervical cancer over the next decade.

—*World Health Organization*, 2013

HPV is especially common in young people, with some of the highest rates of infection among Canadians under the age of 25 (see the In Focus box). Many young women contract HPV infection within three months of becoming sexually active; it is estimated that 2 percent of sexually active young women have genital warts.

Human papillomaviruses cause many types of human warts. There are more than 100 different strains of HPV, and different strains infect specific locations. More than 30 types are likely to cause genital infections, and five of these are often implicated in cervical cancer; other strains are linked to anal, penile, and other genital cancers. The HPV strains that cause most visible genital warts are less likely to cause cancer than some of the other strains. A person can be infected with several different strains.

Genital HPV infection is quite contagious. Most people who carry HPV have no visible warts or any other symptoms and are not aware that they are infected and contagious to others. The strains of HPV that are linked with cancer are especially stealthy in that they generally do not cause warts or any obvious signs of their presence.

Two HPV vaccines—Gardasil® and Cervarix®—have been approved by Health Canada. Gardasil protects against four types of HPV that together account for 90 percent of genital and anal warts and 70 percent of cervical cancers; it has also been shown to prevent cancers of the vagina, vulva, and anus. Cervarix offers protection against two types of HPV but not against the type that causes genital warts. Some studies indicate that Cervarix may be more effective and may provide longer-lasting protection against the viral strains that cause cervical cancer.

Gardasil was originally approved for girls and women, but in 2010 it was also approved for boys and men ages 9–26 to prevent genital warts. In 2011, Gardasil was approved for use in women up to the age of 45 and for the prevention of anal cancer in males and females ages 9–26. Cervarix was approved in 2010 for girls and women ages 10–25. All provinces and territories now offer school-based immunization programs, in which girls (in Grades 4, 5, 6, 7, or 8 depending on the province or territory) are vaccinated against HPV. The pre-adolescent/adolescent age range was chosen because the vaccine is most effective when given prior to exposure to genital HPV, and this virus is so common that many young people will be exposed to it shortly after becoming sexually active. Each of the vaccines requires three injections over a period of six months. (For more about HPV, see Chapter 8).

The use of the vaccine for HPV has been limited by political and moral considerations. Some parents have opted not to vaccinate their daughters at least in part because they want their daughters to choose abstinence and fear that giving the vaccine will be viewed as an endorsement for premarital sexual activity. Public health experts generally believe that giving the vaccine has little effect on girls' sexual choices and that the vaccine offers the opportunity to prevent the majority of cases of cervical cancer.

Symptoms

HPV-infected tissue often appears normal; it may also look like anything from a small bump on the skin to a large, warty growth. Depending on location and size, genital warts are sometimes painful. Untreated warts can grow together to form a cauliflower-like mass. In males, they appear on the penis and often involve the urethra, appearing first at the opening and then spreading inside. The growths may cause irritation and bleeding, leading to painful urination and a urethral discharge. Warts may also appear around the anus or within the rectum. In women, warts may appear on the labia or vulva and may spread to the perineum, the area between the vagina and the rectum. They may also appear on the cervix.

The incubation period ranges from one month to two years from the time of contact. People can be infected with the virus and be capable of transmitting it to their sex partners without having any symptoms at all. The vast majority of people with HPV infection have no visible warts or symptoms of any kind.

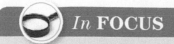

In FOCUS

Post-secondary Students and STIs

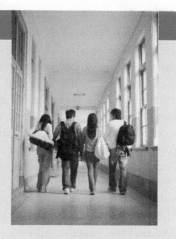

Why Do Post-secondary Students Have High Rates of STIs?

- Risky sexual behaviour is common. One study of university students found that fewer than half used condoms consistently and one-third had had 10 or more sex partners. Another study found that 19 percent of male students and 33 percent of female students had consented to sexual intercourse simply because they felt awkward refusing.
- University students underestimate their risk of STIs. Although students may have considerable knowledge about STIs, they often feel the risks do not apply to them—a dangerous assumption. One study of students with a history of STIs showed that more than half had unprotected sex while they were infected, and 25 percent of them continued to have sex without ever informing their partner(s).
- Many students are infected but don't know it. A 2006 study of asymptomatic college women revealed that nearly 10 percent were infected with chlamydia.

What Effect Does Alcohol or Drug Use Have on My Likelihood of Getting an STI?

- Between one-third and one-half of university students report participating in sexual activity as a direct result of being intoxicated. All too often, sexual activity while intoxicated leads to unprotected intercourse.
- Students who binge-drink are more likely to have multiple partners, use condoms inconsistently, and delay seeking treatment for STIs than students who drink little or no alcohol. Sexual assaults occur more frequently when either the perpetrator or the victim has been drinking.

What Can Students Do to Protect Themselves Against STIs?

- Choose to not have sex. Abstinence, if used consistently, is 100 percent effective in preventing STIs. Many people choose to abstain from sex at various times in their lives for a number of different reasons. In fact, some suggest that abstinence encourages partners to experience intimacy on levels beyond the physical, in ways that are meaningful and satisfying for both individuals.
- If you are sexually active, limit the number of sex partners. Even people who are always in a monogamous relationship can end up with extensive potential exposure to STIs if, over the years, they have numerous relationships.
- Use condoms consistently, and don't assume it's safe to stop after you have been with a partner for several months. HIV infection, HPV infection, herpes, and chlamydia can be asymptomatic for months or years and can be transmitted at any time. If you haven't been using condoms with your current partner, start now.
- Enjoy sexuality on your own terms. Don't let the expectations of friends and partners cause you to ignore your own feelings. Let your own wellness be your first priority. If you choose to be sexually active, learn about safer sex practices.
- Get to know your partner, and talk to him or her before becoming intimate. Be honest about yourself, and encourage your partner to do the same. But practise safer sex no matter what.

Genital warts sometimes grow very large during pregnancy and can occasionally be large enough to make vaginal delivery difficult. However, most pregnant women with HPV infection can deliver vaginally. HPV infection is infrequently transmitted to an infant during delivery but can occasionally cause warts to form on the infant's vocal cords.

Diagnosis

Genital warts are usually diagnosed based on the appearance of the lesions. Sometimes an examination with a special magnifying instrument or a biopsy is done to evaluate suspicious lesions. HPV infection of the cervix is often detected on routine Pap tests. Special tests are now available to detect the presence of HPV infection and to distinguish among the more common strains of HPV, including those that cause most cases of cervical cancer.

Treatment

Treatment of genital HPV infection depends on whether the infection manifests as genital warts or as a cancerous or precancerous condition. Treatment of genital warts focuses on reducing the number and size of warts, although most warts eventually disappear, even without treatment. The currently available treatments do not eradicate HPV infection. Warts may be removed by cryosurgery (freezing), electrocautery (burning), or laser surgery. Direct applications of podophyllin or other cytotoxic acids may also be used. The success rates of methods vary, and warts often recur despite initial improvement. Warts are more likely to persist and become severe in people with an impaired immune system. Cervical abnormalities that are cancerous or precancerous are treated surgically or with other techniques such as electrical excision, freezing, and laser. See Chapter 8 for more information about cervical cancer.

Even after treatment and the disappearance of visible warts, the individual may continue to carry HPV in healthy-looking tissue and can probably still infect others. Anyone who has ever had HPV infection should inform all partners and use condoms, even though they do not provide total protection. Whether or not they have had the vaccine, all women should have regular pelvic exams and Pap tests. Women who have regular screening exams almost never develop full-blown cervical cancer.

Genital Herpes

Along with HPV, HIV, and Hepatitis B, genital herpes is a viral STI. Because herpes simplex virus (HSV) infection is not a reportable STI in Canada, the annual incidence of **genital herpes** is unknown (see the In Focus box earlier in this chapter). However, recent data from a random sample of thousands of Canadians aged 14 to 59 showed that nearly 14 percent tested positive for genital herpes. The vast majority (94 percent) did not know they were infected. Worldwide, genital herpes is extremely common and is a major factor in the transmission of HIV. Most people with HIV are also infected with one form of herpes (HSV 2) and their herpes lesions contain large amounts of HIV, making it more likely that the virus will be transmitted. The presence of herpes lesions in an individual who is HIV-negative increases the likelihood that she or he will be infected by a partner who is infected with HIV. Genital herpes may also interact with HPV infection to increase the risk of cervical cancer.

> **genital herpes**
> A sexually transmitted infection caused by the herpes simplex virus.

Two types of herpes simplex viruses, HSV 1 and HSV 2, cause genital herpes and oral-labial herpes (cold sores). Many people assume that they are unlikely to pick up an STI if they limit their sexual activity to oral sex, but this is not true, particularly in the case of genital herpes. Oral sex is a common way of acquiring herpes infections, particularly among young people. HSV can also cause rectal lesions, usually transmitted through anal sex. Infection with HSV is generally lifelong. After infection, the virus lies dormant in nerve cells and can reactivate at any time. The type of virus may determine how frequently genital outbreaks occur. Individuals with HSV 2 genital infections tend to have more frequent outbreaks of genital lesions and shed more virus without having symptoms compared to individuals with HSV 1 infections.

HSV 1 infection is so common that an estimated 50 percent of Canadians have antibodies to HSV 1 (which indicates previous exposure to the virus); most were exposed during childhood. HSV 2 infection is more common in women than it is in men. In Canada, 2009–2011 statistics indicate that 16 percent of females have antibodies to HSV 2, in comparison to 11 percent of males. Based on this sample, Canadian women ages 35 to 49 appear to have the highest rates of genital herpes.

HSV 2 is almost always sexually transmitted. The infection spreads readily whether people have active sores or are

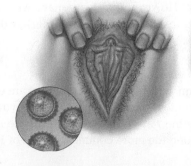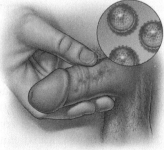

completely asymptomatic. Because new HSV 2 infections are asymptomatic in about 60 percent of people, the infection is often acquired from a person who does not know that he or she is infected.

If you have ever had an outbreak of genital herpes, you should consider yourself always contagious and inform your partners. Avoid intimate contact when any sores are present, and use condoms during all sexual contact. One study showed that using condoms for every act of intercourse results in a 30 percent decrease in the transmission of herpes compared with no condom use. Condoms are more effective in preventing the transmission of STIs than for herpes, but this study shows that they can make a significant difference in preventing the spread of genital herpes.

Newborns can occasionally be infected with HSV, usually during passage through the birth canal of an infected mother (or through an HSV infection acquired by the mother during the third trimester of pregnancy). Without treatment, 65 percent of newborns with HSV will die, and most who survive will have some degree of brain damage. The risk of mother-to-child HSV transmission during pregnancy and delivery is low (less than 1 percent) in women with long-standing herpes infection. Blood tests to screen pregnant women and their sexual partners for herpes could substantially reduce neonatal herpes infections. If an uninfected pregnant woman's partner carries HSV, abstinence or the use of condoms could prevent infection during pregnancy.

Pregnant women who have been exposed to genital herpes should inform their health care providers so that appropriate precautions can be taken to protect the baby from infection. These precautions sometimes include a Caesarean section if active lesions are present at the time of delivery.

Symptoms

A large number of people who are infected with HSV have no symptoms. Those that do develop symptoms often first notice them within 2–20 days of having sex with an infected partner. (However, it is not unusual for the first outbreak to occur months or even years after initial exposure.) The first episode of genital herpes frequently causes flu-like symptoms in addition to genital lesions. The lesions tend to be painful or itchy and can occur anywhere on the genitals, inner thighs, or anal area. Depending on their location, they can cause considerable pain with urination. Lymph nodes in the groin may become swollen and tender. The lesions usually heal within three weeks

On average, newly diagnosed people will experience five to eight outbreaks per year, with a decrease in the frequency of outbreaks over time. Recurrent episodes are usually less severe than the initial one, with fewer and less painful sores that heal more quickly. Outbreaks can be triggered by stress, illness, fatigue, sun exposure, sexual intercourse, and menstruation (see the Mind Body Spirit box).

Diagnosis

Genital herpes is often diagnosed on the basis of symptoms; a sample of fluid from the lesions may also be sent to a laboratory for culture. This test is helpful if the specimen is obtained within about two days of the lesion's development. If the lesion has been around for longer than two days, the culture will often be negative even if the person has genital herpes.

Several tests can detect the presence of HSV antibodies in the blood. Older tests don't distinguish between HSV 1 and HSV 2. Tests can also distinguish between HSV 1 and HSV 2 infection. This knowledge may help prevent transmission of HSV in couples where one partner is infected and the other is not (particularly important for uninfected women who are pregnant).

Treatment

There is no cure for herpes. Once infected, a person carries the virus for life. Antiviral drugs, such as acyclovir, can be taken at the beginning of an outbreak to shorten the severity and duration of symptoms. A person on suppressive therapy can still transmit HSV to an uninfected partner, but the risk appears to be reduced by about half. Using condoms consistently and taking suppressive medication is a reasonable way to reduce the risk of passing herpes to an uninfected sexual partner. Support groups are also available to help people learn to cope with herpes. There is no vaccine to prevent herpes, but research is ongoing. It is always important to inform a sexual partner if you have genital herpes.

Mind *Body* **SPIRIT**

Stress and Genital Herpes

Patients and health care workers alike have long suspected that stress and genital herpes outbreaks are related. Research into this potential link has yielded mixed results. One study of women with genital herpes found that persistent stressors (those lasting more than a week) and persistent high levels of anxiety were associated with increased outbreaks. Short-term stress, mood changes, and brief negative life experiences did not influence the rate of herpes outbreaks.

Experts suspect that stress has a negative impact on the immune system. Studies have shown that immune function and antibody levels may drop in response to psychological stress. Perhaps herpes viruses that are usually dormant in nervous system tissue become activated when immune function declines because of stress.

Still to be investigated is whether stress-reduction techniques, such as meditation or exercise, result in reduced rates of herpes outbreaks. Until such research becomes available, it makes sense for people who suffer recurrent genital herpes outbreaks to do what they can to reduce stress, especially long-term stress and anxiety (see Chapter 3). If you have herpes, joining a support group may help reduce your stress and improve your ability to cope with this chronic disease. If you have several outbreaks a year, or if you have recently had your first episode of genital herpes, talk to your health care provider about suppressive antiviral medication, which can reduce outbreaks substantially. Keep in mind that regardless of stress level, genital herpes outbreaks naturally tend to become less and less frequent over time. Knowing that your outbreaks are likely to diminish may, in and of itself, help reduce your feelings of stress.

HIV Infection and AIDS

The **human immunodeficiency virus (HIV)** causes **acquired immune deficiency syndrome (AIDS)**, a disease that, without treatment, kills most of its victims. AIDS originated in Africa sometime during the early twentieth century but was not recognized or named until 1981. The disease spread rapidly throughout the world and is now a leading cause of death globally.

human immunodeficiency virus (HIV)
The virus that causes HIV infection and AIDS.

acquired immune deficiency syndrome (AIDS)
A generally fatal, incurable, sexually-transmitted viral infection.

An estimated 75 million people have been infected since the epidemic began—approximately 1 percent of the world's population—and tens of millions of those people have died (see the Dimensions of Diversity box). Currently, about 35 million people are infected with HIV/AIDS worldwide, with nearly 71 percent of them living in sub-Saharan Africa.

For the first time in the history of the AIDS epidemic, the number of people worldwide that are living with HIV infection has begun to level off. Many experts believe that the global HIV epidemic peaked in the late 1990s, at about 3.5 million new infections per year, compared with an estimated 2.1 million new infections in 2013. Despite a slowing of the epidemic, however, AIDS remains a primary cause of death in Africa and continues to be a major cause of mortality around the world.

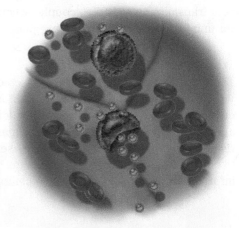

In Canada, more than 76 000 positive HIV tests have been reported since 1985 (when HIV reporting began). The first death attributed to AIDS in Canada occurred in 1983; since then, more than 13 000 Canadians have died from AIDS. In 2012, 2062 new HIV infections were reported—the lowest number of annual HIV cases since 1985 and a decrease of almost 8 percent from the number of

Dimensions *of* DIVERSITY

HIV/AIDS Around the World

In 2016, the world will mark the 35th year since AIDS, a previously unknown disease, was diagnosed in five young gay men in Los Angeles. HIV is now a worldwide scourge (see Figure 13.1), with approximately 75 million people infected and 36 million deaths since the epidemic began. Because of the many promising developments and efforts to address the epidemic, experts have suggested that the world has turned the corner in the fight against HIV. Worldwide, there has been a 38 percent decrease in new HIV infections since 2001, and a 35 percent decrease in AIDS-related deaths since 2005.

The vast majority of HIV cases—95 percent—occur in developing countries, where heterosexual contact is the primary means of transmission and is responsible for 85 percent of all adult infections. HIV continues to be a disease that disproportionately affects the poor and ethnic minorities. Worldwide, women are the fastest-growing group of newly infected people; half of adults living with HIV in 2013 were women. In sub-Saharan Africa, the region most heavily burdened with HIV, 59 percent of adults living with HIV in 2013 were women. About 3.2 million children were living with HIV in 2013, and more than 90 percent of these children were living in sub-Saharan Africa.

Despite the ongoing tragedy of the HIV epidemic, strides have been made in treatment and prevention measures. In 2006, 90 percent of individuals living with HIV were not receiving antiretroviral treatment; by the end of 2013, that percentage had decreased to 63 percent. In 2013, 67 percent of pregnant women received treatment to prevent transmission of HIV to their babies, up from 32 percent in 2008. Treating HIV with effective drugs not only prolongs life and decreases suffering, it also has a major impact in reducing the spread of the virus because individuals who have been treated are generally much less infections than those who have not been treated.

FIGURE 13.1

Approximate Number of Adults and Children Living with HIV in 2012

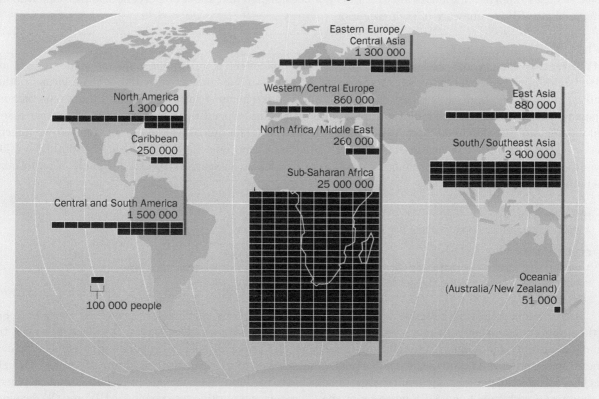

Source: Data from Joint United Nations Programme on HIV/AIDS (UNAIDS). 2013. Global Report: *UNAIDS Report on the Global AIDS Epidemic 2013.* Geneva: Joint United Nations Programme on HIV/AIDS (UNAIDS), http://www.unaids.org/en/media/unaids/contentassets/documents/epidemiology/2013/gr2013/UNAIDS_Global_Report_2013_en.pdf (retrieved October 25, 2015).

The HIV epidemic seems to have stabilized in many parts of the world. Rates of new infections have remained steady or have even dropped in a few regions. Though sub-Saharan Africa remains the hardest-hit area of the world, there was a 33 percent decrease in the number of new infections and a 39 percent drop in AIDS-related deaths between 2005 and 2013. The expanded availability of antiretroviral medications to this region has contributed significantly to these declining rates. Still, two-thirds of all adults and children with HIV live in sub-Saharan Africa, and nearly three-quarters of all deaths due to AIDS in 2013 occurred there.

Eastern Europe and parts of Asia have also been hit by HIV. In many of these areas, HIV infection is seen in intravenous drug users and their sexual partners.

Efforts to combat HIV/AIDS are complicated by political, economic, and cultural barriers. Education and prevention programs are often hampered by resistance from social and religious institutions and by the taboo related to openly discussing sexual issues. Condoms are not commonly used in many countries, and women in many societies do not have sufficient control over their lives to demand that men use condoms during sex. Empowering women is a crucial priority in reducing the spread of HIV. In particular, reducing sexual violence against women, promoting financial independence, and increasing women's education and employment opportunities are essential.

Successful prevention approaches include STI treatment and education, public education campaigns about safer sex, and syringe exchange programs for injection drug users. Efforts are ongoing to improve access to barrier protective devices such as condoms. Other measures have included male circumcision, which has been shown to reduce HIV transmission in some studies.

In developed nations such as Canada, new drugs are easing AIDS symptoms and lowering viral levels dramatically for some patients. In the past few years, a growing number of people in poor countries have gained access to antiviral drugs because of the introduction of inexpensive generic drugs and increasing international funding for HIV treatment. Still, far too many people with HIV remain untreated, and far too many new infections are occurring.

positive cases reported in Canada in 2011. Today, it is estimated that about 25 percent of Canadians who are infected with HIV are unaware of their condition.

What Is HIV Infection?

HIV infection is a chronic disease that progressively damages the body's immune system, making an otherwise healthy person less able to resist a variety of infections and disorders. Normally, when a virus or other pathogen enters the body, it is targeted and destroyed by the immune system. But HIV attacks the immune system itself, invading and taking over **CD4 T cells** (a type of helper T cell), macrophages, and other essential elements of the immune system (see Chapter 9). HIV enters a human cell and converts its own genetic material, RNA, into DNA. It then inserts this DNA into the chromosomes of the host cell. The viral DNA takes over the CD4 cell, causing it to produce new copies of HIV; it also makes the CD4 cell incapable of performing its immune functions.

HIV infection
A chronic, progressive viral infection that damages the immune system.

CD4 T cell
A type of white blood cell that helps coordinate the activity of the immune system; the primary target for HIV infection. The decrease in the number of these cells correlates with the risk and severity of HIV-related illness.

Immediately following infection with HIV, billions of infectious particles are produced every day. For a time, the immune system keeps pace, also producing billions of new cells. Unlike the virus, however, the immune system cannot make new cells indefinitely; as long as the virus keeps replicating, it wins in the end. The destruction of the immune system is signalled by the loss of CD4 T cells (see Figure 13.2). As CD4 cells decline, an infected person may begin to experience mild to moderately severe symptoms. In Canada, a person is diagnosed with full-blown AIDS when he or she (1) receives a positive test result for HIV and (2) develops one or more of the illnesses defined as markers for AIDS. In the United States, an individual must also have a CD4 count that it is less than 200 cells per cubic millimetre of blood (200/ĩL) to be diagnosed with AIDS; this indicates a severely damaged immune system. AIDS represents the most severe form of HIV infection. People with AIDS are vulnerable to a number of serious **opportunistic (secondary) infections**. The infections that most often prove deadly for people with HIV are seldom serious in people with a healthy immune system. Opportunistic infections are usually caused by organisms that are common in the environment and generally do not cause illness in healthy people. Figure 13.2 provides an overview of the general pattern of untreated HIV infection, from the *primary/acute infection* phase through to the *chronic asymptomatic* (symptom-free) stage and the final *chronic symptomatic phase.*

> **opportunistic (secondary) infection**
> An infection caused when organisms take the opportunity presented by a primary (initial) infection to multiply and cause a new, different infection.

Transmitting the Virus

HIV lives only within cells and body fluids, not outside the body. It is transmitted by blood and blood products, semen, vaginal and cervical secretions, and breast milk. It cannot live in air, in water, or on objects or surfaces, such as toilet seats, eating utensils, or telephones. A person is not at risk of getting HIV infection by being in the same classroom, dining room, or even household with someone who is infected. The three main routes of HIV transmission are from (1) specific kinds of sexual contact, (2) direct exposure to infected blood, and (3) contact between an HIV-infected woman and her child during pregnancy, childbirth, or breastfeeding.

FIGURE 13.2

The General Pattern of Untreated HIV Infection

The blue line represents the number of CD4 cells in the blood, a marker for the status of the immune system. The orange line shows the amount of HIV RNA in the blood.

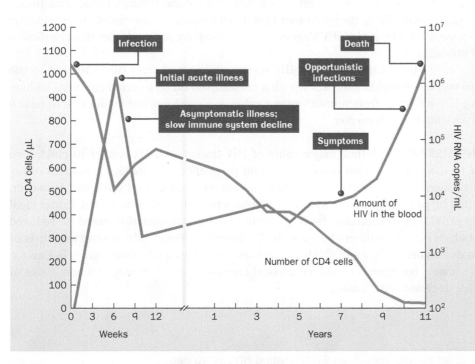

During the initial acute illness, CD4 levels fall sharply and HIV RNA levels increase; 60–90 percent of infected people experience flulike symptoms during this period. Antibodies to HIV usually appear 2–12 weeks after the initial infection. During the asymptomatic phase that follows, CD4 levels gradually decline, and HIV RNA levels again increase. Because of declines in immunity, infected individuals eventually begin to experience symptoms; when CD4 levels drop very low, people become vulnerable to serious opportunistic infections characteristic of full-blown AIDS. Chronic or recurrent illnesses continue until the immune system fails and death results.

Source: Adapted from A. S. Fauci and Giuseppe Pantaleo, 1996, "Immunopathogenic Mechanisms of HIV infection," *Annals of Internal Medicine* 124(7), 654–663, Figure 1. Reprinted with permission of the American College of Physicians.

SEXUAL CONTACT   HIV is more likely to be transmitted by unprotected anal or vaginal intercourse than by other sexual activities. HIV has been found in pre-ejaculatory fluid, so transmission can occur before ejaculation. Being the receptive partner during unprotected anal intercourse is the riskiest of all sexual activities. Oral-genital contact carries some risk of transmission, although less than anal or vaginal intercourse. HIV can be transmitted through tiny tears, traumatized points, or irritated areas in the lining of the vagina, cervix, penis, anus, mouth, and throat, and through direct infection of cells in these areas. Sexual assault is an important factor in the transmission of HIV both in Canada and throughout the world. Protection is almost never used during sexual assault, and tissue trauma is generally greater than in unforced sexual activity.

The presence of lesions, blisters, or inflammation from other STIs in the genital, anal, or oral areas makes it two to nine times easier for the virus to be passed. Spermicides may also cause irritation and increase the risk of HIV transmission, and recent studies have shown that some commonly used lubricants can also cause rectal irritation.

The risk of HIV transmission during oral sex is generally considered to be low but may be increased if a person has oral sores or other damage to the gums or tissues in the mouth.

Studies in developing nations with high rates of HIV infection have found that circumcised males have a lower risk of HIV infection than uncircumcised males. Circumcision is uncommon in most parts of the world, but these findings are heightening interest in the practice. In Canada, where circumcision is fairly common and HIV infection rates are much lower, circumcision does not appear to offer any significant protection against HIV.

DIRECT CONTACT WITH INFECTED BLOOD   Direct contact with the blood of an infected person is another major route of HIV transmission. Needles used to inject drugs (including heroin, cocaine, and anabolic steroids) are usually contaminated with the user's blood. If needles are shared, small amounts of one person's blood are directly injected into another person's bloodstream. HIV may be transmitted through subcutaneous and intramuscular injection as well, from needles or blades used in acupuncture, tattooing, body piercing, and ritual scarring.

In the past, before effective screening was available, some people were infected with HIV through blood transfusions and other medical procedures involving blood products. In Canada, blood donors have been screened for HIV infection since 1985. Since then, the estimated risk of infection through blood transfusion has been reduced substantially. Unfortunately, the blood supply is much less safe in the rest of the world. The WHO estimates that about 5 percent of all cases of HIV infection worldwide have resulted from the transfusion of infected blood and blood products.

A small number of health care workers have acquired HIV on the job; most of these cases involve needle sticks, in which a health care worker is accidentally stuck with a needle used on an infected patient. The likelihood of a patient acquiring HIV infection from a health care worker is almost negligible; the risk to health care workers from infected patients is much greater.

MOTHER-TO-CHILD TRANSMISSION   The final major route of HIV transmission is mother to child, also called *vertical* or *perinatal transmission*, which can occur during pregnancy, childbirth, or breastfeeding. Without intervention, the likelihood of HIV transmission from mother to child is 20–45 percent. However, transmission may be prevented by providing antiretroviral medications to both mother and child. Under ideal conditions of treatment and providing replacement feeding, mother-to-child transmission could be reduced to fewer than 2 percent of babies born to mothers living with HIV infection. Worldwide, about two-thirds of vertical transmission occurs during pregnancy and childbirth and one-third through breastfeeding. In Canada and other developed countries, new treatments to reduce vertical transmission are in use, and new cases of this type of HIV infection have declined significantly.

QUICK STATS

Worldwide, more than 1 million people acquire an STI (including HIV) every day.
—World Health Organization, 2013

Populations of Special Concern for HIV Infection

Among Canadians with AIDS, the most common means of HIV exposure is sexual activity between men; heterosexual contact and injection drug use are the next most common, as shown in Figure 13.3. In 2011, men who have sex with men (MSM) accounted for nearly half (46.7 percent) of all HIV infections, even though they are estimated to represent less than 2 percent of the Canadian population. Young men in particular are at risk, in part because they tend to engage in unsafe sexual practices such as unprotected anal intercourse. Use of methamphetamine and club drugs, as well as the recreational use of erectile dysfunction drugs, has also been associated with risky health behaviour and HIV infection in MSM.

Disproportionately high rates of infection in certain groups are tied to social, cultural, and economic factors. HIV in Canada is increasingly becoming a disease that affects ethnic minorities, women, and poor people. Women, especially Aboriginal women, make up an increasingly large proportion of all Canadian cases of HIV infection. Overall, Aboriginal people made up 12.2 percent of the reported new HIV infection cases in 2011, with approximately half occurring in Aboriginal women. See the Dimensions of Diversity box for more on these trends.

These patterns of HIV infection reflect complex social, economic, and behavioural factors. Reducing the rates of HIV transmission and AIDS death in minorities, women, and other groups at risk requires addressing problems of poverty, discrimination, and drug abuse. HIV prevention programs must be tailored to meet the special needs of minority communities and include testing, education, and equal access to health care.

Symptoms

Within a few days or weeks of infection with HIV, most people will develop symptoms of primary (also called acute) HIV infection. These can include fever, fatigue, rashes, headache, swollen lymph nodes, body aches,

FIGURE 13.3

Estimated Number of New HIV Infections and Routes of Transmission Among Canadians

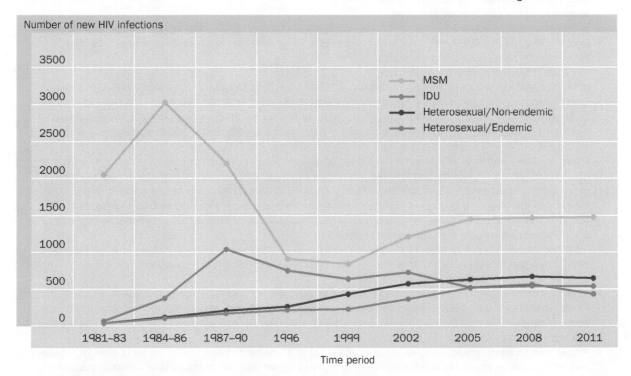

MSM = Men who have sex with men; IDU = Persons who inject drugs; Heterosexual/Non-endemic = Heterosexual contact with a person who is either HIV-infected or at risk for HIV as the only identified risk; Heterosexual/Endemic = Origin in a country where HIV is endemic.

Source: Public Healthy Agency of Canada, 2012. *Summary: Estimates of HIV Prevalence and Incidence in Canada, 2011.* Reproduced with permission from the Minister of Health, 2015. All rights reserved. (http://www.phac-aspc.gc.ca/aids-sida/publication/survreport/estimat2011-eng.php; retrieved October 25, 2015)

Dimensions *of* DIVERSITY

HIV/AIDS: Canada's At-Risk Populations

HIV does not discriminate; it affects males and females of all ages, religions, education and income levels, and ethnicities. However, the reality is that in Canada, specific populations are disproportionately affected by HIV and AIDS.

- *Aboriginal peoples:* Individuals who identify themselves as Aboriginal (including First Nations, Inuit, and Métis) continue to be over-represented in the HIV epidemic in Canada (see Figure 13.4). In 2011, an estimated 6380 Aboriginal people in Canada were living with HIV, a 17.3 percent increase from the 2008 estimate of 5440. Injection drug use has been identified as a primary mode of HIV transmission in the Aboriginal community.
- *Canadians of African ancestry:* Black Canadians make up a growing percentage of positive HIV reports and reported AIDS cases (see Figure 13.4). Heterosexual exposure accounts for more than 80 percent of positive HIV test reports in Canadians of African ancestry. Again, about half of the positive HIV test reports in this group are in women.
- *Injection drug users (IDU) and men who have sex with men (MSM):* As was shown in Figure 13.3, men who have sex with

FIGURE 13.4

Distribution of Positive HIV Test Reports in Canada, by Ethnic Status

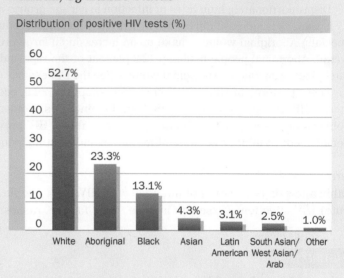

Distribution of positive HIV tests (%)

White 52.7%
Aboriginal 23.3%
Black 13.1%
Asian 4.3%
Latin American 3.1%
South Asian/West Asian/Arab 2.5%
Other 1.0%

Note: In 2012, approximately 62 percent of positive HIV reports in Canada included race/ethnicity information; as such, data should be interpreted with caution.

Source: Public Health Agency of Canada. 2012. *At a Glance - HIV and AIDS in Canada: Surveillance Report to December 31st, 2012.* Reproduced with the permission of the Minister of Health.

men represent the largest category of positive HIV test reports in Canada. Interestingly, although injection drug use represents a large exposure category in Canada, the number of HIV infections in this group appears to be decreasing. The overall heterosexual exposure category (including individuals from HIV-endemic and non-endemic countries) now represents a growing number of positive HIV tests, surpassing injection drug use as the second-largest exposure category.

- *Prison inmates:* Rates of HIV infection in Canadian prisons appear to be considerably higher than in the general population. In federal prisons, the prevalence of HIV among women is higher than among men. It is probable that some offenders infected with HIV engaged in risky behaviours before going to prison; however, some inmates also engage in high-risk behaviours while in prison, including needle-sharing, tattooing, and unprotected sex. The potential for HIV transmission is great in penitentiaries, with possible infection of spouses and partners once inmates are released.
- *Youth:* Approximately one-quarter of the positive HIV cases in 2012 were among youth ages 20–29. Studies have shown that homeless or street-involved youth, those who inject drugs, and young men who have sex with men are particularly vulnerable to HIV infection.
- *Women:* Women represent an increasing proportion of reported HIV and AIDS cases in Canada. In 2012, the Public Health Agency of Canada estimated that approximately 23 percent of Canadians infected with HIV were women, compared to less than 10 percent before 1995. Heterosexual exposure and injection drug use are the two main risk behaviours for HIV infection in women.
- *People from countries where HIV is endemic:* In 2011, about 17 percent of new HIV test reports were for individuals from countries where HIV is endemic, a rate nine times higher than that in the general Canadian population.

   A continued focus on new and effective approaches to prevention and treatment are needed to combat the high incidence of HIV/AIDS among the populations discussed above. HIV prevention messages need to communicate effectively with the populations most at risk. For those who are already living with HIV, other resources such as peer networks, legal assistance, and on-site child care at clinics may help improve treatment access and success.

The Federal Initiative to Address HIV/AIDS in Canada represents a government commitment to increased HIV/AIDS funding and several other areas of action, with a particular focus on some of the populations discussed above. The use of population-specific approaches is essential to developing culturally appropriate strategies that can address the myriad of complex social, economic, and environmental factors that contribute to infection in these at-risk groups.

Some of the factors that increase a person or group's risk of HIV infection include stigma and discrimination, homophobia, gender inequity, poverty, limited access to education and health services, substance use, lack of HIV/AIDS awareness, high prevalence of HIV infection in a community, and low perceptions of risk. When such factors are present, individuals may be less likely to seek testing, prevention, and treatment services, and more likely to engage in unsafe behaviours such as unprotected sex or the use of contaminated needles.

Sources: Health Canada. 2012. *Federal Initiative to Address HIV/AIDS in Canada*, http://www.phac-aspc.gc.ca/aids-sida/fi-if/index-eng.php (retrieved September 25, 2015); Public Health Agency of Canada. 2007. *Populations at Risk—Federal Initiative to Address HIV/AIDS in Canada*, http://www.phac-aspc.gc.ca/aids-sida/populations-eng.php (retrieved February 21, 2015); Public Health Agency of Canada. 2008. *Canadian Guidelines on Sexually Transmitted Infections*, http://www.phac-aspc.gc.ca/std-mts/sti-its/index-eng.php (retrieved February 10, 2015); Public Health Agency of Canada. 2013. *At a Glance - HIV and AIDS in Canada: Surveillance Report to December 31st, 2012*, http://www.phac-aspc.gc.ca/aids-sida/publication/survreport/2012/dec/index-eng.php (retrieved October 20, 2015); Public Health Agency of Canada. 2010. *HIV/AIDS Epi Updates. July 2010*, http://www.phac-aspc.gc.ca/aids-sida/publication/epi/2010/4-eng.php (retrieved October 20, 2015); Public Health Agency of Canada. 2012. *Summary: Estimates of HIV Prevalence and Incidence in Canada, 2011*, http://www.phac-aspc.gc.ca/aids-sida/publication/survreport/estimat2011-eng.php (retrieved September 30, 2015); Public Health Agency of Canada. 2010. *Population-Specific HIV/AIDS Report: Aboriginal Peoples*, http://www.phac-aspc.gc.ca/aids-sida/publication/ps-pd/aboriginal-autochtones/pdf/pshasrap-revspda-eng.pdf (retrieved October 25, 2015).

night sweats, sore throat, nausea, and ulcers in the mouth. Because the symptoms of primary HIV infection are similar to those of many common viral illnesses, the condition often goes undiagnosed.

Other than the initial flu-like symptoms, most people have few if any symptoms in the first months or years of HIV infection. As the immune system weakens, however, a variety of symptoms can develop, such as persistent swollen lymph nodes; lumps, rashes, sores, or other growths on or under the skin or the mucous membranes; persistent yeast infections; unexplained weight loss; fever and drenching night sweats; dry cough and shortness of breath; persistent diarrhea; easy bruising and unexplained bleeding; profound fatigue; memory loss; difficulty with balance; tremors or seizures; changes in vision, hearing, taste, or smell; changes in mood and other psychological symptoms; and persistent or recurrent pain. Obviously, many of these symptoms can also occur with a variety of other illnesses. Because the immune system is weakened, people with HIV infection are also highly susceptible to a number of opportunistic infections, both common and uncommon, as noted earlier.

QUICK STATS

93% of new HIV infections occur in low- and middle-income countries.

—World Health Organization, 2013

Diagnosis

The most commonly used screening tests for HIV are **HIV antibody tests**. Standard testing involves an initial test called an **ELISA**. If it is positive, a second test—either a **Western blot** or immunoflourescence assay—is done to confirm the results (see the Critical Consumer box).

HIV antibody test
A blood test to determine whether a person has been infected by HIV; becomes positive within weeks or months of exposure.

ELISA (enzyme-linked immunosorbent assay)
A blood test that detects the presence of antibodies to HIV.

Western blot
A blood test that detects the presence of HIV antibodies; a more accurate and expensive test used to confirm positive results from an ELISA test.

Critical CONSUMER

Getting an HIV Test

You should strongly consider being tested for HIV if any of the following apply to you or any past or current sexual partners:

- You have had unprotected sex (vaginal, anal, or oral) with more than one partner or with a partner who was not in a mutually monogamous relationship with you.
- You have had sex while under the influence of alcohol or drugs (you might not have used protection).
- You have used or shared needles, syringes, or other paraphernalia for injecting drugs (including steroids).
- You have exchanged sex for drugs or money.
- You have had tattooing, piercing, or acupuncture with unsterilized equipment.
- You received a transfusion of blood or blood products before 1986.
- You have ever been diagnosed with an STI.

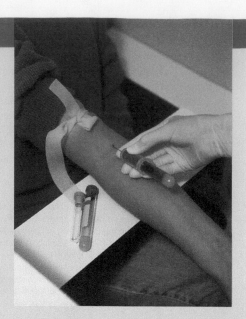

Physician or Clinic Testing

Your physician, student health clinic, public health department, or local AIDS association can arrange your HIV test. Before you take the test, a nurse or counsellor will ask you why you want to take the test, when and how you think you were exposed to HIV, and whether you have any questions. This is also a good time to obtain accurate information about HIV and AIDS and to talk about the implications of the test result, especially if it is positive. It is your choice to get tested, and you must give your consent in writing.

The standard test involves drawing a sample of blood that is sent to a laboratory, where it is checked for antibodies. If the first stage of testing is positive, the test is repeated. This standard test takes one to two weeks, and you will be asked to phone or come in personally to obtain your results, which should also include appropriate counselling. In Canada, HIV testing is not automatically anonymous. Although anonymous testing may encourage more people to get tested for HIV, it is not available in all provinces and territories.

Home Testing

Using an HIV home test kit requires an individual to prick his or her finger with a supplied lancet, blot a few drops of blood onto blotting paper, and mail it to a laboratory. In about a week, the test result is retrieved over the telephone. Anyone who tests positive is connected to a trained counsellor, who can provide emotional and medical support. These results are anonymous.

While home test kits have been available in the United States since 1996, these kits have not been approved for use in Canada. Both Canadian and U.S. governments have warned individuals about the dangers of purchasing unapproved HIV home test kits sold over the Internet. On several occasions, Health Canada has issued recalls for and advised consumers not to use HIV home test kits as they have not been authorized for use and may provide false results.

Understanding the Results

A negative test result means that no antibodies were found in your sample. However, it usually takes at least three months after exposure to HIV (and possibly as long as six months in some people) for antibodies to appear. Therefore, an infected person may receive a false-negative result. In patients with a negative HIV test result and a high risk of infection, repeat testing is recommended.

A positive result means that you are infected. It is important to seek medical care and counselling immediately. Rapid progress is being made in treating HIV, and treatments are potentially much more successful when started early.

For more information about HIV testing and a list of AIDS service organizations in your region, visit the Canadian AIDS Society Web site (http://www.cdnaids.ca). You can also find a testing centre in your area (including anonymous test sites) by calling your provincial or territorial HIV/AIDS hotline. These numbers are listed on the Public Health Agency of Canada's website (http://www.phac-aspc.gc.ca/aids-sida/info/4-eng.php#find).

Antibodies may not appear in the blood for weeks or months after infection, so people who are newly infected are likely to have a negative antibody test. In its early stages, the infection can be detected with an HIV RNA assay, which directly measures the presence of the virus in the blood.

If a person is diagnosed as **HIV-positive**, the next step is to determine the disease's severity to plan appropriate treatment. The immune system's status can be gauged by measuring CD4 T cells every few months. The infection itself can be monitored by tracking the viral load (the amount of virus in the body) through the **HIV RNA assay**.

> **HIV-positive**
> A diagnosis resulting from the presence of HIV in the bloodstream; also referred to as *seropositive*.
>
> **HIV RNA assay**
> A test used to determine the viral load (the amount of HIV in the blood).

Many people are not aware that rapid HIV tests are now available in Canada. These tests must be performed by a health care professional in a setting where HIV counselling is available. Results are typically obtained within 15 minutes. Whereas a negative test result is considered accurate (and no further testing is necessary), an initially positive (or "initially reactive") test result requires another test at an approved HIV-testing laboratory for confirmation.

Anyone who was recently exposed to HIV and has a negative antibody test should have the test repeated in a few months. Periodic routine testing is the best way for anyone to find out if the person has HIV. The Public Health Agency of Canada recommends that anyone who engages in risky behaviour should be tested and that the consideration and discussion of HIV testing be included as part of routine medical care for all patients (refer to the Critical Consumer box for a list of risky behaviours). These recommendations were advanced in hopes that routine HIV testing will help to normalize the practice and increase the likelihood that people with HIV will be diagnosed earlier.

In Canada, all diagnosed cases of HIV or AIDS must be reported to public health authorities (refer to the In Focus box earlier in this chapter). Despite efforts to safeguard confidentiality and prohibit discrimination, mandatory reporting of HIV infection remains controversial. If people believe they are risking their jobs, friends, or social acceptability, they may be less likely to be tested. At the same time, it is essential that enough information be disclosed to monitor the epidemic. People living with HIV (or a health care professional) must also notify all of their sexual partners and other contacts that may have been exposed in the past. Partner notification is a prevention process through which at-risk individuals are identified, located, assessed, and treated if necessary. In 2012, the Supreme Court of Canada ruled that individuals living with HIV have a legal obligation to disclose their HIV status with partners before sexual relations, except when HIV transmission risk is considered to be low, such as when the person living with HIV has a low viral load and wears a condom.

Treatment

Although there is no known cure for HIV infection, medications can significantly alter the course of the disease and extend life. On average, with the best treatment currently available, someone with HIV infection will live 20 to 30 years or more after diagnosis. In fact, the drop in the number of deaths in Canada from AIDS since 1996 is in large part due to the increasing use of combinations of new and effective drugs. For most people worldwide, however, this progress is irrelevant; adequate treatment is not available and/or affordable, and most infected people die within 10 years following diagnosis.

The main types of antiviral drugs used against HIV/AIDS are reverse transcriptase inhibitors, protease inhibitors, integrase inhibitors, and entry inhibitors. These drugs either block HIV from replicating itself or prevent it from infecting other cells. Research has shown that using combinations of antiviral drugs can sometimes reduce HIV in the blood to undetectable levels. More than 30 drugs are now available to treat HIV. However, people on antiviral drugs can still transmit the infection, and concerns are growing that even these very aggressive treatments are starting to fail and that drug-resistant strains of HIV are developing rapidly. In addition to antiviral drugs, most patients with low CD4 T cell counts take a variety of antibiotics to help prevent opportunistic infections. A person with advanced HIV infection may need to take 20 or more pills every day. Medication side effects can become severe when so many drugs are used in combination.

The cost of treatment for HIV continues to be an area of major concern. Costs are tremendous even for relatively wealthy countries, and given that the vast majority of people with HIV infection live in developing countries, treatments are unlikely to be available to anyone except the wealthiest few. Pharmaceutical companies, the World Bank, and the international community are working to lower drug costs and provide aid for developing regions.

Prevention

The best hope for stopping the spread of HIV worldwide is the development of a safe, effective, and inexpensive vaccine. Many different approaches to the development of an HIV vaccine are currently under investigation. One that appears to hold promise was developed by researchers at Western University in London, Ontario. Results of recent (Phase I) clinical trials with humans have been successful and have shown no adverse effects on patients. If the next phases of clinical trials demonstrate positive results, the vaccine could be commercially available within the next five years.

Researchers are also making progress in producing a **microbicide** that could be used to prevent HIV and other STIs. A microbicide in the form of a cream, gel, sponge, or suppository could function as a kind of chemical condom.

---

microbicide
An agent that destroys microorganisms; also known as an *antiseptic*.

QUICK STATS

In 39 countries, the incidence of HIV infection decreased by more than 25% between 2001 and 2011.
—UNAIDS, 2012

How Can You Protect Yourself?

Although AIDS cannot be cured, infection can be prevented. You can protect yourself by avoiding behaviours that may bring you into contact with HIV. This means making careful choices about sexual activity and not sharing needles if you inject drugs.

In a sexual relationship, the current and past behaviours of you and your partner determine the amount of risk involved. If you are uninfected and in a mutually monogamous relationship with another uninfected person, you are not at risk for HIV.

For anyone not involved in a long-term, mutually monogamous relationship, abstinence from any sexual activity that involves the exchange of body fluids is the only sure way to prevent HIV infection (see Figure 13.5).

Anal and vaginal intercourse are the sexual activities associated with the highest risk of HIV infection. If you have intercourse, always use a condom. Use of a condom reduces the risk of transmitting HIV during all forms of intercourse. Condoms are not perfect, and they do not provide risk-free sex; however, when used properly, a condom provides a high level of protection against HIV. Experts also suggest the use of latex squares and dental dams, rubber devices that can be used as barriers during oral-genital or oral-anal sexual contact. Avoid using nonoxynol-9 lubricants because of the risk of tissue irritation, which can make STI transmission more likely.

QUICK STATS

HIV and tuberculosis (TB) represent a "dual epidemic"; the risk of acquiring TB is 12–20 times greater in people living with HIV than among those not infected.
—World Health Organization, 2014

FIGURE 13.5

What's Risky and What's Not: The Approximate Relative Risk of HIV Transmission of Various Sexual Activities

High Risk

Unprotected anal sex is the riskiest sexual behaviour, especially for the receptive partner.

Unprotected vaginal intercourse is the next riskiest, especially for women, who are much more likely to be infected by an infected male partner than vice versa.

Oral sex is probably considerably less risky than anal and vaginal intercourse but can still result in HIV transmission.

Sharing of sex toys can be risky because they can carry blood, semen, or vaginal fluid.

Use of a condom reduces risk considerably but not completely for any type of intercourse. Anal sex with a condom is riskier than vaginal sex with a condom; oral sex with a condom is less risky, especially if the man does not ejaculate.

Hand-genital contact and deep kissing are less risky but could still theoretically transmit HIV; the presence of cuts or sores increases risk.

Sex with only one uninfected and totally faithful partner is without risk, but effective only if both partners are uninfected and completely monogamous.

Activities that don't involve the exchange of body fluids carry no risk: hugging, massage, closed-mouth kissing, masturbation, phone sex, and fantasy.

Abstinence is completely without risk. For many people, it can be an effective and reasonable method of avoiding HIV infection and other STIs during certain periods of life.

No Risk

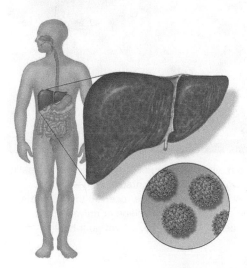

People who inject drugs should avoid sharing needles, syringes, filters, or anything that might have blood on it. Needles can be decontaminated with a solution of bleach and water, but it is not a fool-proof procedure, and HIV can survive in a syringe for a month or longer. HIV can also survive boiling.

As described in Chapter 14, obtaining sterile syringes through a syringe exchange program is much more effective than attempting to sterilize used syringes. Many prominent health organizations, including the Joint United Nations Programme on HIV/AIDS (UNAIDS) and the Canadian Public Health Association, support syringe exchange programs, but these programs are unavailable or illegal in many other parts of the world.

Until an effective vaccine and a cure are found, HIV infection will remain one of the biggest challenges of this generation. Confronting the complex environmental and socioeconomic factors that contribute to this devastating epidemic, as well as focusing on education and individual responsibility, can lead the way to controlling the spread of HIV (see the Take Charge box).

Hepatitis B

Hepatitis (inflammation of the liver) can cause serious and sometimes permanent damage to the liver, which can result in death in severe cases. One of the many types of hepatitis is caused by hepatitis B virus (HBV). HBV is somewhat similar to HIV in that it is found in most body fluids, including blood and blood products, semen, saliva, urine, and vaginal secretions.

HBV is much more contagious than HIV. It is easily transmitted through any sexual activity that involves the exchange of body fluids.

The primary risk factors for acquiring HBV are sexual exposure and injection drug use; having multiple partners greatly increases risk. HBV can also be transmitted through non-sexual close contact, including the use of contaminated needles, razor blades, toothbrushes, and eating utensils.

Other forms of viral hepatitis can also be sexually transmitted. Hepatitis A is of particular concern for people who engage in anal sex. A vaccine is available and is recommended for all people at risk. Less commonly, hepatitis C can be transmitted sexually. Experts believe that traumatic sexual activity that causes tissue damage is most likely to transmit hepatitis C. See Chapter 9 for more about these forms of hepatitis.

Take CHARGE

Preventing STI Infection

For those who aren't in a long-term monogamous relationship with an uninfected partner, abstinence is the only truly safe option for avoiding STIs. Remember that it's OK to say no to sex and drugs.

If you choose to be sexually active, talk with potential partners about STIs, safer sex, and the use of condoms before you begin a sexual relationship. The following guidelines can also help you avoid infection:

- Don't drink alcohol or use drugs in sexual situations. Mood-altering drugs can affect your judgment and make you more likely to take risks. Having sex when intoxicated significantly increases the risk of exposure to STIs.
- Limit the number of partners. Avoid sexual contact with people who have HIV or an STI or who have engaged in risky behaviours in the past, including unprotected sex and injection drug use.
- Use condoms during every act of intercourse and oral sex. Condoms do not provide perfect protection, but they greatly reduce your risk of contracting an infection. Multiple studies show that regular condom use can reduce the risk of several diseases, including HIV, chlamydia, gonorrhea, HPV, and genital herpes.
- Use condoms properly to obtain maximum protection; follow the condom use guidelines listed in Chapter 11.
- Avoid sexual contact that could cause cuts or tears in the skin or tissue.
- Get periodic screening tests for STIs and HIV. Sexually active young women should be tested for STIs at least annually. Canadian guidelines suggest that women should have a Pap test within three years of becoming sexually active or by age 21, and annually thereafter. Once a woman has two normal test results in a row, it is recommended that she has a Pap test once every three years.
- Get vaccinated. Talk to your health-care provider about vaccinations against hepatitis A, hepatitis B, and HPV.
- Get prompt treatment for any STIs you contract. Make sure your partner gets treated, too. Don't have sex until both of you have completed your treatment.

If you inject drugs of any kind, don't share needles, syringes, or anything that might have blood on it. If your community has a syringe exchange program, use it. Seek treatment, and stop using injectable drugs.

Symptoms

Many people infected with HBV never develop symptoms; they have what are known as silent infections. The normal incubation period is 30–180 days. Mild cases of hepatitis cause flu-like symptoms, such as fever, body aches, chills, and loss of appetite. As the illness progresses, people may experience nausea, vomiting, dark-coloured urine, abdominal pain, and jaundice. Some people with hepatitis also develop a skin rash and joint pain or arthritis. Acute hepatitis B can sometimes be severe, resulting in prolonged illness or even death.

Most adults who have acute hepatitis B recover completely within a few weeks or months. But about 5 percent of adults who are infected with HBV become chronic carriers of the virus, capable of infecting others for the rest of their lives. Some chronic carriers remain asymptomatic, while others develop chronic liver disease. Chronic hepatitis can cause cirrhosis, liver failure, and a deadly form of liver cancer. Hepatitis B kills about 100 Canadians each year; worldwide, the annual death toll exceeds 600 000.

Diagnosis and Treatment

Hepatitis B is diagnosed by blood tests used to analyze liver function, detect the infecting organism, and detect antibodies to the virus. While there are currently no specific treatment options for acute infections, antiviral drugs and immune system modulators may be used for cases of chronic HBV infection.

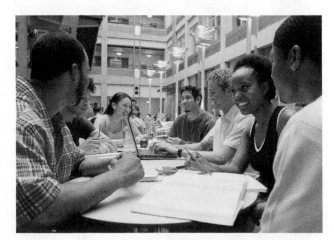

Hepatitis B is a highly contagious STI that can spread easily among people who live in close contact with one another. In Canada, all students should have received the Hepatitis B immunization prior to starting college or university. If you have not received the vaccine, inform your health care provider.

Hepatitis B is a potentially fatal disease with no cure, but an effective vaccine is available. In Canada, routine vaccination of children has drastically reduced the number of cases of acute hepatitis B. In addition, mother-to-child transmission has been greatly reduced because of routine HBV screening of pregnant women.

Preventive measures for hepatitis B are similar to those for HIV infection: Avoid sexual contact that involves sharing body fluids, including saliva; use condoms during sexual intercourse; and don't share needles. If you have tattooing or body piercing done, make sure all needles and equipment are sterile.

Other STIs

A number of other infections are also transmitted sexually.

Trichomoniasis (often called *trich*) is a common STI among young women. The single-celled organism that causes trich, *Trichomonas vaginalis*, thrives in warm, moist conditions, making women particularly susceptible to these infections in the vagina. Women who become symptomatic with trich develop a greenish, foul-smelling vaginal discharge and severe itching and pain in the vagina. Men usually have no symptoms, but may have mild irritation after urinating, or a slight discharge. Prompt treatment with metronidazole is important because studies suggest that trich may increase the risk of HIV transmission and, in pregnant women, premature delivery.

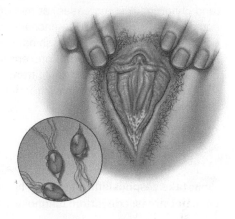

trichomoniasis
A protozoal infection caused by *Trichomonas vaginalis*, transmitted sexually and externally.

Bacterial vaginosis (BV) is the most common cause of abnormal vaginal discharge in women of reproductive age. BV occurs when healthy bacteria that normally inhabit the vagina become displaced by unhealthy species. BV is usually, but not always, associated with sexual activity and often occurs after a change in partners. Symptoms of BV include vaginal discharge with a fishy odour and sometimes vaginal irritation. BV can place women at risk for other STIs, complications after some gynecological surgical procedures, and complications during pregnancy. BV is treated with topical and oral antibiotics.

bacterial vaginosis (BV)
A condition linked to sexual activity that is caused by an overgrowth of certain bacteria inhabiting the vagina.

Pubic lice (commonly known as *crabs*) and **scabies** are highly contagious parasitic infections. They are usually treated with topical medicines, but oral medications are sometimes needed as well. Lice infestation can require repeated treatment.

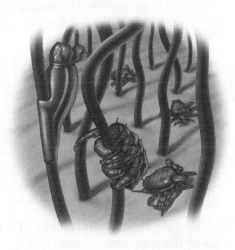

pubic lice
Parasites that infest the hair of the pubic region, commonly called *crabs*.

scabies
A contagious skin disease caused by a type of burrowing parasitic mite.

THINKING ABOUT THE ENVIRONMENT

In some parts of the world, the human environment is far more responsible than the natural one for the spread of STIs. As has been mentioned in this chapter, people in remote and poverty-stricken areas typically have little access to health care resources, information on safer sex practices, and barrier devices, such as condoms. Without access to medical testing and treatment, whole populations have little means for preventing or dealing with STIs of any kind.

Making matters worse is the harsh male-dominated sexual environments found in some regions. Whether these circumstances are based on local religious or social mores, they often place women (and children, in some cases) at risk of exploitation and greatly increase the risks of STIs. For example, some cultures allow or even encourage male infidelity. In many parts of the world, women have little or no say in their sexual relationships, meaning they may not be able to use protective measures against STIs. Often, the cultures that prevent women from protecting themselves shun or punish women who become infected with a sexually transmitted infection.

See Chapter 21 for more information on the environment and environmental health.

What You Can Do

You can take responsibility for your health and contribute to a general reduction in the incidence of STIs in three major areas: education, diagnosis and treatment, and prevention.

Education

Many schools, universities, and colleges have STI counselling and education programs. These programs allow students a chance to practise communicating with potential sex partners and negotiating safer sex, among other skills. You can find information about STIs online and at health clinics and physicians' offices. National hotlines provide free, confidential information and referral services to callers anywhere in the country (see the "For More Information" section at the end of the chapter).

Educational campaigns about HIV/AIDS and other STIs have paid off in changing attitudes and sexual behaviours. Levels of awareness about HIV infection among the general population are quite high, although some segments of the population are harder to reach and continue to engage in high-risk behaviours. Learning about STIs is still up to every person individually, as is applying that knowledge to personal situations. Once you know about STIs—their symptoms, how they are transmitted, and how they can be prevented—you are in a position to educate others. Providing information to your friends and partners, whether in casual conversation or in more serious decision-making discussions, is an important way that you can make a difference in both your own wellness and that of others.

QUESTIONS FOR CRITICAL THINKING AND REFLECTION

Have you ever had sex and regretted it later? If so, what were the circumstances, and what influenced you to engage in the behaviour? Were there any negative consequences? Based on this chapter, are there any steps you could take now to avoid possible negative consequences? What preventive strategies can you use in the future to make sure it doesn't happen again?

Diagnosis and Treatment

Early diagnosis and treatment of STIs can help you and your sex partner(s) avoid complications and help prevent the spread of infection.

Get Vaccinated

Every young, sexually active person should be vaccinated for hepatitis B; vaccines are available for all age groups. In Canada, immunization against hepatitis A is recommended for anyone at risk for infection, including people who plan to travel internationally, men who have sex with men, and those who use drugs. Men and women ages 9–26 should also be vaccinated for HPV.

Be Alert for Symptoms

If you are sexually active, be alert for any sign or symptom of infection, such as a rash, a discharge, sores, or pain. Although only a physician can make a proper diagnosis of an STI, you can perform *genital self-examinations* between checkups to look for early warning signs of infection. Use a mirror to view your entire genital area. Remember, though, that many STIs can be asymptomatic, so a professional exam and testing are recommended following any risky sexual encounter.

Get Tested

If you are sexually active, be sure to get periodic STI checks, even if you have no symptoms. If you have a risky sexual encounter, see a physician as soon as possible (see the Take Charge box for more information).

 Take **CHARGE**

Don't Wait—Early Treatment of STIs Really Matters

If you have had a recent risky sexual encounter, visit your physician, student health centre, or local STI clinic and ask for testing. Don't wait for symptoms to develop—you may never have any. Permanent damage from STIs, including infertility, can occur even if you have no symptoms. Treating some STIs, such as chlamydia and gonorrhea, within a few days of infection is very likely to prevent complications, such as PID and infertility. You will also be much less likely to pass the infection on to anyone else.

Unsafe sex with a person who is infected with HIV meets the criteria for post-exposure prophylaxis (PEP) treatment, which involves taking antiviral medication as soon as possible. If you are treated within 72 hours of possible exposure, PEP will significantly reduce your risk of HIV infection. If you develop flulike symptoms in the days or weeks following risky sexual or drug-taking behaviour, see your physician immediately. If HIV treatment is started within the first weeks of the infection, there is still a good chance that damage to the immune system can be reduced or even prevented. Many physicians will not think of primary HIV infection when you describe flu-like symptoms, so be sure to speak up about your recent risky activities and your concerns about HIV.

If tests come back positive for a particular STI, you need to be tested for others, including HIV infection. Infection with any STI means that you are at higher risk for all others. Women should also have a pelvic exam and a Pap test. If you are given medication to treat an STI, take all of it as directed. Incomplete treatment can result in an incomplete cure, thereby contributing to the development of drug-resistant organisms.

Do not have sexual intercourse until your treatment—and your partner's treatment—is complete. If your partner still carries the infection, you are likely to be reinfected when you resume sexual activity. If you have an incurable STI, such as herpes or HPV infection, always use a condom and make sure your partner is fully informed of the potential risks of being intimate with you, even if you are using condoms.

Inform Your Partners

Telling a partner that you have exposed him or her to an STI isn't easy. Despite the awkwardness and difficulty, it is crucial that your sex partner(s) be informed and urged to seek testing and/or treatment as quickly as possible. You can get help telling your partner if you need it. Public health departments will notify sex partners of their possible exposure while maintaining your confidentiality and anonymity.

Get Treated

Generally speaking, treatments for STIs are safe and (with the exception of AIDS treatments) fairly inexpensive. If you are being treated, follow instructions carefully and take all the medication as prescribed. Don't stop taking the medication just because you feel better or your symptoms have disappeared. Above all, don't give any of your medication to anyone else, including your partner. If you have an STI, your partner needs to be tested and, if necessary, treated. Taking a few of your pills is unlikely to cure your partner, and may make your treatment incomplete, leaving you both at risk for reinfection.

Prevention

STIs *are* preventable. As discussed earlier, the only sure way to avoid exposure to STIs is to abstain from sexual activity. But if you choose to be sexually active, the key is to think about prevention *before* you have a sexual encounter or find yourself in the heat of the moment. To iden-

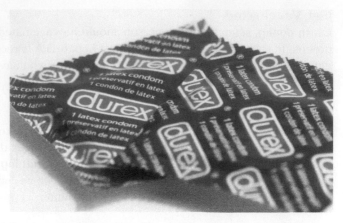

Condoms protect against STIs and should be used even if another form of contraception, such as birth control pills or an IUD, is being used.

tify your STI risk factors, see the Assess Yourself box at the beginning of this chapter. Find out what your partner thinks before you become sexually involved.

Most people don't want to think, talk, or ask questions about STIs for a variety of reasons. They may think it detracts from the appeal and excitement of the moment, that it takes away from the spontaneity of the experience, or that it will be perceived as a personal insult. For others, simply not knowing how to talk about STIs and safer sex may prevent them from bringing up the issue with a partner. (For advice on communicating with potential sex partners, see the Take Charge box.)

You may find that your partner is just as concerned as you are. By thinking and talking about responsible sexual behaviour, you are expressing a sense of caring for yourself, your potential partner, and your future children.

QUESTIONS FOR CRITICAL THINKING AND REFLECTION

Have you ever thought about where you get your behaviours and habits related to STIs? Many factors can influence our behaviours and habits, some not as obvious as others. Did you have comprehensive sex education in high school? Do the significant people in your peer group use condoms and practice safer sex? Have you been influenced by a partner who didn't want to use protection?

 Take **CHARGE**

Talking About Condoms and Safer Sex

The only sure way to prevent STIs, including HIV infection, is to abstain from sexual activity. If you choose to be sexually active, you should do everything possible to protect yourself from STIs. This includes good communication with your sex partner(s). The time to talk about safer sex is before you begin a sexual relationship. But even if you have been having unprotected sex with your partner, you can still practise safer sex now.

There are many ways to bring up the subject of safer sex and condom use with your partner. Be honest about your concerns and stress that protection against STIs means that you care about yourself and your partner. You may find that your partner shares your concerns and also wants to use condoms. He or she may be happy and relieved that you have brought up the subject of safer sex.

However, if your partner resists the idea of using condoms, you may need to negotiate. Stress that you both deserve to be protected and that sex will be more enjoyable when you aren't worrying about STIs (see the suggestions that follow). If you and your partner haven't used condoms before, buy some and familiarize yourselves with how to use them. Once you feel more comfortable handling condoms, you will be able to use them correctly and incorporate them into your sexual activity. Consider trying the female condom as well.

If your partner still won't agree to use condoms, think carefully about whether you want to have a sexual relationship with this person. Maybe he or she is not the right person for you.

If your partner says ...	Try saying ...
"They're not romantic."	"Worrying about STIs isn't romantic, and with condoms we won't have to worry." OR "If we put one on together, a condom could be fun."
"You don't trust me."	"I do trust you, but how can I trust your former partners or mine?" OR "It's important to me that we're both protected."
"I don't have any diseases. I've been tested."	"I'm glad you've been tested, but tests aren't foolproof for all diseases. To be safe, I always use condoms."
"I forgot to bring a condom. But it's OK to skip it just this once."	"I'd really like to make love with you, but I never have sex without a condom. Let's go get some."
"I don't like the way they feel."	"They might feel different, but let's try." OR "Sex won't feel good if we're worrying about diseases." OR "How about trying the female condom?"
"I don't use condoms."	"I use condoms every time." OR "I don't have sex without condoms."
"But I love you."	"Being in love can't protect us from diseases." OR "I love you, too. We still need to use condoms."
"But we've been having sex without condoms."	"I want to start using condoms now so we won't be at any more risk." OR "We can still prevent infection or reinfection."

Source: Dialogue from San Francisco AIDS Foundation. 1998. *Condoms for Couples* (IMPACT AIDS, 3692 18th Street, San Francisco, CA 94110). Copyright © 1998 San Francisco AIDS Foundation. All rights reserved. Used with permission.

SUMMARY

- Chlamydia causes epididymitis and urethritis in men; in women, it can lead to pelvic inflammatory disease (PID) and infertility if untreated.
- Untreated gonorrhea can cause pelvic inflammatory disease (PID) in women and epididymitis in men, leading to infertility. In infants, untreated gonorrhea can cause blindness.
- PID, a complication of untreated gonorrhea or chlamydia, is an infection of the uterus and oviducts that may extend to the ovaries and pelvic cavity. It can lead to infertility, ectopic pregnancy, and chronic pelvic pain.
- Syphilis is a highly contagious bacterial infection that can be treated with antibiotics. If left untreated, it can lead to deterioration of the central nervous system and death.
- Human papillomavirus (HPV) causes genital warts and cervical cancer. Treatment does not eradicate the virus, which can be passed on by asymptomatic people.
- Genital herpes is a common incurable infection that can cause painful blisters on the genitals. The virus remains in the body for life and may cause recurrent outbreaks.
- HIV affects the immune system, making an otherwise healthy person less able to resist a variety of infections.
- HIV is carried in blood and blood products, semen, vaginal and cervical secretions, and breast milk. HIV is transmitted through the exchange of these fluids.
- There is currently no cure or commercially available vaccine for HIV infection. Drugs have been developed to slow the course of the disease and to prevent or treat certain secondary infections.
- HIV infection can be prevented by making careful choices about sexual activity, not sharing drug needles, and learning how to protect yourself from HIV.

- Hepatitis B is an inflammation of the liver caused by one of the many types of hepatitis viruses. It is transmitted through both sexual and nonsexual contact. Following an initial infection, most people recover; but some become carriers and may develop serious complications.
- Other infections that can be transmitted sexually or are linked to sexual activity include trichomoniasis, bacterial vaginosis, pubic lice, and scabies. Any STI that causes sores or inflammation can increase the risk of HIV transmission.
- Individuals can contribute to a reduction in the incidence of STIs by educating themselves, being diagnosed and treated for any infections, and practicing preventive strategies.

FOR MORE INFORMATION

BOOKS

Grimes, J. A., Apffel Smith, L., and Fagerberg, K. 2013. *Sexually Transmitted Disease: An Encyclopedia of Diseases, Prevention, Treatment, and Issues*. Greenwood. An overview of the scientific and historical background of sexually transmitted infections, as well as information about their transmission, diagnosis, and treatment.

Hyde, J. S., and J. D. DeLamater. 2013. *Understanding Human Sexuality*, 12th ed. New York: McGraw-Hill. A comprehensive, multidisciplinary introduction to human sexuality, including material on STIs.

Moore, E. A. 2008. *Encyclopedia of Sexually Transmitted Diseases*, Illustrated ed. Jefferson, N.C.: McFarland. A variety of information about STIs in an easy-to-use format.

Pepin, J. 2011. *The Origin of AIDS*. Cambridge, UK: Cambridge University Press. A highly readable investigation into the perplexing evolutionary origin and early epidemiology of the AIDS virus.

ORGANIZATIONS, HOTLINES, AND WEBSITES

The Internet addresses listed here were accurate at the time of publication.

Action Canada for Sexual Health & Rights. Promotes sexual and reproductive health and rights in Canada and internationally. Provides information pertaining to STIs, pregnancy, and contraception.
   http://www.sexualhealthandrights.ca/

The Body: The Complete HIV/AIDS Resource. Provides information about prevention, testing, and treatment and includes an online risk assessment.
   http://www.thebody.com

Canadian AIDS Society. Provides information about a variety of topics, including AIDS-related events, HIV and poverty, and harm reduction, as well as other resources (including links, hotline information, and online discussion groups).
   http://www.cdnaids.ca

Canadian AIDS Treatment Information Exchange. Provides free, confidential information about all aspects of HIV, including prevention, medications, nutrition, supplements, side effects, and complementary therapies.
   http://www.catie.ca

Canadian Foundation for Women's Health. Provides information about research and resources related to women's sexual and reproductive health. Founded by the Society of Obstetricians and Gynaecologists of Canada.
   http://www.cfwh.org

Canadian Public Health Association. Provides information and resources related to public health issues in Canada, with links to provincial and territorial public health associations.
   http://www.cpha.ca

Federal Initiative to Address HIV/AIDS in Canada. Provides information on HIV/AIDS funding and the use of population-specific approaches to develop culturally appropriate strategies to reduce HIV/AIDS transmission in at-risk groups.
   http://www.phac-aspc.gc.ca/aids-sida/fi-if/

Health Canada: Sexually Transmitted Infections. Offers information on prevention and control of STIs, along with links to resources statistics, educational materials, and support programs.
    http://www.hc-sc.gc.ca/hc-ps/dc-ma/sti-its-eng.php

Joint United Nations Programme on HIV/AIDS (UNAIDS). Provides statistics and information on the international HIV/AIDS situation.
    http://www.unaids.org

The NAMES Project Foundation AIDS Memorial Quilt. Includes the story behind the quilt, images of quilt panels, and information and links relating to HIV infection.
    http://www.aidsquilt.org

Public Health Agency of Canada: Sexual Health and Sexually Transmitted Infections. Provides a wealth of credible and up-to-date information on sexual health and sexually transmitted infections.
    http://www.phac-aspc.gc.ca/std-mts/index-eng.php

SexualityandU. Provides information and education on sexual health for teens, adults, parents, teachers, and health professionals. Administered by the Society of Obstetricians and Gynaecologists of Canada.
    http://www.sexualityandu.ca

Society of Obstetricians and Gynaecologists of Canada. Provides information, research, and resources related to women's health issues and clinical practice guidelines.
    http://www.sogc.org

WHO: Sexually Transmitted Infections. Provides information on international statistics and prevention efforts.
    http://www.who.int/topics/sexually_transmitted_infections/en

See also the listings for Chapters 9 and 11.

SELECTED BIBLIOGRAPHY

Agot, K. E., et al. 2004. Risk of HIV-1 in rural Kenya: A comparison of circumcised and uncircumcised men. *Epidemiology* 15(2): 157–163.

Alary, M. 1997. Gonorrhea: Epidemiology and control strategies. *Canadian Journal of Human Sexuality* 6(2): 151–159.

AVERT. 2009. *The Origin of AIDS and HIV and The First Cases of AIDS,* http://www.avert.org/origins.htm; (retrieved October 27, 2015).

Brown, D. R., et al. 2005. A longitudinal study of genital human papillomavirus infection in a cohort of closely followed adolescent women. *Journal of Infectious Diseases* 191(2): 182–192.

Canadian Public Health Association. 2005. *Leading Together: Canada Takes Action on HIV/AIDS (2005–2010),* http://www.leadingtogether.ca/pdf/Leading_Together.pdf (retrieved October 27, 2015).

Cohen, M. 2004. HIV and sexually transmitted diseases: A lethal synergy. *Topics in HIV Medicine* 12(4):104–107.

Crosby, R., and R. J. DiClemente. 2004. Use of recreational Viagra among men having sex with men. *Sexually Transmitted Infections* 80(6): 466–468.

Erbelding, E. J., and J. M. Zenilman. 2005. Toward better control of sexually transmitted diseases. *New England Journal of Medicine* 352(7): 720–721.

Gupta, R., et al. 2004. Valacyclovir and acyclovir for suppression of shedding of herpes simplex virus in the genital tract. *Journal of Infectious Diseases* 190(8): 1374–1381.

Hampton, T. 2006. High prevalence of lesser-known STDs. *Journal of the American Medical Association* 295(21): 2467.

Health Canada. 2009. *A statistical profile of First Nations in Canada: Self-rated health and selected conditions, 2002 to 2005,* http://www.hc-sc.gc.ca/fniah-spnia/pubs/aborig-autoch/2009-stats-profil-vol3/index-eng.php; (retrieved October 27, 2015).

Health Canada. 2009. *Health Canada Is Warning Canadians Not to Use Clean Testing HIV Home Test Kit, or Any Home HIV Test Kit,* http://www.healthycanadians.gc.ca/recall-alert-rappel-avis/hc-sc/2009/13392a-eng.php (retrieved October 27, 2015).

Health Canada. 2011. Unlicensed HIV Home Test Kit: Accu-HIV 1 & 2 Saliva Test, http://www.canadiensensante.gc.ca/recall-alert-rappel-avis/hc-sc/2011/13543a-eng.php (retrieved October 27, 2015).

Health Canada. 2012. *CuraHerbDistributor.com Selling Unlicensed Home-Use HIV and STDs Test Kits,* http://www.healthycanadians.gc.ca/recall-alert-rappel-avis/hc-sc/2012/15051a-eng.php?_ga=1.7637042.1446590054.1411654512 (retrieved October 27, 2015).

Health Canada. 2012. *First Nations and Inuit Health: HIV and AIDS,* http://www.hc-sc.gc.ca/fniah-spnia/diseases-maladies/aids-sida/index-eng.php (retrieved October 27, 2015).

Huppert, J. S. 2006. New detection methods for trichomoniasis may help curb more serious STIs. *Patient Care for the Nurse Practitioner* 40(5): 32–36.

Immunize Canada. 2013. *Hepatitis A,* http://www.immunize.ca/en/diseases-vaccines/hepatitis-a.aspx (retrieved October 27, 2015).

Joint United Nations Programme on HIV/AIDS (UNAIDS). 2010. *UNAIDS Report on the Global AIDS Epidemic 2010.* Geneva: UNAIDS, http://www.unaids.org/globalreport/Global_report.htm (retrieved October 27, 2015).

Kimberlin, D., and D. Rouse. 2004. Genital herpes. *New England Journal of Medicine* 350(19): 1970–1977.

Lexum. *Judgments of the Supreme Court of Canada: R. v. Mabior,* https://scc-csc.lexum.com/scc-csc/scc-csc/en/item/10008/index.do (retrieved October 27, 2015).

Mathers, C. D., and Loncar, D. 2006. Projections of global mortality and burden of disease from 2002 to 2030. Public Library of Science, *Medicine* 3(11): 2011–2030.

Merson, M. 2006. The HIV-AIDS pandemic at 25—The global response. *New England Journal of Medicine* 354(23): 2414–2417.

Miller, W. C., et al. 2004. Prevalence of chlamydial and gonococcal infections among young adults in the United States. *Journal of the American Medical Association* 291(18): 2229–2236.

Money, D., and M. Steben. 2008. Genital herpes: Gynaecological aspects. *Journal of Obstetrics and Gynaecology Canada* 30(4): 347–353.

Options for Sexual Health. 2009. *Abstinence,* https://www.optionsforsexualhealth.org/birth-control-pregnancy/birth-control-options/natural-methods/abstinence (retrieved October 27, 2015).

Public Health Agency of Canada. 2010. *HIV/AIDS Epi Updates. July 2010,* http://www.phac-aspc.gc.ca/aids-sida/publication/epi/2010/4-eng.php (retrieved October 27, 2015).

Public Health Agency of Canada. 2012. *Human Immunodeficiency Virus HIV Screening and Testing Guide,* http://www.catie.ca/sites/default/files/EN_HIV-Screening-Guide-2013.pdf (retrieved October 27, 2015).

Public Health Agency of Canada. 2012. *Report on Sexually Transmitted Infections in Canada: 2010,* http://publications.gc.ca/collections/collection_2013/aspc-phac/HP37-10-2010-eng.pdf (retrieved October 27, 2015).

Public Health Agency of Canada. 2012. *Summary: Estimates of HIV Prevalence and Incidence in Canada, 2011,* http://www.phac-aspc.gc.ca/aids-sida/publication/survreport/estimat2011-eng.php (retrieved October 27, 2015).

Public Health Agency of Canada. 2013. *At a Glance – HIV and AIDS in Canada: Surveillance Report to December 31st, 2012,* http://www.phac-aspc.gc.ca/aids-sida/publication/survreport/2012/dec/index-eng.php (retrieved October 27, 2015).

Public Health Agency of Canada. 2013. *Canadian Guidelines on Sexually Transmitted Infections,* http://www.phac-aspc.gc.ca/std-mts/sti-its/ (retrieved October 27, 2015).

Public Health Agency of Canada. 2013. *Canadian Guidelines on Sexually Transmitted Infections: Gonococcal Infections Chapter,* http://www.phac-aspc.gc.ca/std-mts/sti-its/cgsti-ldcits/assets/pdf/section-5-6-eng.pdf (retrieved October 27, 2015).

Public Health Agency of Canada. 2013. *The Chief Public Health Officer's Report on the State of Public Health in Canada, 2013. Infectious Disease—The Never-ending Threat,* http://www.phac-aspc.gc.ca/cphorsphc-respcacsp/2013/sti-its-eng.php (retrieved October 27, 2015).

Rodriguez, B., et al. Predictive value of plasma HIV RNA level on rate of CD4 T-cell decline in untreated HIV infection. *Journal of the American Medical Association* 296(12): 1498–1506.

Sanders, G. D., et al. 2005. Cost-effectiveness of screening for HIV in the era of highly active antiretroviral therapy. *New England Journal of Medicine* 352(6): 570–585.

Sepkowitz, K. 2006. One disease, two epidemics—AIDS at 25. *New England Journal of Medicine* 354(23): 2411–2414.

Statistics Canada. 2004. *The Daily: Canadian Community Health Survey,* http://www.statcan.gc.ca/daily-quotidien/040615/dq040615b-eng.htm (retrieved October 27, 2015).

Statistics Canada. 2013. *Prevalence of Chlamydia trachomatis and herpes simplex virus type 2: Results from the 2009 to 2011 Canadian Health Measures Survey,* http://www.statcan.gc.ca/pub/82-003-x/2013004/article/11777-eng.htm (retrieved October 27, 2015).

UNAIDS. 2014. *The Gap Report,* http://www.unaids.org/en/media/unaids/contentassets/documents/unaidspublication/2014/unaids_gap_report_cn.pdf (retrieved October 27, 2015).

Wang, C., et al. 2004. Mortality in HIV-seropositive versus seronegative persons in the era of highly active antiretroviral therapy: Implications for when to initiate therapy. *Journal of Infectious Diseases* 190(6): 1046–1054.

Western News. 2013. *HIV vaccine produces no adverse effects in trials,* http://communications.uwo.ca/western_news/stories/2013/September/hiv_vaccine_produces_no_adverse_effects_in_trials.html (retrieved October 27, 2015).

World Health Organization. 2007. *Post-exposure Prophylaxis to Prevent HIV Infection: Joint WHO/ILO Guidelines on Post-exposure Prophylaxis (PEP) to Prevent HIV Infection,* http://www.who.int/hiv/pub/guidelines/PEP/en/ (retrieved October 27, 2015).

World Health Organization. 2012. *Global Report: UNAIDS report on the global AIDS epidemic 2012,* http://www.unaids.org/en/media/unaids/contentassets/documents/epidemiology/2012/gr2012/20121120_UNAIDS_Global_Report_2012_with_annexes_en.pdf (retrieved October 27, 2015).

World Health Organization. 2013. *Sexually Transmitted Infections (STIs),* http://apps.who.int/iris/bitstream/10665/82207/1/WHO_RHR_13.02_eng.pdf?ua=1 (retrieved October 27, 2015).

World Health Organization. 2013. *Sexually Transmitted Infections (STIs): Fact sheet N°110,* http://www.who.int/mediacentre/factsheets/fs110/en/ (retrieved October 27, 2015).

World Health Organization. 2014. *HIV/AIDS: Tuberculosis and HIV,* http://www.who.int/hiv/topics/tb/about_tb/en/ (retrieved October 27, 2015).

World Health Organization. 2014. *HIV/AIDS: Fact sheet N°360,* http://www.who.int/mediacentre/factsheets/fs360/en/ (retrieved October 27, 2015).

World Health Organization. n.d. *Global Health Observatory: HIV/AIDS,* http://www.who.int/gho/hiv/en/ (retrieved October 27, 2015).

Yeni, P. G., et al. 2004. Treatment for adult HIV infection. *Journal of the American Medical Association* 292(2): 251–265.

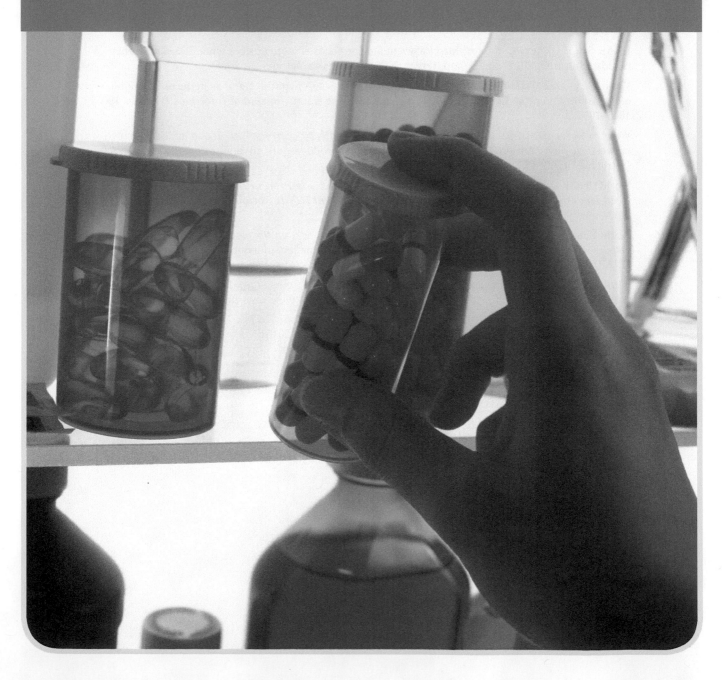

CHAPTER 14

Drug Abuse and Addiction

LOOKING AHEAD

After you have read and studied this chapter, you should be able to:

LO1 Define and discuss the concepts of addictive behaviour, substance abuse, and substance dependence

LO2 Explain factors contributing to drug abuse and addiction

LO3 List the major categories of psychoactive drugs and describe their effects, methods of use, and potential for abuse and addiction

LO4 Discuss social issues related to psychoactive drug abuse and its prevention and treatment

LO5 Evaluate the role of drugs and other addictive behaviours in your life and identify your risk factors for abuse or addiction

TEST YOUR KNOWLEDGE

1. **The most recent *Diagnostic and Statistical Manual of Mental Disorders* (DSM-5) released by the American Psychiatric Association includes the categories *substance abuse* and *substance dependence*.**
   True or false?

2. **Which of the following is the most widely used illegal drug among Canadian university and college students?**
   a. hallucinogens b. marijuana c. opioids

3. **Caffeine use can produce physical dependence.**
   True or false?

4. **Which of the following drugs is most addictive?**
   a. marijuana b. nicotine c. LSD

5. **About what percentage of Canadians reported using cocaine in 2012?**
   a. 1 percent b. 10 percent c. 25 percent

ANSWERS

1. FALSE. The *Diagnostic and Statistical Manual of Mental Disorders* (DSM-5) no longer includes the substance abuse and substance-dependence categories; they have been combined to represent a single condition, ranging from mild to severe, called substance use disorder.

2. b. Marijuana ranks first, followed by hallucinogens and then opioids. Alcohol remains by far the most popular drug among post-secondary students.

3. TRUE. Regular users of caffeine develop physical tolerance, needing more caffeine to produce the same level of alertness. Many experience withdrawal symptoms, such as headaches and irritability, when they decrease their caffeine intake.

4. b. Nicotine is believed to be the most highly addictive psychoactive drug.

5. a. The prevalence of past-year cocaine use among the general Canadian population was 1.1 percent in 2012; this percentage was down slightly from the 1.6 percent reported in 2008.

The use of **drugs** for both medical and social purposes is widespread in Canada, as shown in Table 14.1. Many people believe that every problem has or should have a chemical solution. For fatigue, many turn to caffeine; for insomnia, sleeping pills; for anxiety or boredom, prescription medication, alcohol, or other recreational drugs. Advertisements, social pressures, and the human desire for quick solutions to difficult problems all contribute to the prevailing attitude that drugs can ease all pain. But benefits often come with the risk of harmful consequences, and drug use can—and often does—pose serious or even life-threatening risks.

> **drug**
> Any chemical other than food intended to affect the structure or function of the body.

The most serious risks are abuse and addiction. The drugs most often associated with abuse are **psychoactive drugs**—those that alter a person's experiences or consciousness. In the short term, psychoactive drugs can cause **intoxication**, a state in which sometimes unpredictable physical and emotional changes occur. A person who is intoxicated may experience potentially serious changes in physical functioning. The individual's emotions and judgment may be affected in ways that lead to uncharacteristic and unsafe behaviour. In the long term, recurrent drug use can have profound physical, emotional, and social effects.

> **psychoactive drug**
> A chemical that can alter a person's consciousness or experience.
>
> **intoxication**
> The state of being mentally affected by a chemical (literally, a state of being poisoned).

TABLE 14.1

Non-medical Drug Use Among Canadians, 2012

	Percentage Using Substance in the Past Year	
	Young Adults (ages 15–24)	All Canadians (ages 15 and older)
Tobacco (cigarettes*)	15.6	16.1
Alcohol	70.0	78.4
Exceeds Canada's low-risk drinking guidelines (weekly)[a]	17.0	14.4
Exceeds Canada's low-risk drinking guidelines (single occasion)[b]	12.5	9.9
Cannabis (marijuana and hashish)	20.3	10.2
Cocaine/crack	N/A	1.1
Methamphetamine/crystal meth	N/A	N/A
Hallucinogens	4.8	1.1
Ecstasy	2.6[†]	0.6
Speed	N/A	0.5[†]
Abuse of pharmaceuticals	1.5	4.9

Sources: Butt, P., D. Beirness, L. Gliksman, C. Paradis, and T. Stockwell. (2011). *Alcohol and health in Canada: A summary of evidence and guidelines for low-risk drinking.* Ottawa, ON: Canadian Centre on Substance Abuse; Health Canada. 2014. *Canadian Alcohol and Drug Use Monitoring Survey (CADUMS): Summary of Results for 2012,* http://www.hc-sc.gc.ca/hc-ps/drugs-drogues/stat/_2012/summary-sommaire-eng.php (retrieved October 29, 2015); Health Canada. 2012. *Canadian Alcohol and Drug Use Monitoring Survey (CADUMS): Summary of Results for 2011,* http://www.hc-sc.gc.ca/hc-ps/drugs-drogues/stat/_2011/tables-tableaux-eng.php#t1 (retrieved October 29, 2015); and Health Canada. 2013. *Canadian Tobacco Use Monitoring Survey (CTUMS) 2012,* http://www.hc-sc.gc.ca/hc-ps/tobac-tabac/research-recherche/stat/ctums-esutc_2012-eng.php (retrieved November 8, 2015).

*Percentage of Canadians who identified themselves as a "current smoker" in 2012.
[a] A person who, in the last 7 days, has consumed more than 10 drinks a week for women (more than 2 drinks a day most days) and 15 drinks a week for men (more than 3 drinks a day most days).
[b] A person who, in the last 7 days, has consumed more than 3 drinks (for women) or 4 drinks (for men) on any single occasion.
[†] Most recent data available are from 2011.
N/A = data are not reportable.

This chapter introduces the concept of abuse and addiction, then focuses on the major classes of psychoactive drugs, their effects, their potential for abuse and addiction, and other issues related to their use. Alcohol and nicotine—two of the most widely used and most harmful psychoactive drugs—are discussed in Chapters 15 and 16.

Addictive Behaviour

Although addiction is most often associated with drug use, many experts now extend the concept of addiction to other behaviours. **Addictive behaviours** are habits that become out of control, with resulting negative effects on a person's health. The Canadian Society of Addiction Medicine defines **addiction** as a chronic disease that disrupts brain systems that regulate motivation, reward, and memory. The most characteristic feature of addiction is behavioural—a nearly uncontrollable pursuit of physical or psychological reward and/or relief through substance use or behaviours. Addiction involves craving and the inability to recognize significant risk or other problems with behaviours, interpersonal relationships, and emotional response. Like other chronic diseases, addiction often involves cycles of relapse and remission. Without treatment, addiction is progressive and can result in disabling or deadly health consequences. Looking at the nature of addiction and a range of addictive behaviours can help us understand similar behaviours when they involve drugs.

> **addictive behaviours**
> Any habit that becomes out of control, resulting in a negative effect on a person's health.
>
> **addiction**
> A chronic disease that disrupts the brain's system of motivation, reward, and memory; characterized by a compulsive desire and increasing need for a substance or behaviour, and by harm to the individual and/or society.

What Is Addiction?

Today scientists view addition as a chronic disease that involves disruption of the brain's systems related to reward, motivation, and memory. Dysfunction in these systems leads to biological, psychological, and social effects associated with pathologically pursuing pleasure or relief by substance use and other behaviours.

Historically, the term *addiction* was applied only when the habitual use of a drug produced chemical changes in the user's body. Though experts now agree that addiction is more fully defined by behavioural characteristics, they also agree that changes in the brain underlie the disease. One such change is **tolerance**, in which the body adapts to a drug so that the initial dose no longer produces the original emotional or psychological effects. This process means the user has to take larger and larger doses of the drug to achieve the same high. The concept of addiction as a disease process, one based in identifiable changes to brain cells and brain chemistry rather than a moral failing, has led to many advances in the understanding and treatment of drug addiction.

> **tolerance**
> A physical state in which the body adapts to a drug so that the initial dose no longer produces the original physical or psychological effects.

Some scientists think that other behaviours may share some of the chemistry of drug addiction. They suggest that some activities, such as gambling, eating, exercising, and sex, trigger the release of brain chemicals that cause a pleasurable rush in much the same way that psychoactive drugs do. The brain's own chemicals thus become the "drug" that can cause addiction. These theorists suggest that all addictions—whether to drugs or to pleasurable activities—have a common mechanism in the brain. In this view, addiction is partly the result of our own natural wiring.

The view that addiction is based in our brain chemistry does *not* imply that people are not responsible for their addictive behaviour. Many experts believe that it is inaccurate and counterproductive to think of all bad habits and excessive behaviours as diseases. All addictions involve an initial voluntary step, and other factors such as lifestyle and personality traits, as well as social and economic conditions, play key roles in the development of addiction.

Characteristics of Addiction

Experts have identified some general characteristics typically associated with addictive behaviours:

- *Reinforcement:* Addictive behaviours reinforce themselves. Reinforcement can be positive—the activity or situation reliably results in pleasure or reward. It can also be negative—avoiding the drug or activity results in stress, anxiety, discomfort, or depression.
- *Compulsion or craving:* The individual feels a strong compulsion—a compelling need or irresistible "hunger"—to engage in the behaviour. Craving is often associated with environmental cues and accompanied by obsessive planning for the next opportunity to perform it.
- *Loss of control:* The individual loses control over the behaviour and cannot block the impulse to do it.
- *Escalation:* Addiction often involves a pattern of escalation in response to tolerance. More and more of the substance or activity is required to produce its desired effects.
- *Negative consequences:* The behaviour continues despite serious negative consequences, such as problems with academic or job performance, personal relationships, and health; legal or financial troubles are also typical.

The Development of Addiction

We all engage in activities that are potentially addictive. Some of these activities can be good for you if they are done appropriately and in moderation. But if a behaviour starts to be excessive, it may become an addiction.

An addiction often starts when a person does something to bring pleasure or avoid pain. The activity may be drinking a beer, using the Internet, playing the lottery, or shopping. If it works, the person is likely to repeat it. Reinforcement leads to an increasing dependence on the behaviour. Tolerance—caused by physical changes to brain cells and reward pathways in the brain—develops, and the person needs more of the behaviour to feel the expected effect. Eventually, the behaviour becomes a central focus of the person's life, and there is a deterioration in other areas, such as academic or job performance or relationships. The behaviour no longer brings pleasure, but repeating it is necessary to avoid **withdrawal**, which is the physical and mental pain that results from going without it. Something that started as a seemingly innocent way of feeling good has triggered physiological changes in the brain that create a behavioural prison.

> **withdrawal**
> A set of symptoms including anxiety, pain, irritability, sweating, tremors, vomiting, and insomnia.

Although many common behaviours are potentially addictive, most people who engage in them do not develop problems. The reason lies in the combination of factors that are involved in the development of addiction, including personality, lifestyle, heredity, the social and physical environment, and the nature of the substance or behaviour in question. For addiction to develop, these diverse factors must come together in a certain way. For example, nicotine (the psychoactive drug in tobacco) has very high potential for physical addiction. Genetic factors make some individuals much more likely to develop dependence and addiction if they start smoking. Other factors—family, social, or cultural—play a role in determining if someone takes a first puff and if so, whether the individual continues smoking and becomes addicted. Like other addictions, addiction to nicotine begins with a voluntary and seemingly inconsequential "yes or no" choice that spirals catastrophically out of control.

Characteristics of People with Addictions

The causes and course of an addiction are extremely varied, but people with addictions seem to share some characteristics. Many use a substance or an activity as a substitute for healthier coping strategies. People vary in their ability to manage their lives, and those who have the most trouble dealing with stress and painful emotions may be more susceptible to addiction.

Some people may have a genetic predisposition to addiction to a particular substance based on a variation in brain chemistry. People with addictive disorders usually have a distinct preference for a particular addictive behaviour. They also often have problems with impulse control and self-regulation, and tend to be risk takers.

Examples of Addictive Behaviours

Behaviours that are not related to drugs can become addictive for some people. Such behaviours can include eating, gambling, and playing video games. Any substance or activity that becomes the focus of a person's life at the expense of other needs and interests can be damaging to health. Like addiction to drugs, behavioural or non-drug addiction involves symptoms such as craving, loss of control over the behaviour, tolerance, withdrawal, and a repeating pattern of recovery and relapse.

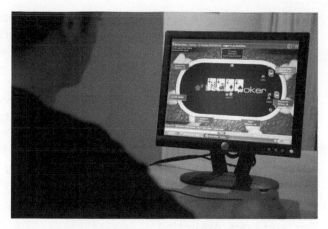

In early 2015, Ontario joined British Columbia, Manitoba, Quebec, and the Atlantic Provinces in offering a government-sponsored online gambling website. Critics argue that increasing the convenience of gambling carries potential risks for many Canadians.

Gambling Disorder

Individuals who are affected by moderate and severe problem gambling cannot control the urge to gamble, even in the face of ruin. The consequences of compulsive gambling are not just financial; the Canada Safety Council estimates that more than 200 people with compulsive gambling problems take their own lives every year. It has been estimated that approximately 3 percent of adults in Canada are affected by moderate to severe problem gambling. More than 60 percent of youth (ages 15–24) in Canada have reported gambling at least once in the past year, and about 2 percent have reported problem gambling. Young men tend to have higher rates of gambling problems than young women.

The American Psychiatric Association (APA), an organization composed of mental health professionals from around the world, now recognizes *gambling disorder* as a behavioural addiction in the "Substance-Related and Addictive Disorders" category. The APA lists nine characteristic behaviours associated with gambling disorder, including preoccupation with gambling, unsuccessful efforts to quit, gambling when feeling distressed, and lying to conceal the extent of involvement with gambling.

QUICK STATS

Approximately 2% of youth ages 15–24 in Canada are affected by moderate-risk or problem gambling.
—Huang and Boyer, 2007

Compulsive Exercising

When taken to a compulsive level, even healthy activities may develop into harmful addictions. For example, compulsive exercising is now recognized as a serious departure from normal behaviour. Compulsive exercising is often accompanied by more severe psychiatric disorders, such as anorexia nervosa and bulimia (discussed in Chapter 4). Traits frequently associated with compulsive exercising include an excessive preoccupation and dissatisfaction with body image, the use of laxatives or vomiting to lose weight, and the development of other obsessive-compulsive symptoms.

Work Addiction

The term *workaholic* is often used to describe individuals with an excessive preoccupation with work and work-related activities. Work addiction, however, is actually based on a set of specific symptoms:
- An intense work schedule
- The inability to limit one's own work schedule

- The inability to relax, even when away from work
- Failed attempts at curtailing the intensity of work (in some cases)

Work addiction is a serious concern for various reasons. Someone suffering from this addiction is likely to neglect other areas of his or her life. For example, work addicts may exercise less, spend less time with family and friends, and avoid social activities.

Work addiction typically coincides with a well-known risk factor for cardiovascular disease—the type A personality (see Chapter 7). Traits associated with type A personality include competitiveness, ambition, drive, time urgency, restlessness, hostility, and hyperalertness.

Many researchers see work addiction as a culture-bound disorder arising from a workplace that encourages these harmful behavioural patterns. The changing landscape of the modern workplace is likely to make work addiction a source of disability for a growing number of people.

Sex and Love Addiction

More controversial is the notion of addiction to sex or love. Behaviours associated with sex addiction include having an extreme preoccupation with sex, a compulsion to have sex repeatedly in a given period of time, spending a great deal of time and energy looking for partners or engaging in sex, using sex as a means of relieving painful feelings, and suffering negative emotional, personal, and professional consequences as a result of sexual activities. The online world represents a more novel means through which people can engage in sexual behaviour, either passively (downloading and watching pornography) or interactively (exchanging sexual content with others). Research has shown that for some people, engaging in online sexual behaviours can result in Internet sex addiction, defined as a sub-form of both Internet addiction (discussed below) and real life or "offline" sex addiction. Not surprisingly, this form of sex addiction is also associated with several negative consequences.

Some experts are reluctant to call compulsive sexual activity a true addiction. However, even therapists who challenge the concept of sex addiction recognize that some people become overly preoccupied with sex, cannot seem to control their sex drive, and act in potentially harmful ways to obtain satisfaction. This pattern of sexual behaviour seems to meet the criteria for addictive behaviours discussed earlier.

Compulsive Buying or Shopping

A compulsive buyer repeatedly gives in to the impulse to buy more than he or she needs or can afford. Compulsive spenders usually buy luxury items rather than daily necessities. Compulsive shoppers are usually distressed by their behaviour and its social, personal, and financial consequences. Some experts link compulsive shopping with neglect or abuse during childhood; it also seems to be associated with eating disorders, depression, and bipolar disorder.

Internet Addiction

In the years since the Internet became widely available, millions of Canadians have become compulsive Internet users. To spend more time online, Internet addicts skip important school, social, or recreational activities. In addition, compulsive Internet users often spend their work time online, a fact that has led many employers to adopt strict Internet usage policies.

Despite negative financial, social, or academic consequences, compulsive Internet users don't feel

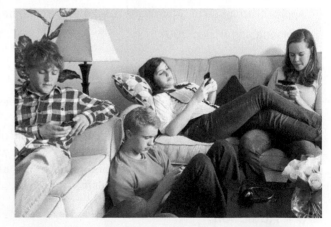

Because the Internet provides easy access to so many different kinds of content, many Canadians experience Internet addiction.

able to stop. As with other addictive behaviours, online addicts may be using their behaviour to alleviate stress or avoid painful emotions (see the Assess Yourself box).

Generally speaking, studies have shown that up to 10 percent of Internet users may experience Internet addiction. One study showed that Internet addicts spent an average of 38 hours online every week. There is concern that the number of Internet addicts will continue to grow as the Internet becomes more accessible and affordable.

 Assess YOURSELF

Is Internet Use a Problem for You?

To assess the extent to which your Internet use is creating problems in your life, answer the following questions using this point scale:

Rarely	1 point
Occasionally	2 points
Frequently	3 points
Often	4 points
Always	5 points

_____ 1. How often do you find that you stay online longer than you intended?

_____ 2. How often do you neglect household chores to spend more time online?

_____ 3. How often do you prefer the excitement of the Internet to intimacy with your partner?

_____ 4. How often do you form new relationships with fellow online users?

_____ 5. How often do others in your life complain about the amount of time you spend online?

_____ 6. How often do your grades or schoolwork suffer because of the amount of time you spend online?

_____ 7. How often do you check your email before something else that you need to do?

_____ 8. How often does your job performance or productivity suffer because of the Internet?

_____ 9. How often do you become defensive or secretive when someone asks you what you do online?

_____ 10. How often do you block out disturbing thoughts about your life with soothing thoughts about the Internet?

_____ 11. How often do you find yourself anticipating when you will go online again?

_____ 12. How often do you fear that life without the Internet would be boring, empty, and joyless?

_____ 13. How often do you snap, yell, or act annoyed if someone bothers you while you are online?

_____ 14. How often do you lose sleep due to late-night log-ins?

_____ 15. How often do you feel preoccupied with the Internet when offline or fantasize about being online?

_____ 16. How often do you find yourself saying "just a few more minutes" when online?

_____ 17. How often do you try to cut down on the amount of time you spend online and fail?

_____ 18. How often do you try to hide how long you've been online?

_____ 19. How often do you choose to spend more time online over going out with others?

_____ 20. How often do you feel depressed, moody, or nervous when you are offline, which goes away once you are back online?

Add the points associated with your responses to get your final score. The higher your score, the more problems your Internet usage is causing you. Here's a general scale to help you evaluate your score:

20–49 points: You are an average online user. You may surf the web a bit too long at times, but you have control over your usage.

50–79 points: You are experiencing occasional or frequent problems because of the Internet. You should consider their full impact on your life.

80–100 points: Your Internet usage is causing significant problems in your life. You should evaluate the impact of the Internet on your life and start thinking about how to address the problems.

Source: Netaddiction.com. *Internet Addiction Test,* http://netaddiction.com/internet-addiction-test/ (retrieved November 3, 2015). Reprinted by permission of Dr. Kimberly S. Young.

QUESTIONS FOR CRITICAL THINKING AND REFLECTION

Have you ever repeatedly or compulsively engaged in a behaviour that had negative consequences? What was the behaviour, and why did you continue? Did you ever worry that you were losing control? Were you able to bring the behaviour under control?

The Drug Tradition

Drugs are chemicals other than food that are intended to affect the structure or function of the body. They include prescription medicines, such as antibiotics and antidepressants; non-prescription or over-the-counter (OTC) substances, such as alcohol, tobacco, and caffeine products; and illegal substances, such as LSD and heroin. Using drugs to alter consciousness is an ancient and universal pursuit. People have used alcohol for celebration and intoxication for thousands of years. People in all parts of the world have exploited the psychoactive properties of various local plants, such as the coca plant in South America and the opium poppy in the Far East.

In the nineteenth century, chemists began extracting the active chemicals from medicinal plants, such as morphine from the opium poppy and cocaine from the coca leaf. This was the beginning of modern **pharmacy**, the art of compounding drugs, and of **pharmacology**, the science and study of drugs. It was also the start of the era of human-made psychoactive drugs, from codeine to methamphetamine, which continues to the present.

pharmacy
The art of compounding drugs from various substances.

pharmacology
The science and study of drugs.

Drug addiction among middle-class Europeans and North Americans was more common by 1900 than at any time before or since. Concerns about drug addiction and the need to regulate drug sales and manufacture led to the passage of harsh federal drug laws in Canada in the early 1900s. Middle-class use of regulated drugs dropped, and drug use became increasingly identified with criminal subcultures.

Non-medical (recreational) drug use expanded in Canada during the 1960s and 1970s and then declined until the early- to mid-1990s, when drug use rates began to rise in certain high-risk segments of the Canadian population. From 2004 to 2011, the prevalence of past-year cannabis and other illicit drug use among Canadians decreased steadily. However, drug use among young adults ages 15–24 remains substantially higher than that reported by Canadians 25 years and older: three times higher for cannabis use and almost five times higher for the use of other illicit drugs (cocaine or crack, ecstasy, heroin, speed, or hallucinogens). With regard to gender differences, Canadian data show that in 2012, the rate of self-reported illicit drug use (for any drug) among people ages 15 and older was nearly two times higher for males (15.2 percent) than for females (7.7 percent).

Substance Use Disorder

As mentioned earlier, Canadian mental health professionals use the American Psychiatric Association's (APA) *Diagnostic and Statistical Manual of Mental Disorders*. It is the authoritative reference for defining all sorts of behavioural disorders, including those related to drugs. The most recent diagnostic manual (DSM-5) combines the previously-defined categories of substance abuse and substance dependence into a single condition called *substance use disorder*. A diagnosis of *mild* substance use disorder requires that an individual displays 2–3 symptoms from a list of 11 possible criteria. For a diagnosis of *moderate* or *severe* substance use disorder, individuals must exhibit 4–5 symptoms or 6–11 symptoms, respectively. The list of criteria is as follows:

1. Developing tolerance to the substance. When a person requires increased amounts of a substance to achieve the desired effect or notices a markedly diminished effect with continued use of the same amount, the person has developed tolerance.

2. Experiencing withdrawal. In an individual who has maintained prolonged, heavy use of a substance, a drop in its concentration within the body can result in unpleasant physical and cognitive withdrawal

symptoms. Withdrawal symptoms are different for different drugs. For example, nausea, vomiting, and tremors are common for alcohol, opioids, and sedatives. Some drugs have no significant withdrawal symptoms.

3. Taking the substance in larger amounts or over a longer period than was originally intended.
4. Craving, or a strong desire or urge to use a substance.
5. Making unsuccessful efforts to cut down or regulate substance use.
6. Spending a great deal of time obtaining the substance, using the substance, or recovering from its effects.
7. Giving up or reducing important social, school, work, or recreational activities because of substance use.
8. Continuing to use the substance in spite of recognizing that it is contributing to a psychological or physical problem.
9. Using the substance repeatedly, resulting in failure to fulfill obligations at work, school, or home.
10. Using the substance repeatedly, resulting in hazardous situations.
11. Continuing to use the substance despite social or interpersonal problems.

QUICK STATS

The annual cost of hospitalizing individuals with substance use disorders in Canada increased from $219 million in 2006 to $267 million in 2011.

—Canadian Centre on Substance Abuse, 2014

Who Uses Drugs?

The use and abuse of drugs occur at all income and education levels, among all ethnic groups, and at all ages (see the In Focus box). Society is concerned with the casual or recreational use of illegal drugs because it is not really possible to know when drug use will lead to addiction. Some casual users develop substance-related problems; others do not. Some drugs are more likely than others to lead to addiction, but some users of even heroin or cocaine do not meet the APA's criteria for substance use disorder.

It isn't possible to accurately predict which drug users will become addicted, but young people at a high risk of *trying* drugs share certain characteristics:

- *Being male:* Males are twice as likely as females to abuse drugs.
- *Being a troubled adolescent:* Teens are more likely to try drugs if they have poor self-image or self-control, use tobacco, or suffer from certain mental or emotional problems.
- *Being a thrill-seeker:* A sense of invincibility is a factor in drug experimentation.
- *Being in a dysfunctional family:* A chaotic home life or parental abuse increases the risk of drug use. The same is true for children from a single-parent home or whose parents didn't complete high school.
- *Being in a peer group that accepts drug use:* Young people who are uninterested in school and receive poor grades are more likely to try drugs.
- *Being poor:* Young people who live in disadvantaged areas are more likely to be around drugs at a young age.
- *Dating young:* Adolescent girls who date boys two or more years older than themselves are more likely to use drugs.

What about people who *don't* use drugs? As a group, non-users also share some characteristics. Not surprisingly, people who perceive drug use as risky and who disapprove of it are less likely to use drugs than those who believe otherwise. Drug use is also less common among people who have positive self-esteem and self-concept and who are assertive, independent thinkers who are not controlled by peer pressure. Self-control, social competence, optimism, academic achievement, and regular church attendance are also linked to lower rates of drug use (see the Mind Body Spirit box).

Home environments are also influential: Coming from a strong family, one that has a clear policy on drug use, is another characteristic of people who don't use drugs. Young people who communicate openly with their parents and feel supported by them are also less likely to use drugs.

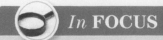

In FOCUS

Drug Use Among Post-Secondary Students

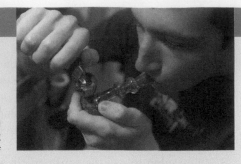

Drug use in college and university has long been recognized as a significant health problem that affects many students. According to data collected in 2009 from more than 8000 undergraduates at eight post-secondary institutions across Canada, 17.5 percent of students reported the use of marijuana in the past 30 days, while 3.5 percent reported using other illicit drugs. These numbers represent a slight increase from 2004, when 16.7 percent of undergraduate students reported the use of cannabis (marijuana or hashish or both) in the past 30 days, and 2.2 percent reported the use of other illicit drugs. Together, these data show that recreational drug use is fairly common among college and university students. For example, in 2004, 5.6 percent of university students reported using hallucinogens at least once in the past year, while another 5 percent reported using opioids and 2.5 percent reported using ecstasy. Finally, 2.1 percent said they had used cocaine at least once in the past year, and 2.6 percent reported using amphetamines.

Drug use on college and university campuses has been examined extensively, and many experts believe that no single factor can explain the widespread impact of this phenomenon. Family history, peer pressure, depression, anxiety, low self-esteem, and the dynamics of post-secondary life (for example, the drive to compete and distorted perceptions of drug use among peers) have been suggested as potential explanations for drug use among college and university students.

Excessive alcohol use often accompanies illicit drug use. In fact, the term *AOD* (alcohol and other drug) has been coined to refer to this type of substance use among college and university students. Further, AOD use and depression and/or anxiety are generally recognized as coexisting conditions that require a comprehensive approach to prevention and treatment. Despite the growing awareness among counsellors and other health professionals who work with post-secondary students, it is not entirely clear whether anxiety and depression precede the onset of alcohol and drug use, or whether early exposure to alcohol and drug use before college or university exacerbates more serious psychiatric disorders by the time a student enters post-secondary. A third line of research suggests that AOD use, depression, and anxiety share common causes, such as genetic predisposition or family history.

However, one aspect of drug use among college and university students remains clear: AOD use has dramatic consequences for the educational, family, and community life of students. Poor academic performance has been linked with AOD use. Further, driving while intoxicated remains one of the most dangerous outcomes associated with AOD use affecting families and communities. Fortunately, several AOD prevention programs are now under way at campuses across Canada.

Sources: Adlaf, E. M., et al. (eds.). 2005. *Canadian Campus Survey 2004*. Toronto: Centre for Addiction and Mental Health; and Kwan, M. Y. W., G. E. J. Faulkner,, K. P. Arbour-Nicitopolous, and J. Cairney. (2013). Prevalence of health-risk behaviours among Canadian post-secondary students: Descriptive results from the National College Health Assessment. *BMC Public Health* 13: 548–553.

Why Do People Use Drugs?

Young people may be drawn to drugs by the allure of the exciting and illegal. They may be curious, rebellious, or vulnerable to peer pressure. Young people may want to imitate adult models in their lives or in the movies. Most people who take illicit drugs do so experimentally, typically trying the drug one or more times but not continuing. The main factors in the initial choice of a drug are whether it is available and whether peers are using it.

Although some people use drugs because they have a desire to alter their mood or are seeking a spiritual experience (as discussed in the Mind Body Spirit box), others are motivated primarily by a desire to escape boredom, anxiety, depression, feelings of worthlessness, or other distressing symptoms of psychological problems. They use drugs as a way to cope with the difficulties they are experiencing in life. The common practice in our society of seeking a drug solution to every problem is a factor in the widespread reliance on both illicit and prescription drugs.

For people living in poverty, many of these reasons for using drugs are magnified. The problems are more devastating, and the need for escape is more compelling. Furthermore, the buying and selling of drugs provide access to an unofficial, alternative economy that may seem like an opportunity for success.

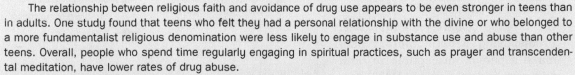

 Mind *Body* SPIRIT

Spirituality and Drug Abuse

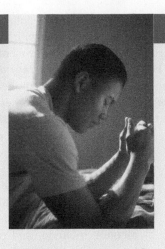

Although religious viewpoints on drug use are diverse, many religions infer some link between psychoactive drugs and spirituality. Some religions use drugs in the quest for spiritual transcendence: for example, Polynesian, African, and other indigenous religions have used psychoactive drugs, such as peyote, khat, alcohol, and hashish, for expanding consciousness and developing personal spirituality. Other religions view psychoactive drugs as a threat to spirituality. In Islam, for example, the consumption of alcohol and certain other drugs is strictly forbidden.

Research with teens and adults has shown that spiritual or religious involvement is generally associated with a lower risk of trying psychoactive drugs and, for those who do use drugs, a lower risk of heavy use and addiction. The mechanism for this protective effect is unclear; possibilities include the adoption of a strict code of behaviour or set of principles that rejects drug use, the presence of a social support system for abstinence or moderation, and the promotion of values that include avoidance of drug use.

The relationship between religious faith and avoidance of drug use appears to be even stronger in teens than in adults. One study found that teens who felt they had a personal relationship with the divine or who belonged to a more fundamentalist religious denomination were less likely to engage in substance use and abuse than other teens. Overall, people who spend time regularly engaging in spiritual practices, such as prayer and transcendental meditation, have lower rates of drug abuse.

People with substance addiction tend to have lower rates of religious affiliation and involvement and lower levels of spiritual wellness, characterized by a lack of a sense of meaning in life. One of the hallmarks of substance use disorder is spending increasing amounts of time and energy obtaining and using drugs; such a pattern of behaviour inevitably reduces the resources an individual puts toward developing physical, emotional, and spiritual wellness.

Among people in treatment for addiction, higher levels of religious faith and spirituality may contribute to the recovery process. A study of people recovering from alcohol or other drug abuse found that spirituality and religiousness were associated with better coping skills, greater optimism about life, greater resilience to stress, and greater perceived social support.

More research is needed to clarify the relationships among spirituality, religion, drug use, and recovery. One of the difficulties in conducting research in this area is the difficulty in defining and measuring spirituality and religious involvement. Spirituality is a complex part of human nature, involving behaviour, belief, and experience. And although some behaviours, such as the spiritual practices of prayer or meditation, can be measured, it is more difficult to determine what such practices mean to an individual and her or his overall sense of self.

Sources: Brown, A. E., et al. 2006. Alcohol recovery and spirituality: Strangers, friends, or partners? *Southern Medical Journal* 99(6): 654–657; Substance Abuse and Mental Health Network. 2004. Religious beliefs and substance use among youths. *NSDUH Report*, January; and Dunn, M. S. 2005. The relationship between religiosity, employment, and political beliefs on substance use among high school seniors. *Journal of Alcohol and Drug Education* 49(1): 73.

Risk Factors for Addiction

Why do some people use psychoactive drugs without becoming addicted, whereas others are not as lucky? The answer seems to be a combination of physical, psychological, and social factors. Research indicates that some people may be born with certain characteristics of brain chemistry or metabolism that make them more vulnerable to drug addiction. Other research suggests that people who were exposed to drugs while still in the womb may have an increased risk of abusing drugs themselves later in life.

Psychological risk factors for substance use disorders include difficulty controlling impulses and a strong need for excitement, stimulation, and immediate gratification. Feelings of rejection, hostility, aggression, anxiety, or depression are also associated with drug abuse. People may turn to drugs to blot out their emotional pain. Social factors that may influence drug dependence include growing up in a family in which a parent or sibling abused drugs, belonging to a peer group that emphasizes or encourages drug abuse, and living in poverty. Because they have easy access to drugs, health care professionals are also at a higher risk.

Lastly, people with mental illnesses have a very high risk of substance use disorder. Research shows that about one-third of people with psychological disorders also have a substance-dependence problem and about one-third of those have another mental disorder. People with two or more coexisting mental disorders are referred to as having *dual (co-occurring) disorders*. Diagnosing psychological problems among people with substance use disorder can be very difficult because drug intoxication and withdrawal can mimic the symptoms of a mental illness. Although drug use disorders commonly occur with other mental illnesses, this does not mean that one caused the other, even if one appeared first. Research suggests the following possibilities for this common co-occurrence:

- *Drug abuse may bring about symptoms of another mental illness.* Increased risk of psychosis in vulnerable marijuana users suggests this possibility.
- *Mental disorders can lead to drug abuse*, possibly as a means of "self-medication." Patients suffering from anxiety or depression may rely on alcohol, tobacco, and other drugs to temporarily alleviate their symptoms.

These disorders could also be caused by shared risk factors, such as:

- *Overlapping genetic vulnerabilities:* Predisposing genetic factors may make a person susceptible to both addiction and other mental disorders or to having a greater risk of a second disorder once the first appears.
- *Overlapping environmental triggers:* Stress, trauma (such as physical or sexual abuse), and early exposure to drugs are common environmental factors that can lead to addiction and other mental illnesses.
- *Involvement of similar brain regions:* Brain systems that respond to reward and stress, for example, are affected by drugs of abuse and may show abnormalities in patients with certain mental disorders.
- *Drug use disorders and other mental illnesses are developmental disorders:* That means they often begin in the teen years or even younger—periods when the brain experiences dramatic developmental changes. Early exposure to drugs may change the brain in ways that increase the risk for mental disorders. Also, early symptoms of a mental disorder may indicate an increased risk for later drug use.

Other Risks of Drug Use

Addiction is not the only serious potential consequence of drug use. In 2011, substance use disorders were responsible for close to 35 000 hospital stays in Canada (see Figure 14.1).

FIGURE 14.1

Number of Hospital Stays with Primary Diagnosis of Mental and Behavioural Disorder Due to Drug Use

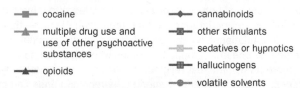

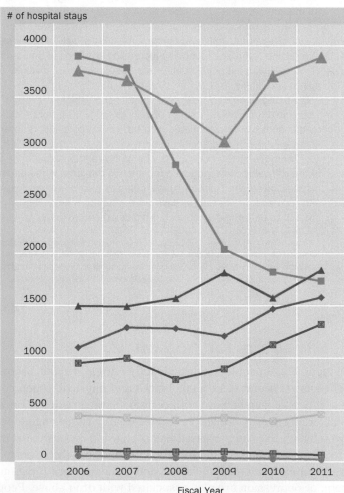

Source: Young, M. M., and R. J. Jesseman. (2014). *The impact of substance use disorders on hospital use.* Ottawa, ON: Canadian Centre on Substance Abuse, http://www.ccsa.ca/Resource%20Library/CCSA-Substance-Use-Hospital-Impact-Report-2014-en.pdf. Reproduced with permission from the Canadian Centre on Substance Abuse.

Intoxication

People who are under the influence of drugs—intoxicated—may act in uncharacteristic and unsafe ways because both their physical and their mental functioning are impaired. They are more likely to be injured from a variety of causes, including falls, drowning, and automobile crashes; to engage in unsafe sex, increasing their risk for sexually transmitted infections and unintended pregnancy; and to be involved in incidents of aggression and violence, including sexual assault.

Unexpected Side Effects

Psychoactive drugs have many physical and psychological effects beyond the alteration of consciousness. These effects range from nausea and constipation to paranoia, depression, and heart failure. Some drugs also carry the risk of fatal overdose.

Unknown Drug Constituents

There is no quality control in the illegal drug market, so the composition, dosage, and toxicity of street drugs is highly variable. Studies indicate that half of all street drugs don't contain their promised primary ingredient. In some cases, a drug may be present in unsafe dosages or mixed with other drugs to boost its effects. Makers of street drugs aren't held to any safety standards, so illicit drugs can be contaminated or even poisonous.

Risks Associated with Injection Drug Use

Heroin is the most commonly injected drug, but individuals can also inject cocaine, amphetamines, and other drugs. Many people who inject drugs share or reuse needles, syringes, and other injection equipment, which can easily become contaminated with the user's blood. Small amounts of blood can carry enough human immunodeficiency virus (HIV) and hepatitis C virus (HCV) to be infectious. In 2011, injection drug use (IDU) accounted for almost 14 percent of all new HIV/AIDS cases in Canada. IDU also accounts for the majority of Hepatitis C (HCV) infections reported in Canada. Unsterile injection practices can cause skin and soft tissue infections, which can progress to gangrene and be fatal if untreated. Other risks include endocarditis (infection of the heart valves), tuberculosis, and tetanus.

The surest way to prevent diseases related to IDU is never to inject drugs. Those who inject drugs should use a new needle and syringe with each injection and should use sterile water and other equipment to prepare drugs. Bleach or boiling water may kill some viruses and bacteria, but they are not foolproof sterilization methods. Many viruses can survive in a syringe for a month or more.

Syringe (or needle) exchange programs—where people who inject drugs can trade a used syringe for a new one—have been advocated to help slow the spread of HIV and reduce the rates and cost of other health problems associated with IDU. Opponents of syringe exchange programs argue that supplying injection drug users with syringes gives them the message that illegal drug use is acceptable and could thus exacerbate the nation's drug problem. However, studies have shown that well-implemented syringe exchange programs do not increase the use of drugs, and most offer AIDS counselling and provide referrals to drug-treatment programs. Getting people off drugs is clearly the best solution, but there are far more people who inject drugs than treatment facilities can currently handle.

Legal Consequences

Many psychoactive drugs are illegal, so using them can result in large fines or imprisonment. According to Statistics Canada, the rate of police-reported drug offences reached 310 incidents per 100 000 Canadians in 2013—a 13 percent increase over the past decade. This trend is likely related to a number of factors, including police policies, charging practices, and available resources. For example, targeted initiatives to crack down on drugs may result in more incidents being identified by police, rather than more incidents actually occurring.

QUICK STATS

More than 17 000 youth in Canada were accused of a drug violation in 2013—81% involved possession of cannabis.

—Statistics Canada, 2014

QUESTIONS FOR CRITICAL THINKING AND REFLECTION

Have you ever tried a psychoactive drug for fun? What were your reasons for trying it? Who were you with, and what were the circumstances? What was your experience like? What would you tell someone else who was thinking about trying a drug?

How Drugs Affect the Body

The drugs discussed in this chapter have complex and variable effects, many of which can be traced to changes in brain chemistry. However, the same drug may affect different people differently or the same person in different ways under different circumstances. Beyond a fairly predictable general change in brain chemistry, the effects of a drug may vary depending on drug factors, individual factors, and social factors.

Changes in Brain Chemistry

Psychoactive drugs produce most of their key effects by acting on brain chemistry in a characteristic fashion. Before any changes in brain chemistry can occur, however, molecules of the drug have to be carried to the brain through the bloodstream via a particular route of administration. A drug that is taken by mouth has to dissolve in the stomach, be absorbed into the bloodstream through the lining of the small intestine, and then pass through the liver, heart, and lungs before returning to the heart to be carried via arteries to the brain. A drug that is already dissolved and is injected directly into the bloodstream will reach the brain in much less time, and drugs that are inhaled and absorbed by the lungs travel to the brain even more rapidly. The faster a drug reaches the brain, the more likely the user is to become addicted.

Once a psychoactive drug reaches the brain, it acts on one or more **neurotransmitters**, either increasing or decreasing the neurotransmitters' concentration and actions. Cocaine, for example, affects dopamine, a neurotransmitter thought to play a key role in the process of reinforcement—the brain's way of telling itself "That's good; do the same thing again." When a neurotransmitter is released by one neuron, it travels across a gap, called a *synapse*, to signal another neuron. The signaling is controlled in part by removing the neurotransmitter molecules from the synapse by a process called resorption. Some drugs, such as cocaine, inhibit the resorption of dopamine, thereby extending or intensifying their action (see Figure 14.2). The euphoria produced by cocaine is thought to be a result of its effect on dopamine. Heroin, nicotine, alcohol, and amphetamines also affect dopamine levels.

neurotransmitter
A brain chemical that transmits nerve impulses.

The duration of a drug's effect depends on many factors and may range from 5 minutes (crack cocaine) to 12 or more hours (LSD). As drugs circulate through the body, they are metabolized by the liver and eventually excreted by the kidneys in urine. Small amounts may also be eliminated in other ways, including in sweat, in breast milk, and via the lungs.

FIGURE 14.2

Effect of Cocaine on Brain Chemistry

Under normal circumstances, the amount of dopamine at a synapse is controlled in part by the reuptake of dopamine by the transmitting neuron. Cocaine blocks the removal of dopamine from a synapse; the resulting buildup of dopamine causes continuous stimulation of the receiving neurons.

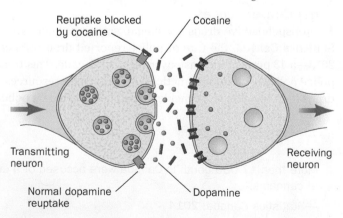

Reuptake blocked by cocaine

Cocaine

Transmitting neuron

Receiving neuron

Normal dopamine reuptake

Dopamine

Factors That Influence a Drug's Effect

When different drugs or dosages produce different effects, the differences are usually caused by one or more of five different drug factors:

1. The **pharmacological properties** of a drug are its overall effects on a person's body chemistry, behaviour, and psychology. The pharmacological properties also include the amount of a drug required to exert various effects, the time course of these effects, and other characteristics, such as a drug's chemical composition.

pharmacological properties
The overall effects of a drug on a person's behaviour, psychology, and chemistry.

2. The **dose-response function** is the relationship between the amount of drug taken and the type and intensity of the resulting effect. Many psychological effects of drugs reach a plateau in the dose-response function, and increasing the dose does not increase the effect any further. With LSD, for example, the maximum changes in perception occur at a certain dose, and no further changes in perception take place if higher doses are taken. However, all drugs have more than one effect, and the dose-response functions usually are different for different effects. This means that increasing the dose of any drug may begin to result in additional effects, which are likely to be increasingly unpleasant or dangerous at high doses.

dose-response function
The relationship between the amount of a drug taken and the intensity and type of the resulting effect.

3. The **time-action function** is the relationship between the time elapsed since a drug was taken and the intensity of its effect. The effects of a drug are greatest when concentrations of the drug in body tissues are changing fastest, especially if they are increasing.

time-action function
The relationship between the time elapsed since a drug was taken and the intensity of its effect.

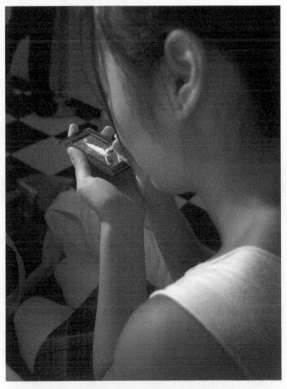

4. The person's *drug use history* may influence the effects of a drug. A given amount of alcohol, for example, will generally affect a habitual drinker less than an occasional drinker. Tolerance to some drugs, such as LSD, builds rapidly. To experience the same effect, a user has to abstain from the drug for a time before that dosage will again exert its original effects.

5. The *method of use (or route of administration)* has a direct effect on how strong a response a drug produces. Methods of use include ingestion, inhalation, injection, and absorption through the skin or tissue linings. Drugs are usually injected in one of three ways: intravenously (IV, or mainlining), intramuscularly (IM), or subcutaneously (SC, or skin popping).

Physical Factors

Certain physical and psychological characteristics also help determine how a person will respond to a drug. Body

The method of use (or route of administration) is one variable in the overall effect of a drug on the body.

mass is one variable. The effects of a certain dose of a drug on a 50-kilogram person will be twice as great as on a 100-kilogram person. Other variables include general health and genetic factors. For example, some people have an inherited ability to rapidly metabolize a cough suppressant called dextromethorphan, which also has psychoactive properties. These people must take a higher-than-normal dose to get a given cough-suppressant effect.

If a person's biochemical state is already altered by another drug, this too can make a difference. Some drugs intensify the effects of other drugs, as is the case with alcohol and sedatives. Some drugs block the effects of other drugs, such as when a tranquilizer is used to relieve anxiety caused by cocaine. Interactions between drugs, including many prescription and over-the-counter (OTC) medications, can be unpredictable and dangerous.

One physical condition that requires special precautions is pregnancy. It can be risky for a woman to use any drugs at all during pregnancy, including alcohol and common OTC preparations like cough medicine. The risks are greatest during the first trimester, when the fetus's body is rapidly forming and even small biochemical alterations in the mother can have a devastating effect on fetal development (see Chapter 12). Even later, the fetus is more susceptible than the mother to the adverse effects of any drugs she takes. The fetus may even become physically dependent on a drug being taken by the mother and suffer withdrawal symptoms after birth.

Psychological Factors

Sometimes a person's response to a drug is strongly influenced by the individual's expectations about how he or she will react (the psychological *set*). With large doses, the drug's chemical properties seem to have the strongest effect on the individual's response. But with small doses, psychological (and social) factors are often more important. When people strongly believe that a given drug will affect them a certain way, they are likely to experience those effects regardless of the drug's pharmacological properties. In one study, regular users of marijuana reported a moderate level of intoxication (**high**) after using a cigarette that smelled and tasted like marijuana but contained no THC, the active ingredient in marijuana. This is an example of the **placebo effect**—when a person receives an inert substance yet responds as if it were an active drug. In other studies, participants who smoked low doses of real marijuana that they believed to be a placebo experienced no effects from the drug. Clearly, the person's expectations had a greater effect than the drug itself.

high
The subjectively pleasing effects of a drug, usually felt quite soon after the drug is taken.

placebo effect
A response to an inert or innocuous medication given in place of an active drug.

QUESTIONS FOR CRITICAL THINKING AND REFLECTION

Has an over-the-counter medication (such as a decongestant) ever made you feel strange, drowsy, or even high? Did you expect to react to the medication that way? Do such reactions influence the way you use OTC drugs?

Social Factors

The *setting* is the physical and social environment surrounding the drug use. If a person uses marijuana at home with trusted friends and pleasant music, the effects are likely to be different from the effects if the same dose is taken in an austere experimental laboratory with an impassive research technician. Similarly, the dose of alcohol that produces mild euphoria and stimulation at a noisy, active cocktail party might induce sleepiness and slight depression when taken at home while alone.

THINKING ABOUT THE ENVIRONMENT

A number of addiction researchers have focused on interpersonal and intrapersonal characteristics associated with an individual's drug use. Recently, however, there has been increasing interest in environmental factors that may influence substance abuse. For example, the proximity of commercial outlets selling alcohol has been suggested as an important determinant of heavy alcohol use.

Spatial and spatially-related features of the environment—such as land use, urban sprawl, quality of housing, neighbourhood characteristics, and density of particular commercial outlets—are emerging topics in addiction research. The term *built environment* has been used to refer to attributes of an area or neighbourhood (such as parks, schools, buildings, roads, and sidewalks) that individuals use and encounter regularly, which may be associated with substance use.

For more information on the environment and health, see Chapter 21.

Representative Psychoactive Drugs

The following sections introduce six representative groups of psychoactive drugs (see Figure 14.3): opioids, central nervous system depressants, central nervous system stimulants, marijuana and other cannabis products, hallucinogens, and inhalants. Some of these drugs are classified according to how they affect the body. Others—the opioids and the cannabis products—are classified according to their chemical makeup.

Opioids

Also called *narcotics*, **opioids** are natural or synthetic (laboratory-made) drugs that relieve pain, cause drowsiness, and induce **euphoria**. Opium, morphine, heroin, methadone, codeine, hydrocodone, oxycodone, meperidine, and fentanyl are opioids. When taken at prescribed doses, opioids have beneficial medical uses, including pain relief and cough suppression. Opioids tend to reduce anxiety and produce lethargy, apathy, and an inability to concentrate. People who use opioids become less active and less responsive to frustration, hunger, and sexual stimulation. These effects are more pronounced in novice users; with repeated use, many effects diminish.

> **opioids**
> Any of several natural or synthetic drugs that relieve pain and cause drowsiness or euphoria; examples are opium, morphine, and heroin; also called a *narcotic*.
>
> **euphoria**
> An exaggerated feeling of well-being.

Opioids are typically injected. They can also be absorbed into the body from the stomach, intestines, nasal membranes (from snorting or sniffing), or lungs (from smoking). Effects depend on the method of administration. If brain levels of the drug change rapidly, more immediate effects will result. Although the euphoria associated with opioids is an important factor in their abuse, many people experience a feeling of uneasiness when they first use these drugs. People who use opioids also often feel nauseated and vomit, and they may have other unpleasant sensations. Even so, the abuse of opioids often results in addiction. Tolerance can develop rapidly and be pronounced. Withdrawal symptoms include cramps, chills, sweating, nausea, tremors, irritability, and feelings of panic.

Rates of heroin use have always been low, but there are periodic episodes of increased use among some groups. In Canada, about twice as many males as females use heroin. Whereas first-time users are often young (typically in their teens or 20s), most people who use heroin regularly are over the age of 30. Heroin use among youth remains low but has increased in some locations, mostly through increased rates of sniffing or smoking the drug. The potentially high but variable purity of street heroin poses a risk of unintentional

FIGURE 14.3

Commonly Abused Drugs and their Effects

Category	Representative drugs	Street names	Appearance	Methods of use	Short-term effects
Opioids 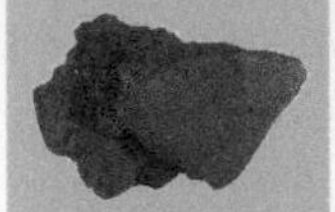	Heroin	Dope, H, junk, brown sugar, smack	White / dark brown powder; dark tar or coal-like substance	Injected, smoked, snorted	Relief of anxiety and pain; euphoria; lethargy, apathy, drowsiness, confusion, inability to concentrate; nausea, constipation, respiratory depression
	Opium	Big O, black stuff, hop	Dark brown or black chunks	Swallowed, smoked	
	Morphine	M, Miss Emma, monkey, white stuff	White crystals, liquid solution	Injected, swallowed, smoked	
	Oxycodone, codeine, hydrocodone	Oxy, O.C., killer, Captain Cody, schoolboy, vike	Tablets, powder made from crushing tablets	Swallowed, injected, snorted	
Central nervous system depressants 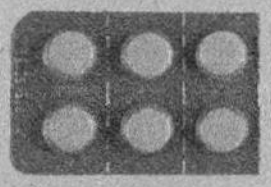	Barbiturates	Barbs, reds, red birds, yellows, yellow jackets	Coloured capsules	Swallowed, injected	Reduced anxiety, mood changes, lowered inhibitions, impaired muscle coordination, reduced pulse rate, drowsiness, loss of consciousness, respiratory depression
	Benzodiazepines (e.g., Valium, Xanax, Rohypnol)	Candy, downers, tranks, roofies, forget-me pill	Tablets	Swallowed, injected	
	Methaqualone	Ludes, quad, quay	Tablets	Injected, swallowed	
	Gamma hydroxy-butyrate (GHB)	G, Georgia home boy, grievous bodily harm	Clear liquid, white powder	Swallowed	
Central nervous system stimulants 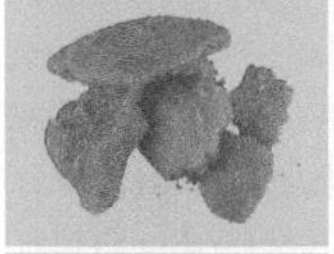	Amphetamine, methamphetamine	Bennies, speed, black beauties, uppers, chalk, crank, crystal, ice, meth	Tablets, capsules, white powder, white crystals	Injected, swallowed, smoked, snorted	Increased heart rate, blood pressure, metabolism; increased mental alertness and energy; nervousness, insomnia, impulsive behaviour; reduced appetite
	Cocaine, crack cocaine	Blow, C, candy, coke, flake, rock, toot	White powder, beige pellets or rocks	Injected, smoked, snorted	
	Ritalin	JIF, MPH, R-ball, Skippy	Tablets	Injected, swallowed, snorted	
Marijuana and other cannabis products 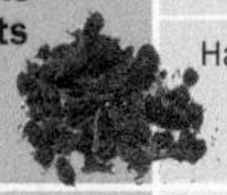	Marijuana	Dope, grass, joints, Mary Jane, reefer, skunk, weed	Dried leaves and stems	Smoked, swallowed	Euphoria, slowed thinking and reaction time, confusion, anxiety, impaired balance and coordination, increased heart rate
	Hashish	Hash, hemp, boom, gangster	Dark, resin-like compound formed into rocks or blocks	Smoked, swallowed	
Hallucinogens 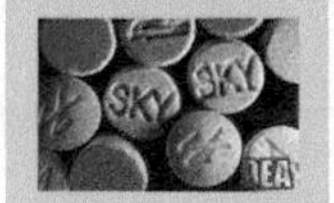	LSD	Acid, boomers, blotter, yellow sunshines	Blotter paper, liquid, gelatin tabs, pills	Swallowed, absorbed through mouth tissues	Altered states of perception and feeling; nausea; increased heart rate, blood pressure; delirium; impaired motor function; numbness, weakness
	Mescaline (peyote)	Buttons, cactus, mesc	Brown buttons, liquid	Swallowed, smoked	
	Psilocybin	Magic mushrooms, shrooms, mushies, fungus delight	Mushrooms, light to dark brown; available fresh, dried, or powdered	Swallowed (eaten raw or cooked, or steeped in hot water)	
	Ketamine	K, special K, cat valium, vitamin K	Clear liquid, white or beige powder	Injected, snorted, smoked	
	PCP	Angel dust, hog, love boat, peace pill	White to brown powder, tablets	Injected, swallowed, smoked, snorted	
	MDMA (ecstasy)	X, peace, clarity, Adam	Tablets	Swallowed	
Inhalants 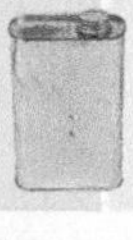	Solvents, aerosols, nitrites, anaesthetics	Laughing gas, poppers, snappers, whippets	Household products, sprays, glues, paint thinner, petroleum products	Inhaled through nose or mouth	Stimulation, loss of inhibition, slurred speech, loss of motor coordination, loss of consciousness

Sources: Partnership for Drug-Free Kids. 2015. *Drug Guide for Parents: Learn the Facts to Keep Your Teen Safe,* http://www.drugfree.org/wp-content/uploads/2014/03/drug_chart.pdf (retrieved January 19, 2015); and U.S. Department of Justice Drug Enforcement Administration. 2011. *Drugs of abuse, 2011 edition: A DEA resource guide,* http://www.dea.gov/docs/drugs_of_abuse_2011.pdf (retrieved January 19, 2015).

overdose. Symptoms of overdose include respiratory depression, coma, and constriction of the pupils; death can also result.

Non-medical use of prescription pain relievers that contain oxycodone and hydrocodone, including Oxycontin and Vicodin, is now recognized as a serious public health concern in Canada. When taken as prescribed in tablet form, these drugs treat moderate to severe chronic pain and do not typically lead to abuse. However, like other opioids, use of prescription painkillers can lead to abuse and addiction. Oxycodone and hydrocodone can be abused orally; the long-acting form of oxycodone is also sometimes crushed and snorted or dissolved and injected, providing a powerful heroin-like high. When taken in large doses or combined with other drugs, oxycodone and hydrocodone can cause fatal respiratory depression.

In response to the growing problem of non-medical use of prescription drugs across the country, the Canadian Centre on Substance Abuse, in partnership with the National Advisory Council on Prescription Drug Misuse, developed a pan-Canadian strategy entitled *First Do No Harm: Responding to Canada's Prescription Drug Crisis* (available at http://www.ccsa.ca/Resource%20Library/Canada-Strategy-Prescription-Drug-Misuse-Report-en.pdf). The strategy, released in 2013, outlined a 10-year plan aimed at reducing the harms (including addiction) associated with prescription drug abuse. The first annual report, published in 2014, documented the progress that has been made since the strategy was released, as well as the momentum that seems to be building with regard to this landmark initiative and its 58 recommendations.

QUICK STATS

Following the United States, Canada is the 2nd largest per capita consumer of prescription opioids worldwide.

—International Narcotics Control Board, 2013

Central Nervous System Depressants

Central nervous system **depressants**, also known as **sedative-hypnotics**, slow down the overall activity of the **central nervous system (CNS)**. The result can range from mild **sedation** to death, depending on the various factors involved—which drug is used, how it's taken, how tolerant the individual who is using the drug is, and so on. CNS depressants include alcohol (see Chapter 15), barbiturates, and other sedatives.

depressants or sedative-hypnotics
Drugs that decrease nervous or muscular activity, causing drowsiness or sleep.

central nervous system (CNS)
The brain and spinal cord.

sedation
The induction of a calm, relaxed, often sleepy state.

Types

The various types of barbiturates are similar in chemical composition and action, but they differ in how quickly and how long they act. People who use drugs call barbiturates "downers" or "downs" and refer to specific brands by names that describe the colour and design of the capsules. People usually take barbiturates in capsules, but they may also inject them.

Antianxiety agents, also called sedatives or **tranquilizers**, include the benzodiazepines, such as Xanax, Valium, Librium, clonazepam (Klonopin), and flunitrazepam (Rohypnol, also called *roofies*). Other CNS depressants include methaqualone (Quaalude), ethchlorvynol (Placidyl), chloral hydrate, and gamma hydroxy butyrate (GHB).

tranquilizers
Central nervous system depressants that reduce tension and anxiety.

Effects

CNS depressants reduce anxiety and cause mood changes, impaired muscular coordination, slurring of speech, and drowsiness or sleep. Mental functioning is also affected, but the degree varies from person to person and also depends on the kind of task the person is trying to do. Most people become drowsy with small doses, although a few become more active.

Medical Uses

Barbiturates, antianxiety agents, and other sedative-hypnotics are widely used to treat insomnia and anxiety disorders and to control seizures. Some CNS depressants are used for their calming properties in combination with **anaesthetics** before operations and other medical or dental procedures.

> **anaesthetics**
> Drugs that produce a loss of sensation with or without a loss of consciousness.

From Use to Abuse

People are usually introduced to CNS depressants either through a medical prescription or through peers who use drugs. The use of Rohypnol and GHB is often associated with dance clubs and raves (see the In Focus box). The abuse of CNS depressants by a medical patient may begin with repeated use for insomnia and progress to dependence through increasingly larger doses at night, coupled with a few capsules at stressful times during the day.

Most CNS depressants, including alcohol, can lead to addiction. Tolerance, sometimes for up to 15 times the usual dose, can develop with repeated use. Tranquilizers can produce physical dependence even at ordinary prescribed doses. Withdrawal symptoms can be more severe than those accompanying opioid dependence and are similar to the DTs of alcoholism (see Chapter 15). They may begin as anxiety, shaking, and weakness, but may turn into convulsions and possibly cardiovascular collapse and death.

While intoxicated, people on depressants cannot function well. They are confused and are frequently obstinate, irritable, and abusive. Long-term use of depressants, such as alcohol, can lead to poor health and brain damage, with impaired ability to reason and make judgments.

 In FOCUS

Club Drugs

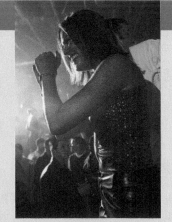

Some people refer to club drugs as soft drugs because they see them as recreational—for the casual, weekend user—rather than as addictive. But club drugs have many potential negative effects and are particularly potent and unpredictable when mixed with alcohol. Substitute drugs are often sold in place of club drugs, putting users at risk for taking dangerous combinations of unknown drugs.

MDMA (methylenedioxymethamphetamine), when taken in pill form, is a stimulant with mildly hallucinogenic and amphetamine-like effects. Users may experience euphoria, increased energy, and a heightened sense of belonging. In club settings, using MDMA can produce a dangerously high body temperature and potentially fatal dehydration; some users experience confusion, depression, anxiety, paranoia, muscle tension, involuntary teeth clenching, blurred vision, nausea, and seizures. Even low doses can affect concentration, judgment, and driving ability. Tolerance can develop, leading users to take the drug more frequently, to use higher doses, or to combine MDMA with other drugs to enhance the drug's effects. At high doses or when mixed with other drugs, MDMA is extremely dangerous; most deaths linked to MDMA have occurred as a result of multidrug toxicity or traumatic injuries.

LSD (lysergic acid diethylamide) is a potent hallucinogen that is sold in tablets or capsules, in liquid form, or on small squares of paper called blotters. LSD increases heart rate and body temperature and may cause nausea, tremors, sweating, numbness, and weakness.

Ketamine is a veterinary anaesthetic that can be taken in powdered or liquid form, and may cause hallucinations and impaired attention and memory. At higher doses, ketamine can cause delirium, amnesia, high blood pressure, and potentially fatal respiratory problems. Tolerance to ketamine develops rapidly.

GHB (gamma hydroxybutyrate) can be produced in clear liquid, white powder, tablet, and capsule form. GHB is a central nervous system depressant that in large doses or when taken in combination with alcohol or other depressants can cause sedation, loss of consciousness, respiratory arrest, and death. GHB may cause prolonged and potentially life-threatening withdrawal symptoms. GHB is often produced clandestinely, resulting in widely varying degrees of purity; it has been responsible for many poisonings and deaths.

Rohypnol (flunitrazepam) is a sedative that is 10 times as potent as Valium. Its effects, which are magnified by alcohol, include reduced blood pressure, dizziness, confusion, gastrointestinal disturbances, and loss of consciousness. Users of Rohypnol may develop physical and psychological dependence on the drug. Rohypnol and some other club drugs are used as "date rape drugs" or to facilitate sexual assault. Because they can be added to beverages surreptitiously, these drugs may be unknowingly consumed by intended rape victims. In addition to depressant effects, some drugs also cause *anterograde amnesia*, the loss of memory of things occurring while under the influence of the drug. Rohypnol can be fatal if combined with alcohol.

Overdosing with CNS Depressants

Too much depression of the central nervous system slows respiration and may stop it entirely. CNS depressants are particularly dangerous in combination with another depressant, such as alcohol. People who combine depressants with alcohol account for numerous emergency room visits and overdose deaths each year.

Central Nervous System Stimulants

CNS **stimulants** speed up the activity of the nervous or muscular system. Under their influence, the heart rate accelerates, blood pressure rises, blood vessels constrict, the pupils of the eyes and the bronchial tubes dilate, and gastric and adrenal secretions increase. There is greater muscular tension and sometimes an increase in motor activity. Small doses usually make people feel more awake and alert, less fatigued and bored. The most common CNS stimulants are cocaine, amphetamines, nicotine (discussed in Chapter 16), ephedrine, and caffeine.

stimulants
Drugs that increase nervous or muscular activity.

Cocaine

Usually derived from the leaves of coca shrubs that grow high in the Andes in South America, cocaine is a potent CNS stimulant. For centuries, natives of the Andes have chewed coca leaves both for pleasure and to increase their endurance. For a short time during the nineteenth century, some physicians were enthusiastic about the use of cocaine to cure alcoholism and addiction to the painkiller morphine. Enthusiasm waned after the drug's adverse side effects became apparent.

Cocaine quickly produces a feeling of euphoria, which makes it a popular recreational drug. Cocaine use surged in popularity during the early 1980s, when the drug's high price made it a status drug. The introduction of crack cocaine during the 1980s made the drug available in smaller quantities and at lower prices to more people. The typical recreational user shifted rapidly from wealthy professionals snorting powdered cocaine to poor inner-city smokers of crack cocaine. The prevalence of cocaine use among the general population in Canada in 2012 was 1.1 percent; this percentage is slightly lower than the rate of use reported in 2008.

METHODS OF USE Cocaine is usually snorted and absorbed through the nasal mucosa or injected intravenously, providing rapid increases of the drug's concentration in the blood and therefore fast, intense effects. Another method of use involves processing cocaine with baking soda and water, yielding the ready-to-smoke form of cocaine known as crack. Crack is typically available as small beads or pellets that are smoked in glass pipes. The tiny but potent beads can be handled more easily than cocaine powder and marketed in smaller, less expensive doses.

EFFECTS The effects of cocaine are usually intense but short-lived. The euphoria lasts from 5 to 20 minutes and ends abruptly, to be replaced by irritability, anxiety, or slight depression. When cocaine is absorbed via the lungs, by either smoking or inhalation, it reaches the brain in about 10 seconds, and the effects are particularly intense. This is part of the appeal of smoking crack. The effects from IV injections occur almost as quickly—in about 20 seconds. Since the mucous membranes in the nose briefly slow absorption, the onset of effects from snorting takes 2–3 minutes. Heavy users may inject cocaine intravenously every 10–20 minutes to maintain the effects.

The larger the cocaine dose and the more rapidly it is absorbed into the bloodstream, the greater the immediate—and sometimes lethal—effects. Sudden death from cocaine is most commonly the result of excessive CNS stimulation that causes convulsions and respiratory collapse, irregular heartbeat, extremely high blood pressure, blood clots, and possibly heart attack or stroke. Although rare, fatalities can occur in healthy young people; among people ages 18–59, people who use cocaine are seven times as likely as non-users to have a heart attack. Chronic cocaine use produces inflammation of the nasal mucosa, which can lead to persistent bleeding and ulceration of the septum between the nostrils. The use of cocaine may also cause paranoia and aggressiveness.

When steady cocaine users stop taking the drug, they experience a sudden "crash" characterized by depression, agitation, and fatigue, followed by a period of withdrawal. Their depression can be temporarily relieved by taking more cocaine, so its continued use is reinforced. A binge cocaine user may go for weeks or months without using any cocaine and then take large amounts repeatedly. Although he or she may not be physically dependent, a binge cocaine user who misses work or school and risks serious health consequences is clearly abusing the drug.

Because cocaine rapidly passes from a mother's bloodstream into the placenta, a woman who uses cocaine during pregnancy is at higher risk for miscarriage, premature labour, and stillbirth. She is more likely to deliver a low-birth-weight baby who has a small head circumference. Her infant may be at increased risk for defects of the genitourinary tract, cardiovascular system, central nervous system, and extremities. It is difficult to pinpoint the effects of cocaine because many women who use cocaine also use tobacco or alcohol or both.

Infants whose mothers use cocaine may also be born intoxicated. They are typically irritable and jittery and do not eat or sleep normally. These characteristics may affect their early social and emotional development because it may be more difficult for adults to interact with them. Cocaine also passes into breast milk and can intoxicate a breastfeeding infant.

Amphetamines

Amphetamines (uppers) are a group of synthetic chemicals that are potent CNS stimulants. Some common drugs in this family are amphetamine (Benzedrine), dextroamphetamine (Dexedrine), and methamphetamine (Methedrine or "meth"). Meth is more addictive and dangerous than most forms of amphetamine because it is more toxic and its effects last longer. Once taken, the drug causes the brain to release high amounts of dopamine, a key neurotransmitter. Methamphetamine is highly addictive; many casual users rapidly become regular users. Crystal methamphetamine ("crystal meth" or "ice"), a smokable, high-potency form of methamphetamine, is popular in some cities across Canada. Easy to manufacture, crystal meth is cheaper than crack and produces a similar but longer-lasting euphoria. The use of crystal meth can quickly lead to addiction.

EFFECTS Small doses of amphetamines usually make people feel more alert. Amphetamines generally increase motor activity but do not measurably alter a normal, rested person's ability to perform tasks calling for challenging motor skills or complex thinking. When amphetamines do improve performance, it is primarily by counteracting fatigue and boredom. In small doses, amphetamines increase heart rate and blood pressure and change sleep patterns.

Amphetamines are sometimes used to curb appetite, but after a few weeks the user develops tolerance and higher doses are necessary. When people stop taking the drug, their appetite usually returns, and they gain back the weight they lost unless they have made permanent changes in eating behaviour.

Short-term effects associated with methamphetamine use can include euphoria, rapid breathing, increased body temperature (hyperthermia), insomnia, tremors, anxiety, and convulsions. In the long term, methamphetamine's effects can be devastating. Severe weight loss, heart attack, stroke, hallucinations, violence, paranoia, and psychotic behaviour have all been linked to meth addiction. Meth use causes extensive tooth decay and tooth loss, a condition referred to as "meth mouth." The drug takes a severe toll on the heart, increasing heart rate and blood pressure, damaging blood vessels, and causing irregular heartbeat. Such damage can be fatal.

ABUSE AND ADDICTION   Much amphetamine abuse begins as an attempt to cope with a temporary situation. A student cramming for an exam or an exhausted long-haul truck driver can go a little longer by taking amphetamines, but the results can be disastrous. The likelihood of making bad judgments significantly increases. The stimulating effects may also wear off suddenly, and the individual may precipitously feel exhausted or fall asleep ("crash").

Another problem is **state dependence**, the phenomenon whereby information learned in a certain drug-induced state is difficult to recall when the person is not in that same physiological state. Test performance may deteriorate when students use drugs to study and then take tests in their normal, non-drug state. (Users of antihistamines may also experience state dependence.)

---

state dependence
A situation in which information learned in a drug-induced state is difficult to recall when the effect of the drug wears off.

Repeated use of amphetamines, even in moderate doses, often leads to tolerance and the need for increasingly larger doses. The result can be severe disturbances in behaviour, including a temporary state of paranoid **psychosis**, with delusions of persecution and episodes of unprovoked violence. If injected in large doses, amphetamines produce a feeling of intense pleasure, followed by sensations of vigour and euphoria that last for several hours. As these feelings wear off, they are replaced by feelings of irritability and vague uneasiness. Long-term use of amphetamines at high doses can cause paranoia, hallucinations, delusions, and incoherence.

---

psychosis
A severe mental disorder characterized by a distortion of reality; symptoms might include delusions or hallucinations.

Methamphetamine is more addictive than other forms of amphetamine. It is also more dangerous because it is more toxic and its effects last longer. Meth use has also been linked to high-risk sexual activity and increased rates of STIs, including HIV infection (see Chapter 13).

Methamphetamine users have signs of brain damage similar to those seen in individuals with Parkinson's disease that appear to persist even after drug use ceases, causing impaired memory and motor coordination. Withdrawal symptoms may include muscle aches and tremors, profound fatigue, deep depression, despair, and apathy. Chronic high-dose use is often associated with pronounced psychological cravings and obsessive drug-seeking behaviour.

Women who use amphetamines during pregnancy risk premature birth, stillbirth, low birth weight, and early infant death. Babies born to mothers who use amphetamines have a higher incidence of cleft palate, cleft lip, and deformed limbs. They may also experience symptoms of withdrawal.

Ritalin

A stimulant with amphetamine-like effects, Ritalin (methylphenidate) is used to treat attention deficit hyperactivity disorder (ADHD). When taken orally at prescribed levels, it has little potential for abuse. When injected or snorted, however, addiction can rapidly result. There is growing concern that more and more young people are abusing these drugs for various reasons, including appetite suppression, increased focus, and euphoria. In fact, the non-prescription use of so-called "study drugs" (stimulants such as Ritalin and Adderall, another prescription medication used to treat ADHD) is gaining in popularity among post-secondary students; experts have estimated that 5–35 percent of university and college students have abused these medications in an attempt to increase academic performance through enhanced alertness and concentration. Most evidence, however, suggests that stimulants are *not* associated with cognitive improvements in healthy people. Rather, there are serious and potentially life-threatening risks associated with the misuse of these drugs, including death, cardiovascular complications, addiction (similar to that of cocaine), overdoses, and depression, among others. Because it is illegal to buy or use such medications without a prescription, and to sell one's own prescription, students can also experience serious legal ramifications. In addition to dispelling myths and providing students with credible information about the dangers associated with the abuse of stimulants, increased attention and resources should be devoted to combatting this issue on university and college campuses. It is crucial that institutions both acknowledge and identify ways to reduce the problem before it escalates further.

QUICK STATS

4% of students in grades 7 to 12 across Canada reported using at least one prescription drug for non-medical purposes in 2012–2013.

—*Youth Smoking Survey, 2012–2013*

Ephedrine

Although somewhat less potent than amphetamine, ephedrine produces stimulant effects. Ephedrine has been linked to heart arrhythmia, stroke, psychotic reactions, seizures, and some deaths, and it may be particularly dangerous at high doses or when combined with another stimulant, such as caffeine. Health Canada has issued several warnings to consumers about the dangers of using unauthorized products containing ephedra or ephedrine, either alone or in combination with other stimulants, for weight loss, body building, or increased energy.

Caffeine

Caffeine is probably the most popular psychoactive drug and also one of the most ancient. It is found in coffee, tea, cocoa, soft drinks, headache remedies, and OTC preparations. (Table 14.2 lists typical levels of caffeine in several popular beverages.) In ordinary doses, caffeine produces greater alertness and a sense of well-being. It also decreases feelings of fatigue or boredom, so using caffeine may enable a person to keep at physically tiring or repetitive tasks longer. Such use is usually followed, however, by a sudden letdown. Caffeine does not noticeably influence a person's ability to perform complex mental tasks unless fatigue, boredom, or other factors have already affected normal performance.

TABLE 14.2

Caffeine Content of Popular Beverages

	Serving Size	Typical Caffeine Level (mg)*
Coffee		
Regular coffee, brewed	237 mL (1 cup)	135
Regular coffee, instant	237 mL	76–106
Tim Horton's original blend	414 mL (Medium)	205
Starbucks coffee	473 mL (Grande)	330
Decaffeinated coffee, brewed	237 mL	5
Decaffeinated coffee, instant	237 mL	5
Tea		
Regular tea, brewed	237 mL	43
Decaffeinated tea	237 mL	0
Green tea	237 mL	30–60
Tim Horton's steeped tea	414 mL (Medium)	90
Starbucks Tazo Chai Tea Latte	473 mL (Grande)	95
Nestea	355 mL (1 can)	17
Herbal tea, brewed	237 mL	0
Cola Beverages		
Diet Coke	355 mL (1 can)	47
Dr. Pepper, Diet Dr. Pepper	355 mL	41
Pepsi	355 mL	38
Coca-Cola Classic, Diet Pepsi	355 mL	35
A&W Crème Soda	355 mL	29
Barq's Root Beer	355 mL	23
Energy Drinks		
NoDoz Energy Shots	55 mL	115
Monster Energy, Rockstart	473 mL	160
Redline Energy Drink	236 mL	316
Starbucks Refreshers, Can	354 mL	50
Red Bull	250 mL	80
Cocoa Products		
Chocolate milk	237 mL	8
Hot-cocoa mix, 1 envelope	237 mL	5
Candy, milk chocolate	28 g	7
Chocolate cake	80 g	36

Sources: Center for Science in the Public Interest. 2014. *Caffeine Content of Food & Drugs,* http://www.cspinet.org/new/cafchart.htm (retrieved January 19, 2015); Health Canada. 2012. *Food and Nutrition: Caffeine in Food,* http://www.hc-sc.gc.ca/fn-an/securit/addit/caf/food-caf-aliments-eng.php (retrieved January 19, 2015); and Tim Horton's Caffeine Content, http://www.timhortons.com/ca/en/pdf/CAFFEINE_CONTENT_-_Canada_-_August2014.pdf (retrieved January 19, 2015).

*Caffeine levels vary greatly by brand of product, manner of preparation, and amount consumed. The amounts shown here are averages based on tests conducted by a variety of organizations. To find the exact amount of caffeine in any product, check the product's label.

Caffeine mildly stimulates the heart and respiratory system, increases muscular tremor, and enhances gastric secretion. Higher doses may cause nervousness, anxiety, irritability, headache, disturbed sleep, and gastric irritation or peptic ulcers. In people with high blood pressure, caffeine can cause blood pressure to rise even further above normal; in people with type 2 diabetes, caffeine may cause glucose and insulin levels to rise after meals. Some people, especially children, are quite vulnerable to the adverse effects of caffeine. They become hyperactive and overly sensitive to any stimulation in their environment. In rare instances, the disturbance is so severe that they experience misperceptions of their surroundings—a toxic psychosis.

Drinks containing caffeine are rarely harmful for most people, but some tolerance develops, and withdrawal symptoms of irritability, headaches, and even mild depression do occur. Thus, although we don't usually think of caffeine as a dependence-producing drug, for some people it is. People can usually avoid problems by simply decreasing their daily intake of caffeine; if intake is decreased gradually, withdrawal symptoms can be reduced or avoided. For the general population of healthy adults, Health Canada advises an intake of no more than 400 milligrams of caffeine per day.

Marijuana and Other Cannabis Products

Marijuana is the most widely used illegal drug in Canada. According to the 2012 *Canadian Alcohol and Drug Use Monitoring Survey*, more than 40 percent of Canadians have tried marijuana at least once in their lifetime; among 15–24-year-olds, almost 35 percent have tried marijuana.

Marijuana is a crude preparation of various parts of the Indian hemp plant *Cannabis sativa*, which grows in most parts of the world. THC (tetrahydrocannabinol) is the main active ingredient in marijuana. Based on THC content, the potency of marijuana preparations varies widely. Marijuana plants that grow wild often have less than 1 percent THC in their leaves. When selected strains are cultivated by separation of male and female plants (*sinsemilla*), the bud leaves from the flowering tops may contain 7–8 percent THC. Hashish, a potent preparation made from the thick resin that exudes from the marijuana leaves, may contain up to 14 percent THC.

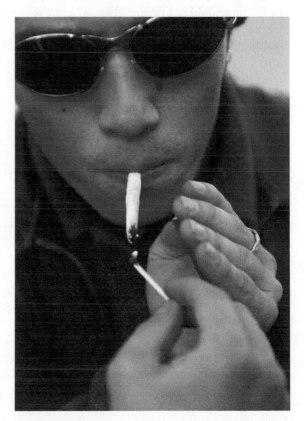

These various preparations have all been known and used for centuries, so the frequently heard claim that today's marijuana is more potent than the marijuana of the 1970s is not strictly true. However, a greater proportion of the marijuana sold today is the higher-potency (and more expensive) sinsemilla; hence, the average potency of street marijuana has increased.

Marijuana is usually smoked, but it can also be ingested. The classification of marijuana is a matter of some debate. For this reason, it is treated separately here.

Short-Term Effects and Uses

As is true with most psychoactive drugs, the effects of a low dose of marijuana are strongly influenced both by the individual's expectations and by past experiences. At low doses, people who use marijuana typically experience euphoria, a heightening of subjective sensory experiences, a slowing down of the perception of passing time, and a relaxed, laid-back attitude. These pleasant effects

Marijuana is the most widely used illegal drug in Canada.

are the reason this drug is so widely used. With moderate doses, these effects become stronger, and the user can also expect to have impaired memory function, disturbed thought patterns, lapses of attention, and feelings of **depersonalization**, in which the mind seems to be separated from the body.

> **depersonalization**
> A state in which a person loses the sense of reality or perceives his or her body as unreal.

At higher doses, the effects of marijuana are determined mostly by the drug itself rather than by the individual's expectations and setting. Very high doses produce feelings of depersonalization, as well as marked sensory distortion and changes in body image (such as a feeling that the body is very light). Inexperienced users sometimes think these sensations mean they are going crazy, and they become anxious or even panicky. Unexpected reactions are the leading reason for emergency room visits by users of marijuana or hashish.

Physiologically, marijuana increases heart rate and dilates certain blood vessels in the eyes, which creates the characteristic bloodshot eyes. Individuals who use marijuana may also feel less inclined toward physical exertion and may feel particularly hungry or thirsty. Because THC affects parts of the brain controlling balance, coordination, and reaction time, marijuana use impairs driving performance. The combination of alcohol and marijuana is even more dangerous: even a low dose of marijuana, when combined with alcohol, significantly impairs driving performance and increases crash risk.

Some compounds in marijuana may have legitimate medical use. For example, marijuana has been shown to ease pain, reduce nausea, and increase appetite. These benefits led Health Canada to approve the use of "medical marijuana" by extremely ill patients, in situations where conventional treatments are not appropriate or do not provide adequate relief. Despite these benefits, Health Canada warns that the use of medical marijuana should not be confused with the legalization of marijuana in Canada. Marijuana remains an illegal and controlled substance; therefore, it is not legal to grow or possess marijuana except with permission from Health Canada. The ethical debates over medical marijuana use continue, as do court cases.

QUICK STATS

In 2011, nearly 18% of Canadians who reported using cannabis said they did so for medical reasons.
—Canadian Alcohol and Drug Use Monitoring Survey, 2011

Long-Term Effects

The most probable long-term effect of smoking marijuana is respiratory damage, including impaired lung function and chronic bronchial irritation. Although no evidence links marijuana use to lung cancer, it may cause changes in lung tissue that promote cancer growth. Individuals who use marijuana may be at increased risk for emphysema and cancer of the head and neck; among people with chronic conditions, such as cancer and AIDS, marijuana use is associated with increased risk of fatal lung infections. Heavy users may experience learning problems, as well as subtle impairments of attention and memory that may or may not be reversible following long-term abstinence. Long-term use may also decrease testosterone levels and sperm counts and increase sperm abnormalities.

Heavy marijuana use during pregnancy may cause impaired fetal growth and development, low birth weight, and increased risk of ectopic pregnancy. Marijuana may act synergistically with alcohol to increase the damaging effects of alcohol on the fetus. THC rapidly enters breast milk and may impair an infant's early motor development.

Addiction

Regular users of marijuana can develop tolerance, and some develop addiction. In fact, it has been suggested that 1 in 9 people who use marijuana will become addicted. Withdrawal symptoms may occur in the majority of addicted or heavy users. Common symptoms include anger or aggression, irritability, nervousness or restlessness, sleep difficulties, and decreased appetite or weight loss.

Hallucinogens

Hallucinogens are a group of drugs whose predominant pharmacological effect is to alter perceptions, feelings, and thoughts. Hallucinogens include the following:

- LSD (lysergic acid diethylamide)
- Psilocybin
- STP (4-methyl-2,5-dimethoxyamphetamine)
- DMT (dimethyltryptamine)
- MDMA (3,4-methylenedioxymethamphetamine)
- Ketamine
- PCP (phencyclidine)

These drugs are most commonly ingested or smoked.

hallucinogens
Drugs that alter perception, feelings, or thoughts; examples are LSD and PCP.

QUICK STATS

Almost 5% of Canadians ages 15–24 have tried hallucinogens at least once in the past year.
—Health Canada, 2014

LSD

LSD is one of the most powerful psychoactive drugs. Tiny doses will produce noticeable effects in most people, such as an altered sense of time, visual disturbances, an improved sense of hearing, mood changes, and distortions in how people perceive their bodies. Dilation of the pupils and slight dizziness, weakness, and nausea may also occur. With larger doses, individuals may experience a phenomenon known as **synaesthesia**, feelings of depersonalization, and other alterations in the perceived relationship between the self and external reality.

synaesthesia
A condition in which a stimulus evokes not only the sensation appropriate to it but also another sensation of a different character, such as when a colour evokes a specific smell.

Many hallucinogens induce tolerance so quickly that after only one or two doses their effects decrease substantially. The user must then stop taking the drug for several days before his or her system can be receptive to it again. Typically, these drugs cause little drug-seeking behaviour and no physical dependence or withdrawal symptoms.

The immediate effects of low doses of hallucinogens are largely determined by expectations and setting. Many effects are hard to describe because they involve subjective and unusual dimensions of awareness—the **altered states of consciousness** for which these drugs are famous. For this reason, hallucinogens have acquired a certain aura not associated with other drugs. People have taken LSD in search of a religious or mystical experience or in the hope of exploring new worlds. During the 1960s, some psychiatrists gave LSD to their patients to help them talk about their repressed feelings.

altered states of consciousness
Profound changes in mood, thinking, and perception.

A severe panic reaction, which can be terrifying in the extreme, can result from taking any dose of LSD. It is impossible to predict when a panic reaction will occur. Some LSD users report having had hundreds of pleasurable and ecstatic experiences before having a bad trip, or "bummer," however a tranquil experience is never guaranteed.

Even after the drug's chemical effects have worn off, spontaneous flashbacks and other psychological disturbances can occur. **Flashbacks** are perceptual distortions and bizarre thoughts that occur after the drug has been entirely eliminated from the body. Although they are relatively rare phenomena, flashbacks can be extremely distressing. They are often triggered by specific psychological cues associated with the drug-taking experience, such as certain mood states or even types of music.

flashbacks
Perceptual distortions or bizarre thoughts that recur after the chemical effects of a drug have worn off.

Other Hallucinogens

Most other hallucinogens have the same general effects as LSD, but there are some variations. For example, a DMT or ketamine high does not last as long as an LSD high; an STP high lasts longer. MDMA has both hallucinogenic and amphetamine-like properties. Tolerance to MDMA develops quickly, and high doses can cause anxiety, delusions, and paranoia. (Refer back to the In Focus box for more on MDMA.)

PCP reduces and distorts sensory input, especially proprioception, the sensation of body position and movement; it creates a state of sensory deprivation. PCP was initially used as an anaesthetic but was unsatisfactory because it caused agitation, confusion, and delirium (loss of contact with reality). Because it can be easily made, PCP is often available illegally and is sometimes used as an inexpensive replacement for other psychoactive drugs.

The effects of ketamine are similar to those of PCP—confusion, agitation, aggression, and lack of coordination—but they tend to be less predictable. Tolerance to either drug can develop rapidly.

Hallucinogenic effects can also be obtained from certain mushrooms (psilocybin, or "magic mushrooms"), certain morning glory seeds, nutmeg, jimsonweed, and other botanical products, but unpleasant side effects, such as dizziness, have limited the popularity of these products.

Inhalants

Inhaling certain chemicals can produce effects ranging from heightened pleasure to delirium and death. Inhalants fall into several major groups:

- Volatile solvents, which are found in many products, such as paint thinner, glue, and gasoline
- Aerosols, which are sprays that contain propellants and solvents
- Nitrites, such as butyl nitrite and amyl nitrite
- Anaesthetics, which include nitrous oxide (laughing gas)

Inhalant use tends to be highest among younger adolescents and declines with age. It is estimated that 3–5 percent of Canadian adolescents have tried inhalants, although this statistic does not take into consideration the growing and rampant problem of inhalant use in some remote Inuit and First Nations communities across Canada.

Inhalant use is difficult to control because inhalants are easy to obtain. They are present in a variety of seemingly harmless products—from dessert-topping sprays to underarm deodorants—that are both inexpensive and legal. Using the drugs also requires no illegal or suspicious paraphernalia. People who use inhalants get high by

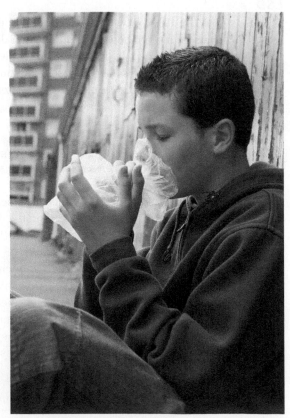

Inhalant use is difficult to monitor and control because inhalants are found in many inexpensive and legal products.

sniffing, snorting, "bagging" (inhaling fumes from a plastic bag), or "huffing" (placing an inhalant-soaked rag against the mouth).

Although different in makeup, nearly all inhalants produce effects similar to those of anaesthetics, which slow down body functions. Low doses may cause people to feel slightly stimulated; at higher doses, people may feel less inhibited and less in control. Sniffing high concentrations of the chemicals in solvents or aerosol sprays can cause a loss of consciousness, heart failure, and death. High concentrations of any inhalant can also cause death from suffocation by displacing the oxygen in the lungs and central nervous system. Deliberately inhaling from a bag or in a closed area greatly increases the chances of suffocation. Other possible effects of the excessive or long-term use of inhalants include damage to the nervous system (impaired perception, reasoning, memory, and muscular coordination); hearing loss; increased risk of cancer; and damage to the liver, kidneys, and bone marrow.

QUESTIONS FOR CRITICAL THINKING AND REFLECTION

Do you know anyone who may be at risk for using inhalants? If so, would you try to intervene in some way? What would you tell a person to convince him or her to stop inhaling chemicals?

Synthetic Recreational Drugs

In recent years, herbal or synthetic recreational drugs have become increasingly available. These "designer drugs" are intended to have pharmacological effects similar to those of illicit drugs, but to be chemically distinct from them and therefore either legal or impossible to detect in drug screening. The drugs fall into two main groups. One group is marketed as synthetic marijuana and sold as "herbal incense," or "herbal highs," with names such as Spice, K2, Genie, and Nice Guy. The other group is marketed as stimulants with properties like those of cocaine or amphetamine, and is sold as "bath salts" with names such as Zoom, Ivory Wave, and White Rush.

Spice and other synthetic mimics of THC are distributed in the form of dried leaves or powder. They are typically smoked, using a pipe or by rolling in a cigarette paper, but can also be ingested as an infusion such as tea, or inhaled. The active ingredients in Spice and similar products are synthetic cannabinoids that act on brain cells to produce effects similar to those of THC, such as physical relaxation, changes in perception, elevated mood, and mild euphoria. These drugs may seem new to adults, but young people in Canada appear to be using them; almost 2 percent of Ontario students in Grades 7–12 reported using synthetic marijuana in the prior year, according to the 2013 *Ontario Student Drug Use and Health Survey.*

Spice and similar products have not been included in any wide-scale animal or human studies, and little information is available in international medical databases. The blends of ingredients vary widely, but these products typically contain more than a dozen different plant-derived compounds, which give rise to a wide variety of drug combinations. Calls to poison control centres for exposure to synthetic marijuana are common, with patients describing symptoms that include rapid heart rate, vomiting, agitation, confusion, and hallucinations.

"Bath salts," marketed as cocaine or methamphetamine substitutes, contain the synthetic stimulants mephedrone, methylone, or methylenedioxypyrovalerone (MDPV). Relatively new and similar in effect to MDMA ("Ecstasy"), MDPV is a synthetic version of the active ingredient found in the stimulant khat, which is widely used in countries of the Middle East. The products are sold in small packets of salt-like crystals with warnings like "novelty only" and "not for human consumption." Bath salts are highly addictive and can be ingested by smoking, eating, or injecting, or by crushing them and snorting the powder. The speed of onset is up to 15 minutes depending on how the drug is ingested, and the effects may last as long as six hours. The effects of bath salts can be severe and include combative violent behaviour, extreme agitation, confusion, hallucinations, hypertension, chest pain, and suicidal thoughts. From 2010 to 2012, Health Canada's Drug Analysis Service (DAS) reported a total of 549 cases in which bath salts were seized by law enforcement agencies.

Drug Use: The Decades Ahead

Drug research will undoubtedly provide new information, new treatments, and new chemical combinations in the decades ahead. New psychoactive drugs may present unexpected possibilities for therapy, social use, and abuse. Making honest and unbiased information about drugs available to everyone, however, may cut down on their abuse.

Although the use of some drugs, both legal and illegal, has declined dramatically since the 1970s, the use of others has held steady or increased. Mounting public concern has led to great debate and a wide range of opinions about what should be done. Efforts to combat the problem include workplace drug testing, tougher law enforcement and prosecution, and treatment and education. With drugs entering the country on a massive scale from a variety of countries and being distributed through tightly controlled drug-smuggling organizations and street gangs, it remains to be seen how effective any program will be.

The Costs of Substance Abuse

The economic cost of drug abuse is staggering. According to the Canadian Centre on Substance Abuse, the justice-related cost to society of illicit drug use, including police, courts, and correctional services, is $2 billion annually. That figure expands substantially when combined with the costs of alcohol and tobacco use and when other expenses, such as health care costs and lost productivity, are taken into account. But the costs are more than just financial; they are also paid in human pain and suffering.

Drug abuse is a health care issue for society. In Canada, illegal drug use leads to more than 47 000 deaths and thousands more injuries and disabilities each year. Although it is in the best interest of society to treat people who want help, not nearly enough space is available in treatment facilities to help the vast number of Canadians who need immediate treatment. Individuals who are addicted to drugs and who want to quit, especially those among the urban poor, often have to wait a year or more for acceptance into a residential care or other treatment program.

Drug abuse also takes a toll on individuals and families. Children born to women who use drugs, such as alcohol, tobacco, or cocaine, may have long-term health problems. Drug use in families can become a vicious cycle. Observing adults around them using drugs, children assume it is an acceptable way to deal with problems. Problems, such as abuse, neglect, lack of opportunity, and unemployment, become contributing factors to drug use and serve to perpetuate the cycle.

QUICK STATS

More than 1700 Canadians are in jail abroad; approximately one-third of them have been arrested for drug-related offences.

—Government of Canada, 2014

Legalizing Drugs

Pointing out that many of the social problems associated with drugs are related to prohibition rather than to the effects of the drugs themselves, some people have argued for various forms of drug legalization or decriminalization. Proposals range from making some drugs, such as marijuana and heroin, available by prescription, to allowing licensed dealers to sell some of these drugs to adults. Proponents argue that legalizing some currently illicit drugs—but putting controls on them similar to those used for alcohol, tobacco, and prescription drugs—could eliminate many of the problems related to drug use.

Opponents of drug legalization argue that allowing easier access to drugs would expose many more people to possible abuse and addiction. Drugs would be cheaper and easier to obtain, and drug use would be more socially acceptable. Legalizing drugs could cause an increase in drug use among children and teenagers.

Opponents point out that alcohol and tobacco are major causes of disease and death in our society and that they should not be used as models for other practices.

Treatment for Drug Addiction

Treatment for drug addiction often is characterized by discrete episodes of short-term abstinence and relapse. Regardless of the therapeutic approach used for drug dependence, many individuals undergoing treatment will often slide back into their drug habits. Often, this backsliding results in worsening of the original substance abuse problem. For some substances, the period from abstinence to relapse occurs within one year after treatment.

Preventing relapse and maintaining long-term cessation of drug use is an exceedingly complex medical goal. Medical interventions based on pharmaceutical aids to enhance the individual's long-term commitment to change and stay drug-free remain an elusive goal. Relapse prevention research is instead increasingly focusing on the need to expand the behavioural repertoire of skills needed to decrease the risk of recidivism among individuals receiving drug-treatment services.

Medication-Assisted Treatment

Medications are increasingly being used in addiction treatment to reduce the craving for the abused drug or to block or oppose its effects. Perhaps the best-known medication for drug abuse is methadone, a synthetic drug used as a substitute for heroin. Use of methadone prevents withdrawal reactions and reduces the craving for heroin; it enables dependent people to function normally in social and vocational activities, although they remain dependent on methadone. The narcotic buprenorphine, approved by Health Canada in 2007 for treatment of opioid addiction, also reduces cravings. Many other medications are under study; drugs used specifically in the treatment of nicotine and alcohol dependence are discussed in Chapters 15 and 16.

Medication therapy is relatively simple and inexpensive and is therefore popular among patients and health care providers. However, the relapse rate is high. Combining drug therapy with psychological and social services improves success rates, underscoring the importance of psychological factors in drug dependence.

Treatment Centres

Treatment centres offer a variety of short-term and long-term services, including hospitalization, detoxification, counselling, and other mental health services. The therapeutic community is a specific type of centre, a residential program run in a completely drug-free atmosphere. Administered by ex-addicts, these programs use confrontation, strict discipline, and unrelenting peer pressure to attempt to resocialize individuals with addictions with a different set of values. Halfway houses, transitional settings between a 24-hour-a-day program and independent living, are an important phase of treatment for some people. Strategies for evaluating programs are given in the Critical Consumer box.

 Critical CONSUMER

Choosing a Drug-Treatment Program

When evaluating different facilities or programs for drug treatment, consider the following issues:
- *What type of treatment or facility is most appropriate?* Intensive outpatient treatment is available through many community mental health centres, as well as through specialized drug-treatment facilities. Such programs typically require several sessions per week, combining individual therapy, group counselling, and attendance at 12-step meetings. Residential, or in-patient, facilities may be associated with a medical facility, such as a hospital, or they may be freestanding programs that focus solely on substance-abuse treatment. Some residential treatment programs last longer or cost more per week than some health insurance plans will cover.
- *How will treatment be paid for?* Many services are covered by provincial or territorial health insurance plans. However, additional fees may be incurred for services, which may be covered in part, or in full, by workplace extended health benefits plans or other private insurance health care plans.

- *Is there likely to be a need for medical support?* Chronic alcoholics or abusers of other central nervous system depressants may experience life-threatening seizures or other withdrawal symptoms during the first few days of detoxification. Malnutrition is common among substance abusers, and people who inject drugs may suffer from local infections and blood-borne diseases, such as hepatitis or HIV infection. Any medical problems, such as these, are best handled in an inpatient program with good medical support.
- *What is the level of professional training of the staff?* Is there a medical doctor on-site or making frequent visits? Are there trained nurses? Licensed psychologists or social workers? Many successful programs are staffed primarily by recovering alcoholics or drug users. Do those staff members have training and certification as addiction specialists or some other licence or certificate?
- *Does the program provide related services, such as family and job counselling and post-treatment follow-up?* These types of services are extremely important for the long-term success of drug-abuse treatment.
- *Can you visit the facility and speak with the staff and clients?* A prospective client and his or her family should be allowed to visit any treatment centre or program.

Groups and Peer Counselling

Groups such as Alcoholics Anonymous (AA) and Narcotics Anonymous (NA) have helped many people. People treated in drug-substitution programs or substance-abuse treatment centres are often urged or required to join a support group as part of their recovery. These groups follow a 12-step program. Group members' first step is to acknowledge that they have a problem over which they have no control. Peer support is a critical ingredient of these programs, and members usually meet at least once a week. Each member is paired with a sponsor to call on for advice and support if the temptation to relapse becomes overwhelming. With such support, thousands of substance-dependent people have been able to recover, remain abstinent, and reclaim their lives. Chapters of AA and NA meet on some university campuses; community-based chapters are typically listed online and in local newspapers.

Many colleges and universities also have peer counselling programs, in which students are trained to help other students who have drug problems. A peer counsellor's role may be as limited as referring a student to a professional with expertise in substance dependence for an evaluation, or as involved as helping arrange a leave of absence from school for participation in a drug-treatment program. Most peer counselling programs are founded on principles of strict confidentiality. Peer counsellors may also be able to help students who are concerned about a classmate or loved one with an apparent drug problem (see the Take Charge box). Information about peer counselling programs is usually available from the student health centre.

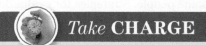

Take CHARGE

If Someone You Know Has a Drug Problem

Changes in behaviour and mood in someone you know may signal a growing dependence on drugs. Signs that a person's life is beginning to focus on drugs include the following:

- Sudden withdrawal or emotional distance
- Rebellious or unusually irritable behaviour
- A loss of interest in usual activities or hobbies
- A decline in school or work performance
- A sudden change in the chosen group of friends
- Changes in sleeping or eating habits
- Frequent borrowing of money or stealing
- Secretive behaviour about personal possessions, such as a backpack or the contents of a drawer
- Deterioration of physical appearance

If you believe a family member or friend has a drug problem, obtain information about resources for drug treatment available on your campus or in your community. Communicate your concern, provide the person with information about treatment options, and offer your support during treatment. If the person continues to deny having a problem, you may want to talk with an experienced counsellor about setting up an intervention—a formal, structured confrontation designed to end denial by having family, friends, and other caring individuals present their concerns to the person using drugs. Participants in an intervention would indicate the ways in which the individual is hurting others as well as himself or herself. If your friend or family member agrees to treatment, encourage him or her to attend a support group, such as Narcotics Anonymous or Alcoholics Anonymous. And finally, examine your relationship with the individual who is using drugs for signs of codependency. If necessary, get help for yourself; friends and family of people who use drugs can often benefit from counselling.

Harm-Reduction Strategies

Because many attempts at treatment are at first unsuccessful, some experts advocate the use of harm-reduction strategies. The goal of harm reduction is to minimize the negative effects of drug use and abuse; a common example is the use of designated drivers to reduce alcohol-related motor vehicle crashes. Drug-substitution programs such as methadone maintenance are a form of harm reduction; although participants remain drug dependent, the negative individual and social consequences of their drug use is reduced. Syringe or needle exchange programs, designed to reduce transmission of HIV and hepatitis C, are another harm-reduction approach. Some experts have also suggested free testing of street drugs for purity and potency to help people who use drugs avoid unintentional toxicity or overdose.

Codependency

Many treatment programs also offer counselling for those who are close to people who abuse drugs. Drug abuse takes a toll on friends and family members, and counselling can help people work through painful feelings of guilt and powerlessness. **Codependency**, in which a person close to the individual who abuses drugs is controlled by the abuser's behaviour, sometimes develops. Codependent people may come to believe that love, approval, and security are contingent on their taking care of the person who abuses drugs. People can become codependent naturally because they want to help. They may assume that their good intentions will persuade the individual to stop using drugs.

codependency
A relationship in which a partner or family member who does not abuse drugs or alcohol is controlled by the abuser's behaviour; codependent people frequently engage in enabling behaviours.

Codependent people often engage in behaviours that remove or soften the effects of drug use on the user—so-called *enabling* behaviours. However, the habit of enabling can inhibit an addicted person's recovery because the person never has to experience the consequences of his or her behaviour. Often, the enabler is dependent, too—on the patterns of interaction in the relationship. People who need to take care of people often marry people who need to be taken care of. Children in these families often develop the same behaviour pattern as one of their parents, by either becoming helpless or becoming a caregiver. For this reason, many treatment programs involve the whole family.

Have you ever been an enabler in a relationship? You may have, if you have ever done any of the following:
- Given someone one more chance to stop abusing drugs, then another, and another...
- Made excuses or lied for someone to his or her friends, teachers, or employer
- Joined someone in drug use and blamed others for your behaviour
- Loaned money to someone to continue drug use
- Stayed up late waiting for or gone out searching for someone who uses drugs
- Felt embarrassed or angry about the actions of someone who uses drugs
- Ignored the drug use because the person became defensive when you brought it up
- Not confronted a friend or relative who was obviously intoxicated or high on a drug

If you come from a codependent family or see yourself developing codependency relationships or engaging in enabling behaviours, consider acting now to make changes in your patterns of interaction. Remember, you cannot cause or cure substance abuse or addiction in another person.

Preventing Drug Abuse

Obviously, the best solution to drug abuse is prevention. Government attempts at controlling the drug problem often focus on stopping the production, importation, and distribution of illegal drugs. Creative effort also has to be put into stopping the demand for drugs. Developing persuasive anti-drug educational programs offers the best hope for solving the drug problem in the future. Indirect approaches to prevention involve building young people's self-esteem, improving their academic skills, and increasing their recreational opportunities. Direct approaches involve giving information about the adverse effects of drugs and teaching tactics that help students resist peer pressure to use drugs in various situations. Developing strategies for resisting peer pressure is one of the more effective techniques.

Prevention efforts need to focus on the different motivations individuals have for using and abusing specific drugs at different ages. For example, grade-school children seem receptive to programs that involve their parents or well-known adults, such as professional athletes. Adolescents in high school are often more responsive to peer counsellors. Many young adults tend to be influenced by efforts that focus on health education. For all ages, it is important to provide non-drug alternatives—such as recreational facilities, counselling, greater opportunities for leisure activities, and places to socialize—that speak to the individual's or group's specific reasons for using drugs. Reminding young people that most people, no matter what age, are *not* users of illegal drugs, do *not* smoke cigarettes, and do *not* get drunk frequently is a critical part of preventing substance abuse.

QUESTIONS FOR CRITICAL THINKING AND REFLECTION

Do you know someone who may have a drug problem? What steps, if any, have you taken to help that person? If you were using drugs and felt that things were out of control, what would you want your friends to do for you?

Take CHARGE

Changing Your Drug Habits

This strategy focuses on one of the most commonly used drugs: caffeine. If you are concerned about your use of a different drug or another type of addictive behaviour, you can devise your own plan based on this one and on the steps outlined in Chapter 1.

Because caffeine supports certain behaviours that are characteristic of our culture, such as sedentary, stressful work, you may find yourself relying on coffee (or tea, chocolate, or cola) to get through a busy schedule. Such habits often begin in college or university. Fortunately, it's easier to break a habit before it becomes entrenched as a lifelong dependency.

When you are studying for exams, the forced physical inactivity and the need to concentrate even when fatigued may lead you to overuse caffeine. But caffeine doesn't help unless you are already sleepy. And it does not relieve any underlying condition (you are just more tired when it wears off). How can you change this pattern?

Self-Monitoring
Keep a log of how much caffeine you eat or drink. Use a measuring cup to measure coffee or tea. Using Table 14.2, convert the amounts you drink into an estimate expressed in milligrams of caffeine. Be sure to include all forms, such as chocolate bars and over-the-counter medications, as well as caffeine candy, colas, hot chocolate, chocolate cake, tea, and coffee.

Self-Assessment
At the end of the week, add up your daily totals and divide by seven to get your daily average in milligrams. How much is too much? At more than 250 milligrams per day, you may well be experiencing some adverse symptoms. If you are experiencing at least five of the following symptoms, you may want to cut down:
  • Restlessness

- Nervousness
- Excitement
- Insomnia
- Flushed face
- Excessive sweating
- Gastrointestinal problems
- Muscle twitching
- Rambling thoughts and speech
- Irregular heartbeat
- Periods of inexhaustibility
- Excessive pacing or movement

Set Limits
Can you restrict your caffeine intake to a daily total and stick to this contract? If so, set a cutoff point, such as one cup of coffee. Pegging it to a specific time of day can be helpful, because then you won't confront a decision at any other point (and possibly fail). If you find you cannot stick to your limit, you may want to cut out caffeine altogether; abstinence can be easier than moderation for some people. If you experience caffeine withdrawal symptoms (headache, fatigue), you may want to cut your intake more gradually.

Find Other Ways to Keep Up Your Energy
If you are fatigued, it makes sense to get enough sleep or exercise more, rather than drowning the problem in coffee or tea. Different people need different amounts of sleep; you may also need more sleep at different times, such as during a personal crisis or an illness. Also, exercise raises your metabolic rate for hours afterward—a handy fact to exploit when you want to feel more awake and want to avoid an irritable caffeine jag. And if you have been compounding your fatigue by not eating properly, try filling up on complex carbohydrates, such as whole-grain bread or crackers, instead of candy bars.

Tips on Cutting Out Caffeine
Here are some more ways to decrease your consumption of caffeine:
- Keep some uncaffeinated drinks on hand, such as decaffeinated coffee, herbal teas, mineral water, bouillon, or hot water.
- Alternate between hot and very cold liquids.
- Fill your coffee cup only halfway.
- Avoid the school lunchroom or cafeteria and the chocolate sections of the grocery store. (Often people drink coffee or tea and eat chocolate simply because they are available.)
- Read labels of over-the-counter medications to check for hidden sources of caffeine.

SUMMARY

- Addictive behaviours are self-reinforcing. People with addictions experience a strong compulsion for the behaviour and a loss of control over it; an escalating pattern of abuse with serious negative consequences may result.
- The sources or causes of addiction include heredity, personality, lifestyle, and environmental factors. People may use an addictive behaviour as a means of alleviating stress or painful emotions.
- Many common behaviours are potentially addictive, including gambling, shopping, sexual activity, Internet use, eating, and working.
- Drug abuse is a maladaptive pattern of drug use that persists despite adverse social, psychological, or medical consequences.
- Substance use disorder involves taking a drug compulsively, which includes neglecting constructive activities because of it and continuing to use the drug despite experiencing adverse effects resulting from its use. Tolerance and withdrawal symptoms are often present.

- Reasons for using drugs include the lure of the illicit; curiosity; rebellion; peer pressure; and the desire to alter one's mood or escape boredom, anxiety, depression, or other psychological problems.
- Psychoactive drugs affect the mind and body by altering brain chemistry. The effect of a drug depends on the properties of the drug and how it's used (drug factors), the physical and psychological characteristics of the individual (individual factors), and the physical and social environment surrounding the drug use (social factors).
- Opioids relieve pain, cause drowsiness, and induce euphoria; they reduce anxiety and produce lethargy, apathy, and an inability to concentrate.
- Central nervous system depressants slow down the overall activity of the nerves; they reduce anxiety and cause mood changes, impaired muscular coordination, slurring of speech, and drowsiness or sleep.
- Central nervous system stimulants speed up the activity of the nerves, causing acceleration of the heart rate, a rise in blood pressure, dilation of the pupils and bronchial tubes, and an increase in gastric and adrenal secretions.
- Marijuana usually causes euphoria and a relaxed attitude at low doses; very high doses produce feelings of depersonalization and sensory distortion. The long-term effects may include chronic bronchitis and cancer; use during pregnancy may impair fetal growth.
- Hallucinogens alter perception, feelings, and thought and may cause an altered sense of time, visual disturbances, and mood changes.
- Inhalants are present in a variety of harmless products; they can cause delirium. Their use can lead to loss of consciousness, heart failure, suffocation, and death.
- Economic and social costs of drug abuse include the financial costs of law enforcement, treatment, and health care, and the social costs of crime, violence, and family problems. Drug testing and drug legalization have been proposed to address some of the problems related to drug abuse.
- Approaches to treatment include medication, treatment centres, self-help groups, and peer counselling; many programs also offer counselling to family members.

FOR MORE INFORMATION

BOOKS

Nelson, D. 2010. *Teen Drug Abuse (Opposing Viewpoints)*. San Diego: Greenhaven Press. Explores key issues relating to drug use and abuse by teenagers.

Hanson, G. R., et al. 2011. *Drugs and Society*, 11th ed. Boston: Jones & Bartlett. Discusses the impact of drug abuse on individuals' lives and on the broader society.

Hart, C. L., and C. Ksir. 2012. *Drugs, Society, and Human Behavior*, 15th ed. New York: McGraw-Hill. Examines drugs and behaviour from the behavioural, pharmacological, historical, social, legal, and clinical perspectives.

ORGANIZATIONS, HOTLINES, AND WEBSITES

The Internet addresses listed here were accurate at the time of publication.

Canadian Centre on Substance Abuse. Provides information relating to substance-abuse issues; contains a number of links and resources.
    http://www.ccsa.ca

Center for Online Addiction. Contains information about Internet and cybersex addiction.
    http://netaddiction.com

Centre for Addiction and Mental Health. Provides information and resources pertaining to clinical care, research, education, policy development, and health promotion in relation to mental health and addiction.
    http://www.camh.net

ClubDrugs.Org. Provides information on drugs commonly classified as "club drugs."

http://www.clubdrugs.org

Gamblers Anonymous. Includes questions to help diagnose gambling problems and provides resources for getting help.

http://www.gamblersanonymous.org

Health Canada: Drug and Alcohol Statistics. Offers information and statistics on alcohol and drug use in Canada, including findings from the *Canadian Alcohol and Drug Use Monitoring Survey 2008*, the Not4Me Youth Drug Prevention Program.

http://www.hc-sc.gc.ca/hc-ps/drugs-drogues/stat/index-eng.php

Higher Education Center for Alcohol, Drug Abuse, and Violence Prevention. Gives information about alcohol and drug abuse on campus and links to related sites.

http://www.edc.org/projects/higher_education_center_alcohol_drug_abuse_and_violence_prevention

Narcotics Anonymous. Similar to Alcoholics Anonymous, NA sponsors 12-step meetings and provides other support services for drug abusers.

http://www.na.org

There are also 12-step programs that focus on specific drugs:

Cocaine Anonymous

http://www.ca.org

Marijuana Anonymous

http://www.marijuana-anonymous.org

National Anti-Drug Strategy (Government of Canada). Offers information and news related to three identified priority areas: preventing illicit drug use, treating illicit drug dependency, and combatting the production and distribution of illicit drugs. Also offers resources related to youth drug prevention for parents.

http://www.nationalantidrugstrategy.gc.ca

Responsible Gambling Council. Creates awareness programs related to problem gambling prevention; provides information on problem gambling, treatment, and warning signs, as well as other resources, such as brochures and videos.

http://www.responsiblegambling.com

See also the listings for Chapters 15 and 16.

SELECTED BIBLIOGRAPHY

Adams, G. R., et al. 2007. A study of differences in Canadian university students' gambling and proximity to a casino. *Journal of Gambling Issues* 19: 9–17, http://jgi.camh.net/doi/pdf/10.4309/jgi.2007.19.1 (retrieved April 1, 2015).

Adlaf, E. M., et al. (eds.). 2005. *Canadian Campus Survey 2004*. Toronto: Centre for Addiction and Mental Health.

American Psychiatric Association. 2013. *Diagnostic and Statistical Manual of Mental Disorders*, 5th ed. Washington, D.C.: American Psychiatric Association.

Boak, A., H. A. Hamilton, E. M. Adlaf, and R. E. Mann. 2013. Drug use among Ontario students, 1977–2013: Detailed OSDUHS findings (CAMH Research Document Series No. 36). Toronto, ON: Centre for Addiction and Mental Health.

Butt, P., D. Beirness, L. Gliksman, C. Paradis, and T. Stockwell. 2011. *Alcohol and health in Canada: A summary of evidence and guidelines for low-risk drinking.* Ottawa, ON: Canadian Centre on Substance Abuse.

Canadian Centre on Substance Abuse. 2014. *First do no harm: Responding to Canada's prescription drug crisis: annual report, 2013–2014.* Ottawa, ON: Author, http://www.ccsa.ca/Resource%20Library/CCSA-Canada-Strategy-Prescription-Drug-Misuse-Annual-Report-2014-en.pdf (retrieved January 19, 2015).

Canadian Society of Addiction Medicine. 2014. *Policy Statements,* http://www.csam-smca.org/about/policy-statements/ (retrieved November 8, 2015).

Center for Science in the Public Interest. 2014. *Caffeine Content of Food & Drugs,* http://www.cspinet.org/new/cafchart.htm (retrieved January 19, 2015).

Delaney-Black, V., et al. 2004. Prenatal cocaine: Quantity of exposure and gender moderation. *Journal of Developmental and Behavioral Pediatrics* 25(4): 254–263.

Government of Canada. 2014. *The National Anti-Drug Strategy,* http://www.nationalantidrugstrategy.gc.ca/nads-sna.html (retrieved January 19, 2015).

Griffiths, M. D. (2011). Internet sex addiction: A review of empirical research. *Addiction Research and Theory* 20(2): 111–124.

Health Canada. 2008. *Health Canada Reminds Canadians Not to Use Ephedra/Ephedrine Products,* http://www.healthycanadians.gc.ca/recall-alert-rappel-avis/hc-sc/2008/13279a-eng.php (retrieved January 19, 2015).

Health Canada. 2012. *Food and Nutrition: Caffeine in Food,* http://www.hc-sc.gc.ca/fn-an/securit/addit/caf/food-caf-aliments-eng.php (retrieved January 19, 2015).

Health Canada. 2013. *Canadian Tobacco Use Monitoring Survey (CTUMS) 2012,* http://www.hc-sc.gc.ca/hc-ps/tobac-tabac/research-recherche/stat/ctums-esutc_2012-eng.php (retrieved November 8, 2015).

Health Canada. 2014. *Canadian Alcohol and Drug Use Monitoring Survey (CADUMS): Summary of Results for 2012,* http://www.hc-sc.gc.ca/hc-ps/drugs-drogues/stat/_2012/summary-sommaire-eng.php (retrieved October 29, 2015).

Huang, J. H. and R. Boyer. 2007. Epidemiology of youth gambling problems in Canada: A national prevalence study. *The Canadian Journal of Psychiatry* 52 (10): 657–664, http://publications.cpa-apc.org/media.php?mid=528&xwm=true (retrieved November 10, 2015).

Hurd, Y. L., et al. 2005. Marijuana impairs growth in mid-gestation fetuses. *Neurotoxicology and Teratology* 27(2): 221–229.

Iannone, M., et al. 2006. Electrocortical effects of MDMA are potentiated by acoustic stimulation in rats. *BMC Neuroscience* 7: 13.

Johnston, L. D., et al. 2012. *Monitoring the Future: Overview of Key Findings, 2011.* Ann Arbor, MI: Institute for Social Research, The University of Michigan.

Kim, S. W., et al. 2006. Pathological gambling and mood disorders: Clinical associations and treatment implications. *Journal of Affective Disorders* 92(1): 109–116.

Kwan, M. Y. W., G. E. J. Faulkner,, K. P. Arbour-Nicitopolous, and J. Cairney. 2013. Prevalence of health-risk behaviours among Canadian post-secondary students: Descriptive results from the National College Health Assessment. *BMC Public Health* 13: 548–553.

Mahowald, M. L., J. A. Singh, and P. Majeski. 2005. Opioid use by patients in an orthopedics spine clinic. *Arthritis and Rheumatology* 52(1): 312–321.

Messinis, L., et al. 2006. Neuropsychological deficits in long-term frequent cannabis users. *Neurology* 66(5): 737–739.

National Advisory Committee on Prescription Drug Misuse. (2013). *First do no harm: Responding to Canada's prescription drug crisis.* Ottawa: Canadian Centre on Substance Abuse, http://www.ccsa.ca/resource%20library/canada-strategy-prescription-drug-misuse-report-en.pdf (retrieved January 19, 2015).

National Council on Problem Gambling. 2014. *What Is Problem Gambling?* http://www.ncpgambling.org/help-treatment/faq/ (retrieved January 19, 2015).

National Institute on Drug Abuse. 2011. *DrugFacts: Comorbidity: Addiction and Other Mental Disorders,* http://www.drugabuse.gov/publications/drugfacts/comorbidity-addiction-other-mental-disorders (retrieved January 19, 2015).

Opioid abuse. 2004. *Journal of the American Medical Association* 291(11): 1394.

Parrott, A. C. 2005. Chronic tolerance to recreational MDMA (3,4-methylenedioxymethamphetamine) or ecstasy. *Journal of Psychopharmacology* 19(1): 71–83.

Porter, R. S., et. al. 2011. *The Merck Manual of Diagnosis and Therapy*, 19th ed. New York: Wiley.

Public Health Agency of Canada. 2011. Supportive Environments for Physical Activity: How the Built Environment Affects Our Health, http://www.phac-aspc.gc.ca/hp-ps/hl-mvs/be-eb-eng.php (retrieved January 19, 2015).

Public Health Agency of Canada. 2012. *Summary: Estimates of HIV Prevalence and Incidence in Canada, 2011,* http://www.phac-aspc.gc.ca/aids-sida/publication/survreport/estimat2011-eng.php (retrieved January 19, 2015).

Rehm, J., et al. 2006. The *Costs of Substance Abuse in Canada, 2002: Highlights.* Ottawa: Canadian Centre on Substance Abuse, http://www.ccsa.ca/Resource%20Library/ccsa-011332-2006.pdf (retrieved January 19, 2015).

Ren, S., et al. 2006. Effect of long-term cocaine use on regional left ventricular function as determined by magnetic resonance imaging. *American Journal of Cardiology* 97(7): 1085–1088.

Rosenfeld, D., P. C. Hébert, and M. B. Stanbrook. 2011. Time to address stimulant abuse on our campuses. *Canadian Medical Association Journal* 183(12): 1345.

Savoca, M. R., et al. 2005. Association of ambulatory blood pressure and dietary caffeine in adolescents. *American Journal of Hypertension* 18(1): 116–120.

Singer, L. T., et al. 2004. Cognitive outcomes of preschool children with prenatal cocaine exposure. *Journal of the American Medical Association* 291(20): 2448–2456.

Statistics Canada. 2009. *Perspectives on Labour and Income: Gambling,* http://www.statcan.gc.ca/pub/75-001-x/topics-sujets/pdf/topics-sujets/gambling-jeuxdehasard-2009-eng.pdf (retrieved January 19, 2015).

Statistics Canada. 2014. *Police-Reported Crime Statistics in Canada, 2013,* http://www.statcan.gc.ca/pub/85-002-x/2014001/article/14040-eng.htm?fpv=2693#a6 (retrieved January 19, 2015).

Substance Abuse and Mental Health Services Administration. 2005. Nonmedical oxycodone users: A comparison with heroin users. *The NSDUH Report,* January.

U.S. Department of Justice Drug Enforcement Administration. 2011. *Drugs of abuse, 2011 edition: A DEA resource guide,* http://www.dea.gov/docs/drugs_of_abuse_2011.pdf (retrieved January 19, 2015).

Wareing, M., et al. 2005. Visuo-spatial working memory deficits in current and former users of MDMA ("ecstasy"). *Human Psychopharmacology* 20(2): 115–23.

Waska, R. 2006. Addictions and the quest to control the object. *American Journal of Psychoanalysis* 66(1): 43–62.

Weir, E. 2001. Inhalant use and addiction in Canada. *Canadian Medical Association Journal* 164(3): 397.

Young, M. M., & Jesseman, R. J. (2014). *The impact of substance use disorders on hospital use.* Ottawa, ON: Canadian Centre on Substance Abuse, http://www.ccsa.ca/Resource%20Library/CCSA-Substance-Use-Hospital-Impact-Report-2014-en.pdf (retrieved January 19, 2015).

Zakzanis, K. K., and Z. Campbell. 2006. Memory impairment in now abstinent MDMA users and continued users: A longitudinal follow-up. *Neurology* 66(5): 740–741.

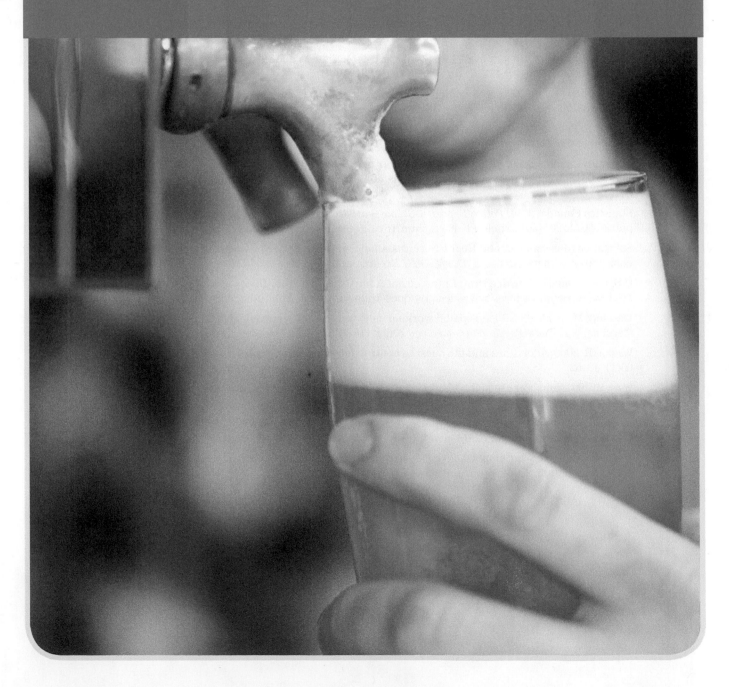

CHAPTER 15

Alcohol Use and Alcoholism

LOOKING AHEAD

After you have read and studied this chapter, you should be able to:

LO1 Explain how alcohol is absorbed and metabolized by the body

LO2 Describe the immediate and long-term effects of drinking alcohol

LO3 Define low-risk alcohol consumption and discuss its possible benefits

LO4 Describe alcohol use disorder and its consequences

LO5 Evaluate the role of alcohol in your life, and list strategies for using it responsibly

TEST YOUR KNOWLEDGE

1. **According to Canadian guidelines, "low-risk" drinking is having four or fewer drinks per day.**
   True or false?

2. **If a man and a woman of the same weight drink the same amount of alcohol, the woman will become intoxicated more quickly than the man.**
   True or false?

3. **Drinking too much alcohol in too short a time can cause death from alcohol poisoning.**
   True or false?

4. **Drinking coffee will help you sober up.**
   True or false?

ANSWERS

1. FALSE.   Canada's Low-Risk Alcohol Drinking Guidelines recommend no more than two drinks per day for women and no more than three drinks per day for men.

2. TRUE.   Women are usually smaller than men, have a higher percentage of body fat, and have a less active form of a stomach enzyme that breaks down alcohol. These factors cause them to become intoxicated more quickly and to a greater degree.

3. TRUE.   Consuming several drinks over a period of several hours is likely to cause intoxication, followed by a hangover; chugging the same amount in an hour or less can be lethal.

4. FALSE.   Once alcohol has been absorbed by the body, nothing speeds its metabolism.

Throughout history, alcohol has been more popular than any other psychoactive drug in the Western world, despite numerous prohibitions against it. Alcohol has a somewhat contradictory role in human life. It carries cultural significance for many, and when used in moderation alcohol can enhance social occasions by loosening inhibitions and creating a pleasant feeling of relaxation. But alcohol use can also be unhealthy. Like other drugs, alcohol has physiological effects on the body that can impair functioning in the short term and cause devastating damage in the long term. For some people, alcohol use becomes an addiction, leading to a lifetime of recovery or, for a few, to debilitation and death.

The use of alcohol is a complex issue, one that demands conscious thought and informed decisions. In our society, some people choose to drink in moderation while some choose not to drink at all. Still others realize too late that they have made an unwise choice—when they become addicted to alcohol, are involved in an alcohol-related car crash, or simply wake up to discover they have done something they regret.

This chapter discusses the complexities of alcohol use and provides information that will help you make choices that are right for you.

The Nature of Alcohol

If you have ever been around people who are drinking, you probably noticed that alcohol seems to affect different people in different ways. One person may seem to get drunk after just a drink or two, while another appears to tolerate a great deal of alcohol without becoming intoxicated. These differences make alcohol's effects on the body seem mysterious and help explain why there are many misconceptions about alcohol use. The following sections describe how alcohol works in the body.

Alcoholic Beverages

Technically speaking, there are many kinds of **alcohol**, and each is an organic compound. In this text, however, the term *alcohol* refers only to ethyl alcohol (or ethanol, often abbreviated as ETOH). Several kinds of alcohol are similar to ethyl alcohol, such as methanol (wood alcohol) and isopropyl alcohol (rubbing alcohol), but they are highly toxic; if consumed, these forms of alcohol can cause serious illness, blindness, and even death.

> **alcohol**
> The intoxicating ingredient in fermented or distilled beverages; a colourless, pungent liquid.

Common Alcoholic Beverages

Alcoholic beverages come in several basic types, and ethanol is the psychoactive ingredient in each of them.
- Beer is a mild intoxicant brewed from a mixture of grains. By volume, beer usually contains 3–6 percent alcohol. Ales and malt liquors, which are similar to beer, typically contain 6–8 percent alcohol by volume.
- Wines are made by fermenting the juices of grapes or other fruits. During *fermentation*, sugars from the fruit react with yeast to create ethanol and other by-products. In table wines, the concentration of alcohol is about 9–14 percent. A more potent type of wine, called *fortified wine*, is so called because extra alcohol is added during its production. Fortified wines—such as sherry, port, and Madeira—contain about 20 percent alcohol.
- Hard liquor—such as gin, rye, rum, tequila, vodka, and liqueur—is made by *distilling* brewed or fermented grains or other plant products. Hard liquors usually contain 35–50 percent alcohol but can be much stronger.

In Canada, any beverage containing 1.1 percent or more alcohol by volume is considered an alcoholic beverage. By law, all labels on alcoholic beverages must include the amount of alcohol in the product.

Standard Drinks Versus Actual Servings

When discussing alcohol consumption, the term **one drink** (or *a standard drink*) means the amount of a beverage that typically contains 13.6 grams of "pure" alcohol. Figure 15.1 shows the amounts of some popular beverages that are considered to be one standard drink, based on their alcohol content.

one drink
The amount of a beverage that typically contains 13.6 grams of alcohol; also called a *standard drink*.

People don't always limit themselves to one drink. In fact, a typical serving of most alcoholic beverages is larger (sometimes significantly larger) than a single standard drink. This is particularly true of mixed drinks, which often include more than one type of hard liquor. In addition, alcoholic beverages are usually purchased in packages that contain multiple servings. In Canada, companies are not required to list the number of standard drinks on alcohol labels; as such, it is important for individuals to have some awareness about what a standard drink is, and how many "drinks" may be in one bottle/container of alcohol.

FIGURE 15.1

One Drink of Various Alcoholic Beverages

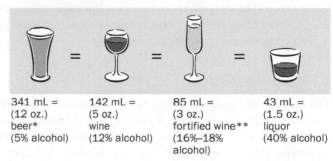

341 mL = (12 oz.) beer* (5% alcohol)

142 mL = (5 oz.) wine (12% alcohol)

85 mL = (3 oz.) fortified wine** (16%–18% alcohol)

43 mL = (1.5 oz.) liquor (40% alcohol)

*Regular beers have an average alcohol content of 5%, but some have as much as 6% or 7%, making them stronger than a "standard" drink. "Light" beers have an average alcohol content of 4%.

**Such as sherry, port, or vermouth.

Source: Centre for Addiction and Mental Health. 2012. *Alcohol,* http://www.camh.ca/en/hospital/health_information/a_z_mental_health_and_addiction_information/alcohol/Pages/alcohol.aspx (retrieved February 2, 2015).

Caloric Content

Alcohol provides 7 calories per gram, and the alcohol in one standard drink (14–17 grams) supplies about 100–120 calories. As noted above, many beverages are larger than one standard drink, and most also contain some carbohydrate, so, for example, one beer provides about 140 total calories. The "light" in light beer refers to calories; a light beer typically has close to the same alcohol content as a regular beer and about 99 calories. A 145-millilitre glass of wine has about 100 calories. An 85-millilitre margarita supplies 157 calories, a 175-millilitre cosmopolitan has 143 calories, and a 175-millilitre rum and cola contains about 180 calories (including the mix). The number of calories in other common alcoholic beverages is provided in Table 15.1. Consuming alcohol on a regular basis can add plenty of extra calories to one's diet and could lead to weight gain and other potential health problems. Experts have suggested several strategies for cutting back on alcohol, including not drinking every day, spacing drinks at least one hour apart, and replacing alcoholic beverages with "virgin" or half-alcohol substitutes.

TABLE 15.1

Estimated Number of Calories in Common Alcoholic Beverages

Beverage	Serving/Container Size	Approximate No. of Calories
Light beer (4 percent alcohol)	341 mL (12 oz.) – 1 bottle	99
Regular beer (5 percent alcohol)	341 mL (12 oz.) – 1 bottle	140
Non-alcoholic beer (0.5 percent alcohol)	350 mL – 1 can	210
Daiquiri	207 mL (7 oz.)	260
Pina Colada	133 mL (4.5 oz.)	245
Vodka	44 mL (1.5 oz.) – 1 "shot"	100
Wine (11.5 percent alcohol)	145 mL (5 oz.)	100

Source: Dietitians of Canada. 2015. *Alcohol and Nutrition,* http://www.eatrightontario.ca/en/Articles/Alcohol/Alcohol-and-Nutrition.aspx#.VM5kB6Mo6po (retrieved February 2, 2015).

Absorption

When a person ingests alcohol, about 20 percent is rapidly absorbed from the stomach into the bloodstream, and about 75 percent is absorbed through the upper part of the small intestine. Any remaining alcohol enters the bloodstream further along the gastrointestinal tract. Once in the bloodstream, alcohol produces feelings of intoxication. The rate of absorption is affected by a variety of factors. For example, the carbonation in a beverage like champagne increases the rate of alcohol absorption. Artificial sweeteners (commonly used in drink mixers) have been shown to have the same effect. Food in the stomach slows the rate of absorption, as does the drinking of highly concentrated alcoholic beverages, such as hard liquor. But remember: *All* alcohol a person consumes is eventually absorbed.

Metabolism and Excretion

The circulatory system quickly transports alcohol throughout the body. Because alcohol easily moves through most biological membranes, it is rapidly distributed throughout most body tissues. The main site of alcohol **metabolism** is the liver, though a small amount of alcohol is metabolized in the stomach. Alcohol can be metabolized by several processes. Most is converted first to acetaldehyde, then to acetate, which is ultimately burned for energy or converted to fat. The enzymes needed for this process vary slightly among individuals, creating differences in how people react to alcohol. (See the Dimensions of Diversity box.)

> **metabolism**
> The chemical transformation of food and other substances in the body into energy and wastes.

Dimensions *of* DIVERSITY

Metabolizing Alcohol: Our Bodies Work Differently

Do you notice that you react differently to alcohol than some of your friends do? If so, your reactions may be affected by genetic differences in alcohol metabolism associated with ethnicity. Alcohol is metabolized mainly in the liver, where it is converted by an enzyme, alcohol dehydrogenase, into a toxic substance called acetaldehyde. Acetaldehyde is responsible for many of alcohol's noxious effects. Ideally, it is quickly broken down to a less active by-product, acetate, by another enzyme, acetaldehyde dehydrogenase (ALDH). Acetate can then separate into water and carbon dioxide and easily be eliminated.

Some people, primarily those of Asian descent, inherit ineffective or inactive variations of that latter enzyme, ALDH. Other people, including some of African descent and some Jewish population groups, have forms of alcohol dehydrogenase that metabolize alcohol to acetaldehyde very quickly. In either case, the result is a buildup of acetaldehyde when these people drink alcohol. They experience a reaction called *flushing syndrome*. Their skin feels hot, their heart and respiration rates increase, and they may get a headache, vomit, or break out in hives. The severity of their reaction is affected by the inherited form of their alcohol-metabolizing enzymes. Drinking makes some people so uncomfortable that they are unlikely to develop alcohol addiction.

The body's response to acetaldehyde is the basis for treating alcohol abuse with disulfiram (Antabuse), which inhibits the action of ALDH. When a person taking disulfiram ingests alcohol, acetaldehyde levels increase rapidly, and he or she develops an intense flushing reaction along with weakness, nausea, vomiting, and other disagreeable symptoms.

How people behave in relation to alcohol is influenced in complex ways by many factors, including social and cultural ones. But in this case at least, individual choices and behaviour are strongly influenced by specific genetic characteristics.

About 2–10 percent of ingested alcohol is not metabolized in the liver or other tissues but is excreted unchanged by the lungs, kidneys, and sweat glands. Excreted alcohol causes the telltale smell on a drinker's breath and is the basis of breath and urine analyses for alcohol levels. Although such analyses do not give precise measurements of alcohol concentrations in the blood, they provide a reasonable approximation if done correctly.

Alcohol readily enters the human brain, crossing the restrictive layer of cells that ordinarily shields that organ. There, alcohol affects neurotransmitters, the chemicals that carry messages between brain cells. The ability of brain cells to receive these messages is changed, and networks within the brain that connect different brain regions are disrupted. These changes are temporary, creating many of the immediate effects of drinking alcohol.

With chronic heavy usage, however, alcohol's effects become permanent, resulting in lasting disruption of brain function and changes in brain structure. Alcohol interferes with the production of new brain cells in unborn children, young children, adolescents, and young adults in whom the brain continues to develop until about age 21. Even in mature adults, new brain cells are produced to replace damaged ones, and alcohol is likely to affect that process as well.

Alcohol Intake and Blood Alcohol Concentration

Blood alcohol concentration (BAC) is the ratio of alcohol in a person's blood by weight, expressed as the percentage of alcohol measured in a decilitre of blood. BAC is affected by the amount of alcohol consumed in a given amount of time and by individual factors:

- *Body weight:* In most cases, a smaller person develops a higher BAC than a larger person after drinking the same amount of alcohol (see Figure 15.2). A smaller person has less overall body tissue into which alcohol can be distributed.
- *Percentage of body fat:* A person with a higher percentage of body fat will usually develop a higher BAC than a more muscular person of the same weight. Alcohol does not concentrate as much in fatty tissue as in muscle and most other tissues, in part because fat has fewer blood vessels.
- *Sex:* Women metabolize less alcohol in the stomach than men do because the stomach enzyme that breaks down alcohol before it enters the bloodstream is four times as active in men as in women. This means that more unmetabolized alcohol is released into the bloodstream in women. Because women are also generally smaller than men and have a higher percentage of body fat, women will have a higher BAC than men after consuming the same amount of alcohol. Hormonal fluctuations may also affect the rate of alcohol metabolism, making a woman more susceptible to high BACs at certain times during her menstrual cycle (usually just before the onset of menstruation).

> **blood alcohol concentration (BAC)**
> The amount of alcohol in the blood expressed as the percentage of alcohol in a decilitre of blood; used as a measure of intoxication.

FIGURE 15.2

Approximate Blood Alcohol Concentration and Body Weight

This chart illustrates the BAC an average person of a given weight would reach after drinking the specified number of drinks in the time shown. In Canada, it is a criminal offence to drive with a BAC of 0.08 percent, or 80 milligrams of alcohol in 100 millilitres of blood; for drivers in a graduated licensing system, most provinces have zero-tolerance laws that set BAC limits at 0 percent.

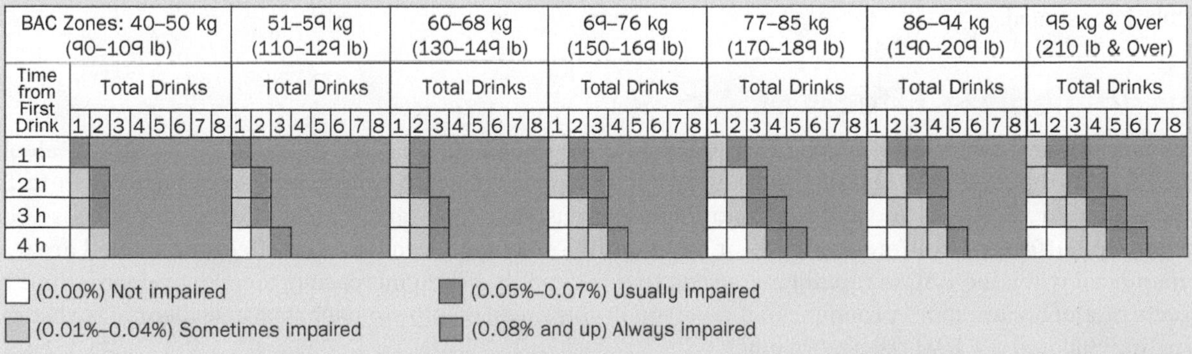

BAC Zones: 40–50 kg (90–109 lb)		51–59 kg (110–129 lb)		60–68 kg (130–149 lb)		69–76 kg (150–169 lb)		77–85 kg (170–189 lb)		86–94 kg (190–209 lb)		95 kg & Over (210 lb & Over)	
Time from First Drink	Total Drinks		Total Drinks		Total Drinks		Total Drinks		Total Drinks		Total Drinks		Total Drinks
	1 2 3 4 5 6 7 8		1 2 3 4 5 6 7 8		1 2 3 4 5 6 7 8		1 2 3 4 5 6 7 8		1 2 3 4 5 6 7 8		1 2 3 4 5 6 7 8		1 2 3 4 5 6 7 8
1 h													
2 h													
3 h													
4 h													

☐ (0.00%) Not impaired   ▨ (0.05%–0.07%) Usually impaired

☐ (0.01%–0.04%) Sometimes impaired   ■ (0.08% and up) Always impaired

BAC also depends on the balance between the rate of alcohol absorption and the rate of alcohol metabolism. A man who weighs 69 kilograms and has normal liver function metabolizes 6.8 grams of alcohol per hour, the equivalent of about half a 341-millilitre bottle of beer or a 145-millilitre glass of wine.

The rate of alcohol metabolism varies among individuals and is largely determined by genetic factors and drinking behaviour. Chronic drinking activates enzymes that metabolize alcohol in the liver, so people who drink frequently metabolize alcohol at a more rapid rate than non-drinkers. Although the rate of alcohol absorption can be slowed by factors like food, the metabolic rate *cannot* be influenced by exercising, breathing deeply, eating, drinking coffee, or taking other drugs. The rate of alcohol metabolism is the same whether a person is asleep or awake.

If a person absorbs slightly less alcohol each hour than he or she can metabolize in an hour, the BAC remains low. People can drink large amounts of alcohol this way over a long period without becoming noticeably intoxicated. Regardless, they run the risk of significant long-term health hazards (described later in the chapter). If a person drinks alcohol more quickly than it can be metabolized, the BAC will steadily increase, and he or she will become increasingly drunk, as described in Table 15.2. Think of a quantity of alcohol drunk over two or three hours—enough to cause intoxication and a hangover the next day. Now imagine chugging that same amount in an hour or less. Drinking that much alcohol so quickly could be lethal.

TABLE 15.2

The Effects of Alcohol

BAC (percent)	Common Behavioural Effects	Hours Required to Metabolize Alcohol
0.00–0.05	Slight change in feelings, usually relaxation and euphoria. Decreased alertness.	2–3
0.05–0.10	Emotional instability, with exaggerated feelings and behaviour. Reduced social inhibitions. Impairment of reaction time and fine motor coordination. Increasingly impaired during driving. Legally drunk at 0.08 percent and subject to license suspensions at 0.05 percent and over.	3–6
0.10–0.15	Unsteadiness in standing and walking. Loss of peripheral vision. Driving is extremely dangerous.	6–10
0.15–0.30	Staggering gait. Slurred speech. Pain and other sensory perceptions greatly impaired.	10–24
More than 0.30	Stupor or unconsciousness. Anaesthesia. Death possible at 0.35 percent and above. Can result from rapid or binge drinking with few earlier effects.	More than 24

Alcohol and Health

The effects of alcohol consumption on health depend on the individual, the circumstances, and the amount of alcohol consumed.

The Immediate Effects of Alcohol

BAC is a primary factor determining the effects of alcohol (see Table 15.2). At low concentrations, alcohol tends to make people feel relaxed and jovial, but at higher concentrations people are more likely to feel angry, sedated, or sleepy. Alcohol is a central nervous system depressant, and its effects vary because body systems are affected to different degrees at different BACs. At any given BAC, the effects of alcohol are more pronounced when the BAC is rapidly increasing than when it is slowly increasing, steady, or decreasing. The effects of alcohol are more pronounced if a person drinks on an empty stomach, because alcohol is absorbed more quickly and the BAC rises more quickly.

Low Concentrations of Alcohol

The effects of alcohol can first be felt at a BAC of about 0.03–0.05 percent. These effects may include light-headedness, relaxation, and a release of inhibitions. Most drinkers experience mild euphoria and become more sociable. When people drink in social settings, alcohol often seems to act as a stimulant, enhancing conviviality or assertiveness. This apparent stimulation occurs because alcohol depresses inhibitory centres in the brain.

Higher Concentrations of Alcohol

At higher concentrations, the pleasant effects tend to be replaced by more negative ones, including interference with motor coordination, verbal performance, and intellectual functions. The drinker often becomes irritable and may be easily angered or given to crying. When the BAC reaches 0.1 percent, most sensory and motor functioning is reduced and many people become sleepy. Vision, smell, taste, and hearing become less acute. At 0.2 percent, most drinkers are completely unable to function, either physically or psychologically, because of the pronounced depression of the central nervous system, muscles, and other body systems. Coma usually occurs at a BAC of 0.35 percent, and any higher level can be fatal.

Small doses of alcohol may improve sexual functioning for individuals who are especially anxious or self-conscious, but higher doses often have negative effects, such as reduced erectile response. Effects of chronic heavy drinking include reduction of testosterone levels and impairment of sperm production.

Alcohol causes blood vessels near the skin to dilate, so drinkers often feel warm; their skin flushes, and they may sweat more. Flushing and sweating contribute to heat loss, however, so the internal body temperature falls. High doses of alcohol may impair the body's ability to regulate temperature, causing it to drop sharply, especially if the surrounding temperature is low. Drinking alcoholic beverages to keep warm in cold weather does not work and can even be dangerous.

Since alcohol is a sedative, it induces sleepiness. But for those using alcohol as a sleep aid, its utility is short lived, because people quickly build up a tolerance to it. Moreover, large amounts of alcohol disturb normal sleep patterns. The sleep that follows drinking becomes poor quality after some hours, fitful and unrefreshing as the person dreams, awakens, and often stays wakeful. Alcohol can also cause or worsen sleep apnea, a breathing disorder in which the air passage at the back of the mouth narrows or closes during sleep. Sleep and sleep disorders are discussed in Chapter 3.

Alcohol Hangover

Alcohol's effects wear off slowly, and anyone who has experienced a severe hangover knows they are not fun. The symptoms include headache, shakiness, nausea, diarrhea, fatigue, and impaired mental functioning. But even after sobering up, at high BACs the resulting hangover can continue to leave a person impaired for several hours.

A hangover is probably caused by a combination of the toxic products of alcohol breakdown, dehydration, and hormonal effects. During a hangover, heart rate and blood pressure increase, making some individuals more vulnerable to heart attacks. Electroencephalography or EEGs (brain wave measurement) shows diffuse slowing of brain waves for up to 16 hours after BAC drops to zero. Studies of pilots, drivers, and skiers all indicate that coordination and cognition are impaired in a person with a hangover, increasing the risk of injury.

The best treatment for hangover is prevention. Nearly all men can expect a hangover if they drink more than four to five standard drinks; for women, the approximate number is three to four drinks. Drinking less, drinking slowly, eating food, and drinking plenty of non-alcoholic liquids decrease the risk of hangover. If you get a hangover, remember that your driving ability is impaired, even after your BAC returns to zero.

 QUESTIONS FOR CRITICAL THINKING AND REFLECTION

Have you ever had a hangover or watched someone else suffer through one? Did the experience affect your attitude about drinking? In what way?

Alcohol Poisoning

Acute alcohol poisoning occurs much more frequently than most people realize, and all too often it causes death. Drinking large amounts of alcohol in a short time can rapidly raise the BAC into the lethal range. Alcohol, either alone or in combination with other drugs, is responsible for more toxic overdose deaths than any other drug.

Death from alcohol poisoning may be caused either by central nervous system and respiratory depression or by inhaling fluid or vomit into the lungs. The amount of alcohol it takes to make a person unconscious is dangerously close to a fatal dose. Although passing out may prevent someone from drinking more, BAC can keep rising during unconsciousness, because the body continues to absorb ingested alcohol into the bloodstream. Special care should be taken to ensure the safety of anyone who has been drinking heavily, especially if he or she passes out (see the Take Charge box).

 Take CHARGE

Dealing with an Alcohol Emergency

Remember: Being very drunk is potentially life threatening. If you aren't sure what to do, call 911. Helping a drunken friend could save a life.

- Be firm but calm. Don't engage the person in an argument or discuss his or her drinking behaviour while the person is intoxicated.
- Get the person out of harm's way. Don't let him or her drive, wander away, or drink any more alcohol. Reduce stimuli and create a safe, quiet place.
- If possible without distressing the person, try to find out what and how much the person drank, and when; and what other drugs or medications he or she took, how much, and when.
- If the person is unconscious, don't assume he or she is just "sleeping it off." Place your friend on his or her side with the knees up. This position will help prevent choking if the person vomits.
- Monitor airway, breathing, and circulation (check pulse).
- Stay with the person. You need to be ready to help if he or she vomits or stops breathing.
- Don't try to give the person anything to eat or drink, including coffee or other drugs. Don't give cold showers or try to make your friend walk around. None of these things help people to sober up, and they can be dangerous.

Call 911 immediately in any of the following instances:
- You can't wake the person even with shouting or shaking.
- The person is taking fewer than eight breaths per minute or the breathing pattern seems shallow or irregular.
- You think the person took other drugs with alcohol.
- The person has had an injury, especially a blow to the head.
- The person drank a large amount of alcohol within a short time and then became unconscious. Death caused by alcohol poisoning most often occurs when the blood alcohol level rises very quickly due to rapid ingestion of alcohol.

Using Alcohol with Other Drugs

Alcohol–drug combinations are a leading cause of drug-related deaths. Using alcohol while taking a medication that can cause central nervous system depression increases the effects of both drugs, potentially leading to coma, respiratory depression, and death. Such drugs include barbiturates, Valium-like drugs, narcotics such as codeine, and over-the-counter antihistamines such as Benadryl. For people who consume approximately three or more drinks per day, use of over-the-counter pain relievers, such as Aspirin, ibuprofen, or acetaminophen increases the risk of stomach bleeding or liver damage. Some antibiotics and diabetes medications can also interact dangerously with alcohol.

Many illegal drugs are especially dangerous when combined with alcohol. Life-threatening overdoses occur at much lower doses when heroin and other narcotics are combined with alcohol. When cocaine and alcohol are used together, a toxic substance called cocaethylene is formed; this substance is responsible for more than half of all cocaine-related deaths.

A growing trend among young drinkers in Canada and elsewhere is mixing alcoholic beverages with caffeinated ones, especially highly caffeinated energy drinks. Caffeinated alcoholic beverages (CABs) are available premixed, but many people make their own by mixing a favourite energy drink with some type of alcohol, such as vodka. CABs are a growing cause of concern because of their popularity with underaged drinkers and because the combined effects of alcohol and caffeine can be dangerous (see the In Focus box). Some provinces have taken action to limit the level of caffeine in CABs.

The safest strategy is to avoid combining alcohol with any other drug—prescription, over-the-counter, or illegal. If in doubt, ask your pharmacist or doctor before combining any drug with alcohol. Better, just don't do it.

 In FOCUS

Alcoholic Energy Drinks: The Dangers of Being "Drunk and Wide Awake"

Over the past decade, the practice of blending alcoholic beverages with highly caffeinated energy drinks has grown increasingly popular, particularly among young adults and underage drinkers. According to a report published in 2012 by the Canadian Centre on Substance Abuse, approximately 11 percent of 18 to 24-year-olds reported drinking caffeinated alcoholic beverages (CABs), also known as alcoholic energy drinks (AEDs), in the 30 days prior to the survey. Other studies of students attending Canadian post-secondary institutions have shown higher rates of CAB drinking, ranging from 23 percent in the past 30 days to 75 percent in their lifetime. The caffeine in a CAB masks the depressant effects of the alcohol, producing a "drunk and wide awake" state of alert intoxication, potentially leading drinkers to consume more alcohol than they would otherwise. Caffeine does nothing to speed the metabolism of the alcohol by the liver.

In addition to consuming more alcohol, a growing body of evidence suggests that college and university students who consume CABs face much higher risks of negative alcohol-related consequences than those who consume regular alcoholic beverages. For example, studies have reported the following:

- Being in a "drunk/awake" state can lead to risky behaviours such as drunk driving, unplanned sex or sexual assault, and aggression.
- CAB drinkers are three times more likely than non-CAB drinkers to binge-drink.
- CAB drinkers are about twice as likely as non-CAB drinkers to report being taken advantage of sexually, taking advantage of someone sexually, or riding with a driver who was under the influence of alcohol.
- Emerging evidence indicates that CAB use, especially by adolescents, may lead to an increased risk of alcohol or drug addiction later in life.

Cashing in on the lucrative energy drink market and CAB trend, alcoholic beverage manufacturers typically target a youth market, emphasizing the "energy boost" the products can provide. These concerns and others led the Liquor Control Board of Ontario (LCBO) to establish a maximum level of caffeine (30 mg) per serving on all products containing alcohol sold in Ontario. As of 2009, this meant that the allowable amount of caffeine in CABs would be similar to that in a soft drink (30–35 mg) and lower than that in a typical cup of coffee (100–120 mg). Since then, other provincial liquor boards (including the Nova Scotia Liquor Corporation) have followed the LCBO's lead on maximum levels of caffeine allowable in alcoholic beverages. As a result of such policies, many CAB manufacturers have reformulated their products to reduce caffeine levels. In the United States, two producers of CABs voluntarily removed their products from the market and committed to discontinuing production of such beverages permanently. In light of these developments, and skepticism among scientists that CABs can be proven safe, the CAB market may start to shrink—if not disappear altogether—in the near future.

Sources: Brache, K., G. Thomas, and T. Stockwell. 2012. *Caffeinated alcoholic beverages in Canada: Prevalence of use, risks and recommended policy responses.* Ottawa, ON: Canadian Centre on Substance Abuse; Brache K., and T. Stockwell. 2011. Drinking patterns and risk behaviours associated with combined alcohol and energy drink consumption. *Addictive Behaviours* 36(12): 1133–1140; Centers for Disease Control and Prevention. 2010. *Alcohol and Public Health: Caffeinated Alcoholic Beverages,* http://www.cdc.gov/alcohol/factsheets/cab.htm; O'Brien, M., T. McCoy, S. Rhodes, A. Wagoner, and M. Wolfson. 2008. Caffeinated cocktails: Energy drink consumption, high-risk drinking, and alcohol-related consequences among college students. *Academic Emergency Medicine* 15(5): 453–460; Price, R., C. Hilchey, C. Darredeau, H. Fulton, and S. Barrett. 2010. Brief communication: Energy drink co-administration is associated with increased reported alcohol ingestion. *Drug & Alcohol Review* 29(3): 331–333; and Thombs, D., R. O'Mara, M. Tsukamoto, M. Rossheim, R. Weiler, M. Merves, and B. Goldberder. 2010. Event-level analyses of energy drink consumption and alcohol intoxication in bar patrons. *Addictive Behaviours* 35(4): 325–330.

Alcohol-Related Injuries and Violence

The combination of impaired judgment, weakened sensory perception, reduced inhibitions, impaired motor coordination, and increased aggressiveness and hostility that characterizes alcohol intoxication can be dangerous. Through alcohol-related health issues, homicide, suicide, automobile crashes, and other traumatic incidents, alcohol use has been linked to an estimated 6700 deaths in Canada each year. In addition, the majority of people who attempt suicide have been drinking. Among suicide-related deaths, alcohol use is common; a recent analysis of 5550 suicide deaths found that one-third involved alcohol. Alcohol use more than triples the chances of fatal injuries during leisure activities, such as swimming and boating, and more than half of all fatal falls and serious burns happen to people who have been drinking.

QUICK STATS

50% of impaired driving incidents happen between 11p.m. and 4 a.m., and are more likely to take place on weekends.
—Statistics Canada, 2013

Alcohol and Aggression

Worldwide, alcohol is associated with more acts of aggression and violence than any other legal or illegal drug. In fact, alcohol use contributes to more than 50 percent of all murders, assaults, and rapes. It is frequently found in the bloodstream of victims as well as perpetrators. However, only some people become violent under alcohol's influence. These people are often predisposed to aggressive behaviour and are highly impulsive. In some cases they may have an underlying psychiatric condition called *antisocial personality disorder*. Their destructive behaviour—repeated criminal acts, deceitfulness, impulsiveness, repeated fights or assaults, and disregard for the safety of others—worsens under alcohol's influence. They are also more likely to become addicted to alcohol. However, all drinkers under alcohol's influence are subject to unpredictable and injurious consequences.

In 2012, approximately one in seven Canadians ages 15 years and older reported experiencing some type of harm due to someone else's alcohol use in the previous year. Verbal abuse was reported most often (8.9 percent), followed by being emotionally hurt or neglected (7.1 percent), feeling threatened (6.3 percent), and being physically hurt (2.2 percent).

Alcohol abuse can wreak havoc on home life. The presence of a parent or close relative with alcohol use disorder affects the health and well-being of all members of the household. Marital discord and domestic violence often exist in the presence of excess alcohol. Family members are frequently the target of the person's verbal or physical abuse and all too often have their own problems with alcohol. Non-drinking female spouses of heavy drinkers often experience high levels of psychological distress. A recent study found that both adults and children in the households of alcohol abusers had more medical problems than people from households without alcohol abusers and, not surprisingly, also incurred greater health care costs. For a child growing up in a household where alcoholism exists, family life can take a painful toll. Whether the alcoholic is a parent, a sibling, or another relative living with the family, the dysfunctional environment's effects start in childhood and can last throughout adulthood. Heavy drinking by parents is associated with abuse of their children, often emotional or psychological abuse. Links between parental drinking and physical or sexual abuse are not found consistently, but when such mistreatment does take place, the damaging effect is often long lasting and associated with alcohol misuse in the grown child.

Alcohol and Sexual Decision Making

Alcohol seriously impairs a person's ability to make wise decisions about sex. A recent survey of university students revealed that frequent binge drinkers were five times more likely to engage in unplanned sexual activity and five-and-a-half times more likely to have unprotected sex as non-binge drinkers. Heavy drinkers are also more likely to have multiple sex partners and to engage in other forms of high-risk sexual behaviour. For all these reasons, rates of sexually transmitted infections (including HIV) and unwanted pregnancy are higher among people who drink heavily than among people who drink moderately or not at all.

Women who binge-drink are at increased risk for rape and other forms of non-consensual sex. The laws regarding sexual consent are clear: A person who is very drunk or passed out cannot consent to sex. Having sex with a person who is drunk or unconscious is sexual assault.

Drinking and Driving

In Canada, drinking and driving remains the single largest criminal cause of death. According to Mothers Against Drunk Driving (MADD) Canada, more than 42 percent of the 2541 crash fatalities in 2010 (the most recent year for which data are available) were impairment related. In fact, MADD estimates that three to four Canadians die each day as a result of impairment-related crashes. Impaired driving is particularly problematic among young Canadians. In 2010, 16–25-year-olds represented only 13.6 percent of the population but were involved in 33.4 percent of Canada's alcohol-related traffic deaths. The highest rate of impaired driving deaths occurs at age 19. Close to 64 000 Canadians were injured in alcohol-related car crashes in 2010—approximately 175 people per day. According to a 2014 survey conducted by the Traffic Injury Research Foundation, 17.4 percent of Canadians admitted to drinking alcohol before driving in the past 30 days. Meanwhile, more than 68 percent of Canadians say they are "concerned" or "very concerned" about drinking and driving.

People who drink are unable to drive safely because their judgment is impaired, their reaction time is slower, and their coordination is reduced. Some driving skills are affected at BACs of 0.02 percent and lower; at 0.05 percent, visual perception, reaction time, and certain steering tasks are all impaired. Any amount of alcohol impairs your ability to drive safely, and fatigue augments alcohol's effects.

The *dose-response function* (see Chapter 14) is the relationship between the amount of alcohol or drug consumed and the type and intensity of the resulting effect. Higher doses of alcohol are associated with a much greater probability of automobile crashes, as shown in Figure 15.3. A person driving with a BAC of 0.14 percent is more than 40 times more likely to be involved in a crash as someone with no alcohol in his or her blood. For those with a BAC above 0.14 percent, the risk of a fatal crash is estimated to be 380 times higher. The risks for young drivers are even greater, even at very low BACs. Younger drivers have less experience with both driving and alcohol, which results in significant impairment with BACs as low as 0.02 percent.

In addition to an increased risk of injury and death, driving while intoxicated can have serious legal consequences. Drunk driving is against the law. Since 1969, the legal limit for driving a vehicle has been a BAC of 0.08 percent, or 80 milligrams of alcohol in 100 millilitres of blood, in all provinces and territories. There are stiff penalties for drunk driving, including fines, loss of licence, confiscation of vehicle, and jail time. Drivers with lower BACs may also be punishable by law and are dealt with under provincial and territorial traffic acts. Researchers have found that drivers with a BAC of 0.05 percent may experience difficulties with vision, a reduced ability to perform simple motor tasks, slower reaction times, and less accurate responses—even if they don't appear to be intoxicated. All these problems negatively affect driving performance and lead to an increased risk of collision. For this reason, many provinces have implemented legal consequences, such as licence suspensions, for individuals who are caught driving with a BAC between 0.05 percent and 0.08 percent (known as the "warn range").

FIGURE 15.3

The Dose-response Relationship Between BAC and Automobile Crashes

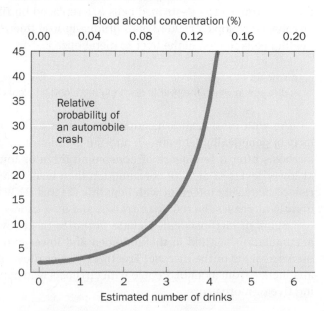

Additionally, under current zero-tolerance laws in most provinces, drivers with a graduated licence must maintain a 0 percent BAC while driving.

If you are out of your home and drinking, find alternative transportation or have a *designated driver* who doesn't drink and can provide safe transportation home. The responsibility can be rotated for different occasions. Remember, you risk more than your own life when you drink and drive. Causing serious injury or death results in lifelong feelings of sadness and guilt for the driver and grief for friends and families of victims.

It's more difficult to protect yourself against someone else who drinks and drives. It's reasonable to insist on not being driven by anyone who drinks and drives. Learn to be alert to the erratic driving that signals an impaired driver. The following behaviours can indicate that someone is driving while drunk:

- Wide, abrupt, and illegal turns
- Straddling the centre line or lane marker
- Driving against traffic
- Driving on the shoulder
- Weaving, swerving, or nearly striking an object or another vehicle
- Following too closely
- Erratic speed
- Driving with the headlights off at night
- Driving with the window down in very cold weather.

If you see any of these signs in another driver, avoid that vehicle by pulling off the road or turning safely at the nearest intersection. Report the driver to the police.

The Effects of Chronic Abuse

Because alcohol is distributed throughout most of the body, it can affect many different organs and tissues, as shown in Figure 15.4. Problems associated with chronic or habitual excessive use of alcohol include diseases of the digestive and cardiovascular systems and some cancers. Drinking during pregnancy risks the health of both the woman and the developing fetus.

The Digestive System

Even in the short term, alcohol can alter the functioning of the liver. Within just a few days of heavy alcohol consumption, fat begins to accumulate in liver cells, resulting in the development of "fatty liver." If drinking continues, inflammation of the liver can occur, resulting in alcoholic hepatitis, a frequent cause of hospitalization and death in people with alcoholism. Both fatty liver and alcoholic hepatitis are potentially reversible if the person stops drinking. With continued alcohol use, however, liver cells are progressively damaged and then destroyed. The destroyed cells are replaced by fibrous scar tissue, a condition known as **cirrhosis**. As cirrhosis develops, drinkers may gradually lose thier capacity to tolerate alcohol, because fewer and fewer healthy cells remain in the liver to metabolize it.

cirrhosis
A disease in which the liver is severely damaged by alcohol, other toxins, or infection.

As with most health hazards, the risk of cirrhosis depends on an individual's susceptibility, which is largely genetically determined, and the amount of alcohol consumed over time. Some people show signs of cirrhosis after a few years of consuming three or four drinks per day. Women generally develop cirrhosis at lower levels of alcohol consumption than men. Heavy drinkers who also inject drugs place themselves at risk of acquiring infection with hepatitis C virus (HCV); the combination of alcohol abuse and HCV infection greatly increases the risk for cirrhosis and liver cancer.

Signs of cirrhosis can include *jaundice* (a yellowing of the skin and white part of the eyes) and the accumulation of fluid in the abdomen and lower extremities. Some people with cirrhosis have no obvious outward signs of the disease. Treatment for cirrhosis includes correcting nutrient deficiencies and complete abstinence from alcohol. People with cirrhosis who continue to drink have only a 50 percent chance of surviving five or more years.

FIGURE 15.4

The Immediate and Long-term Effects of Alcohol Abuse

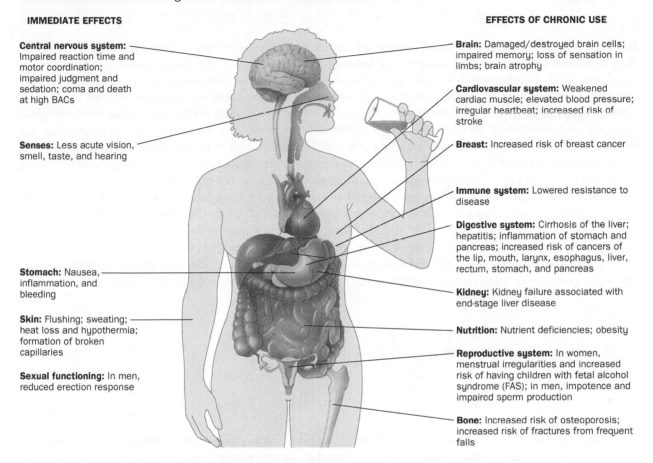

IMMEDIATE EFFECTS

Central nervous system: Impaired reaction time and motor coordination; impaired judgment and sedation; coma and death at high BACs

Senses: Less acute vision, smell, taste, and hearing

Stomach: Nausea, inflammation, and bleeding

Skin: Flushing; sweating; heat loss and hypothermia; formation of broken capillaries

Sexual functioning: In men, reduced erection response

EFFECTS OF CHRONIC USE

Brain: Damaged/destroyed brain cells; impaired memory; loss of sensation in limbs; brain atrophy

Cardiovascular system: Weakened cardiac muscle; elevated blood pressure; irregular heartbeat; increased risk of stroke

Breast: Increased risk of breast cancer

Immune system: Lowered resistance to disease

Digestive system: Cirrhosis of the liver; hepatitis; inflammation of stomach and pancreas; increased risk of cancers of the lip, mouth, larynx, esophagus, liver, rectum, stomach, and pancreas

Kidney: Kidney failure associated with end-stage liver disease

Nutrition: Nutrient deficiencies; obesity

Reproductive system: In women, menstrual irregularities and increased risk of having children with fetal alcohol syndrome (FAS); in men, impotence and impaired sperm production

Bone: Increased risk of osteoporosis; increased risk of fractures from frequent falls

Alcohol can inflame the pancreas, causing nausea, vomiting, abnormal digestion, and severe pain. Acute alcoholic pancreatitis generally occurs in binge drinkers. Unlike cirrhosis, which usually occurs after years of fairly heavy alcohol use, pancreatitis can occur after just one or two severe binge-drinking episodes. Acute pancreatitis is often fatal; in survivors it can develop into a chronic condition.

Overuse of alcohol is a common cause of bleeding in the gastrointestinal tract. Cirrhosis frequently results in development of enlarged, fragile esophageal and rectal veins, which can easily burst or tear with potentially fatal results. Enlarged esophageal veins are especially vulnerable when the drinker vomits after an alcoholic binge. Even a relatively small amount of alcohol can cause painful irritation of the lining of the stomach.

The Cardiovascular System

The effects of alcohol on the cardiovascular system depend on the amount of alcohol consumed. Moderate doses of alcohol—one drink or less a day for women and one to two drinks a day for men—may reduce the risk of heart disease and heart attack in some people. (The possible health benefits of alcohol are discussed later in this chapter.)

However, higher doses of alcohol have harmful effects on the cardiovascular system. In some people, more than two drinks a day will elevate blood pressure, making stroke and heart attack more likely. Some individuals with alcohol use disorder show a weakening of the heart muscle, a condition known as **cardiac myopathy**. Binge drinking can cause "holiday heart," a syndrome characterized by serious abnormal heart rhythms, which usually appear within 24 hours of a binge episode.

cardiac myopathy
Weakening of the heart muscle through disease.

Cancer

Both the International Agency for Research on Cancer and the United States Department of Health and Human Services have identified alcohol as a known human carcinogen. The Canadian Cancer Society suggests that alcohol consumption is a risk factor for the development of cancers of the breast, colon, rectum, esophagus, larynx, liver, mouth, and pharynx. (Some of these cancers are also associated with use of tobacco, with which alcohol frequently acts as a co-carcinogen.) Five or six daily drinks, especially combined with smoking, increase risk of these cancers by a factor of 50 or more. Alcohol also is largely responsible for the most common form of liver cancer, and continued heavy drinking in people with hepatitis accelerates progression to this cancer. In all alcohol-related cancers, however, genetics and other biological factors play important roles and help explain why some chronic alcohol abusers do not get cancer.

As mentioned above, alcohol increases the risk of breast cancer, but quantifying the risk is complicated. A recent study shows that regularly drinking even a small quantity of alcohol—three to six drinks per week—could significantly increase the risk of breast cancer. The kind of alcohol does not seem to matter. Binge drinking, but not frequency of drinking, was associated with breast cancer risk after controlling for cumulative alcohol intake. Women at otherwise increased risk of breast cancer (for example, those with a family history of breast or ovarian cancer) should carefully weigh the risks of even moderate drinking.

QUICK STATS

The incidence rate of liver cancer has tripled in men and doubled in women in Canada since 1970.
—Canadian Cancer Society, 2013

Brain Damage

Brain damage from chronic alcohol abuse is also tempered by an individual's physiology and genetics. Imaging studies document that many people with alcoholism experience brain shrinkage with loss of both grey and white matter, reduced blood flow, and slowed metabolic rates in some brain regions. To some extent, brain shrinkage can be reversed over time with abstinence from alcohol. Individuals who are dependent on alcohol often have cognitive impairments, ranging from mild to severe. These include memory loss, dementia, and compromised problem-solving and reasoning abilities. Even mild-to-moderate drinking can negatively affect certain mental activities that involve acquiring, storing, retrieving, and using information. Additionally, malnutrition, particularly thiamine deficiency, contributes to severe brain damage.

Mortality

Alcohol consumption is related to more than 200 conditions, diseases, and injuries, and causes approximately 6 percent of all deaths worldwide each year. Excessive alcohol consumption is also a factor in several of the leading causes of death for Canadians. A study published in 2012 showed that nearly 4000 deaths in Canada were attributable to alcohol consumption in 2005; this represented almost 8 percent of all deaths among Canadians between the ages of 0 and 64. In general, average life expectancy among people with alcoholism is about 15 years less than among non-alcoholics. About half the deaths caused by alcohol are due to chronic conditions such as cirrhosis and cancer; the other half are due to acute conditions or events such as car crashes, falls, and suicide. Because many deaths from acute conditions occur in Canadian youths, alcohol is responsible for thousands of years of potential life lost each year.

Alcohol Use During Pregnancy

During pregnancy, alcohol and its metabolic product acetaldehyde readily cross the placenta, potentially harming the developing fetus. Damage to the fetus depends on the amount of alcohol consumed and the stage of the pregnancy. Early in pregnancy, heavy drinking can cause spontaneous abortion or miscarriage. Alcohol in early pregnancy, during critical fetal development periods, can also cause a range of disabilities known as *fetal alcohol spectrum disorder (FASD)*. The most severe diagnosis of FASD is **fetal alcohol syndrome (FAS)**, which was discussed in Chapter 12. Children with FAS have a characteristic mixture of deformities that can include a small head, abnormal facial structure, heart defects, and other physical abnormalities. Their physical and mental growth is slower than normal, and most have a mental disability.

> **fetal alcohol syndrome (FAS)**
> A characteristic group of birth defects caused by alcohol consumption by the mother, including facial deformities, heart defects, and physical and mental disabilities.

Because rapid brain development continues throughout pregnancy, the fetal brain stays vulnerable to alcohol use until birth. Although effects of drinking later in pregnancy do not typically cause the characteristic physical deformities of FAS, getting drunk just once during the final three months of pregnancy can damage a fetal brain.

FASD is a permanent, incurable condition that causes lifelong disability; it is among the most common preventable causes of intellectual disability in the Western world. It is estimated that more than 3000 babies are born with FASD each year in Canada. Research also suggests that rates of FASD are significantly higher in Aboriginal populations and in rural, remote, and Northern communities.

In comparison to FAS, about three times as many babies are born with **alcohol-related neurodevelopmental disorder (ARND)**, also on the fetal alcohol spectrum. Children with ARND appear physically "normal" but often have significant learning and behavioural disorders. As adults, they are more likely to develop substance abuse problems and to have criminal records. No one is sure exactly how much alcohol causes FAS or ARND. Like other untoward effects of alcohol, genetics and individual differences in metabolism, along with environmental factors such as diet, are thought to affect vulnerability. One study found that children born to mothers who drank as little as one and a half alcoholic drinks per week during their pregnancy weighed less and were shorter at age 14 years than children of mothers who drank nothing during pregnancy. The children's smaller size may be a marker for subtle, persistent alcohol damage. Therefore, no amount of alcohol during pregnancy is considered safe.

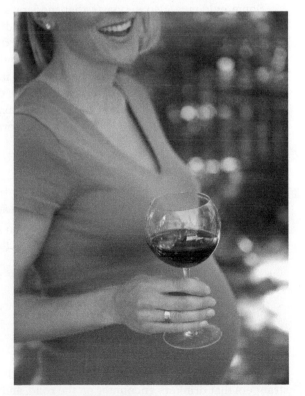

> **alcohol-related neurodevelopmental disorder (ARND)**
> Cognitive and behavioural problems seen in people whose mothers drank alcohol during pregnancy.

Women who are trying to conceive, or who are sexually active without using effective contraception, should abstain from alcohol to avoid inadvertently harming their baby in the first few days or weeks of pregnancy, before they know they are expecting. Binge drinking among women of childbearing age is a particular concern.

In the United States, labels on alcoholic beverages are required to carry a warning on the dangers of drinking during pregnancy. In Canada, only Yukon and the Northwest Territories have adopted the use of similar alcohol warning labels. In 2014, the Alberta government announced that establishments that sell alcohol, including liquor stores, bars, and restaurants, are required to post signs related to FASD prevention.

Any alcohol consumed by a nursing mother quickly enters the breast milk. What impact this has on the child

Experts warn that there is no safe level of alcohol consumption during pregnancy.

or on the mother's milk production is a matter of controversy. Dosage may again be the key issue. However, many physicians advise nursing mothers to abstain from drinking alcohol because of the belief that any amount may have negative effects on the baby's brain development.

QUICK STATS

The proportion of women in Canada who reported consuming alcohol during their pregnancy dropped from 15.5% in 2001–2004 to 10.7% in 2005–2008.

—*Public Health Agency of Canada*, 2013

Possible Health Benefits of Alcohol

The risks and benefits of drinking alcohol vary considerably with the age of the drinker. If you are 35 or younger, your odds of dying *increase* in direct proportion to the amount of alcohol you drink. Among people under age 35, even light drinkers have slightly higher mortality rates than non-drinkers. In other words, young adults who drink *any* amount of alcohol are more likely to die than non-drinkers of the same age. By contrast, alcohol consumption appears to confer certain health benefits primarily to older individuals.

The clearest evidence of benefit relates to coronary heart disease (CHD). The lowest rates of CHD deaths occur with moderate alcohol use, which in studies had a positive effect on both healthy people and individuals at risk for CHD. (CHD is discussed in detail in Chapter 7.) Moderate drinking may improve heart health by raising blood levels of HDL (the beneficial form of cholesterol), by thinning the blood, and by reducing inflammation and the risk of dangerous blood clots, all of which can contribute to the risk of a heart attack. Individuals with heart disease or with strong risk factors should talk with their doctors about the possible health benefits of moderate drinking.

Some evidence also suggests that moderate drinkers may be less likely to develop or better able to manage a variety of other conditions, including diabetes, high blood pressure, strokes, arterial blockages in the legs, cognitive decline (including Alzheimer's disease), and benign prostate enlargement. It is still unclear if these effects are due to the alcohol itself or to the non-alcoholic components of alcoholic drinks (the substances that give each different kind of beverage its distinctive character).

Research is under way to determine whether the apparent health benefits of wine are due to the alcohol or to some other substance found in wine. Some experts believe that the apparent benefit of wine may merely reflect the fact that wine drinkers tend to be more affluent and to have healthier lifestyles than those who don't drink wine.

QUESTIONS FOR CRITICAL THINKING AND REFLECTION

Have you ever witnessed or been involved in an alcohol emergency? Did you think the situation was urgent at the time? What were the circumstances surrounding the event? How did the people involved deal with it?

Alcohol Use

Abuse of and addiction to alcohol affect more than just the drinker. Friends, family members, co-workers, strangers that drinkers encounter on the road, and society as a whole pay the physical, emotional, and financial costs of the misuse of alcohol.

Alcohol Use and Canada's Low-Risk Alcohol Drinking Guidelines

Although most Canadians who consume alcohol do so responsibly, alcohol misuse is still far too prevalent. In fact, recent data have shown a 14 percent increase in per capita alcohol consumption among Canadians since 1996. According to the 2013 Canadian Tobacco, Alcohol and Drugs Survey (CTADS), about 76 percent of Canadians in general (ages 15 and older), 60 percent of minors (ages 15–19 years), and 83 percent of youths (ages 20–24) drink alcohol, whether infrequently or routinely. Heavy drinkers account for more than half of all the alcohol consumed, as well as a disproportionate amount of the social burden of alcohol abuse including productivity losses, health care costs, and law enforcement costs.

On the basis of this evidence, and in consultation with experts from government, non-government, academic, and industry settings, the first ever set of national low-risk alcohol drinking guidelines were launched by the Canadian Centre on Substance Abuse (CCSA) in 2011. Canada's Low-Risk Alcohol Drinking Guidelines (see Figure 15.5) were developed using the best available scientific evidence and consist of five guidelines and several tips designed to provide Canadians with information about minimizing the risks associated with alcohol consumption.

Canada's Low-Risk Alcohol Drinking Guidelines are comprised of the following aims and recommendations:

1. The first guideline aims to reduce the long-term (chronic) risk of diseases and conditions caused by several years of alcohol consumption (e.g., liver disease, some cancers). It recommends that women

FIGURE 15.5

Canada's Low-risk Alcohol Drinking Guidelines

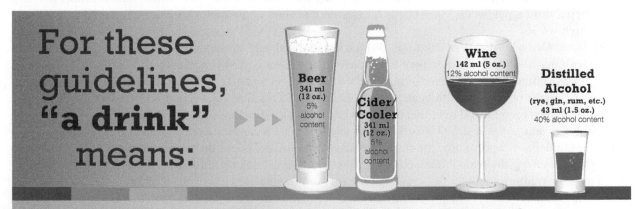

For these guidelines, "a drink" means: ▶ ▶ ▶

Beer 341 ml (12 oz.) 5% alcohol content

Cider/Cooler 341 ml (12 oz.) 5% alcohol content

Wine 142 ml (5 oz.) 12% alcohol content

Distilled Alcohol (rye, gin, rum, etc.) 43 ml (1.5 oz.) 40% alcohol content

Your limits

Reduce your long-term health risks by drinking no more than:

2 3
- 10 drinks a week for women, with no more than 2 drinks a day most days
- 15 drinks a week for men, with no more than 3 drinks a day most days

Plan non-drinking days every week to avoid developing a habit.

Special occasions

Reduce your risk of injury and harm by drinking no more than 3 drinks (for women) or 4 drinks (for men) on any single occasion.

Plan to drink in a safe environment. Stay within the weekly limits outlined above in *Your limits*.

When zero's the limit

Do not drink when you are:

- driving a vehicle or using machinery and tools
- taking medicine or other drugs that interact with alcohol
- doing any kind of dangerous physical activity
- living with mental or physical health problems
- living with alcohol dependence
- pregnant or planning to be pregnant
- responsible for the safety of others
- making important decisions

Pregnant? Zero is safest

If you are pregnant or planning to become pregnant, or about to breastfeed, the safest choice is to drink no alcohol at all.

Delay your drinking

Alcohol can harm the way the body and brain develop. Teens should speak with their parents about drinking. If they choose to drink, they should do so under parental guidance; never more than 1–2 drinks at a time, and never more than 1–2 times per week. They should plan ahead, follow local alcohol laws and consider the *Safer drinking tips* listed in this brochure.

Youth in their late teens to age 24 years should never exceed the daily and weekly limits outlined in *Your limits*.

Sources: Canadian Centre on Substance Abuse. 2013. *Canada's Low-Risk Alcohol Drinking Guidelines* [brochure], http://www.ccsa.ca/Resource%20Library/2012-Canada-Low-Risk-Alcohol-Drinking-Guidelines-Brochure-en.pdf (retrieved February 2, 2015); Reference cited in brochure: Butt, P., D. Beirness, L. Gliksman, C. Paradis, and T. Stockwell. 2011. *Alcohol and health in Canada: A summary of evidence and guidelines for low-risk drinking.* Ottawa, ON: Canadian Centre on Substance Abuse.

should not exceed more than 10 drinks a week, with no more than 2 drinks a day most days. Men should not exceed more than 15 drinks a week, with no more than 3 drinks a day on most days. It also includes a suggestion that everyone should plan non-drinking days every week.

2. The second guideline aims to reduce the short-term (acute) risk of injury, harm, and/or acute illness from drinking alcohol. It recommends that women consume no more than three drinks, and men consume no more than four drinks, on any *single occasion* (defined as "special occasions that occur infrequently and certainly no more than once a week").

3. The remaining three guidelines identify populations (including youth and pregnant women) and situations (such as when driving or taking medication) where alcohol should be avoided altogether. Tips are provided to help further reduce the risk of alcohol-related harms.

As previously mentioned, Canada's Low-Risk Alcohol Drinking Guidelines were developed for Canadians who *choose to drink*. Age-specific recommendations have also been created.

*   *Youth (before age 18/19 years, depending on provincial/territorial alcohol laws)*: It is recommended that youth delay drinking at least until their late teens. Alcohol can harm the healthy physical and mental development of children and adolescents. It is important to remember many young people choose not to drink. However, if youth decide to drink, they should do so in a safe environment under parental guidance, never have more than one to two drinks at a time, and never drink more than one to two times per week. They should plan ahead, follow local alcohol laws, and consider the safer drinking tips provided in Canada's Low-Risk Alcohol Drinking Guidelines.

*   *Young adults (age 18/19 to 24 years)*: From their late teens to age 24, women should never exceed 2 drinks per day or 10 drinks per week. Young men should never have more than 3 drinks per day or 15 drinks per week. Again, it is suggested that men and women should have non-drinking days each week.

*   *Older Canadians (older than age 65)*: Older adults should never exceed the recommendations presented in the guidelines. As people advance in age, their bodies process alcohol more slowly so they may become more sensitive to the effects of alcohol, increasing their risk of accidents, falls, and the worsening of some health issues. Also, many older Canadians have multiple prescriptions and the guidelines recommend avoiding alcohol while taking medications.

Estimates suggest that if all Canadians who drink alcohol were to adhere to Canada's Low-Risk Alcohol Drinking Guidelines, approximately 4600 alcohol-related deaths could be prevented each year. Currently, many Canadians consume alcohol in excess of these guidelines. In 2013, among those who consumed alcohol in the past year, approximately 21 percent exceeded the first guideline (for long-term or chronic effects) and 15 percent exceeded the second guideline (for short-term or acute effects). More males than females reported drinking patterns that exceeded both guidelines. The guidelines were exceeded by youth ages 20 to 24 years at higher rates than by adults aged 25 years and older; almost 29 percent and 23 percent of youth drinkers in Canada exceeded the first and second guidelines respectively, whereas approximately 20 percent and 14 percent of adult drinkers exceeded these guidelines.

Alcohol Use Disorder

As explained in Chapter 14, the 5th edition of the American Psychiatric Association's *Diagnostic and Statistical Manual of Mental Disorders (DSM-5)* has combined the previously distinct categories of alcohol abuse and alcohol dependence into a single condition called **alcohol use disorder**. Because alcohol use disorder is a subcategory within the broader substance use disorder category (see Chapter 14), the diagnostic criteria are similar. That is, a diagnosis of *mild* alcohol use disorder requires that an individual displays 2–3 symptoms from a list of 11 possible criteria within a 12-month period. For a diagnosis of *moderate* alcohol use disorder, individuals must exhibit 4–5 symptoms within the same 12-month period, whereas a diagnosis of *severe* alcohol use disorder requires that a person displays 6 or more symptoms.

alcohol use disorder

A disorder that first appeared in the DSM-5, combining the *previously distinct categories of alcohol abuse* and alcohol dependence; diagnosed as mild, moderate, or severe depending on the number of criteria an individual meets over a 12-month period.

The list of specific criteria is as follows:

1. Consuming alcohol in larger amounts or over a longer period than was intended
2. Having a persistent desire or making unsuccessful efforts to cut down or control alcohol use
3. Spending a great deal of time in activities necessary to obtain alcohol, use alcohol, or recover from its effects
4. Craving, or a strong desire or urge to use alcohol
5. Recurrent alcohol use resulting in a failure to fulfill major role obligations at work, school, or home
6. Continued alcohol use despite having persistent or recurrent social or interpersonal problems caused or exacerbated by the effects of alcohol
7. Giving up or reducing important social, school, work, or recreational activities because of alcohol use
8. Recurrent alcohol use in situations in which it is physically hazardous
9. Continued alcohol use despite knowledge of having a persistent or recurrent physical or psychological problem that is likely to have been caused or worsened by alcohol
10. Developing **tolerance** to alcohol, as defined by a need to consume increased amounts of alcohol to achieve the desired effect, or a markedly diminished effect with continued use of the same amount of alcohol
11. Experiencing alcohol withdrawal resulting in unpleasant physical and cognitive symptoms (such as nausea/vomiting, insomnia, seizures, etc.) or consuming alcohol (or another substance) to reduce or avoid withdrawal symptoms

Alcoholism, previously known as alcohol dependence, has typically been characterized by tolerance to alcohol and withdrawal symptoms. However, everyone who drinks—even those who are not addicted to alcohol—develops tolerance after repeated alcohol use. As a result of the revised diagnostic criteria for mild, moderate, and severe alcohol use disorder, some experts have argued that a larger number of people could now be diagnosed with alcoholism, resulting in a skewed portrait of the problem and the potential for misdirected resources. Still others have suggested that identifying people with mild alcohol use disorder could result in early treatment and the prevention of longer-term problems and costs.

Patterns and Prevalence

People of all ethnic groups and at all socioeconomic levels can develop an alcohol use disorder. The stereotype of the homeless, impoverished alcoholic actually accounts for fewer than 5 percent of all people with an alcohol use disorder and usually represents the final stage of a drinking career that began years earlier.

Once established, individuals with an alcohol use disorder often exhibit a pattern of exacerbations and remissions. The person may stop drinking and abstain from alcohol for days or months after a frightening problem develops. After a period of abstinence, people who are addicted to alcohol often attempt controlled drinking, which almost inevitably leads to an escalation in drinking and more problems. Alcohol addiction is not hopeless, however; many individuals do achieve permanent abstinence.

Health Effects

Tolerance and withdrawal can have a serious impact on health. As described in Chapter 14, *tolerance* means that a drinker needs more alcohol to achieve intoxication or the desired effect, that the effects of continued use of the same amount of alcohol are diminished, or that the drinker can function adequately at doses or a BAC that would produce significant impairment in a casual user. Heavy users of alcohol may need to consume about 50 percent more than they originally needed to experience the same degree of intoxication.

When individuals addicted to alcohol stop drinking or sharply decrease their intake, they experience *withdrawal*. Symptoms include trembling hands (shakes or jitters), a rapid pulse and accelerated breathing rate, insomnia, nightmares, anxiety, and gastrointestinal upset. These symptoms usually begin 5–10 hours after alcohol intake is decreased and improve after four to five days. After a week, most people feel much better, but occasionally anxiety, insomnia, and other symptoms persist for six months or more.

More severe withdrawal symptoms occur in about 5 percent of people with an alcohol use disorder. These include seizures (sometimes called *rum fits*), confusion, and **hallucinations**. Still less common is **delirium tremens** (the **DTs**), a medical emergency characterized by severe disorientation, confusion, epileptic-like seizures, and vivid hallucinations, often of vermin and small animals. The mortality rate from DTs can be as high as 15 percent, especially in very debilitated people with preexisting medical illnesses.

hallucinations
False perceptions that do not correspond to external reality, such as seeing visions or hearing voices that are not there.

delirium tremens (DTs)
A state of confusion brought on by the reduction of alcohol intake in a person addicted to alcohol; other symptoms are sweating, trembling, anxiety, hallucinations, and seizures.

Individuals with an alcohol use disorder face all the physical health risks associated with intoxication and chronic drinking described earlier in the chapter. Some of the damage is compounded by nutritional deficiencies that often accompany addiction to alcohol. A mental problem associated with alcohol use is profound memory gaps (commonly known as blackouts), which are sometimes filled by conscious or unconscious lying.

The specific health effects of alcohol addiction tend to vary from person to person. For example, one individual may suffer from problems with memory and central nervous system defects and have no liver or gastrointestinal problems. Another person with a similar drinking and nutritional history may have advanced liver disease but no memory gaps.

Social and Psychological Effects

Alcohol use causes more serious social and psychological problems than all other forms of drug abuse combined. For every person who is addicted to alcohol, another three or four people are directly affected. Alcohol is a major source of trouble in many families.

People with an alcohol use disorder frequently have mental disorders in addition to their substance addiction. They are also much more likely than non-alcoholics to experience clinical depression, panic disorder, schizophrenia, borderline personality disorder, and antisocial personality disorders. People with anxiety or panic attacks may try to use alcohol to lessen their anxiety, even though alcohol often makes these disorders worse. Individuals with an alcohol use disorder also often have other substance-abuse problems.

QUICK STATS

It is estimated that 4 to 5 million Canadians engage in high-risk drinking.
—Health Canada, 2014

Causes

The precise causes associated with the development of an alcohol use disorder are unknown, but many factors are probably involved. Studies of twins and adopted children clearly demonstrate the importance of genetics. If one of a pair of fraternal twins is addicted to alcohol, then the other has about twice the risk of becoming addicted. For the identical twin of a person with an alcohol use disorder, the risk of addiction is about four times that of the general population. These risks persist even when the twins have little contact with each other or their biological parents. Similarly, adoption studies show an increased risk among children of parents with an alcohol use disorder, even if they were adopted at birth into non-drinking families. Alcohol addiction in adoptive parents, contrarily, doesn't make individuals more or less likely to become addicted to alcohol. Some studies suggest that as much as 50–60 percent of a person's risk for an alcohol use disorder is determined by genetic factors.

Not all children of parents with an alcohol use disorder become addicted to alcohol, however, and it is clear that other factors are involved. A person's risk of developing an alcohol addiction may be increased by certain personality disorders, having grown up in a violent or otherwise troubled household, and imitating the alcohol abuse of peers and other role models. People who begin drinking excessively in their teens are especially prone to binge drinking and alcohol problems later in life. Common psychological features of individuals who abuse alcohol are denial ("I don't have a problem") and rationalization ("I drink because I need to socialize with my customers"). Certain social factors have also been linked with heavy drinking, including urbanization, disappearance of the extended family, a general loosening of kinship ties, increased mobility, and changing values.

QUICK STATS

The average age of first use of alcohol among Canadian youth is 16.2 years.
—Health Canada, 2014

Treatment

Some people with an alcohol use disorder recover without professional help. How often this occurs is unknown, but possibly as many as one-third stop drinking on their own or reduce their drinking enough to eliminate problems. Often these spontaneous recoveries are linked to an alcohol-related crisis, such as a blackout or alcohol-related automobile crash, a health problem, or the threat of being fired. Not all people who are addicted to alcohol must hit bottom before they are motivated to stop. People vary markedly in what induces them to change their behaviour.

Most people with an alcohol use disorder, however, require a treatment program of some kind to stop drinking. Many different kinds of programs exist. No single treatment works for everyone, so a person may have to try different programs before finding the right one. Although treatment is not successful for everyone, considerable optimism has replaced the older view that nothing could be done. Many people suffering with an alcohol addiction have patterns of drinking that fluctuate widely over time. These fluctuations indicate that their alcohol abuse is a response to environmental factors, such as life stressors or social pressures, and therefore may be influenced by treatment.

One of the oldest and best-known recovery programs is Alcoholics Anonymous (AA). AA consists of self-help groups that meet several times each week and follow a 12-step program. Important steps for people in these programs include recognizing that they are "powerless over alcohol" and must seek help from a "higher power" to regain control of their lives. Many AA members have a sponsor of their choosing who is available by phone 24 hours a day for individual support and crisis intervention. AA convincingly shows the individual that abstinence can be achieved and also provides a sober peer group of people who share the same identity—that of recovering alcoholics. Many AA members find that it works best in combination with counselling and medical care.

Other recovery approaches are available. Some, like Rational Recovery and Women for Sobriety, deliberately avoid any emphasis on higher spiritual powers. A more controversial approach to problem drinking is offered by the group Moderation Management, which encourages people to manage their drinking behaviour by limiting intake or abstaining.

Al-Anon is a companion program to AA for families and friends of people with alcohol addictions. In Al-Anon, spouses and others explore how they enabled the family member or friend to drink by denying, rationalizing, or covering up his or her drinking and how they can change this codependent behaviour. Alateen is a part of Al-Anon dedicated to young people, typically teenagers, whose lives have been affected by another individual's drinking. Similar to Al-Anon groups, Alateen members meet regularly to share experiences and learn effective coping mechanisms. Employee assistance programs and school-based programs represent another treatment approach. These programs can deal directly with work and campus issues, often important sources of stress for the person who is abusing alcohol. They encourage effective coping responses for internal and external stressors.

In-patient hospital rehabilitation is useful for some people with an alcohol use disorder, especially if they have serious medical or psychological problems or if life stressors threaten to overwhelm them. When the person returns to the community, however, it is critical that there be some form of active, continuing, long-term treatment. Patients who return to a spouse or family often need to address issues involving those significant others, and to establish new routines and shared recreational activities that do not involve drinking.

Several medical treatments are available for alcohol use disorders. All of these work best in combination with counselling or other non-pharmacological programs:

- *Disulfiram* (Antabuse) inhibits the metabolic breakdown of acetaldehyde and causes patients to flush and feel ill when they drink, thus theoretically inhibiting impulse drinking. However, disulfiram is potentially dangerous if the user continues to drink.

- *Naltrexone* (ReVia, Depade) binds to a brain pleasure centre that reduces the craving for alcohol and decreases its pleasant, reinforcing effects. When taken correctly, naltrexone usually does not make the user feel ill.
- *Injectable naltrexone* (Vivtrol) acts the same as oral naltrexone, but it is a single monthly shot administered by a health professional. Compliance with a monthly regimen may be better for some people.
- *Acamprosate* (Campral) helps people maintain abstinence after they have stopped drinking. It is unclear how acamprosate works, but it appears to act on brain pathways related to alcohol abuse.

A variety of other drugs to treat alcohol addiction are undergoing clinical trials—alone, in combination, or in combination with counselling therapies.

In people who abuse alcohol and have significant depression or anxiety, the use of antidepressant or antianxiety medication can improve both mental health and drinking behaviour. In addition, other drugs, such as diazepam (Valium), are sometimes prescribed to replace alcohol during initial stages of withdrawal. Such chemical substitutes are usually useful for only a week or so, because people with alcoholism are at particularly high risk for developing dependence on other drugs.

Alcohol treatment programs are successful in achieving an extended period of sobriety for about half of those who participate. Success rates of conventional treatment programs are about the same for men and women and for people from different ethnic groups. Women, minority group members, and the poor often face major economic and social barriers to receiving treatment. Many in-patient treatment programs are financially out of reach for people of low income or those without insurance coverage. AA remains the mainstay of treatment for most people and is often a component of even the most expensive treatment programs.

Gender, Setting, and Population Differences

People with an alcohol use disorder come from all socioeconomic levels and cultural groups, but notable differences exist in patterns of drinking between men and women, across provinces and territories, and among Canadian populations. Table 15.4 provides an overview of the rates of past-year alcohol use, as well as the percentage exceeding Canada's Low-Risk Alcohol Drinking Guidelines, for males and females and across provinces.

Men

In 2012, a greater percentage of Canadian males than females reported drinking patterns that exceeded Canada's low-risk drinking guidelines for both chronic and acute effects. Among white Canadian men, excessive drinking often begins in the teens or 20s and progresses gradually through the 30s until individuals are clearly identifiable as people with alcoholism by the time they are in their late 30s or early 40s. Other men remain controlled drinkers until later in life, sometimes becoming alcoholic in association with retirement, the loss of friends and loved ones, boredom, illness, or psychological disorders. (See the Gender Matters box.)

TABLE 15.3

Users of Alcohol in Canada, by Gender and Province, 2012

	Past Year Prevalence (percentage)	Exceeding Low-Risk Drinking Guidelines (percentage)	
		Chronic	Acute
Men	82.7	17.3	12.9
Women	74.4	11.8	7.2
Province			
Newfoundland and Labrador	76.0	16.1	13.4
Prince Edward Island	74.0	12.3	9.2
Nova Scotia	72.3	13.0	10.1
New Brunswick	73.8	15.0	10.4
Quebec	82.1	16.1	10.4
Ontario	77.7	14.5	9.9
Manitoba	79.5	13.6	8.6
Saskatchewan	78.5	14.6	11.3
Alberta	76.2	11.9	8.8
British Columbia	78.1	13.5	9.9
Total Population	**78.4**	**14.4**	**9.9**

Source: Public Healthy Agency of Canada, 2008. *Canadian Alcohol and Drug Use Monitoring Survey: Summary of Results, 2008.* Adapted and reproduced with permission from the Minister of Health, 2015.

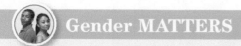

Gender MATTERS

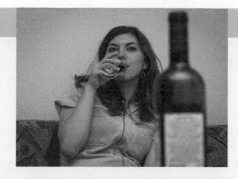

Gender and Alcohol Use and Abuse

Men are more likely than women to drink alcohol, to abuse alcohol, and to have alcohol use disorder. In Canada, men account for the majority of alcohol-related deaths and injuries. Most alcohol-related deaths and injuries among men result from incidents involving intoxication, such as motor vehicle crashes, falls, drowning, suicide, and homicide.

A variety of factors contribute to the higher rates of alcohol use among men. Traditional or stereotypic gender roles and ideas regarding masculinity and drinking behaviour may promote excessive alcohol consumption among men. Young men in particular are also more likely to engage in all types of risky health behaviours. Men drive more kilometres, drive more dangerously, and are more likely to drive while intoxicated. They tend to have greater access to firearms, contributing to their increased rates of suicide and homicide. Men may also be more likely than women to use alcohol to cope with stress and other life challenges.

Generally speaking, 73–77 percent of Canadian women have reported using alcohol in the past year since 2004. Women are not immune to alcohol problems. Whether a woman is a "social drinker," a binge drinker, or a heavy daily user, the impact of alcohol on her will be different from and generally greater than the impact of comparable use on a man. And due in part to the social stigma attached to problem drinking, particularly among women, women are less likely to seek early treatment.

Women become intoxicated at lower doses of alcohol than men, and they tend to experience the adverse physical effects of chronic drinking sooner and at lower levels of alcohol consumption than men. They develop alcohol liver disease and alcohol-related brain damage after a comparatively shorter period of heavy drinking and a lower level of drinking than men. Some alcohol-related health problems are unique to women, including an increased risk of breast cancer, menstrual disorders, infertility, and, in pregnant women, giving birth to a child with FASD.

Women from all walks of life and all ethnic groups can develop alcohol problems, but those who have never married or are divorced are more likely to drink heavily than married or widowed women. Women who have multiple life roles, such as parent, worker, and spouse, are less vulnerable to alcohol problems than women who have fewer socially connecting roles.

Women

Compared with men, more Canadian women abstain from alcohol completely or are low-risk drinkers. The progression of alcoholism in women is usually different than it is in men. Women tend to become addicted to alcohol at a later age and with fewer years of heavy drinking. It is not unusual for women in their 40s or 50s to become alcoholic after years of controlled drinking. Women who abuse alcohol develop cirrhosis and other medical complications somewhat more often and after a shorter period of heavier drinking than men, and have higher death rates—including deaths from cirrhosis—than men with alcoholism.

Provincial and Territorial Differences

According to the *Canadian Alcohol and Drug Use Monitoring Survey*, some notable differences in drinking patterns emerged across provinces in 2012. The overall rate of drinking in the year before the survey was about 74 percent, with Quebec having the highest rate in the country and Nova Scotia having the lowest rate (refer back to Table 15.4). In terms of exceeding Canada's low-risk "chronic" drinking guidelines, Quebec and Newfoundland and Labrador had the highest rates at approximately 16 percent, and Alberta had the lowest rate at about 12 percent. For the low-risk "acute" drinking guidelines, Newfoundland and Labrador also had the highest rate in Canada, while Manitoba had the lowest.

The prevalence of heavy drinking is higher in the Northwest Territories than in the provinces. According to the 2009 *Northwest Territories Addiction Survey*, almost half of the respondents who indicated that they had consumed alcohol in the previous year reported that they had consumed five or more drinks on a single occasion at least once a month. Among youth ages 15–24, 64 percent reported drinking more than five drinks on a single occasion on the days they consumed alcohol in the previous year. Similar to those in the rest of Canada, heavy drinkers in the Northwest Territories are more likely to be males than females.

The legal drinking age is 19 in Canada, except in Alberta, Manitoba, and Quebec, where it is 18.
—Canadian Centre on Substance Abuse, 2014

First Nations Communities

Alcohol abuse is a widespread and severe health problem in many First Nations communities, especially for adolescents and young adults. Unfortunately, data are limited with regard to the use of alcohol among Aboriginal peoples in Canada; however, the 2002–2003 *First Nations Regional Longitudinal Health Survey* revealed that the overall frequency of alcohol use was actually lower among First Nations adults than it was for the general population. However, there was a greater proportion of heavy drinkers (defined as those who drink five or more alcoholic beverages on one occasion) among First Nations adults. The highest-risk group included young males ages 18–29.

The Canadian Centre on Substance Abuse identified several issues, such as poverty, low education levels, unstable family lives, unemployment, physical and mental abuse, poor social support, and problems with the law, as factors that are related to alcohol abuse within First Nations communities. From a historical and cultural perspective, alcohol and substance abuse problems are (and have been) compounded by discrimination, the effects of residential schools, and barriers to health care. As a result, it has been suggested that treatment and prevention efforts in First Nations communities would be more effective if cultural and historical components are included. Many First Nations communities have succeeded in preventing or reducing alcohol and substance use problems among their people by applying community-based, culturally appropriate solutions to the issues noted above.

Binge Drinking

Although many different definitions can be found in the literature, **binge drinking** has recently been defined as a pattern of alcohol use that brings a person's BAC up to 0.08 percent or above (typically five drinks for men or four drinks for women), consumed within about two hours. Binge drinking is also referred to as *heavy drinking* or *heavy episodic drinking*. Statistics Canada defines "heavy drinking" as having five or more drinks on one occasion for males, and four or more drinks on one occasion for females, at least once a month over the past year. A 2013 survey estimated that close to 20 percent of Canadians (about 5.5 million people) over the age of 12 were classified as heavy drinkers; males were more likely than females to report heavy drinking.

binge drinking
Periodically drinking alcohol to the point of severe intoxication; about four drinks (for women) and five drinks (for men) consumed within a period of about two hours.

Among university- and college-aged Canadians, drinking often takes place in the form of a binge, which has a profound effect on students' lives (see the In the News box). In 2013, almost 40 percent of 18–19-year-old males and 30 percent of 18–19-year-old females reported binge drinking at least once per month over the past year. Binge drinking is associated with a number of negative alcohol-related consequences. For example, frequent binge drinkers are three to seven times more likely than non-binge drinkers to engage in unplanned or unprotected sex, to drive after drinking, and to get hurt or injured. Binge drinkers are also more likely to miss classes, fall behind in schoolwork, and argue with friends. The more frequent the binges, the more problems these students encounter.

Helping Someone with an Alcohol Problem

Helping a friend or relative with an alcohol problem requires skill and tact. Start by making sure you are not enabling someone to continue excessively using alcohol. Enabling takes many forms, such as making excuses for the person who is abusing alcohol—for example, saying "he has the flu" when it is really a hangover.

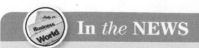 **In *the* NEWS**

Campus Binge Drinking

Although binge drinking among post-secondary students has been a serious problem for decades, it has recently come under a harsh spotlight due largely to highly publicized alcohol-related tragedies on campuses across Canada and worldwide. Deaths from alcohol overdose (sometimes as a result of binge-drinking games), alcohol-related injuries (including motor vehicle crashes), violent crimes, student riots, and serious vandalism have all drawn attention to the epidemic of heavy drinking on university and college campuses.

To many people, heavy drinking is considered a normal and integral part of campus life. But research has shown that heavy drinking has had a devastating impact on far too many students—drinkers and non-drinkers alike—as well as on their families and communities.

Drinking on campus is pervasive. More than 80 percent of Canadian undergraduate students drink alcohol; that's more than use cigarettes, marijuana, and cocaine combined. Much of the current data on college and university drinking in Canada comes from the *National College Health Assessment*, conducted in 2009. This survey includes the responses of more than 8000 undergraduate students from eight Canadian post-secondary institutions. Results show that more than half of students binge-drink; 60 percent of students reported consuming five or more drinks on a single occasion in the last 15 days. Interestingly, students at smaller institutions (less than 20 000 students) reported higher rates of binge drinking than those at larger schools (≥ 20 000 students).

The consequences of campus drinking are serious. The most common alcohol-related harms reported by students include experiencing a hangover, memory loss, and regrets, and missing classes because of a hangover. The negative effects associated with excessive alcohol consumption are also experienced by those around the drinker; secondary alcohol-related harms include study or sleep disruptions, serious arguments, being pushed or assaulted, and experiencing sexual harassment as a result of someone else's drinking.

Post-secondary students in Canada have reported taking advantage of low-priced promotions at campus bars, attending happy hour events, taking advantage of special promotions by beer companies, and attending events that included unlimited drinking for a cover charge. Generally speaking, students who have identified themselves as frequent drinkers have found their campus environments to be conducive to drinking.

Working together, students, faculty, administrators, parents, and the community are beginning to put an end to the destructive culture of heavy drinking on campuses. Social events held during orientation week on many Canadian campuses are becoming "dry" or alcohol free, and at some institutions, incoming students are required to take online classes about alcohol. Peer health education programs are also being offered, and there is stricter punishment for underage drinking and public drunkenness on some campuses. In recent years, student requests for alcohol-free living on some Canadian campuses have increased dramatically. And, at some institutions, rather than targeting the elimination of alcohol, *harm reduction efforts* are being implemented. Examples of such efforts include allowing students living in residences to drink in a common area (rather than alone or behind closed doors) with a restriction on the number of drinks permitted, and maintaining open lines of communication with local bar and restaurant owners.

In response to the increasing alcohol-related problems on university campuses, experts on a U.S. Task Force of the National Advisory Council on Alcohol Abuse and Alcoholism issued a "call to action" for post-secondary institutions. According to the Task Force, efforts and resources must focus on three levels:

1. Ultimately each *student* is accountable and must take responsibility for his or her own behaviour. Programs are needed that encourage and support development of healthy attitudes toward alcohol. These programs should target students at increased risk of developing alcohol problems including first-year students, fraternity and sorority members, and athletes. Treatment should be readily available for problem drinkers.

2. The *student body as a whole* must work to discourage excessive alcohol consumption. These efforts include promoting alcohol-free activities, reducing availability of alcohol, and avoiding social and commercial promotion of alcohol on campus. There should be an environment of acceptance of students who choose to abstain, and disapproval of students who drink to excess. Fraternities, sororities, eating clubs, and other campus organizations should be held accountable for inappropriate alcohol use, especially involving underage students, that takes place on their premises.

3. *Universities and surrounding communities* must cooperate to discourage excessive drinking. Administrators, law enforcement, government officials, bar and restaurant owners, residents who live near campus, and the court system must all do their part to reduce the availability of cheap alcohol and to enforce existing laws. Those who enable students to drink irresponsibly must be held accountable.

Sources: Adlaf, E. M., et al. (eds.). 2005. *Canadian Campus Survey 2004*. Toronto: Centre for Addiction and Mental Health, http://www.camh.ca/en/research/research_areas/social-epi-research/Documents/CCS_2004_report.pdf (retrieved February 2, 2015); and Kwan, M. Y. W., G. E. J. Faulkner, K. P. Arbour-Nicitopolous, and J. Cairney. 2013. Prevalence of health-risk behaviours among Canadian post-secondary students: Descriptive results from the National College Health Assessment. *BMC Public Health* 13: 548–553.

Another important step is open, honest labelling: "I think you have a problem with alcohol." Such explicit statements usually elicit emotional rebuttals and may endanger a relationship. However, you are not helping your friends by allowing them to deny their problems with alcohol or other drugs. Taking action shows that you care.

Even when problems are acknowledged, people are usually reluctant to get help. You can't cure a friend's drinking problem, but you can guide him or her to appropriate help. Your best role might be to obtain information about the available resources and persistently encourage their use. Consider making an appointment for your friend at the student health centre and then go with him or her to the appointment. Most student health centres will be able to recommend local options for treatment. You can also check the Internet or community resources for local chapters of AA and other groups (see the For More Information section at the end of the chapter). And don't underestimate the power of families to help. An honest phone call to your friend's parents could save a life if your friend is in serious trouble with alcohol.

QUESTIONS FOR CRITICAL THINKING AND REFLECTION

Do you know anyone with a serious alcohol problem? What effects, if any, has this person's problem had on your life? Have you thought about getting support or help?

Drinking Behaviour and Responsibility

Responsible use of alcohol means keeping your BAC low, so that your behaviour is always under your control. In addition to controlling your own drinking, you can promote responsible alcohol use in others.

QUICK STATS

Past-year alcohol use among Canadians ages 20–24 decreased from approximately 83% in 2004 to 70% in 2012.

—*Health Canada*, 2014

Examine Your Drinking Behaviour

When you want to drink responsibly, it's helpful to know, first of all, why you drink. The following are common reasons given by university students:

- "It lets me go along with my friends."
- "It makes me less self-conscious and more social."
- "It makes me less inhibited."
- "It relieves depression, anxiety, tension, or worries."
- "It enables me to experience a different state of consciousness."

If you drink alcohol, what are your reasons for doing so?

After examining your reasons for drinking, take a closer look at your drinking behaviour. Is it low-risk and responsible? Or do you frequently overindulge and suffer negative consequences? The Take Charge box at the end of the chapter explains how to keep and analyze a record of your drinking. The *CAGE* screening test can help

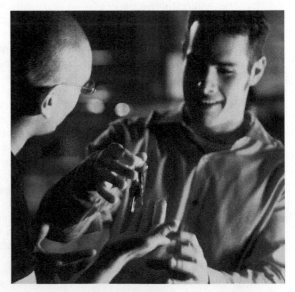

By choosing a designated driver, these men are ensuring a safe trip home.

you determine whether you, or someone close to you, may have a drinking problem. Answer yes or no to the following questions:

- *Have you ever felt you should...*
  Cut down on your drinking?
- *Have people...*
  Annoyed you by criticizing your drinking?
- *Have you ever felt bad or...*
  Guilty about your drinking?
- *Have you ever had an...*
  Eye-opener (a drink first thing in the morning to steady your nerves or get rid of a hangover)?

One "yes" response suggests a possible alcohol problem; if you answered yes to more than one question, it is highly likely that a problem exists. For a more detailed evaluation of your drinking habits, complete the AUDIT questionnaire in the Assess Yourself box. If the results of either assessment test indicate a potential problem, or you feel that you could benefit from some assistance, get help right away.

THINKING ABOUT THE ENVIRONMENT

Our attitudes about alcohol use are usually based on our experiences and observations of the world around us. For example, you may not think of alcohol as being an important part of life if you grew up in a household where alcohol was served only at special events or as an occasional accompaniment to dinner.

Conversely, if your parents or other family members drank heavily or made a big deal of having alcohol on hand for most occasions, then you may have a similar view of alcohol and be more inclined to use it frequently.

The college or university environment can play an important role in shaping students' attitudes about drinking. Does it seem as if everyone at your school drinks? Do you feel pressure to drink, even when you don't want to? Many students feel pressured to use alcohol or illegal drugs. But even though it may seem like everyone drinks, about 10 percent of post-secondary students are non-drinkers. Remember: The majority of Canadian adults drink lightly or not at all. Perceptions about the drinking habits of others can be misleading.

Drink Moderately and Responsibly

Sometimes people lose control when they misjudge how much they can drink. At other times, they set out deliberately to get drunk. The following are some strategies for keeping your drinking and your behaviour under control:

- *Drink slowly.* Sip your drinks rather than gulp them. Do not drink alcoholic beverages to quench your thirst. Avoid drinks made with carbonated mixers, especially if you are thirsty; you will be more likely to gulp them down.
- *Space your drinks.* Drink non-alcoholic drinks at parties, or alternate them with alcoholic drinks. Learn to refuse a round: "I've had enough for right now." Parties are easier for some people if they hold a glass of something non-alcoholic that has ice and a twist of lime floating in it so it looks like an alcoholic drink.
- *Eat before and while drinking.* Avoid drinking on an empty stomach. Food in your stomach will not prevent the alcohol from eventually being absorbed, but it will slow down the rate somewhat and lower the peak BAC. In restaurants, order your food before you order a drink. Try to have something to eat before you go out to a party where alcohol will be served.
- *Know your limits and your drinks.* Learn how different BACs affect you. In a safe setting, such as your home, with your roommate, friend, or family member, see how a set (and reasonable) amount— say, two drinks in an hour—affects you. A good test is walking heel to toe in a straight line with your eyes closed or standing with your feet crossed and trying to touch your finger to your nose with your eyes closed.

Assess YOURSELF

Do You Have a Problem with Alcohol?

The Alcohol Use Disorders Test (AUDIT) is a screening tool for problem drinking. It can also be used for self-assessment. For each question, choose the answer that best describes your behaviour. Then total your scores.

Questions	Points					Your Score
	0	1	2	3	4	
1. How often do you have a drink containing alcohol?	Never	Monthly or less	2–4 times a month	2–3 times a week	4 or more times a week	_____
2. How many drinks containing alcohol do you have on a typical day when you are drinking?	1 or 2	3 or 4	5 or 6	7–9	10 or more	_____
3. How often do you have six or more drinks on one occasion?	Never	Less than monthly	Monthly	Weekly	Daily or almost daily	_____
4. How often during the past year have you found that you were not able to stop drinking once you had started?	Never	Less than monthly	Monthly	Weekly	Daily or almost daily	_____
5. How often during the past year have you failed to do what was normally expected because of drinking?	Never	Less than monthly	Monthly	Weekly	Daily or almost daily	_____
6. How often during the past year have you needed a first drink in the morning to get yourself going after a heavy drinking session?	Never	Less than monthly	Monthly	Weekly	Daily or almost daily	_____
7. How often during the past year have you had a feeling of guilt or remorse after drinking?	Never	Less than monthly	Monthly	Weekly	Daily or almost daily	_____
8. How often during the past year have you been unable to remember what happened the night before because you had been drinking?	Never	Less than monthly	Monthly	Weekly	Daily or almost daily	_____
9. Have you or someone else been injured as a result of your drinking?	No	Yes, but not in the past year (2 points)		Yes, during the past year (4 points)		_____
10. Has a relative, friend, doctor, or other health worker been concerned about your drinking or suggested you cut down?	No	Yes, but not in the past year (2 points)		Yes, during the past year (4 points)		_____
					Total	_____

A total score of 8 or more indicates a strong likelihood of hazardous or harmful alcohol consumption. Even if you score below 8, if you are encountering drinking-related problems with your academic performance, job, relationships, health, or the law, you should consider seeking help.

Source: Sanders, J. B. et al. 1993, *Development of the Alcohol Use Disorders Identification Test (AUDIT)*: WHO collaborative project on early detection of persons with harmful alcohol consumption-II. *Addiction* 88(6): Appendix, 803. Copyright © 2006, 1993 Society for the Study of Addiction to Alcohol and Other Drugs. Reprinted by permission of Blackwell Publishers.

Be aware that in different settings your performance, and especially your ability to judge your behaviour, may change. At a given BAC, you will perform less well when surrounded by activity and boisterous companions than you will in a quiet test setting with just one or two other people. This impairment results partially because alcohol reduces your ability to perform when your brain is bombarded by multiple stimuli.

QUICK STATS

Canadians spent $21.4 billion on alcoholic beverages in 2012–2013, up 2.2% from the previous year.
—Statistics Canada, 2014

Promote Responsible Drinking

Although you cannot completely control the drinking behaviour of others, you can do things to help promote responsible drinking.

Encourage Responsible Attitudes

Our society teaches us attitudes toward drinking that contribute to alcohol-related problems. Many of us have difficulty expressing disapproval about someone who has drunk too much, and we are amused by the antics of a funny drunk. We accept the alcohol industry's linkage of drinking with virility or sexuality (see the Critical Consumer box). And many people treat non-drinkers as non-conformists in social settings. Recognize that the choice to abstain is neither odd nor unusual. More than 20 percent of Canadian adults do not drink at all or have not had an alcoholic beverage in the past year. Most adults are capable of enjoying their leisure time without alcohol or drugs. In hazardous situations, such as driving or operating machinery, abstinence is the only appropriate choice.

 Critical CONSUMER

Alcohol Advertising

To be a careful and informed health consumer, you need to consider the effects that advertisements have on you.

Alcohol manufacturers spend millions of dollars every year on advertising and promotions in Canada. They claim that the purpose of their advertising is to persuade adults who already drink to choose a certain brand. But in reality, ads cleverly engage young people and children—never overtly suggesting that young people should drink, but clearly linking alcohol and good times.

Alcohol ads are common during televised sporting events and other shows popular with young adults. Studies show that the more TV adolescents watch, the more likely they are to take up drinking in their teens. New alcoholic drinks geared to the tastes of young people are heavily promoted. "Hard lemonade" and other fruity or sweetened drinks have been described by teens as a way to get drunk without suffering the bitter taste of most alcoholic beverages.

Alcohol manufacturers also reach out to young people at youth-oriented activities, such as concerts and sporting events. Product logos are heavily marketed through sales of T-shirts, hats, and other items, and many colleges and universities allow alcohol manufacturers to advertise at campus events.

What is the message of all these advertisements? Think about the alcohol ads you have seen. Many give the impression that drinking alcohol is a normal part of everyday life and good times. This message seems to work well on the young, many of whom believe that heavy-duty drinking at parties is normal and fun. The use of famous musicians, athletes, or actors in commercials increases the appeal of alcohol by associating it with fame, wealth, sex, and popularity. Many beer advertisements, for example, portray beer drinking as a critical part of success in finding an attractive mate.

What ads don't show is the darker side of drinking. You never see hangovers, car crashes, slipping grades, or violence. Although some ads include a brief message, such as "know when to say when," the impact of such cautions is small compared with that of the image of happy, attractive young people having fun while drinking.

The next time you see an advertisement for alcohol, take a critical look. What is the message of the ad? What audience is being targeted, and what is the ad implying about alcohol use? Be aware of its effect on you.

Be a Responsible Host

When you are the host, serve non-alcoholic beverages as well as alcohol. Have only enough alcohol on hand for each guest to have a moderate amount. Don't put out large kegs of beer, as these invite people to overindulge. For parties hosted by a dorm, fraternity or sorority, or other campus group, don't allow guests to have unlimited drinks for a single admission fee, as this also encourages binge drinking.

Always serve food along with alcohol, and stop serving alcohol an hour or more before people will leave. If possible, arrange carpools with designated non-drinking drivers in advance. Remind your guests with a graduated licence about the zero-tolerance laws—even a single drink can result in an illegal BAC. Insist that guests who drink too much take a taxi, ride with someone else, or stay overnight rather than drive.

Plan social functions with no alcohol at all. Outdoor parties, hikes, and practically every other type of social occasion can be enjoyable without alcohol. If that doesn't seem possible to you, then examine your own drinking patterns and attitudes toward alcohol. If you can't have fun without drinking, you may have a problem with alcohol.

Hold the Drinker Responsible

The individual who consumes alcohol must take full responsibility for his or her behaviour. Pardoning unacceptable behaviour fosters the attitude that the behaviour is caused by the drug. The drinker is thereby excused from responsibility and learns to expect minimal adverse consequences for bad behaviour. The opposite approach—holding the individual fully accountable—is a more effective policy. For example, alcohol-impaired drivers who receive strict penalties have fewer subsequent rearrests than those who receive only mandatory treatment. Other people's drunkenness can impinge on your living or study environment. Speak up against this behaviour—and insist on your rights.

Take Community Action

Consider joining an action group, such as Ontario Students Against Impaired Driving. Through education, training, and an annual conference centered around leadership and the responsible use of alcohol, OSAID helps students avoid the dangers of drinking, impaired driving, and other destructive choices.

QUESTIONS FOR CRITICAL THINKING AND REFLECTION

Are you aware of the campus and community resources that can help someone overcome an alcohol problem? For example, does your college or university offer alternatives to keg parties or other events where alcohol is traditionally provided? Are there dorms, organizations, or clubs whose members agree to abstain from alcohol? Are counselling services readily available to students?

Take CHARGE

Developing Responsible Drinking Habits

How much do you drink? Is it the right amount for you? You may know the answer to this question already, or you may not have given it much thought. Many people learn through a single unpleasant experience how alcohol affects them. Others suffer ill effects but choose to ignore or deny them.

To make responsible and informed choices about using alcohol, consider, first, whether there is any history of alcohol abuse in your family. If someone in your family is addicted to alcohol, you have a higher-than-average likelihood of becoming addicted too. Second, consider whether you are addicted to other substances or behaviours. Do you smoke, drink strong coffee every day, or use other drugs regularly? Does some habit control your life? Some people have more of a tendency to become addicted than others, and a person with one addiction is often likely to have other addictions as well. If this is the case for you, again you may need to be more cautious with alcohol.

Keep a Record

Find out more about your alcohol-related behaviour by keeping track of your drinking for two weeks in a health journal. Keep a daily alcohol behaviour record like the one illustrated in Chapter 1 for eating behaviour. Include information on the following:

- *The drinking situation*, including number of drinks, type of drink, time of day, how fast you drank it/them, where you were, and what else you were doing.
- *Your internal state*, including what made you want to drink and your feelings, thoughts, and concerns at the time. Note how others influenced you.
- *The consequences of drinking*, including any changes in your feelings or behaviour while or after you were drinking, such as silliness, assertiveness, aggressiveness, or depression.

Analyze Your Record

Next, analyze your record to detect patterns of feelings and environmental cues. Do you always drink when you're at a certain place or with certain people? Do you sometimes drink just to be sociable, when you don't really want a drink and would be satisfied with a non-alcoholic beverage? Refer to the list of warning signs of alcohol use disorder given in the text. Are any of them true for you? For example, do you feel uncomfortable in a social situation if alcohol is *not* available?

Set Goals

Now that you have analyzed your record, think about whether you want to change any of your behaviours. Would you do better academically if you drank less? Has drinking had a negative impact on any of your relationships? Have you risked infection and unplanned pregnancy by having unprotected sex while drunk? Do you depend on alcohol to have a good time? Have you been injured while drinking? If you drink and drive or if you feel you are becoming dependent on alcohol, it is time to change your drinking behaviour. Decide on goals that will give you the best health and safety returns, such as a beer or a glass of wine with dinner, one drink per hour at a party, or no alcohol at all.

Devise a Plan

Refer to your health journal to see what kinds of patterns your drinking falls into and where you can intervene to break the behaviour chain. If you have determined that your life would be improved if you changed your drinking habits, now is the time to make changes. For some people, simple changes in the environment, such as stocking the refrigerator with alternative beverages like juices or sparkling water, can be helpful. If you feel self-conscious about ordering a non-alcoholic drink when you're out with a group, try recruiting a friend to do the same. If it's too difficult to avoid drinking in some situations, such as at a bar or a beer party, you may decide to avoid those situations for a time.

Examine your friendships. If drinking is becoming a problem for you and some of your friends drink heavily, you may need to think about letting those relationships go. If you find support groups helpful, check with your campus health clinic; most schools sponsor peer group activities for those who are working to change their drinking habits. Local chapters of AA and other organizations may have groups geared toward university-age people.

Instead of drinking, try other activities that produce the same effect. For example, if you drink to relieve anxiety or tension, try adding 20–30 minutes of exercise to your schedule to help manage stress. Or try doing a relaxation exercise or going for a brisk walk to help reduce anxiety before a party or date. If you drink to relieve depression or to stop worrying, consider finding a trustworthy person (perhaps a professional counsellor) to talk to. If you drink to feel more comfortable sexually, consider ways to improve communication with your partner so you can deal with sexual issues more openly. When these activities are successful, they will reinforce your responsible drinking decisions and make it more likely that you will make the same decisions again in the future.

For other ways to monitor and control your drinking behaviour, see the suggestions in the section "Drinking Behaviour and Responsibility."

Reward Yourself and Monitor Your Progress

If changing your drinking behaviour turns out to be difficult, it may be a clue that drinking is becoming a problem for you—all the more reason to get it under control now. Be sure to reward yourself as you learn to drink responsibly (or not at all). You may lose weight, look better, feel better, and have higher self-esteem as a result. Keep track of your progress in your health journal, and use the strategies described in Chapter 1 for maintaining your program. Remember, when you establish sensible drinking habits, you're planning not just for this week or month—but for your whole life.

SUMMARY

- Although alcohol has long been a part of human celebrations, it is a psychoactive drug capable of causing addiction.
- After being absorbed into the bloodstream in the stomach and small intestine, alcohol is transported throughout the body. The liver metabolizes alcohol as blood circulates through it.
- If people drink more alcohol each hour than the body can metabolize, blood alcohol concentration (BAC) increases. The rate of alcohol metabolism depends on a variety of individual factors.
- Alcohol is a central nervous system depressant. At low doses, it tends to make people feel relaxed.
- At higher doses, alcohol interferes with motor and mental functioning; at very high doses, alcohol poisoning, coma, and death can occur. Effects may be increased if alcohol is combined with other drugs.
- Alcohol use increases the risk of injury and violence; drinking before driving is particularly dangerous, even at low doses.
- Continued alcohol use has negative effects on the digestive and cardiovascular systems and increases cancer risk and overall mortality.
- Pregnant women who drink risk giving birth to children with a cluster of birth defects known as fetal alcohol spectrum disorder (FASD). Even occasional drinking during pregnancy can cause brain injury in the fetus.
- Moderate or low-risk drinking may decrease the risk of coronary heart disease in some people.
- Individuals can now be diagnosed with alcohol use disorder, a category that first appeared in the DSM-5 and combines the *alcohol abuse* and alcohol dependence categories that were in the DSM-IV. Alcohol use disorder can be diagnosed as mild, moderate, or severe depending on the number of criteria an individual meets over a 12-month period.
- Binge drinking is common on university and college campuses and has negative effects on both drinking and non-drinking students.
- Physical consequences of alcohol addiction include the direct effects of tolerance and withdrawal, as well as all the problems associated with chronic drinking. Psychological problems include memory loss and additional mental disorders, such as depression.
- Treatment approaches include mutual support groups like AA, job- and school-based programs, inpatient hospital programs, and pharmacological treatments.
- Helping someone with alcohol use disorder means avoiding being an enabler and obtaining information about available resources and persistently encouraging their use.
- Strategies for keeping drinking under control include examining attitudes about drinking and drinking behaviour, drinking slowly, spacing drinks, eating before and while drinking, and knowing one's limits.
- Strategies for promoting responsible drinking in others include encouraging responsible attitudes, being a responsible host, holding the drinker responsible for his or her actions, learning about prevention programs, and taking community action.

FOR MORE INFORMATION

BOOKS

Auth, J. 2010. *Emmy's Question*. St. Augustine, Fla.: Morningtide Press. A young girl's experience growing up in a household with alcoholism; for children ages 9–12.

Chrzan, J. 2013. *Alcohol: Social Drinking in Cultural Context*. Routledge. Alcohol-related practices and beliefs across cultures; allows students to examine their own thoughts about and use of alcohol.

Kinney, J. 2014. *Loosening the Grip: A Handbook of Alcohol Information,* 11th ed. New York: McGraw-Hill. A fascinating book about alcohol, including information on physical effects, abuse, alcoholism, and cultural aspects of alcohol use.

Seaman, B. 2006. *Binge: Campus Life in an Age of Disconnection and Excess*. New York: Wiley. An exploration of campus life at 12 residential colleges and universities, with discussions on the effects of student isolation, peer pressure, and drinking on students.

ORGANIZATIONS, HOTLINES, AND WEBSITES

The Internet addresses listed here were accurate at the time of publication.

Al-Anon Family Group Headquarters. Provides information and referrals to local Al-Anon and Alateen groups. The website includes a self-quiz to determine if you are affected by someone's drinking.
    888-4AL-ANON   http://www.al-anon.alateen.org

Alcoholics Anonymous (AA) World Services. Provides general information on AA, literature on alcoholism, and information about AA meetings and related 12-step organizations.
    http://www.aa.org

AlcoholScreening.Org. Provides information about alcohol and health, referrals for treatment and support groups, and a drinking self-assessment.
    http://www.alcoholscreening.org

Betty Ford Center. Provides information about the residential treatment program, along with symposia, newsletters, and programs for children of individuals with alcoholism.
    http://www.bettyfordcenter.org

Canadian Centre on Substance Abuse. Provides information relating to substance-abuse issues; contains a number of links and resources.
    http://www.ccsa.ca

Centre for Addiction and Mental Health. Provides information and resources about clinical care, research, education, policy development, and health promotion in relation to mental health and addiction.
    http://www.camh.net

Drug and Alcohol Helpline. Provides information about drug and alcohol addiction services in Ontario, as well as a confidential and free hotline, email, and web chat service that is available 24/7.
    1-800-565-8603   http://www.drugandalcoholhelpline.ca

Higher Education Center for Alcohol, Drug Abuse, and Violence Prevention. Provides support for campus alcohol and illegal drug prevention efforts; gives information about alcohol and drug abuse on campus and links to related sites.
    http://www.edc.org/projects/higher_education_center_alcohol_drug_abuse_and_violence_prevention

Mothers Against Drunk Driving Canada. Supports efforts to develop solutions to the problems of drunk driving and underage drinking; provides news, information, and brochures about many topics, including a guide to understanding and avoiding alcohol liability when hosting a party.
    http://www.madd.ca

Ontario Students Against Impaired Driving. Provides information and resources, and hosts an annual conference related to the risks associated with drinking and driving.
    http://www.osaid.org

U.S. National Council on Alcoholism and Drug Dependence. Provides information and resources.
    http://www.ncadd.org

See also the listings for Chapter 14.

SELECTED BIBLIOGRAPHY

Addolorato, G., et al. 2006. Baclofen: A new drug for the treatment of alcohol dependence. *International Journal of Clinical Practice* 60(8): 1003–1008.

Adlaf, E. M., et al. (eds.). 2005. *Canadian Campus Survey 2004*. Toronto: Centre for Addiction and Mental Health.

American Psychiatric Association. 2013. *Diagnostic and Statistical Manual of Mental Disorders*, 5th ed. Washington, D.C.: American Psychiatric Association.

Anton, R. F., et al. 2006. Combined pharmacotherapies and behavioral interventions for alcohol dependence: The COMBINE study: A randomized controlled trial. *Journal of the American Medical Association* 295(17): 2003–2017.

Aronson, K. 2003. Alcohol: A recently identified risk factor for breast cancer. *Canadian Medical Association Journal* 168(9): 1147–1148, http://www.cmaj.ca/content/168/9/1147.full (retrieved May 5, 2015).

Brache K., and T. Stockwell. 2011. Drinking patterns and risk behaviours associated with combined alcohol and energy drink consumption. *Addictive Behaviours* 36(12): 1133–1140.

Brache, K., G. Thomas, and T. Stockwell, T. 2012. *Caffeinated alcoholic beverages in Canada: Prevalence of use, risks and recommended policy responses.* Ottawa, ON: Canadian Centre on Substance Abuse.

Butt, P., D. Beirness, L. Gliksman, C. Paradis, and T. Stockwell. 2011. *Alcohol and health in Canada: A summary of evidence and guidelines for low-risk drinking.* Ottawa, ON: Canadian Centre on Substance Abuse.

Callahan, M. 2006. Cocktail confidential. *Health,* June, 169–171.

Canadian Cancer Society. 2009. *Alcohol,* http://www.cancer.ca/en/prevention-and-screening/live-well/alcohol/?region=on (retrieved February 13, 2015).

Canadian Centre on Substance Abuse. 2009. *First Nations, Inuit and Métis People,* http://www.ccsa.ca/Eng/topics/First-Nations-Inuit-and-Metis/Pages/default.aspx (retrieved February 13, 2015).

Canadian Centre on Substance Abuse. 2012. *Canada's low-risk alcohol drinking guidelines: Frequently asked questions.* Ottawa, ON: Canadian Centre on Substance Abuse, http://www.ccsa.ca/Resource%20Library/2012-FAQs-Canada-Low-Risk-Alcohol-Drinking-Guidelines-en.pdf (retrieved February 2, 2015).

Canadian Centre on Substance Abuse. 2013. *Canada's Low-Risk Alcohol Drinking Guidelines* [brochure], http://www.ccsa.ca/Resource%20Library/2012-Canada-Low-Risk-Alcohol-Drinking-Guidelines-Brochure-en.pdf (retrieved February 2, 2015).

Canadian Food Inspection Agency. 2009. *Guide to Food Labelling and Advertising: Chapter 10—Guide to the Labelling of Alcoholic Beverages,* http://www.inspection.gc.ca/english/fssa/labeti/guide/ch10e.shtml (retrieved May 3, 2015).

Centers for Disease Control and Prevention. 2010. *Alcohol and Public Health: Caffeinated Alcoholic Beverages,* http://www.cdc.gov/alcohol/fact-sheets/cab.htm (retrieved February 2, 2015).

Clifasefi, S. L., et al. 2006. Blind drunk: The effects of alcohol on inattentional blindness. *Applied Cognitive Psychology* 20(5): 697–704.

College Drinking Prevention. 2007. *A Snapshot of Annual High-Risk College Drinking Consequences,* http://www.collegedrinkingprevention.gov/StatsSummaries/snapshot.aspx (retrieved February 4, 2015).

Collins, G. B., et al. 2006. Drug adjuncts for treating alcohol dependence. *Cleveland Clinic Journal of Medicine* 73(7): 641–644.

Costello, R. M. 2006. Long-term mortality from alcoholism: A descriptive analysis. *Journal of Studies on Alcohol* 67(5): 694–699.

Department of Health and Human Services. 2007. *The Surgeon General's Call to Action to Prevent and Reduce Underage Drinking.* Washington, D.C.: Department of Health and Human Services, Office of the Surgeon General.

Dietitians of Canada. 2015. *Alcohol and Nutrition,* http://www.eatrightontario.ca/en/Articles/Alcohol/Alcohol-and-Nutrition.aspx#.VM5kB6Mo6po (retrieved February 2, 2015).

First Nations Centre. 2005. *First Nations Regional Longitudinal Health Survey (RHS) 2002/03: Results for Adults, Youth and Children Living in First Nations Communities,* http://fnigc.ca/sites/default/files/ENpdf/RHS_2002/rhs2002-03-technical_report.pdf (retrieved February 2, 2015).

Gruenewald, P. J., and L. Remer. 2006. Changes in outlet densities affect violence rates. Alcoholism: *Clinical and Experimental Research* 30(7): 1184–1193.

Health Canada. 2014. *Canadian Alcohol and Drug Use Monitoring Survey: Summary of Results for 2013,* http://healthycanadians.gc.ca/science-research-sciences-recherches/data-donnees/ctads-ectad/tables-tableaux-2013-eng.php#t12 (retrieved February 2, 2015).

Heilig, M., and M. Egli. 2006. Pharmacological treatment of alcohol dependence: Target symptoms and target mechanisms. *Pharmacology and Therapeutics* 111(3): 855–876.

Hingson, R., et al. 2005. Magnitude of alcohol-related mortality and morbidity among U.S. college students ages 18–24. *Annual Review of Public Health* 26: 259–279.

Hingson, R. W., et al. 2006. Age at drinking onset and alcohol dependence: Age at onset, duration, and severity. *Archives of Pediatrics and Adolescent Medicine* 160(7): 739–746.

Holahan, C. J., et al. 2010. Late-life alcohol consumption and 20-year mortality. *Alcohol: Clinical and Experimental Research* 34(11): 1961–1971.

Krampe, H., et al. 2006. Follow-up of 180 alcoholic patients for up to 7 years after outpatient treatment: Impact of alcohol deterrents on outcome. *Alcohol: Clinical and Experimental Research* 30(1): 86–95.

Kwan, M. Y. W., G. E. J. Faulkner, K. P. Arbour-Nicitopolous, and J. Cairney. 2013. Prevalence of health-risk behaviours among Canadian post-secondary students: Descriptive results from the National College Health Assessment. *BMC Public Health* 13: 548–553.

Mayo Clinic. 2006. Pain relievers and alcohol: A potentially risky combination. *Mayo Clinic Health Letter,* May.

McCaig, L. F., and E. N. Nawar. 2006. National Hospital Ambulatory Medical Care Survey: 2004 emergency department summary. Advance Data from *Vital and Health Statistics* No. 372. Hyattsville, Md.: National Center for Health Statistics.

Mercer, G. 2009. *Estimating the Presence of Alcohol and Drug Impairment in Traffic Crashes and Their Costs to Canadians: 1999 to 2006.* Vancouver: Applied Research and Evaluation Services.

Miller, T. R., et al. 2006. Societal costs of underage drinking. *Journal of Studies on Alcohol* 67(4): 519–528.

Monti, P. M., et al. 2005. Adolescence: Booze, brains, and behavior. *Alcoholism: Clinical and Experimental Research* 29(2): 207–220.

Mothers Against Drunk Driving (MADD). 2013. *Estimating the number and cost of impairment-related traffic crashes in Canada: 1999 to 2010,* http://madd.ca/media/docs/estimating_presence.pdf (retrieved February 2, 2015).

National Center for Health Statistics. 2008. Deaths: Preliminary data for 2006. *National Vital Statistics Reports* 56(16).

National Institute on Alcohol Abuse and Alcoholism. 2006. *Young Adult Drinking. Alcohol Alert No. 68.* Bethesda, Md.: National Institute on Alcohol Abuse and Alcoholism.

National Institute on Alcohol Abuse and Alcoholism. 2013. *Alcohol Use Disorder: A comparison between DSM-IV and DSM-5.* NIH Publication No. 13–7999, http://pubs.niaaa.nih.gov/publications/dsmfactsheet/dsmfact.pdf (retrieved February 2, 2015).

Nelson, T. F., et al. 2005. The state sets the rate: The relationship of college binge drinking rates and selected state alcohol control policies. *American Journal of Public Health* 95(3): 441–446.

Northwest Territories Health and Social Services. 2010. *NTW Addictions Report: Prevalence of alcohol, illicit drug, tobacco use and gambling in the Northwest Territories,* http://www.hss.gov.nt.ca/sites/default/files/nwt_addictions_report.pdf (retrieved February 2, 2015).

O'Brien, M., McCoy, T., Rhodes, S., Wagoner, A., & Wolfson, M. (2008) Caffeinated cocktails: Energy drink consumption, high-risk drinking, and alcohol-related consequences among college students. *Academic Emergency Medicine, 15*(5), 453–460.

Osiowy, M., T. Stockwell, J. Zhao, K. Thompson, and S. Moore. 2014. How much did you actually drink last night? An evaluation of standard drink labels as an aid to monitoring personal consumption. *Addiction Research and Theory: Early Online,* 1–7.

Perreira, K. M., and K. E. Cortes. 2006. Explaining race/ethnicity and nativity differences in alcohol and tobacco use during pregnancy. *American Journal of Public Health,* 27 July [epub].

Price, R., C. Hilchey, C. Darredeau, H. Fulton, and S. Barrett. 2010. Brief communication: Energy drink co-administration is associated with increased reported alcohol ingestion. *Drug & Alcohol Review* 29(3): 331–333.

Rehm, J., J. Patra, and S. Popova. 2006. Alcohol-attributable mortality and potential years of life lost in Canada 2001: Implications for prevention and policy. *Addiction* 101(3): 373–384.

Rehm, J., and K. D. Shield. (2014). Global alcohol-attributable deaths from cancer, liver cirrhosis, and injury in 2010. *Alcohol Research: Current Reviews* 35(2): 174–183.

Shield, K. D., B. Taylor, T. Kehoe, J. Patra, and J. Rehm. 2012. Mortality and potential years of life lost attributable to alcohol consumption in Canada in 2005. *BMC Public Health* 12: 91.

Slutska, W. S. 2005. Alcohol use disorders among US college students and their non-college-attending peers. *Archives of General Psychiatry* 62(3): 321–327.

Thombs, D., R. O'Mara, M. Tsukamoto, M. Rossheim, R. Weiler, M. Merves, and B. Goldberder. 2010. Event-level analyses of energy drink consumption and alcohol intoxication in bar patrons. *Addictive Behaviours* 35(4): 325–330.

Traffic Injury Research Foundation. 2014. *The Road Safety Monitor 2014: Drinking and Driving in Canada,* http://www.tirf.ca/publications/PDF_publications/RSM_2014_Drinking_Driving_Eng_2.pdf (retrieved February 2, 2015).

Willford, J., et al. 2006. Moderate prenatal alcohol exposure and cognitive status of children at age 10. *Alcoholism: Clinical and Experimental Research* 30(6): 1051–1059.

CHAPTER 16

Toward a Tobacco-Free Self and Society

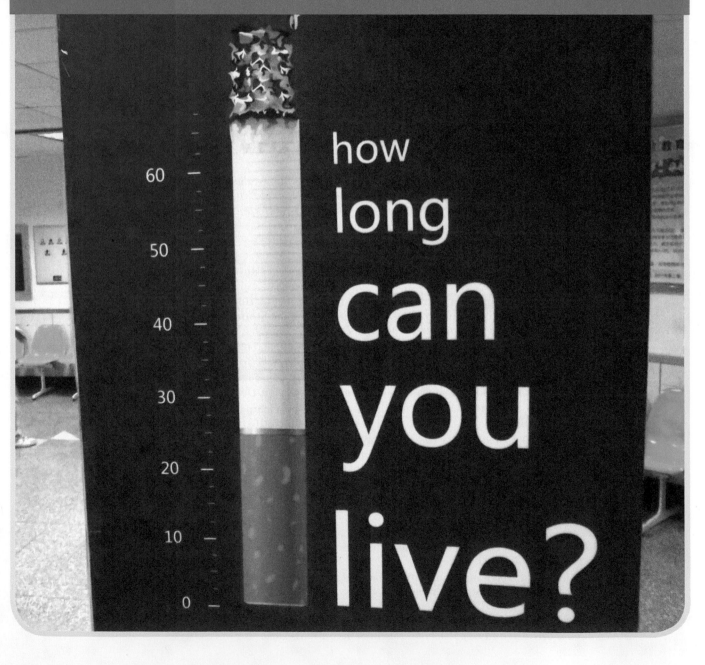

LOOKING AHEAD

After you have read and studied this chapter, you should be able to:

LO1   List the reasons people start using tobacco and why they continue to use it

LO2   Explain the short- and long-term health risks associated with tobacco use

LO3   Discuss the effects of environmental tobacco smoke on non-smokers

LO4   Describe the social costs of tobacco and list actions that have been taken to combat smoking in the public and private sectors

LO5   Prepare plans to stop using tobacco and to avoid environmental tobacco smoke

TEST YOUR KNOWLEDGE

1. **"Light" or low-tar cigarettes are safer than regular cigarettes.**
   True or false?

2. **Which of the following substances is/are found in tobacco smoke?**
   a. acetone (nail polish remover) b. ammonia (cleaner) c. hexamine (lighter fluid) d. toluene (industrial solvent)

3. **Each year in Canada, the equivalent of the population of a small city dies from tobacco use.**
   True or false?

4. **The risk for which of the following conditions is/are increased by cigarette smoking?**
   a. facial wrinkling b. miscarriage c. impotence

5. **A person who quits smoking now will reduce his or her risk of lung cancer within 10 years.**
   True or false?

ANSWERS

1. FALSE.   Smokers who choose light or low-tar cigarettes do not reduce tar intake or smoking-related disease risks, nor is there any evidence that switching to light cigarettes helps smokers quit.

2. ALL FOUR.   Tobacco contains thousands of chemical substances, including many that are poisonous or are linked to the development of cancer.

3. TRUE.   Approximately 47 500 Canadians die each year from tobacco-related causes.

4. ALL THREE.   Cigarette smoking reduces quality of life and is the leading preventable cause of death in Canada.

5. TRUE.   The lung cancer risk of a former smoker is 50 percent of that of a continuing smoker within 10 years of quitting.

Smoking is a leading cause of preventable death in Canada. In fact, each year nearly 37 000 Canadians die prematurely from tobacco-related causes. Tobacco use accounts for nearly one of every five deaths in Canada. The percentage of Canadians who smoke varies widely by province/territory, with the highest rates observed in Nunavut and the lowest rates in British Columbia (see Figure 16.1).

Smoking is the main risk factor for three top causes of death in Canada: cancer, cardiovascular disease, and lung disease. Approximately half of all smokers die from smoking-related illnesses. Smoking affects the health of people at all stages of life and from all walks of life. The life expectancy of an adult smoker on average is reduced from 87 to 73 years. However, the earlier a smoker quits the greater the health benefits; specifically, quitting before 30 years of age avoids 90 percent of lung cancer mortality. It is important to note that non-smokers also suffer, especially the children of parents who smoke. Exposure to environmental tobacco smoke (ETS) kills thousands of non-smokers every year.

In spite of these facts—and despite increasing public and private efforts to restrict smoking—approximately 5.9 million Canadians are smokers, with thousands more joining their ranks each year. This chapter discusses the reasons people use tobacco, the negative impact of smoking, and the measures being taken to stop this public health threat.

Who Uses Tobacco?

According to the 2012 *Canadian Tobacco Use and Monitoring Survey* (CTUMS), 20.3 percent of the Canadian population reported using a tobacco product at least once in the preceding month. Twenty-five percent of

FIGURE 16.1

Smokers by Sex, Province and Territory, 2013

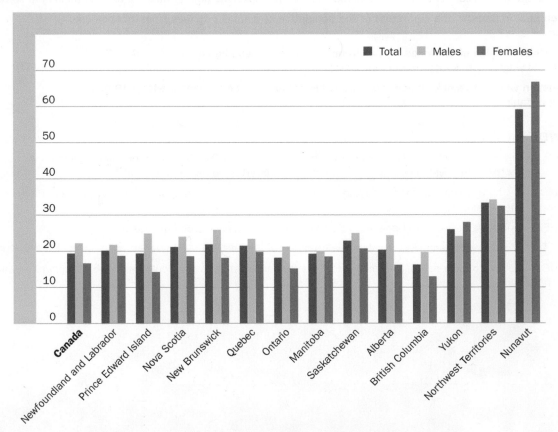

Source: Statistics Canada, CANSIM, table 105-0501 and Catalogue no. 82-221-X, http://www.statcan.gc.ca/tables-tableaux/sum-som/l01/cst01/health74b-eng.htm.

all university students described themselves as current smokers, meaning they smoke cigarettes every day or most days. Smoking rates reported in such surveys are essentially unchanged from those reported in 2000, suggesting that a decades-long decline in smoking prevalence has stalled. Until early 2005, smoking rates had dropped steadily from a high of roughly 49 percent in 1964, when the surgeon general's report linked smoking and lung cancer.

In 2012, 23.1 percent of men and almost 17.5 percent of women smoked cigarettes. Rates of smoking vary based on gender, age, ethnicity, and education level (see Figure 16.2 and the Dimensions of Diversity box). By 2012, adults with less than a Grade 12 education were much more likely to smoke cigarettes than those with a post-secondary education. The reverse is true for cigars; cigar smoking is most common among the affluent and those with high educational attainment.

FIGURE 16.2

Percentage who Smoke Daily or Occasionally, by Age Group and Sex, 2012

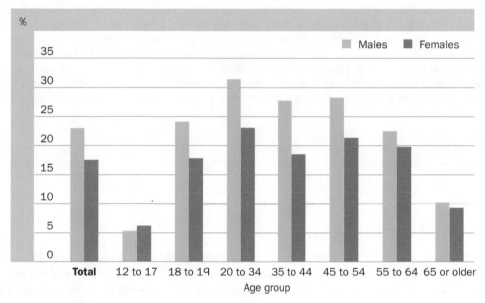

Source: Statistics Canada. Canadian Community Health Survey, 2012, http://www.statcan.gc.ca/pub/82-625-x/2013001/article/11844-eng.htm.

For more than a decade, there has been a gradual increase in the number of *occasional* smokers (people who smoke on some days but not daily). Most such smokers are young adults ages 18–25 who say they smoke only at parties or when they are with friends who smoke. Health officials warn that occasional smokers are as vulnerable as other smokers to the health dangers of tobacco. Occasional smokers are also less likely to try to quit.

Most current smokers, however, seem to understand the risks of tobacco use. For example, more than 80 percent of adult smokers believe tobacco will shorten their life and would like to stop smoking. Each year, approximately 1 million smokers quit; however, 43 percent will relapse. It takes the average smoker 3.2 quit attempts before quitting successfully.

 Dimensions *of* DIVERSITY

Smoking Among Canadian Aboriginal Populations

The overall rate of tobacco use among Canadians ages 12 and older was 20.3 percent in 2012; on average, any group of a dozen people is likely to include three or four who use tobacco. But averages include wide variations among populations, and ethnic differences appear in the earliest stages of tobacco use. Similar to a number of health-related issues, ethnicity and cultural background serve as determinants of tobacco use.

Wide ethnic variations also exist among smokers over 18 years old. Almost 72 percent of Inuit and 52 percent of Métis adults are smokers, a rate that is almost double that of the general population. Within broad ethnic categories, even greater variation occurs. Among people grouped under the broad category of Aboriginal people, which represents only 4.4 percent of the total population, 60 percent smoke. The health-related implications of such a high Aboriginal smoking rate results in an adjusted smoking attributable mortality rate almost 1.5 times as high as in the general population. This means that approximately one in five adult deaths among Aboriginal people is tobacco related. The staggering smoking rate of Aboriginal people is not restricted to adults: Smoking rates of Aboriginal youth are double that of the smoking rate of other Canadian youth.

The variations between and within ethnic populations reflect a complex interplay of social, environmental, and cultural factors. For example, tobacco is used in important Aboriginal spiritual ceremonies, specifically, sweat lodges, pipe ceremonies, and smudges. Tobacco is used in cleansing rituals to enable communication with spirits as a way of seeking the Creator.

The substantial tobacco use among Aboriginal people requires culturally sensitive quitting initiatives. Canada's Aboriginal culture gravitates toward a four-body approach when confronting health issues. The four-body approach encompasses the physical, mental, emotional, and spiritual aspects of the individual in relation with the health concern. As such, initiatives would need to address not only the physical addiction, but also the other three components of the four-body approach. More specifically, cessation efforts may be more successful if they address the mental relationship of tobacco use in spiritual ceremonies as compared with that in tobacco misuse; the emotional aspect of dealing with smoking habits that are encouraged through role modelling; and the spiritual aspect of an individual for whom the misuse of tobacco can negatively affect the effectiveness of communicating with the spirits.

Sources: McKennit, D. 2007. A smoking prevention program for Aboriginal youth. *First Peoples Child and Family Review* 3(2): 52–55; and Reading, J., and Y. Allard. 1999. The tobacco report. First Nations and Inuit Regional Health Survey, National Steering Committee. In The Health of Ontario First Nations People: Results from the Ontario First Nations Regional Health Survey, *Canadian Journal of Public Health*, Vol. 94, No. 3.

Young People and Tobacco

Although all provinces and territories ban the sale of tobacco to anyone younger than 18 years of age, at least 1.6 billion cigarettes are consumed by minors each year, resulting in retail sales of approximately $330 million. Fifty-five percent of youth reported obtaining cigarettes from retail sources, and one-third reported obtaining cigarettes from social sources such as parents or friends.

Of those Canadians in Grade 6 to 9 in 2011, 15.5 percent reported trying cigarettes and 2.2 percent were current smokers. However, there was significant variation across provinces/territories, with a higher prevalence reported in Quebec and Saskatchewan (4.3 percent of students reported being current smokers). Of those smokers, 8.1 percent smoked cigarettes, and 7.5 percent smoked cigars/cigarillos. Moreover, 70 percent of students in Grades 6 to 9 reported trying to quit. In addition, about 11.8 percent of youth ages 15 to 19 years described themselves as "current cigarette users" in 2013. Of those, youth men were more likely to smoke than women, with smoking rates of 13.0 percent and 10.5 percent, respectively.

The use of smokeless tobacco products in high school is not nearly as prevalent as cigarette use. Only 1 percent of students ages 15 and older reported using smokeless tobacco products. All of this is particularly worrisome given that one out of two lifetime smokers will die from tobacco use.

Tobacco and Other Drugs

Men and women with other drug abuse problems frequently use tobacco. For example, studies show that roughly 70 percent of alcoholics and more than 90 percent of heroin addicts are heavy smokers.

Smoking also is two to four times as prevalent among people with mental health diagnoses, including major depression, social phobias, and generalized anxiety disorder, as it is in the general population. Such findings suggest that underlying psychological or physiological traits may predispose people to drug use, including tobacco.

QUESTIONS FOR CRITICAL THINKING AND REFLECTION

Do any of your friends or family members smoke or use smokeless tobacco? What effect has it had on their health and relationships? Have you ever discussed their tobacco use with them? Why or why not?

Why People Use Tobacco

Although people start smoking for a variety of reasons, they usually become long-term smokers after becoming addicted to nicotine—the key psychoactive ingredient in tobacco smoke.

Nicotine Addiction

The primary reason people continue to use **tobacco** is that they have become addicted to a powerful psychoactive drug: **nicotine**. Although the tobacco industry long maintained that nicotine had not been proven to be addictive, scientific evidence overwhelmingly shows that nicotine is highly addictive. Many researchers consider nicotine to be the most physically addictive of all the psychoactive drugs.

> **tobacco**
> The leaves of cultivated tobacco plants prepared for smoking or chewing or for use as snuff.
>
> **nicotine**
> A poisonous, addictive substance found in tobacco and responsible for many of the effects of tobacco.

Some neurological studies indicate that nicotine acts on the brain in much the same way as cocaine and heroin. Nicotine reaches the brain via the bloodstream seconds after it is inhaled or, in the case of spit tobacco, it is absorbed through membranes of the mouth or nose. It triggers the release of powerful chemical messengers in the brain, including epinephrine, norepinephrine, and dopamine. But unlike street drugs, most of which are used to achieve a high, nicotine's primary attraction seems to lie in its ability to modulate everyday emotions.

At low doses, nicotine acts as a stimulant. It increases heart rate and blood pressure, and in adults, nicotine can enhance alertness, concentration, rapid information processing, memory, and learning. The opposite effect occurs in teens who smoke, however; they show impairment in memory and other cognitive functions.

In some circumstances, nicotine acts as a mild sedative. Most commonly, nicotine relieves withdrawal symptoms, such as anxiety, irritability, and mild depression, in tobacco users who are trying to quit. Some studies have shown that high doses of nicotine and rapid smoking cause increases in levels of glucocorticoids and endorphins, chemicals that act in the brain to moderate moods and reduce stress. Tobacco users are able to fine-tune nicotine's effects and regulate their moods by increasing or decreasing their intake of the drug. Studies have shown that smokers experience milder mood variation than non-smokers while performing long, boring tasks or while watching emotional movies, for example.

All tobacco products contain nicotine, and the use of any of them can lead to addiction (see the Assess Yourself box). Nicotine addiction fulfills the criteria for substance dependence described in Chapter 14, including loss of control, tolerance, and withdrawal.

Loss of Control

Half of all Canadian smokers would like to quit smoking. Canadian cessation programs are considered successful if 15 percent of smokers are able to quit. Of the people who try to quit smoking, 60 percent typically relapse in the first three months and 75 percent relapse within six months. This relapse rate is similar to rates for alcoholics and heroin addicts. Quitting may be even harder for smokeless users. For example, in one study, only 1 of 14 spit tobacco users who participated in a tobacco-cessation clinic was able to stop for more than four hours.

Regular tobacco users live according to a rigid cycle of need and gratification. On average, they can go no more than 40 minutes between doses of nicotine, otherwise, they begin feeling edgy and irritable and have trouble concentrating. If ignored, nicotine cravings build until getting tobacco becomes a paramount concern,

Assess YOURSELF

Nicotine Dependence: Are You Hooked?

Answer each question in the list below, giving yourself the appropriate number of points.

_____ 1. How soon after you wake up do you have your first cigarette?
   a. within 5 minutes (3)
   b. 6–30 minutes (2)
   c. 31–60 minutes (1)
   d. after 60 minutes (0)

_____ 2. Do you find it difficult to refrain from smoking in places where it is forbidden, such as the library, a theatre, or a doctor's office?
   a. yes (1)
   b. no (0)

_____ 3. Which cigarette would you most hate to give up?
   a. the first one in the morning (1)
   b. any other (0)

_____ 4. How many cigarettes a day do you smoke?
   a. 10 or less (0)
   b. 11–20 (1)
   c. 21–30 (2)
   d. 31 or more (3)

_____ 5. Do you smoke more frequently during the first hours after waking than during the rest of the day?
   a. yes (1)
   b. no (0)

_____ 6. Do you smoke if you are so ill that you are in bed most of the day?
   a. yes.(1)
   b. no (0)

_____ TOTAL

A total score of 7 or more indicates that you are very dependent on nicotine and are likely to experience withdrawal symptoms when you stop smoking. A score of 6 or less indicates low to moderate dependence.

Source: Heatherton, T. F., et al. 1991. The Fagerstrom Test for Nicotine Dependence: A revision of the Fagerstrom Tolerance Questionnaire. *British Journal of Addictions* 86(9): 1119–1127.

crowding out other thoughts. Tobacco users may plan their daily schedule around opportunities to satisfy their nicotine cravings. This loss of control and personal freedom can affect all the dimensions of wellness (see the Mind Body Spirit box).

Tobacco users become adept, therefore, at keeping a steady amount of nicotine circulating in the blood and going to the brain. In one experiment, smokers were given cigarettes that looked and tasted alike but varied in nicotine content. The subjects automatically adjusted their rate and depth of inhalation so that they absorbed their usual amount of nicotine. In other studies, heavy smokers were given nicotine without knowing it, and they cut down on their smoking without a conscious effort. Spit tobacco users maintain blood nicotine levels as high as those of cigarette smokers.

Tolerance and Withdrawal

Using tobacco builds tolerance. Where one cigarette may make a beginning smoker nauseated and dizzy, a long-term smoker may have to chain-smoke a pack or more to experience the same effects. For most regular tobacco users, sudden abstinence from nicotine produces predictable withdrawal symptoms. These symptoms, which come on several hours after the last dose of nicotine, can include severe cravings, insomnia, confusion, tremors, difficulty concentrating, fatigue, muscle pains, headache, nausea, irritability, anger, and depression.

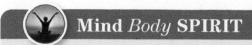

Mind *Body* SPIRIT

Tobacco Use and Religion: Global Views

Religious traditions can best help adult smokers by reminding them of two principles: the value of liberation from any form of slavery, and respect for life out of deference to their god. Most religions regard the human body as the dwelling place of the spirit; as such, it deserves care and respect.

Tobacco Use as a Violation of Religious Principles

The Baha'i faith, for example, strongly discourages smoking as unclean and unhealthy. Some Protestant churches consider tobacco use a violation of the body. For Hindus, smoking goes against one of the primary spiritual practices, the care of the body. The Roman Catholic Church endorses the age-old adage "a sound mind in a sound body." For Muslims, one of the five essential principles on which religious law is based is protection of the integrity of the individual. In Judaism, people are urged to "choose life" and to choose whatever strengthens the capacity to live. Buddhists believe that the body doesn't belong to the person at all—even suicide is considered murder—and a person must do nothing to harm it.

Most religions also contend that dependence and addiction run counter to ideas of freedom, choice, and human dignity. Buddhism teaches a path of freedom—a way of life without dependence on anything. Hindus regard tobacco use as a dependence that is not necessary for the preservation of health. Protestant churches caution that any form of dependence is contrary to the notion of Christian freedom.

Another argument against tobacco use is the immorality of imposing second-hand smoke on non-smokers, which is seen as inflicting harm on others. In Hinduism, harming others is sinful. In the Jewish tradition, those who force non-smokers to breathe smoke jeopardize the lives of others, and to do so is to jeopardize the whole universe.

The Role of Individual Responsibility

Most religions focus on the role of individual responsibility in overcoming dependence on tobacco. In Buddhism, for example, people must assume responsibility for their habits; they practise introspection to understand the cause of problems within themselves and the effects of their actions on others. The principles of Islam are based on notions of responsibility and protection; you are responsible for your body and health.

Religion and Tobacco Control

Different religions share common views on how the problem of tobacco use should be approached. The Islamic view is that the campaign to control tobacco use must be based on awareness, responsibility, and justice. Developing awareness means providing information on the global problem. Fostering responsibility means helping people understand what they need to do to attain well-being. Emphasizing social and human justice means helping the farmers and societies that depend on tobacco cultivation to find alternative crops.

According to the Geneva Interreligious Platform (a project involving Hindus, Buddhists, Jews, Christians, Muslims, and Baha'is), the best approach is prevention. Here, the rights of non-smokers clearly prevail over the freedom of smokers. In support of this position, the common religious exhortation not to do unto others what you would not have them do unto you can be invoked. Further, adequate information should be provided to counter the deceptive images projected by tobacco industry advertising, especially where minors are concerned. Protection of the weak and denunciation of dishonesty are underlying values of all religious traditions.

Users undergo measurable changes in brain waves, heart rate, and blood pressure, and they perform poorly on tasks requiring sustained attention. Although most of these symptoms of physical dependence pass in two or three days, the craving associated with addiction persists. Many ex-smokers report intermittent, intense urges to smoke for years after quitting.

Social and Psychological Factors

Why do tobacco users have such a hard time quitting even when they want to? Social and psychological forces combine with physiological addiction to maintain the tobacco habit. Many people, for example, have established habits of smoking while doing something else—while talking, working, drinking, and so on. The spit tobacco habit is also associated with certain situations, such as studying, drinking coffee, or playing sports. It is difficult for people to break their habits because the activities they associate with tobacco use continue to trigger their urge. Such activities are called **secondary reinforcers**; they act together with the physiological addiction to keep the user dependent on tobacco.

> **secondary reinforcers**
> Stimuli that are not necessarily pleasurable in themselves but that are associated with other stimuli that are pleasurable.

QUICK STATS

Daily smokers in Canada smoked an average of 14.4 cigarettes per day.
—Propel, 2013

Genetic Factors

Inherited characteristics play an important role in some aspects of tobacco use. Genetic factors may be more important than social and environmental factors in smoking initiation and in the development of nicotine dependence.

For example, a gene that influences the way in which nicotine is metabolized, or broken down in the body, helps regulate the activity of an enzyme called CYP2A6. When people with slow CYP2A6 metabolism use tobacco, the nicotine remains in their blood longer than in people who have the gene for a faster metabolizing form of the enzyme. The slow metabolizers are more likely to feel nausea or dizziness when they first use tobacco, are less likely to continue smoking if they try it, and find it easier to quit if they do become regular smokers.

Scientists have also shown that a gene called *DRD2* (associated with the brain chemical dopamine, which plays a key role in the pleasurable effects of nicotine) appears to influence the progression of smoking in adolescence. Among students in Grade 10 who took one puff of a cigarette, those with one form of the gene were more than three times as likely as those with the other form to have become regular smokers when they finished Grade 11.

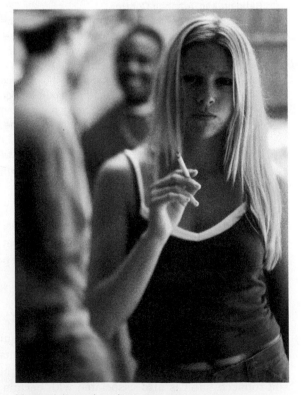

Why Start in the First Place?

By Grade 4, students are thinking about smoking, and by Grade 6, students are likely to start experimenting with smoking. Almost 85 percent of all smokers started smoking before they were 18 years old. Children—especially girls—are beginning to experiment with tobacco at ever-younger ages. The earlier people begin smoking, the more likely they are to become heavy smokers—and to die of tobacco-related disease.

Not all young people are equally vulnerable to the lure of tobacco. According to Health Canada's *Youth Smoking Survey*, fewer Canadian youth are starting to smoke and more are never smokers in recent years (see Figure 16.3). Research suggests that the more the following characteristics apply to a child or adolescent, the more likely he or she is to use tobacco:

- A parent or sibling uses tobacco.
- Peers use tobacco.
- The child comes from a blue-collar family.

Most adult smokers began as teenagers.

- The child comes from a low-income home.
- The family is headed by a single parent.
- The child performs poorly in school.
- The child drops out of school.
- The child has positive attitudes about tobacco use.

Young people start using tobacco for a variety of reasons. Some young, male athletes, for example, begin using spit tobacco to emulate their favourite professional athletes. Young women commonly take up smoking because they think it will help them lose weight or stay thin. Most often, however, young people start smoking simply because their peers are already doing it; smoking gives them a way to fit in with a crowd or to look cool. However, there is good news: If someone has not started smoking by age 20, this is a strong indication of future abstinence.

Rationalizing the Dangers

Making the decision to smoke requires minimizing or denying both the health risks of tobacco use and the tremendous pain, disability, emotional trauma, family stress, and financial expense involved in tobacco-related diseases, such as cancer and emphysema. A sense of invincibility, characteristic of many adolescents and young adults, also contributes to the decision to use tobacco. Young people may persuade themselves they are too intelligent, too lucky, or too healthy to be vulnerable to tobacco's dangers. "I'm not dumb enough to get hooked," they may argue. "I'll be able to quit before I do myself any real harm."

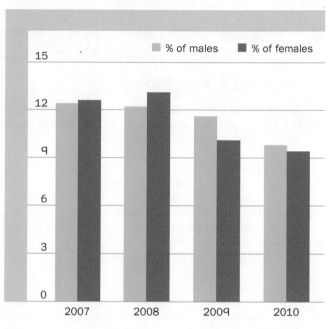

FIGURE 16.3

Daily or Occasional Smokers among Children and Youth in Canada, 2007–2010

Note: Population ages 12 to 19 years

Source: Statistics Canada, CANSIM table 105-0501, http://www.statcan.gc.ca/pub/11-402-x/2012000/chap/c-e/tbl/tbl09-eng.htm.

Many teenagers believe they will be able to stop smoking when they want. In fact, adolescents are more vulnerable to nicotine than are older tobacco users. Compared with older smokers, adolescents become heavy smokers and develop dependence after fewer cigarettes. Nicotine addiction can start within a few days of smoking and after just a few cigarettes. More than half of teenagers who try cigarettes progress to daily use, and about half of those who ever smoke daily progress to nicotine dependence. In surveys, about 70 percent of smoking teens state they wish they had never started. Another survey revealed that a majority high school smokers predicted they would quit at the end of high school or college/university; however, close to 75 percent were smoking seven to nine years later.

Emulating Smoking in the Media

Researchers have found that smoking in movies has increased significantly since 1990, to levels not seen since 1960. Historically, between 1998 and 2000, smoking in PG-13 movies increased by 50 percent. Half the tobacco shots in the top movies from 2002 to 2003 were in G, PG, and PG-13 movies. The World Health Organization (WHO), U.S. Center for Disease Control, and other leading health and public health authorities are pushing an adult rating policy for any movie with tobacco contact. However, progress is slow. The Ontario Film Review Board recorded tobacco use in 52 of the 69 movies released in 2012, and noted an adult rating was inconsistently applied in the content advisories, with only 5 of 16 movies with 50+ tobacco incidents being assigned an advisory.

The portrayal of smoking in films does not reflect Canadian patterns of tobacco use. The prevalence of smoking among lead characters is three to four times that among comparable Canadians. Films typically show the smoker as white, male, well educated, successful, and attractive. In reality, smokers tend to be poor and to have less education. In the top-grossing films in the early 2000s, smoking was portrayed in more than

73 percent of the films, including 82 percent of PG-13 films; smoking was often shown positively as a means to relieve tension or as something to do while socializing. Negative consequences resulting from tobacco use were depicted for only 3 percent of the major characters who used tobacco. By showing smoking in an unrealistically positive light, films may be acting as advertisement (see the Critical Consumer box).

 Critical CONSUMER

Tobacco Advertising

Advertising is a powerful influence. In 2012, the tobacco industry spent more than $8.37 billion on advertising that portrayed users as confident, popular, fit, and sexually attractive. That same year, approximately 37 000 people died from tobacco-related causes.

Youth Appeal

Young people were a prime target of tobacco ads because nicotine addiction can lead to a lifetime of purchasing tobacco. The tobacco industry also understood that young smokers are most likely to buy familiar brands. The most heavily advertised cigarettes were the choice of 90 percent of teen smokers. In the 1980s and 1990s, for example, R.J. Reynolds Tobacco Company's promotion of the Camel brand recruited millions of new smokers. In surveys, more than 90 percent of six-year-olds recognized the Camel character ("Joe Camel"), who became as familiar to children as Mickey Mouse.

Limits on Ads

In Canada, tobacco companies must adhere to the Canadian Tobacco Act (enacted October 1, 2003), which regulates the manufacturing, sale, labelling, and promotion of tobacco products. The act specifically prohibits the following:

- Testimonials in favour of tobacco use
- Displaying cigarettes on the shelves in stores
- Brand stretching to products and services associated with young people
- All forms of promotion except those explicitly stated in the act, which include the following:
  - A mailed publication addressed to an adult who is identified by name
  - A publication with an adult readership of not less than 85 percent
  - Signage in locations where young persons are not permitted by law

Regardless, the tobacco industry continues to spend millions of dollars annually to promote its product. Much of this money is spent on print ads and coupons, but a great deal is also given to retailers to help offset ever-increasing taxes levied on tobacco products by provinces and territories.

Does smoking on-screen affect real-life smoking habits? Studies of adolescents have consistently found a strong association between seeing tobacco use in films and trying cigarettes. Adolescents who see more smoking in films or whose favourite movie stars frequently use tobacco on-screen have more positive attitudes about smoking and are as much as three times as likely to have tried smoking as teens with less exposure to films. Teens may be particularly sensitive to on-screen portrayals of smoking because they are in the process of developing adult identities; during this period, they may try out different personas, including those of their favourite movie stars.

Some groups suggest an automatic R rating for any film that shows tobacco use, equating smoking with violence, strong language, sexuality, and nudity in determining a film's rating.

QUICK STATS

In 2012, 53% of smokers identified themselves as light smokers.

—Statistics Canada, 2012

QUESTIONS FOR CRITICAL THINKING AND REFLECTION

What has influenced your decision to smoke, not to smoke, or to quit smoking? Have you ever felt that images or messages in the media were encouraging you to use tobacco? How do you react to such messages?

Health Hazards

Tobacco adversely affects nearly every part of the body, including the brain, stomach, mouth, and reproductive organs.

Tobacco Smoke: A Toxic Mix

Tobacco smoke contains hundreds of damaging chemical substances, including acetone (nail polish remover), ammonia, hexamine (lighter fluid), and toluene (industrial solvent). Smoke from a typical unfiltered cigarette contains about 5 billion particles per cubic millimetre—50 000 times as many as are found in an equal volume of smoggy urban air. These particles, when condensed, form a brown, sticky mass called **cigarette tar**.

> **cigarette tar**
> A brown, sticky mass created when the chemical particles in tobacco smoke condense.

Carcinogens and Poisons

At least 43 chemicals in tobacco smoke are linked to the development of cancer. Some, such as benzo(a)-pyrene and urethane, are **carcinogens** and directly cause cancer. Other chemicals, such as formaldehyde, are **cocarcinogens**. They do not themselves cause cancer, but combine with other chemicals to stimulate the growth of certain cancers, at least in laboratory animals. Other substances in tobacco cause health problems because they damage the lining of the respiratory tract or decrease the lungs' ability to fight off infection.

> **carcinogen**
> Any substance that causes cancer.
>
> **cocarcinogen**
> A substance that works with a carcinogen to cause cancer.

Tobacco also contains poisonous substances, including arsenic and hydrogen cyanide. In addition to being an addictive psychoactive drug, nicotine is a poison and can be fatal in high doses. Many cases of nicotine poisoning occur each year in toddlers and infants who pick up and eat cigarette butts they find at home or on the playground.

Cigarette smoke contains carbon monoxide, the deadly gas in automobile exhaust, in concentrations 400 times as high as is considered safe in industrial workplaces. Not surprisingly, smokers often complain of breathlessness when they require a burst of energy to climb stairs or lift something. Carbon monoxide displaces oxygen in red blood cells, depleting the body's supply of oxygen needed for extra work. Carbon monoxide also impairs visual acuity, especially at night.

QUICK STATS

Nicotine levels increased more than 1% per year in major cigarette brands from 1998 to 2005. Cigarettes today deliver higher levels of nicotine, with 1.65 mg/cig in 1999 compared to 1.89 mg/cig in 2011.

—Harvard School of Public Health, 2007; Li, 2013

Additives

Tobacco manufacturers use additives to manipulate the taste and effect of cigarettes and other tobacco products. Additives account for roughly 10 percent, by weight, of a cigarette, and include sugars and other flavouring agents, humectants (compounds that keep tobacco from drying out), and chemicals that enhance the addicting properties of nicotine.

Added sugars—including liquorice, cocoa, and honey—have a dual role. As flavour enhancers, sugars mask the harsh, bitter taste of tobacco so smokers can inhale more smoke and absorb more nicotine. When sugars burn, they produce acetaldehyde, a chemical that enhances the addictive effect of nicotine and is a carcinogen. Other flavour components, such as the obromine and glycyrrhizin, act as bronchodilators, opening the lungs' airways and making it easier for nicotine to get into the bloodstream.

Ammonia plays a complex role in tobacco products, but its chief purpose is to boost the amount of addictive nicotine delivered by cigarettes. Ammonia reduces the acidity of tobacco smoke and releases nicotine in the form of a base (alkaline) rather than a salt (acid) bound to other acid components of smoke. As a free base, nicotine is more readily absorbed into the blood.

Some additives are intended to make **sidestream smoke** (the uninhaled smoke from a burning cigarette) less obvious and objectionable. For example, potassium citrate, aluminum, and clay are added to cigarette wrappers to convert particulate ash into an invisible gas with less irritating odour than would be given off by a conventional paper wrapper. These additives serve no purpose in making cigarettes more desirable and addicting to the smoker; instead, they are intended to reduce social pressures from non-smokers.

sidestream smoke
The uninhaled smoke from a burning cigarette.

Nearly 600 chemicals, approved as safe when used as food additives, are used in manufacturing cigarettes. Canada is a world leader in cigarette testing. In 1998, British Columbia became the first jurisdiction to successfully demand disclosure of the chemicals in cigarette smoke from tobacco companies. Canadian tobacco manufacturers now must disclose all additives in their products.

The Results of Inhaling Tobacco Smoke

All smokers absorb some gases, tar, and nicotine from cigarette smoke, but smokers who inhale bring most of these substances into their bodies and keep them there. In one year, a typical pack-a-day smoker takes in 50 000 to 70 000 puffs. Smoke from a cigarette, pipe, or cigar directly assaults the mouth, throat, and respiratory tract. The nose, which normally filters about 75 percent of foreign matter we breathe, is completely bypassed.

In a cigarette, the unburned tobacco itself acts as a filter. As a cigarette burns down, there is less and less filter. Thus, more chemicals are absorbed into the body during the last third of a cigarette than during the first. A smoker can cut down on the absorption of harmful chemicals by not smoking cigarettes down to short butts. Any gains, of course, will be offset by smoking more cigarettes, inhaling more deeply, or puffing more frequently.

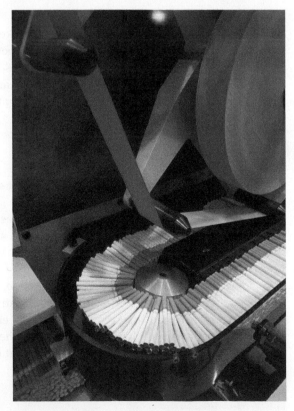

Cigarette making is an elaborate process involving industrial machinery and chemistry. Dozens of compounds may be added to tobacco to produce a specific brand of cigarette.

"Light" and Low-tar Cigarettes

Some smokers switch to low-tar, low-nicotine, or filtered cigarettes because they believe them to be healthier alternatives. But there is no such thing as a safe cigarette, and smoking behaviour is a more important factor in tar and nicotine intake than the type of cigarette smoked. Smokers who switch to a low-nicotine brand often compensate by smoking more cigarettes, inhaling more deeply, taking larger or more frequent puffs, or blocking ventilation holes with lips or fingers to offset the effects of filters.

Studies have found that people who smoke "light" cigarettes inhale up to eight times as much tar and nicotine as printed on the label. Studies also show that smokers of light cigarettes are less likely to quit than smokers of regular cigarettes, probably because of the misperception that light cigarettes are safer. Use of light and low-tar cigarettes does not reduce the risk of smoking-related illnesses.

Menthol Cigarettes

Concerns have also been raised about menthol cigarettes. Menthol is a bronchodilator; as mentioned earlier, bronchodilators open the lungs' airways and make it easier for nicotine to enter the bloodstream. Younger smokers are using more menthol cigarettes than are older smokers. Studies have found that 44 percent of current smokers ages 12–17 years have tried menthol cigarettes, compared with 31 percent of smokers ages 18 and older. The anaesthetizing effect of menthol, which may allow smokers to inhale more deeply and hold smoke in their lungs for longer, may be partly responsible for these differences. Research is needed to determine the relationship between menthol cigarettes and illnesses, such as cancer and cardiovascular disease.

The Immediate Effects of Smoking

The beginning smoker often has symptoms of mild nicotine poisoning: dizziness; faintness; rapid pulse; cold, clammy skin; and sometimes nausea, vomiting, and diarrhea. The seasoned smoker occasionally suffers these effects of nicotine poisoning, particularly after quitting and then returning to a previous level of consumption. The effects of nicotine on smokers vary, depending greatly on the size of the nicotine dose and how much tolerance previous smoking has built up. Nicotine can either excite or tranquilize the nervous system, depending on dosage.

Nicotine has many other immediate effects, as shown in Figure 16.4. It stimulates the part of the brain called the **cerebral cortex**. It also stimulates the adrenal glands to discharge adrenaline. Nicotine inhibits the formation of urine; constricts the blood vessels, especially in the skin; accelerates the heart rate; and elevates blood pressure. Higher blood pressure, faster heart rate, and constricted blood vessels require the heart to pump more blood. In healthy people, the heart can usually meet this demand, but in people whose coronary arteries are damaged enough to interfere with the flow of blood, the heart muscle may be strained.

cerebral cortex
The outer layer of the brain, which controls complex behaviour and mental activity.

Smoking depresses hunger contractions and dulls the taste buds; smokers who quit often notice that food tastes much better. Smoking is not useful for weight loss, however. Smoking for decades may lessen or prevent age-associated weight gain for some smokers, but for people under 30, smoking is not associated with weight loss.

The Long-term Effects of Smoking

Smoking is linked to many deadly and disabling diseases. Research indicates that the total amount of tobacco smoke inhaled is a key factor contributing to disease. People who smoke more cigarettes per day, inhale

FIGURE 16.4

The Short-term Effects of Smoking a Cigarette

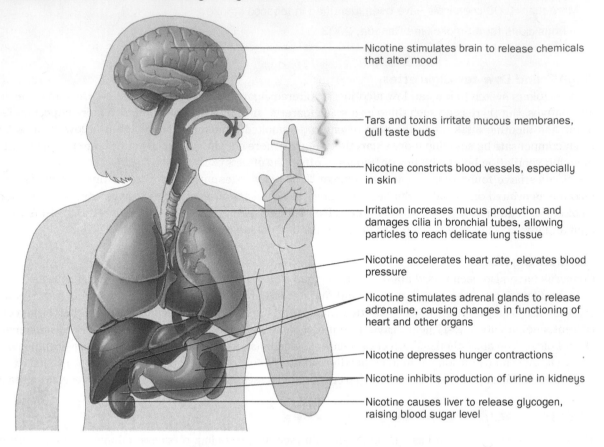

Nicotine stimulates brain to release chemicals that alter mood

Tars and toxins irritate mucous membranes, dull taste buds

Nicotine constricts blood vessels, especially in skin

Irritation increases mucus production and damages cilia in bronchial tubes, allowing particles to reach delicate lung tissue

Nicotine accelerates heart rate, elevates blood pressure

Nicotine stimulates adrenal glands to release adrenaline, causing changes in functioning of heart and other organs

Nicotine depresses hunger contractions

Nicotine inhibits production of urine in kidneys

Nicotine causes liver to release glycogen, raising blood sugar level

deeply, puff frequently, smoke cigarettes down to the butts, or begin smoking at an early age run a greater risk of disease than do those who smoke more moderately or who do not smoke at all.

As more research is done, even more diseases associated with smoking are being uncovered. The costliest ones—to society as well as to the individual—are cardiovascular diseases; respiratory diseases, such as emphysema and lung cancer; and other cancers.

Cardiovascular Disease

Although lung cancer tends to receive the most publicity, one form of cardiovascular disease, coronary heart disease (CHD), is actually the most widespread single cause of death for cigarette smokers. CHD often results from atherosclerosis, a condition in which fatty deposits called plaques form on the inner walls of heart arteries, causing them to narrow and stiffen. Smoking and exposure to environmental tobacco smoke (ETS) permanently accelerate the rate of plaque accumulation in the coronary arteries—50 percent for smokers, 25 percent for ex-smokers, and 20 percent for people regularly exposed to ETS. The crushing chest pain of angina pectoris, a primary symptom of CHD, results when the heart muscle, or myocardium, does not get enough oxygen. Sometimes a plaque forms at a narrow point in a main coronary artery. If the plaque completely blocks the flow of blood to a portion of the heart, that portion may die. This type of heart attack is called a **myocardial infarction**.

myocardial infarction
A heart attack caused by the complete blockage of a main coronary artery.

CHD can also interfere with the heart's electrical activity, resulting in disturbances of the normal heart-beat rhythm. Sudden and unexpected death is a common result of CHD, particularly among smokers. (See Chapter 7 for a more extensive discussion of cardiovascular disease.)

Smokers have a death rate from CHD that is 70 percent higher than that of non-smokers. Deaths from CHD associated with cigarette smoking are most common in people ages 40–50. (In contrast, deaths from lung cancer caused by smoking are most likely to occur in 60–70-year-olds.) Among people *under* age 40, smokers are five times as likely as non-smokers to have a heart attack. Cigar and pipe smokers run a lower risk than cigarette smokers.

We do not completely understand how cigarette smoking increases the risk of CHD, but researchers are beginning to shed light on the process. Smoking reduces the amount of good cholesterol (high-density lipoprotein, or HDL) in the blood, and creates lesions or roughness in arterial walls, which promote plaque deposit. Smoking may also increase tension in heart muscle walls, speeding up the rate of muscular contraction and accelerating the heart rate. The workload of the heart thus increases, as does its need for oxygen and other nutrients. Carbon monoxide produced by cigarette smoking combines with hemoglobin in the red blood cells, displacing oxygen and thus providing less oxygen to the heart. One study showed that the additional blood supply available to the heart during stress was 21 percent less in smokers than in non-smokers. This reduced blood flow is an early indicator of future heart attacks or strokes.

The risks of CHD decrease rapidly when a person stops smoking; this is particularly true for younger smokers, whose coronary arteries have not yet been extensively damaged.

Lung Cancer and Other Cancers

Cigarette smoking is the primary cause of lung cancer (see Figure 16.5). A recent study identified the precise mechanism: Benzo(a)pyrene, a chemical found in tobacco smoke, causes genetic mutations in lung cells that are identical to those found in many patients with lung cancer. Those who smoke two or more packs of cigarettes a day have lung cancer death rates 12–25 times the rates of non-smokers. The dramatic rise in lung cancer rates among women in the past 40 years clearly parallels the increase of smoking in this group; lung cancer now exceeds breast cancer as the leading cause of cancer deaths among women. The risk of developing lung cancer increases with the number of cigarettes smoked each day, the number of years of smoking, and the age at which the person started smoking.

QUICK STATS

85% of lung cancer deaths are attributable to smoking.
—Canadian Cancer Society, 2012

Cigarette smoking has been linked to other cardiovascular diseases, including the following:

- *Stroke*, a sudden interference with the circulation of blood in a part of the brain, resulting in the destruction of brain cells
- *Aortic aneurysm*, a bulge in the aorta caused by a weakening in its walls
- *Pulmonary heart disease*, a disorder of the right side of the heart, caused by changes in the blood vessels of the lungs

Although cigar and pipe smokers have a higher risk of lung cancer than non-smokers do, the risk is lower than that for cigarette smokers. Smoking filter-tipped cigarettes slightly reduces health hazards, unless the smoker compensates by smoking more, as is often the case.

Evidence suggests that after one year without smoking, the risk of lung cancer decreases substantially. After 10 years, the risk of lung cancer among ex-smokers is 50 percent lower than that of continuing smokers.

FIGURE 16.5

Estimated Canadian Lung Cancer Statistics, 2014

Category	Males	Females
New cases	13 400	12 700
Incidence rate (for every 100 000 people)*	59	48
Deaths	10 800	9 700
Death rate (for every 100 000 people)*	47	36
5-year relative survival (estimates for 2006–2008)	14 percent	20 percent

*Age-standardized to the 1991 Canadian Standard Population. Age-standardization is a statistical method that removes the effect of age on the calculated rate. It allows rates to be compared over time or across provinces and territories.

Source: Canadian Cancer Society. *Lung Cancer Statistics,* http://www.cancer.ca/en/cancer-information/cancer-type/lung/statistics/?region=on.

Research has also linked smoking to cancers of the trachea, mouth, pharynx, esophagus, larynx, pancreas, bladder, kidney, breast, cervix, stomach, liver, colon, and skin. For more information on cancer, see Chapter 8.

Chronic Obstructive Pulmonary Disease

The lungs of a smoker are constantly exposed to dangerous chemicals and irritants, and they must work harder to function adequately. The stresses placed on the lungs by smoking can permanently damage lung function and lead to *chronic obstructive pulmonary disease (COPD)*, also known as chronic obstructive lung disease (COLD), or chronic lower respiratory disease. COPD is the fourth leading cause of death in Canada. This progressive and disabling disorder consists of several different but related diseases; emphysema and chronic bronchitis are two of the most common.

Cigarette smokers are up to 18 times as likely as non-smokers to die from emphysema and chronic bronchitis. (Pipe and cigar smokers are more likely to die from COPD than are non-smokers, but they have a smaller risk than cigarette smokers.) A 2012 study estimated that 4 percent of the Canadian population has COPD. The risk rises with the number of cigarettes smoked and falls when smoking ceases. In 80–90 percent of COPD cases in Canada, cigarette smoking is the main cause; however, air pollution also plays a role and exposure to both is more dangerous than exposure to either by itself.

EMPHYSEMA Smoking is the primary cause of **emphysema**, a disabling condition in which the walls of the lungs' air sacs lose their elasticity and are gradually destroyed. The lungs' ability to obtain oxygen and remove carbon dioxide is impaired. A person with emphysema is breathless, is constantly gasping for air, and has the feeling of drowning. The heart must pump harder and may become enlarged. People with emphysema often die from a damaged heart. There is no known way to reverse this disease. In its advanced stage, the person is bedridden and severely disabled.

> **emphysema**
> A disease characterized by a loss of lung tissue elasticity and breakup of the air sacs, impairing the lungs' ability to obtain oxygen and remove carbon dioxide.

CHRONIC BRONCHITIS Persistent, recurrent inflammation of the bronchial tubes characterizes **chronic bronchitis**. When the cell lining of the bronchial tubes is irritated, it secretes excess mucus. Bronchial congestion is followed by a chronic cough, which makes breathing more and more difficult. If smokers have chronic bronchitis, they face a greater risk of lung cancer, no matter how old they are or how many cigarettes they smoke. Chronic bronchitis seems to be a shortcut to lung cancer.

> **chronic bronchitis**
> Recurrent, persistent inflammation of the bronchial tubes.

Other Respiratory Damage

Even when the smoker shows no signs of lung impairment or disease, cigarette smoking damages the respiratory system. Normally the cells lining the bronchial tubes secrete mucus, a sticky fluid that collects particles of soot, dust, and other substances in inhaled air. Mucus is carried up to the mouth by the continuous motion of the cilia, hairlike structures that protrude from the inner surface of the bronchial tubes (see Figure 16.6). If the cilia are destroyed or impaired, or if the pollution of inhaled air is more than the system can remove, the protection provided by cilia is lost.

Cigarette smoke first slows and then stops the action of the cilia. Eventually it destroys them, leaving delicate membranes exposed to injury from substances inhaled in cigarette smoke or from the polluted air in which the person lives or works. Special cells, called *macrophages*, a type of white blood cell, also work to remove foreign particles from the respiratory tract by engulfing them. Smoking appears to make macrophages work less efficiently. This interference with the functioning of the respiratory system often leads rapidly to the conditions known as smoker's throat and smoker's cough, as well as to shortness of breath. Even smokers of high school age show impaired respiratory function when compared with non-smokers of the same age. Other respiratory effects of smoking include a worsening of allergy and asthma symptoms and an increase in the smoker's susceptibility to colds.

Although cigarette smoking can cause many respiratory disorders and diseases, the damage is not always permanent. Once a person stops smoking, steady improvement in overall lung function usually takes place. Chronic coughing subsides, mucus production returns to normal, and breathing becomes easier. The likelihood of lung disease drops sharply. People of all ages, even those who have been smoking for decades, improve after they stop smoking.

Additional Health, Cosmetic, and Economic Concerns

Smoking has many effects and plays a role in the following health, aesthetic, and economic problems:

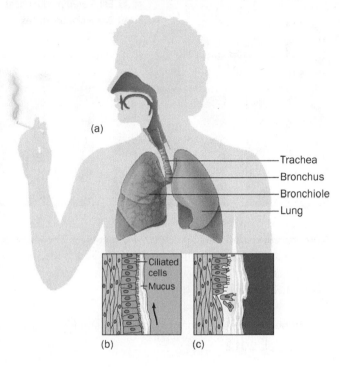

FIGURE 16.6

Damage to the Lungs Caused by Smoking

(**a**) The respiratory system. (**b**) The inside of a bronchiole of a non-smoker. (**c**) The inside of a bronchiole of a smoker.

Trachea
Bronchus
Bronchiole
Lung

Ciliated cells
Mucus

(b)   (c)

- *Ulcers:* People who smoke are more likely to develop peptic ulcers and are more likely to die from them (especially stomach ulcers) because smoking impairs the body's healing ability. Smoking also increases the risk of gastroesophageal reflux, which causes heartburn and can, if severe, raise the risk of esophageal cancer.
- *Impotence:* Smoking affects blood flow in the veins and arteries of the penis, and it is an independent risk factor for impotence. In one recent study, smokers were twice as likely as non-smokers to experience erectile dysfunction (impotence).
- *Reproductive health problems:* Smoking is linked to reduced fertility in both men and women. A study of 18-year-old men who smoked found that they had a significantly higher proportion of abnormally shaped sperm and sperm with genetic defects than non-smokers. In women, smoking can contribute to menstrual disorders, early menopause, and complications of pregnancy.
- *Dental diseases:* Smokers are at increased risk for tooth decay and gum and periodontal diseases, with symptoms appearing by the mid-20s.
- *Diminished physical senses:* Smoking dulls the senses of taste and smell. Over time, it increases the risk for hearing loss, and for macular degeneration and cataracts (both serious eye conditions that can result in partial or total blindness; see Chapter 17).
- *Injuries:* Smokers have higher rates of motor vehicle crashes, fire-related injuries, and back pain.
- *Cosmetic concerns:* Smoking can cause premature skin wrinkling, premature baldness, stained teeth, discoloured fingers, and a persistent tobacco odour in the smoker's clothes and hair.
- *Economic costs:* In 2012, the average per-pack price of cigarettes was between $8 and $12 dollars. A pack-a-day habit costs approximately $3600 each year for cigarettes alone. In Canada, $21.03 of the cost per 200 cigarettes is federal excise tax and anywhere from $25 to $58 is provincial excise tax. Then GST/PST or HST is added to the cost (for a costing breakdown of cigarettes, see Figure 16.7).

In addition, smoking contributes to osteoporosis, increases the risk of complications from diabetes, and accelerates the course of multiple sclerosis. Further research may link tobacco use to still other disorders.

FIGURE 16.7

Taxes on Cigarettes in Canadian Jurisdictions

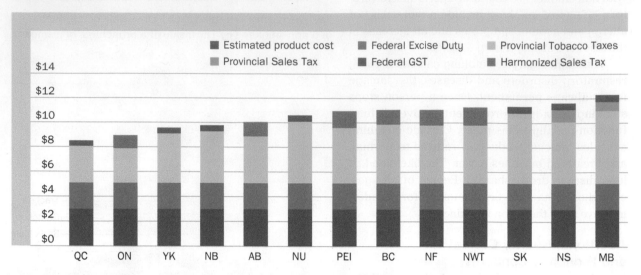

■ Estimated product cost　　■ Federal Excise Duty　　■ Provincial Tobacco Taxes
■ Provincial Sales Tax　　■ Federal GST　　■ Harmonized Sales Tax

Source: Physicians for a Smoke-Free Canada, http://www.smoke-free.ca/factsheets/pdf/taxrates.pdf.

QUICK STATS

The health-related economic costs of smoking are $17 billion annually.
—Propel, 2012

Cumulative Effects

The cumulative effects of tobacco use fall into two general categories. The first category is reduced life expectancy. A male who takes up smoking before age 15 and continues to smoke is only half as likely to live to age 75 as a male who never smokes. Females who have similar smoking habits also have a reduced life expectancy. The second category involves quality of life. A long-term study shows that smokers take an average of eight additional sick days away from their jobs because of illness than non-smokers. Female smokers spend 17 percent more days sick in bed than female non-smokers. Lost workdays because of smoking number in the millions.

Both men and women smokers show a greater rate of acute and chronic disease than people who have never smoked (see the Gender Matters box). Smokers become disabled at younger ages than non-smokers and have more years of unhealthy life as well as a shorter life-span. In Canada, it is estimated 1 person in 20 has chronic bronchitis; smoking accounts for 90 percent of those cases.

 Gender MATTERS

Gender and Tobacco Use

Canadian men are currently more likely than women to smoke, but women younger than age 17 are becoming smokers at a faster rate than any other population segment. As the rate of smoking among women approaches that of men, so do rates of tobacco-related illness and death. More Canadians women now die each year from lung cancer than from breast cancer.

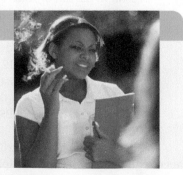

Although overall risks of tobacco-related illness are similar for women and men, gender appears to make a difference in some diseases. Women, for example, are more at risk for smoking-related blood clots and strokes than are men, and the risk is even greater for women who use oral contraceptives. Among men and women with the same smoking history, the odds for developing three major types of cancer, including lung cancer, is 1.2–1.7 times as high in women as in men. Women may also have a greater biological vulnerability to lung cancer.

For both men and women, tobacco use is associated with increased incidence of sex-specific health problems. Men who smoke increase their risk of erectile dysfunction and infertility because of reduced sperm density and motility. Women who smoke also have risks associated with reproduction and the reproductive organs. Smoking is associated with greater menstrual bleeding, greater duration of painful menstrual cramps, and more variability in menstrual cycle length. Smokers have a more difficult time becoming pregnant, and they reach menopause on average a year or two earlier than non-smokers. When female smokers become pregnant, they face increased chances of miscarriage or placental disorders that lead to bleeding and premature delivery; rates of ectopic pregnancy, preeclampsia, and stillbirth are also higher among women who smoke. Smoking is a risk factor for cervical cancer. Women who smoke also have higher rates of osteoporosis (a bone-thinning disease that can lead to fractures), thyroid-related diseases, and depression.

When women decide to try to stop smoking, they are more likely than men to join a support group. Overall, though, women are less successful than men in quitting. Women report more severe withdrawal symptoms when they stop smoking and are more likely than men to report cravings in response to social and behavioural cues associated with smoking. For men, relapse to smoking is often associated with work or social pressure, while women are more likely to relapse when sad or depressed or concerned about weight gain. Women and men also respond differently to medications: Nicotine replacement therapy appears to work better for men, whereas the non-nicotine medication bupropion appears to work better for women.

Other Forms of Tobacco Use

Many smokers have switched from cigarettes to other forms of tobacco, such as spit (smokeless) tobacco, cigars, cigarillos, and pipes, and clove cigarettes and bidis. These alternatives, however, are far from safe. Among students and teenagers, cigarillos (little cigars) were the most popular tobacco product after cigarettes. Figure 16.8 shows the percentage of individuals who reported using flavoured tobacco products in the last 30 days.

Spit (Smokeless) Tobacco

Spit tobacco use has increased in recent years and is especially common among Aboriginal and rural Canadians, adolescent males, and male athletes. Geographically, use of spit tobacco is higher in the Prairies than in other parts of Canada. About 17 percent of Canadians will experiment with spit tobacco some time in their life.

FIGURE 16.8

Percentage of Adults who Use Flavoured Tobacco Products, by Product Type, 2011 and 2012

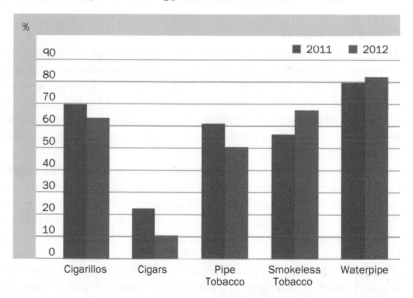

Data sources: Canadian Tobacco Use Monitoring Survey, 2011; Canadian Tobacco Use Monitoring Survey, 2012.

Graph source: Tobacco Use in Canada: Patterns and Trends. Special Supplement: Flavoured Tobacco Use. 2014 Edition. Propel Centre for Population Health Impact, http://tobaccoreport.ca/2014/TobaccoUseinCanada_2014_FlavourSupplement.pdf.

Spit tobacco comes in two major forms: snuff and chewing tobacco (chew). In snuff, the tobacco leaf is processed into a coarse, moist powder and mixed with flavourings. Snuff is usually sold in small tins. Users place a "pinch," "dip," or "quid" between the lower lip or cheek and gum and suck on it. In chewing tobacco, the tobacco leaf may be shredded ("leaf"), pressed into bricks or cakes ("plugs"), or dried and twisted into ropelike strands ("twists"). Chew is usually sold in pouches. Users place a wad of tobacco in their mouth and then chew or suck it to release the nicotine. All types of smokeless tobacco cause an increase in saliva production, and the resulting tobacco juice is spit out or swallowed. A recent innovation in smokeless tobacco, called *snus*, comes in a tiny pouch that is placed between the lip and gum. Snus does not require the user to spit, as do other forms of smokeless tobacco.

The nicotine in spit tobacco—along with flavourings and additives—is absorbed through the gums and lining of the mouth. Holding an average-size dip in the mouth for 30 minutes delivers about the same amount of nicotine as two or three cigarettes. Because of its nicotine content, spit tobacco is highly addictive. Some users keep it in their mouth even while sleeping.

Although not as dangerous as smoking cigarettes, the use of spit tobacco carries many health risks. Changes can occur in the mouth after only a few weeks of use. Gums and lips become dried and irritated and may bleed. White or red patches may appear inside the mouth; this condition, known as *leukoplakia*, can lead to oral cancer. About 25 percent of regular spit tobacco users have *gingivitis* (inflammation), recession of the gums, and bone loss around the teeth, especially where the tobacco is usually placed. The senses of taste and smell are usually dulled. In addition, other people find the presence of wads of tobacco in the mouth, stained teeth, bad breath, and behaviours, such as frequent spitting, to be unpleasant.

One of the most serious effects of spit tobacco is an increased risk of oral cancer—cancers of the lip, tongue, cheek, throat, gums, roof and floor of the mouth, and larynx. Spit tobacco contains at least 28 chemicals known to cause cancer, and long-term snuff use may increase the risk of oral cancer by as much as 50 times. Surgery to treat oral cancer is often disfiguring and may involve removing parts of the face, tongue, cheek, or lip.

Dipping and chewing tobacco produce blood levels of nicotine similar to those in cigarette smokers. Other chemicals in spit tobacco are believed to pose risks to developing fetuses.

Cigars and Pipes

After decades of decline, in 2012 cigar smoking rates were double those in the 1990s. The popularity of cigars is highest among white males ages 25–44 with higher-than-average income and education, but women are also smoking cigars in record numbers. Cigar use is also growing among young people: In government surveys, 4 percent of Canadians 15 years and older reported having smoked at least one cigar in the previous month. Moreover, 10 percent of Canadians 15 years and older, mostly males who also smoke cigarettes, are water-pipe smokers. Of water-pipe smokers, 27 percent erroneously believe that water-pipe smoking is less harmful than cigarettes.

Cigars are made from rolled whole tobacco leaves; pipe tobacco is made from shredded leaves and often flavoured. Because cigar and pipe smoke are more alkaline than cigarette smoke, users of cigars and pipes do not need to inhale to ingest nicotine; instead, they absorb nicotine through the gums and lining of the mouth. Cigars contain more tobacco than cigarettes and so contain more nicotine and produce more tar when smoked. Large cigars may contain as much tobacco as a whole pack of cigarettes and take one to two hours to smoke.

The smoke from cigars contains many of the same toxins and carcinogens as the smoke from cigarettes, some in much higher quantities. The health risks of cigars depend on the number of cigars smoked and whether the smoker inhales. Because most cigar and pipe users do not inhale, they have a lower risk of cancer and cardiovascular and respiratory diseases than cigarette smokers. However, their risks are substantially higher than those of non-smokers. For example, compared with non-smokers, people who smoke one or two cigars per day without inhaling have six times the risk of cancer of the larynx. The risks are much higher for cigar smokers who inhale: They have 27 times the risk of oral cancer and 53 times the risk of cancer of the larynx compared with non-smokers, and their risk of heart and lung diseases approaches that of cigarette smokers. Smoking a cigar immediately impairs the ability of blood vessels to dilate, reducing the amount of oxygen delivered to tissues, including the heart muscle, especially during times of stress. Pipe and cigar smoking are also risk factors for pancreatic cancer, which is almost always fatal.

Nicotine addiction is another concern. Most adults who smoke cigars do so only occasionally, and there is little evidence that suggests that use of cigars by adults leads to addiction. The recent rise in cigar use among young adults has raised concerns, however, because nicotine addiction almost always develops in the teen or young adult years. More research is needed to determine if cigar use by teens will develop into nicotine addiction and frequent use of either cigarettes or spit tobacco. In July 2000, the Canadian government announced an agreement to put warning labels on cigar packages, 34 years after warning labels first appeared on cigarette packages.

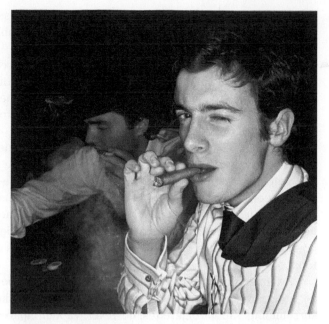

Occasional cigar smoking may be more likely to lead to nicotine addiction in teens than in adults.

QUESTIONS FOR CRITICAL THINKING AND REFLECTION

Do you know anyone who has had an illness related to tobacco use? If so, what problems did that person face? What was the outcome? Did the experience have any effect on your views about using tobacco?

Clove Cigarettes and Bidis

Clove cigarettes, also called *kreteks* or *chicartas*, are made of tobacco mixed with chopped cloves; they are imported primarily from Indonesia and Pakistan. Clove cigarettes contain almost twice as much tar, nicotine, and carbon monoxide as conventional cigarettes and so have all the same health hazards. Some chemical constituents of cloves may also be dangerous. For example, eugenol, an anaesthetic compound found in cloves, may impair the respiratory system's ability to detect and defend against foreign particles. A number of serious respiratory injuries and deaths have resulted from the use of clove cigarettes.

Bidis, or *beadies*, are small cigarettes imported from India that contain species of tobacco different from those used by North American cigarette manufacturers. The tobacco in bidis is hand-rolled in Indian ebony leaves (tendu) and then often flavoured; clove, mint, chocolate, and fruit varieties are available. Bidis contain up to four times as much nicotine and twice as much tar as North American cigarettes. Use of bidis has been growing among teens, possibly because of the flavourings they contain or because they look and smell somewhat like marijuana cigarettes (*joints*); they do not produce the same effects as marijuana, however.

An estimated 4 percent of Canadians have tried clove cigarettes or bidis. Neither is a safe or healthy alternative to conventional tobacco cigarettes.

E-Cigarettes

The electronic cigarette, also known as an *e-cig*, is a battery-powered device that resembles a real cigarette. Instead of containing tobacco, the device uses a changeable filter that contains one or more chemicals, such as nicotine, flavourings, and other compounds. The user "smokes" an e-cig by sucking the filtered end; the device's battery heats the chemicals to create an inhalable vapour. During use, the device's tip even glows like the burning end of a real cigarette.

Although electronic cigarettes have been advertised as a way to help smokers quit smoking, there has been no evidence submitted to Health Canada supporting this claim. No electronic smoking product has yet been authorized for sale in Canada. Some research in the United States by the FDA found that the vapour from electronic cigarettes contains carcinogens and other toxic chemicals, such as diethylene glycol, which is a toxic chemical found in antifreeze.

Marketers of e-cigs have claimed that the devices deliver only nicotine, making them a safe cigarette that does not cause cancer and can serve as an alternative to other nicotine replacement products such as gum and patches. According to the FDA, however, not all e-cigs actually contain nicotine. Further, the FDA has warned consumers not to purchase or use e-cigs because analysis of nearly 20 e-cig cartridges revealed that they contained carcinogens, including at least one of the same carcinogens found in real cigarettes. In issuing its warning, the FDA noted that some varieties of e-cigs are flavoured, apparently to make them appeal to youngsters and other first-time smokers. The products do not carry the same types of warnings required on tobacco products.

An emerging type of e-cigarettes that is gaining popularity is vapour cigarettes. Vapour cigarettes have been marketed in recent years as alternatives to traditional smoking devices. There is a lack of evidence surrounding vapour cigarettes; however, vapour cigarettes are typically marketed as a "safer" alternative to traditional smoking. One study that tested 12 different brands of vapour cigarettes for known carcinogens found toxin levels anywhere from 9 to 450 times lower than that of traditional cigarette smoke. Despite this decrease, research is still unclear on the safety of vapour cigarettes. More research into the health and long terms effects of vapour cigarettes is merited.

The Effects of Smoking on the Non-smoker

Tobacco users aren't the only ones who suffer ill effects from their habits. Tens of thousands of non-smokers die each year because of excess exposure to second-hand smoke. Further, the medical and societal costs of tobacco use are enormous.

Environmental Tobacco Smoke

Environmental tobacco smoke (ETS)—more commonly called second-hand smoke—has been designated a Class A carcinogen and is a known human carcinogen. These designations put ETS in the same category as notorious cancer-causing agents such as asbestos. No level of exposure to ETS is safe; even brief exposure can cause serious harm.

environmental tobacco smoke (ETS)
Smoke that enters the atmosphere from the burning end of a cigarette, cigar, or pipe, as well as smoke that is exhaled by smokers; also called *second-hand smoke*.

ETS consists of mainstream smoke and sidestream smoke. Smoke exhaled by smokers is referred to as **mainstream smoke**. Sidestream smoke enters the atmosphere from the burning end of a cigarette, cigar, or pipe. Nearly 85 percent of the smoke in a room where someone is smoking comes from sidestream smoke. Undiluted sidestream smoke, because it is not filtered through either a cigarette filter or a smoker's lungs, has twice as much tar and nicotine, three times as much benzo(a)pyrene, almost three times as much carbon monoxide, and three times as much ammonia.

mainstream smoke
Smoke that is inhaled by a smoker and then exhaled into the atmosphere.

In rooms where people are smoking, levels of carbon monoxide can exceed those deemed acceptable by the Canadian Environmental Protection Act for outside air. In a typical home with the windows closed, it takes about six hours for 95 percent of the airborne cigarette smoke particles to clear. The carcinogens in the second-hand smoke from a single cigar exceed that of three cigarettes, and cigar smoke contains up to 30 times as much carbon monoxide.

ETS Effects

Non-smokers subjected to ETS frequently develop coughs, headaches, nasal discomfort, and eye irritation. Other symptoms range from breathlessness to sinus problems. People with allergies tend to suffer the most (see the Take Charge box).

ETS causes 330 lung cancer deaths and about 2000 deaths from heart disease each year in people who do not smoke. As described earlier, exposure to ETS is associated with a 20 percent increase in the progression of atherosclerosis. ETS also aggravates asthma and increases the risk for breast and cervical cancers.

Scientists have been able to measure changes that contribute to lung tissue damage and potential tumour promotion in the bloodstreams of healthy young test subjects who spend just three hours in a smoke-filled room. After just 30 minutes of exposure to ETS, the function in the coronary arteries of healthy non-smokers is reduced to the same level as that of smokers. And non-smokers can still be affected by the harmful effects of ETS hours after they have left a smoky environment. Carbon monoxide, for example, lingers in the bloodstream five hours later.

Take CHARGE

Avoiding ETS

Given the health risks of exposure to ETS, try these strategies to keep the air around you safe:

- *Speak up tactfully.* Smokers may not know the dangers they are causing or may not know it bothers you.
- *Display reminders.* Put up signs asking smokers to refrain in your home, work area, and car.
- *Don't allow smoking in your home or room.* Get rid of ashtrays and ask smokers to light up outside.
- *Open a window.* If you cannot avoid being in a room with a smoker, at least try to provide some ventilation.
- *Discuss quitting strategies.* Social pressure is a major factor in many former smokers' decisions to quit. Help the smokers in your life by sharing quitting strategies with them.

Infants, Children, and ETS

Recent studies have found three times as many infants die from sudden infant death syndrome (SIDS) related to second-hand smoke as from child abuse or homicide. Children under five years of age whose primary caregiver smokes 10 or more cigarettes per day have measurable blood levels of nicotine and tobacco carcinogens. Chemicals in tobacco smoke also show up in breast milk, and breastfeeding may pass more chemicals to the infant of a smoking mother than direct exposure to ETS.

ETS triggers approximately 115 000 cases of bronchitis, pneumonia, and other respiratory infections in Canadian children annually, resulting in more than 200 000 visits to physicians. Older children suffer, too. ETS is a risk factor for asthma in children who have not previously displayed

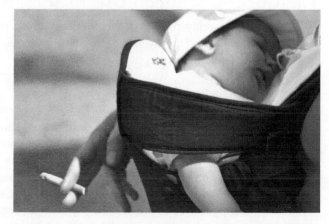

About 1.6 million Canadian infants and children are regularly exposed to environmental tobacco smoke.

symptoms of the disease, and it aggravates the symptoms of children who already have asthma. ETS is also linked to reduced lung function and fluid buildup in the middle ear, a contributing factor in middle-ear infections, a leading reason for childhood surgery. Children and teens exposed to ETS score lower on tests of reading and reasoning. Later in life, people exposed to ETS as children are at increased risk for lung cancer, emphysema, and chronic bronchitis.

QUICK STATS

1000 non-smokers will die in Canada this year due to tobacco use.

—Statistics Canada, 2008

Smoking and Pregnancy

Smoking almost doubles a pregnant woman's chance of having a miscarriage, and it significantly increases her risk of ectopic pregnancy. Maternal smoking causes an estimated 100 infant deaths in the Canada each year, primarily because of premature delivery and smoking-related problems with the placenta. Maternal smoking is a major factor in low birth weight, which puts newborns at high risk for infections and other serious problems. If a non-smoking mother is regularly exposed to ETS, her infant is also at greater risk for low birth weight. Recent studies have also shown that babies whose mothers smoked during pregnancy had higher rates of colic, clubfoot, cleft lip and palate, and impaired lung function; they may also have genetic damage.

Babies born to mothers who smoke more than two packs a day perform poorly on developmental tests in the first hours after birth, compared with babies of non-smoking mothers. Later in life, obesity, hyperactivity, short attention span, and lower scores on spelling and reading tests all occur more frequently in children whose mothers smoked during pregnancy than in those born to non-smoking mothers. Prenatal tobacco exposure has also been associated with behavioural problems in children, including immaturity, emotional instability, physical aggression, and hyperactivity. Other research shows that teenagers whose mothers smoked during pregnancy have lower scores on tests of general intelligence and poorer performance on tasks requiring auditory memory than do children who were not exposed to cigarette smoke before birth. Males born to smoking mothers have higher rates of adolescent and adult criminal activity, suggesting that maternal smoking may cause brain damage that increases the risk of criminal behaviour. Nevertheless, in Canada, almost 9 percent of pregnant women reported smoking regularly during pregnancy in 2009.

The Cost of Tobacco Use to Society

The annual health-related costs of smoking in Canada exceed $17 billion. These costs far exceed the tax revenues that are collected on the sale of tobacco products, even though the average cigarette tax was 70 percent of the cost per pack in 2009.

Tobacco Legislation in Canada

A major step in regulating tobacco in Canada occurred in 1999 when the National Strategy on Tobacco Control was adopted by both the federal and the provincial and territorial governments. Since then, although the strategy's name has changed several times, the focus remains on protection, prevention, cessation, and harm reduction (see the In the News box).

The Tobacco Act, enacted in 1997, regulates the manufacture, sale, labelling, and promotion of tobacco in Canada through a variety of methods, including legislation and fines for non-compliance. For example, in Ontario, selling cigarettes to minors has a graduated penalty structure with fines up to $25 000 for infractions.

Canada is considered to be at the forefront of anti-smoking legislation, with bans on smoking in public places being enacted across all provinces and territories over the last decade (see Table 16.1). Canada passed Bill C-32, An Act to Amend the Tobacco Act, in 2009, which bans flavours in cigarillos, cigarettes, and blunts (tobacco rolling papers). This bill also prohibits advertising of tobacco products in both newspapers and magazines. Bill C-32 came about as new research in tobacco use among youth in Canada from the *Youth Smoking*

Survey (2006–2007) found high rates of cigarillo use by youth. With the removal of tobacco advertising in print resources, the Canadian government hopes to reduce youths' exposure to tobacco products and reduce their tobacco use.

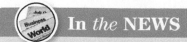

In *the* NEWS

Regulation of Tobacco

Tobacco kills more Canadians annually than motor vehicle accidents, accidental falls, murders, suicides, and alcohol combined. Given the danger associated with tobacco, Canada has imposed regulations in an attempt to regulate tobacco products. The Tobacco Reporting Regulation was created to better control the tobacco industry. This regulation requires that Canadian tobacco companies and tobacco importers in Canada provide annual reports to the federal minster of health. The information that is required in the reports includes the following:

- Tobacco sales
- Ingredients in all tobacco products
- Toxic constituents (20 are identified that require reporting)
- Toxic emissions (40 are identified that require reporting)
- Research activities
- Promotional initiatives

The regulation further details the methods that must be used when analyzing and evaluating the ingredients in tobacco products and the toxic emissions for various types of smoke and tobacco. The Canadian government has clearly outlined sets of rules for mainstream smoke, sidestream smoke, and whole tobacco testing, along with specific guidelines for testing the various components of tobacco. For example, each ingredient in tobacco, including ammonia, carbon monoxide, mercury, tar, and nicotine, must be tested for and reported.

TABLE 16.1

Bans on Smoking in Public Places in Canada

- Prince Edward Island banned smoking in public places and workplaces in 2003.
- Manitoba banned smoking in any indoor location where children or youth where present in 2002, and subsequently banned smoking in public areas in 2004.
- New Brunswick banned smoking in public places in 2004.
- Nunavut and the Northwest Territories banned smoking in business and work sites in 2004.
- Saskatchewan banned smoking in bars, casinos, and restaurants in 2002, and in all public places in 2005.
- Newfoundland and Labrador amended the Smoke-Free Environment Act in 2005 to ban smoking in all public places.
- Alberta banned smoking in public places in 2006.
- Quebec made restaurants, bars, clubs, casinos, and shelters smoke-free in May 2006, and subsequently banned smoking in all public places in June 2006.
- In Halifax, Nova Scotia, smoking was restricted in 2009 in outdoor venues where children are present (i.e., parks, rinks, and sports fields).
- Ontario banned smoking in public places in various cities between 2001 and 2006, banned tobacco displays in 2008, and banned smoking in vehicles carrying children in 2009.
- British Columbia banned smoking in public places in 2008 and smoking in vehicles with minors in 2009.
- Yukon was the last jurisdiction to ban smoking in public places in 2009.

Court Cases

Much of Canada's legal action against tobacco companies is modelled after the Tobacco Master Settlement Agreement of 1998 from the United States. In this class action, 46 U.S. states took four large tobacco companies to court, winning a payment of $206 billion over 25 years. In 2009, the Ontario government launched a $50 billion lawsuit against big tobacco companies, seeking damages for both past and ongoing health-care costs associated with tobacco-related illnesses from 1955 to 2009. As the attorney general in charge of prosecution stated, "the tax payers of the province of Ontario have paid a lot of money for health-care costs directly related to tobacco use over the decades."

In 2009, the government passed the Tobacco Damages and Health Care Costs Recovery Act, which allows provinces to sue for the recovery of past, present, and continuing tobacco-related damages. This legislation is consistent with legislation in other parts of the world. The Imperial Tobacco Company, the largest manufacturer of tobacco in Canada, was named in the lawsuit, along with 14 other Canadian-, American-, and British-based tobacco companies.

The first successful lawsuit against tobacco companies concluded in 1999 in California. Patricia Henley, a woman diagnosed with inoperable lung cancer, was awarded $51.5 million from the Philip Morris tobacco company. Appeals over seven years reduced the award to $10.5 million. Henley died in 2009. (See Figure 16.9 for key dates in Canada's legal anti-smoking campaign.)

FIGURE 16.9

Canada's Legal Anti-smoking Campaign

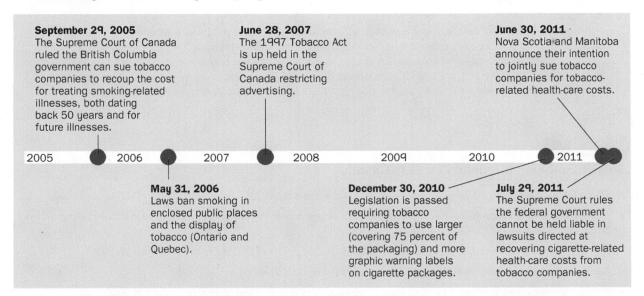

September 29, 2005
The Supreme Court of Canada ruled the British Columbia government can sue tobacco companies to recoup the cost for treating smoking-related illnesses, both dating back 50 years and for future illnesses.

June 28, 2007
The 1997 Tobacco Act is up held in the Supreme Court of Canada restricting advertising.

June 30, 2011
Nova Scotia and Manitoba announce their intention to jointly sue tobacco companies for tobacco-related health-care costs.

May 31, 2006
Laws ban smoking in enclosed public places and the display of tobacco (Ontario and Quebec).

December 30, 2010
Legislation is passed requiring tobacco companies to use larger (covering 75 percent of the packaging) and more graphic warning labels on cigarette packages.

July 29, 2011
The Supreme Court rules the federal government cannot be held liable in lawsuits directed at recovering cigarette-related health-care costs from tobacco companies.

THINKING ABOUT THE ENVIRONMENT

The buildings in which you live, work, and learn are important parts of your environment, as are the skies and oceans. The health and safety of indoor air are threatened by second-hand smoke, just as the outside air is threatened by other forms of pollution.

Physicians for a Smoke-Free Canada estimate that anywhere from 1000 to 7500 non-smokers die annually from exposure to tobacco smoke. They report the following facts:

- Children exposed to second-hand smoke are more likely to die of sudden infant death syndrome and to develop severe infections.
- Adults exposed to second-hand smoke experience immediate harmful effects to the cardiovascular system and increased risk of coronary heart disease and lung cancer.
- No level of exposure to second-hand smoke is safe.
- Completely eliminating indoor smoking is the only way to fully protect non-smokers from exposure to second-hand smoke. Ventilating buildings or separating smokers from non-smokers is not sufficient.

For more information on the environment and environmental health, see Chapter 21.

QUESTIONS FOR CRITICAL THINKING AND REFLECTION

What are your views on the government's role in regulating tobacco products? Is there currently enough regulation, or should the government go further in controlling the production and marketing of these products? What events or experiences have shaped your views on this issue?

What Can Be Done?

Many things can be done to act against this public health threat. Action can take place at various levels, including individual, local, private sector, provincial/territorial, federal, and international.

Action at the Individual Level

Health activists warn that the influence of the tobacco industry remains strong. However, non-smokers have the right not only to breathe clean air, but also to take action to help solve one of society's most serious public health threats. Here are just some of the many ways in which individuals can help support tobacco prevention and stop-smoking efforts:

- When a smoker violates a no-smoking designation, complain.
- If you see children buying tobacco, report this illegal activity to the facility manager or the police.
- Learn more about addiction and tobacco cessation so you can better support the tobacco users you know. (See "Helping a Friend or Partner Stop Using Tobacco" on ⊟ connect.)
- Vote for candidates who support anti-tobacco measures; contact local, provincial or territorial, and national representatives to express your views.
- Cancel your subscriptions to magazines that carry tobacco advertising; send a letter to the publisher explaining your decision. (Canada bans tobacco advertising in magazines, however many U.S. magazines still include these types of ads.)
- Voice your opinion about other positive representations of tobacco use. (A recent study found that more than two-thirds of children's animated feature films depicted tobacco or alcohol use with no clear message that such practices were unhealthy.)
- Volunteer with the Canadian Lung Association, the Canadian Cancer Society, or the Heart and Stroke Foundation of Canada.

Action at the Local Level

Since the 1980s, local government agencies have been passing ordinances designed to discourage smoking in public places. Thousands of local ordinances across Canada now restrict or ban smoking in restaurants, stores, workplaces, and even public outdoor areas.

Action in the Private Sector

The information available about the negative effects of second-hand smoke gave employers reason to worry about workers' compensation claims and lawsuits based on exposure to workplace smoke. Most provinces have enacted smoke-free workplaces legislation.

Action at the Provincial/Territorial Level

Provinces and territories support tobacco control strategies through the use of strategic taxation, which has been identified as a contributing factor for declining smoking rates between 1999 and 2008. There have also been bans on second-hand smoke, such as in public places and vehicles, which are designed to protect non-smokers.

Action at the Federal Level

The federal government has implemented several strategies to reduce the ability of tobacco companies to market and attract new smokers, as well as several educational campaigns about the effects of smoking. These initiatives include: protecting youth by banning flavours and additives to tobacco products, restricting advertising of tobacco products (e.g., bans on retail displays and requiring plain packaging), health warning messages (e.g., pictorial warnings on packages were required in 2000 and must cover 75 percent of package), and targeting contraband cigarettes through the RCMP Contraband Tobacco Enforcement Strategy, which was launched in May 2008.

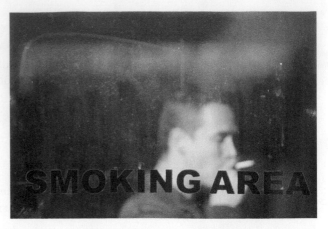

Smokers can light up only in designated smoking areas, which are outdoors and a specified distance from building entrances.

Action at the International Level

Many countries restrict smoking. Smoking is now banned on many international air flights, as well as in many restaurants and hotels and on public transportation in some countries. The World Health Organization has taken the lead in international anti-tobacco efforts by sponsoring the Framework Convention on Tobacco Control. World No Tobacco Day (observed on May 31) encourages smokers to stop smoking for one day. A smoker who successfully takes the first step of quitting for a day may be encouraged enough to follow through on the commitment and become a permanent non-smoker. With more than 1 billion smokers worldwide, addressing the global impact of tobacco use will require a massive coordinated effort.

QUICK STATS

In 2011, 65–78% of the cost per pack of cigarettes was tax (depending on the province/territory).

—Non-Smokers' Rights Association, 2011

QUESTIONS FOR CRITICAL THINKING AND REFLECTION

What anti-smoking ordinances are in effect in your community? Does your school prohibit smoking on campus? Do you think these rules have been effective in reducing smoking or exposure to ETS? Do you support such regulations? Why or why not?

How a Tobacco User Can Quit

Giving up tobacco is a long-term, intricate process. Heavy smokers who say they have just stopped cold turkey often don't tell of the struggling and mental processes that contributed to their final victory over this powerful addiction. Research shows that tobacco users move through predictable stages—from being uninterested in stopping, to thinking about change, to making a concerted effort to stop, to finally maintaining abstinence. But most attempt to quit several times before they finally succeed. Relapse is a normal part of the process.

The Benefits of Quitting

Giving up tobacco provides immediate health benefits to men and women of all ages (see Table 16.2). People who quit smoking find that food tastes better and their sense of smell is sharper. Circulation improves, heart rate and blood pressure drop, and lung function and heart efficiency increase. Ex-smokers can breathe more easily, and their capacity for exercise improves. Many ex-smokers report feeling more energetic and alert. They experience fewer headaches. Even their complexion may improve.

Quitting also has a positive effect on long-term disease risk. From the first day without tobacco, ex-smokers begin to decrease their risk of cancer of the lung, larynx, mouth, pancreas, bladder, cervix, and other sites. Risk of heart attack, stroke, and other cardiovascular diseases drops quickly, too.

The younger people are when they stop smoking, the more pronounced the health improvements. And these improvements gradually but invariably increase as the period of nonsmoking lengthens. It's never too late to quit, though. People who quit smoking, regardless of age, live longer than people who continue to smoke. Even smokers who have already developed chronic bronchitis or emphysema may show some improvement when they quit.

Options for Quitting

Half of tobacco users want to quit, and half of those who want to quit will make an attempt this year. What are their options? No single method works for everyone, but each does work for some people some of the time. Health Canada offers online resources to help smokers quit, as well as information on pharmacological interventions, including nicotine replacement therapy, which can serve as a valuable aid for some people. Health Canada's website also provides behavioural strategies to aid in cessation, along with a toll-free number for people who want more information. The Smoker's Helpline is one such Canadian initiative designed to help people quit smoking through the use of Motivational Interviewing, a cognitive behaviour change strategy aimed at helping smokers increased motivation to quit by decreasing ambivalence and eliciting change talk. The Smoker's Helpline is a national initiative available to all Canadians.

Choosing to quit requires developing a strategy for success (see the Take Charge box). Some

TABLE 16.2

Benefits of Quitting Smoking

Within 20 minutes of your last cigarette
• You stop polluting the air. • Blood pressure drops to normal. • Pulse rate drops to normal. • Temperature of hands and feet increases to normal.
8 hours
• Carbon monoxide level in blood drops to normal. • Oxygen level in blood increases to normal.
24 hours
• The chance of heart attack decreases.
48 hours
• Nerve endings start regrowing. • Ability to smell and taste is enhanced.
2–3 months
• Circulation improves. • Walking becomes easier. • Lung function increases up to 30 percent.
1–9 months
• Coughing, sinus congestion, fatigue, and shortness of breath all decrease.
1 year
• Heart disease death risk is half that of a smoker.
5 years
• Stroke risk drops nearly to the risk for non-smokers.
10 years
• Lung cancer death risk drops to 50 percent of that of a continuing smoker. • Incidence of other cancers (mouth, throat, larynx, esophagus, bladder, kidney, and pancreas) decreases. • Risk of ulcer decreases.
15 years
• Risk of lung cancer is about 25 percent of that of continuing smokers. • Risks of heart disease and death are close to those for non-smokers.

Sources: American Lung Association, 2015, *Benefits of Quitting,* http://www.lung.org/stop-smoking/i-want-to-quit/benefits-of-quitting.html; and American Cancer Society, 2015, *When Smokers Quit - What are the Benefits Over Time?,* http://www.cancer.org/healthy/stayawayfromtobacco/guidetoquittingsmoking/guide-to-quitting-smoking-benefits.

Take CHARGE

Building Motivation to Quit Smoking

A common misconception among smokers is that a few cigarettes a day aren't enough to cause harm. Among post-secondary students who smoke, many describe themselves as casual smokers, smoking ten or fewer cigarettes a day. These smokers are ignoring the very real health risks of even one cigarette. One strategy to enhance motivation to quit is the 5Rs. If you are a smoker or are trying to help one, think about these areas of concern and see if they help develop a desire and readiness to make a real attempt at quitting.

Relevance: Think about the personal relevance of quitting tobacco use. What would the effects be on your family and friends? How would your daily life improve? What is the most important way that quitting would change your life?

Risks: Smokers face immediate risks, such as shortness of breath, infertility, and impotence, and long-term risks, including cancer, heart disease, and respiratory problems. Remember, smoking is harmful to you and you extend that risk to anyone exposed to your smoke.

Rewards: The list of the rewards of quitting is almost endless, including improving immediate and long-term health, saving money, and feeling better about yourself. You can also stop worrying about quitting and set a good example for others.

Roadblocks: What are the potential obstacles to quitting? Are you worried about withdrawal symptoms, weight gain, or lack of support? How can these barriers be overcome?

Repetition: Revisit your reasons for quitting and strengthen your resolve until you are ready to prepare a plan. Most people make several attempts to quit before they succeed. Relapsing once does not mean that you will never succeed.

Sources: Rigotti, N. A., J. E. Lee, and H. Wechsler. 2000. U.S. college students' use of tobacco products. *Journal of the American Medical Association* 284(6): 699–705; Fiore, M. C., et al. 2000. *Treating Tobacco Use and Dependence.* Clinical Practice Guidelines. Rockville, Md.: U.S. Department of Health and Human Services.

---

people quit cold turkey, whereas others taper off slowly. There are over-the-counter and prescription products that help many people (see the In Focus box for more on these options). Behavioural factors that have been shown to increase the chances of a smoker's permanent smoking cessation are support from others and regular exercise. Support can come from friends and family or formal group programs sponsored by organizations, such as the Canadian Cancer Society and the Canadian Lung Association, or by your campus health centre or community hospital. Programs that combine group support with nicotine replacement therapy have rates of continued abstention as high as 35 percent after one year.

QUICK STATS

In 2012, of the over half of Canadian smokers who tried to quit, only 1/10 were still smoke free six months later.

—Propel, 2012

Free telephone quitlines are emerging as a popular strategy to help people stop smoking. Quitlines are staffed by trained counsellors who help each caller plan a personal quitting strategy, usually including a combination of nicotine replacement therapy, changes in daily habits, emotional support, and Motivational Interviewing/readiness to quit. Counsellors provide printed materials that match the smoker's needs and

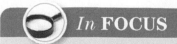 *In* FOCUS

Smoking Cessation Products

Each year, tens of thousands of Canadians visit their doctors in the hope of finding a drug that can help them stop smoking. Although pharmacological options are limited, the few available drugs have proved successful.

Champix (Varenicline)

The newest smoking cessation drug, marketed under the name Champix, works in two ways: It reduces nicotine cravings, easing the withdrawal process, and it blocks the pleasant effects of nicotine. The drug acts on neurotransmitter receptors in the brain.

Six clinical trials, which included more than 3600 long-term, chronic smokers, demonstrated that Champix is an effective smoking cessation aid. In one of the studies, nearly 25 percent of Champix users stopped smoking for a full year. Results varied with the dosage and duration of treatment.

Unlike most smoking cessation products currently on the market, Champix is not a nicotine replacement. For this reason, smokers may be advised to continue smoking for the first few days of treatment, to avoid withdrawal and to allow the drug to build up in their system. The approved course of treatment is 12 weeks, but the duration and recommended dosage depend on several factors, including the smoker's general health and the length and severity of his or her nicotine addiction.

Side effects reported with Champix include nausea, headache, vomiting, sleep disruptions, and change in taste perception. People with kidney problems or who take certain medications should not take Champix, and it is not recommended for women who are pregnant or nursing. In early 2008, Health Canada issued a public health advisory warning that some Champix users had experienced adverse reactions, such as behavioural changes, agitation, depression, suicidal thoughts, and attempted suicide. Anyone taking Champix should immediately notify his or her doctor of any sudden change in mood or behaviour.

Zyban (Bupropion)

Bupropion is an antidepressant (prescribed under the name Wellbutrin) as well as a smoking cessation aid (prescribed under the name Zyban). As a smoking cessation aid, bupropion eases the symptoms of nicotine withdrawal and reduces the urge to smoke. Like Champix, it acts on neurotransmitter receptors in the brain.

Bupropion is not a nicotine replacement, so the user may need to continue smoking for the first few days of treatment. A nicotine replacement product, such as a patch or gum, may be recommended to further ease withdrawal symptoms after the user stops smoking.

Bupropion users have reported an array of side effects, but they are rare. Side effects may be reduced by changing the dosage, taking the medicine at a different time of day, or taking it with or without food. Bupropion is not recommended for people with specific physical conditions or who take certain drugs. Zyban and Wellbutrin should not be taken together.

Nicotine Replacement Products

The most widely used smoking cessation products replace the nicotine that the user would normally get from tobacco. The user continues to get nicotine, so withdrawal symptoms and cravings are reduced. Although still harmful, nicotine replacement products provide a cleaner form of nicotine, without the thousands of poisons and tars produced by burning tobacco. Less of the product is used over time, as the need for nicotine decreases.

Nicotine replacement products come in several forms, including patches, gum, lozenges, nasal sprays, and inhalers. They are available in a variety of strengths and can be worked into many different smoking cessation strategies. Most are available without a prescription.

The nicotine patch is popular because it can be applied and forgotten until it needs to be removed or changed, usually every 16 or 24 hours. Placed on the upper arm or torso, it releases a steady stream of nicotine, which is absorbed through the skin. The main side effects are skin irritation and redness. Nicotine gum and nicotine lozenges have the advantage of allowing the smoker to use them whenever he or she craves nicotine. Side effects of nicotine gum include mouth sores and headaches; nicotine lozenges can cause nausea and heartburn. Nicotine nasal sprays and inhalers are available only by prescription.

Although all these products have proven to be effective in helping users stop smoking, experts recommend them only as one part of a complete smoking cessation program. Such a program should include regular professional counselling and physician monitoring.

schedule phone counselling sessions for key days after a smoker quits. Smokers can schedule sessions to fit their schedule, and some quitlines may provide stop-smoking medications at reduced prices. Almost all smokers make more than one attempt to stop before they succeed in quitting for good. Quitline counsellors can help smokers understand what leads to relapse, review their reasons for wanting to quit, and make a better plan for the next attempt. The goal is for smokers to find a support system and techniques that work for them. Visit Health Canada's website for toll-free quitlines in most provinces and territories.

Most smokers in the process of quitting experience both physical and psychological effects of nicotine withdrawal, and exercise can help with both. For many smokers, tobacco use is associated with certain times and places—following a meal, for example. Resolving to walk after dinner instead of lighting up provides a distraction from cravings and eliminates the cues that trigger a desire to smoke. In addition, many people worry about weight gain associated with quitting. Although most ex-smokers do gain a kilogram or so, at least temporarily, incorporating exercise into a new tobacco-free routine lays the foundation for healthy weight management. The health risks of adding a kilogram are far outweighed by the risks of continued smoking; it's estimated that a smoker would have to gain 35–45 kilograms (75–100 pounds) to equal the health risks of smoking a pack a day.

As with any significant change in health-related behaviour, giving up tobacco requires planning, sustained effort, and support. It is an ongoing process, not a one-time event. The Take Charge box describes one set of steps that some successful quitters follow.

 Take **CHARGE**

Kicking the Tobacco Habit

You can look forward to a longer and healthier life if you join the millions of Canadians who have quit using tobacco. The steps for quitting described below are discussed in terms of the most popular tobacco product in Canada—cigarettes—but they can be adapted for all forms of tobacco.

Gather Information

Collect personal smoking information in a detailed journal about your smoking behaviour. Write down the time you smoke each cigarette of the day, the situation you are in, how you feel, where you smoke, and how strong your craving for the cigarette is, plus any other information that seems relevant. Part of the job is to identify patterns of smoking that are connected with routine situations (for example, the coffee break smoke, the after-dinner cigarette, the tension-reduction cigarette). Use this information to discover the behaviour patterns involved in your smoking habit.

Make the Decision to Quit

Choose a date in the near future when you expect to be relatively stress-free and can give quitting the energy and attention it will require. Don't choose a date right before or during finals week, for instance. Consider making quitting a gift: Choose your birthday as your quit date, for example, or make quitting a Father's Day or Mother's Day present. You might also want to coordinate your quit date with a friend—a fellow tobacco user who wants to quit or a non-smoker who wants to give up another bad habit or begin an exercise program. Tell your friends and family when you plan to quit. Ask them to offer encouragement and help hold you to your goal.

Decide which approach to quitting will work best for you. Will you go cold turkey, or will you taper off? Will you use nicotine patches or gum? Will you join a support group or enlist the help of a friend? Prepare a contract for quitting, as discussed in Chapter 1. Set firm dates and rewards, and sign the contract. Post it in a prominent place.

Prepare to Quit

One of the most important things you can do to prepare to quit is to develop and practise non-smoking relaxation techniques. Many smokers find that they use cigarettes to help them unwind in tense situations or to relax at other times. If this is true for you, you will need to find and develop effective substitutes. It takes time to become proficient at relaxation techniques, so begin practising before your quit date. Refer to the detailed discussion of relaxation techniques in Chapter 3.

Other things you can do to help prepare for quitting include the following:

- Make an appointment to see your physician.
- Ask about OTC and prescription aids for tobacco cessation and whether one or more might be appropriate for you.
- Make a dentist's appointment to have your teeth cleaned the day after your target quit date.
- Start an easy exercise program, if you are not exercising regularly already.
- Buy some sugarless gum. Stock your kitchen with low-calorie snacks.
- Clean out your car, and air out your house. Send your clothes out for dry cleaning.
- Throw away all your cigarette-related paraphernalia (ashtrays, lighters, etc.).
- The night before your quit day, get rid of all your cigarettes. Have fun with this—get your friends or family to help you tear them up.
- Make your last few days of smoking inconvenient: Smoke only outdoors and when alone. Don't do anything else while you smoke.

Quitting

Your first few days without cigarettes will probably be the most difficult. It's hard to give up such a strongly ingrained habit, but remember that many other Canadians have done it—and you can, too. Plan and rehearse the steps you will take when you experience a powerful craving. Avoid or control situations that you know from your journal are powerfully associated with your smoking (see the table). If your hands feel empty without a cigarette, try holding or fiddling with a small object, such as a paper clip or pencil.

Social support can also be a big help. Arrange with a friend to help you with your weak moments, and call him or her whenever you feel overwhelmed by an urge to smoke. Tell people you have just quit. You may discover many inspiring former smokers who can encourage you and reassure you that it's possible to quit and lead a happier, healthier life. Find a formal support group to join if you think it will help.

Maintaining Non-smoking

The lingering smoking urges that remain once you have quit should be carefully tracked and controlled because they can cause relapses if left unattended. Keep track of these urges in your journal to help you deal with them. If certain situations still trigger the urge for a cigarette, change something about the situation to break past associations. If stress or boredom causes strong smoking urges, use a relaxation technique, take a brisk walk, have a stick of gum, or substitute some other activity for smoking.

Don't set yourself up for a relapse. If you allow yourself to get overwhelmed at school or work or to gain weight, it will be easier to convince yourself that now isn't the right time to quit. This is the right time. Continue to practise time-management and relaxation techniques. Exercise regularly, eat sensibly, and get enough sleep. These habits will not only ensure your success at remaining tobacco-free but also serve you well in stressful times throughout your life. In fact, former smokers who have quit for at least three months report reduced stress levels, probably because quitting smoking lowers overall arousal.

Watch out for patterns of thinking that can make non-smoking more difficult. Focus on the positive aspects of not smoking, and give yourself lots of praise—you deserve it. Stick with the schedule of rewards you developed for your contract.

Keep track of the emerging benefits that come from having quit. Items that might appear on your list include improved stamina, an increased sense of pride at having kicked a strong addiction, a sharper sense of taste and smell, no more smoker's cough, and so on. Keep track of the money you are saving by not smoking, and spend it on things you really enjoy. And if you do lapse, be gentle with yourself. Lapses are a normal part of quitting. Forgive yourself, and pick up where you left off.

Strategies for Dealing with High-risk Smoking Situations

Cues and High-risk Situations	Suggested Strategies
Waking up in morning	Brush your teeth as soon as you wake up. Take a shower or bath.
Drinking coffee or tea	Do something else with your hands. Drink another beverage instead.
Eating meals	Get up from the table right after eating, and start another activity. Brush your teeth right after eating.
Driving a car	Have the car cleaned when you quit smoking. Chew sugarless gum or eat a low-calorie snack. Take public transportation or ride your bike. Turn on the radio and sing along.
Socializing with friends who smoke	Suggest non-smoking events (movies, theatre, shopping). Tell friends you have quit and ask them not to smoke around you, offer you cigarettes, or give you cigarettes if you ask for them.
Drinking alcohol	Try to take a non-smoker with you or associate with non-smokers. Let friends know you have just quit. Moderate your intake of alcohol (it can weaken your resolve).
Encountering stressful situations	Practise relaxation techniques. Take some deep breaths. Get out of your room or house. Go somewhere that doesn't allow smoking. Take a shower, chew gum, call a friend, or exercise.

Source: Strategies adapted with permission from *Postgraduate Medicine* 90(I), July 1991.

SUMMARY

- Smoking is the largest preventable cause of ill health and death in the Canada. Nevertheless, millions of Canadians continue to use tobacco.
- Regular tobacco use causes physical dependence on nicotine, characterized by loss of control, tolerance, and withdrawal. Habits can become associated with tobacco use and trigger the urge for a cigarette.
- People who begin smoking are usually imitating others or responding to seductive advertising. Smoking is associated with low education level and the use of other drugs.
- Tobacco smoke is made up of hundreds of different chemicals, including some that are carcinogenic or poisonous or that damage the respiratory system.
- Nicotine acts on the nervous system as a stimulant or a depressant. It can cause blood pressure and heart rate to increase, straining the heart.
- Cardiovascular disease is the most widespread cause of death for cigarette smokers. Cigarette smoking is the primary cause of lung cancer and is linked to many other cancers and respiratory diseases.
- Cigarette smoking is linked to ulcers, impotence, reproductive health problems, dental diseases, and other conditions. Tobacco use leads to shorter life expectancy and to a diminished quality of life.
- The use of spit tobacco leads to nicotine addiction and is linked to oral cancers.
- Cigars, pipes, clove cigarettes, and bidis are not safe alternatives to cigarettes.
- Environmental tobacco smoke (ETS) contains high concentrations of toxic chemicals and can cause headaches, eye and nasal irritation, and sinus problems. Long-term exposure to ETS can cause lung cancer and heart disease.

- Infants and young children take in more pollutants than adults do; children whose parents smoke are especially susceptible to respiratory diseases.
- Smoking during pregnancy increases the risk of miscarriage, stillbirth, congenital abnormalities, premature birth, and low birth weight. SIDS, behaviour problems, and long-term impairments in development are also risks.
- The overall cost of tobacco use to society includes the cost of both medical care and lost worker productivity.
- Individuals and groups can use many avenues to act against tobacco use. Non-smokers can use social pressure and legislative channels to assert their rights to breathe clean air.
- Giving up smoking is a difficult and long-term process. Although most ex-smokers quit on their own, some smokers benefit from stop-smoking programs, OTC and prescription medications, and support groups.

FOR MORE INFORMATION

BOOKS

Canadian Cancer Society. 2007. *One Step at a Time: For Smokers Who Want to Quit.* Toronto: Canadian Cancer Society. Information on how to quit smoking, what not to do, and how to help a smoker quit.

Heart and Stroke Foundation. 2005. *Just Breathe: Becoming and Remaining Smoke Free.* Ottawa: Heart and Stroke Foundation. Information on heart disease associated with smoking as well as the benefits of becoming smoke free.

Government of Ontario. 2008. *Quit: You Have It in You.* Ottawa: Queen's Printer for Ontario. Information for quitters on how to quit smoking, the benefits of cessation, and links to other resources.

Program Training and Consultation Centre. 2003. *Smoke-Free Homes.* Toronto: Government of Ontario. Information on how to make your home smoke free.

ORGANIZATIONS, HOTLINES, AND WEBSITES

The Internet addresses listed here were accurate at the time of publication.

Canadian Cancer Society: The Tobacco Act: An Overview. Provides information on current tobacco legislation, youth and tobacco, and national partnerships in tobacco control.
> http://www.cancer.ca

Health Canada: Canadian Tobacco Use Monitoring Survey. Provides information and statistics on current and past tobacco use in Canada.
> http://www.hc-sc.gc.ca/hc-ps/tobac-tabac/research-recherche/stat/index-eng.php

Health Canada: Second-Hand Smoke. Provides information on the impact of second-hand smoke on Canadians.
> http://www.hc-sc.gc.ca/hc-ps/pubs/tobac-tabac/second-guide/index-eng.php

Non-Smokers' Rights Association. Provides a wide variety of information on the control of tobacco products.
> http://www.nsra-adnf.ca/cms/index.cfm

Physicians for a Smoke-Free Canada. Provides information and links for tobacco facts, research papers, second-hand smoke, policies, and the legislation of tobacco products.
> http://www.smoke-free.ca

Public Health Agency of Canada: Chronic Obstructive Pulmonary Disease. Provides information and links on COPD and smoking.
> http://www.phac-aspc.gc.ca/cd-mc/crd-mrc/copd-mpoc-eng.php

Smoke-Free Living: Resources for Teachers. Provides information on youth smoking habits and smoking in grade schools and ways for teachers to include this information in their curriculum.
   http://www1.toronto.ca/wps/portal/contentonly?vgnextoid=051c62ca69902410VgnVCM10000071d60f89RCRD

World Health Organization: Tobacco-Free Initiative. Promotes the goal of a tobacco-free world.
   http://www.who.int/tobacco/en

World No Tobacco Day. Provides information on the annual worldwide event to encourage people to quit smoking, and general information about tobacco use and testimonials of ex-smokers.
   http://www.who.int/tobacco/communications/events/wntd/en/

Youth Smoking Survey. Provides information and statistics on current and past youth tobacco use in Canada.
   http://www.yss.uwaterloo.ca

See also the listings for Chapters 7, 8, and 14.

SELECTED BIBLIOGRAPHY

Canadian Lung Association. 2010. *Smoking and Tobacco,* http://www.lung.ca/protect-protegez/tobacco-tabagisme_e.php (retrieved May 3, 2011).

Collot, N. (writer/dir.). 2009. *The Tobacco Conspiracy.* Montreal: National Film Board of Canada [documentary].

Crow, M. E. 2005. The human rights responsibilities of multinational tobacco companies. *Tobacco Control* 14(2): 14–18.

D'Avernas, J. R., et al. 1997. *Cigarette Packaging and Event Marketing Increases the Attractiveness of Smoking: A Study of Youth.* Toronto: Ontario Tobacco Research Unit.

Daynard R. 2003. Why tobacco litigation? *Tobacco Control* 12: 1–2.

Edwards, R. 2004. ABCs of smoking cessation: The problem of tobacco smoking. *British Medical Journal* 328(7433): 217–219.

Fagerstrom, K. 2002. The epidemiology of smoking: Health consequences and benefits of cessation. *Drugs* 62 (2): 1–9.

Fair Air Association of Canada. 2006. *McGuinty Government's Addiction to Anti-Smoking Lobby Will Result in Smuggling, Job and Business Losses, Tax Hikes and Drastic Revenue Shortfalls* [press release], http://www.smokersclubinc.com/modules.php?name=News&file=article&sid=2440 (retrieved May 3, 2011).

Health Canada. 2007. *Federal Tobacco Control Strategy,* http://www.hc-sc.gc.ca/hl-vs/tobac-tabac/res/news-nouvelles/ftcs-sflt_e.html (retrieved January 26, 2008).

Health Canada. 2007. *Youth Smoking Survey 2006–2007,* http://www.hc-sc.gc.ca/hl-vs/tobac-tabac/research-recherche/stat/_survey-sondage_2006–2007/result-eng.php (retrieved December 12, 2009).

Health Canada. 2010. Government of Canada Ban on Flavoured Tobacco Products now in Full Force [News Release 2010-112], http://www.hc-sc.gc.ca/ahc-asc/media/nr-cp/_2010/2010_112-eng.php.

Health Canada. 2012. *Tobacco Control Program, Supplementary Tables, CTUMS Annual 2012 (February–December 2006),* http://www.hc-sc.gc.ca/hc-ps/tobac-tabac/research-recherche/stat/_ctums-esutc_2012/ann-table5-eng.php (retrieved May 3, 2011).

Johnson, E. O., and S. P. Novak. 2009. Onset and persistence of daily smoking: The interplay of socio-economic status, gender, and psychiatric disorders. *Drug and Alcohol Dependence* 104: S50–S57.

Kelton, M. H., and M. S. Givel. 2008. Public policy implications of tobacco industry smuggling through Native American reservations into Canada. *International Journal of Health Services* 38(3): 471–487.

Leatherdale, S. T. 2005. Predictors of different cigarette access behaviours among occasional and regular smoking youth. *Canadian Journal of Public Health* 96(5): 348–352.

Makomaski Illing, E. M., and M. J. Kaiserman. 2004. Mortality attributable to tobacco use in Canada and its regions. *Canadian Journal of Public Health* 95(1): 38–44.

McKennitt, D. 2007. A smoking prevention program for Aboriginal youth. *First Peoples Child and Family Review* 3(2): 52–55.

Olser, M., et al. 1999. Gender and determinants of smoking cessation: A longitudinal study. *Preventive Medicine* 29(1): 57–62.

Ontario Tobacco Research Unit. 2006. Toward smoke-free Ontario strategy objectives, 2005–2006. *Special Reports: Monitoring and Evaluation Series, 2005–2006* 12(1). Toronto: Ontario Tobacco Research Unit.

Ontario Tobacco Research Unit. 2011. Tobacco Taxes: Monitoring Update. Toronto: Ontario Tobacco Research Unit, http://otru.org/wp-content/uploads/2012/06/taxes2011.pdf.

Perez, C. E. 2004. Second-hand smoke exposure: Who's at risk? *Health Reports* 16(3): 19–36.

Physicians for a Smoke-Free Canada. 2011. *Tobacco in Canada,* http://www.smoke-free.ca/pdf_1/ TOBACCOINCANADA2003.pdf (retrieved July 20, 2014).

Reading, J., and Y. Allard. 1999. *The Tobacco Report: Report of the FNIRHS.* Ottawa: First Nations and Inuit Health Survey National Steering Committee.

Reid J.L., Hammond, D., Burkhalter, R., Ahmed, R. 2012. Tobacco Use in Canada: Patterns and Trends, 2012 Edition. Waterloo, ON: Propel Centre for Population Health Impact, University of Waterloo.

Royal Canadian Mounted Police. 2008. 2008 Contraband Tobacco Enforcement Strategy. Ottawa: RCMP, http://www.rcmp-grc.gc.ca/ce-da/tobacco-tabac-strat-2008-eng.htm (retrieved September 20, 2008).

Science Daily. 2009. *Smoking Gun: Just One Cigarette Has Harmful Effects on the Arteries of the Young and Healthy,* http://www.sciencedaily.com/releases/2009/10/091027085300.htm (retrieved May 3, 2011).

Shields, M. 2005. The journey to quitting smoking. *Health Reports* 16(3): 19–36.

Shields, M. 2007. Smoking-prevalence, bans and exposure to second hand smoke. *Health Reports* 18(3): 67–85.

Statistics Canada. 2010. *Canadian Tobacco Use Monitoring Survey, 2008,* http://www.hc-sc.gc.ca/hl-vs/ tobac-tabac/research-recherche/stat/_ctums-esutc_2008/wave-phase-1_summary-sommaire-eng.php (retrieved January 6, 2010).

Wardman, D., and Khan, N. 2004. Smoking-attributable mortality among British Columbia's First Nations populations. *International Journal of Circumpolar Health* 63: 81–92.

Wardman, D., and Khan, N. 2005. Registered Indians and tobacco taxation: A culturally appropriate strategy? *Canadian Journal of Public Health* 96: 451–453.

World Health Organization. 2008. *The Global Tobacco Crisis,* http://www.who.int/tobacco/mpower/ mpower_report_tobacco_crisis_2008.pdf (retrieved September 27, 2008).

CHAPTER 17

Aging: A Vital Process

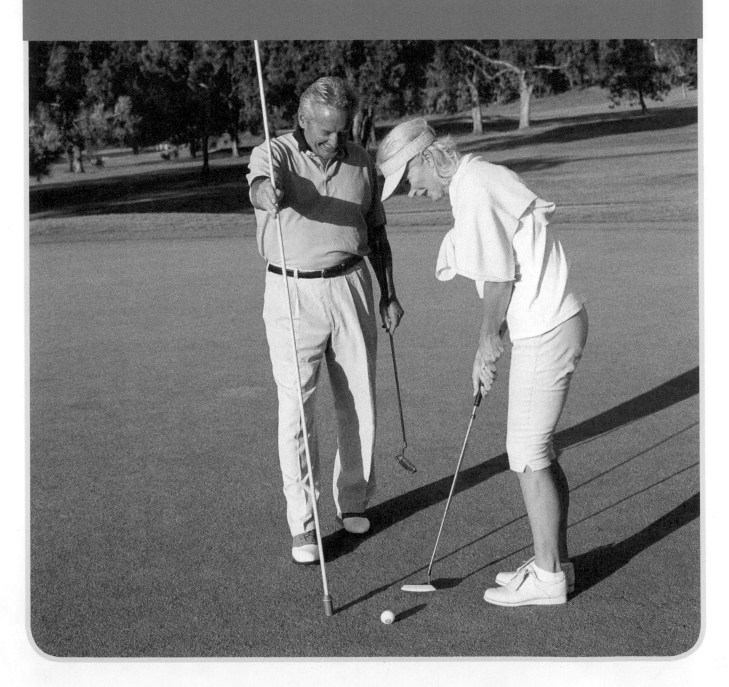

LOOKING AHEAD

After you have read and studied this chapter, you should be able to:

LO1 List strategies for healthy aging

LO2 Identify key physical, social, and mental changes that may accompany aging and discuss how people can best confront these changes

LO3 Describe practical considerations for older adults and caregivers, including housing, finances, health care, communication, and transportation

TEST YOUR KNOWLEDGE

1. **Exercise is beneficial for older people because it:**
   a. Protects against osteoporosis b. Maintains alertness and intelligence c. Prevents falls

2. **The abuse of alcohol is rare among older adults.**
   True or false?

3. **What is the leading cause of vision loss in Canada?**
   a. Glaucoma b. Cataracts c. Age-related macular degeneration (AMD)

4. **Women do not need to take preventive measures against osteoporosis until after menopause.**
   True or false?

ANSWERS

1. ALL THREE.   Even for people over 80, exercise can improve physical functioning and balance and reduce falls and injuries.

2. FALSE.   The abuse of alcohol affects about 6–10 percent of older adults. It often goes undetected because its symptoms may mimic those of other conditions, such as Alzheimer's disease.

3. c.   According to the Canadian National Institute for the Blind, age-related macular degeneration affects approximately 1.4 million Canadians and is the leading cause of vision loss in Canada.

4. FALSE.   All people—but especially women—need to pay attention to diet and exercise in younger years in order to build bone mass.

Aging is the process of becoming older, a process that is genetically determined but profoundly affected by a person's environment. Your grandparents or great-grandparents may be examples of how these two determinants play a role in the aging process.

Aging does not begin at some specific point in life, and there is no precise age at which a person becomes "old." Rather, aging is a normal process of development that occurs throughout life. It happens to everyone, but at different rates for different people. Some people are "old" at 25, and others are still "young" at 75.

Although youth is not entirely a state of mind, your attitude toward life and your attention to your health significantly influence the satisfaction you will get from life. This is especially true when new physical, mental, and social challenges occur in later years. If you optimize wellness during young adulthood, you can exert great control over the physical and mental aspects of aging, and you can better handle your response to events that might be out of your control.

This chapter discusses the aging process and describes some of the major effects increasing age can have on our lives.

Generating Vitality as We Age

As we age, physical and mental changes occur gradually, over a lifetime. Biological aging includes all the normal, progressive, irreversible changes to the body that begin at birth and continue until death. Psychological aging and social aging usually involve more abrupt changes in circumstance and emotion: relocating, changing homes, losing a spouse and friends, retiring, having a lower income, and changing roles and social status. These changes represent opportunities for growth throughout life.

Not all of these changes happen to everybody, and their timing varies, partly depending on how we have prepared for our later years. Some people never have to leave their homes and appear to be in good health until the day they die. Others have tremendous adjustments to make—to entirely new surroundings with fewer financial resources, to new acquaintances, to the changing physical condition of their bodies and new health problems, and possibly to loneliness and loss of self-esteem.

Successful aging requires preparation. People need to establish good health habits in their teens and twenties. During their twenties and thirties, they usually develop important relationships and settle into a particular lifestyle. By their mid-forties, they generally know how much money they need to support the lifestyle they have chosen. At this point, and perhaps even earlier, individuals must assess their financial status and perhaps adjust their savings to continue enjoying their lifestyle after retirement. In their mid-fifties, it is important for adults to reevaluate their financial and retirement plans; in their sixties and seventies people might also start to think about retirement housing. In their seventies and beyond, many older adults focus on the ways in which they can share their legacy with the next generation. Throughout life, people should cultivate interests and hobbies they enjoy, both alone and with others.

What Happens as We Age?

In comparison to younger age groups, a large number of older Canadians describe themselves as being in fair or poor health (see Figure 17.1). Many of the characteristics associated with aging, however, are not due to aging at all. Rather, they result from the neglect and abuse of our bodies and minds. These assaults lay the foundation for later psychological problems and chronic conditions, such as arthritis, heart disease, diabetes, hearing loss, and hypertension. We sacrifice our health by smoking, ignoring our nutrition needs, overeating, abusing alcohol and drugs, bombarding our ears with excessive noise, and exposing our bodies to too much ultraviolet radiation from the sun. We also jeopardize

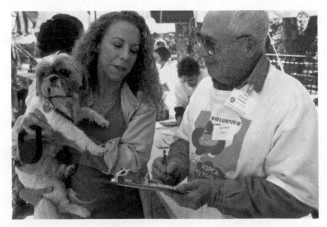

Some individuals defy all preconceived ideas about age and continue to live vigorous and productive lives into their seventies, eighties, and beyond.

our bodies through inactivity and sedentary behaviours, encouraging our muscles and even our bones to wither and deteriorate. And we endure abuse from the toxic chemicals in our environment.

But even with the healthiest behaviour and environment, aging inevitably occurs. It results from biochemical processes we don't yet fully understand. The physiological changes in organ systems are caused by a combination of gradual aging and impairment from disease. Because of redundancy in most organ systems, the body's ability to function is not affected until damage is fairly extensive. Studies of healthy people indicate that functioning remains essentially constant until after age 70. Further research may help pinpoint the causes of aging and aid in the development of therapies to repair damage to aging organs.

Life-Enhancing Measures: Age-Proofing

You can prevent, delay, lessen, or even reverse some of the changes associated with aging through good habits. Simple things you can do daily will make a vast difference to your level of energy and vitality—your overall wellness. The following suggestions have been mentioned throughout this text. But because they are profoundly related to health in later life, we highlight them here.

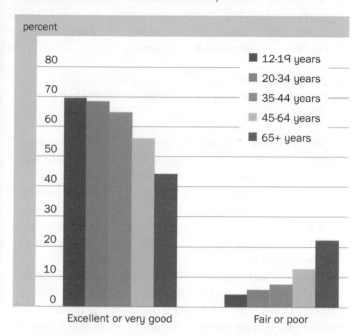

FIGURE 17.1

Self-rated Health of Canadians, 2012

Legend:
- 12-19 years
- 20-34 years
- 35-44 years
- 45-64 years
- 65+ years

Source: Statistics Canada. 2012. Table 105-0501, Health indicator profile, annual estimates, by age group and sex, Canada, provinces, territories, health regions (2012 boundaries) and peer groups, occasional, CANSIM (database), http://www4.hrsdc.gc.ca/.3ndic.lt.4r@-eng.jsp?iid=10 (retrieved February 16, 2015).

Challenge Your Mind

Numerous studies show that older adults who stay mentally active have lower levels of the brain protein linked to Alzheimer's and dementia. Reading, doing puzzles, learning language, and studying music are good ways to stimulate the brain. The more complex the activity, the more protective it may be.

Develop Physical Fitness

Exercise significantly enhances both psychological and physical health. The benefits of exercise are not only observed among individuals who are considered to be *healthy*. In fact, a 2013 review of more than 300 randomized controlled trials showed that exercise interventions may be as beneficial as drug interventions in terms of reducing the odds of mortality in people with coronary heart disease, stroke, and prediabetes. Generally speaking, the positive effects of exercise include the following:

- Lower blood pressure and healthier cholesterol levels
- Better protection against heart attacks and an increased chance of survival should one occur
- Sustained or increased lung capacity
- Maintenance of strength, flexibility, and balance
- Weight control through less accumulation of fat
- Improved sleep
- Longer life expectancy
- Protection against osteoporosis and type 2 diabetes
- Increased effectiveness of the immune system
- Maintenance of mental agility and flexibility, response time, memory, and hand–eye coordination

The stimulus that exercise provides also seems to protect against the loss of **fluid intelligence**, the ability to find solutions to new problems. Fluid intelligence depends on rapidity of responsiveness, memory, and alertness. Individuals who exercise regularly are also less susceptible to depression and dementia.

> **fluid intelligence**
> The ability to develop a solution when confronted with a new problem.

Regular physical activity also fends off *sarcopenia*, which is age-related loss of muscle mass, strength, and function (see Chapter 6). The weaker a person becomes, the less he or she can do; this condition can rob an individual of self-sufficiency and lead to greater dependence on others. The muscle wasting that occurs in sarcopenia also leads to weight gain because muscle burns more calories than fat, even at rest.

Regular physical activity is essential for healthy aging, as it is throughout life. The Canadian Physical Activity Guidelines for Older Adults—65 Years & Older recommend that people over the age of 65 should accumulate at least 150 minutes of moderate- to vigorous-intensity aerobic physical activity each week, in increments of at least 10 minutes each. In addition, these guidelines sug-

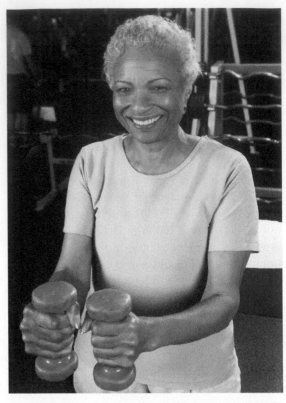

Regular exercise is a key to successful, healthy aging.

gest that older adults should engage in strength training activities that use major muscle groups at least twice per week. It is also recommended that people with poor mobility should perform physical activities that focus on balance and preventing falls. Older individuals who have been sedentary should be encouraged to become more active. It's never too late to start exercising; the more physical activity people engage in, the greater the health benefits. Even in people over 80, endurance and strength training can improve balance, flexibility, and physical functioning and reduce the potential for dangerous falls (see the In Focus box).

 In FOCUS

Falls Among Older Adults

According to Health Canada, the primary cause of injury among older Canadians is falls. The 2014 *Seniors' Falls in Canada: Second Report* provides a wealth of information related to injuries and falls among older Canadians, including the following statistics:

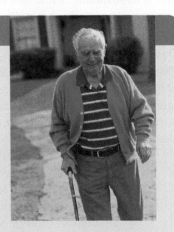

- An estimated 20–30 percent of older adults report injuries as a result of falls each year.
- Approximately 85 percent of injury-related hospitalizations for older adults are the result of falls.
- Older adults with fall-related injuries remain in the hospital an average of nine days longer than those hospitalized for other causes.
- Falls cause about 95 percent of hip fractures in older adults; 20 percent of these older adults die within a year of the fracture.

In Canada, women typically sustain more injuries from falls, although the rate of fall-related injuries among men appears to be increasing. Older women are also at greater risk than older men for breaking a bone as a result of a fall, in part because of lower bone density after menopause and higher rates of osteoporosis. Canadians who have experienced fall-related injuries are also more likely to be older (aged 85+) and less likely to be married than those without such injuries.

Among older Canadians, fall-related injuries not only threaten health, independence, and quality of life but can also lead to permanent residence in long-term care facilities and even death. Even if a fall does not result in an injury, it can result in negative mental health outcomes including fear of falling, as well as a reduction in daily activities (such as regular exercise), both of which can negatively affect health and function and increase the risk for future falls.

Preventing Fall-Related Injuries

Although it is obvious that preventing falls and fall-related injuries is essential for older adults to remain active, healthy, and independent, it is not as easy as telling people to be careful. Fall-related risk factors are numerous and complex, and they typically interact on a number of levels, including biological/intrinsic, behavioural, environmental, and social/economic:

- *Biological/intrinsic risk factors* include advanced age, impaired mobility, muscle weakness, balance and gait deficits, and the presence of diseases such as heart disease, Parkinson's disease, diabetes, and arthritis.
- *Behavioural risk factors* include risky behaviours (such as climbing up an insecure ladder), a history of falling, fear of falling, the use of multiple medications, excessive alcohol consumption, inappropriate use of assistive devices, and inadequate diet, exercise, and/or sleep.
- *Environmental risk factors* include home hazards, such as poorly placed furniture. Half of all falls resulting in hospitalizations among older adults occur in the home. Outside the home, environmental risk factors can include potholes in sidewalks and roads and poor lighting. Institutional hazards can include poorly designed buildings and noncompliance with safety and building standards, codes, or regulations.
- *Social/economic risk factors* include low income levels, which may affect an older adult's access to safe housing, adequate nutrition, and appropriate health and social services. Additionally, low education and low health literacy can reduce the likelihood that individuals will benefit from printed or online resources related to fall prevention. There is also growing evidence showing the protective effects that marriage and strong family and social networks may have against falling among older adults.

Costs and Savings Associated with Falls

Fall-related injuries among older Canadians have been estimated to cost $2 billion a year for expenses related to hospitalization, medication, treatment, and rehabilitation. By 2031, it is estimated that more than $4 billion will be spent per year on health care costs resulting from fall-related injuries sustained by older adults. The Public Health Agency of Canada has estimated that a 20 percent reduction in falls could result in 7500 fewer hospitalizations and 1800 fewer older Canadians with permanent disabilities. These decreases would result in a savings of approximately $138 million annually.

Promising Practices

A number of prevention strategies have been shown to be effective in reducing falls and fall-related injuries among older adults in home, community, and long-term care settings. These include exercise programs consisting of balance, gait, and weight training components; routine medical assessments and physician visits; healthy eating; appropriate home and environment modifications; proper footwear; and the distribution of information about falls prevention. To reduce or eliminate the burden of fall-related injuries among older Canadians, additional research is needed to identify the effectiveness (including the cost effectiveness) of specific falls-prevention interventions alone and in combination. In addition, novel approaches that utilize emerging technology to reduce the impact of falling, such as compliant flooring, should also be further investigated.

Sources: Accreditation Canada/The Canadian Institute for Health Information/The Canadian Patient Safety Institute. 2014. *Preventing Falls: From Evidence to Improvement in Canadian Health Care,* http://www.accreditation.ca/sites/default/files/falls-joint-report-2014-en.pdf (retrieved February 20, 2015); Public Health Agency of Canada. 2014. *Seniors' Falls in Canada: Second Report,* http://www.phac-aspc.gc.ca/seniors-aines/publications/public/injury-blessure/seniors_falls-chutes_aines/index-eng.php (retrieved February 20, 2015); Public Health Agency of Canada. 2006. *Healthy Aging in Canada: A New Vision, A Vital Investment, from Evidence to Action,* http://www.health.gov.nl.ca/health/publications/vision_rpt_e.pdf (retrieved February 20, 2015); Public Health Agency of Canada. 2005. *Report on Seniors' Falls in Canada,* http://publications.gc.ca/collections/Collection/HP25-1-2005E.pdf (retrieved February 20, 2015).

Eat Wisely

Good health at any age is enhanced by eating a varied diet full of nutrient-rich foods. As noted in Chapter 5, *Eating Well with Canada's Food Guide* outlines recommendations that aim to assist Canadians with food choices that provide enough essential nutrients and help to maintain a healthy weight. For many adults, that means eating more fruits, vegetables, and whole grains while eating fewer foods high in saturated and trans fats and added sugars. Additional recommendations for older adults include the following:

- Take a vitamin D supplement. Health Canada recommends that in addition to following *Eating Well with Canada's Food Guide*, adults over the age of 50 should take a daily vitamin D supplement of 400 IU.
- Make sure that you are getting an adequate amount of calcium. According to Osteoporosis Canada, the daily calcium requirement for Canadians over the age of 50 is 1200 milligrams from both foods and supplements.
- Limit sodium intake to 1300 mg (ages 51–70) or 1200mg (ages 71+) per day, and get enough potassium (4700 mg per day). Older adults tend to have higher blood pressure and to be salt-sensitive.
- Eat foods rich in dietary fibre and drink plenty of water to help prevent constipation. A diet rich in whole grains, vegetables, and fruits can meet the recommended goals for fibre.
- Pay special attention to food safety. Older adults are often more susceptible to food-borne illness.

Maintain a Healthy Weight

Weight management is especially difficult if you have been overweight most of your life. While a sensible program of expending more calories through exercise, cutting calorie intake, or a combination of both will work for many people who want to lose weight, there are a number of additional factors—genetic, environmental, social, medical—that also contribute to overweight and obesity. Rising rates of obesity can be seen among Canadians of all ages, including older adults; in 2013, the incidence of self-reported obesity among Canadian females and males ages 65 or older was approximately 19 percent and 20 percent, respectively.

Control Drinking and Overdependence on Medication

The abuse of alcohol ranks with depression as a commonly hidden health problem. It affects 6–10 percent of older adults. (The ability to metabolize alcohol decreases with age.) The problem is often not identified because the effects of alcohol or drug dependence can mimic disease, such as Alzheimer's disease. Signs of potential alcohol or drug dependence include unexplained falls or frequent injuries, forgetfulness, depression, and malnutrition. Older people who retire or lose a spouse are especially at risk. Problems can be avoided by not using alcohol to relieve anxiety or emotional pain and not taking medication when safer forms of treatment are available.

QUICK STATS

Approximately 66% of Canadians ages 65 and older reported using five or more types of prescription drugs in 2012.
—Canadian Institute for Health Information, 2014

Don't Smoke

The average pack-a-day smoker can expect to live about 13–14 fewer years than a non-smoker. Furthermore, smokers suffer more illnesses that last longer, and they are subject to respiratory disabilities that limit their total vigour for many years before their death. Premature balding, skin wrinkling, and osteoporosis have been linked to cigarette smoking. Individuals who smoke at age 50 often have wrinkles resembling those of a person of 60.

Schedule Physical Examinations to Detect Treatable Diseases

When detected early, many diseases, including hypertension, diabetes, and many types of cancer, can be successfully controlled by medication and lifestyle changes. Regular testing for **glaucoma** after age 40 can prevent blindness from this eye disease. Recommended screenings and immunizations can protect against preventable chronic and infectious diseases. (See Chapters 4 and 7–9 for screening and immunization guidelines.)

> **glaucoma**
> A disease in which fluid inside the eye is under abnormally high pressure; can lead to the loss of peripheral vision and blindness.

Recognize and Reduce Stress

Stress-induced physiological changes increase wear and tear on your body. Cut down on the stresses in your life. Don't wear yourself out through lack of sleep, substance abuse or misuse, or overwork. Take a few minutes every so often throughout the day to close your eyes and focus on your breathing. Practise relaxation using the techniques described in Chapter 3. If you contract a disease, consider it your body's attempt to interrupt your life pattern; reevaluate your lifestyle, and perhaps slow down.

The health behaviours you practise *now* are more influential in determining how long and how well you will live than your behaviours at a later age. Retiring from your life's occupation with a physically healthy body will allow far more options for enjoying yourself than will retiring with frail health or disabilities. Preventable poor health drains finances, emotions, and energy and contributes to poor psychological health. By enhancing your wellness today, you are ensuring some wellness for the future.

QUESTIONS FOR CRITICAL THINKING AND REFLECTION

How do you feel about the prospect of growing old? Would you say that you look forward to it, or are you anxious about it? What influences have shaped your feelings about aging?

Dealing with the Changes of Aging

Just as you can act now to prevent or limit the physical changes of aging, you can also begin preparing yourself psychologically, socially, and financially for the many changes—both positive and negative—that may occur later in life. If you have aging parents, grandparents, and friends, the following information may give you insight into their lives and encourage you to begin cultivating appropriate and useful behaviours now.

Planning for Social Changes

Retirement marks a major change in the second half of life. As Canadians' longevity has increased, people have begun spending a larger proportion of their lives—an average of 20 years or more if they retire at age 65—in retirement. This has implications for reestablishing important relationships, developing satisfying interests outside work, and saving for an adequate retirement income. People who have well-developed leisure pursuits adjust better to retirement than those with few interests outside of work. Some Canadians also choose to continue working in their later years; in 2014, 13 percent of older adults were participating in the work force.

Changing Roles and Relationships

Changes in social roles are a major feature of middle age. Children become young adults and leave home, putting an end to daily parenting in the home environment. Parents experiencing this empty-nest syndrome must adapt to changes in their customary responsibilities and personal identities. And although retirement may be a desirable milestone for most people, it may also be viewed as a threat to prestige, purpose, and self-respect—the loss of a valued or customary role—and will probably require some adjustment.

Retirement and the end of child rearing also bring about changes in the relationship between spouses and partners. The amount of time a couple spends together will increase and activities will change. Couples may need a period of adjustment in which they get to know each other as individuals again. Discussing what types of activities each partner enjoys can help couples set up a mutually satisfying routine of shared and independent activities.

Increased Leisure Time

Although retirement confers the advantages of leisure time and freedom from deadlines, competition, and stress, many people do not plan for or know how to spend their free time. If you have developed diverse interests, retirement can be a joyful and fulfilling period of your life. It can provide opportunities for expanding your horizons by giving you the chance to try new activities, take classes, and meet new people. Volunteering in your community can enhance self-esteem and allow you to be a contributing member of society (see the Mind Body Spirit box). In Canada, 80 percent of older adults participate in one or more social activities on a regular basis (at least monthly) and 36 percent engage in some type of volunteer work.

 Mind *Body* **SPIRIT**

Help Yourself by Helping Others

Choosing to help others—whether as a volunteer for a community organization or through spontaneous acts of kindness—can enhance emotional, social, spiritual, and physical wellness at any age. Surveys and studies indicate that the sense of purpose and service and the feelings of generosity and kindness that go with helping others may be as important a consideration for wellness as good nutrition and regular exercise. Volunteer activities result in many of the same benefits as regular exercise, such as increased energy and vitality. Older adults who volunteer have higher levels of emotional and social wellness and lower rates of death.

In a survey of volunteers from all fields, helpers reported the following benefits:

- Helper's high—physical and emotional sensations, such as sudden warmth, a surge of energy, and a feeling of euphoria that occur immediately after helping
- Feelings of increased self-worth, calm, and relaxation
- A perception of greater physical health
- Fewer colds and headaches, improved eating and sleeping habits, and some relief from the pain of chronic diseases, such as asthma and arthritis

Just how might helping benefit the health of the helper? By helping others, we focus on things other than our own problems, and we get a special kind of attention from the people we help. Helping others can be effective at banishing a bad mood or a case of the blues. Helping others can also expand our perspective and enhance our appreciation for our own lives. Helping may benefit physical health by providing a temporary boost to the immune system and by combating stress and hostile feelings linked to the development of chronic diseases.

Helping others doesn't require a huge time commitment or a change of career. To get the most out of helping, keep the following guidelines in mind:

- *Make contact.* Choose an activity that involves personal contact.
- *Help as often as possible.* If your schedule allows, volunteer at least once a week. Any amount of time helping is better than none.
- *Make helping voluntary.* Voluntary helping has positive results, whereas obligatory helping situations can actually increase stress.
- *Volunteer with others.* Working with a group enables you to form bonds with other helpers who can support your interests and efforts. The health benefits of volunteering are strongest for people who otherwise have low levels of social interaction.
- *Focus on the process, not the outcome.* We can't always measure or know the results of our actions.
- *Practise random acts of kindness.* Smile, let people go ahead of you in line, pay for a stranger's coffee, pick up litter, and so on.
- *Avoid burnout.* Recognize your own limits, pace yourself, and try not to feel guilty or discouraged. Take pride in being a volunteer or caregiver.

The Economics of Retirement

Retirement is usually accompanied by a new economic situation. It may mean a severely restricted budget or possibly even financial disaster if you don't take stock of your finances and plan ahead. The majority of older Canadians live with fixed sources of income, such as pensions. In fact, in 2013–2014, more than $41 billion in Old Age Security (OAS) benefits were distributed to 5.4 million Canadians. It is vital to plan for an adequate retirement income, and this financial planning should begin early in life. People in their twenties and thirties should estimate how much money they need to support their standard of living, calculate their projected income, and begin a savings program. The earlier people begin such a program, the more money they will have at retirement.

QUICK STATS

The percentage of Canadian seniors considered to be "low-income" decreased from 21.4% in 1980 to 5.2% in 2011, one of the lowest rates worldwide.

—Government of Canada, 2014

Adapting to Physical Changes

As described earlier in the chapter, people can do many things to avoid or minimize the effects of the physical changes associated with aging. However, some changes in physical functioning are inevitable, and successful aging involves anticipating and accommodating these changes. Adapting, rather than giving up, favourite activities is one potentially effective strategy for dealing with physical limitations. For example, if arthritis interferes with playing an instrument, a person can continue to enjoy music by taking up a different instrument or attending concerts.

Hearing Loss

Although not inevitable, the loss of hearing is a common physical change that can have a particularly strong effect on the lives of older adults. Some people lose their hearing slowly as they age—a condition known as *presbycusis*. Hearing loss affects a person's ability to interact with others and can lead to depression and a sense of isolation. Hearing loss should be assessed and treated by a health care professional; in some cases, hearing can be completely restored by dealing with the underlying cause of hearing loss. In other cases, hearing aids may be prescribed.

Protect your hearing by avoiding exposure to noises above 90 decibels, such as lawn mowers, motorcycles, gun shots, and loud music (see Chapter 21 for more information). Wear ear plugs when you must be around loud noises, limit your time of exposure, and stay as far as possible from the sound's source.

Vision Changes

Vision usually declines with age. For some individuals this can be traced to physical conditions, such as **glaucoma** or **age-related macular degeneration (AMD)** that can be

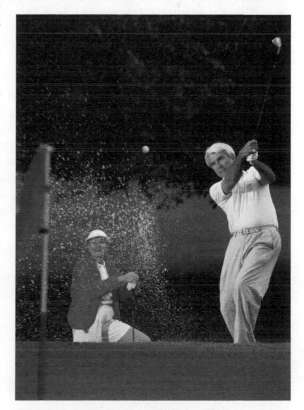

The retirement years can be the best part of one's life socially, with increased opportunities to meet and interact with new and different people.

treated medically. For others, the effects of a decline in vision can be managed by using strategies to make the most of remaining vision.

glaucoma
An increase in pressure in the eye due to fluid buildup that can result in loss of side vision and, if left untreated, blindness.

age-related macular degeneration (AMD)
A deterioration of the macula (the central areas of the retina) that leads to blurred vision and sensitivity to glare; some cases can lead to blindness.

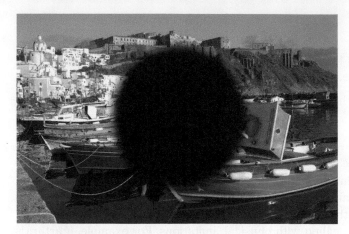

Age-related macular degeneration (AMD) makes many daily tasks difficult or impossible. This photo shows how things look to someone with AMD.

Glaucoma is caused by increased pressure within the eye cause by a buildup of fluid. The optic nerve can be damaged by this increased pressure, resulting in a loss of side vision and, if untreated, blindness. Medication can relieve the pressure by decreasing the amount of fluid produced or by helping it drain more efficiently. Laser and conventional surgery are other options. Glaucoma affects approximately 1 in 100 Canadians over the age of 40; because it often has no symptoms, however, it is estimated that only half of all individuals with glaucoma know that they have it. Being over the age of 40, near-sighted, diabetic, of African, Asian, or Hispanic descent, and having a family history of glaucoma are some of the known risk factors for this disease.

AMD is a slow disintegration of the *macula*, the tissue at the centre of the retina where fine, straight-ahead detail is distinguished. AMD affects approximately 1.4 million Canadians and is the leading cause of blindness and vision loss in Canada. Losing this vision makes it difficult to read, drive, or perform other close-up activities. Risk factors for AMD are age, gender (women may be at higher risk than men), smoking, elevated cholesterol levels, and family history. Some cases of AMD can be treated with laser surgery. Both glaucoma and AMD can be detected with regular screening.

Vision can also be affected by conditions that are products of aging. By the time they reach their forties, many people have developed **presbyopia**, a gradual decline in the ability to focus on objects close to them. This occurs because the lens of the eye no longer expands and contracts as readily. **Cataracts**, a clouding of the lens caused by lifelong oxidation damage (a by-product of normal body chemistry), may dim vision by the sixties.

presbyopia
The inability of the eyes to focus sharply on nearby objects, caused by the loss of elasticity of the lens that occurs with advancing age.

cataracts
Opacity of the lens of the eye that impairs vision and can cause blindness.

QUICK STATS

AMD is the third leading cause of blindness worldwide, after cataracts and glaucoma.
—World Health Organization, 2015

Arthritis

Approximately 4.6 million Canadian adults—one in six over the age of 15—are estimated to have some form of **arthritis**. This degenerative disease causes joint inflammation leading to chronic pain, swelling, and loss of mobility. Its warning signs include swelling, pain, redness, warmth, tenderness, changes in joint mobility, early-morning stiffness, and unexplained weight loss, fever, or weakness in combination with joint pain. Arthritis is a disease that affects people of all ages, although it affects older adults and women more often.

> **arthritis**
> Inflammation and swelling of a joint or joints, causing pain and swelling.

There are more than 100 different types of arthritis; osteoarthritis (OA) is by far the most common. (Rheumatoid arthritis, an autoimmune disorder, is described in Chapter 9.) In a person with OA, the cartilage that caps the bones in joints wears away, forming sharp spurs (see Figure 17.2). It most often affects the hands and weight-bearing joints of the body—the knees, ankles, and hips.

Strategies for reducing the risk of arthritis and, for those who already have OA, for managing it, include exercise, weight management, and avoidance of heavy or repetitive muscle use. Weakness of the muscles around joints is linked to arthritis. This is why exercising is helpful. Exercise lubricates joints and strengthens the muscles around them, protecting them from further damage. Swimming, walking, cross-country skiing, cycling, and tai chi are good low-impact exercises; knitting and crocheting are excellent for the hands. Maintaining an appropriate weight is important to avoid placing stress on the hips, knees, and ankles. Assistive devices, such as kitchen utensils and repair tools with large handles, can also help.

It is also important to visit a physician as soon as arthritis symptoms occur so appropriate treatment can be started to reduce pain and swelling, keep joints moving safely, and prevent further joint damage. If joints are severely damaged and activity is limited, surgery to repair or replace joints may be considered, but medication is usually the first treatment. Many people with OA take medication to relieve inflammation and reduce pain. Because arthritis is a chronic condition, researchers are trying to find medications that are safe and effective when used long-term. Non-steroidal anti-inflammatory drugs like ibuprofen can help but can also irritate the digestive tract; prescription drugs that relieve pain without damaging the stomach have been found to have other potentially dangerous side effects. Acetaminophen can also reduce pain without upsetting the stomach, but exceeding the recommended dosage can cause liver damage.

FIGURE 17.2

Osteoarthritis

When cartilage wears away within a joint, sharp spurs form and the amount of fluid increases, causing pain and swelling.

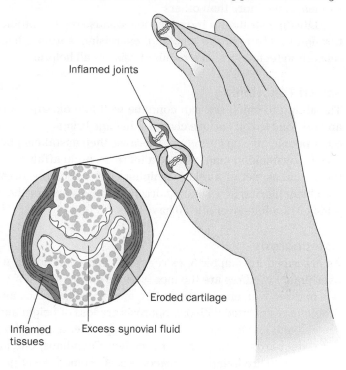

Inflamed joints

Eroded cartilage

Inflamed tissues

Excess synovial fluid

Source: Clayman, C. (ed.). 1995. *The Human Body: An Illustrated Guide to Its Structure, Function, and Disorders.* New York: DK.

QUICK STATS

Approximately 1 in 5 Canadians are expected to have arthritis by 2036.
—The Arthritis Society, 2015

Menopause

The natural process of menopause usually occurs during a woman's forties or fifties. The ovaries gradually stop functioning, estrogen levels drop, and eventually menstruation ceases. Several years before a woman stops menstruating, her periods usually become irregular, and she may experience hot flashes, vaginal dryness, sleep disturbances, and mood swings. This time, called *perimenopause*, can be troublesome for many women, some more than others.

Lifestyle strategies to reduce menopause-related problems include many of the healthy habits discussed throughout the text; not smoking, exercising, eating a healthy diet, losing excess weight, and engaging in relaxation techniques on a regular basis are all helpful.

Sexual Functioning

The ability to enjoy sex can continue well into old age, particularly if people make the effort to understand and respond to the various changes that age brings to the natural pattern of the sexual response. All too often, older people give up intercourse because they mistakenly interpret these changes as signs of impending impotence. Lovemaking may become a more leisurely affair as a couple gets older, but the benefits of maintaining the sexual aspect of a relationship into old age can be great. It is important for older adults, some of whom may be exploring new sexual horizons after divorce or the death of a spouse, to practise safe sex. A growing number of adults over age 50 have STIs.

Osteoporosis

As described in Chapter 5, *osteoporosis* is a condition in which bones become dangerously thin and fragile over time. Fractures are the most serious consequence of osteoporosis; in Canada, it has been estimated that one in three women and one in five men will experience an osteoporotic fracture during their lifetime. Other problems associated with osteoporosis are loss of height and a stooped posture caused by vertebral fractures, severe back and hip pain, and breathing problems caused by changes in the shape of the skeleton.

Osteoporosis affects about 2 million Canadians; one in four women and roughly one in eight men over the age of 50 are living with osteoporosis. Women are at greater risk than men for osteoporosis because they have 10–25 percent less bone in their skeleton. As they lose bone mass with age, women's bones become dangerously thin sooner than men's bones (although more men will probably develop osteoporosis in the future as they live into their eighties and nineties). Bone loss accelerates in women during the first 5–10 years after the onset of menopause because of the drop in estrogen production. (Estrogen improves calcium absorption and reduces the amount of calcium the body excretes.) No single cause for osteoporosis has been identified, however being over the age of 65, having an existing medical condition that can lead to fractures or bone loss (such as chronic liver disease or celiac disease among others), smoking, a family history of osteoporosis, early menopause (before age 45), abnormal or irregular menstruation, a history of anorexia, and a thin, small frame are all considered risk factors. Regular consumption of more than two alcoholic drinks a day increases the risk of osteoporosis, possibly because alcohol can interfere with the body's ability to absorb calcium. Thyroid medication, corticosteroid drugs for arthritis or asthma, and long-term use of certain contraceptives can also have a negative effect on bone mass.

Preventing osteoporosis requires building as much bone as possible when you are young and then maintaining it as you age. In fact, Osteoporosis Canada notes that the condition has been called a "pediatric disease with geriatric consequences," as peak bone mass is typically achieved between ages 16–20 in women and ages 20–25 in men. Diet and exercise play key roles; it is important to eat foods rich in calcium and vitamin D and to get adequate exercise. Weight-bearing aerobic activities must be performed regularly throughout life to have lasting effects. Strength training improves bone density, muscle mass, strength, and balance, protecting against both bone loss and falls, a major cause of fractures. Even for people in their seventies, low-intensity strength training has been shown to improve bone density.

Two other lifelong strategies for reducing the effects of osteoporosis are avoiding tobacco use and managing depression and stress. Smoking reduces the body's estrogen levels and is linked to earlier menopause and more rapid postmenopausal bone loss. Some women with depression experience significant bone loss. Researchers have not identified the reason, but it may be linked to increases in the stress hormone cortisol.

Bone mineral density testing is the most accurate diagnostic test for osteoporosis and can be used to gauge an individual's risk of fracture and help determine if treatment is needed. Below-normal bone density may be classified as *osteopenia*, which is usually treated with medication, exercise, and nutrition. A greater loss of bone mass is classified as full-blown osteoporosis and is often treated with medications.

QUICK STATS

At least 80% of fractures in Canadians over the age of 50 are related to osteoporosis.
—Osteoporosis Canada, 2015

Handling Psychological and Mental Changes

Many people associate old age with forgetfulness, and slowly losing one's memory was once considered an inevitable part of growing old. However, we now know that most older adults in good health remain mentally alert and retain their full capacity to learn and remember new information. Occasional confusion or forgetfulness may indicate only a temporary information overload, fatigue, or response to medications. Many people become more intelligent as they become older and more experienced.

Dementia

Dementia is a loss of brain function that occurs with certain diseases. It affects memory, thinking, language, judgment, and behaviour. Close to 15 percent of people aged 65 and older in Canada have some degree of dementia, and that number will increase over the next few decades with the aging of the population. Early symptoms include slight disturbances in a person's ability to grasp the situation he or she is in. As dementia progresses, memory failure becomes apparent, and the person may forget conversations, the events of the day, or how to perform simple tasks. It is important to have any symptoms evaluated by a health care professional because some of the more than 50 known causes of dementia are treatable (for example, depression, dehydration, malnutrition, vitamin B12 deficiency, alcoholism, and misuse of medications).

> **dementia**
> Deterioration of mental functioning (including memory, concentration, and judgment) resulting from a brain disorder; often accompanied by emotional disturbances and personality changes.

The most common forms of dementia among older people—**Alzheimer's disease**, Lewy body dementia, and multi-infarct dementia—are irreversible. The most common, Alzheimer's disease, is a progressive brain disorder that damages and eventually destroys brain cells, leading to loss of memory, thinking, and other brain functions (see the In Focus box). Lewy body dementia is an umbrella term for a form of dementia that resembles Alzheimer's disease but has two or more distinctive features. Symptoms that differentiate Lewy body dementia from Alzheimer's include unpredictable levels of cognitive ability, attention, or alertness; changes in walking or movement; and a sleep disorder called REM sleep behaviour disorder, in which people physically act out their dreams. Multi-infarct dementia results from a series of small strokes or changes in the brain's blood supply that deprive the brain of oxygen and destroy brain tissue. Symptoms may appear suddenly and worsen with additional strokes; they include disorientation in familiar locations; walking with rapid, shuffling steps; incontinence; laughing or crying inappropriately; difficulty following instructions; and problems handling money. High blood pressure, cigarette smoking, and high cholesterol are some of the risk factors for stroke that may be controlled to prevent vascular dementia. Even for these incurable forms of dementia, treatment can improve an affected person's quality of life.

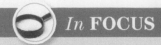 *In* FOCUS

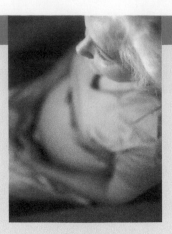

Alzheimer's Disease

Alzheimer's disease (AD) is a fatal brain disorder that causes physical and chemical changes in the brain. As the brain's nerve cells are destroyed, the system that produces the neurotransmitter acetylcholine breaks down, and communication among parts of the brain deteriorates. Autopsies reveal that the interiors of the affected neurons are filled with clusters of proteins known as *tangles*: the spaces between the neurons are filled with protein deposits called *amyloid plaques*.

Approximately 750 000 Canadians have Alzheimer's disease or a related dementia, and that number is expected to increase to 1.4 million by 2031. AD usually occurs in people over age 60, but it can occur in people as young as 40.

Symptoms

The first symptoms of AD are forgetfulness and inability to concentrate. A person may have difficulty performing familiar tasks at home and work and have problems with abstract thinking. As the disease progresses, people experience severe memory loss, especially for recent events. They may vividly remember events from their childhood but be unable to remember the time of day or their location. Depression and anxiety are also common.

In the later stages, people with AD are disoriented and may even hallucinate; some experience personality changes—becoming very aggressive or very docile. Eventually, they lose control of physical functioning and are completely dependent on caregivers. On average, a person will survive eight years after the development of the first symptoms.

Causes

Scientists do not yet know what causes AD. Age is the main risk factor, although about 10 percent of cases seem tied to inherited gene mutations. Inherited familial AD generally strikes people before age 65, while the more common late-onset AD occurs in people 65 and older. Some evidence suggests that many of the same factors that affect heart disease risk also apply to AD. In women, low levels of estrogen in the brain may contribute to AD. A mutation of the protein apolipoprotein E, which can destroy neural cells, may be a cause of the disease in some people.

A great deal of research is focusing on the role of a peptide molecule known as amyloid-beta, which may play a role in the development of plaques in the brain. Scientists are looking for genetic factors that cause certain people to develop high levels of amyloid-beta.

People who regularly take non-steroidal anti-inflammatory drugs (NSAIDs) like ibuprofen (often to control arthritis) and people who regularly consume fish rich in omega-3 fatty acids appear to have lower rates of AD, indicating a possible protective effect of substances that reduce inflammation. Some studies indicate that vitamin E and other antioxidants may reduce risk for AD or slow the progress of the disease, suggesting that oxidative stress caused by free radicals may also play a role.

Diagnosis and Treatment

Currently, the only certain way to diagnose AD is to examine brain tissue during an autopsy. In most cases, physicians use a combination of medical history, neurological and psychological tests, physical exams, blood and urine tests, and a brain-imaging scan. Good early results have also been seen by using a test that measures levels of a specific protein in spinal fluid; less invasive blood tests to measure the same proteins are under development.

For people with AD, several drugs can provide modest improvements in memory, language, thinking ability, and motor skills. Some medications help maintain cognitive function by inhibiting the breakdown of the neuro-transmitter acetylcholine but do not alter the course of the disease. Medications approved in Canada include Aricept (donepezil), Exelon (rivastigmine), Reminyl (galantamine), and Ebixa (memantine).

Scientists are also investigating new treatments that may stop Alzheimer's progress before it can cause too much damage. Non-pharmacological options such as music therapy, pet therapy, and massage may also benefit some individuals with AD. Due to a lack of research in the area, the Alzheimer Society of Canada is currently funding research that aims to identify effective alternative therapies for people with AD.

Sources: Alzheimer Society of Canada. 2015. *Dementia Numbers in Canada,* http://www.alzheimer.ca/en/About-dementia/What-is-dementia/Dementia-numbers (retrieved June 17, 2015); and Alzheimer Society of Canada. 2014. *Treatment Options,* http://www.alzheimer.ca/en/About-dementia/Treatment-options (retrieved June 23, 2015).

Alzheimer's disease
A disease characterized by a progressive loss of mental functioning (dementia), caused by a degeneration of brain cells.

Evidence suggests that some cases of dementia are hereditary, but experts say genetics are not always a sure sign that a person will develop the disease. You can also take lifestyle steps to help ward off dementia, such as controlling weight and blood pressure, eating a balanced diet (including adequate B vitamins and omega-3 fatty acids), exercising, not smoking, moderating your use of alcohol, practising stress reduction techniques, maintaining social contacts, and cultivating a variety of mental pursuits, such as doing crossword puzzles. Strong evidence links the Mediterranean diet with reduced risk of these diseases.

Grief

Another psychological and emotional challenge of aging is dealing with grief and mourning. While these challenges can occur at any age, aging is often associated with increased loss—the loss of friends, peers, physical appearance, possessions, and health. Grief is the process of getting through the pain of loss, and it can be one of the loneliest and most intense times in a person's life. It can take a year or two or more to completely come to terms with the loss of a loved one. (See Chapter 18 for more information about responses to loss and how to support a grieving person.)

Unresolved grief can have serious physical and psychological or emotional health consequences and may require professional help. Signs of unresolved grief include hostility toward people connected with the death (physicians or nurses, for example), talking about the death as if it occurred yesterday, and unrealistic or harmful behaviour (such as giving away all of one's own belongings). Many people become depressed after the loss of a loved one or when confronted with retirement or a chronic illness. But after a period of grieving, people are generally able to resume their lives.

Depression

Unresolved grief can lead to depression, a common problem in older adults (see Chapter 2). If you notice the signs of depression in yourself or someone you know, consult a mental health professional. A marked loss

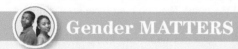 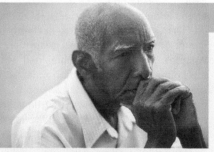

Gender MATTERS

Suicide Among Older Canadians

One group of Canadians is more likely to commit suicide than any other. From mass media accounts, you might imagine this group to be adolescents; according to the Centre for Suicide Prevention, however, people over the age of 65—and men in particular—have the highest suicide rate among Canadians.

Why is this so? One possible explanation is that some older adults may believe they are a burden to their family and/or caregivers. With regard to older men specifically, it has been suggested that aging and retirement could represent a relatively greater "loss" in terms of power, status, and contributions to society in comparison to older women. Another theory is that men tend to have weaker social ties than women, and as they retire their increasing social isolation leads to depression and suicide.

In contrast to younger Canadians, suicidal attempts among older adults—both male and female—are more likely to result in completed suicides. This may be because older adults choose more lethal methods to end their lives, they may display fewer warning signs, and they are also more likely to be physically frail and thus not able to recover from self-inflicted injury. Social isolation also contributes to the increased likelihood of death among older adults by reducing the chance that they will be found by others in the time needed to receive medical attention.

See Chapter 2 for more on risk and protective factors for suicide.

Source: Centre for Suicide Prevention. 2014. *Plus 65: At The End of the Day [Resource Toolkit]*, https://suicideinfo.ca/LinkClick. aspx?fileticket=cmFwRL4DMJw= (retrieved June 23, 2015).

of interest in usually pleasurable activities, decreased appetite, insomnia, fatigue, and feelings of worthlessness are signs of depression. Listen carefully when an older friend or relative talks about being "down" or depressed; it may be a request for help. Suicide rates are relatively high among older adults, and depression should be taken seriously (see the Gender Matters box).

Aging and Life Expectancy

Life expectancy is the average length of time we can expect to live. It is calculated by averaging mortality statistics—the ages at death of a group of people over a certain period. In 2013, life expectancy was 80 years for Canadian men and 84 years for Canadian women (see the Gender Matters box). Those who reach age 65 can expect to live even longer because they have already survived hazards to life in the younger years. Life expectancy also varies among ethnic groups; reasons for these differences include socioeconomic, genetic, and lifestyle factors.

> **life expectancy**
> The average length of time a person is expected to live.

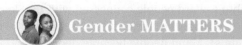

Gender MATTERS

Why Do Women Live Longer?

Women live longer than men in most countries around the world, even in places where maternal mortality rates are high. In Canada, women on average can expect to live about four years longer than men (see the table). Among Canadians over age 100, women outnumber men about five to one.

Generally speaking, the probability of dying is lower at all ages for women than it is for men. The reason for the gender gap in life expectancy is not entirely understood but may be influenced by biological, social, and lifestyle factors. Estrogen production and other factors during a woman's younger years may protect her from early heart disease and from age-related declines in the pumping power of the heart. Women may have lower rates of stress-related illnesses because they cope more positively with stress by seeking social support.

The news for women is not all good, however, because not all their extra years are likely to be healthy years. They are more likely than men to suffer from chronic conditions, such as arthritis and osteoporosis. Women's longer lifespan, combined with the facts that men tend to marry younger women and that widowed men remarry more often than widowed women, means there are many more single older women than men. Older men are more likely to live in family settings, whereas older women are more likely to live alone. Older women are also less likely to be covered by a pension or to have retirement savings, so they are more likely to experience financial challenges.

Increased male mortality can be traced in part to higher rates of unhealthful behaviours, such as smoking and alcohol and drug abuse. Testosterone production may be partly responsible in that it is linked to aggressive and risky behaviour and to unhealthy cholesterol levels. Men have much higher rates of death than women from car crashes and other unintentional injuries, firearm-related deaths, homicide, suicide, AIDS, and early heart attack. Gender roles that promote risky behaviour among young men are a factor in many of these causes of death. Indeed, among people who have made it to age 65, the gender longevity gap is smaller.

Social and behavioural factors may be more important than physiological causes in explaining the gender gap; for

Life Expectancy in Canada (in Years)

Year	Men	Women
At birth		
1971	69.6	76.6
1991	74.6	81.0
2000–2002	77.0	82.0
2009–2011	79.3	83.6
At age 65		
1971	13.9	17.7
1991	15.8	20.0
2000–2002	17.0	20.5
2009–2011	18.8	21.7

example, among the Amish, a religious sect that has strict rules against smoking and drinking, men usually live as long as women. This suggests that the longevity gap could be substantially narrowed through lifestyle changes.

Sources: Statistics Canada. 2014. Centenarians in Canada, https://www12.statcan.gc.ca/census-recensement/2011/as-sa/98-311-x/98-311-x2011003_1-eng.cfm (retrieved July 20, 2015); Statistics Canada. 2000. *Report on the Demographic Situation in Canada*, http://www.statcan.gc.ca/pub/91-209-x/91-209-x2000000-eng.pdf (retrieved July 20, 2015); Statistics Canada. 2010. *Table 1: Life Expectancy at Birth and at Age 65 by Sex, Canada*, http://www.statcan.gc.ca/daily-quotidien/100223/t100223a1-eng.htm (retrieved July 20, 2015); and Statistics Canada. 2013. *Table 4: Life Expectancy at Birth and at Age 65, Canada, Provinces and territories, 2009–2011*, http://www.statcan.gc.ca/pub/91-209-x/2013001/article/11867/tbl/tbl4-eng.htm (retrieved July 20, 2015).

Life expectancy in Canada increased dramatically in the twentieth century, as described in Chapter 1. This does not mean that every Canadian lives longer now than in 1900; rather, far fewer people die young now because childhood and infectious diseases are better controlled and diet and sanitation are much improved.

How long can humans expect to live in the best of circumstances? It now seems possible that our maximum potential **lifespan** is 100–120 years. Our **health span**, by contrast, is the period of life when we are generally healthy and free from chronic or serious disease. The major difference between lifespan (how long we live) and health span (how long we stay healthy) is freedom from chronic or disabling disease. Failure to achieve a positive health span results to some degree from destructive environmental and behavioural factors—factors over which we can exert considerable control. Longevity appears to be influenced very little by genetics. Studies of identical twins and other research suggest that lifespan is only about 3 percent heritable, meaning that the age at which our parents die has only a 3 percent effect on our own age at death.

lifespan
A theoretically projected length of life based on the maximum potential of the human body in the best environment.

health span
The period of life when a person is generally healthy and free from chronic or serious disease.

Long life does not necessarily mean a longer period of disability, either. People often live longer because they have been well longer. A healthy old age is very often an extension of a healthy middle age. However, behaviour changes cannot extend the maximum human lifespan, which seems to be built into our genes.

No one really knows how and why people change as they get older. Different theories claim that aging is caused by accumulated injuries from ultraviolet light, wear and tear on the body, by-products of metabolism, and so on. Other theories view aging as a predetermined, genetically programmed process. No theory, however, sufficiently explains all the changes of the aging process. Aging is complex and varies in how it affects different people and even different organs. Most gerontologists (scientists who study aging and its effects) feel that aging is the cumulative result of the interaction of many lifelong influences, including heredity, environment, culture, diet, exercise and leisure, past illnesses, and many other factors.

QUICK STATS

Canadian men who reach 65 years of age can expect to live about 19 years longer than the life expectancy calculated from birth; Canadian women who reach 65 years of age can expect to live 22 years longer.

—Statistics Canada, 2012

Life in an Aging Canada

As life expectancy increases, a larger proportion of the population will be in their later years. This change will necessitate new government policies and changes in our general attitudes toward older adults.

People over 65 were a minority in the Canadian population at almost 16 percent of the total population in 2014. As the baby boomers age, the older adult population is expected to reach 24–28 percent of the population by 2063. The proportion of the oldest Canadians is growing rapidly; in 2012, approximately 4 percent of Canadians were 80 years of age or older—more than twice as many as in 1982. According to Statistics Canada projections, an unprecedented event will likely take place as early as 2015: Older adults will outnumber youth under the age of 15 in Canada (see Figure 17.3). Despite the fact that many Canadians are now enjoying longer lives, life expectancy among some distinct populations in our country—Inuit seniors, for example—is still much lower than the rest of the population.

FIGURE 17.3

Proportion of Canadian Population Ages < 15 Years and ≥ 65 Years, 1982–2036

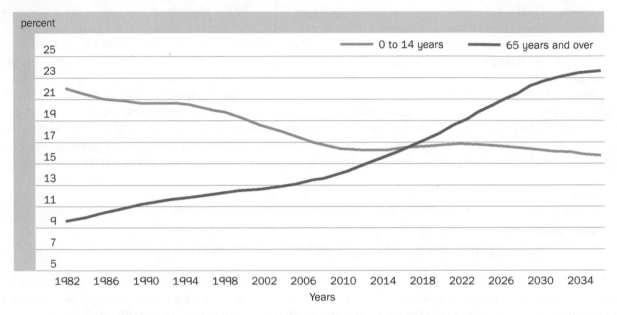

Source: Statistics Canada. 2013. *Proportion of population aged less than 15 years old and 65 years old and over, 1982 to 2036, Canada,* http://www.statcan.gc.ca/pub/91-215-x/2012000/ct008-eng.htm (retrieved July 20, 2015).

Today, low fertility rates (1.6 children per woman currently versus three or more children per woman in the mid-1940s to the 1960s), longer life expectancy, and the effects of the baby boom generation are some of the factors contributing to Canada's aging population (see the In the News box).

 In *the* NEWS

Baby Boomers: Redefining Age and Retirement

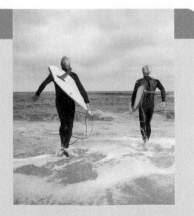

If you are a post-secondary student between the ages of 18 and 24, chances are good that one or both of your parents are members of the *baby boom* generation—people born between 1946 and 1965. In 2011, the first members of the baby boom generation turned 65, which means that Canada is now experiencing what some call the "retirement boom." However, despite the fact that the boomers in your life will likely be reaching retirement age in the near future, this doesn't mean that they will actually retire.

Living Longer, Living Younger

In general, baby boomers are living longer than their parents did. As a result, the average boomer's retirement period is longer. Near the beginning of the twentieth century, the average 65-year-old Canadian could expect to live another 13 years; today, that number has been extended to about 20 years. And it's becoming increasingly common for people to live into their eighties and nineties. Boomers "live younger" than their parents, too, meaning they tend to be healthier than their parents and enjoy better long-term prospects for good health.

Redefining Notions of Age

What are baby boomers doing with all that extra time and health? As it turns out, they have big plans for retirement, including retiring early and continuing an active lifestyle. Baby boomers don't necessarily consider age 60 or 65 to be the start of their "golden years." As they reach age 60 and beyond, boomers are re-inventing themselves and their lives, leaving long-held notions of aging in the dust.

A Shift in Thinking

Traditional views of retirement are starting to change, primarily because of the cost of retiring. Most Canadians do not save enough money to fund 20 or more years of leisure time. According to the 2014 Canadian Financial Capability Survey, approximately one-third of adults are not preparing financially for retirement, either on their own or through an employer pension plan. In addition, close to 30 percent of Canadian adults reported being "not very confident" or "not at all confident" that their income will be enough for them to maintain their standard of living during retirement. Additionally, an earlier Statistics Canada report showed that about one-third of Canadians aged 55 and over retired with some form of debt with a median amount owing of $19 000.

Some reports suggest that not all baby boomers downsize their lifestyles in retirement. In fact, some Canadians may even plan to maintain or even increase their standard of living in retirement. This plan has led many older Canadians to practise what experts call *revolving* or *cycling retirement*: periods of work interspersed with extended periods of leisure. Following this strategy, older people can work only as required to support their lifestyle. When not working, they can pursue other interests.

Of course, this scenario can play out only if people stay relatively healthy. Although older Canadians are fitter than ever, continued good health is not a given. If current positive trends continue, however, baby boomers may be just the first of many generations not only to live longer but to put off retirement altogether. It appears as though the early boomers (people born between 1946 and 1955) will be both trend setters and game changers in the new retirement landscape in Canada, while the late boomers (born between 1956 and 1965) and the gen-Xers (born between 1966 and 1979) will be able to observe and learn from their experiences.

The enormous increase in the aging population is markedly affecting our stereotypes of what it means to grow old. The misfortunes associated with aging—frailty, forgetfulness, poor health, isolation—occur in fewer people in their sixties and seventies and are shifting instead to burden the very old, those over 85.

The financial situation of older adults in Canada has improved over the past quarter century. In many cases, the living expenses of older adults are lower after retirement because they no longer support children and have fewer work-related expenses; they also consume and buy less food. They are more likely to continue practising their expertise for years after retirement: Thousands of retired consultants, teachers, technicians, and craftspeople work until their middle and late seventies. They also receive government assistance, including the **Old Age Security (OAS) pension**, and often have greater net worth from lifetime savings. Unfortunately, the highest incidence of low-income among older adults in Canada occurs among women who live alone.

Old Age Security (OAS) pension

A monthly benefit available to Canadians 65 years of age and older who have lived in Canada for at least 10 years; financed through taxes paid by Canadians.

QUICK STATS

In 2014, more than 1.7 million Canadian men and women were widowed.

—Statistics Canada, 2014

As the aging population increases proportionately, however, the number of older people who are ill and dependent rises. Additionally, the need for medications, medical equipment, and health services—and the costs associated with them—are often substantial. On average, older Canadians visit physicians much more often than younger Canadians. In 2009, the proportion of older adults who visited their family physician frequently (10 times per year or more) was almost double the proportion of younger adults who were also frequent visitors. Older adults are also hospitalized more frequently and are higher users of prescription drugs than the general (non-senior) adult population. In 2009, provincial and territorial governments spent an average of $1311 per older adult compared with $170 per adult aged 20 to 64 for prescription drugs. In Canada, the difference in prescription drug costs can be partially explained by older adults' greater reliance on public sources of financing, in comparison to younger adults who are more likely to use private insurance and out-of-pocket payments.

Health care policy planners hope that rising medical costs for older adults will shrink dramatically through education and prevention. Health

TABLE 17.1

Percentage of Older Canadians (65+) with Chronic Conditions

Condition	Percentage
Heart disease	57
Stroke	54
Cancer	40
Emphysema or Chronic Obstructive Pulmonary Disease (COPD)	40
High blood pressure	39
Diabetes	37
Arthritis	31
Asthma	18
Chronic pain	17
Depression	14

Source: Canadian Institute for Health Information. 2011. *Seniors and the health care system: What is the impact of multiple chronic conditions?*, https://secure.cihi.ca/free_products/air-chronic_disease_aib_en.pdf (retrieved July 20, 2015).

care professionals, including **gerontologists** and **geriatricians**, are beginning to practise preventive medicine, just as pediatricians do. They advise older people about how to avoid and, if necessary, how to manage diseases and disabilities. In Canada, most older people have at least one chronic condition; many have more than one. Table 17.1 lists some of the most commonly reported conditions among older adults in Canada.

gerontologist
A person who studies the biological, psychological, and social phenomena associated with aging and old age.

geriatrician
A physician specializing in the diseases, disabilities, and care of older adults.

QUESTIONS FOR CRITICAL THINKING AND REFLECTION

Have you ever thought about growing old? Is it a topic that you have discussed with others, or is it one that you avoid? What do you think are the most important dimensions of wellness for older adults? What health behaviours will you focus on as you move from youth to middle age to old age? What behaviour change strategies might be helpful?

Family and Community Resources for Older Adults

With help from friends, family members, and community services, people in their later years can remain active and independent. According to the 2011 census, 92 percent of Canadians over the age of 65 live in private households, either alone or with others. Only 7 percent live in collective dwellings, such as long-term care hospitals or nursing homes, but among those over age 85, almost 30 percent live in special care facilities. Figure 17.4 shows the breakdown by sex.

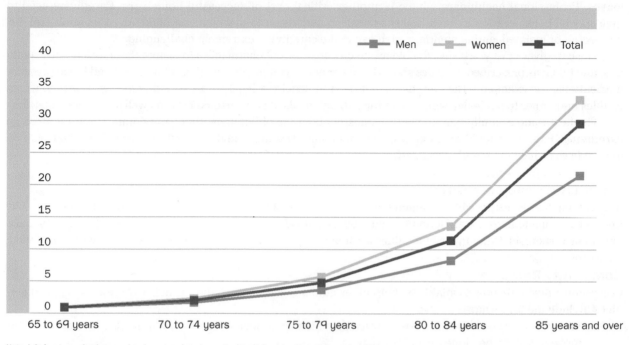

FIGURE 17.4

Percentage of Older Canadians Living in Special Care Facilities, by Age Group and Sex

Note: I. Refers to nursing homes, chronic care or long-term care hospitals and residences for senior citizens.

Source: Statistics Canada. 2013. *Percentage of the population aged 65 and over linving in special care facilities, by age group, Canada, 2011,* http://wwwl2.statcan.ca/census-recensement/2011/as-sa/98-312-x/2011003/fig/fig3_4-4-eng.cfm (retrieved July 20, 2015).

THINKING ABOUT THE ENVIRONMENT

Both the natural and human-made environments pose many threats to the well-being of older adults.

Particulate air pollution and ozone, for example, aggravate breathing-related conditions, such as asthma and chronic obstructive pulmonary disease (COPD). In older people with such disorders, even brief exposure to dirty air can result in hospitalization. Indoor air can be just as hazardous, especially if it contains lingering mould or dust particles.

Environmental factors can be a special concern for older adults with diabetes. When a person with diabetes is exposed to hot weather, for example, the body can lose its ability to regulate its temperature—a condition that can be fatal. Air pollution can affect the ability of the blood vessels of a person with diabetes to control blood flow. Several types of air pollution have been associated with an increased risk of cardiovascular problems in people with diabetes.

For more information on the environment and environmental health, see Chapter 21.

The living arrangements of older Canadians appear to be related to the overall well-being of these individuals. Although many factors influence a person's level of happiness, compared with older adults who live with a spouse or other family members, those living alone are less likely to describe themselves as very happy. Interestingly, the proportion of older adults who report being divorced or separated has increased from 4 percent to 12 percent from 1981 to 2011.

Family Involvement in Caregiving

Studies show that in about three out of four cases, a spouse, a grown child, or a daughter- or son-in-law assumes a caregiving role for older relatives. With more parents living into their eighties and with fewer children per family, many people, and women in particular, will face the dilemma of how best to care for an aging relative.

Caregiving can be rewarding, but it is also hard work. If the experience is stressful and long-term, family members may become emotionally exhausted. Corporations are increasingly responsive to the needs of their employees who are family caregivers by providing helpful services, such as referrals, flexible schedules, and leaves. Professional health care advice is another critical part of successful home care. Caregivers need to give special consideration to such issues as hearing and vision loss, which can make an older adult feel disconnected or isolated, and dementia, which can make caregiving extremely challenging.

The caregiver must work with the older person's doctors and pharmacists to ensure that medication is available and taken as prescribed. (Studies show that older adults commonly skip their cholesterol and blood pressure medications, for example.) The caregiver may need to acquire a legal status called *power of attorney*, which enables him or her to make decisions about the patient's medical and personal care, as well as financial matters.

The best thing a family can do is talk honestly about the obligations, time, and commitment required by caregiving. Families should also explore the community resources and professional assistance that may be available to reduce the stress in this difficult job.

Other Living and Care Options

If living together is not possible for aging parents and adult children, other living and care options are available. Retirement communities are an option for individuals in good health and with a good income who want to maintain home ownership. Other types of facilities are available for people who need more assistance with daily living.

Community Resources

Community resources are available to help older adults remain active and in their own homes. Typical services include the following:

- *Senior centres or adult daycare centres* provide meals, social activities, and health care services for those unable to be alone during the day.
- *Homemaker services* offer housekeeping, cooking, errand running, and escorting to appointments.
- *Visiting nurses* provide basic health care.
- *Household services* perform household repairs.
- *Friendly visitor or daily telephone reassurance services* provide contacts, medication and other reminders, and friendly conversation for older people who live alone.
- *Home food delivery services* such as "Meals on Wheels" provide meals to homebound people.
- *Adult day hospital care* provides daycare plus physical therapy and treatment for chronic illnesses.
- *Low-cost legal aid* helps manage finances and health care.
- *Transportation services* offer rides at low rates.
- *Case management* helps older adults navigate confusing health care services.

Transportation

Older drivers usually have safe driving records compared with young adults because they tend to be more cautious; however, crashes in the older age group are more likely to be fatal. The decision to stop driving is an extremely difficult one for older adults, their family members, and their physicians. In Canada, most provinces and territories require physicians to report patients who are medically unfit to drive. Other regulations relating to driver's licences held by older adults vary across jurisdictions. In Ontario, for example, the Senior Driver's Licence Renewal Program requires that adult drivers ages 80 years and over complete a vision test, undergo a driver record review, take part in a group education session, and complete two in-class screening assignments every two years. Because of changes in vision or other health problems, some older drivers may be required to give up their licence before they feel ready. Many older adults report that the loss of a driver's licence, and the loss of independence it brings, is one of the most severe hardships they face.

Government Aid

Financial well-being is an essential component of health, wellness, and security for all individuals, including older adults. The federal government helps older Canadians through several programs, such as the OAS program and the Canada Pension Plan (CPP) or Quebec Pension Plan (QPP).

The OAS pension is governed by Canada's Old Age Security Act, which came into effect in 1952. This program is Canada's largest public pension program and is financed solely from tax revenues collected by the government. Benefits paid under this act fall into several categories, including the basic OAS pension, the Guaranteed Income Supplement (GIS), the Allowance, and the Allowance for the Survivor. The OAS pension is a monthly benefit available to most Canadians ages 65 and over, regardless of employment history or retirement status. In 2015, the maximum amount was $563.74 per month. The GIS is an additional benefit for Canadians with little or no income other than the OAS. The Allowance and Allowance for the Survivor were established in response to the difficulties experienced by widows and by couples living on one pension. The Allowance provides a monthly benefit to low-income Canadians ages 60–64 whose spouse or common-law partner receives an OAS pension. The Allowance for the Survivor provides money to low-income Canadians ages 60–64 whose spouse or common-law partner has died.

The CPP and QPP are an earnings-related social insurance system that provides a retirement pension to Canadians as early as 60 years of age who have contributed to the plan. Over the past few years, the Canadian government has introduced several modifications to the CPP in an attempt to acknowledge changing retirement trends. For example, Canadians no longer have to stop working to receive CPP, providing older adults with the option to transition into retirement when and how they want to. According to the Government of Canada, the CPP/QPP is designed to replace about 25 percent of an individual's earnings from employment, up to a maximum amount. For example, in 2015, the maximum CPP amount that a Canadian could receive was $1065.00 per month.

Many older Canadians may also have contributed to private pensions and savings, such as Registered Pension Plans (RPPs) and Registered Retirement Savings Plans (RRSPs). In most cases, people have determined how much money they will need in retirement and contributed accordingly. Tax deductions on RPPs and RRSPs are the primary ways that the Canadian government assists individuals in saving for retirement. In Canada, the vast majority of retirement income is received from private pensions, while the remainder is typically composed of income from RRSPs.

Additional government programs for older Canadians who may be eligible include international social security agreements (for older adults who have lived or worked in Canada and in another country), the Assisted Living Program (for First Nations members living on-reserve who have functional limitations because of age, disability, or health problems), and the Home Adaptations for Seniors Independence program (for older adults who are homeowners or landlords and who want to make specific home adaptations).

Between 1980 and 2011, the proportion of older Canadians living with a low income decreased from about 21 percent to 5 percent—a rate lower than most other industrialized countries. This decline has been attributed—in part—to the effectiveness of Canada's retirement income system. For example, one of the many factors that has contributed to the rising incomes of older Canadians has been the growing number of Canadians collecting CPP/QPP. These programs were established in 1966 and the first cohort of Canadians to receive full benefits turned 65 in 1976. With the aging of the Canadian population, the proportion of older adults eligible for full CPP/QPP benefits has increased. In 2012–2013, more than 4 million older adults in Canada received approximately $27 billion in retirement benefits.

QUESTIONS FOR CRITICAL THINKING AND REFLECTION

What do you want your life to be like when you are old? Do you hope to retire or keep working indefinitely? Where would you like to live? How much time do you spend thinking about these questions? Have you done any planning yet for older age?

QUICK STATS

The participation rate of older adults in the Canadian labour force increased from 6% in 2000 to 13% in 2013.

—Government of Canada, 2014

Changes in the Public's View of Aging

Aging people may be one of our least used and least appreciated resources. (For another view, see the Dimensions of Diversity box.) How can we use the knowledge and productivity of our growing numbers of older citizens, particularly those who are retiring early?

To start, we must change our thinking about what aging means. We must learn to judge productivity rather than age. Capacity to function should replace age as a criterion for usefulness. An example of this is the recent abolishment of mandatory retirement in many jobs across most of Canada, allowing Canadians to work beyond the age of 65. Instead of singling out 65 as a magic number, we are now starting to consider ages 50–75 as the third quarter of life. Changes occur around 50 that signal a new era: Children are usually grown and gone, and a person has often achieved a level in career, earnings, and accomplishments that meets his or her ambitions. The upper end of the quarter is determined by the fact that most people today are vigorous, in good health, mentally alert, and capable of making a productive contribution until they are at least in their seventies.

 Dimensions *of* DIVERSITY

Aboriginal Seniors in Canada: The Role of the Elder

The ancient wisdom, the traditions, rituals, languages, and cultural values were passed on and carried forward. In this process, a primary role was played by the Elders, the Old Ones, the Grandmothers and Grandfathers. As individuals especially knowledgeable and experienced in the culture, they were seen as those most closely in touch with the philosophical teachings of life lived in harmony with the Creator and creation.

—Royal Commission on Aboriginal Peoples, 1996

Older adults are revered in many Aboriginal cultures for their knowledge and experiences, along with the integral role that they play in the vitality and well-being of their families, communities, and nations. Aboriginal people view Elders as key sources of traditional knowledge, wisdom, and cultural continuity. In a sense, Elders are experts on life. Their expertise may depend on the nature of their experience, but in one way or another it involves some aspect of traditional knowledge and culture or an interpretation of their experience in traditional terms. They must also be able to communicate that learning to others. Although age is part of being an Elder, it is not the only part. As one Ojibway traditional teacher described it, "Some people say that it isn't a matter of age, but to a certain extent it is when you have experienced enough of the stages of life that you can look back and reflect on them.... Some people have been able to do it more completely than others. When you're 35, you're only about halfway, so you can't talk about all of life, not from experience."

Aboriginal seniors have lived through many changes in their communities, and they are often considered an important link to the teachings of the past. It is not surprising that many people recognized as Elders have lived through difficult times, both personally and politically. Some have had problems with the law, with alcohol, with family separation; some have seen such things happen to others. What they have in common is the fact that they learned something from those experiences, that they turned to the traditional culture for understanding, support, and healing, and that they are committed to helping others, especially those of similar background.

It is clear that Aboriginal seniors play an important role in passing Aboriginal culture and languages on to the next generation. For many Aboriginal children, spending time with Elders on a regular basis has a beneficial outcome. An analysis of participation in extracurricular activities of Aboriginal children living off-reserve revealed that although sports are the most popular extracurricular activities, time spent with Elders ranked second.

In the Aboriginal community, an Elder is not a figurehead or a symbol, but rather someone who is actively involved in the community. A primary role of the Elder is to express the best of tradition and to bring that tradition forward into current times. Although many definitions of an Elder exist, perhaps the most appropriate description is one that has been advanced by the Elders themselves: "We are helpers, that is the highest level we can be. We are part of the family."

Sources: Stiegelbauer, S. M. 1996. What is an Elder? What do Elders do? First Nations Elders as teachers in culture-based urban organizations. *Canadian Journal of Native Studies* 16(1): 37–66, http://www3.brandonu.ca/library/cjns/16.1/Stiegelbauer.pdf (retrieved July 20, 2015); Turcotte, M., and G. Schellenberg. 2007. *A Portrait of Seniors in Canada, 2006,* http://www.statcan.gc.ca/pub/89-519-x/89-519-x2006001-eng.pdf (retrieved July 20, 2015); and Royal Commission on Aboriginal Peoples. 1996. *The Report of the Royal Commission on Aboriginal Peoples.* Ottawa: Minister of Supply and Services Canada.

Aging can have benefits, but they don't come automatically. They require planning and wise choices earlier in life. One octogenarian, Russell Lee, founder of a medical clinic in California, perceived the advantages of aging as growth: "The limitations imposed by time are compensated by the improved taste, sharper discretion, sounder mental and aesthetic judgment, increased sensitivity and compassion, clearer focus— which all contribute to a more certain direction in living.... The later years can be the best of life for which the earlier ones were preparation."

QUESTIONS FOR CRITICAL THINKING AND REFLECTION

Have you watched someone you know grow old? How did the aging process affect that person? In what ways did the person's physical and mental health change? In what ways were you affected, as you watched him or her age?

SUMMARY

- People who take charge of their health during their youth have greater control over the physical and mental aspects of aging.
- Biological aging takes place over a lifetime, but some of the other changes associated with aging are more abrupt.
- A lifetime of interests and hobbies helps maintain creativity and intelligence.
- Exercise and a healthy diet throughout life enhance physical and psychological health.
- Alcohol abuse is a common but often hidden problem, as is overdependence on medications. Tobacco use not only shortens life, but also may cause severe health impairment for many years.
- Regular physical examinations help detect conditions that can shorten life and make old age less healthy.
- Stress increases wear and tear on the body; getting enough sleep, avoiding drugs, and practising relaxation help reduce stress.
- Retirement can be a fulfilling and enjoyable time of life for those who adjust to their new roles, enjoy participating in a variety of activities, and have planned ahead for financial stability.
- Successful aging involves anticipating and accommodating physical changes and limitations.
- Slight confusion and forgetfulness are not signs of a serious illness; however, severe symptoms may indicate Alzheimer's disease or another form of dementia.
- Older adults can be role models for the successful integration of life's experiences and the ability to adapt to challenges.
- People over 65 form a minority in Canada, but the proportion of older adults in Canada is expected to grow substantially over the next few decades, reaching between 24 percent and 28 percent of the population by 2063.
- Family and community resources can help older adults stay active and independent.
- Government aid to older Canadians includes the Old Age Security pension, the Guaranteed Income Supplement, the Allowances, the Canadian Pension Plan/Quebec Pension Plan, and tax deductions on Registered Pension Plans and Registered Retirement Savings Plans.

FOR MORE INFORMATION

BOOKS

Buettner, D. 2011. *Thrive: Finding Happiness the Blue Zones Way.* National Geographic. An exploration of the world in search of those who live the longest and seeks to answer why.

Hyams, J. 2010. *Time to Help Your Parents: A Practical Guide to Recognising Problems and Providing Support*. London: Piatkus. A sympathetic overview of the many challenges facing adult children who must care for their aging parents.

Johns Hopkins Medical Center. 2007. *The Johns Hopkins Medical Guide to Health After 50*. New York: Black Dog & Leventhal. A practical guide to healthy aging for all wellness dimensions.

Weil, A. 2007. *Healthy Aging: A Lifelong Guide to Your Physical and Spiritual Well-Being*. New York: Anchor. One of America's best-known complementary care physicians discusses the aging process and explains methods for maintaining health during the latter years of life.

ORGANIZATIONS AND WEBSITES

The Internet addresses listed here were accurate at the time of publication.

Alliance for Aging Research. Provides medical and psychological research on aging.
http://www.agingresearch.org

Alzheimer Society of Canada. Provides research and news, and offers tips for caregivers and patients on the causes and treatment of Alzheimer's disease and related dementias.
http://www.alzheimer.ca/en

The Arthritis Society. Provides information about arthritis, programs and services, and research updates.
http://www.arthritis.ca

Canadian Centre for Activity and Aging. Promotes physical activity and the well-being of older adults through educational resources and community programs; site provides information about research, conferences and events, leadership training, and physical activity.
http://www.uwo.ca/ccaa/

Canadian National Institute for the Blind. Provides information, resources, and research about eye conditions, care, and safety. Also provides vision support services and works to protect and promote the vision health of all Canadians.
http://www.cnib.ca/en/Pages/default.aspx

CARP. Provides information on all aspects of aging, including health promotion, health care, and retirement planning.
http://www.carp.ca

Menopauseandu.ca. Provides information about menopause symptoms and treatments.
http://www.menopauseandu.ca

Osteoporosis Canada. Provides information on the causes, prevention, detection, and treatment of osteoporosis.
http://www.osteoporosis.ca

Public Health Agency of Canada, Division of Aging and Seniors. Provides information on matters related to healthy aging, including the prevention and control of disease and injury among older Canadians.
http://www.publichealth.gc.ca/seniors

Seniors Canada (Government of Canada). Provides a wide range of information about resources and services for older adults and caregivers in Canada, including financial matters and health and wellness.
http://www.seniors.gc.ca

SELECTED BIBLIOGRAPHY

Accreditation Canada/The Canadian Institute for Health Information/The Canadian Patient Safety Institute. 2014. *Preventing Falls: From Evidence to Improvement in Canadian Health Care*, http://www.accreditation.ca/sites/default/files/falls-joint-report-2014-en.pdf (retrieved February 20, 2015).

Alzheimer Society of Canada. 2009. *Rising Tide: the Impact of Dementia on Canadian Society*, http://www.alzheimer.ca/~/media/Files/national/Advocacy/ASC_Rising_Tide_Full_Report_e.pdf (retrieved July 20, 2015).

Alzheimer Society of Canada. 2014. *Treatment Options,* http://www.alzheimer.ca/en/About-dementia/Treatment-options (retrieved June 23, 2015).

Alzheimer Society of Canada. 2015. *Dementia Numbers in Canada,* http://www.alzheimer.ca/en/About-dementia/What-is-dementia/Dementia-numbers (retrieved June 17, 2015).

Arthritis Society. 2015. *Arthritis Facts and Figures,* http://www.arthritis.ca/facts (retrieved June 17, 2015).

BMO Wealth Institute, 2015 *Retirement planning: How do your retirement plans measure up?,* https://www.bmo.com/pdf/ewp/retirementplan/14-2619-BWI-retirement-report-E04-web.pdf (retrieved July 20, 2015).

Buys, Y. M. 2008. World Glaucoma Day, March 6, 2008—What can you do? *Canadian Journal of Ophthalmology* 43: 1–3, http://www.jgh.ca/uploads/PatientVisitor/international_glaucoma_day.pdf (retrieved July 20, 2015).

Canadian Institute for Health Information. 2011. *Health Care in Canada, 2011: A Focus on Seniors and Aging,* https://secure.cihi.ca/free_products/HCIC_2011_seniors_report_en.pdf (retrieved July 20, 2015).

Canadian Institute for Health Information. 2011. *Seniors and the health care system: What is the impact of multiple chronic conditions?,* https://secure.cihi.ca/free_products/air-chronic_disease_aib_en.pdf (retrieved July 20, 2015).

Canadian Institute for Health Information. 2014. *Drug Use Among Seniors on Public Drug Programs in Canada, 2012,* https://secure.cihi.ca/free_products/Drug_Use_in_Seniors_on_Public_Drug_Programs_EN_web_Oct.pdf (retrieved April 9, 2015).

Canadian National Institute for the Blind. 2015. *About AMD,* http://www.cnib.ca/en/your-eyes/eye-conditions/eye-connect/AMD/About/Pages/default.aspx (retrieved July 20, 2015).

Canadian Ophthalmological Society. nd. *Glaucoma,* http://www.cos-sco.ca/vision-health-information/conditions-disorders-treatments/glaucoma/ (retrieved July 20, 2015).

Canadian Society for Exercise Physiology. 2011. *Canadian Physical Activity Guidelines for Older Adults—65 Years & Older,* http://www.csep.ca/CMFiles/Guidelines/CSEP-InfoSheets-older%20adults-ENG.pdf (retrieved February 16, 2015).

Centre for Addiction and Mental Health. 2009. *Responding to Older Adults with Substance Use, Mental Health and Gambling Challenges,* http://www.camh.net/Publications/Resources_for_Professionals/Older_Adults/rtoa_alcohol_problems.html (retrieved July 20, 2015).

Centre for Suicide Prevention. 2014. *Plus 65: At The End of the Day [Resource Toolkit],* https://suicideinfo.ca/LinkClick.aspx?fileticket=cmFwRL4DMJw= (retrieved June 23, 2015).

Cirillo, D., et al. 2005. Effect of estrogen therapy on gallbladder disease. *Journal of the American Medical Association* 293(3): 330–339.

Federal, Provincial, and Territorial Ministers Responsible for Seniors. 2005. *Planning for Canada's Aging Population.* Ottawa: Division of Aging and Seniors, Public Health Agency of Canada.

Gilmour, H., and Park, J. 2005. Dependency, chronic conditions and pain in seniors. *Health Reports* (16 Suppl.), http://www.statcan.gc.ca/pub/82-003-s/2005000/pdf/9087-eng.pdf (retrieved July 20, 2015).

Government of Canada. 2009. *Canada's Aging Population: Seizing the Opportunity, Special Senate Committee on Aging Final Report,* http://www.parl.gc.ca/40/2/parlbus/commbus/senate/com-e/agei-e/rep-e/AgingFinalReport-e.pdf (retrieved July 20, 2015).

Government of Canada. 2013. *Sodium: The Basics,* http://healthycanadians.gc.ca/eating-nutrition/healthy-eating-saine-alimentation/sodium/basics-savoir-eng.php (retrieved February 20, 2015).

Government of Canada. 2014. *Action for Seniors Report,* http://www.seniors.gc.ca/eng/report/index.shtml (retrieved April 9, 2015).

Harvard Medical School. 2006. Minding your mind: 12 ways to keep your brain young with proper care and feeding. *Harvard Men's Health Watch* 10(10): 1–4.

Health Canada. 2004. *Aboriginal Health,* http://www.hc-sc.gc.ca/hcs-sss/delivery-prestation/fptcollab/2004-fmm-rpm/fs-if_02-eng.php (retrieved July 20, 2015).

Health Canada. 2012. *Food and Nutrition: Men and Women Over the Age of 50,* http://www.hc-sc.gc.ca/fn-an/food-guide-aliment/choose-choix/advice-conseil/adult50-eng.php (retrieved February 20, 2015).

Heyn, P. C., et al. 2008. Endurance and strength training outcomes on cognitively impaired and cognitively intact older adults: A meta-analysis. *Journal of Nutrition, Health and Aging* 12(6): 401–409.

Jager, R. D., et al. 2008. Age-related macular degeneration. *New England Journal of Medicine* 258(24): 2606–2617.

Kado, D. M., et al. 2005. Homocysteine versus the vitamins folate, B6, and B12 as predictors of cognitive function and decline in older high-functioning adults: MacArthur Studies of Successful Aging. *American Journal of Medicine* 118(2): 161–167.

Kirkwood, T. 2010. Why women live longer: stress alone does not explain the longevity gap. *Scientific American* October 1, 2010, http://www.scientificamerican.com/article/why-women-live-longer/ (retrieved July 20, 2015).

Kolata, G. 2006. Live long? Die young? Answer isn't just in genes. *New York Times,* 31 August.

Lanza, R., and N. Rosenthal. 2004. The stem cell challenge. *Scientific American,* June.

Marshall, K. 2011. Retiring with debt. Component of Statistics Catalogue no. 75-001-X, http://www.statcan.gc.ca/pub/75-001-x/2011002/pdf/11428-eng.pdf (retrieved July 20, 2015).

Mudge, A. M., et al. 2008. Exercising body and mind: An integrated approach to functional independence in hospitalized older people. *Journal of the American Geriatrics Society* 56(4): 630–635.

Naci, H., and J. P. A. Ioannidis. 2013. Comparative effectiveness of exercise and drug interventions on mortality outcomes: Metaepidemiological study. *British Medical Journal* 347: f5577.

Nelson, H. D., et al. 2006. Nonhormonal therapies for menopausal hot flashes: Systematic review and meta-analysis. *Journal of the American Medical Association* 295(17): 2057–2071.

Ontario Ministry of Transportation. 2015. *Senior Driver's Licence Renewal Program,* http://www.mto.gov.on.ca/english/driver/senior-driver-licence-renewal-program.shtml (retrieved July 20, 2015).

Osteoporosis Canada. 2015. *Calcium: An Important Nutrient That Builds Stronger Bones,* http://www.osteoporosis.ca/osteoporosis-and-you/nutrition/calcium-requirements/ (retrieved February 20, 2015).

Osteoporosis Canada. 2015. *Facts and Statistics,* http://www.osteoporosis.ca/osteoporosis-and-you/osteoporosis-facts-and-statistics/ (retrieved June 17, 2015).

Public Health Agency of Canada. 2006. *Healthy Aging in Canada: A New Vision, A Vital Investment, From Evidence to Action,* http://www.health.gov.nl.ca/health/publications/vision_rpt_e.pdf (retrieved February 20, 2015).

Public Health Agency of Canada. 2010. *Life with Arthritis in Canada: A Personal and Public Health Challenge,* http://www.phac-aspc.gc.ca/cd-mc/arthritis-arthrite/lwaic-vaaac-10/9-eng.php#Int6 (retrieved July 20, 2015).

Public Health Agency of Canada. 2014. *Report on Seniors' Falls in Canada: Second Report,* http://www.phac-aspc.gc.ca/seniors-aines/publications/public/injury-blessure/seniors_falls-chutes_aines/assets/pdf/seniors_falls-chutes_aines-eng.pdf (retrieved July 20, 2015).

Rosengren, A., et al. 2005. Body mass index, other cardiovascular risk factors, and hospitalization for dementia. *Archives of Internal Medicine* 165(3): 321–326.

Scarmeas, N., et al. 2006. Mediterranean diet, Alzheimer disease, and vascular mediation. *Archives of Neurology* 63: 1709–1717.

Service Canada. 2014. *Canada Pension Plan,* http://www.servicecanada.gc.ca/eng/services/pensions/cpp/index.shtml?utm_source=vanity+URL&utm_medium=print+publication,+ISPB-185,+ISPB-341&utm_term=/CPP&utm_content=Mar+2013,+eng&utm_campaign=OAS+Pension+2013,+Benefits+for+Low+-Income+Seniors (retrieved July 20, 2015).

Service Canada. 2015. *Old Age Security,* http://www.servicecanada.gc.ca/eng/services/pensions/oas/index.shtml?utm_source=vanity+URL&utm_medium=print+publication,+ISPB-185,+ISPB-341&utm_term=/oas&utm_content=Mar+2013,+eng&utm_campaign=OAS+Pension+2013,+Benefits+for+Low+Income+Seniors (retrieved July 20, 2015).

Society of Obstetricians and Gynaecologists of Canada. 2009. Menopause and osteoporosis update 2009. *Journal of Obstetrics and Gynaecology Canada* 31(1 Suppl.), http://sogc.org/wp-content/uploads/2013/01/Menopause_JOGC-Jan_09.pdf (retrieved July 20, 2015).

Sorrell, J. M. 2008. As good as it gets? Rethinking old age. *Journal of Psychosocial Nursing and Mental Health Services* 46(5): 21–24.

Statistics Canada. 2007. A portrait of seniors. *The Daily*, February 27, http://www.statcan.gc.ca/daily-quotidien/070227/dq070227b-eng.htm (retrieved July 20, 2015).

Statistics Canada. 2013. *Percentage of the population aged 65 and over living in special care facilities, by age group, Canada, 2011*, http://www12.statcan.ca/census-recensement/2011/as-sa/98-312-x/2011003/fig/fig3_4-4-eng.cfm (retrieved July 20, 2015).

Statistics Canada. 2013. *Proportion of population aged less than 15 years old and 65 years old and over, 1982 to 2036, Canada*, http://www.statcan.gc.ca/pub/91-215-x/2012000/ct008-eng.htm (retrieved July 20, 2015).

Statistics Canada. 2014. *Overweight and Obese Adults (Self-Reported), 2013*, http://www.statcan.gc.ca/pub/82-625-x/2014001/article/14021-eng.htm (retrieved February 20, 2015).

Statistics Canada. 2014. *Centenarians in Canada*, https://www12.statcan.gc.ca/census-recensement/2011/as-sa/98-311-x/98-311-x2011003_1-eng.cfm (retrieved July 20, 2015).

Statistics Canada. 2014. *Canadian Financial Capability Survey, 2014*, http://www.statcan.gc.ca/daily-quotidien/141106/dq141106b-eng.htm (retrieved July 20, 2015).

Stiegelbauer, S. M. 1996. What is an Elder? What do Elders do? First Nations Elders as teachers in culture-based urban organizations. *Canadian Journal of Native Studies* 16(1): 37–66, http://www2.brandonu.ca/library//CJNS/16.1/Stiegelbauer.pdf (retrieved May 26, 2010).

Stern, C., and Z. Munn. 2010. Cognitive leisure activities and their role in preventing dementia: a systematic review. *International Journal of Evidence-Based Healthcare* 8(1): 2–17.

Suicide Information and Education Centre. 1998. *Suicide Among the Aged*, http://www.suicideinfo.ca/csp/assets/alert28.pdf (retrieved May 1, 2011).

Syed, F. A., and A. C. Ng. 2010. The pathophysiology of the aging skeleton. *Current Osteoporosis Reports* 8(4): 235–240.

Tufts University. 2006. Pendulum swings on estrogen and women's heart health risk. *Tufts University Health & Nutrition Letter* 24(3): 1–2.

Ward, E. M. 2006. A weekly to-do list to help delay or prevent dementia. *Environmental Nutrition* 29(5): 2.

Welland, D. 2006. Keeping an eye on your diet may help save your sight. *Environmental Nutrition* 29(5): 1, 6.

Whitmer, R. A., et al. 2005. Midlife cardiovascular risk factors and risk of dementia in late life. *Neurology* 64(2): 277–281.

Wilson, R. S., et al. 2005. Proneness to psychological distress and risk of Alzheimer disease in a biracial community. *Neurology* 64(2): 380–382.

Wolfe, M. S. 2006. Shutting down Alzheimer's. *Scientific American* 294(5): 72–79.

World Health Organization. 2015. *Prevention of Blindness and Visual Impairment: Priority Eye Diseases*, http://www.who.int/blindness/causes/priority/en/index7.html (retrieved June 17, 2015).

Yuhas, D. 2012. Cracks in the plaques: Mysteries of Alzheimer's slowly yielding to new research. *Scientific American*: February.

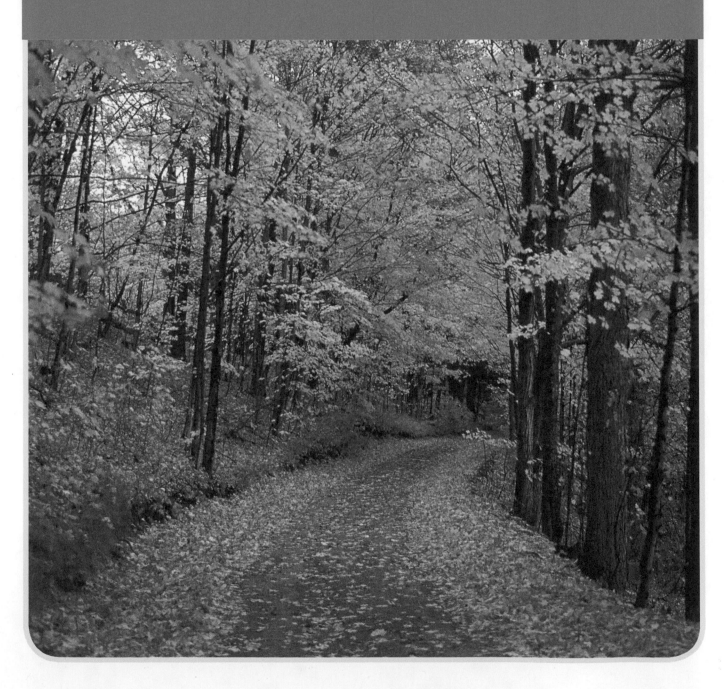

CHAPTER 18

Dying and Death

LOOKING AHEAD

After you have read and studied this chapter, you should be able to:

LO1 Identify the physical, mental, social, behavioural, and spiritual dimensions of dying and death

LO2 Describe various ways of defining death and the components of a mature concept of death

LO3 Understand personal considerations in preparing for death, including making a will, assessing choices for end-of-life care, and making arrangements for a funeral or memorial service

LO4 Describe the experience of living with a life-threatening illness and list ways to support a person who is dying

LO5 Explain the grieving process and how support can be offered to adults and children who have experienced a loss

TEST YOUR KNOWLEDGE

1. Approximately how many Canadians do not have a signed will?
a. 23 percent b. 56 percent c. 75 percent

2. Physician-assisted death is illegal in all provinces and territories in Canada.
True or false?

3. If you die in a car crash, your organs will automatically be donated to people waiting for transplants.
True or false?

4. Approximately how many people are waiting for organ transplants in Canada?
a. 1500 b. 4500 c. 11 500

5. The best way to help a friend who is grieving is to distract her or him from the loss by talking about sports, gossip, or other lighthearted topics.
True or false?

ANSWERS

1. b. If an individual dies without leaving a will, the deceased person's estate is distributed according to provincial or territorial law, which may not reflect what the person would have wanted.

2. TRUE. Currently, physician-assisted death is illegal in all parts of Canada. In February 2015, however, the Supreme Court of Canada ruled in favour of physician-assisted death in specific cases, giving the federal government 12 months to create legislation in response to this landmark ruling.

3. FALSE. For your organs to be donated, you must have authorized it before your death (for example, by registering your intent to donate online), *and* the donation must be authorized by relatives at the time of your death.

4. b. Approximately 4500 Canadians are on the waiting list for an organ transplant in Canada. In 2012, 256 people died while waiting for a needed organ. The number of patients waiting for organs continues to be several times greater than the number of organs donated each year.

5. FALSE. Most people who are grieving need to talk about their loss, and a friend who will let them talk freely is very valuable. The best strategy is simply to be a good listener and to follow your grieving friend's lead.

Whether it is a powerful earthquake killing thousands in Nepal, a man collapsing with a heart attack in a crowded restaurant, or a woman in her 90s dying peacefully with her family close by, images of death are easy to envision. Nevertheless, very rarely do we think about the inevitability of death in our own lives. Accepting and dealing with death are important tasks that present unique challenges to our sense of self, our relationships with others, and our understanding of the meaning of life itself.

Although pain and distress may accompany the dying process, facing death also presents an opportunity for growth and affirmation of the preciousness of simple aspects of our daily lives. Dealing with the death of a loved one can tear families apart, but it can also bring them together, healing old wounds in the process. The way we choose to confront death can greatly influence how we live our lives.

This chapter discusses some of the many questions surrounding the end of life. The following sections explain steps individuals can take to make their own death a bit easier for their loved ones and describe tasks you may need to consider in preparing for your own passing. This chapter also examines the process of grieving and provides advice that can help in dealing with the death of a loved one.

Why is There Death?

Ultimately, there is no completely satisfying answer to the question of why death exists. When we look at the big picture, we see that death promotes variety through the evolution of species. The average human life is long enough to allow us to reproduce and ensure that our species continues. Yet it is brief enough to allow for new genetic combinations, thereby providing a means of adaptation to changing conditions in the environment. From the perspective of species survival, the cycle of life and death makes sense.

Senescence, the biological process of aging, is a complex process rooted in genetics and is universal in all mammals, including humans. Organisms age on both a cellular and whole-organism level, ultimately resulting in death. Although scientific understanding of senescence is progressing, and average life spans are increasing, death remains an inevitable event for humans.

senescence
The biological process of aging.

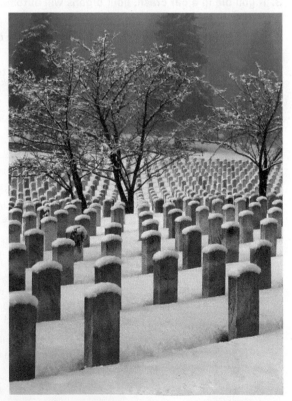

From a personal point of view, death challenges our emotional and intellectual security. We may acknowledge the fact that all living things eventually die and that this is nature's way of renewal, but this recognition offers little comfort when death touches our own lives. Questions about the meaning of death and what happens when we die are central concerns of the great religions and philosophies. Some promise a better life after death. Others teach that everyone is evolving toward perfection or divinity, a goal reached after successive rounds of death and rebirth. Some suggest that it is not possible to know what happens—if anything—after death and that any judgment about life's worth must be made on the basis of satisfactions or rewards that we create for ourselves in our lifetime.

It is worth noting that, even in modern secular societies, religion plays a major role in shaping our attitudes and behaviours toward death. Religion offers solace to the extent that it suggests some meaning in dying. The mourning ceremonies associated with various religious practices ease the pangs of grief for many people. Dying and death are more than biological events; they have

Given the inevitability of death, accepting and dealing with dying and death are difficult but important tasks.

social and spiritual dimensions. Our beliefs—religious or philosophical—can be a key to how we relate to the prospect of our own death as well as the deaths of others.

Understanding Dying and Death

Death forces us to puzzle out an understanding of its meaning in our lives. We may choose not to think about some issues, such as the possibility of an afterlife, but we cannot keep from facing the reality of dying and death. Regardless of our explanations or efforts to minimize its effects, death can be challenging and painful—both to the person who is dying and to those left behind. However, it also offers an opportunity for remarkable growth and an appreciation of our relationships with other people and myriad other aspects of life itself.

Defining Death

Paradoxically, as our scientific understanding of death increases, defining death has become increasingly difficult. Traditionally, death has been defined as cessation of the flow of vital body fluids. This occurs when the heart stops beating and breathing ceases. These traditional signs are adequate for determining death in most cases. However, over the last several decades the use of cardiopulmonary resuscitation and other medical techniques have brought many "dead" people (by the traditional definition) back to life. The use of ventilators, artificial heart pumps, and other **life-support systems** allow many body functions to be artificially sustained. In such cases, making a determination of death can be difficult and often controversial. The concept of **brain death** was developed to determine whether a person is alive or dead when the traditional signs are inadequate because of supportive medical technology.

life-support systems
Medical technologies, such as a ventilator, that allow vital body functions to be artificially sustained.

brain death
A medical determination of death as the cessation of brain activity indicated by various diagnostic criteria, including a flat electroencephalogram (EEG) reading.

According to standards published by a Harvard Medical School committee, brain death involves four characteristics: (1) lack of receptivity and response to external stimuli, (2) absence of spontaneous muscular movement and spontaneous breathing, (3) absence of observable reflexes, and (4) absence of brain activity, as signified by a flat **electroencephalogram (EEG)**. The Harvard criteria require a second set of tests to be performed after 24 hours have elapsed, and they exclude cases of hypothermia (body temperature below 32°C) and situations involving central nervous system depressants, such as barbiturates. In Canada, the legal definition of brain death includes the standard of "according to accepted medical practice," a potentially problematic scenario given that practices and policies often differ from hospital to hospital.

electroencephalogram (EEG)
A record of the electrical activity of the brain (brain waves).

In contrast to **clinical death**, which is determined by either the cessation of heartbeat and breathing or the criteria for establishing brain death, **cellular death** refers to a gradual process that occurs when heartbeat, respiration, and brain activity have stopped. It encompasses the breakdown of metabolic processes and results in complete non-functionality at the cellular level. In a biological sense, therefore, death can be defined as the cessation of life because of irreversible changes in cell metabolism.

clinical death
A determination of death made according to accepted medical criteria.

cellular death
The breakdown of metabolic processes at the level of the body's cells.

The way death is defined has potential legal and social consequences in a variety of areas, including criminal prosecution, inheritance, taxation, treatment of the corpse, and even mourning. It also affects the practice of organ transplantation, because some organs—hearts, most obviously—must be harvested from a human being who is legally determined to be dead. Timing is critical in removing a heart from someone who has been declared dead and transplanting it into a person whose life can thereby be saved. Safeguards are necessary to ensure that the determination of death occurs without regard to any plans for subsequent transplantation of the deceased's organs.

Learning About Death

Our understanding of death changes as we grow and mature, as do our attitudes toward it. Very young children view death as an interruption and an absence, but their lack of a mature time perspective means that they do not understand death as final and irreversible. A child's understanding of death evolves greatly from about age 6 to age 9. During this period, most children come to understand that death is final, universal, and inevitable. A child who consciously recognizes these facts is said to possess a **mature understanding of death**. This understanding of death is further refined during the years of adolescence and young adulthood by considering the impact of death on close relationships and contemplating the value of religious or philosophical answers to the enigma of death.

> **mature understanding of death**
> The recognition that death is universal and irreversible, that it involves the cessation of all physiological functioning, and that there are biological reasons for its occurrence.

Based on a body of work done by Mark Speece and Sandor Brent, a formal understanding of the empirical, or observable, facts about death includes four components:

1. *Universality:* All living things eventually die. Death is all-inclusive, inevitable, and unavoidable (although unpredictable with respect to its exact timing). The bottom line is that we know we will die, but we don't know when.
2. *Irreversibility:* Organisms that die cannot be made alive again.
3. *Non-functionality:* Death involves the cessation of all physiological functioning or signs of life.
4. *Causality:* There are biological reasons for the occurrence of death.

It is important to add, however, that individuals who possess a mature understanding of death commonly hold non-empirical ideas about it as well. Such non-empirical ideas—that is, ideas not subject to scientific proof—deal mainly with the notion that human beings survive in some form beyond the death of the physical body. What happens to an individual's personality after he or she dies? Does the self or soul continue to exist after the death of the physical body? If so, what is the nature of this afterlife? Developing personally satisfying answers to such questions, which involve what Speece and Brent term **non-corporeal continuity**, is also part of the process of acquiring a mature understanding of death.

> **non-corporeal continuity**
> The notion that human beings survive in some form after the death of the physical body.

QUICK STATS

A 2014 survey revealed that approximately 42% of Canadians believe in life after death.

—Angus Reid Institute/University of Lethbridge, 2015

Denying Versus Acknowledging Death

Understanding death in a mature fashion does not imply that we never experience anxiety about the deaths of those we love or about the prospect of our own death. The news of a friend's or loved one's serious illness can shock us into an encounter with mortality that creates a need to cope not only with the painful reality of our friend's or loved one's illness, but also with our own eventual death. Our ability to find meaning and comfort in the face of mortality depends not only on our having an understanding of the facts of death, but also on our attitudes toward it.

Many people seek to avoid any thought or mention of death. The sick and old are often isolated in hospitals and nursing homes. Relatively few Canadians have been present at the death of a loved one. Where the reality of death is concerned, "out of sight, out of mind" often appears to be the rule of the day. Instead of facing death directly, we tend to be inundated with unrealistic portrayals in movies, television, and video games.

The fictitious deaths of characters we barely know do not cause us to confront the reality of death as it is experienced in real life. Moreover, such faked death is often presented as reversible. Children watch a daily fare of superhuman heroes, invincible to bullets and other weapons. In their games, they reenact these false ideas about death—falling down dead and jumping up again unharmed. Cartoons and video games present death in a two-dimensional world where one can die and then be reborn to play seconds later.

Our attitudes about death in our culture are also shaped by a sense that death is "creepy." Most people find dead bodies frightening, and many believe that the dead can come back to haunt us. Ghost stories and horror movies capitalize on the irrational fears that surround death. These fears can prevent us from being truly close to our loved ones as they die, and can impair our ability to say our goodbyes without being constrained by superstitious ideas about death and dead bodies.

Although some commentators characterize the predominant attitude toward death in North America as "death denying," others are reluctant to generalize so broadly. People often maintain conflicting or ambivalent attitudes toward death. Those who come to view death as a relief or release from insufferable pain may have at least a partial sense of welcoming death. Few people wholly avoid or wholly welcome death. Problems can arise, however, when avoidance or denial fosters the notion that death happens to others, but not to you or me. (For another perspective, see the Dimensions of Diversity box.)

In the last several decades, attitudes toward death in our culture have slowly begun to change. The hospice movement (discussed later in this chapter) has provided the support and guidance for many families to be present during the dying process of their loved ones, often in their own homes. Dying in a home setting fulfills the wishes of many patients and can also be a great comfort to friends and family.

Dimensions *of* DIVERSITY

El Día de los Muertos: The Day of the Dead

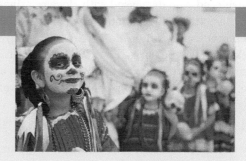

Not all cultures are reluctant to publicly acknowledge death. Traditional Mexican culture honours the dead by remembering them often and even including them in family activities. In the Mexican worldview, death is another phase of life, and those who have passed into it remain accessible. Ancestors are not forever lost, nor is the past dead. This sense of continuity has its roots in the culture of the Aztecs, for whom regeneration was a central theme. When the Spanish came to Mexico in the sixteenth century, their beliefs about death, along with symbols, such as skulls and skeletons, were absorbed into the native culture.

Mexican artists and writers confront death with humour and even sarcasm, depicting it as the inevitable fate that all—even the wealthiest—must face. At no time is this attitude toward death livelier than at the beginning of each November on the holiday known as *Día de los Muertos*, "the Day of the Dead." This holiday coincides with All Souls' Day, the Catholic commemoration of the dead, and represents a unique blending of indigenous ritual and religious dogma.

The celebration in honour of the dead typically spans two days—one day devoted to children who have passed, and one to adults. It reflects the belief that the dead return to Earth in spirit once a year to rejoin their families and partake of holiday foods prepared especially for them. The fiesta usually begins at midday on October 31, with flowers and food—candies, cookies, honey, milk—set out on altars in each house for the family's dead. The next day, family groups stream to the graveyards, where they have cleaned and decorated the graves of their loved ones, to celebrate and commune with the dead. They bring games, music, and special food.

People sit on the graves, eat, sing, and talk with the departed ones. Tears may be shed as the dead are remembered, but mourning is tempered by the festive mood of the occasion.

During the season of the dead, graveyards and family altars are decorated with yellow candles and yellow marigolds—the "flower of death." In some Mexican villages, yellow flower petals are strewn along the ground, connecting the graveyard with all the houses visited by death during the year.

Keeping death in the forefront of consciousness may provide solace to the living, reminding them of their loved ones and assuring them that they themselves will not be forgotten when they die. Yearly celebrations and remembrances may help people keep in touch with their past, their ancestry, and their roots. The festive atmosphere may help dispel the fear of death, allowing people to look at it more directly. Although it is possible to deny the reality of death even when surrounded by images of it, such practices as *Día de los Muertos* may help people face death with more equanimity.

Sources: Adapted from DeSpelder, L., and A. Strickland. 2007. *The Last Dance*, 8th ed. New York: McGraw-Hill; Puente, T. 1991. Día de los Muertos. *Hispanic*, October; and Milne, J. 1965. *Fiesta Time in Latin America*. Los Angeles: Ward Ritchie Press.

QUESTIONS FOR CRITICAL THINKING AND REFLECTION

What situations or events make you think seriously about your own mortality? Is this something you consider often, or do you avoid thinking about death? What has influenced your willingness or reluctance to think about death?

Planning for Death

Acknowledging the inevitability of death allows us to plan for it. Adequate planning can help ensure that a sudden, unexpected death is not made even more difficult for survivors. Even when death is not sudden, individuals with a debilitating illness may become unable to make decisions. Many decisions can be anticipated, considered, and discussed with close relatives and friends.

Basic tasks in planning for death include making a will, anticipating medical care needs and expressing preferences for end-of-life care, considering whether to become an organ donor, and helping survivors plan tasks that will be carried out after we die. It is reasonable to begin such planning during the university years, particularly with regard to organ donation, and to periodically review and revise your decisions throughout life. Young people can also help their older relatives by urging them to complete these important tasks.

Making a Will

Surveys indicate that more than half—56 percent—of adult Canadians do not have a signed will. Common reasons for not leaving a will include not wanting to deal with a "depressing subject," wanting to avoid the expense of legal services, and the idea that "I don't need a will because I don't have much money." Whatever the reason, dying without a will can lead to unnecessary hardships for survivors, even when an estate is modest in size.

A **will** is a legal instrument expressing a person's intentions and choices for the disposition of his or her property after death. It is a declaration of how one's **estate**—that is, money, property, and other possessions—will be distributed after death. During the life of the **testator** (the person making the will), a will can be changed, replaced, or revoked. On the testator's death, it becomes a legal instrument governing the distribution of the testator's estate.

will
A legal instrument expressing a person's intentions and wishes for the disposition of his or her property after death.

estate
The money, property, and other possessions belonging to a person.

testator
The person who makes a will.

When a person dies **intestate**—that is, without having left a valid will—property is distributed according to rules set up by the province or territory. The failure to execute a will may result in a distribution of property that is not compatible with a person's wishes or best suited to the interests and needs of heirs. If you have a will, consider whether it needs to be updated in response to a key life event such as marriage, the birth of a child, divorce, or the purchase of a home. In making a will, it is generally advisable to involve close family members to prevent problems that can arise when actions are taken without the knowledge of those who will be affected.

> **intestate**
> Referring to the situation in which a person dies without having made a legal will.

Individuals can also help family members by completing a *testamentary letter*; this document includes information about an individual's personal affairs, such as bank accounts, credit cards, the location of documents and keys, the names of professional advisers, the names of people who should be notified of the death, and so on.

You may feel that you are too young to be thinking about your own will, and if you are a young student that may be reasonable. But this is a good time to be courageous and broach the subject with family members. Do your parents have a will? Do you know where they keep their important information should something happen to them? Let your family members know that their efforts to plan ahead and keep you informed are greatly appreciated.

Considering Options for End-of-Life Care

The timeline of dying has changed radically over the last several generations. Not only do we, on average, tend to live longer, but we also are much more likely to live with chronic disease and disability for months or years before we pass away, compared to past generations who tended to be relatively healthy to nearly the end of life, and die over a short period of time of an acute illness. Most of us will need some sort of care during our last days, weeks, months, or even years of life.

As life draws to a close, care may involve a combination of home care, hospital stays, and hospice or palliative care. By becoming aware of our options, we and our families are empowered to make informed, meaningful choices.

Home Care

Many people express a preference to be cared for at home during the end stages of life. An obvious advantage of home care is the fact that the dying person is in a familiar setting, ideally in the company of family and friends.

Care for a person in the last stage of life is often a 24-hour-a-day job and requires varying degrees of skill, medical knowledge, and physical strength. Family members may or may not be capable of providing the level of care that is needed. Professional at-home caregivers can often make a big difference in allowing a person to continue to live at home.

When a patient requires sophisticated medical procedures, does not have access to qualified caregivers, or intends to be an organ donor, institutional care may be more appropriate. When suitable, however, home care is believed by many to be the most satisfying option for care as a person's life comes to a close. While surveys suggest that most Canadians have expressed a preference for dying at home, the majority—almost 70 percent—of deaths in Canada still take place in hospitals.

Hospital-Based Palliative Care

Although hospitals are primarily organized to provide short-term intensive treatment for acute injury and illness, they are also adopting the principles of **palliative care** for patients who require comprehensive care at the end of life. Unlike acute care, which involves taking active measures to sustain life, palliative care focuses on controlling pain and relieving suffering by caring for the physical, psychological, spiritual, and existential needs of the patient. Although the emphasis is generally placed on comfort care, palliative therapies can be combined with cure-oriented treatment approaches in some cases. In all cases, the goal of palliative care is to achieve the best possible quality of life for patients and their families.

> **palliative care**
> A form of medical care aimed at reducing the intensity or severity of a disease by controlling pain and other discomforting symptoms.

Hospice Palliative Care

As a comprehensive program of care offering a set of services designed to support terminally ill patients and their families, **hospice** is a well-known form of palliative care. Although the term *hospice* sometimes refers to a freestanding medical facility to which terminally ill patients are admitted, Canada has few of these facilities, and consequently, most hospice care takes place in patients' homes with family members as primary caregivers. Entering hospice care usually means affiliating with a hospice program—that is, arranging to receive the services of a local hospice. Such hospices are generally community-based organizations that coordinate a range of palliative care services that may be provided in nursing homes and hospitals, as well as in patients' homes.

> **hospice**
> A program of care for dying patients and their families.

Hospice (and palliative care generally) involves a team-oriented approach to care that typically includes physicians, nurses, social workers, home health aides, pharmacists, chaplains, physical and occupational therapists, and trained volunteers. This team-oriented approach seeks to provide state-of-the-art care to prevent or relieve pain and other distressing symptoms, as well as to offer emotional and spiritual support to both patient and family.

Hospice care allows many people to choose where they die, a comforting fact for patients and families. In addition to helping patients achieve a peaceful death, an important gift of hospice care is the potential to help patients and families discover how much can be shared at the end of life through personal and spiritual connections.

QUICK STATS

In 2012, 13% of Canadians aged 15 and older reported providing end-of-life or palliative care to a family member or friend at some point in their lives.

—Statistics Canada, 2014

Difficult Decisions at the End of Life

The decision to stop doing tests and administering treatments is often a difficult one for patients and their families. Many people owe their lives to the advanced medical technologies now available. Yet a medical stance that strives to keep people alive by all means and at any cost is increasingly being questioned. In addition, medical diagnostic procedures and treatments often cause discomfort and can reduce the quality of life of people who are likely to die soon whether or not they receive further medical intervention.

Modern medicine can sometimes keep the human organism alive despite the cessation of normal heart, brain, respiratory, or kidney function. But should a patient without any hope of recovery be kept alive by means of artificial life support? At what point does such treatment become futile? What if a patient has fallen into a **persistent vegetative state**, a state of profound unconsciousness, lacking any sign of normal reflexes and unresponsive to external stimuli, with no reasonable hope of improvement?

> **persistent vegetative state**
> A condition of profound unconsciousness in which a person lacks normal reflexes and is unresponsive to external stimuli, lasting for an extended period with no reasonable hope of improvement.

Ethical questions about a person's right to die became prominent in Canada in the early 1990s with the landmark case of Sue Rodriguez. Rodriguez, a 42-year-old woman living in British Columbia, suffered from amyotrophic lateral sclerosis (ALS), or Lou Gehrig's disease. She fought for the right to die with the assistance of a physician, taking her case through the British Columbia court system and eventually to the Supreme Court of Canada. She argued that the Canadian ban on physician-assisted death violated the Constitution by dismissing her rights of personal autonomy as outlined in the Charter of Rights and Freedoms. In 1993, the Supreme Court of Canada denied her request, ruling in a five-to-four decision that society's obligation to respect human life outweighed her rights to exercise control over her own death. In 1994, Rodriguez ended her life with the assistance of a physician who remains anonymous.

Withholding or Withdrawing Treatment

The right of a competent patient to refuse unwanted treatment is now generally established in both law and medical practice. The consensus is that no medical or ethical distinction exists between withholding (not starting) a treatment and withdrawing (stopping) a treatment once it has been started. The choice to forgo life-sustaining treatment involves refusing treatments that would be expected to extend life. The right to refuse treatment remains constitutionally protected even when a patient is unable to communicate. Although specific requirements may vary, all provinces and territories authorize some type of written advance directive to honour the decisions of individuals unable to speak for themselves but who have previously recorded their wishes in an appropriate legal document. We discuss advance directives later in this chapter.

Physician-Assisted Death and Active Euthanasia

In contrast to withdrawing or withholding treatment, **physician-assisted death** and **active euthanasia** refer to practices that intentionally hasten the death of a person.

> **physician-assisted death**
> The practice of a physician intentionally providing, at the patient's request, lethal drugs or other means for a patient to hasten death with the understanding that the patient plans to use them to end his or her life.
>
> **active euthanasia**
> A deliberate act intended to end another person's life; voluntary active euthanasia involves the practice of a physician administering—at the request of a patient—medication or some other intervention that causes death.

Physician-assisted death occurs when a physician provides lethal drugs—at the patient's request—with the understanding that the patient plans to use them to end his or her life. The patient chooses if and when he or she wishes to take the fatal dose, usually (but not always) in a home setting without the physician being present.

As of 2015, physician-assisted death continues to be illegal in all Canadian provinces and territories. In February 2015, however—more than 20 years after the Rodriguez case—the Supreme Court of Canada ruled in favour of physician-assisted death in specific cases, allowing the federal government 12 months to create new legislation.

In the United States, Oregon was the first state to legalize physician-assisted death following a citizens' initiative called the Death with Dignity Act, which was passed by Oregon voters in 1994 and again in 1997. Even though physician-assisted death has been legally available in Oregon since 1994, the practice remains rare; in 2013, only 71 deaths occurred in Oregon as a result of physician-assisted death. The states of Washington and Montana have also since chosen to allow physician-assisted death.

Oregon's Death with Dignity Act has many regulations and safeguards that will likely be examined closely in Canada as a result of the recent Supreme Court ruling. Specifically, a patient who wishes to pursue an assisted death must orally request physician-assisted death from his or her physician on two different occasions at least 15 days apart. The request also must be written and signed by two witnesses. Two physicians need to confirm the patient's diagnosis and prognosis, whether the person is capable of making such a decision, and whether the patient may have a mental illness (such as depression). If either physician suspects a psychological disorder, the patient must be referred for a psychological evaluation. The patient must be informed of alternatives to physician-assisted death such as pain control and comfort and hospice care. A patient can rescind a physician-assisted death request at any time, and experience has shown that about one-third of patients who have received lethal medication from their physician have chosen not to use it. Many patients who end up not using the medication have said that merely having the means to end their own suffering gave them great comfort, and in the end they chose to let nature take its own course.

Patients who choose physician-assisted death generally have strong beliefs in personal autonomy and a determination to control the end of their lives. Physician-assisted death is not an option for patients with diseases that affect their mental functioning, such as dementia or psychiatric disorders. In addition, physicians can choose whether they wish to participate in the Death with Dignity Act. In Oregon, physicians employed by the Veteran's Administration and many Catholic hospitals are not allowed to participate in physician-assisted death as terms of their employment.

An issue of importance related to physician-assisted death is the concept of **double effect** in the medical management of pain. The doctrine of double effect states that a harmful effect of treatment, even if it results in death, is permissible if the harm is not intended and occurs as a side effect of a beneficial action. Sometimes the dosages of medication needed to relieve a patient's pain (especially those in the end stage of some diseases) must be increased to levels that can cause respiratory depression, resulting in the patient's death. Thus, the relief of suffering, the intended good effect, may have a potential bad effect, which is foreseen but is not the primary intention. It is generally accepted that such medication for pain, even if it hastens death, is not physician-assisted death if the intent is to relieve suffering.

> **double effect**
> A situation in which a harmful effect occurs as an unintended side effect of a beneficial action, such as when medication intended to control a patient's pain has the unintended result of causing the patient's death.

Unlike physician-assisted suicide, active euthanasia is the intentional act of killing someone who would otherwise suffer from an incurable and painful disease. Active euthanasia can be involuntary, non-voluntary, or voluntary. *Involuntary euthanasia* (or involuntary active euthanasia) refers to the ending of a patient's life by a medical practitioner without the patient's consent. The most notorious example of this is the medical killing programs of the Nazi regime. *Non-voluntary euthanasia* occurs when a surrogate decision maker (not the patient) asks a physician for assistance to end another person's life. *Voluntary euthanasia* (also known as voluntary active euthanasia) is the intentional termination of life at the patient's request by someone other than the patient. In practice, this generally means that a competent patient requests direct assistance to die, and he or she receives assistance from a qualified medical practitioner. Voluntary active euthanasia is legal in Belgium and the Netherlands but is unlawful in North America. Taking active steps to end someone's life is a crime—even if the motive is mercy.

Many people believe that the demand by some patients for physician-assisted death results from inattention to the needs of the dying by the health care system. The advocates of hospice and palliative care have highlighted the need for adequate pain management, not only for patients with terminal illness, but also for all patients with untreated or undertreated pain and suffering. Increasingly, pain is being viewed as a fifth vital sign, one that should be added to the four vital signs—temperature, pulse, respiration, and blood pressure—now recorded and assessed as a standard part of patient care.

Unfortunately there is tremendous variation among health care providers with respect to assessing and managing pain adequately. Even when physicians are aggressive in treating pain, there are times when adequate pain control is difficult to achieve. When a patient is near death and still suffering despite optimal treatment with pain medications, sometimes **palliative sedation** will be used. This involves giving a sedative medication that keeps the patient in an unconscious or semiconscious state until pain is brought under control or the patient dies as a result of his or her underlying disease. Palliative sedation is not meant to hasten death; rather, it is used as a last resort when physician, patient, and family agree that this is the best way to relieve otherwise intractable suffering. Palliative sedation is legal in Canada and is accepted by the Canadian Medical Association and many other medical organizations when used as a last resort in appropriately selected cases.

> **palliative sedation**
> The practice of using a sedative medication to keep a patient in an unconscious or semiconscious state until pain is brought under control or the patient dies as a result of the underlying disease.

Completing an Advance Directive

To make your preferences known about medical treatment, you need to document them through a written **advance directive**. In a general sense, an advance directive is any statement made by a competent person about choices for medical treatment should he or she become unable to make such decisions or communicate them at some time in the future.

advance directive
Any statement made by a competent person about his or her choices for medical treatment should he or she become unable to make such decisions or communicate them in the future.

Two forms of advance directives are legally important. First is the **instructional directive**, or living will, which enables individuals to provide instructions about the kind of medical care they want to receive if they become incapacitated or otherwise unable to participate in treatment decisions. Many people believe that living wills are appropriate only for stating a desire to forgo life-sustaining procedures or to avoid medical heroics when death is imminent; indeed, most standard forms for completing a living will reflect this purpose. In reality, however, a living will can be drafted to express very different ideas about the kinds of treatment a person would or would not want, and they can be written to cover various contingencies.

instructional directive
A type of advance directive that allows individuals to provide instructions about the kind of medical care they want to receive if they become unable to participate in treatment decisions.

The second important form of advance directive is the **proxy directive**, which is also known as a *durable power of attorney for health care*. This document makes it possible to appoint another person to make decisions about medical treatment if you become unable to do so. This person, also known as a **substitute decision maker**, may be a family member, a close friend, or an attorney with whom you have discussed your treatment preferences. The proxy is expected to act in accordance with your wishes as stated in an advance directive or as otherwise made known. Some provinces/territories allow individuals to appoint more than one proxy, so it is important to look into the details in your provincial or territorial legislation. A proxy should be asked in advance whether he or she is willing to take on the responsibility of making potentially difficult decisions for you, and he or she must also be capable of making these decisions. For advance directives to be of value, you must do more than complete the paperwork. Discuss your wishes ahead of time with caregivers and family members as well as with your proxy and physician.

proxy directive
A type of advance directive that allows an individual to appoint another person as an agent in making health care decisions in the event he or she becomes unable to participate in treatment decisions; also known as a *durable power of attorney for health care*.

substitute decision maker
The agent appointed by a person to act on his or her behalf by means of a proxy directive.

Planning ahead means different things at different stages of life. For older adults, or those with a potentially terminal illness, making specific plans for what lies ahead becomes an urgent matter. For most students reading this text, specific planning for your eventual death is probably not a priority. But thinking about some of these issues now will help you down the road both in dealing with your own life, as well as helping your loved ones as they near the end of their lives. Completing an advance directive is appropriate at any age. If you fill out an advance directive and share it with your parents (or grandparents), they may be encouraged to follow your example.

Giving the Gift of Life

People at all stages of life should consider the pros and cons of becoming an organ donor. A human body is a valuable resource. Of all the advances in medical techniques for helping patients who were formerly beyond recovery, perhaps the best known is the transplantation of human organs. Yet the demand for organs continues to outpace the number of organ donations. Approximately 4500 Canadians are currently on the waiting list for organ transplants, and in 2012, 256 people died before receiving a transplant. For a visual display of the need, supply, and deaths while waiting for organ transplants in in Canada in 2012, see Figure 18.1.

Organs and tissues that are used for transplant come from several sources. Living donors can donate a single kidney and parts of organs such as the liver, lungs, intestine, and pancreas. Living donors can also donate blood and bone marrow. Deceased donors are the only source of hearts, whole lungs, or other body parts that can't be removed from living donors. Eyes, bone, tendons, skin, and heart valves are some of the tissues that can be donated. Organ and tissue donors are matched with potential recipients based on many factors including blood and tissue types. Generally the most successful transplants occur when the donor and recipient are as genetically similar as possible. To help prevent rejection, transplant recipients often must take powerful drugs to suppress their immune systems.

According to a report by the Canadian Institute for Health Information (CIHI), the number of deceased organ donors in Canada has, for the first time in 10 years, surpassed the number of organ donors who are living. In 2012, approximately three-quarters of the organ transplant procedures performed in Canada were from deceased donors, reflecting an increase of 5 percent over one year and 17 percent over the previous 10 years. While this increase in Canada's deceased donor rate is promising and may be explained at least in part by

FIGURE 18.1

Organs Required by Canadians, 2012

The continuation of current demographic trends (declining birth and death rates and an aging population), combined with the rapidly growing need for transplants and projected organ donation rates, will lead to an ever-widening shortfall between the need for, and supply of, organs for transplantation.

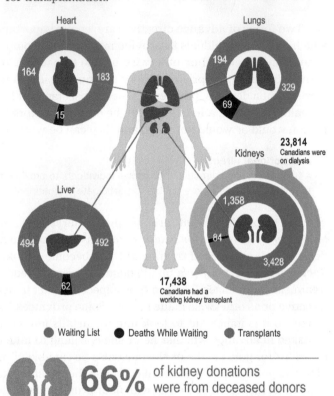

Source: Canadian Institute for Health Information, *Canadian Organ Replacement Register*, 2013. p. 2. (https://www.cihi.ca/en/corr_public_summary_2014_en.pdf; retrieved July 22, 2015).

growing media exposure and social media campaigns, it continues to lack in comparison to that of many other countries. According to the Canadian Transplant Society, while 90 percent of Canadians have indicated that they support organ and tissue donation, less than 25 percent have made plans to donate.

QUICK STATS

One deceased donor can save up to 8 lives through organ donation, and can benefit and improve the quality of 75 more people's lives through tissue donation.

—Canadian Transplant Society, 2014

There are many reasons for the current shortage of donor organs. The number of people in need of transplants is growing because modern medical care tends to keep people with serious health problems alive longer. In addition, as transplant technology improves, more medical conditions can be treated effectively with transplantation. While the need for transplantation grows, the supply of organs has not kept pace. Not enough people register as donors. In addition, improved medical care of the victims of trauma, as well as widespread use of safety devices such as seat belts and motorcycle helmets, have reduced the number of individuals who become brain-dead, who might otherwise have been potential donors of many organs.

People of any age or health status can register as donors. It is crucial that people of all ages, young and old, who are willing to donate organs and tissue, let their families know and register as donors. In particular, it is important that young people consider becoming donors. The sudden unexpected death of a young person, usually due to some form of trauma, is a horrendous tragedy to her or his family, friends, and society as a whole. But some good can come from such a loss by donating organs. Knowing that their loved one saved or improved the lives of many people can be a lasting comfort to grieving family and friends.

There are several long-standing myths and fears about organ donation. A common unfounded fear is that if you are seriously injured, physicians won't work as hard to save your life if they know you are a donor. This is definitely not true! Saving a life is always the first priority. Another common myth is that organ donation disfigures the body and makes an open casket funeral impossible. In fact, donated organs are removed surgically, which does not change the appearance of the body for the funeral service. In addition, some people are

FIGURE 18.2

Ontario's "Be a Donor" Website

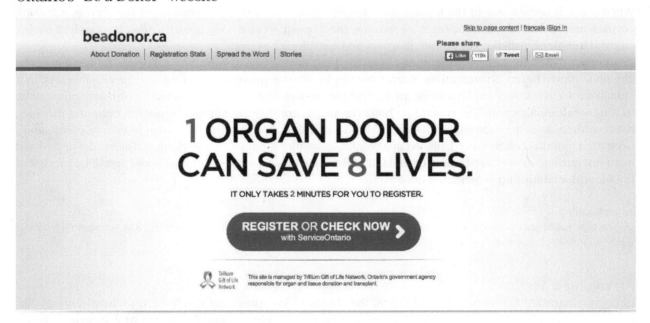

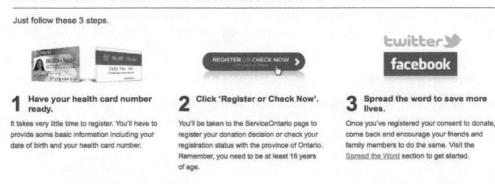

Source: Trillium Gift of Life Network, www.beadonor.ca

concerned that their religion may prohibit organ donation. When in doubt, it always makes sense to discuss this with your clergy; but most major organized religions approve of organ and tissue donation, and many consider it an act of great kindness and charity.

If you decide to become a donor, the first step is to register; the steps one takes to register his or her intent to donate differ by province/territory. Some provinces and territories, including British Columbia and Ontario, have an organ donor registry that residents can join. Ontarians, for example, can register their intent to donate online at http://www.beadonor.ca (see Figure 18.2). Because relatives are called on to make decisions about organ and tissue donation at the time of a loved one's death, your second step is to discuss your decision with your family. Many organs that could be donated are lost each year because potential donors did not make their family members aware of their wishes.

Planning a Funeral or Memorial Service

Funerals and memorial services are rites of passage that commemorate a person's life and acknowledge his or her passing from the community. Funerals and memorials allow survivors to support one another as they cope with their loss and express their grief. The presence of death rites in every human culture suggests that they serve innate human needs.

Disposition of the Body

When a death occurs, one of the immediate concerns of survivors is the disposition of the corpse. Although corpses must be disposed of for sanitary reasons, the disposition of a body is surrounded by a web of social, cultural, religious, psychological, and interpersonal considerations.

People generally have a preference about the final disposition of their body. For most Canadians, the choice is either burial or cremation. *Burial* usually involves a grave dug into the soil or entombment in a mausoleum. *Cremation* involves subjecting a body to intense heat, thereby reducing its organic components to a mineralized skeleton. The remaining bone fragments are then usually put through a cremulator, which reduces them to a granular state, often referred to as ashes (which actually resemble coarse coral sand). Cremated remains can be buried, placed in a columbarium niche, put into an urn kept by the family or interred in an urn garden, or scattered at sea or on land. If the body is to be viewed during a wake or will be present at the funeral, **embalming** is generally done.

> **embalming**
> The process of removing blood and other fluids and replacing them with chemicals to disinfect and temporarily slow deterioration of a corpse.

Arranging a Service

In commemorating a person's life and death, the choice of last rites may involve a traditional funeral ceremony or a simple memorial service. Whereas the casketed body is typically present at a funeral, it is not at a memorial service. In some cases, both a funeral and a memorial service are held, the former occurring within a few days after death and the latter being held sometime later. Although some individuals express a preference for not having any kind of service, in general bereaved relatives and friends can derive important benefits from having an opportunity to honour the deceased and express their grief through ceremony.

QUICK STATS

Approximately 66% of corpse dispositions in Canada were done via cremation in 2013; in the United States, it was approximately 45%.

—Cremation Association of North America, 2015

A funeral or memorial service can be a healing experience that allows loved ones to share memories and support one another. Memorial services can be held almost anywhere, including outdoors, in a home, or in a chapel. The service is often led by clergy, but many non-traditional services are led by a family member or close friend. The more the service fits the personality of the deceased person and meets the practical needs of the family, the better. A memory book or other photo display is common, and this helps bring back cherished memories of the person at different stages in his or her life. A home-based or outdoor service with a potluck meal or snacks afterward can be meaningful and healing while not placing a great financial burden on the grieving family.

People who have a terminal illness sometimes find comfort and satisfaction in helping to plan for their own memorial services. A memorial service can be the joint creation of the dying person and family members who wish to be part of the project. Making at least some plans ahead of time can help ease the burden on survivors, who will undoubtedly face a great number of tasks and decisions when the death occurs (see the Take Charge box).

 Take CHARGE

Tasks for Survivors

Some of the following tasks must be attended to soon after a death occurs, whereas others take weeks or months to complete. Many of these tasks, especially those that need to be dealt with in the first hours and days following the death, can be taken care of by friends and relatives of the immediate survivors. If the deceased person has been served by a hospice, the social worker has likely worked with the patient and family to make many of these plans ahead of time.

- Prepare a list of relatives, friends, and colleagues, and contact them about the death as soon as possible. Friends can help with notifications.
- Find out if the deceased left instructions for disposition of the body or for a funeral or memorial service.
- If no prior plan exists, contact a funeral home, mortuary, or memorial society for help in making arrangements. Clergy, friends, and other family members can be asked to help decide what is most appropriate.
- If flowers are to be omitted from the funeral or memorial service, choose an appropriate charity or other memorial to which gifts can be made.
- Write the obituary. Consider including the deceased's age, birthplace, cause of death, occupation, academic degrees, memberships, military service, accomplishments, names and relationships of nearest survivors, and the time and place of the funeral or memorial service. If a small funeral is planned, and you are notifying people by phone or email, you can wait to write the obituary later, or skip it entirely. You can also use an online obituary website, and even create an online memorial to a loved one.
- Ask friends to help coordinate the supplying of meals for the first few days following the death, as well as the management of other household tasks and child care, if necessary. You can also ask friends to coordinate a potluck or catered meal if you wish to have a gathering after the funeral. Simple snacks and drinks are fine, if you choose.
- If you have relatives and friends who will be coming from out of town for the funeral, ask a friend or family member to help with arrangements for lodging and transportation to and from the airport.
- If a funeral ceremony is planned, choose the individuals who are to be pallbearers, and notify them that you would like their participation.
- Gather photos or other mementos for a memory book, memory board, or memorial website.
- Do you want to have a small booklet with information about the deceased and perhaps a photo or poem to give to mourners at the funeral or memorial service? If so, get help from family members and friends to create the pamphlet and have it printed.

It can be worthwhile to consider such decisions early in life so you can gather information about options and discuss plans with family members (see the Critical Consumer box). Religious and cultural or ethnic traditions play a major role in shaping the way people honour their dead. The diversity of life and death in Canada calls for a diversity of rites. A meaningful funeral or memorial service can be designed in many ways.

Critical CONSUMER

A Consumer Guide to Funerals

A traditional funeral with a casket costs about $7000, and many funerals cost $10 000 or more. When no pre-planning has been done, as often occurs, family members have to make decisions under time pressure and in the grip of strong feelings. As a result, they may make poor decisions and spend more than they need to. To avoid these problems, many Canadian consumers are now making funeral arrangements in advance, comparing prices and services so they can make well-informed purchasing decisions. Many people see funeral planning as an extension of will and estate planning.

Alternatives to traditional funerals exist. In Canada, cremation is a much less expensive (and more common) alternative to a traditional burial. A direct cremation (no service or visitation at the funeral home) can cost as little as $600 in some cities. Cremated remains can be buried in a family plot or placed in a mausoleum, but many people choose to keep the ashes at home or scatter them in a beautiful location. Whole-body donation (usually to a medical school) is another option chosen by many people for altruistic reasons, as well as the fact that there is usually no cost. Another alternative to an expensive traditional funeral is a more personalized, "do-it-yourself" family-centred funeral, with minimal costs because most or all of the tasks needed to care for the deceased person are provided by family and friends.

To ensure that you make the best possible decisions when planning a funeral, follow these guidelines:

- *Plan ahead.* Think about what type of funeral you want, and ask your loved ones about their preferences.
- *Shop around.* If you are going to use a funeral home, look for one that has a good reputation, and compare prices from at least two funeral homes.
- *Ask for a price list.* In most provinces and territories, funeral homes and cemeteries are required to provide families with a detailed cost breakdown of all the products and services they provide. This will enable you to select only those services you require and can afford.
- *Decide on the goods and services you want.* Basic services include planning the funeral and coordinating arrangements with the cemetery or crematory. The price of a casket can easily account for half the total cost of an average funeral service. Prices range from a few hundred dollars for a cloth-covered casket to thousands of dollars for a metal or hardwood casket. You may have to ask to see less expensive caskets, since these are often not on display at funeral homes. Discount casket stores have also opened in some Canadian cities.
- *Consider your options.* In Canada, funeral and burial regulations vary depending on the province or territory. Generally, embalming is not legally required; however, it may be required when transferring remains to another province or territory, or out of the country (unless it is contrary to religious beliefs). In many cases, except in Alberta and Ontario, unless you give instructions to the contrary, funeral homes will automatically go ahead with embalming and charge you for it.
- *Resist pressure to buy goods and services you don't really want or need.* Funeral directors are required to inform you that you need buy only those goods and services you want.
- *Choose a cemetery carefully.* In choosing a cemetery, consider its location; its religious affiliation, if any; the types of monuments allowed; and cost. Visit the cemetery to make sure it's suitable, and ask for a copy of the cemetery's rules and regulations.
- *Commit it to paper.* Once you have made decisions, put them in writing, give copies to family members, and keep a copy accessible. It's a good idea to review your decisions every few years and revise them if necessary.
- *Ask for help.* If you need help dealing with a funeral home, contact your provincial or territorial consumer affairs office or funeral service regulator.

Source: Federal-Provincial-Territorial Consumer Measures Committee. nd. *Canadian Consumer Handbook: Funerals*. Ottawa: Industry Canada, http://www.consumerhandbook.ca/en/topics/products-and-services/funerals#information (retrieved July 20, 2015).

QUESTIONS FOR CRITICAL THINKING AND REFLECTION

Have you ever been involved in a funeral? What role did you play? Did you feel that the service reflected the values and beliefs of the deceased person? Did the experience cause you to think about your own funeral and what it should be like?

THINKING ABOUT THE ENVIRONMENT

Canada has thousands of cemeteries, covering tens of thousands of hectares of land. These burial grounds hold millions of graves, some of which are hundreds of years old.

In the face of long-standing tradition, however, some Canadians are rethinking the notion of burying the dead in sealed caskets, placed in permanent concrete vaults. This practice, say environmentalists, needlessly consumes vast tracts of land, and chemicals from embalmed bodies and caskets slowly leach into the soil and water. Despite the notion that cremation solves these problems, the practice uses a great deal of energy and pollutes the air.

One solution is the natural, or "green," burial. In a green burial, the body is wrapped in cloth or placed in a biodegradable casket made from wood, wicker, or recycled paper, and then buried in the ground. No embalming takes place and no chemicals are used. No pesticides are used on the land either, and grave markers, such as plants, trees, flowers, and boulders, are used in place of traditional gravestones.

In 2008, the first natural burial site in Canada opened in Victoria, British Columbia. In Ontario, the green burial movement is also gaining momentum. Members of the Natural Burial Association in Canada have been working since 2005 to raise awareness about the environmental benefits of natural burials and to facilitate the creation of additional grounds across the country. Currently, there are four natural burial sites in Canada; three in Ontario plus the abovementioned site in British Columbia. There are also several natural burial grounds that, according to the Natural Burial Association, are currently in the planning stages. If all goes well, these sites will provide additional environmentally friendly burial options for a growing number of Canadians in the years ahead.

Coping With Dying

There is no one right way to live with or die of a life-threatening illness. Every disease has its own set of problems and challenges, and each person copes with these problems and challenges in his or her own way. Much of the suffering experienced by people with a life-threatening illness comes from overwhelming feelings of loss on all levels. Besides the emotional havoc, they usually have concerns about medical care, loss of income, hospitalization, and physical pain. How a person copes with such an experience is likely to reflect his or her personality and life history, as well as the nature of family relationships and patterns of interaction in the person's wider social environment. Spiritual strength can be a major factor in how we deal with these losses. The support of loving family, friends, clergy or other spiritual guides, and health care professionals including a hospice team, can make the journey easier to bear.

Awareness of Dying

Living with an illness that is life threatening and incurable can be described as a living-dying experience. From the time discomforting symptoms are first noticed and a person's worst fears are confirmed by a diagnosis, through the ups and downs of treatment, and on to the final days or hours of life, hope and honesty are often delicately balanced—honesty to face reality as it is, hope for a positive outcome. The object of hope changes. The early hope that the symptoms are not really serious gives way to hope that a cure is possible. When the illness is deemed incurable, hope for more time arises. As time begins to run out, the hope changes to a pain-free death, a "good death" (see the Mind Body Spirit box).

Psychiatrist Avery Weisman described this process of coping as involving **middle knowledge**, with patients and their families seeking a balance between sustaining hope and acknowledging the reality. Maintaining a sense of self-worth, setting goals and striving to reach them, engaging in fruitful interactions with the environment—all of these reflect a coping strength that sustains the will to live fully despite a bleak prognosis.

middle knowledge
A state of knowing when a person both acknowledges the reality of a threatening situation and maintains hope for a positive outcome.

Mind *Body* SPIRIT

In Search of a Good Death

Participants in a landmark study were asked to discuss the deaths of family members, friends, or patients and reflect on what made their deaths good or bad. From these discussions, six major themes emerged as components of a good death.

1) *Pain and symptom management:* Many people fear dying in pain, and portrayals of bad deaths usually included inadequate pain management. Every health care provider in the study told regret-filled stories of patients who died in pain. Patients were concerned with pain control; when reassured that pain could be managed, they were less anxious.

2) *Clear decision making:* Both providers and families feared entering a medical crisis without knowing the patient's preferences. Patients and families who had good communication with health care providers and had discussed treatment decisions ahead of time felt empowered, and providers felt they were giving good care. Although all uncertainty about end-of-life decisions cannot be eliminated, tolerance for uncertainty may increase if values and preferences are clarified.

3) *Preparation for death:* Patients expressed satisfaction when they had time to prepare their wills and help plan their funeral arrangements. Many times, providers avoided end-of-life discussions to prevent their patients from losing hope, thus depriving them of the opportunity to plan ahead. Patients and families also wanted to know what to expect during the illness and what physical and psychosocial changes would take place as death approached. It was important for providers and families to have reached some personal comfort with death so they felt prepared when death occurred.

4) *Completion:* The opportunity to review life, to resolve conflicts, to spend time with loved ones, and to say goodbye were also found to be important. Participants confirmed the deep importance of spirituality or meaningfulness at the end of life. Many times, patients were able to view their experience of dying as part of a broader life trajectory and thus continue to grow emotionally and spiritually in their last days. Issues of faith were often mentioned as important to healing, but participants emphasized that the cues about the particular expression of faith must be taken from the patient.

5) *Contributing to others:* Patients wanted to know that they still had something to offer to others, whether it was making someone laugh or lightening the load of someone closer to death. Many patients found that as they reflected on their lives, what they valued most was their personal relationships with family and friends, and they were anxious to impart this wisdom to others.

6) *Affirmation of the whole person:* Patients appreciated empathic health care providers, and family members were comforted by those who treated their loved ones as unique and whole people, rather than as a disease. The quality of dying is related to the acknowledgment that people die in character; that is, as an extension of who they have been in their lives. Health care providers also focused on their personal relationships with patients and family members as important to a satisfying death.

The study affirmed that most people think of death as a natural part of life, not as a failure of technology. Although the biomedical aspects of end-of-life care are crucial, they merely provide a point of departure toward a good death. When pain is properly managed and the practical aspects of dying are taken care of, patients and their families have the opportunity to address the important emotional, psychological, and spiritual issues that all human beings face at the end of life.

The Tasks of Coping

In her groundbreaking 1969 book *On Death and Dying*, Elisabeth Kübler-Ross suggested that the response to an awareness of imminent death involves five psychological stages: denial, anger, bargaining, depression, and acceptance. The notion that these five stages occur in a linear progression has since become a kind of modern myth of how people *ought* to cope with dying. Unfortunately, this can lead to the idea that it is a person's task to move sequentially through these stages, one after another, and that if this is not accomplished, the person has somehow failed. In fact, however, Kübler-Ross said that individuals go back and forth among the stages during an illness, and different stages can occur simultaneously.

The stage-based model devised by Kübler-Ross more than four decades ago has been a stimulus toward a better understanding of how people cope with dying. The notion of stages, however, has been deemphasized in favour of highlighting the tasks that deserve attention in coping with a life-threatening illness. Charles Corr, for example, distinguishes four primary dimensions in coping with dying:

1. *Physical:* Satisfying bodily needs and minimizing physical distress.
2. *Psychological:* Maximizing a sense of security, self-worth, autonomy, and richness in living.
3. *Social:* Sustaining significant relationships and addressing the social implications of dying.
4. *Spiritual:* Identifying, developing, or reaffirming sources of meaning and fostering hope.

Helping a dying person, and her or his loved ones, requires attention to all four of these dimensions. In addition, we must remember that a person's death is as unique as his or her life. Thus, although models can help us gain understanding, they need to be balanced by paying attention to the dying person's own unfolding *life* story. Each person's pathway through life-threatening illness is determined by many factors, such as the specific disease and its course, his or her personality, and the available supportive resources.

People who apparently cope best with life-threatening illness often exhibit a fighting spirit that views the illness not only as a threat, but also as a challenge. These people strive to inform themselves about their illness and take an active part in treatment decisions. They are optimistic and have a capacity to discover positive meaning in ordinary events. Holding to a positive outlook despite distressing circumstances involves creating a sense of meaning that is bigger than the threat. In the context of life-threatening illness, this encompasses a person's ability to comprehend the implications an illness has for the future, as well as for his or her ability to accomplish goals, maintain relationships, and sustain a sense of personal vitality, competence, and power. Although life-threatening illness disrupts virtually all aspects of a person's life, there is a vital link between finding meaning and achieving a sense of mastery.

Supporting a Person in the Last Phase of Life

People often feel uncomfortable in the presence of a person who is in the final stage of life. How should we act? What can we say? Perhaps the most important and comforting thing we can do for a dying person is to simply be present. Sitting quietly and listening carefully, we can take our cues from the person who is dying. If the person is capable of speaking, and wishes to talk, attentive listening is an act of great kindness. If the person doesn't wish to talk, or is not able to, physical touch such as holding hands or putting a hand on the person's shoulder can be the most effective way to express your love and concern.

Attempting to cheer up a dying person by saying something like "you are going to be just fine" or "you can fight this and be well again" can be frustrating for a patient at the end of life, who knows that your words are simply not true. You cannot fix all the difficulties your dying loved one is facing, but you can listen, and show by your loving presence that you care. Speaking simply and from the heart can be a healing experience for us and for the loved one whose time is short.

The level of alertness of a dying person often fluctuates. It is not unusual for a patient who has been non-verbal to have moments of clear speech in the days or hours before death. People with dementia may have lucid periods from time to time. Even if a person appears to be in a coma or deep sleep, he or she may be able to hear what is going on around them. Most experts think that hearing and touch are the last senses to go. Always assume that a dying person can hear what you say; be sure to keep that in mind when you speak to others in the room. Don't hesitate to speak lovingly to a dying person whether or not she or he shows outward signs of hearing you.

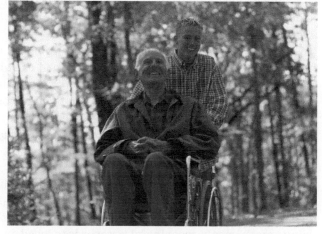

The simple act of listening can be extremely supportive to someone who is facing death.

Besides the loving presence of friends and family, the dying person may need other supportive resources. Trained individuals who have experience with dying patients, such as clergy and palliative care workers, can provide invaluable support for dying people and their families.

The Trajectory of Dying

Our expectations about dying may be quite different from what most people actually experience. The concept of a **trajectory of dying** is useful for understanding patients' experiences as they near death. Although sudden death from an unexpected cause—a massive heart attack or an accident, for example—is one type of dying trajectory, our focus here is on deaths that occur when there is forewarning. Among these, some trajectories involve a steady and fairly predictable decline. This is the case with many cancers, which tend to follow the course of a progressive disease with a terminal phase. Other kinds of advanced, chronic illness involve a long period of slow decline marked by episodes of crisis, the last of which proves to be fatal.

> **trajectory of dying**
> The duration and nature of a person's experience in approaching death as influenced by the underlying cause of dying.

We can also distinguish between different stages in a dying trajectory, namely, a period when a person is known to be terminally ill but is living with a life expectancy of perhaps weeks or months, possibly years, and a later period when dying is imminent and the person is described as actively dying. The way in which such trajectories are estimated—their duration and expected course—can affect both patients and caregivers and influence their actions. Deaths that occur out of time (too quickly or too slowly) may pose special difficulties. A family may experience more shock and guilt if the death occurs before they have had time to "say their goodbyes" and emotionally prepare for the loss of their loved one. When death is slow in coming, and the dying individual lingers for days, weeks, or months longer than anticipated, families and the dying person may become physically, emotionally, and spiritually exhausted. The support of extended family, friends, hospice, and clergy can make the difference between an unbearable situation and one that is tolerable. In the best scenarios, the dying process can be a time when bonds of family and friendship are strengthened, and personal growth occurs for the dying individual and his or her loved ones.

When a person is actively dying, his or her death is expected to occur within hours or, at most, a few days. During the last phase of a fatal illness, a dying person may exhibit irregular breathing or shortness of breath, decreased appetite and thirst, nausea and vomiting, incontinence, restlessness and agitation, disorientation and confusion, and diminished consciousness. These symptoms can usually be managed by skilled palliative care. Pain, if it is present, should be treated aggressively as part of a comprehensive approach to comfort care. Since most patients are more comfortable without eating or drinking at the end of life, forcing food or liquids is usually not beneficial. The stopping of eating and drinking has always been part of the last phase of a terminal condition.

Near the time of death, relaxation of the throat muscles or secretions in the throat may cause the person's breathing to become noisy, resulting in a sound called the death rattle. Other signals may be noticeable as death draws closer. For example, the patient's extremities may feel cold to the touch; lips, fingers, and ears may appear bluish; urination becomes less frequent; or the ability to communicate may be lost. In the final hours, purple blotches (mottling) may appear on the legs or arms. Simple steps—such as repositioning the patient, covering the individual with blankets, dimming the room's lighting, or just holding hands—can provide great relief and reassurance in the last moments. Just before death, the person may take a breath and sigh or shudder.

It is not unusual for a dying person to seem to wait until loved ones have left the room before taking her or his last breath. You should not feel guilty or rejected if you are not present at the moment of death. Some dying people seem to need to be alone in the moment of passing. The Hollywood version of death, where the dying person speaks meaningful last words to loved ones, then dies immediately, is much less common than a period of hours or days of apparent unresponsiveness before death finally comes.

What is your notion of a "good death"? In what setting does it take place, and who is there? In the last days of your life, what do you think you will need to say, and to whom will you want to say it? If you were terminally ill, what would be the most supportive things others could do for you?

Coping With Loss

Even if we have not experienced the death of someone close, we are all survivors of losses that occur in our lives because of changes and endings. The loss of a job, the ending of a relationship, transitions from one school or neighbourhood to another—these are examples of the kinds of losses that occur in all our lives. Such losses are sometimes called little deaths and, in varying degrees, they all involve grief.

For many of us, our first really significant loss is the death of a pet. The intensity of grief after losing a beloved companion animal is often comparable to the grief experienced following the loss of a human loved one. Never assume that the loss of a pet is "no big deal—you can always get another one." The pain following loss of a pet may be made even harder to bear if the experience of the grieving person is belittled. The comments here about grief are relevant to many types of loss, not just the loss of a human friend or relative.

Experiencing Grief

Grief is the reaction to loss. It encompasses thoughts and feelings, as well as physical and behavioural responses. Mental distress may involve disbelief, confusion, anxiety, disorganization, and depression. The emotions that can be present in normal grief include not only sorrow and sadness, but also relief, anger, and self-pity, among others. Bereaved people experience a range of feelings, even conflicting ones. Recognizing that grief can involve many different feelings—not just sadness—makes us more able to cope with it.

> **grief**
> A person's reaction to loss as manifested physically, emotionally, mentally, and behaviourally.

Common behaviours associated with grief include crying, searching for the deceased, and talking incessantly about the deceased and the circumstances of the death. Bereaved people may be restless, as if not knowing what to do with themselves. Physically, grief may involve frequent sighing, insomnia, and loss of appetite. Grief may also evoke a re-examination of religious or spiritual beliefs as a person struggles to make meaning of the loss.

Guilt is a common emotion after the death of a loved one. People may blame themselves in some way for the death, or for not doing enough for the deceased, or for feeling a sense of relief that their loved one is gone. All such manifestations of grief can be present as part of one's total response to **bereavement**—that is, the event of loss.

> **bereavement**
> The objective event of loss.

Mourning is closely related to grief and is often used as a synonym for it. However, mourning refers not so much to the *reaction* to loss but to the *process* by which a bereaved person adjusts to loss and incorporates it into his or her life. How this process is managed is determined, at least partly, by cultural and gender norms for the expression of grief (see the Gender Matters box). Considered jointly, grief and mourning are the means to healing the pain of loss.

> **mourning**
> The process whereby a person actively copes with grief in adjusting to a loss and integrating it into his or her life.

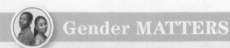

Gender MATTERS

Grief and Gender

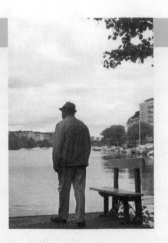

The loss of a loved one generates a broad range of reactions—physical, emotional, and behavioural. But do women and men react differently to the loss of someone close to them? Some clinicians say yes, and studies now support the idea that grief has different gender patterns.

Data suggest that a greater proportion of women may be vulnerable to the more distressing and disruptive symptoms characteristic of severe grief reactions. In general, women have a higher lifetime incidence and prevalence of depressive and anxiety disorders, so it is not surprising that at times of great stress, such as the loss of a loved one, these gender differences would be present.

In a study of gender differences in grief among parents who have lost a child, researchers found that compared with fathers, mothers showed greater feelings of being hurt, cheated, and depressed, while also revealing greater irritability and anger. The women also cried more, experienced greater numbness and confusion, were more preoccupied with thoughts of the deceased, and felt more guilt both for having failed to prevent the death and for having survived. They also experienced more physical symptoms, such as insomnia and loss of appetite.

In a study of people who had lost a spouse, researchers similarly found that women had a higher level of emotional distress in reaction to loss. Women who lost a husband had higher levels of traumatic grief, depression, and anxiety than men who had lost a wife. These findings persisted at least two years following the death of the spouse.

Physiological factors contributing to these gender differences might include hormonal differences, subtle differences in brain chemistry or function, or genetic influences. Gender roles and cultural expectations also likely play a role. Women are often readier to express emotion and seek out social support and opportunities to talk about loss, whereas men may be more reticent to admit to any psychological distress or allow the appearance of excessive emotionality.

Tasks of Mourning

Experiencing grief is part of the process by which a bereaved person integrates a significant loss into his or her life. Psychologist William Worden has identified four tasks that should be attended to:

1. *Accepting the reality* of the loss.
2. *Working through the pain* of grief.
3. *Adjusting to a changed environment* in which the deceased is absent.
4. *Emotionally relocating the deceased* and moving on with life.

Accomplishing the fourth task does not mean dishonouring the deceased's memory or denying normal feelings of connection that persist beyond death. Finding healthy ways to maintain bonds with the deceased is a testimony to the enduring strength of love. When this task is managed successfully, however, the bereaved is not stuck in the past. Making the journey of grief and attending to the various tasks along the way, we come to a place where we learn how to keep a special place for the deceased in our hearts and memories while moving forward with our lives.

The Course of Grief

Grieving, like dying, is highly individual. In the first hours or days following a death, a bereaved person is likely to experience overwhelming shock and numbness, as well as a sense of disbelief. There is often a period of denial—"No! This can't be true!"—especially if the death was unexpected. Consider the ways in which people die: a young child pronounced dead on arrival after a bicycle crash; an aged grandmother dying quietly in her sleep; a despondent executive who commits suicide; a young soldier killed in battle; a chronically ill person who dies a lingering death. The cause or mode of death—natural, accidental, homicide, or suicide—has an influence on how a bereaved person experiences grief (see the In the News box). Even when a death is anticipated, grief is not necessarily diminished when the loss becomes real.

The death of a loved one is frequently a severe physical as well as emotional stressor. For example, the rate of heart attack in the first day after the death of a significant person in one's life increases by as much

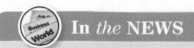

In *the* NEWS

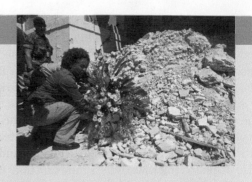

Profound Trauma and Loss

Profoundly traumatic events—the earthquakes in Nepal, Japan, and Haiti, Hurricane Katrina, the 2004 tsunami in Southeast Asia, the terrorist attacks of September 11, 2001, the deaths and destruction resulting from the wars in Iraq and Afghanistan—all represent a category of loss far beyond normal comprehension. Experiencing traumatic loss in such extraordinary circumstances can cause severe and disruptive reactions in emotion and behaviour.

World War I veterans often developed psychological symptoms that collectively were described as shell shock. However, it was not until after the Vietnam War that the medical community became fully aware of how disruptive and enduring the psychological effects could be for those experiencing profound traumatic loss.

It is now widely recognized that significant psychological symptoms can follow when people experience loss in traumatic circumstances. Elements commonly seen in a customary reaction to grief, such as sadness, disbelief, crying, insomnia, and loss of appetite, are frequently exaggerated in the aftermath of profoundly traumatic events and will often include more pronounced symptoms, such as overwhelming distress, numbness, doubt, despair, guilt, and disabling depression and anxiety.

Depending on the severity of exposure and a person's underlying vulnerability, the symptoms can persist long after the original trauma. Memories and images of the event may suddenly pop into the victim's mind, causing anxiety, depression, and anger. Insomnia and nightmares can disrupt the sleep-wake cycle. The person may start avoiding everything that serves as a reminder of the event and, as a kind of self-protection, may begin to become numb, to lose all feelings. Such people may startle easily and have difficulty concentrating. Their work life, social life, and intimate relationships may become markedly impaired. People experiencing these severe symptoms are said to have post-traumatic stress disorder (PTSD), which can persist for months or years.

The events of September 11, 2001, are an example of a profound trauma that caused PTSD in affected people. As described in Chapter 2, PTSD symptoms occurred among survivors, rescue workers, passersby, residents of Manhattan, and some people exposed to the events through repeated television images. Researchers who interviewed residents of Manhattan found that about 7.5 percent reported symptoms consistent with a diagnosis of PTSD and 9.7 percent reported symptoms consistent with new onset of depression; these numbers are about twice as high as the expected rates in surveys of this type. Among people who lived closest to the World Trade Center, the prevalence of PTSD was as high as 20 percent.

Many people experience disabling depression or anxiety but do not meet the full criteria for PTSD. More persistent and severe grief reactions, unexplained physical symptoms, and the increased use of alcohol and drugs are frequent occurrences for people who have undergone such trauma. In addition, family and interpersonal conflict and financial strain are commonly seen. All too frequently, in war or natural disasters, the primary wage earner of the family dies or the family's house and belongings are destroyed.

How long will an individual's symptoms last after experiencing an event like September 11 or witnessing a friend killed by a roadside bomb in Afghanistan? Many factors, such as the severity of the trauma, the individual's proximity to the event, and his or her emotional closeness to those who have died, can all play important roles in the magnitude and duration of the reaction to traumatic loss. In general, though, symptoms will diminish with time, especially in the absence of new threats and traumatic losses. Studies of those who have developed full-blown PTSD suggest that approximately half of the cases resolve within two years, but that nearly a third never fully recover.

Psychological support and treatment can greatly help many of those who suffer from disabling emotional symptoms in reaction to traumatic loss. Building on research and work done with Vietnam veterans in the 1970s and 1980s, clinicians have developed multiple therapeutic strategies involving group therapy, individual psychological support, and pharmacologic intervention to treat persistent symptoms.

Sources: Coker, A. L., et al. 2006. Social and mental health needs assessment of Katrina evacuees. *Disaster Management and Response* 4(3): 88–94; Watanabe, T., et al. 2006. Acute stress syndrome in a victim of the Indian Ocean Tsunami. *Psychiatry and Clinical Neurosciences* 60(5): 644; Galea, S., and H. Resnick. 2005. Posttraumatic stress disorder in the general population after mass terrorist incidents: Considerations about the nature of exposure. *CNS Spectrums* 10(2): 107–115; Galea, S., et al. 2002. Psychological sequelae of the September 11 terrorist attacks in New York City. *New England Journal of Medicine* 346(13): 982–987; Shuster, M., et al. 2001. A national survey of stress reactions after the September 11, 2001, terrorist attacks. *New England Journal of Medicine* 345(20): 1507–1512; and Ornstein, R. D., and R. K. Pitman (section eds.). 2000. Trauma and post-traumatic stress disorder. In *Massachusetts General Hospital Psychiatry Update and Board Preparation*, 2nd ed., T. A. Stern and J. B. Herman (eds.). New York: McGraw-Hill.

as 21 times. The risk gradually decreases over time, but still remains above normal for several months after a loved one dies. After a death, grieving people often have difficulty sleeping, may neglect to eat nourishing food, and may forget to take their usual medications. These factors add to the health risks associated with recent loss. Recent loss also has a cognitive impact on many grievers. People often report that they feel confused and have difficulty concentrating following a significant loss.

After the initial shock begins to fade, the course of grief is characterized by anxiety, apathy, and pining for the deceased. The pangs of grief are felt as the bereaved person deeply experiences the pain of separation. There is often a sense of despair as a person repeatedly goes over the events surrounding the loss, perhaps fantasizing that somehow everything could be undone and be as it was before. During this period, the bereaved person may also begin to look toward the future and take the first steps toward building a life without the deceased.

Psychiatrist Colin Murray Parkes points to three main influences on a person's course of grieving:

1. The urge to look back, cry, and search for what is lost.
2. The urge to look forward, explore the world that emerges out of the loss, and discover what can be carried forward from the past into the future.
3. The social and cultural pressures that influence how the first two urges are inhibited or expressed.

As these influences interact in various ways, at times the bereaved tries to avoid the pain of grief and at other times confronts it. The goal is to achieve a balance between avoidance and confrontation that facilitates coming to terms with the loss. Attaining this goal can be seen as an oscillation between what Margaret Stroebe and Henk Schut call *loss-oriented* and *restoration-oriented* mourning. From this perspective, looking at old photographs and yearning for the deceased are examples of loss-oriented coping, whereas doing what is needed to reorganize life in the wake of the loss—for example, learning to do tasks that the deceased had always managed, such as finances—is part of restoration-oriented coping.

As time goes on, the acute pain and emotional turmoil of grief begin to subside. Physical and mental balance are reestablished. The bereaved person becomes increasingly reintegrated into his or her social world. Sadness doesn't go away completely, but it recedes into the background much of the time. Although reminders of the loss stimulate waves of active grieving from time to time, the main focus is the present, not the past. Adjusting to loss may sometimes feel like a betrayal of the deceased loved one, but it is healthy to engage again in ongoing life and the future (see the Take Charge box).

Social support for the bereaved is as critical during the later course of grief as it is during the first days after a loss. In offering support, we can reassure the grieving person that grief is normal, permissible, and appropriate. The first anniversary and major holidays following a significant loss can be times of renewed grieving when the support of others is important and appreciated. Knowing that others remember the loss and that they take time to connect is usually perceived as comforting.

Bereaved people may find it helpful to share their stories and concerns through organized support groups. Many hospitals and organizations offer bereavement support groups and counselling. Many online and in-person support groups are organized around specific types of bereavement. The Compassionate Friends of Canada, for example, is a nationwide organization composed of parents who have experienced a child's death. This organization provides both local and online support groups. The Canadian Association for Suicide Prevention has an online directory of suicide survivor support centres across the country. Losing a loved one to suicide is an especially traumatic loss that is often best understood by others who have had a similar loss. Suicide support groups are available in most communities. If you have lost a loved one to drugs or alcohol, GRASP (Grief Recovery After Substance Passing) has support groups available in some Canadian communities as well as online support. (See the end of this chapter for web addresses for these groups.)

Supporting a Grieving Person

When a person finds out that a loved one has died, the initial reaction may be profound shock and overwhelming distress. Such a person may initially respond best to the physical comfort of hugging and holding. Later, simply listening may be the most effective way to help. Talking about a loss is an important way that many survivors cope with the changed reality, and they may need to tell their story over and over. The key to being a good listener is to avoid speaking too much and to refrain from making judgments about whether the thoughts and feelings expressed by a survivor are right or wrong, good, or bad. The emotions, thoughts, and

Take **CHARGE**

Coping with Grief

- Recognize and acknowledge your loss.
- React to grief in the way that feels most natural to you. There is no "right" way to grieve.
- Take time for nature's process of healing. The odds are good that you will be functioning well again before long. Be patient with yourself.
- Know that powerful, overwhelming feelings will change with time. Grief is often experienced as a long series of ups and downs, with the intensity of feelings gradually decreasing over time.
- Beware of the lure of drugs and alcohol to reduce the pain of your grief, especially if you have had substance abuse issues in the past. Using alcohol or drugs to numb yourself will ultimately backfire and make your recovery more difficult.
- Honour your loved one in a way that is meaningful to you. Consider creating a small memorial with a photo and flowers, start a scholarship in your loved one's name, plant a memorial tree, or write a song or poem in his or her honour.
- Consider joining a bereavement support group to connect with others who have also had recent losses.
- Surround yourself with life: plants, animals, friends, and family.
- If you are having difficulty functioning at school, work, or home after a few weeks, consider counselling or a support group.
- People who have had a recent loss are at higher risk for suicide. If you are having thoughts of suicide or are feeling hopeless, seek help right away.
- Care for yourself by finding time to eat, sleep, and move your body.
- Don't be afraid to let laughter and joy remain in your life. Experiencing positive feelings during mourning does not indicate a lack of respect or love for the deceased.

Sources: The Centre for Living with Dying (554 Mansion Park Dr., Santa, Clara, CA 95054; 408-980-9801); Rando, T. A. 1993. *The Treatment of Complicated Mourning*. Champaign, Ill.: Research Press.

behaviours evoked by loss may not be the ones we expect, but they can nonetheless be valid and appropriate within a survivor's experience of loss.

If a grieving friend or relative talks about suicide, or seems in danger of causing harm to him or herself or others, seek professional help right away. Most people are resilient and cope well with loss, but keep in mind that the recent loss of a loved one is a major risk factor for suicide and self-harm. Be alert to signs that a grieving person is in serious danger.

While some people respond to loss with a feeling of helplessness, other people may react by taking charge. Making arrangements, taking care of tasks, and generally keeping busy may help them cope. Be aware that some people do not find it helpful to dwell on their feelings or talk a lot about their loss. Find out what *they* want to do—when the time is right, take a walk, go shopping together, go to a ball game, or see a movie. Your companionship while doing everyday activities may be the best gift you can give. Remember also that some grieving people may not appear sad or distressed. This does not mean that they didn't care about the deceased, are "in denial," or have a cold personality. Accept that this is their way of coping with loss and show your support with your loving presence.

When a Young Adult Loses a Friend

Among young people (under the age of 25) in Canada, the three leading causes of death tend to be sudden and unexpected: unintentional injuries, suicide, and cancer. Losing a close friend to an unexpected death can be particularly traumatic. There is usually an outpouring of sympathy and support toward the family of the deceased, but as a friend, you may feel left out and unsupported. Also, it is common to blame yourself in some way for your friend's death or feel that you should have somehow prevented the tragedy. If you lose a friend, be sure to look for support from friends, family, clergy, or health professionals, especially if the intense sadness or guilt feelings last for more than a few days or weeks. Friends can often help each other by working together to create their own way of celebrating the life of their lost friend.

Helping Children Cope with Loss

Children tend to cope with loss in a healthier fashion when they are included as part of their family's experience of grief and mourning. Although adults may be uncomfortable about sharing potentially disturbing or painful news with children, a child's natural curiosity usually negates the option of withholding information. Sudden changes in family communication patterns without any explanation can alarm a child and create anxiety. When children are asked about their experiences of family crises involving death, many say that the most difficult times occurred when they did not know what was happening. Mounting evidence shows that it is best to include children from the beginning—as soon as a terminal prognosis is made, for example—to help them understand what is happening. Children should spend time with the dying person, if possible, to learn, share, and offer and receive comfort. Such visits can be made under the guidance of a mental health professional, working with the child's best interests in mind, if deemed appropriate.

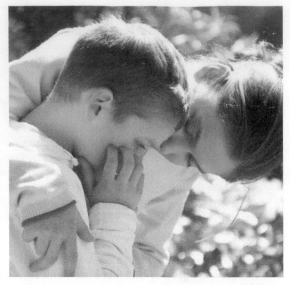

Children are better able to cope with loss when they are included in their family's experience of grief and mourning.

In talking about death with children, the most important guideline is to be honest. Set the explanation you are offering at the child's level of understanding. In general, it's advisable to keep the explanation simple, stick to basics, and verify what the child has understood from your explanation. A child's readiness for more details can usually be assessed by paying attention to his or her questions.

QUESTIONS FOR CRITICAL THINKING AND REFLECTION

Have you ever been in the position of being supportive to a bereaved person? What kind of support did he or she seem to appreciate most? Why do you think that was the case? How did the experience affect you?

Coming to Terms with Death

Although we may wish we could keep death out of view and not make a place for it in our lives, this wish cannot be fulfilled. With the death of a beloved friend or relative, we are confronted with emotions and thoughts that relate not only to the immediate loss, but also to our own mortality. Our encounters with dying and death teach us that relationships are more important than things and that life offers no guarantees. In discovering the meaning of death in our own lives, we find that life is both precious and precarious.

Allowing ourselves to make room for death, we discover that it touches not only the dying or bereaved person and his or her family and friends, but also the wider community of which we are all part. We recognize that dying and death offer opportunities for extraordinary growth in the midst of loss. Denying death, it turns out, results in denying life.

SUMMARY

- Although death makes rational sense in terms of species survival and evolution, there may be no completely satisfying answer to the question of why death exists from a personal point of view.

- Dying and death are more than biological events; they have social and spiritual dimensions.
- The traditional criteria for determining death focus on vital signs such as breathing and heartbeat. Brain death is characterized by a lack of physical responses other than breathing and heartbeat, with absence of brain activity as signified by a flat electroencephalogram (EEG).
- Between ages 6 and 9, most children develop a mature understanding of death; that is, they come to understand death as final, universal, and inevitable.
- A mature understanding of death can include ideas about the survival of the human personality or soul after death. Problems arise when avoidance or denial of death fosters the notion that it happens only to others.
- A will is a legal instrument that governs the distribution of a person's estate after death.
- End-of-life care may involve a combination of home care, hospital stays, and hospice or palliative care.
- Palliative care is devoted to making dying patients comfortable by controlling pain and relieving suffering.
- Hospice programs apply a team-oriented approach to caring for dying patients and their families with the goal of helping people live as fully as possible until the end of their lives.
- Exercising choices about end-of-life care can involve making decisions about attempting to prolong life or choosing to allow natural death with comfort care.
- The practice of withholding or withdrawing potentially life-sustaining treatment is sometimes termed passive euthanasia.
- Physician-assisted death occurs when a physician provides lethal drugs or other interventions, at a patient's request, with the understanding that the patient plans to use them to end his or her life. Voluntary active euthanasia refers to the intentional ending of a patient's life, at his or her request, by someone other than the patient.
- Advance directives, such as living wills and health care proxies, are used to express one's wishes about the use of life-sustaining treatment and how they wish to be treated if they cannot speak for themselves.
- People can donate their bodies or specific organs for transplantation and other medical uses after death. People of all ages can donate their organs and need to let their families know if they wish to be organ donors.
- For Canadians, the decision about what to do with the body after death usually involves either burial or cremation.
- Bereaved people usually benefit from participating in a funeral or other type of memorial service to commemorate a loved one's death.
- Coping with dying involves physical, psychological, social, and spiritual dimensions.
- It is useful for patients and caregivers to understand the trajectory, or course, of dying.
- In offering support to a dying person, the gift of listening can be especially important.
- Grief encompasses thoughts and feelings, as well as physical and behavioural responses.
- Mourning, the process by which a person integrates a loss into his or her life, is determined partly by social and cultural norms for expressing grief.
- Children tend to cope with death in a healthier fashion when they are included in their family's experience of grief and mourning.
- Dying and death offer opportunities for growth in the midst of loss.

FOR MORE INFORMATION

BOOKS

Albom, M. 2005. *Tuesdays with Morrie: An Old Man, A Young Man, and Life's Greatest Lesson.* New York: Anchor. A young man reconnects with an old professor in his last months of life and learns some of the greatest lessons that life has to offer.

Bonanno, G. A. 2009. *The Other Side of Sadness: What the New Science of Bereavement Tells Us about Life after Loss.* New York: Basic Books. Explains modern thinking about grief and resilience, with many vignettes. Very readable and encouraging—highly recommended for anyone who has experienced a recent loss.

DeSpelder, L. A., and A. L. Strickland. 2011. *The Last Dance: Encountering Death and Dying,* 9th ed. New York: McGraw-Hill. A comprehensive and readable text highlighting a broad range of topics related to dying and death.

Karnes, B. 1986, revised 2009. *Gone from My Sight: The Dying Experience.* Vancouver: BK Books. This booklet is distributed to the families of dying patients by many hospices across the country. Hospice workers refer to it simply as "the blue book." By explaining in simple, straightforward terms the process of dying, it is an invaluable resource in helping to alleviate a family's fears of the unknown.

Shannon, J. B. 2006. *Death and Dying Sourcebook,* 2nd ed. Detroit: Omnigraphics. A wide-ranging discussion of topics relating to terminal illness, care for the dying, and the practical realities of death.

Turner, M. 2006. *Talking with Children and Young People about Death and Dying,* 2nd ed. London: Jessica Kingsley Publishers. A workbook designed to help parents explain death, loss, and grief to their children.

ORGANIZATIONS, HOTLINES, AND WEBSITES

The Internet addresses listed here were accurate at the time of publication.

Canadian Virtual Hospice. Provides information and support on palliative and end-of-life care, loss, and grief.
   http://www.virtualhospice.ca

The Canadian Association for Suicide Prevention (CASP). Provides information and help for people who have lost loved ones to suicide. Contains a variety of resources, including a map of support centres across the country.
   http://suicideprevention.ca/

The Compassionate Friends of Canada. Provides grief support after the death of a child, including local chapters and online support groups.
   http://tcfcanada.net/

The Dougy Center. Offers education about childhood bereavement and support groups for bereaved children.
   http://www.dougy.org

GriefNet. Provides an opportunity to communicate with others via email support groups in the areas of death, grief, and major loss.
   http://www.griefnet.org

Grief Recovery After a Substance Passing (GRASP). Provides support for friends and family of people who have died as a result of substance use. Includes information about Canadian and online support groups.
   http://grasphelp.org/

Growth House. Offers an extensive directory of Internet resources relating to life-threatening illness and end-of-life care.
   http://www.growthhouse.org

Natural Burial Association. Provides information about increasing awareness about the environmental benefits of natural burials and how to facilitate the creation of natural burial grounds.
   http://www.naturalburialassoc.ca/

The following organizations provide information about organ donation in Canada, as well as provincial or territorial information pertaining to organ donor requirements and registries.

Beadonor.ca
   https://beadonor.ca

Canadian Blood Services
   https://blood.ca/en/organs-tissues

Canadian Society of Transplantation
http://www.cst-transplant.ca

Canadian Transplant Association
http://organ-donation-works.org

The Kidney Foundation of Canada
http://www.kidney.ca

SELECTED BIBLIOGRAPHY

Angus Reid Institute. 2015. *Three-quarters of Canadians don't completely dismiss the possibility of life after death,* http://angusreid.org/wp-content/uploads/2015/01/2015.01.28-ARI-Life-after-death.pdf (retrieved July 21, 2015).

Baxter, D., and J. Smerdon. 2000. *Donation Matters: Demographics and Organ Transplants in Canada, 2000–2040.* Vancouver: The Urban Futures Institute, http://www.lhsc.on.ca/Patients_Families_Visitors/MOTP/Organ_and_Tissue_Donation/Report46.pdf (retrieved July 22, 2015).

Bender, E. 2005. Palliative care. *Journal of the American Medical Association* 294(14): 1850.

Bonanno, G.A. 2009. *The Other Side of Sadness: What the New Science of Bereavement Tells Us about Life after Loss.* New York: Basic Books.

Canada's Office of Consumer Affairs. nd. *Canadian Consumer Handbook: Funerals.* Ottawa: Industry Canada, http://www.consumerhandbook.ca/en/topics/products-and-services/funerals#information (retrieved July 20, 2015).

Canadian Institute for Health Information. 2007. *Health Care Use at the End of Life in Western Canada.* Ottawa: CIHI.

Canadian Institute for Health Information. 2014. *Organ transplants on the rise,* https://www.cihi.ca/en/types-of-care/specialized-services/organ-replacements/organ-transplants-on-the-rise (retrieved July 22, 2015).

Canadian Medical Association. 2014. *Euthanasia and assisted death (Update 2014)* https://www.cma.ca/Assets/assets-library/document/en/advocacy/EOL/CMA_Policy_Euthanasia_Assistedpercent 20Death_PD15-02-e.pdf (retrieved July 22, 2015).

Canadian Organ Replacement Register. 2013. Canadian Institute for Health Information, https://www.cihi.ca/en/corr_public_summary_2014_en.pdf (retrieved July 22, 2015).

Canadian Press/Leger Marketing. 2001. *How Canadians View Paranormal Phenomena in This Halloween Season: Report,* http://www.legermarketing.com/documents/SPCLM/011022ENG.pdf (retrieved June 14, 2010).

Canadian Press/Leger Marketing. 2002. *Canadians and Death: Report,* http://www.legermarketing.com/documents/spclm/030113eng.pdf (retrieved June 14, 2010).

Canadian Transplant Society. 2014. *Canadian Transplant Society,* http://www.cantransplant.ca/home/ (retrieved July 22, 2015).

Casarett, D., et al. 2005. Making difficult decisions about hospice enrollment: What do patients and families want to know? *Journal of the American Geriatrics Society* 53(2): 249–254.

CBC News. 2012. *The fight for the right to die,* http://www.cbc.ca/news/canada/the-fight-for-the-right-to-die-1.1130837 (retrieved on July 22, 2015).

Chochinov, H. M. 2006. Dying, dignity, and new horizons in palliative end-of-life care. *CA: A Cancer Journal for Clinicians* 56(2): 84–103.

Christ, G. H., and A. E. Christ. 2006. Current approaches to helping children cope with a parent's terminal illness. *CA: A Cancer Journal for Clinicians* 56(4): 197–212.

Collier, R. 2009. Euthanasia debate reignited. *Canadian Medical Association Journal* 181(8): 463–464, http://www.cmaj.ca/content/181/8/463.full (retrieved July 22, 2015).

Corr, C. A., et al. 2008. *Death and Dying: Life and Living.* Florence, KY: Wadsworth Publishing.

Death with Dignity National Center. 2012. *Death with Dignity around the U.S.*, http://www.deathwith dignity.org/advocates/national/.

Doka, K. J., and A. S. Tucci (ed.). 2011. *Beyond Kubler-Ross: New Perspectives on Death, Dying and Grief.* Washington, DC: Hospice Foundation of America.

Donatelli, L. A., et al. 2006. Ethical issues in critical care and cardiac arrest: Clinical research, brain death, and organ donation. *Seminars in Neurology* 26(4): 452–459.

DuBois, J. M., and E. E. Anderson. 2006. Attitudes toward death criteria and organ donation among healthcare personnel and the general public. *Progress in Transplantation* 16(1): 65–73.

Field, N. P. 2006. Unresolved grief and continuing bonds: An attachment perspective. *Death Studies* 30(8): 739–756.

Galante, J. M., et al. 2005. Experience and attitudes of surgeons toward palliation in cancer. *Archives of Surgery* 140(9): 873–878.

Government of Canada. 2015. *Blood, organ and tissue donation*, http://healthycanadians.gc.ca/diseases-conditions-maladies-affections/donation-contribution-eng.php (retrieved July 21, 2015).

Gozalo, P. L., and S. C. Miller. 2006. Hospice enrollment and evaluation of its causal effect on hospitalization of dying nursing home patients. *Health Services Research,* 17 August [online early ed.].

Green Burial Council. 2012. *FAQs and Fictions*, http://www.greenburialcouncil.org/.

Harvard Medical School. 2005. Living wills and health care proxies. *Harvard Health Letter* 30(8): 1–3.

Health Law Institute, Dalhousie University. 2009. *Advance Directives*, http://eol.law.dal.ca/?page_id=231 (retrieved July 22, 2015).

Health Law Institute, Dalhousie University. 2009. *Withholding and Withdrawal of Potentially Life-Sustaining Treatment*, http://eol.law.dal.ca/?page_id=366 (retrieved July 23, 2015).

Ipsos Reid. 2006. *Canadians Willing to Donate Their Organs in the Case of Their Death*, http://www.marketwired.com/press-release/canadians-willing-to-donate-their-organs-in-the-case-of-their-death-603162.htm (retrieved July 23, 2015).

Jansen-van der Weide, M. C., et al. 2005. Granted, undecided, withdrawn, and refused requests for euthanasia and physician-assisted suicide. *Archives of Internal Medicine* 165(15): 1698–1704.

Kohara, H., et al. 2005. Sedation for terminally ill patients with cancer with uncontrollable physical distress. *Journal of Palliative Medicine* 8(1): 20–25.

Konigsberg, R. D. 2011. *The Truth about Grief.* New York: Simon and Schuster.

Lawyers' Professional Indemnity Company/Assurance LawPRO. 2012. *Survey: More than half of Canadians do not have a signed will*, https://www.lawpro.ca/news/pdf/Wills-POAsurvey.pdf (retrieved July 21, 2015).

Lipkin, K. M. 2006. Identifying a proxy for health care as part of routine medical inquiry. *Journal of General Internal Medicine,* 17 July [online early ed.].

Mayo Clinic. 2005. Advance directives: A plan for end of life. *Mayo Clinic Health Letter* 23(2): 6.

Melhem, N. M., et al. 2004. Traumatic grief among adolescents exposed to a peer's suicide. *American Journal of Psychiatry* 161(8): 1411–1416.

Mostofsky, E., et al. 2012. Risk of acute myocardial infarction after the death of a significant person in one's life. *Circulation: Journal of the American Heart Association* 125: 491–496.

Natural Burial Association. 2013. *How it works*, http://www.naturalburialassoc.ca/how-it-works/ (retrieved July 23, 2015).

Onrust, S., et al. 2006. Predictors of psychological adjustment after bereavement. *International Psychogeriatrics,* 14 September, 1–15.

Oregon Health Authority. 2012. *Frequently Asked Questions about the Death with Dignity Act*, http://public.health.oregon.gov/ProviderPartnerResources/EvaluationResearch/DeathwithDignityAct/Pages/faqs.aspx#whatis (retrieved July 23, 2015).

Oregon Public Health Division. 2012. *Death with Dignity Act 2010,* http://public.health.oregon.gov/ProviderPartnerResources/EvaluationResearch/DeathwithDignityAct/Pages/index.aspx (retrieved July 23, 2015).

Organ transplants. 2004. *Mayo Clinic Health Letter Supplement,* October.

Owen, A. M., et al. 2006. Detecting awareness in the vegetative state. *Science* 313(5792): 1402.

Picard, A. 2015. *Canadians deserve stronger response on assisted death.* The Globe and Mail, July 20, 2015, http://www.theglobeandmail.com/globe-debate/we-dont-need-an-outside-panel-to-assess-right-to-die-law/article25594885/ (retrieved July 23, 2015).

Pivar, I. L., and N. P. Field. 2004. Unresolved grief in combat veterans with PTSD. *Journal of Anxiety Disorders* 18(6): 745–755.

Rietjens, J. A., et al. 2006. Terminal sedation and euthanasia: A comparison of clinical practices. *Archives of Internal Medicine* 166(7): 749–753.

Satel, S. 2006. Death's waiting list. *New York Times,* 15 May.

Schulz, R., et al. 2006. Predictors of complicated grief among dementia caregivers: A prospective study of bereavement. *American Journal of Geriatric Psychiatry* 14(8): 650–658.

Searight, H. R., and J. Gafford. 2005. Cultural diversity at the end of life: Issues and guidelines for family physicians. *American Family Physician* 71(3): 515–522.

Sepúlveda, C. et al. 2002. Palliative care: The World Health Organization's global perspective. *Journal of Pain and Symptom Management* 24(2): 91–96, http://www.ncbi.nlm.nih.gov/pubmed/12231124 (retrieved July 22, 2015).

Shemie, S. D., et al. 2006. Brain arrest: The neurological determination of death and organ donor management in Canada. *Canadian Medical Association Journal* 174(6): S1–S12, http://www.cmaj.ca/content/174/6/S1.full (retrieved July 21, 2015).

Siminoff, L. A., et al. 2006. Racial disparities in preferences and perceptions regarding organ donation. *Journal of General Internal Medicine* 21(9): 995–1000.

Statistics Canada. 2013. *CANSIM Table 102-050: Deaths in hospital and elsewhere, Canada, provinces and territories,* http://www5.statcan.gc.ca/cansim/a26?lang=eng&id=1020509 (retrieved July 21, 2015).

Statistics Canada. 2014. *Study: End-of-life care, 2012,* http://www.statcan.gc.ca/daily-quotidien/141003/dq141003c-eng.htm (retrieved July 21, 2015).

Statistics Canada. 2014. *The 10 leading causes of death, 2011,* http://www.statcan.gc.ca/pub/82-625-x/2014001/article/11896-eng.htm (retrieved July 23, 2015).

Steinhauser, K. E., et al. 2000. In search of a good death: patients, families and providers. *Annals of Internal Medicine* 132(10): 825–832.

Stroebe, M., et al. 2007. Health outcomes of bereavement. *The Lancet* 370(9603): 1960–1973.

Supreme Court of Canada. 2012. *Docket: 35591. Lee Carter, et al. v. Attorney General of Canada, et al.,* http://www.scc-csc.gc.ca/case-dossier/info/dock-regi-eng.aspx?cas=35591 (retrieved July 23, 2015).

Supreme Court of Canada. 2015. *Supreme Court Judgements: Carter v. Canada (Attorney General),* http://scc-csc.lexum.com/scc-csc/scc-csc/en/item/14637/index.do (retrieved July 22, 2015).

United Network for Organ Sharing. 2012. *Fact Sheets,* http://www.unos.org/donation/index.php?topic=fact_sheets (retrieved July 23, 2015).

University of Toronto Joint Centre for Bioethics. *Living Will,* http://www.jcb.utoronto.ca/tools/documents/jcb_livingwill.pdf (retrieved July 23, 2015).

Wijdicks, E. F., et al. 2006. Practice parameter: Prediction of outcome in comatose survivors after cardiopulmonary resuscitation (an evidence-based review): Report of the Quality Standards Subcommittee of the American Academy of Neurology. *Neurology* 67(2): 203–210.

Wilson, D. M., et al. 2009. The rapidly changing location of death in Canada, 1994–2004. *Social Science and Medicine* 68: 1752–1758.

CHAPTER 19

Conventional and Complementary Medicine

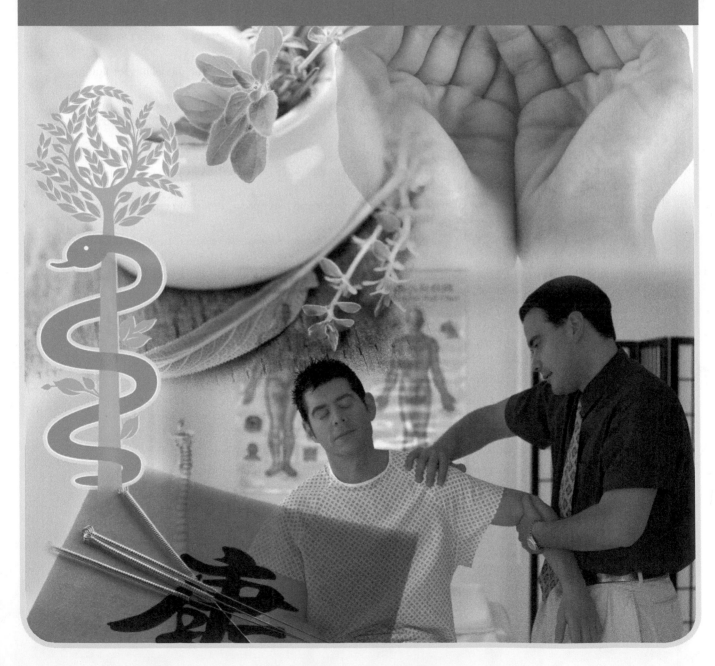

LOOKING AHEAD

After you have read and studied this chapter, you should be able to:

LO1 Explain the different forms of evidence and the meaning of evidence-based health-care decision making

LO2 Describe the basic premises, practices, and providers of conventional medicine

LO3 Describe the basic premises, practices, and providers of complementary and alternative medicine

LO4 Explain how to communicate effectively with health-care providers and to use their input when evaluating different types of treatment

TEST YOUR KNOWLEDGE

1. **The people most likely to use complementary and alternative medicine are those without a conventional primary care physician.**
   True or false?

2. **Which practices or interests are shared by both conventional Western medicine and complementary and alternative medicine?**
   a. careful observation of symptoms
   b. treatment with remedies derived from plants
   c. concern with the patient-physician relationship

3. **The sale and use of herbal remedies and dietary supplements, such as ginkgo biloba and St. John's wort, are not well regulated in Canada.**
   True or false?

4. **Generic drugs are generally less effective than brand-name drugs.**
   True or false?

ANSWERS

1. FALSE.   The more often a person visits a conventional primary care physician, the more likely he or she is to use complementary and alternative medicine.

2. ALL THREE.   Although profound philosophical differences exist between the approaches, they share many characteristics.

3. FALSE.   Under Health Canada's Natural Health Products Regulations, all natural health products require a product licence before they can be sold. Once a product has been assessed and granted market authorization by Health Canada, the product label must have an eight-digit product licence number preceded by the letters NPN (Natural Product Number) or, in the case of a homeopathic medicine, by the letters DIN-HM (Drug Identification Number-Homeopathic Medicine).

4. FALSE.   Price is often the only difference. The generic version of a drug has the same active ingredient as the brand-name drug, but it may have different inactive ingredients.

Today, Canadians as a whole are becoming more empowered and confident in their ability to solve personal health problems on their own. People who manage their own health care gather information and learn skills from a variety of resources; they solicit opinions and advice, make decisions, and take action. They know how to practise safe, effective self-care, and they know how to make decisions about professional medical care, whether conventional Western medicine or complementary and alternative medicine or both. The key to good decision making is using the best evidence to help you choose which actions to take regarding your health care. As the terms *complementary* and *alternative* imply, these forms of medicine can be used as complements or alternatives to conventional medicine.

This chapter will provide basic information for you to consider when making decisions about using the conventional health-care system together with complementary and alternative health-care options.

Self-Care

Effectively managing health and medical problems involves developing several skills. First, you need to learn to be a good observer of your own body and assess your symptoms. You also must be able to decide when to seek professional advice and when you can safely deal with the problem on your own. You need to know how to self-treat common medical problems safely and effectively. Finally, you need to know how to develop a partnership with physicians and other health-care providers and how to carry out treatment plans.

Self-Assessment

Symptoms are often an expression of the body's attempt to heal itself. For example, the pain and swelling that occur after an ankle injury immobilize the injured joint to allow healing to take place. A fever may be an attempt to make the body less hospitable to infectious agents. A cough can help clear the airways and protect the lungs. Understanding what a symptom means and what is going on in your body helps reduce anxiety about symptoms and enables you to practise safe self-care that supports your body's own healing mechanisms.

Carefully observing symptoms also lets you identify those signals that suggest you need professional assistance. You should begin by noting when the symptom began, how often and when it occurs, what makes it worse, what makes it better, and whether you have any associated symptoms. You can also monitor your body's vital signs, such as temperature and heart rate. Medical self-tests for blood pressure, blood sugar, pregnancy detection, and urinary tract infections can also help you make a more informed decision about when to seek medical help and when to self-treat.

QUICK STATS

The top three reasons in 2012–2013 for visiting an emergency department were abdominal/pelvic pain, pain in throat and chest, and acute upper respiratory infection. 9 out of 10 visits for these conditions lasted 8.8, 8.9, and 3.9 hours or less, respectively.

—Canadian Institute for Health Information, 2014

Health Literacy and Evidence-Based Decision Making for Canadians

The *Canadian Public Health Association* defines health literacy as the "skills to enable access, understanding and use of information for health." Making healthy lifestyle choices, finding and interpreting health information, as well as locating proper health services are important decision-making skills for all Canadians. The ability to process document and online information—both text and numbers—has become imperative along with the mass of data publically available on the Internet, through social media, and from a variety of other sources, some of which are, at best, questionable in their authenticity and reliability.

In terms of health literacy, the three most vulnerable populations are seniors, immigrants, and the unemployed. Very likely, the risks for these groups are related either to lack of access to trustworthy information and/or an inability to understand and use that information. Even if you are not part of one of these vulnerable groups, improving health literacy can enhance the quality of life for many Canadians; in turn, such learning could result in significant cost savings for an already heavily-burdened health-care system.

In exploring and becoming knowledgeable about conventional and complementary medicine, part of the issue of health literacy is related to making evidence-based decisions. Evidence-based medicine is a concept generally characterized as using the best currently available research evidence, combined with clinical judgment and experience, to make a medical or health decision. Figure 19.1 shows the intersections of clinical expertise, best evidence, and patient or health consumer values and expectations, which are important for understanding how the public and health-care professionals can work together in making evidence-based decisions. Notice, for example, that all three circles are of the same size; that is, evidence-based decision making is not merely formulaic or objective and/or based merely on research or clinical expertise; people's values and beliefs are a vital part of this process.

Part of the issue in making evidence-based decisions is understanding different kinds of evidence.

FIGURE 19.1

The Evidence-based Medicine Triad

The definition of evidence-based medicine is a systematic approach to clinical problem solving that allows the integration of the best available research evidence with clinical expertise and patient values.

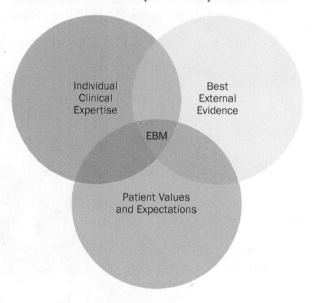

There are literally millions of articles pertaining to research about different health issues; health consumers are able to access these articles from databases (discussed below). Part of health literacy is learning how to interpret the nature and levels of evidence used in health research. In general, the "gold standard" of evidence is equated with what is called the experimental or scientific method. This method uses and relies on experiments that assign subjects (animal and/or human) randomly to an intervention group (to test, for example, a new drug) or to a control group (which usually does not receive the new drug). In the most highly regarded studies, the researchers don't know which group received the intervention and the subjects don't know whether or not they received the drug or the placebo (a harmless drug); in study design terms, this is called "double-blind." Thus, a study that is experimentally randomized, double-blind, and controlled (often abbreviated to RCT study) means that the researchers try in every way possible to be able to come to an objective conclusion about the intervention being studied.

If there are enough subjects in such studies, researchers are able to make statistically strong conclusions about the effectiveness of the intervention in order to provide the best evidence for decision making regarding the use of the new drug. For instance, in an RCT testing a new drug, researchers might be able to conclude statistically that the drug would be effective 95 times out of 100 uses, or, even better, 99 times out of 100, thereby achieving statistical significance. Typically, the primary source of RCTs are published in peer-reviewed (meaning the studies were approved by a panel of experts) science and/or medical journals.

For many practitioners and clinicians in the health-care system, this gold standard type of confirmation is perceived as the bottom line in evidence-based decision making regarding health and medicine. The difficulty is that not all health-care interventions can be subjected to such rigorous scrutiny as the experimental method. One way to think about the nature of evidence is in hierarchical terms, as shown in Figure 19.2. That is, there are various levels of evidence, and understanding these levels is vital in making informed, literate decisions about health care in daily living. At the top of this pyramid are randomized controlled trials (RCTs) as well as systematic reviews; the latter are also known as meta-analyses or interpretations of the best RCTs for any given intervention. One tier down the pyramid from RCTs are cohort studies where two groups or cohorts—say smokers in one cohort and non-smokers in another cohort—are followed over time regarding identified health parameters, and at some point the two groups are evaluated for their health status. There is no form of control as there is in RCTs, and it's difficult to relate all health changes to the impact of smoking.

FIGURE 19.2

Hierarchy of Evidence Pyramid

There are various levels of evidence, and understanding these levels is vital in making informed, literate decisions about health care in daily living. The quality of evidence increases as you go higher in the pyramid.

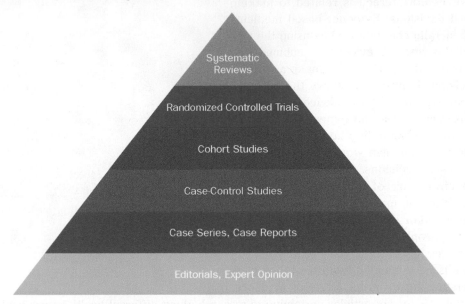

In case control studies, researchers take two groups, for example a group of breast cancer patients and a comparison group of people (same age, gender, ethnicity, etc.) without breast cancer, and examine and analyze their health histories, make comparisons among the groups and cases, and draw conclusions based on this cross-case/group analysis. Case series or case report studies are ones where a researcher or clinician uses individual cases or collections of medical or health-issue reports on the treatment of an individual patient or a number of reports on patients with a similar health issue. Important—sometimes critical—information can be gained from case control, case series, and case report studies that can help guide both clinicians and health-care consumers in making evidence-based decisions based upon similar histories or cases or health issues.

Finally, consumers are bombarded in all forms of media with testimonials, editorials, and other forms of "expert" opinion on health issues, practices, health substances, and health behaviours. Such information may or may not be evidence; it depends on the source of the expertise that is being delivered. For example, "Dr. Mom" is or can be a trusted source for many families because moms might be assumed to be well informed about daily health care, while unsubstantiated claims from questionable providers where the source of expertise is not available are not valid resources for evidence-based decision making. In the same vein, health consumers need to be aware that media outlets, Internet sources, and other public domains may represent second-hand opinions or interpretations of different forms of evidence. (See the Critical Consumer box.)

One of the best single resources for evidence-based decision making for health is the Cochrane Consumer Network (http://consumers.cochrane.org/). This valuable online resource assesses the effects of health-care treatments to provide consumers with information on the risks and benefits of those treatments at a population level. The network is a strong reflector of evidence-based healthcare. It underscores the fact that people differ in their preferences and values, and therefore individuals might make entirely different treatment or health-care choices based upon the same evidence. The network is careful to point out that it does subscribe to the hierarchy of evidence, where expert reports are accorded low quality of evidence status while systematic reviews are deemed to provide the highest evidence.

Critical CONSUMER

Evaluating Health News

Health-related research is now described in popular newspapers and magazines rather than just in medical journals, meaning that more and more people have access to the information. Greater access is certainly a plus, but news reports of research studies may oversimplify or exaggerate both the results and what those results mean to the average person. Researchers do not set out to mislead people, but they must often strike a balance between reporting promising preliminary findings to the public, thereby allowing people to act on them, and waiting 10–20 years until long-term studies confirm (or disprove) a particular finding.

All this can leave you in a difficult position. You cannot become an expert on all subjects, capable of effectively evaluating all the available health news. However, the following questions can help you better assess the health advice that appears in the popular media:

1. *Is the report based on research or on an anecdote?* Information or advice based on one or more carefully designed research studies has more validity than one person's experiences.

2. *What is the source of the information?* A study published in a respected peer-reviewed journal has been examined by editors and other researchers in the field, people who are in a position to evaluate the merits of a study and its results. Many journal articles also include information on the authors and funders of research, alerting readers to any possible conflicts of interest. Research presented at medical meetings should be considered very preliminary because the results have not yet undergone a thorough prepublication review; many such studies are never published. It is also wise to ask who funded a study to determine whether any potential for bias exists. Information from government agencies (Health Canada and provincial or territorial government agencies) and national research organizations (such as Ipsos-Reid) are usually considered fairly reliable.

3. *How big was the study?* A study involving many subjects is more likely to yield reliable results than a study involving only a few subjects. Another important indication that a finding is meaningful is having several other studies yield the same results.

4. *Who were the participants involved in the study?* Research findings are more likely to apply to you if you share important characteristics with the participants in the study. For example, the results of a study on men over age 50 who smoke may not be particularly meaningful for a 30-year-old non-smoking woman. Even less applicable are studies done in test tubes or on animals. Such research should be considered very preliminary in terms of its applicability to humans. Promising results from laboratory or animal research frequently cannot be replicated in human study subjects.

5. *What kind of study was it?* Epidemiological studies (which deal with the study of the causes, distribution, and control of disease in populations) use observation or interviews to trace the relationships among lifestyle, physical characteristics, and diseases. Although epidemiological studies can suggest links, they cannot establish cause-and-effect relationships. Clinical or interventional studies or trials involve testing the effects of different treatments on groups of people who have similar lifestyles and characteristics. They are more likely to provide conclusive evidence of a cause-and-effect relationship. The best interventional studies share the following characteristics:

   - *Controlled:* A group of people who receive the treatment is compared with a matched group of people (called a *control group*) who do not receive the treatment. The matched control group may receive an inert placebo or an established active treatment.
   - *Randomized:* The treatment and control groups are selected randomly.
   - *Double-blind:* Researchers and participants are unaware of who is receiving the treatment.
   - *Multicentre:* The experiment is performed at more than one institution.

   A third type of study, a systematic- or meta-analysis, involves combining the results of individual studies to get an overall view of the effectiveness of a treatment.

6. *What do the statistics really say?* First, are the results described as statistically significant? If a study is large and well designed, its results can be deemed statistically significant, meaning there is less than a 5 percent chance that the findings resulted from chance. Second, are the results stated in terms of relative or absolute risk? Many findings are reported in terms of relative risk—how a particular treatment or condition affects a person's disease risk. Consider the following examples of relative risk:

   - According to some estimates, taking estrogen without progesterone can increase a post-menopausal woman's risk of dying from endometrial cancer by 233 percent.
   - Giving AZT to HIV-infected pregnant women reduces prenatal transmission of HIV by about 90 percent.

The first of these findings seems far more dramatic than the second—until you also consider absolute risk, the actual risk of the illness in the population being considered. The absolute risk of endometrial cancer is 0.3 percent; a 233 percent increase based on the effects of estrogen raises it to 1 percent, a change of 0.7 percent. Without treatment, about 25 percent of infants born to HIV-infected women will be infected with HIV; with treatment, the absolute risk drops to about 2 percent, a change of 23 percent. Because the absolute risk of an HIV-infected mother passing the virus to her infant (25 percent) is so much greater than a woman's risk of developing endometrial cancer (0.3 percent), a smaller change in relative risk translates into a much greater change in absolute risk.

7. *Is new health advice being offered?* If the media report new guidelines for health behaviour or medical treatment, examine the source. Government agencies and national research foundations usually consider a great deal of evidence before offering health advice. Above all, use common sense, and check with your physician before making a major change in your health habits based on news reports.

The Cochrane Consumer Network is one example of what is called a database of research; this particular one is geared specifically to consumer use. For example, a person interested in finding out about the effectiveness of the use of Aspirin for different purposes can just search the site using the word Aspirin and the network provides pages of reviews and evidence-based research articles about Aspirin usage. The network provides both quantitatively-based studies—ones where statistical data or analyses are provided—as well as qualitative studies that include contextual information about behaviours, beliefs, opinions, emotions, social norms, and individual relationships relevant to a particular health concern or question. There are a wide variety of health-care databases, however for basic health information, the Cochrane Network is a great place to start. What will make the network even more important to consumers is its recent undertaking to provide "plain language reviews" that summarize scientific reviews in language that can be understood at a high school level of reading—another clear contribution to elevating health literacy.

Two other resources deserve mention from a Canadian health-care and health literacy perspective. One is the College of Family Physicians (CFPC), available at http://www.cfpc.ca/ForPatients/. This site provides helpful information and resources on common health issues such as weight control, sore throats, and overall patient education. All of the health or medical information is provided via family physician members of the college for reference and information, and there is no intent to replace advice or care from a health-care professional. The CFPC website is funded by the college and does not receive funding from advertising or from the display of commercial content.

Finally, it can be almost as important for health consumers to be literate about what procedures might be avoidable as it is to gather treatment information. Choosing Wisely Canada (CWC) is a nationwide, online campaign (http://www.choosingwiselycanada.org/about/what-is-cwc/) to help physicians and patients engage in conversations about unnecessary tests, treatments, and procedures, and to make smart and effective choices to ensure high-quality care. The CWC campaign has created plain-language and patient-friendly materials to help patients learn about the tests, treatments, or procedures of concern; when they might be necessary and when they might not; and what patients can do to improve their health in terms of these health concerns. Mirroring true evidence-based decision-making practices, doctors, health-care professionals, and the public are advised to use the Choosing Wisely Canada materials to determine an appropriate treatment plan together.

Self-Medication

Self-treatment with non-prescription medications is an important part of health care. One of the very disconcerting issues about medications prescribed in Canada is that our country is now the second-largest per capita consumer of prescription opioids (medications that relieve pain). Globally, North America consumes approximately 80 percent of the world's opioids. Non-prescription or **over-the-counter (OTC) medications** are medicines that Health Canada, through the Food and Drug Act and the Therapeutic Products Programme, has determined are safe for use without a physician's prescription. More than 100 000 OTC drugs are on the market; about 60 percent of all medications are sold over the counter. During any six-month period, about two-thirds of Canadians use one or more OTC drugs.

over-the-counter (OTC) medications
Medications or products that can be purchased by the consumer without a prescription.

Many OTC drugs are highly effective in relieving symptoms and sometimes in curing illnesses. In fact, many OTC drugs were formerly prescription drugs. More than 600 products sold over the counter today use ingredients or dosage strengths available only by prescription 20 years ago. However, with this increased consumer choice comes increased consumer responsibility for using OTC drugs safely. OTC drugs can be sold under a brand name, such as Tylenol, or in a generic form; generic drugs are the same as brand-name drugs in terms of quality, purity, effectiveness, and safety. Generic drugs have to meet the same Health Canada standards as their brand-name counterparts.

Consumers also need to be aware of the barrage of OTC drug advertising aimed at them. The implication of such advertising is that every symptom can and should be relieved by a drug. Although many OTC products are effective, others are unnecessary or divert attention from better ways of coping. Many ingredients in OTC drugs—perhaps 70 percent—have not been proven to be effective. And any drug has risks and side effects. The Drug Information and Research Centre is the leading Canadian provider of evidence-based drug information and the place to turn when you need information. See the For More Information section at the end of the chapter.

Follow these simple guidelines to self-medicate safely:

1. Always read labels and follow directions carefully. The information on most OTC and prescription drug labels appears in a standard format developed by Health Canada. Ingredients, directions for safe use, and warnings are clearly indicated, but if you have any questions, ask a pharmacist or another qualified health-care provider before using a product. Your pharmacist and all health-care providers should also know about all the OTC, prescriptions drugs, and natural health products you are taking. Use a chart, such as the one from Health Canada shown in Figure 19.3, to keep track of your medicines.

   The key to understanding and reading drug labels in Canada is learning about the Drug Identification Number (DIN). A DIN is a computer-generated eight-digit number assigned by Health Canada to a drug product before the drug is marketed. It uniquely identifies all authorized drug products sold in dosage form and is printed on the label of prescription and OTC drug products that are authorized for sale in Canada. The DIN identifies the manufacturer, product name, active ingredient(s), strength(s) of active ingredient(s), pharmaceutical form, and route of administration. Often, non-prescription and prescription drugs are packaged with what is called a monograph, a page containing detailed information for consumers.

2. Do not exceed the recommended dosage or length of treatment unless you discuss this change with your physician.

3. Use caution if you are taking other medications or supplements because OTC drugs and natural health products can interact with some prescription drugs. If you have questions about drug interactions, ask your pharmacist or another qualified health-care provider *before* you mix medicines.

4. Try to select medications with one active ingredient rather than combination products. A product with multiple ingredients is likely to include drugs for symptoms you don't even have. Using single-ingredient products also allows you to adjust the dosage of each medication separately for optimal symptom relief with minimal side effects.

5. When choosing medications, try to buy **generic drugs**, which contain the same active ingredient as the brand-name product but generally at a much lower cost. (Brand-name and generic drugs are discussed in more detail later in the chapter.)

6. Never take or give a drug from an unlabelled container or in the dark when you can't read what the label says.

7. If you are pregnant or nursing or have a chronic condition, such as kidney or liver disease, consult your health-care provider before self-medicating.

8. The expiration date marked on many medications is an estimate of how long the medication is likely to be safe and effective. If a medicine is more than a few months past its expiry date and you need to be certain that the medication is completely effective, buy new medication. You can dispose of old medicine by placing it in a sealed container with coffee grounds or cat litter, but the safest way to get

FIGURE 19.3

Health Canada's Medicine Chart

You can use this chart to keep track of the all the medicines you take. Make sure your pharmacist and all health-care providers have a copy.

Health Canada Santé Canada

It's Your Health

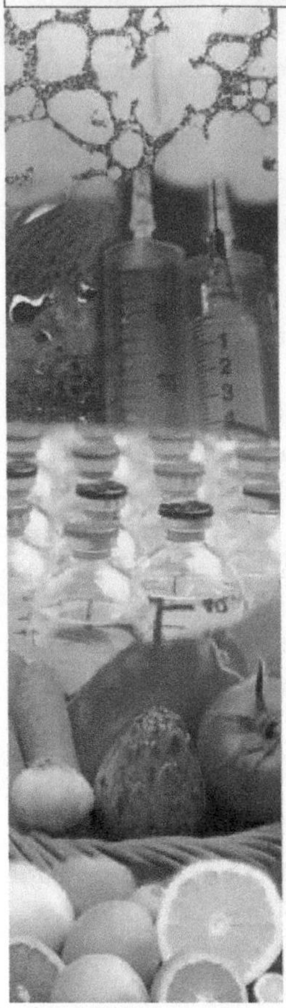

Use Medicines Safely

Use this chart to keep track of the medicines you are taking, including over-the-counter, natural health products and prescription drugs.

Name of Medicine	Dosage	Time when taken	Reason for taking

Family doctor's name: _____

Telephone number: _____

Name of pharmacy: _____

Telephone number: _____

Keep this chart up to date and share it with your doctor and pharmacist. Always use medicine as directed by your doctor or pharmacist. Know when to take it, how often, and for how long. Know when and under what conditions you should stop using a medicine, and what to do if you miss a dose.

Canada

Source: Public Health Agency of Canada, 2006, *Integrated Pan-Canadian Healthy Living Strategy,* and Public Health Agency of Canada, 2013. It's Your Health: Using Medication Safely. Adapted and reproduced with permission from the Minister of Health, 2015. © All Rights Reserved.

rid of outdated medicines is to take them to a pharmacy or hospital. If you have any question about a medicine's expiration date, ask a pharmacist.

9. Store your medications and home medical care kit in a cool, dry place that is out of the reach of children (see Figure 19.4).

10. Use special caution with Aspirin. Because of an association with a rare but serious problem known as Reye's syndrome, Aspirin or its generic counterpart, acetylsalicylic acid (ASA), should not be used by children or adolescents who may have the flu, chicken pox, or any other viral illness. Outdated Aspirin that has an acidic odour should be discarded. Some people are sensitive to the acidity of Aspirin; thus, some manufacturers coat Aspirin with an acid-resistant coating. This means that the Aspirin is absorbed in the colon rather than in the stomach. Enteric-coated Aspirin is less potent than plain Aspirin and therefore perhaps less effective among moderate- and high-risk patients taking Aspirin daily to prevent heart attacks.

generic drug
A drug that is not registered or protected by a trademark; a drug that does not have a brand name.

FIGURE 19.4

Your Home Medical Care Kit

A cool, dark, and dry place, such as the top of a linen closet, preferably in a locked container and out of a child's reach, is best for storing medicines. Showers and baths create heat and humidity that can cause some drugs to deteriorate rapidly. Use your bathroom medicine cabinet for supplies that aren't affected by heat and humidity.

Closet
- Analgesic (relieves pain)
- Antacid (relieves upset stomach)
- Antibiotic ointment (reduces risk of infection)
- Antihistamine (relieves allergy symptoms)
- Antiseptic (helps stop infection)
- Fever reducer (adult and child)
- Hydrocortisone (relieves itching and inflammation)
- Decongestant (relieves stuffy nose and other cold symptoms)

Medicine Cabinet
- Adhesive bandages
- Adhesive tape
- Alcohol wipes
- Calibrated measuring spoon
- Disinfectant
- Gauze pads
- Thermometer
- Tweezers

Source: Lewis, C. 2000. Your medicine cabinet needs an annual checkup, too. *FDA Consumer*, March/April.

QUESTIONS FOR CRITICAL THINKING AND REFLECTION

Do you often self-medicate for common medical problems, such as headaches or colds? If so, how careful are you about reading product labels and following directions? For example, would you know if you were taking two OTC medications that contained the same ingredient (such as ibuprofen) at the same time?

Professional Care

Becoming health literate, seeking self-care, and learning about different health-care resources are important responsibilities for all Canadians. However, it is just as essential to seek professional care when appropriate, whether by going to a hospital emergency room, by scheduling an appointment with your physician, or by accessing some other conventional health care. This system is a broad network of professionals and organizations, including independent practitioners, health-care providers, hospitals, clinics, and public and private insurance programs.

In recent years, many Canadians have also sought health care from practitioners of **complementary and alternative medicine (CAM)**, defined as those therapies and practices that do not form part of conventional, or mainstream, health care and medical practices as taught in most Canadian medical schools and offered in most Canadian hospitals. The most commonly used CAM therapies are relaxation techniques, herbal medicine, massage, and chiropractic (see Table 19.1). People often use CAM therapies in addition to their conventional medical treatments, but many do not tell their physicians about it. In reality, it would be more helpful to professionals and the public to be open to the idea of CAM therapies being another informed, evidence-based choice in partnership with conventional medicine.

complementary and alternative medicine (CAM)
Therapies or practices that are not part of conventional or mainstream health care and medical practice as taught in most Canadian medical schools and available at most Canadian health-care facilities; examples of CAM practices include acupuncture and herbal remedies.

TABLE 19.1

Demographics of Users of Complementary and Alternative Medicine in Canada and the United States

	Canada No. (%)	United States No. (%)
	70 884 (100)	16 400 (100)
Age, years		
15–19	4 449 (6)	1 590 (10)
20–44	34 053 (48)	8 026 (49)
45–64	19 019 (27)	4 339 (27)
≥65	13 363 (19)	2 445 (15)
Male	32 981 (47)	7 709 (47)
White	65 642 (93)	13 486 (82)
High school or higher	50 520 (72)	12 010 (74)
Residence[a]		
East	3 389 (5)	8 903 (54)
Central	40 128 (57)	3 569 (22)
West	27 367 (39)	3 687 (23)
Health status		
Excellent	16 437 (23)	4 951 (30)
Very good	26 988 (38)	4 872 (30)
Good	19 152 (27)	4 117 (25)
Fair	6 237 (9)	1 742 (11)
Poor	2 070 (3)	658 (4)
Problem with instrumental ADLs	8 282 (12)	632 (4)
Problem with ADLs	1 682 (2)	316 (2)
Service use in past 12 months		
MD/DO	56 035 (79)	10 894 (66)
Acupuncturist	800 (1)	101 (1)
Chiropractor	9 074 (13)	573 (4)
Homeopath/naturopath	906 (1)	73 (0.4)
Massage therapist	2 290 (3)	318 (2)
Any CAM provider	11 400 (16)	862 (5)
Only physician (MD or DO)	48 168 (68)	10 316 (63)
Only CAM provider	1 412 (2)	133 (1)
Both CAM and physician	9 979 (14)	729 (4)

Source: McFarland, B., et. al. 2002. Complementary and alternative medicine use in Canada and the United States. *American Journal of Public Health* 92(10): 1616-1618, Table I, p. 1617, retrieved from http://ajph.aphapublications.org/cgi/content/full/92/10/1616.

Note: ADLs = activities of daily living; CAM = complementary and alternative medicine (acupuncture, chiropractic, homeopathy/naturopathy, massage therapy); MD = doctor of medicine; DO = doctor of osteopathy.

[a] East = Atlantic Canada (including Nunavut) and Northeast and South U.S. census divisions; Central = Quebec and Ontario and Midwest U.S. census division; West = remaining Canadian provinces and territories and Western U.S. census division.

Consumers turn to CAM for a large variety of purposes related to health and well-being, such as boosting their immune system, lowering their cholesterol levels, losing weight, quitting smoking, or enhancing their memory. Studies suggest that people with chronic conditions, including cancer, asthma, autoimmune diseases, and HIV infection, are particularly likely to try CAM therapies. Despite their growing popularity, many CAM practices remain controversial, and individuals need to be especially aware of safety issues. In Canada, CAM products are regulated by Health Canada's Natural Health Products division; in 2005, a nationwide survey administered by this division determined that 71 percent of Canadians regularly take what have become known as natural health products (NHPs) such as:

- Vitamins and minerals
- Herbal remedies
- Homeopathic medicines
- Traditional medicines, such as traditional Chinese medicines (TCM)
- Probiotics
- Other products, such as amino acids and essential fatty acids

Through the Natural Health Products Directorate, Health Canada ensures that all Canadians have ready access to natural health products that are safe, effective, and of high quality, while respecting freedom of choice and philosophical and cultural diversity. NHPs must be safe for use as OTC products and not require a prescription to be sold. Products requiring a prescription continue to be regulated under the Canadian Food and Drug Regulations. As for specific CAM therapies, although some CAM practitioners are regulated (e.g., chiropractors) and some are not regulated (e.g., herbalists, homeopaths) in all provinces and territories, others (e.g., naturopathic practitioners, acupuncture/TCM practitioners) are regulated in some jurisdictions but not others. For Canadians seeking such therapies, this means that **evidence-based practice**, decision making, and decision analysis are very important.

> **evidence-based practice**
> The practice of health-care in which the practitioner systematically finds, appraises, and uses the most current and valid research findings as the basis for health-related decisions; the term is sometimes used to denote evidence-based medicine specifically, but can also include other specialties, such as evidence-based nursing, pharmacy, and dentistry.

In the next sections we examine the principles and providers of both conventional medicine—the dominant medical system in North America and Europe, also referred to as standard Western medicine or biomedicine—and complementary and alternative medicine (also referred to as integrative medicine), paying particular attention to consumer issues.

QUESTIONS FOR CRITICAL THINKING AND REFLECTION

What are your views about the use of CAM treatments and therapies? How are those views similar to or different from your perspectives on the use of conventional medicine? What events or information have shaped those views? At this point in your life, would you consider using complementary or alternative medicine?

Conventional Medicine

Referring to **conventional medicine** as *standard Western medicine* draws attention to the fact that it differs from the various medical systems that have developed in China, Japan, India, and other parts of the world. Calling it *biomedicine* reflects conventional medicine's foundation in the biological and physical sciences.

> **conventional medicine**
> A system of medicine based on the application of the scientific method; diseases are thought to be caused by identifiable physical factors and characterized by a representative set of symptoms; also called *biomedicine* or *standard Western medicine*.

Premises and Assumptions of Conventional Medicine

One of the important characteristics of Western medicine is the belief that disease is caused by identifiable physical factors. Western medicine identifies the causes of disease as pathogens (such as bacteria and viruses), genetic factors, and unhealthy lifestyles that result in changes at the molecular and cellular levels. In most cases, the focus is primarily on the physical causes of illness rather than on mental or spiritual imbalance.

Another feature that distinguishes Western biomedicine from other medical systems is the concept that every disease is defined by a certain set of symptoms and that these symptoms are similar in most patients suffering from this disease. Western medicine tends to treat illnesses as isolated biological disturbances that can occur in human beings, rather than as integral in some way to the individual with the illness.

Related to the idea of illness as the result of invasion by outside factors is the strong orientation toward methods of destroying pathogens or preventing them from causing serious infection. The public health measures of the nineteenth, twentieth, and twenty-first centuries—chlorination of drinking water, sewage disposal, food safety regulations, vaccination programs, education about hygiene, and so on—are an outgrowth of this orientation.

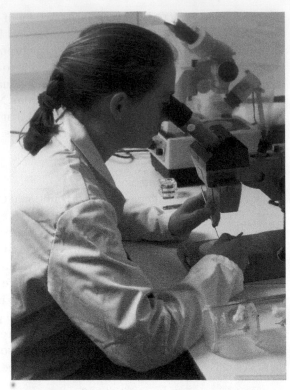

Conventional Western medicine is firmly grounded in scientific explanations resulting from the application of the scientific method to a question or problem.

The implementation of public health measures is one way to control pathogens; another is the use of drugs and surgery. The discovery and development of sulpha drugs, antibiotics, and steroids in the twentieth century, along with advances in chemistry that made it possible to identify the active ingredients in common plant-derived remedies, paved the way for the current close identification of Western medicine with **pharmaceuticals** (medical drugs, both prescription and OTC). Western medicine also relies heavily on surgery and on advanced medical technology to discover the physical causes of disease and to correct, remove, or destroy them.

> **pharmaceuticals**
> Medical drugs, both prescription and over-the-counter.

One technological innovation Canada will soon be implementing is the use of a health information highway. Infoway is a non-profit organization that will collaborate with the provincial and territorial ministries of health, health-care providers, and technology solution providers to accelerate the use of electronic health records (EHRs) in Canada. EHRs are secure electronic records of people's health history that can be accessed and shared through a network of client information management systems. With authorization from a patient, EHRs will enable health-care professionals to view and update essential patient data, such as medications, X-rays, and lab results. Some are skeptical about the use of this system, citing very real concerns about privacy issues for sensitive medical information.

Western medicine is based on the scientific method of obtaining knowledge and explaining health-related phenomena. Scientific explanations have these characteristics:

- *Empirical:* They are based on the evidence of the senses and on objective and systematic observation, often carried out under carefully controlled conditions; they must be capable of verification by others.
- *Rational:* They follow the rules of logic and are consistent with known facts.

- *Testable:* Either they are verifiable through direct observation or they lead to predictions about what should occur under conditions not yet observed.
- *Parsimonious:* They explain phenomena by using the fewest number of causes.
- *General:* They have broad explanatory power.
- *Rigorously evaluated:* They are constantly evaluated for consistency with the evidence and known principles, for parsimony, and for generality.
- *Tentative:* Scientists are willing to entertain the possibility that their explanations are faulty, based on new, better, or connected evidence.

The scientific method is both a way of acquiring knowledge and a way of thinking that involves approaching a problem by carefully defining its parameters, seeking out relevant evidence, and subjecting proposed solutions to rigorous testing.

Western medicine translates the scientific method into practice through the experimental research process, a highly refined and well-established approach to exploring the causes of disease and ensuring the safety and efficacy of treatments. Research ranges from case studies—descriptions of a single patient's illness and treatment—to randomized controlled trials conducted on large populations.

The process of drug development is equally rigorous. Drugs are developed and tested through an elaborate course that begins with preliminary research in the lab and continues through trials with human participants, review and approval by Health Canada, and monitoring of the drugs' effects even after they are on the market.

When results of research studies are published in medical journals, a community of scientists, physicians, researchers, and scholars has the opportunity to read the findings and enter into a dialogue about the subject. Publication of research often prompts further research designed to replicate and confirm the findings, challenge the conclusions, or pursue a related line of thought or experiment. (For guidelines on how to interpret research when it is reported in the popular press, see the Critical Consumer box earlier in this chapter.)

The Providers of Conventional Medicine

Since 1962, Canada has had a government-funded national health-care system founded on the five basic principles of the Canada Health Act to provide a health-care system that is (1) universally available to permanent residents, (2) comprehensive in the services it covers, (3) accessible without income barriers, (4) portable within and outside the country, and (5) publicly administered. Under this system, Canada's provinces and territories are responsible for administering their own health-care plans and must provide residents with prepaid coverage for all medically necessary hospital and physician services. Coverage for other services, such as dental care, prescription drugs, optometric services, hearing aids, and home care, varies by province or territory. For example, Ontario has its own prescription drug plans, the Ontario Drug Benefit Program and the Trillium Drug Program, which help seniors and others in need with the high costs of prescription drugs. These differ from British Columbia's Fair Pharmacare Program and from Alberta's prescription drug plans, which are offered in conjunction with Blue Cross, a private insurer.

A wide range of health-care professionals in Canada practise conventional medicine. Several kinds of professionals are permitted to practise specific fields of medicine independently, including medical doctors, osteopath practitioners, podiatrists, optometrists, and dentists. Although every province and territory governs the qualifications and expectations of health-care professionals, in general, health-care professionals include the following:

- Registered nurses and registered psychiatric nurses
- Licensed practical nurses
- Medical laboratory technologists
- Medical laboratory technicians
- Respiratory therapists
- Medical radiation technologists
- Medical sonographers
- Audiologists/speech-language pathologists
- Physiotherapists
- Occupational therapists
- Dentists
- Dental hygienists and therapists
- Dental assistants
- Ergonomists
- Pharmacists
- Physicians

Medical doctors are practitioners who hold a doctor of medicine (MD) degree from one of 17 accredited Canadian medical schools. Their education in medicine has several stages: three to four years of pre-medical education in university, with an emphasis on the sciences; three to four years of medical school, which teaches basic medical skills and awards the MD degree; graduate medical study, called an internship, and residency lasting from two to five years, during which a specialty (such as obstetrics) is chosen and studied and a medical licence is obtained. Medical certification and practice is regulated by each province and territory. MDs must pursue continuing medical education to keep abreast of advances in medical science.

medical doctors
Independent practitioners who hold a doctor of medicine degree from an accredited medical school.

Doctors of osteopathic medicine (DO) have received an undergraduate medical degree, but their postgraduate training places special emphasis on musculoskeletal problems and manipulative therapy. MDs and DOs are the two types of "complete" physicians in the North America, meaning they are trained and licensed to perform surgery and prescribe medication. DOs are osteopathic graduates of medical schools, which emphasize training students to be primary care physicians and to practise a whole-person approach to medicine. According to the Canadian Osteopathic Association, despite a variety of business websites promoting training and certification in osteopathy within Canada, no government-recognized or accredited colleges of osteopathy exist in Canada. Only graduates of American colleges of osteopathic medicine accredited by the Canadian and American Osteopathic Associations are eligible for licensure in Canada. Some Canadian osteopaths are non-physicians who practise osteopathic manual manipulation after graduation, with a diploma in osteopathic manual practice or DO(MP), from the Canadian College of Osteopathy, which has campuses in Toronto, Vancouver, and Halifax.

doctors of osteopathic medicine
Medical practitioners who have graduated from a medical school in Canada or an osteopathic medical school in the United States; osteopathy incorporates the theories and practices of scientific medicine but focuses on musculoskeletal problems and manipulative therapy.

Podiatrists are practitioners who specialize in the medical and surgical care of the feet. In Canada, the only podiatric medical training is via the Michener Institute for Applied Health Sciences in Toronto. Graduates are called podiatrists or chiropodists (a primary care professional practising podiatric medicine who specializes in the assessment, management, and prevention of diseases and disorders of the foot), and they hold an advanced diploma of health sciences (podiatric medicine). In the United States, eight colleges and universities grant a doctor of podiatric medicine (DPM) degree; the length of training is similar to that of MDs. DPMs can prescribe drugs, perform surgery on the feet, and be licensed to practise in any province and territory in Canada.

podiatrists
Practitioners who hold a doctor of podiatric medicine degree and specialize in the medical and surgical care of the feet.

Optometrists are primary health-care providers trained to examine the eyes, detect eye diseases, and treat vision problems. Prospective optometrists must complete at least three years of prerequisite college or university courses, including those in mathematics and the physical and biological sciences, as well as a four- or five-year university doctor of optometry (OD) degree. To practise, graduates of the OD program must then satisfy the licensing requirements of a provincial or territorial college of optometry. Included in these requirements are the successful completion of a national examination (except in Quebec) and, typically, a province- or territory-specific jurisprudence examination. Canada has only two schools of optometry: one in Waterloo, Ontario, and one in Montreal, Quebec. Canadian optometrists are permitted to prescribe therapeutic pharmaceutical agents (drugs) in only seven jurisdictions nationally. Note that ophthalmologists have an MD followed by a specialization in ophthalmology; in essence, they are eye specialists who care for all types of eye problems and can perform eye surgery. An optician is a specialist in fitting eyeglasses and making lenses to correct vision problems. An optometrist performs eye examinations and writes prescriptions for corrective lenses; an optician fills that prescription.

> **optometrists**
> Practitioners who hold a doctor of optometry degree and are trained to examine the eyes, detect eye diseases, and prescribe corrective lenses.

Dentists specialize in oral hygiene, typically the care of the teeth and mouth. They are graduates of four-year dental schools in seven Canadian provinces and hold a doctor of dental surgery (DDS) degree; specialists (such as endodontists) receive additional education. Dentists can perform surgery and prescribe drugs within the scope of their training. Dental hygienists and dental assistants are trained dental professionals who are granted diplomas from a variety of community colleges and programs across the country.

> **dentists**
> Practitioners who hold a doctor of medical dentistry degree and who specialize in the prevention and treatment of diseases and injuries of the teeth, mouth, and jaws.

In addition to these practitioners, millions of other trained health-care professionals, known as **allied health-care providers**, work in Canada. Some of them are licensed to work independently; others are permitted to work under medical supervision or medical referral. They include registered nurses (RNs), licensed vocational nurses (LVNs), physical therapists, social workers, registered dietitians (RDs), nurse practitioners, and certified nurse midwives.

> **allied health-care providers**
> Health-care professionals who typically provide services under the supervision or control of independent practitioners.

Choosing a Primary Care Physician

Most experts believe it is best to have a primary care physician, someone who gets to know you, who coordinates your medical care, and who refers you to specialists when you need them. Primary care physicians include those certified in family practice, internal medicine, pediatrics, and gynecology. These physicians are able to diagnose and treat the vast majority of common health problems; they also provide many preventive health services. The best time to look for a physician is before you are sick. At all ages, it is important for both men and women to obtain recommended health-care screenings and immunizations. Preventive care throughout life is important to maximize wellness.

To select a physician, begin by making a list of possible choices. If your insurance, beyond Canada's national health-care system, limits the type of health-care providers you can see, check the plan's list first. Ask for recommendations from family, friends, co-workers, local medical societies, and the physician referral service at a local clinic or hospital. Some clinics provide brief biographies of physicians on staff who are taking new patients. If you have a particular health problem, you may want to identify physicians who are board-certified in appropriate specialties. In Canada, only the Royal College of Physicians and Surgeons can certify physicians and surgeons in medical specialties. When you have a list of possible physicians, find out if a consumer or other independent group has rated doctors in your area; this will help you check on the quality of care they provide.

Once you have the names of a few physicians you might want to try, call their offices to find out more information, such as the following:

- Is the physician accepting new patients?
- What are the office hours, and when is the physician or office staff available? What do patients do if they need urgent care or have an emergency?
- Which hospitals does the physician use?
- How many other physicians are available to cover when he or she isn't available, and who are they?
- How long does it usually take to get a routine appointment?
- Does the office send reminders about preventive tests, such as Pap tests?
- Does the physician (or a nurse or physician assistant) give advice over the phone for common problems?

Schedule a visit with the physician you think you would most like to use. During that first visit, you will get a sense of how well matched you are and how well he or she might meet your medical needs. In 2002, Canadians made about 309 million visits to office-based physicians. Typically, females are viewed as more likely than males to visit a health-care provider. Reproductive health-care needs may be one reason for the difference, with women making doctor visits related to prenatal care and childbirth. Women of reproductive age may also need to make health-care visits to obtain prescription contraceptives and have the necessary pelvic exam and Pap test. However, recent evidence in Canada suggests that physician visits and hospitalizations are comparable for both sexes when rates are adjusted to exclude reproductive issues.

Getting the Most Out of Your Medical Care

The key to making the health-care system work for you lies in good communication with your physician and other members of the health-care team. Studies show that patients who interact more with physicians and ask more questions enjoy better health outcomes. Canada's EHR system should help with cross-practitioner sharing of health information.

The Physician–Patient Partnership

The physician–patient relationship is undergoing an important transformation. The image of the all-knowing physician and the passive patient is fading. What is emerging is a physician–patient *partnership*, in which the physician acts more like a consultant and the patient participates more actively. You should expect your physician to be attentive, caring, and able to listen and clearly explain things to you. You also must do your part. You need to be assertive in a firm but non-aggressive manner. You need to express your feelings and concerns, ask questions and, if necessary, be persistent. If your physician is unable to communicate clearly with you despite your best efforts, you probably need to change physicians.

Your Appointment with Your Physician

Physicians are often pressed for time, so prepare for your visit ahead of time. Make a written list of your key concerns and questions, along with notes about your symptoms (when they started, how long they last, what makes them better or worse, what treatments you have already tried, and so on). If you have questions you are uncomfortable about asking, practise discussing them ahead of time. Bring a list of all the medications you are taking—prescription, non-prescription, and herbal. Also bring any medical records or test results your physician may not already have.

Present your concerns at the beginning of the visit to set the agenda. Be specific and concise about your symptoms, and be open and honest about your concerns. Share your hunches with your physician— your guesses can provide vital clues. Ask questions if you don't understand something. Let your physician know if you are taking any drugs, are allergic to any medications, are breastfeeding, or may be pregnant.

At the end of the visit, briefly repeat the physician's diagnosis, prognosis, and instructions. Make sure you understand your next steps, such as making another appointment, phoning for test results, watching for new symptoms, and so on. You may also want to ask about the possibility of using email for follow-up. (See the Take Charge box at the end of the chapter for more information about following physicians' instructions.)

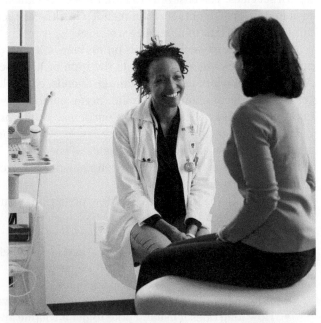

Good communication is a crucial factor in an effective physician–patient partnership.

The Diagnostic Process

The first step in the diagnostic process is the medical history, which includes your primary reason for the visit, your current symptoms, your past medical history, and your social history (job, family life, major stressors, living conditions, and health habits). Keeping up-to-date records of your medical history can help you provide your physician with key facts about your health (see the Assess Yourself box).

The next step is the physical exam, which usually begins with a review of vital signs: blood pressure, heart rate (pulse), breathing rate, and temperature. Depending on your primary concern, your physician may give you a complete physical, or the exam may be directed to specific areas, such as your ears, nose, and throat.

Assess YOURSELF

Personal Health Profile

General Information

Age: _____   Total cholesterol: _____   Blood pressure: _____ / _____   Other: _____

Height: _____   HDL: _____   Triglycerides: _____   _____

Weight: _____   LDL: _____   Glucose: _____   _____

Blood type: _____

Medical Conditions

Check any of the following that apply to you and add other conditions that might affect your health and well-being.

_____ heart disease   _____ back pain   _____ depression, anxiety, or another psychological disorder

_____ lung disease   _____ arthritis   _____ major stressors

_____ diabetes   _____ allergies   _____ other injury or joint problem

_____ eating disorder   _____ asthma   _____ substance abuse problem

_____ other: _____   _____ other: _____

Medications/Treatments

List any drugs you are taking or any medical treatments you are undergoing. Include the name of the substance or treatment and its purpose. Include both prescription and OTC drugs and any vitamin, mineral, herb, or other dietary supplement you are taking.

_____   _____   _____

_____   _____   _____

Health-Care Providers

Primary care physician: name _____   phone _____

Specialist physician: name _____   phone _____

Condition treated: _____

Other health-care provider: name _____   phone _____

Condition treated: _____

To ensure that you get the most out of your medical care, you should also keep a record of your vaccinations and medical screening tests. Chapters 7–9 and 13 describe recommended vaccinations and screening tests for CVD, cancer, and STIs.

Additionally, your physician may order medical tests to complete the diagnosis. Diagnostic testing provides a wealth of information to help solve medical problems. Physicians can order X-rays, biopsies, blood and urine tests, scans, and **endoscopies** to view, probe, or analyze almost any part of the body.

> **endoscopies**
> Medical procedures in which a viewing instrument is inserted into a body cavity or opening.

If your physician orders a test for you, be sure you know why you need it, what the risks and benefits of the test are for you, how you should prepare for it (for example, by fasting or discontinuing medications or herbal remedies), and what the test will involve. Also ask what the test results mean, because no test is 100 percent accurate—**false positives** and **false negatives** do occur—and interpretation of some tests is subjective. Sometimes it is important to get a second opinion on a diagnosis.

> **false positives**
> Test results that incorrectly detect a disease or condition in a healthy person.
>
> **false negatives**
> Test results that fail to correctly detect a disease or condition.

Medical and Surgical Treatments

Many conditions can be treated in a variety of ways; in some cases, lifestyle changes are enough. Make sure you know the possible risks and side effects of each treatment option, as well as the likelihood that it will improve your condition.

PRESCRIPTION MEDICATIONS   In 2008, 453 million prescriptions were filled in the 10 Canadian provinces, up 7.1 percent over the previous year. That's about 14 prescriptions for each man, woman, and child in the country. Health Canada noted in 2002 that drug use among seniors was notably higher compared with the rest of the population; people over 65 take 40 percent of all medications dispensed. Thousands of lives are saved each year by antibiotics, insulin, and other drugs, but we pay a price for having such powerful tools. No specifically Canadian data are available regarding drug-related errors, also called *adverse drug events* or ADEs, but they do occur. ADEs happen for several reasons:

- *Medication errors:* Physicians may overprescribe drugs, sometimes in response to pressure by patients (see the In the News box). Adverse effects can occur if a physician prescribes the wrong drug or a dangerous combination of drugs; such problems are especially prevalent for older adults, who typically take multiple medications. The risk of ADEs increases greatly with the number of medicines you take. At the pharmacy, patients may receive the wrong drug or may not be given complete information about drug risks, side effects, and interactions. Problems can occur because of a physician's poor handwriting, misinterpretation of an abbreviated drug name, or similarities between the names and packaging of different drugs.

- *Off-label drug use:* Another potential problem is off-label use of drugs. Once a drug is approved by Health Canada for one purpose, it can legally be prescribed (although not marketed) for purposes not listed on the label. A recent study revealed that about 20 percent of medications are prescribed for off-label use; three-quarters of those prescriptions are made with little or no evidence supporting such use. Many off-label uses are safe and supported by some research, but both consumers and health-care providers need to take special care with off-label use of medications.

QUICK STATS

Medications are given or prescribed in about 80% of physician office visits.

—Health Canada, 2003

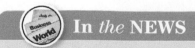

Medical Errors, Adverse Events, and Their Prevention

The Canadian Institute for Health Information estimates that $750 million in extra health-care spending is attributable to medical errors, as are 23 750 deaths per year and 1.1 million days in hospital. The Institute of Medicine (IOM) defines a *medical error* as "the failure to complete a planned action as intended or the use of a wrong plan to achieve an aim," and an *adverse event* as "an injury caused by medical management rather than by the underlying disease or condition of the patient."

Medical errors take many forms, including surgical mismanagement, such as removal of the wrong breast in a mastectomy operation; misdiagnosis leading to incorrect therapy; misinterpretation of or failure to order diagnostic tests; failure to act on abnormal test results; equipment failure; blood transfusion injuries; misinterpretation of physician orders leading to use of the wrong drug or an incorrect dosage; and hospital-acquired infections.

Medication Errors

The U.S. Food and Drug Administration defines a *medication error* as "any preventable event that may cause or lead to inappropriate medication use or patient harm while the medication is in the control of the health-care professional, patient, or consumer." Such events may be related to practice, including prescribing and order communication, or to product labelling, packaging, dispensing, administration, and use. In the absence of Canadian studies, extrapolation from U.S. data suggests that approximately 700 Canadians die each year as a result of medication errors.

Hospital Errors

Hospital-acquired infections are the fourth-leading cause of death in Canada. Each year 220 000–250 000 hospital-acquired infections result in 8000–12 000 deaths. Between 35 percent and 50 percent of these hospital-acquired infections are preventable. Most infections are caused by bacteria that normally inhabit the skin and mucous membranes. The most common infections involve the urinary tract, surgical wounds, the respiratory tract, and skin. Proper handling of equipment and frequent handwashing by providers are the major ways to avoid such infections.

Prevention Within the System

Fortunately, most errors are preventable. Major system improvements proposed in recent reports include the following:

- *The application of standardized procedure and equipment guidelines:* For example, the error rate in anaesthesia was cut by a factor of seven when standardized protocols and equipment were used.
- *Medical rounds that include a pharmacist:* Adding a pharmacist to the team reduces medication error rates by 66 percent.
- *The use of computer technology and barcodes:* In one hospital, wireless computer technology and barcoding reduced medication errors by 70 percent.

In 2001, the National Steering Committee on Patient Safety was created in Canada. One of the recommendations of this committee was the establishment of the Canadian Patient Safety Institute (CPSI). In 2003, the federal government announced the provision of $10 million annually to support patient safety initiatives, including the formation of the CPSI. The mandate of the CPSI is to provide "national leadership in building and advancing a safer Canadian health system." The CPSI's flagship program, Safer Healthcare Now, endorses and promotes six interventions whose implementation has the potential to reduce mortality and morbidity:

- *Rapid response teams:* To prevent deaths in patients who are progressively failing outside the intensive care unit
- *Improved care for acute myocardial infarction:* To prevent deaths among patients hospitalized for acute myocardial infarction by ensuring the reliable delivery of evidence-based care
- *Prevention of ADEs:* To reduce ADEs by using a medication reconciliation process
- *Prevention of central line–associated bloodstream infection:* To reduce central venous catheter-related bloodstream infection and deaths from that infection by using two sets of interventions called the *central line insertion bundle* and the *central line maintenance bundle*
- *Prevention of surgical site infection (SSI):* To prevent SSI and deaths from SSI by using four interventions known as the *SSI bundle* in all surgical patients

- *Prevention of ventilator-associated pneumonia (VAP):* To prevent VAP and deaths from VAP and other complications in patients on ventilators by using a set of interventions known as the *ventilator bundle*

  Studies show that most medical errors are system related and not attributable to negligence or misconduct by individual providers. Patient participation and empowerment may be the best defences against medical errors. As a patient, you can take the following steps to prevent medical errors:

  - *Take all medications exactly as prescribed, for as long as prescribed.* If you don't understand why you are being given a medication, ask your physician or pharmacist to explain.
  - *If you require hospitalization, select your hospital carefully.* Research has shown that patients who choose a hospital with extensive experience treating patients with their condition can expect better results and fewer complications.
  - *When being discharged from a hospital, ask about any special care, precautions, medications, and other procedures that will be required on returning home.* Studies show that physicians assume patients understand more about their discharge instructions than they actually do.
  - *If you have doubts about the care you are getting, recruit a patient advocate.* Choose someone who can give support and speak on your behalf to protect your rights, promote your interests, and assist you in making decisions. An advocate can be a close friend or family member who is tactful and able to take accurate notes.
  - *If you require hospitalization, rely on a hospitalist.* A *hospitalist* is a physician who specializes in the care of hospitalized patients. Hospitalists focus on advocacy and safety, and help remedy the lack of continuity that occurs among hospital providers. Hospitalists manage a patient's course through the hospital, coordinate the providers and consultants, and stay in touch with the patient's family and primary care physician. Hospitalists help remedy many of the problems that lead to medical errors.

- *Online pharmacies:* Although convenient, some online pharmacies may sell products or engage in practices that are illegal in the offline world, putting consumers at risk for receiving adulterated, expired, ineffective, or counterfeit drugs. Consumers should avoid sites that prescribe drugs for the first time without a physical exam, sell prescription drugs without a prescription, or sell medications not approved by Health Canada. You should also avoid sites that do not provide access to a registered pharmacist to answer questions or that do not provide a Canadian address and phone number to contact if there's a problem. Some online services, such as Canadian Pharmacy Online and Online Canada Rx, are not pharmacies themselves, but provide access to pharmacy services from licensed pharmacies. Many experts recommend that consumers use online pharmacies only to obtain medicines prescribed by their usual health-care provider.

- *Costs:* International Marketing Services Health estimates that Canadians spent $21.4 billion on prescription medications in 2008, up from $20.2 billion in 2007. Consumers may be able to lower their drug costs by using generic versions of medications (the dispensed volume for generic drugs grew by 15 percent in 2008); by joining a drug discount program sponsored by a company, an organization, or a local pharmacy; or by investigating reputable mail-order or Internet pharmacies.

Patients also share some responsibility for problems with prescription drugs. Many people don't take their medications properly, skipping doses, taking incorrect doses, stopping too soon, or not taking the medication at all. Consumers can increase the safety and effectiveness of their treatment by carefully reading all prescription labels (see Figure 19.5) and all fact sheets, brochures, or monographs that come with the medication. Whenever a health-care provider gives you a prescription, ask the following questions:

- Are there non-drug alternatives?
- What is the name of the medication, and what is it supposed to do, within what period of time?
- How and when do I take the medication, how much do I take, and for how long? What should I do if I miss a dose?
- What other medications, foods, drinks, or activities should I avoid?
- What are the side effects, and what do I do if they occur?
- Can I take a generic drug rather than a brand-name one?
- Is there written information about the medication?

Remember to store your medications in a cool, dry place, out of direct light. Never share your prescription medications with anyone else, and never use an old prescription for a new ailment.

Reading and Understanding Prescription Medication Labels

Question		Answer
1. What is the name of the pharmacy?	**MANITOBA Pharmacy** 204 Manitoba Street Winnipeg MB M2B 2Y2 Canada Store # 0001 Phone: 204-204-2004	Manitoba Pharmacy
2. What is the address of the pharmacy?	R# 2042042 Ref:0 Dr. Manitoba Toba Man	204 Manitoba Street, Winnipeg, MB, M2B 2Y2
3. What is the store number of the pharmacy?	TAKE 1 CAPSULE THREE TIMES DAILY UNTIL FINISHED (ANTIBIOTIC)	Store: #0001
4. What is the phone number of the pharmacy?	APO-AMOXI 500MG AMOXICILLIN 500MG RED/YEL/ELLIP/APO{500} APX 00628123	Phone: 204-204-2004
5. What is the prescription number?	30 CAP 14 Oct 2015 Total: 21.43 EDS	Rx: #2042042
6. What is the physician's name?	Important: Take this medication for the prescribed duration.	Dr. Manitoba
7. What is the date that the prescription was filled?		October 14, 2015
8. What is the name of the person for whom the drug is prescribed? (Prescription drugs should be used only by the person for whom the drugs were prescribed.)		Toba Man
9. What is the brand name of this drug? (Various manufacturers or companies may make the same generic drug but will call it by their own brand or trade name.)		APO-Amoxi
10. What is the name of the medication or the main ingredient?		Amoxicillin
11. What is the strength of the medication?		500 mg
12. What do the letters APX mean?		The manufacturer's/company's code
13. What does the number listed below the company code represent?		The Drug Identification Number (DIN)
14. How much is in the package?		30 cap (capsules)
15. What are the directions or instructions for taking the medication?		Take 1 capsule three times daily until finished (antibiotic).
16. Are there any cautions or warnings on the label?		Important: Take this medication for the prescribed duration. Keep out of reach of children.
17. Do prescription drug labels often include any additional information that is not on this one?		Expiry date, refill information, and additional information, on stickers, such as "Take with food."

WEB OR INTERNET HEALTH INFORMATION It is important to approach Web-based health information with some skepticism. The information superhighway is a tremendous technological boon, but information presented on the Internet may or may not be true. Here are important questions to consider before you accept any Web-based health information:

- Who runs this site?
- Who pays for this site?
- What is the purpose of this site?
- Where does the information come from?
- What kind of evidence is the information based on?
- How is the information selected?
- How current is the information?
- How does the site choose links to other sites?
- What information about you, if any, does this site collect and why?
- How does the site manage its interactions with visitors?

SURGERY The number of surgeries performed in Canadian hospitals increased by 17 percent between 1995–1996 and 2005–2006, and by another 5 percent in 2007, according to the Canadian Institute for Health Information. In hospitals across the country, more surgeries are being performed in an **outpatient** day surgery setting (an increase of 31 percent over 10 years), while inpatient surgeries have decreased by 17 percent over the past decade.

> **outpatient**
> A person receiving medical attention without being admitted to the hospital.

If a health-care provider suggests surgery for any reason, ask the following questions:
- Why do I need surgery at this time?
- Are any non-surgical options available, such as medicine or physical therapy?
- What are the risks and complications of the surgery?
- Can the operation be performed on an outpatient basis?
- What can I expect before, during, and after surgery?

QUESTIONS FOR CRITICAL THINKING AND REFLECTION

What sort of relationship do you have with your primary physician? Do you think he or she really understands your needs and is familiar enough with your history? What could you do to improve this relationship? Does your primary physician support the integrated use of complementary and alternative forms of medicine?

Complementary and Alternative Medicine

Although *complementary and alternative medicine (CAM)* is the term commonly used in the Western world, some health practitioners instead use the term *integrative medicine* to capture the notion of conceptualizing medicine as allopathic *and* complementary or alternative. Compared with conventional or allopathic medicine, CAM implies the concept of *along with* rather than *instead of*; instead of either/or in choosing between these two systems, it is more a case of both/and. In other words, they complement each other when used from an evidence-based, decision-making approach. Within this framework, all treatments or drugs or remedies need to be evaluated by the health-care practitioner along with the consumer for their effectiveness, potential harm, non-intended side effects, and their utility compared to other healing or medical practices.

Some health-care practitioners phrase the approach to medicine as a question: "Do we treat the disease or do we treat the patient?" But the difference is more subtle. While conventional Western medicine tends to focus on the body, on the physical causes of disease, and on ways to eradicate pathogens to restore health, CAM tends to focus on an integration of mind, body, and spirit in seeking ways to restore the whole person to harmony so that the individual can regain health. Conventional medicine is based primarily on science, and the experimental method and evidence gathered from RCTs, while CAM tends to be based on healing traditions and accumulated experience. The evidence for CAM use tends to be lower on the hierarchy of evidence pyramid because standardizing a treatment such as acupuncture to apply to whole populations or large groups of people is very difficult, if not impossible, to do.

Many alternative medical systems with long-standing traditions have concepts and theories of medicine that once were very different from those of conventional Western medical thought. Some people consider all of CAM quackery and tell you that you can recognize a quack by his or her use of pseudoscientific language. However, the use of some phrases, such as "bringing into harmony with nature" or "enhancing the flow of vital energy" does not necessarily mean that a practitioner is a quack; rather, it may reflect this practitioner's different concept of health and healing. The key for consumers is matching CAM practitioner values with your own and working in partnership with conventional health-care providers.

You might have heard that there are only anecdotal testimonials to support the value of many forms of CAM and that because such reports do not constitute scientific proof of effectiveness, they are meaningless. Although it is correct that anecdotes and testimonials are not, by the standards of RCTs in the experimental method, scientifically reliable evidence, that does not mean that they are meaningless. What is called anecdotal evidence may actually be a form of case report, a valuable and standard form of study in which a researcher describes a single patient, his or her medical history, the treatments administered, and the outcome of the case. Still, case reports alone are not sufficient to prove scientifically the effectiveness of a medical treatment. Caution is in order when choosing any mode of treatment—conventional or unconventional—that has not been carefully evaluated for safety and effectiveness (see the Critical Consumer box).

 Critical CONSUMER

Avoiding Health Fraud and Quackery

According to the U.S. Federal Trade Commission, North American consumers waste billions of dollars on unproven, fraudulently marketed, and sometimes useless health-care products and treatments. Various estimates indicate that 2–10 percent of every health-care dollar spent in North America is lost to fraud. In Canada, health-care spending was estimated at $213 billion in 2013. That would mean that the real cost of health-care fraud could be as much as $18 billion each year. These figures represent enough money to drastically revitalize Canadian medicare and purchase more than 3000 magnetic resonance imaging (MRI) machines. In addition, people with serious medical problems may waste valuable time before seeking proper treatment. Worse yet, some of the products they are buying may cause serious harm. Health fraud is a business that sells false hope. It preys on people with diseases that have no medical cure and on people who want shortcuts to weight loss or improvements to personal appearance.

To check out a particular product, talk to a physician or another health-care professional and to family members and friends. Be wary of treatments offered by people who tell you to avoid talking to others. Check with the Better Business Bureau in Canada (http://www.bbb.org/canada/) or a local legal office to see whether other consumers have lodged complaints about the product or the product's marketer. You can also check with the appropriate health professional group. For example, check with the Canadian Diabetes Association or the Canadian Arthritis Network if the products are promoted for diabetes or for arthritis. Take special care with products and devices sold online; the broad reach of the Internet, combined with the ease of setting up and removing websites, makes online sellers particularly difficult to regulate.

If you think you have been a victim of health fraud or if you have an adverse reaction that you think is related to a particular supplement, you can report it to the Canadian Health Care Anti-fraud Association. You can report suspected health or health-care fraud anonymously. One self-appointed guardian against fraud and staunch advocate of conventional and allopathic medicine is physician Stephen Barrett; via his website, http://www.quackwatch.com, he monitors a wide variety of issues that he labels as quackery. Although his viewpoint is heavily based on the "truth" of the experimental method only, his evidence is worth considering in any health-related, evidence-based decision-making process.

In the Canadian Health Literacy section of this chapter, we noted the importance of using the Cochrane Consumer Network in making evidence-based decisions. In the same vein, the Cochrane Library, a subset of the overall Cochrane Collaboration, provides independent, high-quality evidence for health decision making for both conventional and complementary medicine. Intriguingly, over half the world's population only has access to CAM practices and treatments and no access to Western medicine.

The National Center for Complementary and Alternative Medicine (NCCAM) in the United States conventionally groups CAM practices into five domains: alternative medical systems, mind–body interventions, biological-based therapies, manipulative and body-based methods, and energy therapies (see Figure 19.6). It is impossible to discuss all of these forms fully in a single chapter. Instead, what follows is a general introduction to the types of CAM available and a brief description of some of the more widely used ones.

FIGURE 19.6

The Five Domains of CAM Practices

Domain	Characteristics	Examples
Alternative medical systems	Involve complete systems of theory and practice that have evolved independently of and often long before the conventional biomedical approach	Traditional Chinese medicine; Kampo; ayurveda (India); Native American, Aboriginal, African, Middle-Eastern, Tibetan, Central and South American medical systems; homeopathy; naturopathy
Mind–body interventions	Employ a variety of techniques designed to make it possible for the mind to affect bodily function and symptoms	Meditation, certain uses of hypnosis, prayer, mental healing
Biological-based therapies	Include natural and biologically-based practices, interventions, and products, many of which overlap with conventional medicine's use of dietary supplements	Herbal, special dietary, orthomolecular,* and individual biological therapies
Manipulative and body-based methods	Include methods that are based on manipulation and movement of the body	Chiropractic, osteopathy, massage therapy
Energy therapies	Focus on energy fields within the body (biofields) or from other sources (electromagnetic fields)	Qi gong, Reiki, therapeutic touch, bioelectromagnetic-based therapies

*Orthomolecular therapies are treatments of diseases with varying, but usually high, concentrations of chemicals, including minerals (e.g., magnesium), hormones (e.g., melatonin), or vitamins.

Alternative Medical Systems

Many cultures elaborated complete systems of medical philosophy, theory, and practice long before the current biomedical approach was developed. In fact, Western (or allopathic or conventional) medicine is only about 150 years old; some medical systems—the Indian Ayurvedic system, for example—have been practised for thousands of years and are the only systems available to a large proportion of the world's population. The complete systems that are best known in the North America are probably traditional Chinese medicine

(TCM), chiropractic, naturopathy, and homeopathy. Traditional medical systems have also been developed in many other regions of the world, including North, Central, and South America, the Middle East, India, Tibet, and Australia. In many countries, these medical approaches continue to be used today—frequently alongside Western medicine and quite often by physicians trained in Western medicine. Today, about two-thirds of Canadians use some form of CAM each year. Of interest and importance is the fact that all Canadian medical schools provide at least an introduction to CAM in their curricula; in fact, one of the bestselling textbooks on CAM forms, uses, and supporting evidence—*Fundamentals of Alternative and Complementary Medicine* (Miccozi)—is written almost entirely by physicians. At the very least, this attention of Canadian medical schools and medical practitioners to CAM reflects the perceived importance of CAM to the Canadian public.

Alternative medical systems tend to have concepts in common. For example, the concept of life force or energy exists in many cultures. In TCM, the life force contained in all living things is called *qi* (sometimes spelled chi). Qi resembles the *vis vitalis* (Latin for "life force") of Greek, Roman, and European medical systems, and *prana* of ayurveda, the traditional medical system of India. Most traditional medical systems think of disease as a disturbance or imbalance not just of physical processes, but also of forces and energies within the body, the mind, the spirit, and even within the larger environment. In TCM, for example, the principle of balance is expressed as yin and yang, which are opposites yet complement each other; many apparent, natural dualities—dark and light, female and male, low and high, cold and hot—are viewed in Chinese culture as manifestations of yin and yang (respectively). Disease is seen a disturbance of qi reflecting an imbalance between yin and yang. Treatment aims at reestablishing equilibrium, balance, and harmony.

Because the whole patient, rather than an isolated set of symptoms, is treated in most comprehensive alternative medical systems, it is rare that only a single treatment approach is used. Most commonly, multiple techniques and methods are employed and are continually adjusted according to the changes in the patient's health status that occur naturally or are brought about by the treatment.

Traditional Chinese Medicine

Traditional Chinese medicine (TCM) is based on highly abstract concepts; a sophisticated set of techniques and methods; and individualized diagnosis, treatment, and prevention. No identical diseases exist in TCM. Two patients with the same diagnosis in Western medicine will get different diagnoses in TCM and will be given different treatments. In TCM, the free and harmonious flow of qi produces health—a positive feeling of well-being and vitality in body, mind, and spirit. Illness occurs when the flow of qi is blocked or disturbed. TCM works to restore and balance the flow of blocked qi; the goal is not only to treat illnesses but also to increase energy, prevent disease, and support the immune system. In TCM, diagnosis of each individual is a an extensive, fourfold process of inspection, listening and smelling, inquiry, and palpation; palpation is always the last part of the process.

> **traditional Chinese medicine (TCM)**
> The traditional medical system of China, which views illness as the result of a disturbance in the flow of qi, the life force; therapies include acupuncture, herbal medicine, and massage.

Two of the primary treatment methods in TCM are herbal remedies and acupuncture. Chinese herbal remedies number about 5800 and include plant products, animal parts, and minerals. Herbal remedies, like everything else, have yin and yang properties. When a disease is perceived to be due to a yin deficiency, remedies with more yin characteristics might be used for treatment. The

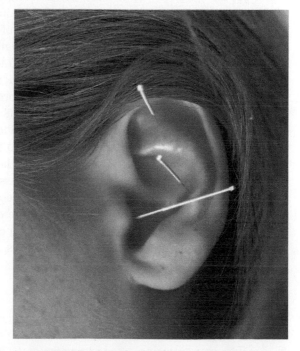

Acupuncture involves the insertion of needles at appropriate points in the skin to restore balance to the flow of qi.

use of a single medicinal botanical is rare in Chinese herbal medicine; rather, several different plants are combined in very precise proportions, often to make a tea or soup. For example, a remedy might include a primary herb that targets the main symptom, a second herb that enhances the effects of the primary herb, a third that lessens side effects, and a fourth that helps deliver ingredients to a particular body site.

Acupuncture works to correct disturbances in the flow of qi through the insertion of thin needles at appropriate points in the skin. Acupuncture needles are blunted, unlike hypodermic needles; that is, inserting an acupuncture needle is like inserting a knitting needle into a skein of wool; the knitting needle does not puncture the wool and so too the acupuncture needle rarely draws blood. Qi is believed to flow through the body along several *meridians*, or pathways, and people have 12–15 meridians and at least 2000 acupuncture points located along these meridians. The certified acupuncturist targets the acupuncture point, based on the diagnosis, and the needle actually moves through body tissue to the designated point. The traditional method consists of inserting the needle and leaving it in place for 20–40 minutes. Other means of stimulating acupuncture points include heat, pressure (called **acupressure**), friction, suction, laser, or electric stimulation. The points chosen for acupuncture are highly individualized for each patient, and they change over the course of treatment as the patient's health status changes. In addition, acupuncture points are named, such as liver 12 or lung 7, but the names are not consistent with the anatomical location on the body. Lung 7, for example, is a site at the wrist.

acupuncture
Insertion of thin needles into the skin at points along meridians, pathways through which qi is believed to flow.

acupressure
The art and science of applying physical pressure on certain acupuncture points.

The World Health Organization has identified more than 40 conditions for which acupuncture may be beneficial. At a recent conference called by the National Institutes of Health, a panel of experts analyzed the available information on the scientific evidence for the efficacy of acupuncture in many of these conditions. These experts found evidence that acupuncture was effective in relieving nausea and vomiting after chemotherapy and pain after surgery, including dental surgery. Newer studies show that acupuncture may help relieve the painful symptoms of fibromyalgia and reduce the joint pain and stiffness of osteoarthritis. There is not yet enough evidence to show conclusively that acupuncture is effective for menstrual cramps, tennis elbow, carpal tunnel syndrome, asthma, or certain other conditions. Western researchers typically use a different framework for understanding the effects of acupuncture. For example, they might explain pain relief not in terms of qi, but rather in terms of altering nervous system pathways and the release of hormones and neurotransmitters. Often such explanations are framed in the context of anatomical acupuncture in efforts to add perceived Western precision to determining acupuncture's efficacy.

Very few negative side effects have been reported in conjunction with acupuncture. Nonetheless, problems can occur from the improper insertion and manipulation of needles and from the use of unsterile needles. If you consider acupuncture, you should ask your practitioner about the relative risks of the procedure and the safety practices he or she observes. Most provinces and territories regulate licensing for acupuncture practitioners, but requirements vary widely. Other regulated health-care professionals, such as naturopaths, physicians, physiotherapists, chiropractors, dentists, and massage therapists, can perform acupuncture treatments when they fulfill educational requirements set up by their regulatory colleges. It is noteworthy that the school (philosophy and approach) and style of acupuncture differs depending on the training of the practitioner. TCM practitioners are trained at specific TCM-training colleges, such as the Academy of Clinical Chinese Medicine of Toronto, or at broad-based community colleges, such as the Grant MacEwan College in Edmonton.

QUICK STATS

About 54% of Canadians have tried some form of CAM. Women are more likely than men to consult alternative practitioners.

—*Fraser Institute Health Survey*, 2006

THINKING ABOUT THE ENVIRONMENT

Several forms of alternative medicine, such as traditional Chinese medicine, rely heavily on remedies made from plant and animal parts. Although millions of people claim that these remedies are beneficial, their production now threatens the very existence of several species. Here are some examples:

- Today fewer than 10 000 tigers live in the wild (and about 5000 are being raised on farms). Despite their dwindling numbers and status as an endangered species, hundreds of tigers are poached every year. The carcasses are sold to purveyors of traditional medicine, who use tiger body parts in some of their remedies.
- Only a few thousand rhinoceros live in the wild today, but they continue to be poached for their horns, which are prized by traditional healers. Rhinos are classified as "critically endangered" and will disappear within a few years unless they are protected.
- Other species, such as seahorses, musk deer, and bears, are being harvested at rates that may put them at risk of extinction soon.

For more than a decade, environmentalists and wildlife protection officials worldwide have been calling for practitioners of traditional medicine to either stop using endangered plants and animals in their remedies, or to support farming of these species as an alternative to harvesting them from the wild. Progress is slow, but according to many organizations, such as the International Fund for Animal Welfare, practitioners have started responding positively.

For more information on the environment and environmental health, see Chapter 21.

Homeopathy

An alternative medical system of Western origin, **homeopathy** is based on two main principles: "Like cures like," and remedies become more effective with greater dilution. "Like cures like" summarizes the concept that a substance that produces the symptoms of an illness in a healthy person can cure the illness when given in very minute quantities. Modern vaccination is based on this same principle, although vaccinations are much more potent dosages than homeopathic remedies. Remedies containing very small quantities of a particular substance are obtained by repeatedly diluting the original solution. The extent of dilution varies, but the final extract is often so diluted that few, if any, of the original molecules are left in it. According to homeopathic thinking, such highly diluted extracts not only retain some form of biological activity, but actually become more potent. As with all forms of CAM, the final dilution of remedy is based on the individual; therefore, it is very difficult to conduct RCTs on one remedy when there is so much variation in dosage.

> **homeopathy**
> An alternative medical system that treats illnesses by giving very small doses of drugs that in larger doses would produce symptoms like those of the illness.

More than 1000 different substances (plant and animal parts, minerals, and chemicals) are used to prepare homeopathic remedies, and each of these substances is thought to have different effects at different dilutions. That means a homeopath must not only choose the correct remedy for a particular patient, but also decide on the specific dilution of that remedy to achieve the desired effect. As noted, and like other traditional systems of medicine, homeopathy constitutes a highly individualized form of therapy; that is, the treatment of each patient is determined by the overall condition of the patient rather than by specific signs and symptoms. To assess a patient's condition, homeopaths generally spend quite a bit of time talking with a patient and assessing his or her physical, psychological, and emotional health before deciding on the correct remedy at the proper dilution. This intensive interaction between the practitioner and the patient might play an important role in the success of the therapy. Indeed, critics of homeopathy often attribute its reported effectiveness to this non-specific placebo effect (see the Mind Body Spirit box). However, when the results of 185 homeopathic trials were analyzed recently, it was concluded that the clinical effects of homeopathy could not be completely explained by the placebo effect. Homeopathy remains one of the most controversial forms of CAM.

Mind *Body* SPIRIT

The Power of Belief: The Placebo Effect

A placebo is a chemically inactive substance or ineffective procedure that a patient believes is an effective therapy for his or her condition. Researchers frequently give placebos to the control group in an experiment testing the efficacy of a particular drug or other treatment. By comparing the effects of the actual treatment with the effects of the placebo, researchers can judge whether the treatment is effective.

The *placebo effect* occurs when a patient improves after receiving a placebo. In such cases, the effect of the placebo on the patient cannot be attributed to the specific actions or properties of the drug or procedure.

Researchers have consistently found that 30–40 percent of all patients given a placebo show improvement. This result has been observed for a wide variety of conditions or symptoms, including coughing, seasickness, depression, migraines, and angina. For some conditions, placebos have been effective in up to 70 percent of patients. In some cases, people given a placebo even report having the side effects associated with an actual drug. Placebos are particularly effective when they are administered by a practitioner whom the patient trusts.

A clear demonstration of the placebo effect occurred in a recent study that examined the effectiveness of a drug used to treat benign enlargement of the prostate. The men who participated in the study were randomly assigned to one of two groups: One group received the medication; the other received a placebo, a look-alike dummy pill. More than half the men who got the placebo pills reported significant relief from their symptoms, including faster urine flow—despite the fact that men on the placebo actually experienced an *increase* in the size of their prostates.

How did the men in the study experience fewer symptoms despite no actual improvement in their condition? Researchers hypothesize that the patients' positive expectations of the medication's effects may have resulted in changes in nerve activity and muscle relaxation affecting the bladder, prostate, and urethra.

Studies on patients with depression and people with Parkinson's disease have found that treatment with an inactive placebo results in changes in brain function. Such changes in the electrical or chemical activity of the brain may help explain the placebo effect. Different forms of CAM are often criticized as being placebo-like in effect simply because the forms cannot be explained by the conventional scientific method. In efforts to counter this claim, studies have been done by using "sham" acupuncture; that is, a trained acupuncturist inserts needles in neutral points instead of normal treatment points; still, these studies are inconclusive at best.

The placebo effect can be exploited by unscrupulous people who sell worthless medical treatments to the scientifically unsophisticated public. But placebo power can also be harnessed for its beneficial effects. When a skilled and compassionate medical practitioner provides a patient with a sense of confidence and hope, the positive aspects of placebo power can boost the benefits of standard medical treatment. Whenever you swallow a pill, you swallow your expectations right along with the medication or herb; imagining how the pill is helping you can stimulate a positive placebo effect. Getting well, like getting sick, is a complex process. Anatomy, physiology, mind, emotions, and the environment are all inextricably intertwined. But the placebo effect does show that belief can have both psychological and physical effects.

Because of the extremely diluted nature of homeopathic remedies, it is generally assumed that they are safe. In Canada, the practice of homeopathic medicine is within provincial and territorial jurisdiction, while the regulation of homeopathic medicines is federal. For example, in June 2007, Ontario passed the Homeopathy Act to regulate the practice of homeopathy. Homeopathic medicines, however, are regulated under the Natural Health Products Regulations, which came into force on January 1, 2004. These regulations are administered by the Natural Health Products Directorate branch of Health Canada. Remedies designed to treat many conditions, such as colds and headaches, can be sold over the counter; products that claim to treat serious conditions, such as heart disease, can be sold only by prescription.

Mind–Body Interventions

Mind-body interventions make use of the integral connection between mind and body and the effect each can have on the other. They include many of the stress-management techniques discussed in Chapter 3, including meditation, yoga, visualization, taijiquan, and biofeedback. Psychotherapy, support groups, prayer, and music, art, and dance therapy can also be thought of as mind-body interventions. In addition, the placebo effect is one of the most widely known examples of mind-body interdependence.

Some forms of **hypnosis** are considered to be CAM therapies. Hypnosis involves the induction of a state of deep relaxation during which the person is more suggestible (more easily influenced). While the individual is in such a hypnotic trance, the practitioner tries to help the individual change unwanted behaviour or deal with pain and other symptoms. Good evidence supports the effectiveness of relaxation techniques and hypnosis in reducing chronic pain stemming from a variety of medical conditions, although subsequent studies have cast some doubt on this conclusion. Hypnosis is sometimes used in smoking cessation programs and as a non-drug approach to anxiety disorders, such as phobias, and chronic conditions, such as irritable bowel syndrome. It has been shown to help some women deal with the pain of childbirth with less medication.

hypnosis
The process by which a practitioner induces a state of deep relaxation in which an individual is more suggestible; commonly used in cases of pain, phobia, and addiction.

Hypnosis can be used by medical professionals (MDs, DOs, DDSs) but is also offered by hypnotherapists. Physicians are certified by their own associations; however, hypnotherapy is not an insured physician service in Canada under the terms of the Medical Care Insurance Act of 1999. A certified clinical hypnotherapist must have a degree or advanced degree from an accredited university, be registered with a professional association approved by the province or territory where the hypnotherapist lives, and have a minimum of 50 class hours of training in hypnosis. There is little regulation of practitioners of other relaxation techniques, but it is very rare that adverse events result from such techniques. Many studies have shown that support groups, friendships, strong family relationships, and prayer can all have a positive impact on health. (See the Mind Body Spirit box for more information).

 Mind *Body* SPIRIT

Expressive Writing and Chronic Conditions

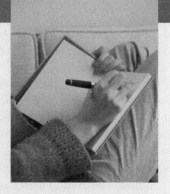

The act of writing down feelings and thoughts about stressful life events has been shown to help people improve their health. In one recent study, people with asthma or rheumatoid arthritis were asked to write down their feelings about the most stressful event in their lives; they wrote for 20 minutes a day for three days. In follow-up exams four months later, nearly half of those who engaged in expressive writing experienced positive changes in their condition, such as improved lung function or reduced joint pain.

Investigators remain unsure why writing about our feelings has beneficial effects. It is possible that expressing feelings about a traumatic event helps people work through the event and put it behind them. The resulting sense of release and control may reduce stress levels and have positive physical effects, such as reduced heart rate and blood pressure and improved immune function. Alternatively, expressive writing may change the way people think about previous stressful events in their lives and help them cope with new stressors. Whatever the cause, it's clear that expressive writing can be a safe, inexpensive, and effective supplement to the standard treatment of certain chronic illnesses.

What about the effects of expressive writing on otherwise healthy individuals? Other studies have, in fact, found a similar benefit: People who wrote about traumatic experiences reported fewer symptoms, fewer days off work, fewer visits to the doctor, improved mood, and a more positive outlook.

If you would like to try expressive writing to help you deal with a traumatic event, set aside a special time—15 minutes a day for four consecutive days, for example, or one day a week for four weeks. Write in a place where you won't be interrupted or distracted. Explore your very deepest thoughts and feelings and why you feel the way you do. Don't worry about grammar or coherence or about what someone else might think about what you are writing; you are writing just for yourself. You may find the writing exercise to be distressing in the short term—sadness and depression are common when dealing with feelings about a stressful event—but most people report relief and contentment soon after writing for several days. If you need help or guidance with expressive or journal writing, see the For More Information section at the end of the chapter.

Biological-Based Therapies

Biological-based therapies include substances derived from plant or animal origin. They consist primarily of herbal therapies or remedies, botanicals, extracts from animal tissues (such as shark cartilage), and dietary supplements. A growing area of such therapies is holistic nutrition whereby patients work one on one with nutritionists for specific dietary needs and issues. Herbal therapies are sometimes referred to as *materia medica*, Latin for "medical matter," a term that can include a much larger variety of compounds than just herbs (which are plants that die down at the end of a growing season and do not produce woody tissue). Some herbal remedies are not technically herbs; the leaves of the *Ginkgo biloba* tree are an example of a remedy commonly termed *herbal*. Other substances that constitute *materia medica* are algae, bacteria, fungi, and minerals. For traditional remedies that are of plant origin, many scientists prefer to use the term *botanicals*.

> **biological-based therapies**
> CAM therapies that include biologically based interventions and products; examples include herbal remedies, extracts from animal tissues, and dietary supplements.

Herbal remedies are a major component of all indigenous forms of medicine; before the development of pharmaceuticals at the end of the nineteenth century, people everywhere in the world relied on materials from nature for pain relief, wound healing, and treatment of a variety of ailments. Herbal remedies are also a common element in most systems of traditional medicine. Much of the **pharmacopoeia** of modern scientific medicine originated in the folk medicine of native peoples, and many drugs used today are derived from plants.

> **pharmacopoeia**
> A collection of descriptions and formulas for drugs and medicinal preparations.

A majority of botanical products are sold as natural health products, that is, in the form of tablets, pills, capsules, liquid extracts, or teas. Like foods, natural health products must carry ingredient labels (see Chapter 5). As with food products, it is the responsibility of the manufacturers to ensure that their natural health products are safe and properly labelled before marketing them. In Canada, the regulation of natural health products is governed and regulated by the Natural and Non-prescription Health Products Directorate (NNHPD) branch of Health Canada, and food regulations are regulated through the Canadian Food Inspection Agency.

Well-designed clinical studies have been conducted on only a small number of biologically-based therapies. A few commonly used botanicals, their uses, and the evidence supporting their efficacy are presented in Table 19.2. Participants in clinical trials with St. John's wort, ginkgo, and echinacea experienced only minor adverse events. However, most clinical trials of this type last for only a few weeks, so the tests did not indicate whether it is safe to take these botanicals for longer times. They also didn't examine the effects of different dosages or how these therapies interact with conventional drugs.

Although most drug-herb interactions are relatively minor compared with conventional drug-drug interactions, some can be potentially serious. An example is the use of herbs that have anticoagulant (anticlotting) properties, such as ginkgo biloba, when used concurrently with the commonly prescribed anticoagulant Coumadin.

Studies have shown that most people do not reveal their use of CAM therapies to their conventional health-care providers, an oversight that can have severe health consequences. Any herbs or drugs used in combination should be evaluated for safety by a knowledgeable health-care provider, such as a pharmacist (see the In Focus box).

Manipulative and Body-Based Methods

Touch and body manipulation are long-standing forms of health care. Manual healing techniques are based on the idea that misalignment or dysfunction in one part of the body can cause pain or dysfunction in that or another part; correcting these misalignments can bring the body back to optimal health.

Manual healing methods are an integral part of physical therapy and osteopathic medicine, now considered a form of conventional medicine. Other physical healing methods include massage, acupressure, Feldenkrais, Rolfing, and numerous other techniques.

TABLE 19.2

Commonly Used Botanicals: Their Uses, Evidence for Their Effectiveness, and Contraindications

Botanical	Use	Evidence	Examples of Adverse Effects and Interactions
Cranberry (*Vaccinium macrocarpon*)	Prevention or treatment of urinary tract disorders	May eliminate and prevent bacteria from infecting the urinary tract	None known
Dandelion (*Taraxacum officinale*)	As a "tonic" against liver or kidney ailments	None yet	May cause diarrhea in some users; people with gallbladder or bile duct problems should not take dandelion
Echinacea (*Echinacea purpurea, E. angustifolia, E. pallida*)	Stimulation of immune functions; to prevent colds and flulike diseases; to lessen symptoms of colds and the flu	Some trials showed that it prevents colds and the flu and helps patients recover from colds faster	Might cause liver damage if taken over long periods of time (more than eight weeks); since it is an immune stimulant, it is not advisable to take it with immune suppressants (e.g., corticosteroids) or during chemotherapy
Evening primrose oil (*Oenothera biennis L.*)	Reduction of inflammation	Long-term supplementation effective in reducing symptoms of rheumatoid arthritis	None known
Feverfew (*Tanacetum parthenium*)	Prevention of headaches and migraines	The majority of trials indicate that it is more effective than placebo	Should not be used by people allergic to other members of the aster family; has the potential to increase the effects of warfarin and other anticoagulants
Garlic (*Allium sativum*)	Reduction of cholesterol	Short-term studies have found a modest effect	May interact with some medications, including anticoagulants, cyclosporine, and oral contraceptives
Ginkgo (*Ginkgo biloba*)	Improvement of circulation and memory	Improves cerebral insufficiency and slows progression of Alzheimer's disease and other types of senile dementia in some patients; improves blood flow in legs	Could increase bleeding time; should not be taken with nonsteroidal anti-inflammatory drugs or anticoagulants; gastrointestinal disturbance
Ginseng (*Panax ginseng*)	Improvement of physical performance, memory, immune function, and glycemic control in diabetes; treatment of herpes simplex 2	No conclusive evidence exists for any of these uses	Interacts with warfarin and alcohol in mice and rats, hence should probably not be used with these drugs; may cause liver damage
St. John's wort (*Hypericum perforatum*)	Treatment of depression	There is strong evidence that it is wort significantly more effective than placebo, is as effective as some standard antidepressants for mild to moderate depression, and causes fewer adverse effects	Known to interact with a variety of pharmaceuticals and should not be taken together with digoxin, theophylline, cyclosporine, indinavir, and serotonin-reuptake inhibitors
Saw palmetto (*Serenoa repens*)	Improvement of prostate health	Early studies showed that it may reduce mild prostate enlargement	Has no known interactions with drugs but should probably not be taken with hormonal therapies
Valerian (*Valeriana officinalis*)	Treatment of insomnia	Appears to help with sleep disorders	Interacts with thiopental and pentobarbital and should not be used with these drugs

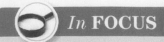

In FOCUS

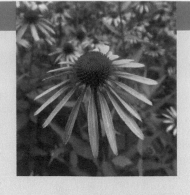

Herbal Remedies: Are They Safe?

Consider the following research findings and advisories:

- St. John's wort interacts with drugs used to treat HIV infection and heart disease; the herb may also reduce the effectiveness of oral contraceptives, antirejection drugs used with organ transplants, and some medications used to treat infections, depression, asthma, and seizure disorders.
- Supplements containing kava kava have been linked to severe liver damage, and anyone who has liver problems or takes medications that can affect the liver are advised to consult a physician before using supplements that contain kava kava.
- In a sample of Ayurvedic herbal medicine products, 20 percent were found to contain potentially harmful levels of lead, mercury, or arsenic.

These findings highlight growing safety concerns about natural health products, which in 2010 had estimated sales of $1.4 billion in Canada.

Drug Interactions

Botanicals may decrease the effects of drugs, making them ineffective, or increase their effects, in some cases making them toxic. Most patients fail to tell their physicians about their use of herbal substances. Botanicals can also interact with alcohol, usually heightening alcohol's effects. Many manufacturers are offering new combinations of botanical preparations without empirical or scientific information about the interactions of the individual products.

Lack of Standardization

Natural health products must have labels that list the name and quantity of each ingredient. However, confusion can result because different plant species—with distinct chemical compositions and effects—may have the same common name. The content of herbal preparations is also variable. Botanicals are naturally grown products. Herb producers do not have complete control over natural processes any more than farmers have control over the vitamin content of fruit.

As an attempt toward standardization, herb producers have identified one or two substances that indicate quality; these substances should be listed on a product's label with their corresponding concentrations, lot numbers, and purity analysis data. Avoid any herbal product whose label is missing this information. Reputable retailers sell only products with this identifying information, and some send qualified inspectors to the site of production to verify the label information.

These self-imposed quality control measures have been adopted by reputable producers and retailers to increase consumer confidence and to help divert additional government-imposed regulation. Today, this level of disclosure and standardization is rarely seen in the production of healthy foods by the agricultural industry.

The most commonly used CAM manual healing method is **chiropractic**, a method that focuses on the relationship between structure, primarily of joints and muscles, and function, primarily of the nervous system, to maintain or restore health. An important therapeutic procedure is the manipulation of joints, particularly those of the spinal column. However, chiropractors also use a variety of other techniques, including exercise, patient education and lifestyle modification, nutritional supplements, and orthotics (mechanical supports and braces) to treat patients. They do not use conventional drugs or surgery.

chiropractic
A system of manual healing most frequently used to treat musculoskeletal problems; the primary treatment is manipulation of the spine and other joints.

Chiropractors, or doctors of chiropractic, train for a minimum of four full-time academic years at accredited chiropractic colleges and can go on to postgraduate training in many countries. Although specifically listed by NCCAM as one of the manipulative and body-based methods of CAM, chiropractic is accepted by many health-care and health insurance providers to a far greater extent than the other types of CAM therapies. Based on research showing the efficacy of chiropractic management in acute low-back pain, spinal manipulation has been included in most provincial and territorial guidelines for the treatment of this condition. In fact, electro-diagnostic tests show that chiropractic is effective in controlling back pain. Promising results have also been reported with the use of chiropractic techniques in treating neck pain and headaches.

A caution is in order regarding chiropractic: Spinal manipulation performed by a person without proper chiropractic training can be extremely dangerous. The Canadian Chiropractic Association, listed in For More Information at the end of the chapter, can help you find a licensed chiropractor near you.

QUICK STATS

Some 15% or 4 million Canadians received chiropractic care in 2009.

—Chiropractic Canada, 2009

Energy Therapies

Energy therapies are forms of treatment that use energy originating either within the body (biofields) or from other sources (electromagnetic fields). Biofield therapies are based on the idea that energy fields surround and penetrate the body and can be influenced by movement, touch, pressure, or the placement of hands in or through the fields. **Qigong**, a component of TCM, combines movement, meditation, and regulation of breathing to enhance the flow of qi, improve blood circulation, and enhance immune function. **Therapeutic touch** is derived from the ancient technique of laying-on of hands; it is based on the premise that healers can identify and correct energy imbalances by passing their hands over the patient's body. **Reiki** is one form of therapeutic touch; it is intended to correct disturbances in the flow of life energy (ki is the Japanese form of the Chinese qi) and enhance the body's healing powers through the use of 13 specific hand positions on the patient.

energy therapies
Forms of CAM treatment that use energy fields originating either within the body or from outside sources to promote health and healing.

qigong
A component of traditional Chinese medicine that combines movement, meditation, and regulation of breathing to enhance the flow of qi, improve blood circulation, and enhance immune function.

therapeutic touch
A CAM practice based on the premise that healers can identify and correct energy imbalances by passing their hands over the patient's body.

Reiki
A CAM practice intended to correct disturbances in the flow of life energy and enhance the body's healing powers through the use of 13 hand positions on the patient.

Bioelectromagnetics is the study of the interaction between living organisms and electromagnetic fields, both those produced by the organism itself and those produced by outside sources. The recognition that the body produces electromagnetic fields has led to the development of many diagnostic procedures in Western medicine, including electroencephalography (EEG), electrocardiography (ECG), and nuclear magnetic resonance (NMR) scans.

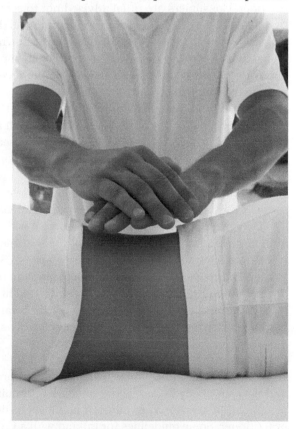

One of several touch therapies, Reiki massage has a spiritual, as well as physical, component.

Bioelectromagnetic-based therapies involve the use of electromagnetic fields to manage pain and to treat many conditions, such as asthma. Some indications suggest that the use of electromagnetic fields might be useful in the areas of bone repair, wound healing, nerve stimulation, immune system stimulation, and modulation of the neuroendocrine (nerve and hormonal) system. Although promising, the available research is still very limited and does not allow firm conclusions about the efficacy of these therapies.

> **bioelectromagnetic-based therapies**
> CAM therapies based on the notion that electromagnetic fields can be used to promote healing and manage pain.

Evaluating Complementary and Alternative Therapies

Because less information is available about complementary and alternative therapies, as well as less regulation of associated products and providers, it is important for consumers to take an active role when they are thinking about using them. It is difficult to appraise CAM methods by using research methods and standards that rely exclusively on traditional scientific, allopathic standards. Instead, decision analysis may provide a more practical framework for evaluating CAM. Decision analysis allows for an explicit estimate of the nature of the evidence and how much evidence is enough evidence for decision making. To recommend a CAM therapy or treatment, the harmfulness of treatment must be lower than the harmfulness of the illness, multiplied by the probability that treatment will be successful. Thus, using both evidence-based decision making along with decision analysis, we consider the effectiveness, potential harm, unintended side effects, and utility of any one therapy versus any other under consideration.

Working with Your Physician

If you are considering a CAM therapy, your first source of information should be your primary health-care provider. Consumers are often advised not to seek complementary therapies without first visiting a conventional health-care provider for an evaluation and diagnosis of their symptoms. It's usually best to discuss and try conventional treatments that have been shown to be beneficial for your condition. If you are thinking of trying any alternative therapies, it is critically important to tell your physician to avoid any dangerous interactions with conventional treatments you are receiving. Areas to discuss with your physician or pharmacist include the following:

- *Safety:* Is there something unsafe about the treatment in general or for you specifically? Are there safety issues you should be aware of, such as drug-herb interactions?
- *Effectiveness:* Is there evidence-based research about the use of the therapy for your condition? What level of evidence is sufficient for your confidence and that of your primary health-care provider in the therapy?
- *Timing:* Is the immediate use of a conventional treatment indicated?
- *Cost:* Is the therapy likely to be very expensive, especially in light of the potential benefit?

If appropriate, schedule a follow-up visit with your physician to assess your condition and your progress after a certain amount of time using a complementary therapy. Keep a symptom diary to more accurately track your symptoms and gauge your progress. (Some symptoms, such as pain and fatigue, are very difficult to recall with accuracy, so an ongoing symptom diary is an important tool.) If you plan to pursue a therapy against your physician's advice, you need to tell him or her.

For natural health products, particularly botanicals, pharmacists can also be an excellent source of information, if they are familiar with other medications you are taking.

Questioning the CAM Practitioner

You can also get information from individual practitioners and from schools, professional organizations, and licensing boards. Ask about education, training, licensing, and certification. If appropriate, check with provincial or territorial regulatory agencies to determine if any complaints have been lodged against the practitioner. Some guidelines for talking with a CAM practitioner include the following:

- Ask the practitioner why he or she thinks the therapy will be beneficial for your condition. Ask for a full description of the therapy and any potential side effects.

- Describe in detail any conventional treatments you are receiving or plan to receive.
- Ask how long the therapy should continue before it can be determined if it is beneficial.
- Ask about the expected cost of the treatment. Does it seem reasonable? Will your health insurance pay some or all of the costs?

If anything an alternative practitioner says or recommends directly conflicts with advice from your physician, discuss it with your physician before making any major changes in any current treatment regimen or in your lifestyle.

Doing Your Own Research

You can investigate CAM therapies on your own by going to the library or doing research online, although caution is in order when using websites for the various forms of CAM. Erroneous information about CAM is rampant among unscientific and "pop" resources. A good place to start is the Cochrane Library, a research database for independent, high-quality evidence for health-care decision making. Other excellent resources are Health Canada's website and the Canadian Natural Health Products' website.

If possible, also talk to people with the same condition you have who have received the same treatment. Remember, though, that patient testimonials should not be used as the sole criterion for choosing a therapy or assessing its safety and efficacy. Controlled scientific trials usually provide the best information and should be consulted whenever possible. The absence of documented danger is not the same thing as proof of safety. Quite often, people working in health food stores are only too willing to give advice and make recommendations, particularly about botanical products. Many of these people are not qualified to give this kind of advice. Ask about qualifications (training or education) before accepting recommendations from anyone. Perhaps more so than for any other consumer products and services, the use of CAM calls for consumer decision-making skills, critical thinking, and caution.

 QUESTIONS FOR CRITICAL THINKING AND REFLECTION

Have you ever considered using a complementary or alternative treatment? If so, was it in addition to conventional treatment, or instead of it? What kind of research did you do before having the treatment? What advice did your primary health-care provider give you about it?

Paying for Health Care

In 2014, total *health-care spending* in this country was projected to exceed $214.9 billion, or $6045 per person. Many factors contribute to the high cost of health care in our country, including the cost of advanced equipment and new technology, the expensive treatments for some illnesses, the aging of the population, the high earnings by some people in the health-care industry, and the demand for profits by investors.

The Current System

Canada's national health insurance program, often referred to as medicare, is designed to ensure that all residents have reasonable access to medically necessary hospital and physician services, on a pre-paid basis. Instead of having a single national plan, we have a national program that is composed of 13 interlocking provincial and territorial health insurance plans, all of which share certain common features and basic standards of coverage. Framed by the Canada Health Act, the principles governing our health-care system are symbols of the underlying Canadian values of equity and solidarity.

The roles and responsibilities for Canada's health-care system are shared between the federal and provincial or territorial governments. Under the Canada Health Act, our federal health insurance legislation, criteria and conditions are specified that must be met by the provincial and territorial health-care insurance plans for them to qualify for their full share of the federal cash contribution, available under the Canada Health Transfer. Provincial and territorial governments are responsible for the management, organization, and delivery of health services for their residents.

Health Insurance

In 2007, out-of-pocket expenses by Canadians represented 15 percent of total health expenditure, or $23.4 billion. Private insurance accounted for 12 percent, or $19.5 billion. Thus, about 73 percent of total health-care costs were paid by the provincial, territorial, and federal governments. Health insurance enables people to receive health care they might not otherwise be able to afford. Hospital care costs hundreds of dollars a day, and surgical fees can cost thousands. Health insurance is important for everyone, especially as health-care costs continue to rise.

Take **CHARGE**

Adherence to Physicians' Instructions

Even though we sometimes have to entrust ourselves to the care of medical professionals, that doesn't mean we give up responsibility for our own behaviour. Following medical instructions and advice often requires the same kind of behavioural self-management that's involved in quitting smoking, losing weight, or changing eating patterns. For example, if you have an illness or injury, you may be told to take medication at certain times of the day, do special exercises or movements, or change your diet.

The medical profession recognizes the importance of patient adherence to physicians' recommendations and instructions and encourages different strategies to support adherence, such as the following:

1. Use reminders placed at home, in the car, at work, on your computer screensaver, or elsewhere that improve follow-through in taking medication and keeping scheduled appointments. To help you remember to take medications:
   - Link taking the medication with some well-established routine, like brushing your teeth or eating breakfast.
   - Use a medication calendar, and check off each pill.
   - Use a medication organizer or pill dispenser.
   - Plan ahead; don't wait until the last pill to get a prescription refilled.
2. Use a journal and other forms of self-monitoring to keep a detailed account of health-related behaviours, such as pill taking, diet, exercise, and so on.
3. Use self-reward systems so that desired behaviour changes are encouraged, with a focus on short-term rewards.
4. Develop a clear image or explanation of how the medication or behaviour change will improve your health and well-being.

If these strategies don't help you stick with your treatment plan, you may need to consider other possible explanations for your lack of adherence. For example, are you confused about some aspect of the treatment? Do you find the schedule for taking your medications too complicated, or do the drugs have bothersome side effects that you would rather avoid? Do you feel that the recommended treatment is unnecessary or unlikely to help? Are you afraid of becoming dependent on a medication or that you will be judged negatively if people know about your condition and treatment? An examination of your attitudes and beliefs about your condition and treatment plan can also help improve your compliance.

SUMMARY

- Health literacy is an essential skill for all Canadians. While gathering and assessing evidence about health issues or symptoms is advisable, it is necessary to see a physician if symptoms are severe, unusual, persistent, or recurrent.

- Self-treatment doesn't necessarily require medication, but OTC drugs can be a helpful part of self-care.
- Conventional medicine is characterized by a focus on the external, physical causes of disease; the identification of a set of symptoms for different diseases; the development of public health measures to prevent disease and of drugs and surgery to treat them; the use of rational, scientific thinking to understand phenomena; and a well-established research methodology.
- Conventional practitioners include medical doctors, doctors of osteopathic medicine, podiatrists, optometrists, and dentists, as well as allied health-care providers.
- The diagnostic process involves a medical history, a physical exam, and medical tests. Patients should ask questions about medical tests and treatments recommended by their physicians.
- Safe use of prescription drugs requires knowledge of what the medication is supposed to do, how and when to take it, and what the side effects are.
- All surgical procedures carry risk; patients should ask about alternatives and get a second opinion from another physician.
- Complementary and alternative medicine (CAM) is defined as those therapies and practices that do not form part of conventional health-care and medical practice as taught in most Canadian medical schools and offered in most Canadian hospitals.
- CAM is characterized by a view of health as a balance and integration of body, mind, and spirit; a focus on ways to restore the individual to harmony so that he or she can fight disease and regain health; and a body of knowledge based on accumulated experience and observations of patient reactions.
- Alternative medical systems, such as traditional Chinese medicine and homeopathy, are complete systems of medical philosophy, theory, and practice.
- Mind-body interventions include meditation, biofeedback, group support, hypnosis, and prayer.
- Biological-based therapies consist of herbal remedies, botanicals, animal-tissue products, and dietary supplements.
- Manipulative and body-based methods include massage and other physical healing techniques; the most frequently used is chiropractic.
- Energy therapies are designed to influence the flow of energy in and around the body; they include qigong, therapeutic touch therapies, and Reiki.
- Because less information available is about CAM and less regulation of its practices and providers, occurs, consumers must be proactive in researching and choosing treatments, using critical thinking and evidence-based decision-analysis skills while exercising caution.

FOR MORE INFORMATION

BOOKS AND REPORTS

Chappell, N. L., and M. J. Penning. 2009. *Understanding Health, Health-Care, and Health Policy in Canada: Sociological Perspectives*. Toronto: Oxford University Press. An examination of topical issues, such as obesity, smoking, homelessness, AIDS, stress, and mental illness, from a sociological debate perspective and in the context of Canadian health policy.

Kliger, B., and R. Lee. 2004. *Integrative Medicine: Principles for Practice*. New York: McGraw-Hill. An integration of CAM with conventional medicine written primarily by physicians. This evidence-based and clinically authoritative guide often is used by family medicine and primary care providers.

Miccozi, Marc S. 2010 (4th edition). *Fundamentals of Alternative and Complementary Medicine*. New York, Saunders. An examination of most aspects and forms of CAM, written by physicians.

Morgan, S., et al. 2008. *Canadian Rx Atlas*, 2nd ed. Vancouver: UBC Centre for Health Services and Policy Research. The first-ever portrait of age-specific patterns of prescription drug use and costs across provinces. It breaks down nearly $20 billion in prescription drug spending by Canadians.

Romanow, R. (Commission on the Future of Health-Care in Canada). 2002. *Building on Values: The Future of Health-Care in Canada,* http://dsp-psd.pwgsc.gc.ca/Collection/CP32-85-2002E.pdf (retrieved June 1, 2015). A comprehensive examination of health care in Canada. Recommendations and findings reflect current thinking and initiatives about the future of health care in Canada.

Thompson, W. G. 2005. *The Placebo Effect and Health: Combining Science and Compassionate Care.* New York: Prometheus Books. An examination of the placebo effect and how it may be used to benefit health.

Whorton, J. C. 2004. Nature *Cures: The History of Alternative Medicine in America.* New York: Oxford University Press. A history of alternative medicine in the United States, including background information on many CAM therapies.

ORGANIZATIONS, HOTLINES, AND WEBSITES

The Internet addresses listed here were accurate at the time of publication.

IN-CAM. Provides evidence-based information on complementary and alternative medicine (CAM) for health-care professionals and the public.
> http://www.incamresearch.ca/content/about-cam *Canada Health Infoway.* Provides information about electronic health records in Canada.
> http://www.infoway-inforoute.ca/lang-en/about-ehr/what-is-ehr

Canada's Food and Drug Act. Outlines the statute about food, drugs, cosmetics, and therapeutic devices.
> http://laws.justice.gc.ca/en/F-27/

Canadian Health-Care Anti-fraud Association. Gives a voice to the public and private sector health-care organizations interested in preventing fraud in the Canadian health-care environment.
> http://www.chcaa.org/report/

Canadian Chiropractic Association. Represents the chiropractic profession in Canada in collaboration with its provincial members.
> http://www.ccachiro.org

Canadian Arthritis Network. Provides information on arthritis research and development in Canada.
> http://www.arthritisnetwork.ca

Canadian Diabetes Association. Provides health-care professionals and people with diabetes with education and services.
> http://www.diabetes.ca

Canadian Institute for Health Information. Provides comprehensive information and resources for a wide variety of health issues in French and English.
> http://www.cihi.ca

Canadian Patient Safety Institute. Performs a coordinating and leadership role across health sectors and systems; promotes leading practices and raises awareness with stakeholders, patients, and the general public about patient safety.
> http://www.patientsafetyinstitute.ca

The Cochrane Library. Provides a collaboration database for health-care decision making.
> http://www.thecochranelibrary.com

Drug Information and Research Centre. Provides comprehensive information on evidence-based drug information for all of Canada by Ontario pharmacists.
> http://www.dirc.ca

First Nations and Inuit Health Branch of Health Canada. Provides information on health issues and resources for Canada's indigenous populations.
> http://www.hc-sc.gc.ca/ahc-asc/branch-dirgen/fnihb-dgspni/index-eng.php

Health Canada Drug Product Database. Contains product specific information on drugs approved for use in Canada. The database is managed by Health Canada and includes human pharmaceutical and biological drugs, veterinary drugs, and disinfectant products. It contains approximately 18 000 products.
> http://www.hc-sc.gc.ca/dhp-mps/prodpharma/databasdon/index-eng.php

Health Canada Compendium of Monographs. Helps speed the evaluation of the safety and efficacy of medicinal ingredients commonly used in natural health products. A monograph is a written description of particular elements on an identified topic.

http://www.hc-sc.gc.ca/dhp-mps/prodnatur/applications/licen-prod/monograph/index-eng.php

Health Canada. Provides information from the federal department responsible for helping Canadians maintain and improve their health, while respecting individual choices and circumstances.

http://www.hc-sc.gc.ca

International Association of Journal Writing. Promotes journal writing through expert advice, programs, and support.

http://www.iajw.org

Natural Health Products Directorate of Health Canada. Explains Canada's regulatory processes regarding vitamins and minerals, herbal products, homeopathic medicines and the like—products that have come to be known as natural health products.

http://www.hc-sc.gc.ca/dhp-mps/prodnatur/index-eng.php

Statistics Canada Health Data Tables and Maps. Provides a database for almost all Canadian health indicators and measures.

http://www.statcan.gc.ca/pub/82-221-x/2008001/tbl-eng.htm

Quackwatch. Provides information on health fraud, quackery, and health decision making.

http://www.quackwatch.org/

U.S. National Center for Complementary and Alternative Medicine. Provides general information packets, answers to frequently asked questions about CAM, consumer advice for safer use of CAM, research abstracts, and bibliographies.

http://nccam.nih.gov

SELECTED BIBLIOGRAPHY

Ernst, E. 2004. Prescribing herbal medications appropriately. *Journal of Family Practice* 53(12): 985–988.

Frazier, S. C. 2005. Health outcomes and polypharmacy in elderly individuals: An integrated literature review. *Journal of Gerontological Nursing* 31(9): 4–11.

Gan, T. J., et al. 2004. A randomized controlled comparison of electro-acupoint stimulation or ondansetron versus placebo for the prevention of postoperative nausea and vomiting. *Anesthesia and Analgesia* 99(4): 1070–1075.

Grzywaca, J. G., et al. 2008. Age-related differences in the conventional health care–complementary and alternative medicine link. *American Journal of Health Behavior* 32(6): 650–663.

Harden, B. L., and C. R. Harden. 1997. *Alternative Health Care: The Canadian Directory.* Toronto: Noble Ages Publishing.

Kaiser Family Foundation. 2005. *Trends and Indicators in the Changing Health Care Marketplace.* Menlo Park, Calif.: Kaiser Family Foundation.

Kondro, W. 2004. Canadian report quantifies the cost of medical errors. *The Lancet* 363(9426): 2059–2065.

Miller, F. G., et al. 2004. Ethical issues concerning research in complementary and alternative medicine. *Journal of the American Medical Association* 291(5): 599–604.

Progoff, I. 1992. *At a Journal Workshop: Writing to Access the Power of the Unconscious and Evoke Creative Ability.* New York: Tarcher.

Rappaport, K. (ed.). 1999. *Directory of Schools for Alternative and Complementary Health Care*, 2nd ed. Phoenix: Oryx Press.

Saper, R. B., et al. 2004. Heavy metal content of Ayurvedic herbal medicine products. *Journal of the American Medical Association* 292(23): 2868–2873.

Wahbeh, H., S. M. Elsas, and B. S. Oken. 2008. Mind-body interventions: Applications in neurology. *Neurology* 70(24): 2321–2328.

Nutritional Resources

Nutritional Content of Popular Items from Fast-Food Restaurants

Although most foods served at fast-food restaurants are high in calories, fat, saturated fat, cholesterol, sodium, and sugar, some items are more healthful than others. If you eat at fast-food restaurants, knowing the nutritional content of various items can help you make better choices. Fast-food restaurants provide nutritional information both online and in print brochures available at most restaurant locations. To learn more about the items you order, visit the restaurants' websites. Here are some popular fast-food restaurants and their web addresses:

Arby's	http://arbys.ca/
Burger King	http://burgerking.ca/
Dairy Queen	http://www.dairyqueen.com/ca-en/
Domino's Pizza	http://www.dominos.ca/
KFC	http://www.kfc.ca/
McDonald's	http://www.mcdonalds.ca/ca/en.html
Pizza Pizza	http://www.pizzapizza.ca/
Starbucks	http://www.starbucks.ca/
Subway	http://w.subway.com/en-ca/
Taco Bell	http://www.tacobell.ca/
Tim Horton's	http://www.timhortons.com/ca/en/index.php
Wendy's	https://www.wendys.com/en-ca

Photo Credits

Index